For Women Only!

For Women Only!

YOUR GUIDE TO HEALTH EMPOWERMENT

Gary Null
Barbara Seaman

seven stories press / new york toronto london

A Seven Stories Press First Edition.

This book is not intended to replace the services of a physician.
Any application of the recommendations set forth in the following pages
is at the reader's discretion. The reader should consult with his or her
own physician concerning the recommendations in this book.

Portions of the "Alternative Treatment Solutions" chapters in *For Women Only!*
have been adapted from the following books by Gary Null:
The Woman's Encyclopedia of Natural Healing and *Get Healthy Now!*

In Canada:
Hushion House, 36 Northline Road, Toronto, Ontario M4B 3E2, Canada

In the U.K.:
Turnaround Publisher Services Ltd., Unit 3, Olympia Trading Estate,
Coburg Road, Wood Green, London N22 6TZ U.K.

Null, Gary.
    For women only!: your guide to health empowerment /
Gary Null and Barbara Seaman. —Seven Stories Press 1st ed.
    p.   cm.
    Includes bibliographical references and index.
    ISBN 1-58322-015-1 (cl.)
    1. Women—Health and hygiene. 2. Women's health services—
Government policy—United States. I. Seaman, Barbara. II. Title.
RA778.N883 1999
613'.04244—dc21   99-39822
                                   CIP

9 8 7 6 5 4 3 2 1

Book design by Cindy LaBreacht

Seven Stories Press
140 Watts Street
New York, NY 10013
http://www.sevenstories.com

Printed in the U.S.A.

This book is dedicated to women who have navigated their way

through our present, byzantine health care system, and towards

returning to patients everywhere their dignity as human beings

Contents

PART II: Health Empowerment for Women
BY BARBARA SEAMAN

"Motherhood" by Elizabeth Cady Stanton
"Why Elizabeth Isn't on Your Silver Dollar" by Barbara Seaman
"Out of Conflict Comes Strength and Healing: Women's Health
    Movements" by Dr. Helen I. Marieskind
"Women Healers in Shamanic Culture" by Suzanne Clores

Publisher's Note

A year ago, as the text of Gary Null's breakthrough *Get Healthy Now!* finally neared readiness, and as we began to recover from the shock of its sheer size—at just under 1,100 large-format pages the largest one-volume title I knew of that wasn't a dictionary or a phone book—Gary proposed that we embark on an even bigger project. Women's health, he said, was the most neglected area of modern medicine and it was about time that women be informed of this fact.

Meanwhile, another Seven Stories author, the distinguished women's health pioneer Barbara Seaman, had been talking to me for several years about a major book she was considering writing, in which the history of the women's health movement could be presented using the parts of a woman's body as its organizational principle.

It occurred to me that these two authors had much in common. Both were fearless patients' rights advocates who had appeared before Congress and in the media as sharp, painful thorns in the paw of the mighty medical establishment. And, as I knew from personal experience, both had the spontaneous, courageous instincts of writer-warriors, the kind of individuals who could stand back to back with you and fight off an army.

I suggested they work together on the project; they agreed; a team of dozens of researchers, editors, and one heroic designer (Cindy LaBreacht of LaBreacht Design), was formed to support their efforts, and it was not long before we had a manuscript of over a million words! Our job then became to reduce the text to a mere 700,000 words to fit in the book's projected 1,600 pages (*Get Healthy Now!* was about to find it had a big sister). Finally, the project reached completion, although not without extra effort, well beyond what could be reasonably expected, from everyone involved. The results, the book's quality and informational content, exceeded our most ambitious expectations.

Of course, alternative health as espoused by Gary, Barbara and their peers does not seek to replace modern medicine, but to complement it—and enlighten it. Ideally, the various traditions will work together and enhance each other's strengths. But until that happens, alternative health practitioners and advocates cannot just sit by and wait to be invited to participate in the health care debate. It is up to patients everywhere, people everywhere, to ask for—demand—nutritional solutions, environmental solutions, alternative solutions, wise solutions.

It has been suggested that a patients' association should be formed, something along the lines of AARP, and like that group, perhaps based around a publication of high quality which all its members would receive, and which would serve as a legislative lobbying body to counterbalance the lobbying that is done by trade groups lobbying on behalf of specific business interests in the health care community. I fervently hope that such an organization is formed.

Daniel Simon, Publisher
Seven Stories Press, New York

Introduction

The idea behind *For Women Only!* is to join together the practical with the spiritual—basic, but hard-to-find, health care information, together with a consumer's, patient's, women's story you may not have heard before. Here is a straight-talking guide packed with alternative approaches to a wide range of health issues, solutions to return you to complete wellbeing. Also, here is a proud history of the women writers, practitioners, and equal rights advocates who for hundreds of years, and especially during our lifetime, have struggled to protect your right to the best health care information and treatments available. These women (and some men) have earned our respect and we honor them in these pages.

A Barnard College senior recently asked Judy Norsigian of *Our Bodies, Ourselves* what she hopes to see when the continuously updated volume celebrates its 50th anniversary in the year 2020. Norsigian answered, "The creation of a health and a medical care system that is far more responsive to women's needs and accessible to all women regardless of age, income, sexual preference, race, etc.... And using technology in the most appropriate way—that is science-based, not profit-based...." People need to be in control of their own health. But in order for that to be possible, they must have information from a trustworthy source.

We asked Cindy Pearson, Executive Director of the National Women's Health Network, what she thinks about patients taking their health into their own hands. "Thirty years ago," Pearson said, "if anyone talked about a bad experience they had with the health care system... the response would usually be, 'You need a better doctor....'" Today, in part through the hard-won battles of consumer advocates, AIDS activists, and the feminist health movement, among others, that isn't the only answer. Pearson continues, "People talked about finding a good doctor, but then realized, good doctors aren't the answer, informed patients are the answer."

We believe that within the yin and the yang of these two thoughtful responses there is to be found the right approach: good science combined with leadership from the patients' point of view. What makes a good doctor these days isn't always easy to say. But if there is one quality we should all be looking for in our doctors it is the willingness to listen seriously to their patients' concerns.

Do you remember the ad—one like many such promotions for products aimed at women—in which a goofy looking foursome of women whispered among themselves while playing cards, as a written message addressed to doctors promoted ways to counteract what it suggested were irresponsible rumors concerning the safety of the birth control pill. At that time, doctors were still declaring the high-dose Pills to be "safe" and unrelated to the blood clots, mainly in the leg and lungs, that were crippling, and sometimes killing, many young women.

Radical mastectomies became the "gold standard" of breast cancer care in the late 1800s. And only recently was it shown that less traumatic operations can be just as effective. In order for that battle to be won it took an activist, Rose Kushner, to get the ear of President Jimmy Carter, after which the government funded the watershed National Cancer Institute (NCI) study by Dr. Bernard Fisher, which led to the acceptance of lumpectomies. Activism led to better science, and ultimately, better patient care.

Not long ago, the conventional medical treatment for diverticulitis included advising patients to exclude roughage from their diet. Today, doctors agree that the old advice was not a cure but a cause of the disease and patients are advised to eat more roughage.

As published on the *New York Times* Op Ed page on June 25, 1995, Sherwin B. Nuland, clinical professor of surgery at Yale School of Medicine, suggests that the very term "medical science" is an oxymoron, a contradiction in terms! And in his essay he cites an estimate made by Dr. David Eddy of the Jackson Hole Group that "no more than 15 percent of medical interventions are supported by reliable scientific evidence."

In fact, with drugs that are widely used—the Pill being one example, Prozac another—patients are often far ahead of their doctors in recognizing adverse reactions.

Who could not admire him—U.S. Surgeon General from 1981-89 and, the polls say, our most trusted health authority—for his campaigns to deter cigarette smoking, to raise AIDS awareness, to convince physicians that wife-beating ("more women are injured by battery than by rape, muggings, and accidents combined," he declared in 1985) demanded their attention. But then in 1999, under the slogan "Your Trusted Health Network," C. Everett Koop opened his popular health information web site, DrKoop.com. The problem wasn't the fabulous wealth he almost immediately acquired, but the seeming conflicts of interest. In the prospectus he filed on June 8 with the Securities and Exchange Commission, he acknowledged that he would receive 2 percent of his web site's revenues "derived from sales of our current products and up to 4 percent of our revenues derived from sales of new products." Such products included prescription drugs, nonprescription drugs, vitamins, nutritional supplements, and health insurance offered by outside parties. Early in 1999, the not-for-profit Koop Foundation accepted a $1 million grant from Schering-Plough and then proceeded to solicit Congress on behalf of legislation that would allow Schering-Plough to extend its patent on Claritin an extra five years—a move expected to produce an additional $6 billion of revenue. Koop also met with members of the House Commerce Committee to defend Schering-Plough's interest in a drug for Hepatitis C. In May 1999, he entered into an agreement with the American Council on Science and Health, an organization that, according to Philip E. Clapp, president of the National Environmental Trust, "has never met a pesticide it didn't like." A medical ethicist at the University of Chicago, Dr. Joshua Hauser, noted that the web site listed fourteen hospitals and health centers, describing them as "the most innovative and advanced health care institutions across the country." As reported in the *New York Times* of September 5, 1999, Dr. Hauser found that each of these fourteen institutions had paid a fee of about $40,000 for inclusion on the Koop web site. Has this "icon"—a term he used recently to describe himself—lost his integrity? We hope not. But, either way, we can console ourselves with the thought that perhaps this is a necessary wake-up call, warning us that medical marketing has spun so out of control that almost no individual is immune. With a new urgency, we must seek out new ways to obtain information we can trust.

This past summer, American Home Products Corporation (of which Wyeth Ayerst is a part) agreed to pay $54 million to settle claims regarding problems with the birth control device Norplant. A month later, the company offered to pay $4 billion to settle lawsuits filed by consumers who say they were injured because of fen-phen, a diet pill that was said to cause heart valve damage, and which was removed from the market in 1997. Eli Lilly and Company joined this dubious party when it was discovered that this pharmaceutical company had misled doctors and patients about the ability of its drug raloxifene hydrochloride (Evista) to prevent breast cancer. This is not to say that prescription drugs are not powerful tools of health care, but rather to suggest that pharmaceutical companies may not be trusted to monitor themselves and that government bodies don't always do the job either. Again, informed patients and patient groups is our best defense.

Since the FDA relaxed its regulations on television and radio direct-to-consumer drug ads in August 1997, pharmaceutical companies have greatly increased their spending on broadcast and print ads. In 1996, they spent $595 million; in 1997, $843 million; and in 1998, a whopping $1.3 billion. Women tend to be their most lucrative market, and are often the targets of such ads. The National Women's Health Network has just launched their Campaign to Stop Deceptive Drug Ads to fight the good fight. So must we all.

To practice good health, to care for one's body, one needs reliable information, but one also needs the confidence—the discernment—to distinguish the reliable and authentic from the sales pitch. We hope that the two parts of this book, the practical and the inspirational, will satisfy both needs. You need both parts to give you the complete picture.

The women's health movement of the 1970s persuaded the FDA to require patient inserts on the Pill and other prescription drugs, made enormous progress in institutionalizing informed consent, prompted the passage of regulations to restrain sterilization abuse against minority women, and secured the ownership of medical records by patients. Today the FDA is much more open to regular consumer participation than it once was. Natural childbirth has been revived, along with midwifery, and labor and delivery is rightfully looked at today as a family event, rather than as an illness. And today, radical mastectomies are no longer the only surgical choice for breast cancer patients and there is an atmosphere where many patients became "partners" in electing their own treatment plans. In recent decades, "medical science" has made many impressive strides, including in imaging technologies, in psychopharmacology, and, finally, in gender medicine, in which there have finally been practical discoveries into the ways in which women and men differ in terms of illness prevention and cure.

Our goal is to build on these accomplishments with new victories. Read, learn, enjoy, and let's talk to one another about what we discover.

Gary Null and Barbara Seaman
October 1999, New York

Acknowledgments

Thanks go out to the following people, each of whom made indispensible contributions toward the creation of this book.

Amy Allina, Jennifer Barbosa, Lori Barer, Louise Bernikow, Rachel Burd, Nancy Cain, Martha Cameron, Carmen Cartagena, Janet Cavallero, Suzanne Clores, Gwen Darien, Mikola De Roo, Gita J. Drury, Victoria Eng, Jim Feast, Barbara Findlen, Andres Garcia, Lisa Renee Garey, Jon Gilbert, Stephanie Golden, Thomas Hartman, Pam Hayashi, Carol Inskip, Gloria Jacobs, Tania Ketenjian, Judith Kletter, Gary Krup, Cindy LaBreacht, Vivien Labatov, Lisa Lomonaco, Connie Long, Eric Lowenbrun, Michael Manekin, Roland Marconi, Bob Marty, William Marty, Joan Michel, Ann Pappert, Joanna Perlman, Tammy Pinkston, Sünje Redies, Amy Richards, Agata Rumprecht, Mei Hwei Astella Saw, Sarah Olu, Dan Simon, Tara Smith, Kofi A. Taha, Jessica Tanne, Jerry Traub, Huy Truong, Maggie Warren, Mitchell Waters, Ethan Young.

Part I

Alternative Treatment Solutions

Gary Null

Chapter 1

Addiction

T he opening shot of the 1990s' film *GirlQuake!*, written and directed by Michael Randall, is of a hamburger frying on a grill. In an Arizona diner, a group of overweight American men are smoking, drinking, and chowing down on burgers, dogs, fries, coffee, and other junk food. They get their comeuppance when they attempt to rape a bevy of fit, quaintly dressed extraterrestial Wonder Women, and the biggest food junkie is smothered to death in a gigantic fruit bowl of raw hamburger meat.

One way to look at this scene is as an ironic commentary on addiction: addictions ill fit us for facing life's sometimes unexpected challenges, and one way or another an addiction will kill you if you don't wise up. The scene also serves as a reminder that we can be addicted to other substances besides drugs—such as sugar and caffeine.

The number of Americans using drugs is skyrocketing, though many drug users don't consider themselves addicts. (For example, some people say they take cocaine because it gives them that extra energy to work longer days.) Tens of millions of Americans use drugs. Aside from the two most popular 12-step programs, Alcoholics Anonymous and Narcotics Anonymous, what other approaches to facing and overcoming substance abuse are out there?

There are in fact a number of alternative approaches to beating addiction, including detoxification, eating natural foods, and hypnosis. Let's start by talking about detoxification, a process whereby the body is cleansed of the toxins created by the addictive substance.

Detoxification

Elson Haas is a practicing integrated medical physician and the director of the Preventive Medical Center in San Rafael, California. He is the author of several best-selling books on health and nutrition, including *The Detox Diet*. Haas describes the best times to detox: "Right now, I'm on day six of my 25th annual spring cleanse, so I've been doing juices and broth. I usually cleanse in spring. That's one of the best times. Seasonal change times are usually more fraught with problems, and a cleanse can help a person. Going into autumn is another good time.

"I live on the West Coast, and even though it's a rainy and lightly cool March day here, back East it's probably colder. Probably a good time out there would be as it warms up into mid-April. Then you can count on a little warmer weather. Because when you do cleansing programs, your body gets a little cooler, so you need to take a little more protection from the cold, and dress warmer. Exercise, keep your body warm and all those things."

Of course, in embarking on a detox program, there are other considerations besides the seasonal. Reasons to begin one include when you experience congestive problems or are having regular headaches or sluggish intestines. Other good times to start are "when allergies are kicking up, when blood pressure is getting too high and the cholesterol is rising. Those are times when I, as a physician, would use detoxification as one of my medical treatments. When I see people who have problems of toxicity and congestion, and other things stemming from or related to addictions, I see that detoxification works better therapeutically than almost anything I can do for them. So we have both the time of the year and also the individual time for people when it's appropriate."

Haas adds, "Anytime you decide to go off any of these substances, you have to get your mind set first. When we are using any of these substances, we are hooked in emotionally. Mentally, we think we need them, and physically, we are slightly dependent on them. This varies with the substance. Nicotine is probably the most addictive, alcohol next, caffeine after that. Sugar is probably the least physically addictive, but emotionally people are really hooked into it."

CHOICE OF PROGRAM

As Haas points out, "There are various levels of detoxification. You can do everything from juice cleanses to changing your diet in certain ways that will allow your detoxification to begin. Even drinking more water and getting more exercise and doing steams or saunas will help in the detoxification process. There are a lot of levels. It doesn't mean just one thing or one program. There are a lot of approaches out there."

Haas's prescription for the type of detox regimen to follow depends on how advanced the person's level of toxicity is. "If you treat somebody too extremely," he explains, "and she has too much toxicity, then she'll have more symptoms come up and more problems. In any kind of diet change—and the detox diet particularly—there's usually a couple of days of transition during which, as you're starting the diet, you may feel headachy, a cold, irritable. Usually by the third day, you start to click in. It's much like aerobic exercise. The first few minutes are difficult, but as soon as you get into that aerobic state, you think, 'Wow, this feels good. I'm moving forward.'"

Note, however, that pregnant women, people who are convalescing from illness, diabetics, hypoglycemics, people with mental problems, those with metabolic imbalances, and people taking medications should not undertake a cleansing program unsupervised. First they must determine that any proposed supplements or juices are not counterindicated by their medical program. Then if the person feels weak, faint, or dizzy, she should have a protein drink made of high-quality soy- or rice-based protein—containing anywhere from 20 to 35 gm of protein. She can also have grains, such as brown rice, millet, or barley, and beans, or a serving of fish while cleansing to maintain blood sugar. Eating these foods does not detract from the cleansing program.

Haas says detox is broadly helpful. "Anybody," he says, "can benefit from a detox program if it is done in the right way at the right time. Each detox depends on where a person is at and what she needs. To me, good medicine connects you with the patient and helps the patient take her next steps. Everybody is in a different state. If the person has a regular job and cannot easily go on a juice cleanse, she may have to go a different way. That's why I wrote *The Detox Diet,* to show people how they can take very simple steps that most anybody can handle. The detox diet provides nutrition for people with fruits and grains and vegetables, which provide many vitamins and minerals. With this diet, you are being nourished while you are detoxing."

CAFFEINE

How can detox help you escape the clutches of caffeine addiction? First, let's make it clear how bad for the body caffeine is and how people come to ignore its negative effects. "If you do something for the first time, such as drink alcohol, smoke a cigarette, or have a cup of coffee," Haas says, "you will be aware of the irritating, stimulating, or sedating effects of the substance." When people start to use any of these substances regularly, however, they tend to overlook those initial effects. They now have an addiction and take the substance not so much to feel the original sensations as to counteract the withdrawal symptoms.

Caffeine is bad for you, particularly over time. In the short term, it raises your blood pressure. It can also make you hyperagitated, increase anxiety, and affect sleep. Over time, because caffeine is a diuretic, it causes the loss of many minerals, such as calcium, magnesium, and potassium, particularly through the urine. The result of these losses is a more permanent increase in blood pressure. Two other long-term effects of caffeine are to weaken bones and to create mineral deficiencies, both of which can lead to a variety of other problems.

In women, Haas notes, caffeine seems to increase the incidence of all kinds of cystic problems, such as fibrocystic breast tumors and uterine fibroids. Studies on the relationship between caffeine use and cancer have produced conflicting results. However, a number of studies suggest that caffeine does increase the risk of certain types of cancer, and Haas believes that is another good reason for minimizing caffeine intake.

He observes that "most people, when they go off caffeine, will have some secondary effects, usually a tension headache, at least for 24 hours. Sometimes they will feel agitated or fatigued. They are going through a short-term withdrawal. If they have a very large habit, it may last 48 hours, but usually it's only 24 hours." Haas says that some people can mitigate the withdrawal headache by taking an over-the-counter aspirin, but thinks it's better to avoid that chemical medication if possible.

He recommends that you begin a detox diet the day before you start getting off caffeine. You can either go cold turkey or try to reduce your intake so that over a week you get down to maybe half a cup a day or less. If you do it gradually in this way, you will have fewer symptoms. According to Haas, "Many of the withdrawal symptoms happen because of elimination of acid from the foods and chemicals that we're cutting out."

"Doing the detox diet will reduce the withdrawal. I advise that you take additional nutrients, as follows: 2,000-10,000 mg vitamin C from calcium ascorbate, 1,200 mg calcium and magnesium from citrate, 400 mg potassium, 400 mg alpha lypoic acid, 200 mg ginkgo, 1,500 mg of essential fatty acids, a 20-mg capsule of cayenne pepper, 200 mg ginseng, 400 IU vitamin E, 500 mcg vitamin B_{12}, and 200 mg non-flush niacin.

"Drinking lots of water helps. Also make sure the bowels move. Some people like caffeine because it gets their bowels to move in the morning. It stimulates the intestine's peristaltic activities. For these people caffeine withdrawal may cause constipation. Now not moving your bowels enough can cause more toxins to back up, and you will feel worse. So it's really important to do what you can about this. Even a day or two after you go off caffeine, you might get something from the natural food store such as laxative tea or laxative tablets or find other means of cleansing the bowels."

ALCOHOL

Drinking alcohol has serious negative nutritional consequences. "Alcohol doesn't have a lot of nutrients in it," Haas explains. "People will say wine has a little bit of vitamin C and some nutrients from grapes. Beer has some B vitamins. Yet the levels aren't really that significant. Alcohol also is a diuretic. It causes loss of nutrients through the urine."

Nevertheless, he is not in favor of teetotaling. "When people have a drink here or there and they are eating a healthy diet, it will not cause a problem. In fact, a recent study showed that people who drink wine tend to have a better, more Mediterranean-like diet" and the associated better health, "whereas people who drink beer and other kinds of alcohol tend not to eat as conscientiously."

He adds, "One thing I've seen over the years is that bad habits tend to multiply. People who tend to abuse any substance, whether sugar, alcohol, nicotine, or caffeine, tend to also be less conscientious about how they take care of their bodies. They have other habits which are undermining their health."

Alcohol also irritates the liver, and people who drink more tend to consume more calories. Haas explains, "Alcohol is a sugar that gets absorbed relatively directly into the body and causes an overstimulation of insulin. Then you are dealing with problems in the whole sugar metabolism. These heavy drinkers then tend to consume less nutrient-rich foods. They get depleted that way. Those are some of the ways that alcohol endangers the body."

What is the best detox program for getting off alcohol? "For alcohol," Haas advises, "you want a nutrient-rich program. If you have been taking a lot of alcohol, you will definitely need professional guidance and intervention to help get through the period of withdrawal." Haas finds that the best daily combination of supplements for getting off alcohol is vitamin B, vitamin C, and a combination of calcium and magnesium, which helps alleviate the agitation that accompanies withdrawal. Chromium is another substance that can help in sugar metabolism. He advises a person to take either chromium picolinate or another form of chromium. "You'll need at least 200 mcg, which is the way they usually come in capsules. Take these a couple times a day to help with processing the sugar."

Another amino acid that can really help is L-glutamine, which affects brain chemistry. "Remember, a lot of the addictions we have are related to the opiate receptors which oversee addiction in the brain. L-glutamine seems to help feed the brain the nourishment it needs. It appears to reduce both sugar cravings and alcohol cravings. It's been used successfully in several alcohol clinics for people with more serious problems. The amount of glutamine that people might use is 500 to 1,000 mg, two to three times a day. If you have cravings, you can take more. It's safe. I never see problems with it."

Haas does suggest that "with any amino acid or any B vitamin, you don't want to use one substance for a long time by itself because you can throw the body off balance a little bit. So if you are using the amino acid or B vitamin for more than a few weeks, you may want to use a whole complex."

Orthomolecular psychiatrist Dr. Abram Hoffer has this advice: "For alcoholism the basic treatment starts with Alcoholics Anonymous. Bill W., the cofounder of Alcoholics Anonymous, first showed that when you added niacin to the treatment of alcoholism you got a major response that you did not see before." Today, there are a large number of very good alcoholism treatment programs in the United States which combine AA's 12-step approach, various social aids, good nutrition, and the right supplements.

SUGAR

Many people may debate whether sugar is addictive in the same way nicotine and alcohol are addictive, but it is definitely a hard habit to break. Haas notes: "When I talk to people about cleaning up sugar because there are so many books out now recommending lowering sugar intake and mentioning the problems with refined sugar, I find that it is an emotional problem above all. People were trained so early on that sugar is a reward. Sugar is sweet. All the love-talk words involve sugar. You're 'sweet on someone,' the person is your 'honey' or 'sweetie.' Sugar is associated with love and reward. So it's hard to break that emotional pattern."

Yet getting rid of sugar improves health. "When women who have problems with their menstrual cycle, who are irregular, who have pain, who have PMS clean that sugar out of their diets, often within a couple of months they are feeling a lot better, as long as they are taking some other nutrients," says Haas.

Not only does sugar affect behavior and moods, it is responsible for quite a few health problems. As Haas tells it, "Although some studies have refuted these findings—studies sponsored by the industry, I might add—researchers have found that sugar causes problems in kids in their focus and behavior. I think it causes increases in candida and parasites. It causes weakness in the digestive tract. Clearly, it's a cause of tooth decay. It has some causal relation to obesity, diabetes, and chronic digestion problems, as well as menstrual irregularities. It also hooks into alcohol abuse."

He has seen psychological problems that he believes had strong roots in the patient's sugar intake. "I've had a number of young women patients who came in. They were on medicine for depression and other low moods. When I interviewed them about their diet, which their psychiatrist never did, it turns out they are drinking a quart of Coke or Pepsi or one of those heavily sweetened beverages a day. So they were getting in the neighborhood of 40 to 50 teaspoons of sugar a day. Those intakes are really influencing their moods. The women who I've gotten to pay attention to their diets and get off sugar have been able to reduce their medicines and be more stable without these psychoactive drugs."

He echoes a theme that recurs throughout this book: "I think there's a lot to be said about how lifestyle and these habits affect our health and sanity. One of the key overall views is that when people don't feel well they need to look at their lifestyle first and see if there are factors in the way they are living that may be contributing to their decline. Then they should look at natural remedies. Lastly, I would tell them to turn to medicines, which I still use in my practice because I think that's part of being an integrated doctor. I use any system that I think is going to be of benefit to my patients. Sometimes people do need prescription medicines to help them get out of trouble. If they lived better, however, they wouldn't be getting into that trouble in the first place."

To really eliminate sugar, he encourages people to read labels and work on cleaning up their diet as a whole. He commonly sees people who have a some form of yeast infection, or candidiasis. They also have problems with moods, energy, and brain function, secondary to the yeast fermentation process in their intestinal tract, which causes toxins to get into their bodies. A key to recovery for such a person is to eliminate alcohols and sugars to stop feeding the yeast:

"Usually, within three or four days of cutting out the sugar, the person will feel a change. She doesn't have any symptoms in the way she would from alcohol withdrawal, but for the first couple of days she may feel headachy and moody. This will only last a day or two.

"Again, if you drink more water and you take your extra Bs and other supplements, you'll have a smoother transition. Typically, by the third day and definitely within the week, you'll notice smoother and more balanced energy and better brain function. After the withdrawal, a person's moods are more stable, she is less reactive. She just starts to feel better quite quickly. Then a week or two later, she will say, 'You know, I had a lapse and I tried some more sugar. I can't believe the stuff I was eating. It's so oversweet that it doesn't taste right to me.'"

Haas is not against sweets per se. Breaking sugar addiction, he says, "doesn't mean we can never eat anything sweet. Fruits are sweet, and they are some of the purest foods that we have. Most sweet foods are based on extracts from either grains, such as corn syrups, or from other plants that are naturally sweet. Overall, we just want to balance out the diet."

Addiction as Ingrained Craving

Jerry Dorsman makes the unusual point that food addictions are harder to kick than drug or alcohol addictions. He's a certified addiction counselor from Oakton, Maryland, and the author of *How to Quit Drinking Without AA* and *How to Quit Drugs for Good*:

"Let me begin by saying that in my clinical experience it is harder to get people to change their diet than to break an addiction to drugs and alcohol," Dorsman says. "I've seen statistics on this recently that show we have a 30 to 40 percent success rate for people breaking addictions to substances; but there is only about a 5 percent success rate for people who are trying to change diet and get away from bad food habits.

"The reason for this, I think, is that we have deeply ingrained addictions to food. Our body has come to expect certain foods in our diets. We have a metabolic expectation. If we don't get those foods, we begin to crave them. If you take a look at it, we've been eating foods since we've been one year old, whereas, typically, drugs or alcohol aren't started until we are in our teens or early twenties. So they have had a shorter period of time in which to change the body. I think it's a longer-term, more deeply ingrained pattern that creates the difficulty in changing diet."

To break food addictions, one has to get a handle on cravings. According to Dorsman, "The more balanced we can make our diet, the healthier it becomes. The addiction causes a certain imbalance in the body. The body has to be constantly prepared to metabolize this substance which it's experiencing over and over. This creates a severe imbalance. Our natural response is to balance it. The place to start is dealing with this physical part of cravings. By changing the diet based on the contractive/expansive as well as the acid/alkaline balances, we can really begin to settle our metabolism and find greater peace based on diet alone. In fact, in my opinion, changing diet is the number one stress-reduction technique available.

"A second way to handle cravings is just wait it out. Most cravings, according to scientific studies, last for only about five to ten minutes. Once we know that up front, that particular piece of knowledge can help us beat these cravings. You can think to yourself, 'Hey, I just have a few minutes here to wait this out and manage it.'"

The basic difficulties in resisting cravings—and this applies to any type of addiction, from food to drugs to alcohol—can, in Dorsman's opinion, "be broken into two categories: problems that substance use caused and problems it concealed. The most common problems that substance use causes are the physical problems, because of the biological effects of the drug or alcohol or food on the body, which are very devastating at the cellular level and to the nerve cells. The problems that are concealed are emotional ones. Those are problems which, when a person drank or used drugs or binged on food, tended to go away, because the person could ignore such things as depression, anxiety, and anger. Those emotional difficulties a person ignored when drinking or drugging or binging will come back up when the person puts down the addictive substances."

Hypnotherapy

Another health practitioner with much experience in dealing with addictions is Michael Ellner, a medical hynotherapist with a private practice at the Chelsea Healing Center and co-author, with Dr. Richard Jamison, of *Quantum Force*.

Ellner begins: "One point I should bring up is that anyone a healer works with is an individual who has her own story about why she does something, her own mythology about why something is important to her and what role it plays in her life." Ellner says, for example, that there are many underlying reasons why a woman might use food as her addiction of choice. "Some use food to fill up the empty feeling they have. Other people have social issues with eating. Such a person might eat wisely when she is at home, but in social situations, just to be part of the crowd, she may indulge in food that ordinarily would not appeal to her. If the person is very active socially, then suddenly it becomes habitual, almost a license to eat junk food.

"Some people use food as a shield. Very often when a relationship ends, a woman puts on 10 to 15 pounds. It provides a cushion, because people are unlikely to hit on her. The woman gets a little bit of space. Very often when she begins to feel better about herself and is ready to go back into the world, it occurs to the woman that it is time to let go of the extra pounds. I can help the person do that very quickly."

THE TREATMENT PROCESS

Explaining his treatment for addiction, Ellner uses tobacco addiction to illustrate. "To deal with any addiction, I use one of two ways. For people with combined physical and psychological addictions, in the case of cigarettes, for instance, I work as an adjunct to an acupuncturist. She helps the person resolve the physical addiction, while I am working to help resolve the psychological addiction. That gives a person a one-two punch in helping her take charge of her life. It makes the overall detox much easier.

"The initial phase of treatment begins when the addict decides she wants a change of behavior. That's the first step. The second step comes with helping her develop the self-confidence and self-esteem necessary to move forward, which means stopping the addictive behavior.

"I use hypnotic conditioning to help the person create a shift. The shift would make the desire to be smoke-free much more important to the person than any impulse to smoke. Ordinarily, the impulse to smoke is much stronger. The hypnosis enables the person to make choices rather than responding to preconditioned reflexes. In other words, there are many things in a day that will trigger the response, 'It's time to light a cigarette.' Most of these responses occur unconsciously, and before the person really thinks about it, she is smoking a cigarette. The hypnosis will interfere with that impulse in such a way that she will have the time to stop and think, 'Do I really want that cigarette?' That's the pause that enables people to break habits and end addictions."

To some people, the very word "hypnosis" has a stigma attached to it. Ellner comments: "If you ask 50 of the leading experts in the world about what hypnosis is, then you'd probably get 50 different answers. When I use the word 'hypnosis,' I'm talking about a way to help a person change neurological patterns. This is done through imagery, metaphor, and the power of suggestion.

"Hypnosis in that context is a communication tool. It helps a person communicate with herself more efficiently, and so she is able to do things that ordinarily she wouldn't think that she could do. "There are a number of practices that are quite popular and are in fact hypnosis, but the practitioners avoid using the word. An example would be guided meditation. Guided imagery and visualization are also forms of hypnosis. Many meditation practices are forms of self-hypnosis. I myself am working very hard to educate the public to understand the word and to appreciate that hypnosis is one of the most powerful self-help tools available.

"If I have a client — I don't have 'patients' and I don't like that word — who is dealing with a smoking addiction, I find it can often be resolved in one session, especially if she has a couple of adjunct sessions with an acupuncturist. Hypnosis is a stand-alone therapy, but I work with an acupuncturist because I want to give my client the ultimate protocol for helping her do what she wants in helping herself. These two systems work very well together to help a person stop smoking very quickly and with little or no withdrawal.

"With food issues, it could take between four and eight sessions. There are a lot of additional areas that have to be worked with that involve building self-esteem, building a better self-image, helping a person gain confidence, and helping her let go of a lot of emotional tension.

"In terms of alcohol and drug addictions, let me say this. My general practice is to get the person involved in something else [another rehab program] and to work with her as an adjunct to support whatever it is she is doing. I will recommend different programs for helping a person stop using drugs and stop drinking. Then the hypnosis would take the edge off. It would give the client a higher quality of motivation.

"A substance abuser very often finds herself stuck in an addictive environment. So, if she can go to rehab, she finds that in that environment, it is pretty simple to stay off the drugs. However, then she gets back home and finds that all the things that contributed to that problem in the first place are again staring her in the face. I could help her address that hypnotically in such a way that she can create space and disassociate from those triggers that ordinarily lead back to the addiction. I can help the woman change the way she responds to those triggers. She can then nullify those triggers and create new responses that are healthy."

He mentions some triggers that may start a person drinking. "We live in a country where the founding principle is freedom of speech. Yet the greatest phobia in America is public speaking. You'd be amazed at how many people develop drinking problems because they have a drink or two before they have to speak. It becomes a ritual. Very often, it diminishes the quality of whatever they're saying, but they can't appreciate that. The speaker feels helpless without that drink or two.

"The situational triggers produce anxiety and the anxiety says, 'Hey, I need a drink. Maybe I need a drink and a cigarette.' With the hypnosis, the same stimuli can now create a relaxation response. Instead of anxiety overwhelming the person in that situation, suddenly the person feels calm and peaceful. Suddenly, speaking to the people in front of her is as natural as taking a deep breath. The person is in the same situation, but the triggers don't provoke the same response, don't produce the old unwanted behavior. In that respect, in conjunction with a program and a support system, most people can turn these behaviors around rather quickly and dramatically. A woman will find that she has the inner resolve to stay on the wagon."

Another adjunct to his counseling is nutrition. "When I am working as an adjunct to the acupuncturist, I have the acupuncturist also do nutritional counseling. If I am not working with her, I would refer the client to a nutritionist, giving her two or three recommendations of nutritionists and suggesting that this be part of her overall program to reclaim life and health. One of the more popular programs I recommend is to join one of Gary Null's study groups, which provides peer support and a firm education about nutritional issues and gives people something to do that is a good use of their time. This is very important in making this kind of change. I take advantage of whatever is out there, and I use hypnosis as an additional way of helping the client accomplish her goals."

TOXIC THINKING

Ellner speaks passionately about how thought processes can have a negative impact. "To me, the biggest and most dangerous addiction is toxic thinking. People are very often addicted to negative beliefs, negative opinions about themselves and the world they live in. This addiction really diminishes one's quality of life. Instead of having fun, life is always a drag. Very often, that primary addiction gives rise to all the secondary addictions that people put all their time and energy into. One of the first things I do is make people aware of the nature of toxic thinking. Then I help them do a mental detox and change the way they think.

"As a part of that I use meditation, creative visualization, and other forms of hypnosis. One of the most engaging forms of hypnosis comes about when a person has some kind of creative pursuit, whether it's strumming a guitar and going into an enhanced state of consciousness, or reading a very exciting book, or taking a walk and having contact with nature. All those things are hypnotic experiences. All those things involve moving from one state of consciousness to another. I encourage a person to get very active in her everyday life."

A Final Note

If you are taking a substance because you are depressed, your depression may be physiologically induced, perhaps due to some form of brain imbalance. You might have an underactive thyroid, for example, or a blood-sugar imbalance— whether high or low blood sugar. Either of these conditions can be manifested as depression. In order to get away from the chronic feeling of emptiness that frequently accompanies depression, people will start to drink.

One of the reasons people drink is that it takes away the feelings: both the highs and the lows. It gives the drinker a sense of being in a never-never land.

The same is true of many drugs. People take drugs because it gives them a euphoria they wouldn't have achieved on their own or that they may have had but could not sustain. So they keep going back to it. Once you get used to that, it's quick and easy to just stick a needle in your arm or put some form of narcotic up your nose. You drink it or ingest it. None of this helps us resolve the underlying conflict, which may be biological, psychological, or a combination of the two.

I have found that the best single way to approach this is to get the person into a systematic cleansing program—and there are many—where the person actually breaks all physical addictions, and not just to one thing like sugar, but also every other thing they could be allergic to. That seems to be a major first step. The person's energy comes back. See, a very big thing about any addiction withdrawal is the lack of energy. So when you substitute for the energy they had been getting from the drug by giving it to the person naturally, through the body's own process of metabolism, the person feels better.

Then you start to rebuild the center of the brain with phosphatidyl serine, 500 mg, acetyl L-carnitine, 500 mg, phosphatidyl choline, 500 mg, and with certain herbs that are known to have an impact like feverfew and green tea. Also flood the body with flavonoids. The person should also juice, juice, juice, taking anywhere from four to six glasses of fresh-made organic vegetable juice a day. Within six months to a year, I have seen people who have been totally addicted clear up about 80 percent, stay off, and not come back.

Consider the alternative: You might end up face down on a slab... of hamburger patties.

Chapter 2

Aging

The idea that aging inevitably means gaining weight and having high blood pressure, high triglycerides, high cholesterol levels, and arthritis is widely accepted. Since so many people have these problems, we think of them as normal. Even doctors are likely to say that when you get to be a certain age, these conditions are to be expected and, since they are irreversible, accepted. The idea that diminished health inevitably accompanies aging is particularly pernicious in a society in which older men and women, and particularly women, are the victims of a pervasive ageism, which holds that sexual attractiveness is the exclusive province of the young.

Fortunately, research over the last decade has given us a better understanding of the causes of aging; in particular, several theories have led to new therapies offering women opportunities not only to improve their health but to actually slow down the aging processes. We now know that it's possible to live to 100 and beyond and to stay healthy throughout our life spans, thus "rectangularizing" the aging curve. Dr. Martin Feldman, a traditionally trained physician who practices complementary medicine, supports this stand. "We need to have optimum energy as we grow old, not accept the diminishment many find encroaching as they grow older." Dr. Feldman cites joint disease as an example of a condition that medicine has accepted as inevitable, a condition that is reversible. There is now an epidemic of joint disease in the United States. The majority of people over 60 have early, moderate, or late osteoarthritis. Conventional doctors call osteoarthritis a wear-and-tear disease, as if the joints wore out like the parts of a car. That sounds plausible, but it is nonsense. The disease is a product of deficiencies and occurs when the joint is not being nourished. A nourished joint will remain healthy. Dr. Feldman has seen marathon runners in their seventies and eighties who use their joints 10-fold or even 50-fold more than a normal person does, yet their joints remain robust.

Causes

FREE RADICAL DAMAGE

It is widely accepted that aging and degenerative diseases are the result of cellular damage brought on by free radicals, molecules that have become unstable after losing one of their orbiting electrons. The unpaired electrons of these molecules make the molecules highly reactive, and in an attempt to restore balance, a free radical will steal electrons from other molecules, causing cellular damage and destruction.

Free radicals are produced through normal metabolism in the body, but increase with exposure to animal fat, alcohol, cigarettes, and other toxic chemicals. Dr. Christopher Calapai, a proponent of complementary medicine who has a medical practice in New York City, gives an example of how this damage can occur: "Free radicals generated by cigarette smoke are huge in number. They steal healthy electrons from the lining of the lungs, thereby oxidizing lung tissue. When lung tissue is oxidized, cells break down and die. As hundreds of thousands of cells become oxidized and damaged, tissues and organs throughout the body are affected. Aging and disease are magnified."

LOW THYROID FUNCTION

Low thyroid functioning can prompt diseases associated with aging. Dr. Ray Peat, a distinguished research scientist from Eugene, Oregon, says that doctors in the first part of the twentieth century were better informed than today's doctors about the importance of correcting this condition: "Most of the basic research on the thyroid was done before World War II. Pharmaceutical companies came in after the war with what they thought was the latest word in understanding the thyroid. It turns out they were wrong. Until 1940, it was accepted that 40 percent of Americans benefited from taking thyroid supplements. After faulty tests were established, it was believed that only 5 percent of Americans needed or benefited from thyroid supplements. In the 1930s indications of hypothyroidism included such things as too much cholesterol in the blood, insomnia, emphysema, arthritis, and failure of the immune system. Many conditions now considered mysterious diseases were recognized as traits of low thyroid. Very often these conditions would simply disappear when thyroid supplements were given.

"When the thyroid is low we have to rely on emergency systems—such as the production of adrenaline and cortisone—to adapt to stress. Cortisone and adrenaline are now recognized as factors that cause damage, setting degenerative diseases in motion and causing damage to the lining of blood vessels and brain cells, but very often people don't realize that it is the thyroid that keeps us from relying excessively on these stress hormones."

BIOLOGICAL CLOCK

Another theory holds that the body has a built-in cellular "biological clock" that is set so that cells self-destruct after a certain amount of time. Dr. Lance Morris, a naturopathic physician from Tucson, Arizona, notes that since the theory was first propounded, the proposed upper limits for the clock's running time have increased. "At this time," he says, "there is a feeling that the top limit is pushing 140 years. Individuals have actually lived to that age, and even longer."

SHRINKING THYMUS GLAND

Another theory relates aging to atrophy of the thymus gland, which plays a role in maintaining a healthy immune system and fighting infection. As Dr. Morris explains it, "When we are born, this gland covers our entire chest. It's huge. As we grow older, it diminishes in size, a process known as thymic involution. One of the theories of aging is that if we could stop thymic shrinking we could stop the aging process altogether."

MERCURY

Dr. Hal A. Huggins of Colorado Springs, Colorado, highlights another cause of premature aging, the mercury in silver amalgam fillings. According to Huggins, the mercury in your fillings does not just sit there—you inhale it and it goes into your lungs. Every time you eat and and chew, minute amounts of mercury get into your stomach and digestive system and from there to cells in all parts of your body, where it can undergo oxidation, forming methyl mercury, a highly toxic substance.

OTHER THEORIES

Dr. Elton Haas, a practicing integrated medicine physician, is director of the Preventive Medical Center in San Rafael, California, and author of *The Staying Healthy Shopper's Guide,* among other best-selling books. In an article on the HealthWorld Online website (www.healthy.net), he summarizes a few other theories of aging: errors in DNA, possibly caused by free radicals; alterations in brain function; imbalance in the hormonal and nervous systems; a breakdown in immune system function; and stress. His own theory, he explains, is that all these processes combine in various ways in each person to result in aging, with the key factor being "stagnation of bioenergy circulation and stagnation of the digestive tract and bowels."

Symptoms

A wide variety of gradual bodily changes are associated with aging, such as an increased susceptibility to weight gain and fatigue. But there is no physiological reason why most people should become obese or get tired more easily as they grow older: these are society's, not nature's, norms. It can be just as natural, for example, for people to eat and sleep a little less as they grow older, compensating for any slowing down of metabolic processes and thus maintaining stable weight and energy levels.

Typical signs of aging also include changes in skin, hair, nails, and connective tissue. Decreases in memory, concentration, and sharpness may also accompany aging. Again, it is not inevitable that these changes take place.

As women (and men) age, they may suffer from elevated blood sugar, an increase in cholesterol and triglycerides, and other chemical imbalances. The risk of contracting degenerative diseases such as cancer and heart disease, and suffering from thyroid dysfunction, musculoskeletal problems, and gastrointestinal disorders, also typically increases with age, for both women and men.

Clinical Experience

DIAGNOSING PROBLEMS

Aging well means being healthy and balanced from within. To check that all systems are running optimally, Dr. Calapai recommends a full spectrum of diagnostic tests, with special attention to adrenal function, vitamin and mineral levels, blood chemistry, pancreatic enzymes, and stool. "The adrenal glands produce our antiaging hormones. With age, some people start producing less. This can be from free radical damage, excessive stress, injuries, and all sorts of reasons. As a result we see changes in memory, concentration, skin, hair, hormonal fluctuations, and energy levels. We start to see problems with immune response and increases in blood sugar, cholesterol, and abdominal deposition of body fat. So we need to look at adrenal function.

"Certainly, tests should look at vitamin and mineral levels to check our digestive and absorptive abilities. Looking at the basic blood chemistry tells us how well we are absorbing protein. We need to look at the fat-soluble vitamins and cholesterol, triglycerides, and the ratio of good HDL cholesterol to bad LDL cholesterol, which can provide information about our fat absorption. I also recommend looking at enzymes of the pancreas to assess function and having a comprehensive stool analysis done to see whether or not there are too many undigested particles in the stool. If parasites are present, this can decrease our absorptive ability. These are some of the main tests we need to perform to get a thorough picture of the individual."

BASIC DIET

An antiaging diet for women of all ages should consist of high-quality organic foods, emphasizing complex carbohydrates such as beans and whole grains, fruits, and vegetables. Adolescents, who are still growing, may need more of certain nutrients, and individual women in specific age groups may have specific nutrient requirements that can be addressed through supplements. But a basic healthy diet will vastly improve the quality of life and reduce the aging process in women of all ages.

Antiaging diets contain few, if any, animal-based proteins; fats are minimized and high-fiber foods are emphasized. High-fiber diets help prevent common afflictions associated with aging, such as constipation, hemorrhoids, pressure in the intestines, ulcers, high blood pressure, colorectal cancer, and overall body toxemia. One of the principles of longevity is eating to the point of being not quite full. As women get older, it is advisable to eat small servings more frequently. Uneaten portions can be frozen for later use.

At least eight 8-oz glasses of water should be drunk daily. Many senior citizens suffer from dehydration because their intake of fluid is inadequate. Dehydration adversely affects the body's electrolytes, which carry electricity and are important for normal functioning of the nervous system. Additionally, fresh juices, which are high in enzymes, should be a regular part of the diet. Recommended intake is two to three 6-oz glasses of fresh, organic mixed vegetable juice per day, with 1-2 mg of buffered vitamin C added to each glass, or up to bowel tolerance.

VEGETARIAN DIETS

A number of doctors stress the benefits of a healthy vegetarian diet. For example, participants in Dr. Martin Feldman's nutritional program, who are on a vegetarian diet, are doing better on lowering cholesterol than any comparable group. He states, "We did not select people to come in to work on cholesterol problems. We are using a total assault on the lifestyle without focusing on cholesterol. The level of reduction is superior to that found in any prior drug study [studies in which drugs were used to cut down on cholesterol]. It is extremely important that we can achieve this reduction without drugs. Drugs are expensive and have side effects. Also, we do not know what long-term problems may arise with them."

Dr. Dean Ornish has shown that a vegetarian diet can help clear the arteries (see Chapter 15 for more information on his program).

SUPPLEMENTS

The first thing to look at as a means of reversing the symptoms of aging is supplements. Most people do not understand the effective use of vitamins and minerals as dietary supplements. Basically, you must follow the law of compensation. If you smoked, used sugar, caffeine, or alcohol, if you were an angry person who held in your anger, if you have not honored the life force, if you have not exercised, if you have felt unfulfilled, you must work to compensate for these deficiencies.

One-a-day supplements are the easy way out. I have met people who say, "I eat meat. I eat sugar. But it's all right because I take my one-a-day vitamin." My friend, that does not work. The body cannot be lied to. After 30 or 40 years of the body's being debilitated by an unhealthy lifestyle and environment, a little pill will not do the trick. You need to detoxify and cleanse the body.

Another illusion is that the "recommended daily dose," or "minimal daily requirement (MDR)," given by drug companies and conventional physicians, is a useful number. This is not a good way to think about health. These recommendations are like the minimum wage. Is that what we are interested in, minimal health? Or do we want optimal health? The supplement dosages given as recommended daily values are very substandard if one wants long-term health through the life span.

You have to know what your bodily state is and plan accordingly. I would suggest one level of usage for healthy people who know they are healthy, and a very different level for those processing diseases. A woman becoming conscious of her health will need to consult a nutritionist who can design a personalized supplement program to meet her individual needs.

The reason that supplements are even more crucial as we get older is that as we age, certain fatty acids, amino acids, and members of the main groups of nutrients are lost. Scientists looking into this issue already know that choline, tyrosine, glutathione, cystine, vitamin E, zinc, and chromium are poorly absorbed and deficient in older people. Meanwhile, as these substances grow scarce, there is a buildup of heavy metals, such as aluminum and lead. These metals can be removed from the body through a process known as chelation. Vitamin C and zinc are also useful in flushing them out. Most importantly, all the nutrients that are lost, for whatever reason, must be restored for optimum physical and mental functioning.

At the same time, the free radicals in our bodies, which grow in number as we age, have to be fought. Remember, when you eat meat, drink alcohol, and are exposed to pollutants, the body creates free radicals. They cause the skin to wrinkle in the sun, and they foster cancer, arthritis, and heart disease. However, nutrients called antioxidants, such as beta carotene and vitamin A, are able to neutralize the effect of the free radicals, slowing down the aging process.

ANTIOXIDANTS

Dr. Morris calls aging a catch-22: "Oxygen is the great substance that sustains and gives life, but unfortunately it is also the substance that destroys us through oxidation." For this reason, antioxidants are essential. Here are the most important ones.

VITAMIN E. 400–1,600 IU of vitamin E, taken at the largest meal. People with herpes, chronic fatigue syndrome, hepatitis, and even AIDS have miraculously improved after taking large doses of this vitamin on a regular basis. Dr. Wilfred Shute, who works with his brother Evan in Canada, has treated over 30,000 patients in his decades of medical practice. He has helped patients with intermittent claudication, diabetes, gangrene, and many other conditions. Vitamin E is best in its natural form (as a mixed tocopherol or d-alphatocopherol). Synthetic vitamin E (dl-alpha) should be avoided.

BETA CAROTENE. 25,000 IU per meal. Beta carotenes can be obtained in all the green, red, and orange fruits and vegetables. They help slow down aging and lessen cancer risk. They are nontoxic, since the body converts beta carotenes into vitamin A and will not convert more than it can use.

VITAMIN A. 1,000–3,000 IU per meal. Blood tests will determine whether or not a person is getting too much vitamin A, which can be toxic.

SELENIUM. 100 mcg per meal. One cause of premature aging and even death, particularly in professional athletes, is cardiomyopathy, an enlargement of the heart. This is usually associated with selenium deficiency. Adequate amounts of this critical nutrient are needed to help the body produce the antioxidant enzyme glutathione peroxidase, which is on the front line of aging defense.

ZINC. 30–90 mg daily. Zinc feeds over 100 enzyme systems in the brain, as well as various systems throughout the body. It is essential in the formation of stomach acid; without sufficient zinc, malabsorption syndrome occurs. Most older people are zinc-deficient.

VITAMIN C. 2,000–5,000 mg daily, higher doses for antiaging protocols and fighting disease (under medical supervision, up to 150,000 mg via intravenous drips). The single most important dietary supplement is vitamin C. Its benefits are multiple. This vitamin is important for the skin, giving it youthful elasticity. This is because it produces collagen, a type of connective tissue that holds the muscles and skin together. It helps the body produce interferon (an antiviral glycoprotein) and increases leukocyte activity. It aids the thymus gland, the liver, and the brain, while acting to prevent arthritis, cataracts, and heart disease.

At the Healing Center of New York City, drips of vitamin C and other nutrients are used to counteract the aging process. Dr. Howard Robins points out that toxins and free radicals are stressful to both the body and mind. A body in pain, fatigued, and under attack from heavy metal and other pollutants, which we come in contact with on a daily basis, is weakened, and the mind is adversely affected. Robins asserts that intravenously administered vitamin C cleanses the body. The Healing Center also uses drips with other nutrients, such as EDTA (ethylenediaminetetra-acetic acid), to cleanse the heavy metals from the body and destroy viruses and keep them from replicating. These drips will also help boost the energy level.

GRAPESEED EXTRACT. 50 mg per day, up to 200 mg per day for people in a disease state. This bioflavonoid has the highest known antioxidant properties of any nutrient.

SUPEROXIDE DISMUTASE. This important antienzyme nutrient is produced by the body. It is not effective when taken orally unless it is enteric-coated. According to Dr. Haas, manganese and copper, together with zinc, support the action of superoxide dismutase.

HORMONES

DHEA: The Mother of All Hormones. Dr. Richard Ash has talked to his large New York City radio audience about the revivifying power of DHEA (dihydroepiandrosterone), which is a key underlying ingredient in the normal functioning of the adrenal gland. He tells us that when the body is under stress, the adrenal gland requires higher amounts of cortisone and adrenaline. If these hormones are overused, they will become depleted as will DHEA, their precursor.

An 80-year-old woman may have only one-twentieth of the DHEA she had at age 20. According to Dr. Ash, this can result in all sorts of negative consequences for the immune system, leading to a weakened capacity to fight diseases. One of the earliest signs of DHEA depletion is an inability to get REM sleep, which can lead to insomnia and chronic fatigue. An uninformed doctor may prescribe sleeping pills for a patient with insomnia, which will not get at the root of the problem. Other symptoms of low DHEA levels are hyperglycemia (an excess of glucose in the blood), palpitations, sweating, confusion, poor concentration, and the inability to cope with everyday stress.

Another effect of low DHEA is a reduction in salivary IgA, an antibody that fights infection in the gastrointestinal (GI) tract. When IgA is depleted or absent, there will be more antigen penetration in this area as well as increased sensitivity reactions to foods and chemicals There may be inflammation of the GI tract, a condition called "leaky gut," in which certain foods and chemicals are not absorbed but pass out into the bloodstream. When the body tries to defend itself against these unexpected intruders, autoimmune disease may arise. Dr. Ash notes that by administering DHEA and building back up salivary IgA, we can diminish food sensitivity, lower toxic load, and repair the GI tract, restoring normal immune system functioning by treating the cause not the symptoms.

PROGESTERONE, ESTROGEN, AND TESTOSTERONE. Dr. Eric Braverman, founder and director of Princeton Associates for Total Health (PATH), in Princeton, New Jersey, has found that counteracting the aging process has to be undertaken on an individual basis. His treatments are personalized on the basis of each patient's specific hormone balance, brain function, attention span, memory capacity, and cardiac and exercise capacities. Once these have been evaluated, the patient's nutritional needs are assessed. He recommends natural yam extract, which contains progesterone, estrogen, and testosterone (PET), the three hormones he considers essential. Progesterone has anticancer properties and helps calm the brain. Estrogen strengthens the bones, has anticancer effects, especially in the colon, aids memory, and gives cardiovascular protection. Testosterone reduces the side effects of other hormones, and helps keep the sex drive vigorous through a person's fifties, sixties, and beyond. For a woman, the ovary produces all three of these substances, but, as Dr. Braverman puts it, "If the ovary dies, you must resurrect it. If you permit an organ to die, you allow yourself to die. We must stop this if we want abundant life. We replace depleted hormones with PET, and missing adrenal with DHEA."

BIOFLAVONOID COMPLEX

Another invaluable supplement is the citrus bioflavonoid complex, which can be obtained from lemons, plums, and oranges, among other fruits. With an orange, one can cut open the skin and right below is the nutrient, the bioflavonoid. Another good bioflavonoid is rutin, which comes from buckwheat. To take the bioflavonoid in pill form, I recommend 300 mg per day for a healthy person, while someone in poor health should take 500 mg. As for the rutin, the proper dosage for a healthy person is 25 mg per day, while the ill person may take up to 50 mg.

BLUEBERRY AND RED CABBAGE EXTRACTS

Blueberry extract is good for the eyes. During World War II, the Royal Air Force gave this to its pilots to improve night vision and strengthen the immune system. Red cabbage extract is also important. There are cultures that lack a variety of foodstuffs, but those peoples eat cabbage and obtain its antibacterial, antiulcer properties. Cabbage, eaten juiced or steamed, is very healthful.

GREEN TEA

If you lived in China, you would probably be drinking green tea and taking green tea extract. We know it has anticancer properties. It is an immune system stimulator. Decaffeinated green tea is very beneficial.

GLUTATHIONE

Glutathione is good for the immune system, but it is not easily assimilated by the body, so it should be taken with something that produces it in the body, such as N-acetylcysteine. The recommended dose is 200 mg a day for the healthy and up to 400 mg for those not in the best of health.

OTHER SUPER SUPPLEMENTS

SEA ALGAE. High in trace elements, antioxidant cofactors, flavonoids, and carotenoid.

COENZYME Q10. Every cell in the body needs this coenzyme to create energy and build stamina.

NADH (nicotinamide adenine dinucleatide). Also known as coenzyme 1, NADH is a naturally occurring substance in the body that supplies energy to the cells, allowing them to live longer.

THYMUS EXTRACT. Pure oral thymus extract enhances immune function and helps reverse the aging process.

TYROSINE. Strengthens the thyroid and adrenal glands, protecting against stress.

DR. HAAS RECOMMENDS A NUMBER OF OTHER SUPPLEMENTS

L-CYSTEINE. This amino acid, which scavenges free radicals, protects the tissues from chemicals and aids detoxification, partly by helping the liver produce and store glutathione. Most often it is taken with vitamin C to prevent the formation of kidney stones of cystine, which is produced when cysteine is metabolized. Take 250 mg with a gram of vitamin C twice a day. When you take L-cysteine on a regular basis, you should also take a formula that contains the other amino acids the body needs.

CALCIUM. Calcium protects against osteoporosis and colon cancer, is important for strong teeth, and helps energy (ATP) production as well as heart and nerve function.

MAGNESIUM. Magnesium supports the cardiovascular system and decreases nervous tension.

CHROMIUM. Chromium supports glucose tolerance, decreasing the craving for sugar, and plays a role in preventing atherosclerosis by helping to lower blood cholesterol.

MOLYBDENUM. Molybdenum is a trace mineral that may help prevent cancer.

NIACIN. Niacin, a form of vitamin B3, decreases cholesterol and helps improve circulation.

VITAMIN B$_{12}$. Vitamin B$_{12}$ boosts energy and protects the fatty sheaths that cover the nerves. It is involved in synthesis of red blood cells and DNA and RNA, which are needed for important rebuilding processes.

FOLIC ACID. Folic acid also helps in RNA, DNA, and red blood cell synthesis, but a dose higher than the 400-mcg RDA is needed, often 1-2 mg twice a day.

RNA. RNA, taken in blue-green algae, spirulina, chlorella, and wheatgrass (all of which also are rich in chlorophyll), can decelerate the aging process.

ESSENTIAL FATTY ACIDS. Essential fatty acids, such as EPA (eicosapentaenoic acid) and DHA (docosahexaenoic acid), diminish the risk of cardiovascular disease. Flaxseed oil is a good source of both omega-3 and omega-6 essential fatty acids.

L-CARNITINE. L-carnitine, a nonessential amino acid involved in fat metabolism, may help reduce fat and weight.

DIGESTIVE AIDS. *Lactobacillus acidophilus,* along with other intestinal bacteria, may be needed occasionally to support the balance of bacteria in the colon. Similarly, supplements of hydrochloric acid and digestive enzymes aid digestion and metabolism of food, and thus prevent both nutritional deficiencies and free-radical formation due to food reactions.

HERBS

Herbs are an important part of any antiaging nutritional protocol, and can be taken as capsules, powders, teas, or tinctures.

FO-TI. *Fo-ti* rejuvenates the endocrine system and is an excellent digestive tonic.

GINKGO BILOBA. The ginkgo tree has survived for hundreds of thousands of years due to its powerful immune system. An extract of the leaf of the tree improves circulation to the microcapillaries of the brain and heart so that needed nutrients and oxygen can get to all the tissues.

GINSENG. Ginseng is the best-known longevity herb. For centuries, the Chinese have revered ginseng for its rejuvenating effects. Research has shown that ginseng can stop the free radical damage associated with aging. It helps people focus better when under stress and increases overall energy levels.

GOTA KOLA. Elephants, which graze on gota kola, are known to have excellent memories and to be long-lived. Gota kola is useful for increasing vitality and endurance, and may lower blood pressure.

HAWTHORN BERRIES. Hawthorn berries support circulation and cardiac function.

MILK THISTLE. Milk thistle protects liver function. The liver releases toxins from the body, promoting health and youthfulness.

YAM. Wild yam supports adrenal gland production of DHEA, a building block for the development of estrogen, progesterone, testosterone, and cortisols, which decrease with age. As an adaptogen, wild yam balances the body's hormonal functions. It has been shown to ameliorate numerous chronic conditions, including heart disease, cancer, arthritis, and autoimmune diseases. DHEA is extremely safe, with no known side effects.

DR. HAAS MENTIONS TWO OTHER BENEFICIAL HERBS: *Capsicum* stimulates elimination and circulation, and its mild diuretic properties help cleanse the kidneys. *Garlic* is antiviral, antibacterial, and antifungal. It boosts energy but—unlike coffee—helps lower cholesterol and blood pressure. Garlic also stimulates liver and colon detoxification and may have anticancer properties.

DETOXIFICATION THERAPIES

The more toxic we are, the faster we age. Cosmetic changes such as face-lifts and hair dye may temporarily make women appear younger, but they do not make a real difference. To keep youthful and healthy, women must address what is happening inside. "Everyone needs detoxification," says Susan Lombardi, founder and president of the We Care Health Center in Palm Springs, California, and author of *Ten Easy Steps for Complete Wellness.* "I am vegetarian, and I take care of myself. Do I still need detoxification? Yes, because the air that we breathe is polluted, the water that we drink is full of chlorine, the clothing we wear is made of artificial fabrics and chemicals, the lotions and shampoos that we use all contain chemicals. Once these chemicals are inside us, we never fully eliminate them unless we go through a detoxification procedure." Lombardi recommends rejuvenating the system from the inside out by limiting food intake to fresh raw vegetable juices once a week, along with the following simple, yet effective, detoxification therapies:

JUICE FASTING

Juice fasting gives the digestive system a rest and speeds up the growth of new cells, which promotes healing. (If you have any medical problems, do not fast without medical approval and supervision.)

On a juice fast, a person abstains from solid foods and drinks juice, water, and herbal teas throughout the day. "We should be drinking every half hour to an hour," advises Lombardi. "If we go for long periods of time without drinking anything, then a little glass of juice will not be able to sustain us. But if we are constantly drinking, the day will go by very smoothly."

Lombardi recommends a combination of the following:

CARROT JUICE. High in the antioxidant beta carotene and full of wonderful enzymes.

CELERY JUICE. HIGH IN SODIUM—not the artificial type poured from the saltshaker, which is bad for you, but the good, natural kind that promotes tissue flexibility.

BEET JUICE. Beets nourish the liver, one of the most important organs in the body, with hundreds of different functions. If your liver is functioning well, most likely everything else in your body will be too.

CABBAGE JUICE. Cabbage juice is high in vitamin C.

Mix the juice from each vegetable in equal proportion and drink this combination throughout the day. A little cayenne, which increases circulation, sending blood to every corner of the body to promote healing, can be added for flavor. Lemon juice in water and different herbal teas——some good ones are parsley and dandelion tea for the liver and kidneys and pau d'arco for blood purification —can be added for variety. "Any herbal tea free of caffeine will be good," Lombardi says. "Since you need to drink on an hourly basis, you don't want to drink the same thing over and over."

CHELATION THERAPY

Martin Dayton, M.D., of Florida, who is board-certified in family medicine, chelation therapy, and clinical nutrition, says that chelation therapy has multiple benefits, and long life is one of them: "Dramatic increases in life span are found with chelation. While there are no longevity studies per se, this conclusion is implied indirectly by studies which show a lessening of killer degenerative diseases. In fact, chelation favorably impacts all four major causes of death in the United States [heart disease, cancer, cerebrovascular disease, and lung disease]."

During the chelation process many beneficial changes occur at the cellular level. A synthetic amino acid called EDTA is administered to the patient via intravenous drip. Once in the bloodstream, EDTA attaches itself to heavy metals such as lead, cadmium, and mercury and holds onto those toxic substances until they exit the body through the urine. Dr. Dayton explains why removal of these substances is vital to good health: "The toxic material prevents normal function and repair. For example, lead prevents normal enzymatic processes so that the body cannot function properly and repair itself. This leads to premature aging and the premature development of disease. Removal of toxic material through chelation keeps the body functioning optimally."

Dr. Dayton notes that an excess even of iron, which is necessary for life, accelerates free radical production and causes harm: "Periodic purging of iron from the body via menstrual bleeding is thought to protect women from hardening of the arteries. However, this protection is lost at menopause with the cessation of menstruation. At this time, arterial clogging accelerates. Chelation removes this excess iron."

Since modern people are overwhelmed by pollutants, Dr. Dayton recommends chelation therapy for anyone over thirty. "Lead is found everywhere, in the air we breathe, the water we drink, the food supply. It is even found at the North Pole. Lead and other toxic pollutants are hard to avoid in today's world. As a matter of fact, the concentration of lead found in the human skeleton now is several hundred times greater than that found in our pre–industrial revolution ancestors. In one study, where lead was thought to be involved, 18 years following chelation therapy a 10-fold decrease in cancer death rate was found for those who had the treatment versus those who had nothing."

Aside from its overall benefits, chelation therapy specifically helps aging individuals by improving brain function. Dr. Dayton cites the following evidence: "Research shows that circulation improves greatly in the brain and to the brain. One study of 15 patients who had 20 infusions of chelation therapy found that 14 out of 15 demonstrated significant cerebral blood flow. Some showed dramatic improvement in cognitive abilities.

"In another study, 30 patients with carotid blockages were given 30 chelation treatments over a 10-month period. The carotid artery extends from the chest through the neck to the brain. It is the brain's main source of blood flow. Blockage decreased between 20 and 40 percent.

"Unclogging carotid blockage is vitally important because the American College of Physicians states that patients with an obstruction of 70 percent or greater are at a high risk for stroke. They even recommend chelation therapy as a preferred treatment. I take that to heart and use chelation therapy on these individuals. People who have carotid artery disease improve as their arteries open up. I see this happen over and over again."

COLON CLEANSING

Colon cleansing is an ancient and time-honored health practice for rejuvenating the system; it was used in Egypt over 4,000 years ago. Later, Hippocrates taught these procedures in his health care system. The large intestine, or colon, is healed, rebuilt, and finally restored to its natural size, normal shape, and correct function.

Colon therapist Anita Lotson explains the procedure and some of its physical and psychological benefits: "There are several stages of therapy. The first segment involves cleansing, a thorough washing of the large intestine. The colon is irrigated by a technique whereby water is gently infused into the large bowel, flowing in and out at steady intervals. Through this method, water is allowed to travel the entire length of the colon, all the way around to the cecum area. The walls of the colon are washed and old encrustations and fecal material are loosened, dislodged, and swept away. This toxic waste material has often been attached to the bowel walls for many, many years. It is laden with millions of bacteria, which set up the perfect environment for disease to take root and entrench itself in the system, wreaking havoc. As this body pollution is eliminated, many conditions—from severe skin disorders to breathing difficulties, depression, chronic fatigue, nervousness, severe constipation, and arthritis—are reduced in severity, providing great relief, especially when augmented with dietary changes and other treatment modalities.

"The next phases are healing, rebuilding, and finally restoration of a healthy colon, functioning at maximum efficiency for the final absorption of nutrients, and the total and timely elimination of all remaining waste materials. During the healing phase, we begin to infuse materials into the bowel that will cool inflamed areas and strengthen weak sections of the colon wall.

Flaxseed tea, white oak bark, and slippery elm bark all soothe, lubricate, and introduce powerful healing agents directly into the large intestine. These herbal teas may be taken orally as well. Simple dietary changes have been made by now, such as the addition of water. This simple measure spells the difference between success and failure in alleviating many bowel conditions. I ask all my clients to double their intake of water.

"I love to see people's change in attitude from the time they come in to the time that they leave. Sometimes people are very irritable when their bowels are backed up. They're often depressed, and sometimes nasty. By the time they leave, you can see a smile and a bounce in their step. It's a different person altogether."

DETOX DRINK. An excellent formula for colon cleansing is a drink made from ground flax seeds, psyllium seeds, and bentonite, which is a liquid clay. "Clay absorbs toxins," says Lombardi. "The seeds expand in the water and become like a brush. They brush the interior tubing, our pipe system. When the pipe system is completely clean, foods are absorbed through our digestive system."

ENZYME THERAPY

Nina Anderson, author of *Over Fifty, Looking Thirty: The Secrets of Staying Young,* attributes slow aging to sufficient enzyme levels: "Many scientists say that people get old before their time due to enzyme exhaustion. Some people are old at 40 because of the lack of enzymes, while others are young at 80 because of an abundance. Above all else, I would advise anybody who is trying to avoid looking and feeling older as they get older to take supplemental enzymes."

She goes on to explain that enzymes allow nutrients to be used. For example, you have enzymes in the heart that allow magnesium to be used. Without those enzymes, magnesium cannot not get to the heart: "Enzymes are molecule catalysts found everywhere in your body. In fact, there are over 1,300 different ones. They make everything happen. In my book I use this analogy: minerals are building blocks of your body. They are the nose, eyes, ears, bones, all the things that hold you together. Something has to build this. Enzymes are the construction workers that facilitate everything in the body going together."

Anderson recommends eating more raw foods, mineral supplements, and digestive plant enzymes to increase enzyme levels. Raw foods are loaded with enzymes. Fruit and vegetable juices are filled with enzymes. When food is processed, the first things taken out are enzymes. Why? Because the enzymes are what allow the food to ripen. However, if the food becomes too ripe, it rots. To stop it from ripening and rotting so that it can be sold longer, these enzymes must be destroyed. But if you destroy the enzymes, you destroy the food's life force. It will have carbohydrates, vitamins, fats, and minerals, but not its life force.

"The mineral supplements to take," Anderson adds, "should be in crystalloid form, with electrolytes. The crystalloid form goes right into the cell walls. This fortifies your body.

"Plant enzymes assist in the digestion of food right on through the intestinal tract. You want to help the digestive process for the whole length of the digestive tract. With supplemental enzymes, you won't have an upset stomach anymore or feel bloated and exhausted after a big meal. The skin will start to improve too. The skin manifests everything that happens inside. If your inner organs start to degenerate, if they are not functioning properly, this kind of stress shows up on your face. The first thing people do when they start getting older is look in the mirror and go, 'Oh my God, I've got wrinkles.' They spend millions trying to get rid of them. But what they have to realize is that wrinkles start from inside. You have to work on the inside to get the outside to reflect that good health.

"Without the proper enzymes, none of the other good things you do matter. For example, the fat-soluble vitamins A, D, E, and K require fat for absorption. That fat has to be broken down by an enzyme, lipase. If lipase is not present in sufficient quantities, that fat will not be broken down. If the fat isn't broken down, the vitamins will not be released. Therefore, you can spend a fortune on vitamin pills, and if you don't have the proper enzymes to release those vitamins into your system, they are just going to be flushed out."

Enzymes can be used externally as well as internally for youthful effects: "There are amazing enzyme treatments for the skin. Papaya enzymes are wonderful. Or you can mix a plant enzyme powder and put it on as a mask. Not only does it take the lines out of your face, but it fills them in and builds up collagen. It can also get rid of age spots and shrink moles. When you use enzymes as a mud pack when you come in from the sun, it fights free radicals that otherwise might foster melanoma."

EXERCISE AND OTHER PHYSICAL TECHNIQUES

When we exercise, we detoxify as we sweat through our skin and exhale from our lungs. Some good exercises include jogging or daily brisk walks, yoga stretches, and jumping on a minitrampoline, which exercises every cell in the body. Exercise slows down the aging process because it stimulates detoxification.

Chiropractor Dr. Mitch Proffman says that traditional cultures have appreciated the connection between physical fitness and longevity, making athletic activities a part of women's ritual ceremonies: "In traditional Navajo society women would run three times daily as a formal part of the four-day rites of passage after the onset of menstruation. The first run was at dawn, and each subsequent run would be for a longer distance. It was believed that the total distance a woman could run would determine her longevity."

He goes on to state that recent research supports the connection between exercise and a longer life: "The *Journal of the American Medical Association* has reported that exercise increases people's life spans. Women walking forty to fifty minutes, three to four times per week, live longer. The same article claims that exercise decreases the chance of dying from all known diseases. This can be attributed to the fact that most major diseases, such as cancer, diabetes, and heart disease, are stress-related, and exercise reduces stress.

"Another important function of exercising is that people's mental abilities improve. In a recent study at the University of Illinois, Dr. William Greenboro, Ph.D., studied four different groups of rats. One group led a sedentary life. Another group played aimlessly on wood and plastic in their cages. A third group was on a special motorized wheel, and a fourth group walked through intricate mazes and ropes. The finding was that all rats that exercised in any manner had more capillaries in their brains and better brain function. This suggests that exercise fuels the brain with more oxygen and increases natural growth factors, in humans as well as in rats."

Dr. Joseph Pizzorno, N.D., president of John Bastyr College of Naturopathic Medicine in Seattle, Washington, says that strengthening exercises are the best defense against the increased frailty women face as they age: "It turns out that the majority of the debility of old age is simply due to people not using their muscles. The full strength of what one had at twenty and thirty is almost completely returned with weight strengthening exercises. There are a lot of different weight training programs out there. I have been doing some research. The one I find most effective, and am now using personally, is something called Super Slow. Weights are used in a very, very controlled, very, very intense way to get maximum effects from the exercise. I am quite impressed with what I have seen."

STRESS RELEASE

"In my personal opinion, the single most important factor influencing aging and disease is stress," says Dr. Morris. "We need to control emotional anxieties and tensions, and learn how to not let life get to us. It is important to learn to let go and enjoy life." Methods Dr. Morris suggests to overcome stress include deep breathing exercises, tai chi, yoga, meditation, qi gong, mantras, massage, Reiki, and biofeedback. "These are things I recommend that all of us do in the pursuit of health, longevity and wellness." Although exercise strengthens muscle and increases suppleness, sometimes bad patterns of movement or chronic tensions create problems in the joints or muscles. One practice that helps eliminate the problem of poor movement habits is the Feldenkrais method.

Since exercise increases oxygenation, it also has the potential to foster free radical damage. To prevent undesirable effects, women may want to combine exercise with sufficient amounts of antioxidants in the diet and/or as dietary supplements. (See "Antioxidants," above.)

BREATHING EXERCISES

Breathing exercises combined with physical activity increase the action of lymphatic cleansing. Detoxification expert Susan Lombardi explains: "For lymphatic cleansing, you want to synchronize your breathing with the movement of your legs and arms. When you are walking or jumping on the trampoline, inhale four times and exhale four times. Move your arms and legs each time you take a little breath. Inhale through your nose and exhale through your nose or mouth.

"This breathing technique was learned from the Taromaro Indians, who live in the northern part of Mexico. They are famous for their fantastic health. They have no need of hospitals or homes for the elderly. They have no disease, no police force, no jails, and no mental institutions."

SKIN BRUSHING

Using a natural brush on dry skin removes dead cells and leaves pores open, so that more toxins can be expelled. Lombardi explains why this is so important: "We are supposed to eliminate two pounds of toxins through the pores of the skin. Due to pollution, smog, the creams we use, the clothes we wear, and so forth, our pores are more closed than open. Always brush toward the heart."

SAUNAS

The sauna is a good follow-up to dry skin brushing because it pushes toxins out through the skin. The main thing to remember with saunas is to be prudent. You want to perspire but not remain there for too long. Nor do you want too much heat. "Follow the directions," says Lombardi. "And wear a cooling drape on your head. You don't want to heat up the brain area."

There are multiple benefits from sauna detoxification, explains Lombardi: "You will look and feel better. Your skin will be clear and you will not have constipation. Your nails will improve as well as your heart and digestive system. It will clear your mind and improve concentration. Nothing will de-stress your body like a sauna."

MAGNETIC HEALING

Susan Bucci is a holistically trained nurse who has spearheaded the development of magnetic healing products. "Magnets oxygenate tissues and allow cell walls to absorb more oxygen," she explains. "They promote mental acuity and normalize pH balance by increasing alkalinity. Restorative sleep is enhanced. Therapeutically, they stop pain, fight infection, and reduce inflammation and fluid retention. Over time, fatty and calcium deposits dissolve and the circulatory system opens up. Put that all together and you've got healing from A to Z. Take that a step further: If you achieve optimal well-being, you can actually live a long, productive life."

In addition to promoting overall well-being, magnets can eliminate many specific signs and symptoms of old age. Bucci reports these antiaging benefits from her own use of magnetic healing techniques: "My energy level has increased. I used to have chronic fatigue in the worst way, but now that's gone. My immune system is functioning much better, so my susceptibility to viruses and colds has decreased dramatically. Allergies are basically gone, and there are no more killer sinus headaches. My circulation has improved so that I withstand weather a whole lot easier. Wounds heal quickly, and my spider veins have disappeared. Also, I was headed for an early menopause, but now my menstrual cycle is very much on track, very regular.

"Hair, skin, and nails have definitely improved. My hair grows faster and has a much better quality to it. Within two weeks of using magnets on a daily basis, I was able to see new, thick, dark hair growing. My grays started falling out and disappearing. I was going to color my hair about four years ago, and I still haven't touched it with an ounce of anything. My skin definitely looks and feels younger. And my nails grow so well that if I break one, it doesn't upset me. I know that it will grow right back."

How can magnets do so much? Simply stated, magnets confer a wide range of benefits because we are magnetic beings who derive energy from the earth's magnetic field. Bucci explains: "One reason we get sick is that the earth has lost a good deal of its magnetism, which leaves the body in an unbalanced state. Additionally, we are bombarded by unhealthy energies." Magnets create overall benefit by restoring internal harmony.

It is important to realize that not just any old magnet will do. The negative pole restores health and good energy to the system, while exposure to the positive pole is detrimental. This has been proved repeatedly in studies where a variety of creatures, from earthworms, mice, and chickens to larger animals, live twice as long as untested control groups when exposed to negative field magnets, and half as long when exposed to positive fields. Bucci recommends unipolar magnets, marked by the Davis and Rawls system with an "N" or the word "negative" and a green label. "That's the healthy side, and that's the one we face toward the body." Negative field ions support biological systems, which help the body to heal itself. "The body is an amazing machine with a remarkable capacity to cure itself," Bucci says. "Give it a boost in the right direction and it does the rest on its own. The negative field is completely safe and risk-free."

Bucci finds that magnets work best when worn on a daily basis. During the day she wears a magnet over her heart to improve circulation and oxygenation. "It keeps the heart open and flowing and sends all that wonderful oxygen throughout my body," she says. At night, she takes the magnet off and sleeps with her head on a magnetic mattress pad. She does this because the most important benefit while sleeping is increased melatonin production from the brain's pineal gland: "People are running out to buy melatonin, but guess what? We can encourage our own melatonin production.

"People ask me how long magnets should be worn. Generally speaking, the longer you wear them, the more healing takes place. You can wear them all night and during the day. Generally, the body will tell you when it has had enough. It also will tell you when a condition has healed, although you should check with a physician just to make sure." Magnets, and more information, can be obtained from Susan Bucci's company, Imaginetics, at (800) 285-3430.

LIVE CELL THERAPY

Live cell therapy involves using living embryonic cells to regenerate tissues. Dr. Lance Morris notes, "Research is being performed on Alzheimer's patients to regenerate brain cell tissue. This is very exciting work. There is also work being done using thymus gland tissue to reverse the aging process. Thymus glands that you get in the health food store are useful in supporting immune function and in helping with the aging process. That's a simple thing that you can do on your own, and it's very safe to do." Live cell therapy enhances immune response by increasing stem cells, cells that can differentiate into a wide variety of immune and blood cells throughout the body.

Brain Aging

One of the most disturbing symptoms of aging in women is diminished brain function, which can cause everything from forgetfulness and loss of concentration to Alzheimer's and other serious diseases. Fortunately, modern research reveals that much can be done to keep the brain in top form your entire life. Below, two experts in antiaging discuss new advances in the field.

Dr. Eric Braverman says that brain aging affects people differently and that brain health is a preventative process. "Even when you feel halfway decent in your fifties, sixties, and seventies, parts of your body may be breaking down," he cautions.

The part of the brain affected determines which symptoms manifest themselves. "Individuals age in all different shapes and forms, just as a face can have wrinkles on the brow or wrinkles under the eye," Braverman says. "The area of the brain that slows down can affect such things as general memory, concentration, and logic."

NUTRITION AND SUPPLEMENTS

Another leading researcher in the field of antiaging, Dr. Ross Pelton of San Diego, author of *Mind, Food, and Smart Pills*, agrees that our brains do not have to deteriorate as we age: "It is simply poor nutrition and abuse that allows this condition to develop. Virtually everyone can enhance their memory, learning capabilities, and intelligence." Dr. Pelton helps his women patients optimize brain functioning with two goals in mind: to slow down or stop the brain aging process and to optimize the function that they do have.

First and foremost, Dr. Pelton recommends building total body health with a healthy diet. An organic vegetarian diet supplies the body with more protective nutrients and healthful fiber, and at the same time decreases toxins. Additionally, Pelton believes that every woman should take a high-potency multivitamin and/or mineral supplement and extra antioxidants with each meal: "We are no longer looking at the Recommended Daily Allowance (RDA) as the level of nutrients appropriate for people. I say RDA stands for Really Dumb Allowance. It's more like the minimum wage, the minimal amount you can get by on. If we want to get into lifestyles of antiaging and life extension, we need to consider not only healthy diets but a program of optimal nutritional supplementation. Antioxidants are among the most important protectors against the aging process in general and against brain aging in particular. They will stop the onset of senility, Alzheimer's disease, and other brain injuries."

Doctor Pelton utilizes the following special nutrients to enhance brain function. Unless otherwise noted, they can be purchased in health food stores.

FLAXSEED OIL

Flaxseed oil, an important brain nutrient, is the greatest source of the essential fatty acid omega-3 (EPA). Omega-3 is converted into another fatty acid, which nourishes the fat cells in the brain. One tablespoon of flaxseed oil is needed daily. It should be refrigerated, not cooked, and taken with the largest meal of the day.

HYDERGINE, PIRACETAM, AND LUCIDRIL

Hydergine (co-dergocrine mesylate) increases oxygen to brain cells and makes a person less susceptible to free radical damage and aging. Dr. Pelton says this is one of the most important substances for preventing brain aging because of its oxygenating capabilities. Hydergine is available in the United States, although as a prescription drug; Lucidril (meclofenoxate hydrochloride) and piracetam, which have similar properties (see below), must be ordered from overseas. Although classified as drugs by the FDA, Hydergine, Lucidril, and piracetam have few, if any, negative side effects, according to Dr. Pelton—only positive effects on memory and the prevention of brain aging. Overseas mail order sources sell Hydergine in 4.5-mg tablets, while in the United States it is available only in 1-mg tablets. The higher dose, taken twice a day, is highly effective in helping people with early signs of memory loss.

Piracetam is not available in the United States; however, it is available in over 85 other countries worldwide, where it is appreciated for its remarkable qualities and its complete lack of toxicity. Like Hydergine, piracetam prevents brain cell destruction caused by a lack of oxygen. Piracetam also can increase the flow of electrical information between the left and right hemispheres of the brain, a process known as superconnecting. It has proven effective in treating the learning disorder dyslexia. When used in conjunction with high-potency lecithin, piracetam is highly effective in helping some Alzheimer's patients improve cognition, memory, and recall.

Lucidril, as its name suggests, makes you more lucid. This exciting drug can actually reverse brain aging. Dr. Pelton explains: "The primary yardstick in brain aging is the buildup of lipofuscin, the result of free radical damage over the years. This buildup is really cellular garbage that collects and coalesces inside the cells into a black, tarlike mass. In elderly people you can see this in the skin as liver spots or age pigment. It is theorized that when 60 to 70 percent of the brain cell is clogged, it breaks down and stops working. That's when the symptoms of senility kick in very quickly. Lucidril actually dissolves and flushes out these garbage deposits from brain cells and restores the brain cell to a much younger state." Lucidril has been shown to extend the life of laboratory animals and to enhance intelligence, learning, and recall.

DEPRENYL

Deprenyl (selegiline hydrochloride) has been shown in animal studies to prevent the destruction of a specific group of neurons in the substantia nigra, the area of the brain that goes bad when people develop Parkinson's disease. Moreover, it helps enhance intelligence and cognition when 5 mg is taken once daily.

MELATONIN

Melatonin is the one substance from the armamentarium of alternative medicine that has attracted attention in the mainstream media recently; you've probably already heard a lot about melatonin. This is a brain hormone produced by the pineal gland, and it diminishes with age. A dose of 3 mg once daily taken at bedtime can help normalize sleep cycles and support the pineal gland.

DMAE

DMAE (dimethylaminoethynol) is a naturally occurring but little-known B vitamin that enhances memory, boosts natural energy, and improves sleep. Additionally, it helps learning problems in children who have short attention spans. DMAE is safe, but if too much is taken, it can produce mild headaches, insomnia, and muscle tension.

Unless otherwise noted, these important brain enhancers can be purchased in health food stores.

BRAIN ELECTRONIC ACTIVITY MAP (BEAM)

Dr. Eric Braverman has mapped brain aging and studied how nutrients influence this process. Using a test called the Brain Electronic Activity Map (or BEAM), a technique developed at Harvard Medical School and refined, strengthened, and expanded by Dr. Braverman, the brain's level of electric activity is studied. This is a crucial area of concern because such things as substance abuse, hormonal imbalance, chronic fatigue, anxiety, hypertension, and even Lyme disease may affect the brain and cause premature aging. Often electroencephalography (EEG) or magnetic resonance imaging (MRI) will show nothing wrong, while the BEAM test reveals that the brain has been suffering from stress. It gives a window on the brain and how it is aging. So, as Braverman says, he is using "the BEAM that lights the path to wellness."

He says that one thing this test registers is the speed of brain cycles, since slowing is a key marker of aging. The normal, healthy rhythm of the brain is 10 cycles per second of alpha waves, considerably faster than the heart's normal rate of one cycle per second. As people age, their brain rhythm decreases to nine, eight, or seven beats per second. There is a decrease in alpha rhythms and an increase in theta waves.

This can occur prematurely for many reasons, including head trauma, Alzheimer's disease, and abuse of such substances as cocaine, marijuana, and alcohol. Any one of these conditions can cause the frontal and temporal lobes to age in an accelerated manner. Aging is also accelerated by whiplash, metabolic disorders, loss of circulation, and "toxic home syndrome," which refers to the damage that can be done to the body by substances, such as cleansers, that vaporize; pesticides; and herbicides found around the house or garden. Add to that possible harm from fluorescent lights and electromagnetic pollution. The latter is caused by the electromagnetic grid that characterizes our environment, surrounded as we all are by digital clocks, VCRs, CD players, computers, electric blankets, cellular phones and beepers, and microwave ovens. These appliances transmit negative electrical resonance—the opposite of what our bodies need—causing damage to our chromosomes and tissues. These stresses hurt us slowly, in small ways, causing cumulative degeneration, creating subtle discrepancies in how the body functions.

Dr. Braverman notes that a computerized spectral analysis will pick up how these factors have affected the brain. A PET (positron emission tomography) scan, which provides data about the metabolism of the brain, can be correlated with a BEAM test, which may record not only weaker brain electrical activity but a loss of metabolism of the neurotransmitters.

OTHER NATURAL THERAPIES

Dr. Braverman believes that each person must be individually tested to determine weak areas of brain function and to devise a program that addresses specific needs. For overall general improvement, he endorses these important therapies.

AMINO ACIDS AND OTHER BRAIN NUTRIENTS

Amino acids build up in particular areas of the brain that need help. The dopamine system responds to the essential amino acids tyrosine and phenylalanine. Choline builds memory, while GABA (gamma-aminobutyric acid) available as GABA-pentin, helps anxiety disorders. Choline, phosphatidyl serine, ginkgo, tryptophan, tyrosine, and phenylalanine all boost brain voltage.

CHELATION THERAPY

As described earlier (see "Other Detoxification Techniques," above), chelation therapy pulls out aluminum and other heavy metals from the bloodstream, resulting in improved memory. It can also reverse or prevent other destructive conditions associated with the aging process, such as arthritis, hardening of the arteries, cataracts, and strokes.

ELECTROSTIMULATION

Amino acids and neurotransmitter precursors are more effective when accompanied by electrostimulation of the brain. A transcutaneous electrical nerve stimulation (TENS) unit, worn on the forehead and left wrist, helps drive these substances along a good pathway. A cranioelectrical stimulation (CES) device also helps electrical fields and enhances the entire neurotransmitter system.

EXERCISE

Research shows that the whole neurotransmitter system of the brain can be improved through exercise. (See "Exercise and Other Physical Techniques," above.)

MEDITATION

Meditation connects the body and mind electrically, creating harmony between the brain and other body systems.

NATURAL HORMONES

Women must get three hormones from natural sources to slow down the aging process: progesterone, testosterone, and estrogen. Without natural estrogen, the hair thins, the vagina dries, the nails break, the bones become porous, and the brain weakens. Estrogen improves the absorption of nutrients into the brain; in particular, it increases dopamine levels. Progesterone protects women from the side effects of estrogen. Additionally, it is calming to the brain and improves sleep. Testosterone enhances the sex drive, builds stronger bones, and provides greater physical strength.

PHYSICAL TOUCH

Neurotransmitters are adversely altered when people are in isolation, when they don't have love in their life.

Patient Stories

Reiki is a type of massage therapy or bodywork in which pressure point tech-niques are used to move energy through the body, achieving balance and har-mony. Reiki therapist Nilsa Vergara reports below on her clients' experiences with Reiki therapy.

My first example is a 59-year-old woman who came to our healing circle feeling old and tired. She suffered from aches and severe pain in her neck and knee from car accidents. She was also going through job changes, and was estranged from her adult son.

Each week she received a 15-minute session, and she quickly began feeling better. She released a lot of emotional toxins via crying and verbal expression of what she was feeling. She decided to take a Reiki class so that she could give herself daily treatments.

Within a month, her changes were quite dramatic. She had a tremendous increase in energy and vigor. She told me she now feels like she is 28. With the Reiki, she now has very little pain. She feels emotional and vital. Her attitude has changed. She feels self-fulfilled and in control of her life. Her relationship with her son has greatly improved. To quote her, "I feel like my whole life is as it should be."

My next client is a 65-year-old woman. When she first came to see us, she was depressed. She had been in therapy for years, but nothing seemed to lift the depression. She felt tired all the time and would catch colds easily. Emotionally, she felt like a victim, and others treated her like one.

After her first 15-minute session she felt immediately better. She knew that something powerful was happening. She returned and eventually studied Reiki. Today, she reports feeling much healthier. She has more energy and an optimistic outlook. She no longer feels like a victim, and if anyone tries to put her in that role, she is no longer afraid to set limits. In addition, she is much more able to tolerate cold weather, which indicates that her body has improved its oxygen intake.

One of my students has an 83-year-old mother who fell and broke her hip bone as well as bones in her wrist and arm. She decided to give her mother Reiki regularly, and her mother responded quite well. She began feeling stronger and stronger. Within 4 weeks she was out of her cast, walking with just the aid of a cane, not a walker. This is pretty remarkable for an 83-year-old, because a broken hip does not always lead to a good outcome. So, as you can see, Reiki really enhances the body's ability to recuperate.

Another client is a 53-year-old woman who had some serious memory problems. Her thinking was scattered; emotionally, she was fearful and guilt-ridden; and she was estranged from her adult children.

I recommended Reiki to her to see if we could work through some of these emotional blockages and change these negative patterns. She took a Reiki class, and within 6 months, her memory improved tremendously. She was much more focused in her thinking, and her job performance improved greatly. She became more insightful and much less fearful. Now she can speak with her adult children and set limits, and she no longer feels anxious and guilt-ridden. In addition to using Reiki, she uses herbal teas for detoxification, drinks vegetable juices, fasts, and gets colonics.

Chapter 3

Anemia

A nemia is a health condition characterized by red blood cells deficient in hemoglobin, the iron-containing portion of the blood. Hemoglobin enables the blood to transport oxygen from the lungs and circulate it throughout the body and to carry away carbon dioxide. The listlessness, pallor, and shortness of breath in an anemic patient reflect a lack of oxygen and buildup of carbon dioxide in the tissues.

Causes

Dr. Dahlia Abraham, a complementary physician from New York City, describes three major classifications of anemia, each of which is associated with a specific cause.

"The first cause of anemia is excessive blood loss. Chronic blood loss can occur in association with menstruation or because of conditions such as hemorrhoids and a slowly bleeding peptic ulcer.

"The second cause of anemia is excessive red blood cell destruction. Normally, old and abnormal red blood cells are removed from the circulation. If the rate of destruction exceeds that of manufacture of new cells, anemia can result. A number of factors can cause excessive red blood cell destruction, such as defective hemoglobin synthesis, injury, and trauma within the arteries.

"The third and most common type of anemia is caused by nutritional deficiencies of iron, vitamin B_{12}, and folic acid. Of these, iron deficiency is the most frequently seen. People require extra iron during growth spurts in infancy and adolescence. Pregnancy and lactation are other times when women need iron supplementation. During the childbearing years, many women experience anemia caused by an iron deficiency.

"Supplementation may not solve the problem because many people have difficulty absorbing iron. They lack enough hydrochloric acid, the stomach acid that helps the body assimilate iron. This is common among the elderly, who generally produce less hydrochloric acid. Another cause of decreased iron absorption is chronic diarrhea.

"Vitamin B_{12} deficiency is most often due to a defect in absorption. Vitamin B_{12} must be liberated from food by hydrochloric acid and bound to a substance called intrinsic factor, which is also secreted in the stomach. For B_{12} to be absorbed, then, an individual must secrete enough hydrochloric acid and enough intrinsic factor. Women with this type of anemia may need to take supplements of vitamn B_{12}, hydrochloric acid, and intrinsic factor.

"Folic acid deficiency may also cause anemia. Folic acid becomes totally depleted in alcoholics. It is also commonly deficient among pregnant women because the fetus demands so much of it. Folic acid is vital for cell production in the growing fetus and prevents birth defects, such as neural tube imperfections. This is why prenatal vitamins must contain this nutrient. In addition, a number of pharmaceutical drugs, such as anticancer drugs and oral contraceptives, can drain the body of folic acid. Women taking either of these agents should supplement their diet with folic acid, especially since this nutrient is difficult to get in foods."

Dr. Pat Gorman, an acupuncturist and educator in New York City, explains anemia and other blood disorders in women from an Asian perspective: "In women, blood has an actual cycle that rises and falls every month. There is a building phase that occurs for about a week after the menstrual period. Then there is a peak phase where the blood reaches its richest moment; that's the moment you ovulate. This is followed by a storage phase. (If you are pregnant, the blood is stored.) A week before the period, you go through a cleansing phase where your organs release toxins into the blood. That's the week before your period, when you can go through a PMS hell if the toxins are not being properly released. Next is the purging of the actual period."

Using this philosophy as her framework, Dr. Gorman holds that women become anemic when they are out of touch with their monthly cycles. In a fast-paced society, one of the major reasons for this condition is that women do not rest at the appropriate times: "Women work all the time. They show no vulnerability and just keep on going no matter what. There is no respect for the actual rhythm of the cycle. I believe that we need to bring back the menstrual hut. When you are bleeding, you need to stop working for a day or two. I know I am saying things that sound impossible, but if you have anemia—and 60 to 70 percent of the women I see do—you need to face the fact and work with it."

She adds that another major reason women become anemic is that they approach pregnancy incorrectly: "There is a law called the one-month, one-year law. After a pregnancy is terminated, whether by abortion, miscarriage, or birth, one month of absolute rest is needed. Women say, 'That's not possible. I just gave birth, but I have other children. I have to take care of things.' The Chinese say this is a straight road to a severe anemic problem.

"The one-year aspect is the avoidance of pregnancy for at least another year. Women who try to conceive and who then miscarry often frantically begin again. They need to build up the blood for an entire year's cycle before trying to conceive again. It is very difficult for me to help anxious patients relax and understand that this is the way to overcome anemia and to have a really healthy baby."

Additionally, Dr. Gorman warns that birth control pills are unhealthy because they disturb the integrity of the blood's cycle. They trick the body into believing that it is continuously pregnant by locking blood into its storage phase. By eliminating the cycle of building, peaking, storing, cleansing, and purging, oral contraceptives create many problems.

Symptoms

The general symptoms of anemia are weakness and a tendency to tire easily. When there is a vitamin B_{12} deficiency, the symptoms may also include paleness; shortness of breath; a sore, red, swollen tongue; diarrhea; heart palpitations; and nervous disturbances.

Clinical Experience

DIAGNOSIS

According to Dr. Abraham, the treatment of anemia is dependent on proper clinical evaluation by a physician. Too often, physicians assume that anemia is caused by an iron deficiency, but this is just one possible reason. "It is absolutely imperative that a comprehensive laboratory analysis of the blood be performed. Do not be satisfied when your physician offers a simple diagnosis of anemia," she warns. "Insist that your doctor investigate the underlying causes.

While Dr. Gorman agrees that clinical studies help confirm the diagnosis, she adds that Asian physicians are trained to detect anemia and other blood disorders through observation: "In Chinese medicine, you examine the body. Look at your tongue. Is it pale? Look at your lips. Are they pale? See if the mucous membranes under the eyes are pale. These signs indicate whether you are anemic."

DIET

Green, leafy vegetables are high in iron and folic acid. It is best to purchase organic vegetables, since pesticides interfere with absorption. Eating vegetables raw or lightly cooked preserves their folic acid content. Soy or shoyu sauce, miso, and tempeh are rich sources of vitamin B_{12}.

Proteins should be eaten every day, preferably vegetarian proteins such as those from grains and legumes such as rice and beans or oatmeal with soy milk. When animal protein is eaten, it should be from fish. Caffeine and alcohol are detrimental to healthy blood and should be eliminated.

SUPPLEMENTS

According to Dr. Abraham, iron, vitamin B_{12}, and folic acid should be prescribed as needed. Additionally, hydrochloric acid and intrinsic factor are often required to aid the absorption of these nutrients.

Naturopath Dr. Tori Hudson, in a column in *Prevention* magazine, advises that iron citrate and iron aspartate are forms of iron supplementation that are less likely to cause constipation. She suggests taking 1,000 to 3,000 mg of vitamin C with the iron to enhance absorption. Herbs that may be helpful for iron deficiency anemia are dandelion root, echinacea, yellow dock, and alfalfa.

HERBS

Janet Zand, a naturopathic physician, acupuncturist, and doctor of oriental medicine in Los Angeles, in an article posted on the HealthWorld Online website (www.healthy.net), suggests an herbal program that anemic women can use to build the blood. It is meant to accompany iron and iron-synergistic nutrient supplementation as directed by a health care practitioner. Dr. Zand bases her herbal regimes for women on the shifting hormonal balance over the four weeks of the menstrual cycle.

During all four weeks of the cycle, red raspberry leaf and *dong quai* are used to build blood and balance hormones. These herbs can be taken as a tea, tincture, capsule, or tablet three times a day. Then, during the specified weeks, one also takes the herbs specified below:

FIRST WEEK. Take yellow dock leaf (*Rumex crispus*) and chlorophyll as a tea or tincture three times a day.

SECOND WEEK. Take American ginseng (*Panax quinquefolius* root), a blood builder, as a tea or tincture three times a day.

THIRD WEEK. Take nettle (*Urtica dioica* leaf) and chlorophyll as a tea or tincture three times a day.

FOURTH WEEK. Take alfalfa (*Medicago sativa* leaf), with chlorophyll as a tea or tincture three times a day.

AYURVEDA

According to Swami Sada Shiva Tirtha, founder of the Ayurveda Holistic Center in Bayville, New York, in an article on the center's website (ayurvedahc.com), practitioners of ayurvedic medicine consider anemia an imbalance of the blood that can have a number of causes. Too many sour, salty, or hot foods; drinking alcohol; poor nutrition; injury; excessive menstruation or bleeding; liver disorders; pregnancy; excessive sexual activity; and fevers are all factors that can cause a disorder in the kidneys, blood, and *ojas* (life force) and lead to anemia.

The symptoms of anemia include paleness, fatigue, lack of energy, a low-grade fever or burning feeling, indigestion, irregular elimination or yellow, scanty urine, vertigo, and fainting. The menstrual blood may be paler than usual, may be sparse, or may stop flowing. When you make a fist for a few seconds and then release it, the palm will stay pale for a long time before the blood returns. Another sign of anemia is paleness instead of redness of the inner part of the lower eyelid.

Swami Sada Shiva recommends certain foods that help build blood. These foods include organic milk, pomegranate or black grape juice, boiled black sesame seeds, molasses, and Sucanat (whole cane sugar). Otherwise, people should follow the diet that is appropriate for their body type, according to ayurvedic guidelines. Ayurveda uses meat as a medication only when anemia is extremely severe.

Women should use blood-building herbs after the menstrual period. To properly assimilate iron supplements, take them with ginger or cinnamon. You can take two or three teaspoonfuls of *chyavan prash* twice daily with warm milk as well as turmeric and ghee.

Aloe vera gel and triphala are very gentle laxatives that regulate the bowels and thus can help remove excess bile from the liver, a common reason for thinning of the blood. Other ayurvedic herbs used to treat anemia are saffron, *shatavari, manjishtha,* and *punarnava.*

Patient Story: Yolanda

I was born in Nicaragua, and I used to be a very healthy person. But in June 1993 I went to the emergency room. My hemoglobin was down to 2.8; the normal count for a woman is between 12 and 14. There I was with aplastic anemia, meaning that my bone marrow was not making any blood cells: no red cells, no white cells, no platelets. I almost had no blood.

The doctor said that my sickness was idiopathic, meaning that they didn't know what caused it. They said that one possible cause was the use of an antibiotic. But the only time I had ever taken one was fifteen years earlier. Another possible cause was exposure to chemicals or pesticides. A lot of towns in Nicaragua are surrounded by cotton plantations where cotton growers use a lot of pesticides to spray their crops.

In July 1993 I was referred to a bone marrow transplant unit and was put on a medication, a kind of chemotherapy. After one month of treatment, the medication failed to work. Then the doctors wanted to do a bone marrow transplant. I have seven siblings, and so I had donors, and one of them was a perfect match. But I had reservations. A bone marrow transplant is very costly. Also, you get bone marrow that is working, but because of the chemotherapy or radiation, your liver, kidneys, pancreas, and so forth, pay a terrible toll.

Before my sickness I was following a macrobiotic diet. I was starting to use Oriental and alternative medicine, and I knew about the power of the body to heal itself. I decided to stay on my macrobiotic diet and was able to more or less clean myself of the chemotherapy. During this time I did not even get a cold. I didn't sneeze through all my sickness.

I was clean, but my blood counts were still very low. I needed a transfusion every 10 days. The transfusions were very helpful, and I was grateful to be able to get them. But through transfusions I was also receiving a lot of genetic and other information completely foreign to my body. I could not control what the person who donated that blood was eating. So I was trying to clean my body of toxins, and I decided to look for help.

I went to a naturopath who helped me a lot. Then I read an article on Ayurveda. It said that Ayurveda is very specific, even with the use of grains and vegetables. There are grains and vegetables that are not appropriate for your body type. In early February 1994 I went to an ayurvedic doctor. He gave me a very gentle treatment consisting of diet, aromatherapy, massage, and meditation. After three weeks of following that treatment, my blood count went up for the first time.

I keep up with this treatment still. My last checkup at the hospital showed normal white cells. Red cells were a little bit low. They were 3.83, and the normal count is 4. But they are increasing day by day. My energy level is excellent. I went back to work three months ago and am now leading a completely normal life. I am very grateful to Ayurveda.

Chapter 4

Arthritis

I n *The Cyborg Manifesto*, the feminist scholar Donna Haraway lays out some of the positive aspects of the human-machine interface represented by the humanoids and half-human–half-robot entities that populate so many science fiction movies and television programs. To her mind, the virtue of these hybrids is that insofar as their animal and machine components cannot be separated, they help break down the binary mind-set that divides the world into opposites: male-female, straight-gay, black-white, and so on. Such a division, we should realize, has always ended up as a hierarchy, with one side classified as inferior to the other. To Haraway, the better types of imagined cyborgs help erase these coercive dyads.

However, she was not talking about the superman cyborgs one finds in Hollywood productions such as the *Terminator* or *Robocop* series, where the human machine is a hyped-up macho Rambo in overdrive whose mechanical enhancements increase his combat skills. Film critics have argued that this type of fantasy comes from a desire to escape the body, to avoid all the illnesses that seem to accompany aging. As in so many of the film industry's imaginative creations, this fantasy is constructed equally of avoidance and ignorance. First, there is avoidance of the real question: How do we create a world in which the practices of daily life promote health instead of premature aging? Second, the ignorance lies in the belief that all the health problems Americans tend to develop as they become older, such as arthritis, are inevitable.

Let me tell you about something that recently happened to me that contrasts the ignorance and arrogance of an ensconced medical practitioner with the more open-minded attitude of a sufferer who was willing to try an alternative.

I was getting some juice made at local health food store when a gentleman came over to me and said, "You're Gary Null, aren't you? I just want to shake your hand."

"What is this all about?" I responded.

He said, "I don't have time to listen to your show, but my wife listens regularly. I have crippling arthritis, very serious. I went to my rheumatologist regularly, with few results. You see, I have very different values from my wife. While she has been an advocate of alternative medical therapies, I have always followed conventional methods and trusted my doctor. My wife, though, listens to your program, Gary, and follows what you have to say.

"She asked me about three months ago to try a different approach. I'd been to my physician, and nothing was working. I was in a lot of pain. All the doctor told was to take the anti-inflammatories, which I chose not to. So I agreed to try this Gary Null program.

"I followed the guidelines. I fasted on distilled water for five days. I had had blood chemistry tested beforehand. I eliminated everything I had had in my diet before and began to eat lots of grains and legumes, fruits, herbs, juices. I have no caffeine, no sugar, no wheat, no meat, no yeast.

"Gary, it was like a miracle, an absolute miracle. So I went back in and had an examination by my rheumatologist. He said, 'My goodness, look at the improvement.' He did a test of a blood antibody marker that was indicative of arthritis. He then said, 'It's dropped by half. I guess the medication is really working.' I didn't say anything.

"A month later it had dropped again. Then I went back a third time, and there was no antibody reaction at all. The doctor shook his head and said, 'You have no arthritis.'

"I said, 'You know, Doctor, I didn't use any of the medicines. I was trying this program that Gary Null had advocated. My wife listened to him on the radio and got me started on it.'

"The doctor interrupted me, insisting, 'That's enough. I don't want to hear any more. It's absolute quackery.'

"I returned, 'It may be quackery, but it worked, while what you were giving me didn't.'

"The doctor kept objecting, 'There's no relation of arthritis to diet; you're just in a remission.'"

The question is: How many other people out there have assumed there is no association between diet and arthritis in terms of cause or treatment? Most rheumatologists are not advocating an approach that works to balance a person's biochemistry. With more than 50 million Americans suffering from arthritis, maybe we should think of something by way of treatment other than simply dulling the pain with drugs or performing dangerous and expensive operations. What can we do to slow down and eventually eliminate the disease in many patients?

What Is Arthritis?

The word "arthritis" means pain and swelling of the joints. A joint is the place where two bones meet. Cartilage covers the end of each bone and prevents the bones from rubbing together. The joint capsule surrounds the joint and protects it. Special membranes surround the joint and cover it with a fluid that lubricates it. Muscles and ligaments around the joint provide support and make it move. When all these parts are working right, the joint moves smoothly and easily, but when something is wrong with the joint, arthritis may develop. In osteoarthritis, the cartilage is worn away so that the bones rub against each other. When the cartilage breaks down, the joint may lose its shape. The ends of the bone may thicken and form spurs. In rheumatoid arthritis, the lining of the joint becomes inflamed and swollen; it feels warm, tender, and puffy. Eventually the bone and cartilage may be destroyed.

Adds Dr. Jason Theodosakis, whose treatment program is profiled later in this chapter: "At a biochemical level, the breakdown of cartilage is happening more rapidly than the buildup of cartilage. That brings up an important point. Cartilage on the end of the bones is not like a pencil eraser, which, once it is rubbed off, is gone. It is constantly breaking down and being replaced."

Besides these two types of arthritis, over 100 other diseases affect the area around the joint, including lupus, fibromyalgia, polymyalgia, gout, scleroderma, juvenile arthritis, and ankylosing spondylitis.

The Arthritis Industry

On August 18, 1985, the *New York Times* ran an article on arthritis in its Sunday business section. The title, "Arthritis: Building an Industry on Pain," together with its placement in the business section (as opposed to the health, lifestyle, or human interest section), gave the article a uniquely realistic point of view. For many people, arthritis is not a health issue per se but a very lucrative growth industry. Although the article is an old one, this view remains prevalent. Using the example of Ann, a fairly typical arthritis sufferer, the article reveals how the symptomatic approach to arthritis that is typical of traditional medicine offers little in the way of health benefits while providing tremendous profit-making opportunities for those involved in the arthritis industry.

Ann began to suffer from arthritis at age 28. She was walking downstairs when her knees suddenly gave out, followed by a sharp burning pain. Ann's doctors diagnosed her as having rheumatoid arthritis and started her on an arduous and expensive journey through the maze of treatments used to battle arthritis in the United States. According to the *Times,* Ann spent more than $200 a year on medication (this is probably a very conservative estimate compared with the amount most arthritis sufferers spent on antiarthritics during that period, and of course, medical costs have increased since 1985). This included a daily dosage of 8 to 10 Ecotrin (aspirin) tablets, a prescription pain reliever, and 5 mg of the steroid prednisone. She visited the doctor at least once a month at $20 to $50 a visit. Even with all this medication and regular medical attention, Ann was physically incapacitated. She found it necessary to acquire a number of new arthritic devices designed to replace her ever-decreasing mobility: $35 for a walker, $25 for a set of canes, $15 for a reacher to get objects from shelves or retrieve them from the floor, and $130 for a padded bathtub seat. Ann also had four joints replaced at a cost of $15,000 per joint. "And so," the article concluded, "Ann is one of the nearly 40 million consumers of the arthritis industry. It may sound odd to label arthritis as an industry, but in fact any disease—cancer, diabetes, AIDS—is not only an affliction, it is an employer. For thousands of people and scores of companies, battling arthritis is a livelihood."

The *Times* estimated that arthritis costs this nation $8 billion to $10 billion annually in medical bills and adds to those figures another $7 billion in lost wages and taxes resulting from absenteeism.

Arthritis medications are one of the pharmaceutical industry's biggest and most lucrative products. In 1982, the *Times* estimated in another article (also in the business section) that the projected $717 million in industry sales that year for prescription arthritis drugs would continue to increase at a phenomenal 20 percent annually. Additionally, according to the *Times:*

"Drug company estimates suggest that arthritis relief accounts for anywhere from one-third to one-half of the $900 million in annual aspirin sales.

"Some arthritis sufferers gulp down as many as 10,000 aspirin tablets a year, 30 a day. The extra-big bottles, with as many as 1,000 tablets, are earmarked for arthritis sufferers.

"It is hard to pinpoint how much drug-makers earn from arthritis because antiarthritis products also are taken for headaches, trick knees, and the many other guises of pain. But when one considers all the drugs that find use in fighting arthritis, the market bulges to something close to $3 billion in retail sales, according to analysts. Over-the-counter sales make up more than half of that total, but the swiftest growth comes from prescription drugs."

According to the 1985 article, a spokesman for Upjohn, the manufacturer of Motrin (ibuprofen), one of the best-selling prescription antiarthritics, says about the market for arthritis products: "Every new drug that comes out seems to expand it. Since no one has a cure for arthritis and it's such a debilitating disease, people seek everything that comes along, hoping and praying that this may be the ticket."

One reason the arthritis industry is still so lucrative is precisely the fact that so many people still have this attitude. According to the Arthritis Foundation, the estimated annual cost of arthritis to the economy is some $72 billion in medical care and a whopping $77 billion in indirect costs such as lost wages. Additionally, according to the foundation, individuals with rheumatic disease average eight doctor visits per year, twice the average number for persons with other conditions.

The arthritis establishment, which includes the pharmaceutical companies, special-interest organizations such as the Arthritis Foundation, and specialized medical personnel such as rheumatologists, physical therapists, and surgeons, has consistently maintained that arthritis is an incurable disease. Therapeutically, this translates into the possible need for physical therapy, ad hoc surgical intervention to replace joints, and a lifetime of medication that, even if it is effective at relieving pain, does nothing to address the cause or arrest the progression of the disease. Economically, addressing arthritis as an incurable disease is a prescription for steady long-term profits.

Causes

Dr. Theodosakis describes various causes of osteoarthritis. The first is injuries, especially in young people. Once a joint is injured and becomes loose with torn ligaments as a result of activities such as skiing, the cartilage will break down more quickly: "There are also several metabolic conditions, including iron overload, that act as factors. People take iron pills without knowing what their iron levels are. This is dangerous because of the possibility of overload, although this is more common in men than in women."

Infections from many different types of agents—viral, fungal, bacterial, and so forth—often trigger the disease, he adds.

Moreover, he states, "Other forms of arthritis can lead to osteoarthritis. So if you have gout, for example, which comes from crystals in the joints due to excessive uric acid, or if you have rheumatoid arthritis, these can lead to osteoarthritis. But with any of these many causes, the joint appearance will be the same."

Dr. Ray Wunderlich practices preventive medicine in St. Petersburg, Florida, and is the author of many books, including ones on arthritis and carpal tunnel syndrome. He says, "Rheumatoid arthritis is a very difficult thing to handle. About 70 percent of people who have rheumatoid arthritis, the kind that is crippling, where the joints are disjointed, have a specific genetic marker, an HLA [human leukocyte antigen] histocompatibility locus antigen, DRw4. So we know there is a genetic component to that illness. We have triggers that turn on the arthritis."

He also points to intestinal disorder as significant: "The big thing here is the gut, as with so many other disorders." He explains that circulating endotoxins from bacteria often have as their target the lining of the joints: "That's something you have to think of right away, especially in the rheumatoid patient. The small intestine in arthritis patients is very often overgrown with bacteria. So we have a spread of these unwanted organisms into areas that should be sterile. There is also the problem of a leaky gut and the issue of allergens and infections." That is, a person may be eating nightshade foods—the family including potatoes, tomatoes, tobacco, and coffee—that inflame the joints or acid foods while also having a low-grade infection.

Wunderlich also notices psychological issues. Arthritis can be triggered when "we have a major loss. For example, my stepmother lost my father, and within three months she had a crippling rheumatoid arthritis."

He continues: "We also see environmental problems. One of my patients was a lady from Sarasota, not that old, in her early sixties. She moved into a new condo and within six weeks had a severe, crippling rheumatoid arthritis. It was a chemical in the new carpet. That was removed, and the arthritis went away, and I'm talking about rheumatoid factor positive, erthrocyte sedimentation rate elevated, C-reactive protein elevated, inflammatory disease, well proven."

Thus, we know that a host of factors are triggers for the genetically susceptible. All in all, arthritis seems to be an accumulation of deficits of which we are unaware. This is Wunderlich's opinion: "We talk about inadequate repairs, inadequate defenses for our body. As we go along with inadequate food, digestion, metabolism, and porosity of gut, we develop increasing levels of immune disturbance, and the joints are a major place where this manifests. That may be because of their movement or because of the tremendous amount of connective tissue around them."

Connective tissue disorders, whether lupus or rheumatoid arthritis, are very common in our society. Connective tissue needs high amounts of vitamin C, glucosamine, and appropriate minerals such as silica, magnesium, zinc, and pantothenic acid. "Without these," says Dr. Wunderlich, "there will be a decline of the connective tissue, which is the glue that keeps our bodies together. As the body sails along through space in our journey through life, we get bombarded with more and more toxins. Rachel Carson was right. It's a toxic planet, and it's not getting any better."

At this point, I want to underline how central environmental stress is to arthritis, as it is to so many other illnesses. There has been an intellectual blind spot on our medical, health, and legislative screens. We look out there and we see herbicides, pesticides, genetically engineered foods, pollution in our water—so much new pollution that government regulators cannot even abide by the old standards, and so they keep raising the allowable amount of toxins in the body.

Once, for example, they said we had to maintain zero tolerance of PCPs. Then they found that many people had 2 parts per million of PCPs in their bodies, and so they just raised the standards and said that was allowable. But then they discovered that people had more that that in their bodies, and so they said 5 parts per million were allowable. Then it went to 10 parts. And people were saying, "Gee whiz, why don't you clean up the environment and stop raising the body's tolerance levels because there are no studies showing that we can actually tolerate this stuff?" There are 100,000 man-made chemicals, and there is no way to understand what's going to happen when they are synergistically mixed in our diet, air, and water.

We always have this risk-benefit ratio in government studies, where the risk is always to the consumer and the benefit is always to the manufacturer. It's never reversed.

Traditional Diagnosis and Treatment

Typically, arthritis is diagnosed on the basis of a patient's symptoms, which most commonly include pain or swelling in the joint areas or some limitation of movement. There are some diagnostic tests and x-rays may show abnormalities in the joints, but often these tests are not accurate. Thus, the patient's symptoms are the central factor in determining the diagnosis.

Because medical students have been taught that there is no cure for arthritis, as doctors they do not look for the cause of the disease but instead focus on alleviating the symptoms. This approach can be very dangerous because many of the drugs used to counteract pain and swelling can have serious side effects. Even aspirin, which is ordinarily considered one of the least toxic medications and normally constitutes the first line of attack in the traditional treatment of arthritis, is not without side effects. In the treatment of arthritis, aspirin is given in large doses on a constant basis. Consequently, arthritis patients have consistently high levels of aspirin in their systems; this can result in dizziness, ringing in the ears, intestinal tract bleeding, and kidney damage.

When aspirin does not work or when an arthritis sufferer develops adverse reactions to it, other medications called nonsteroidal anti-inflammatory drugs (NSAIDs), such as the widely advertised Motrin, are used to control inflammation. Since these drugs are nonsteroidal (i.e., do not contain cortisone), they are less toxic than are some medications commonly used to combat inflammation, but they nevertheless have side effects.

NSAIDs came onto the market as effective alternatives to aspirin, which had caused internal bleeding in many long-term users. Ironically, while the NSAIDs are less effective than aspirin as anti-inflammatories, they also have side effects that include gastrointestinal bleeding and peptic ulcers. Other side effects include dizziness, nervousness, nausea, vomiting, and ringing in the ears. If these drugs are unsuccessful, doctors often prescribe cortisone-derived drugs such as prednisone. These drugs are notorious for their severe toxicity. They interfere with the immune system, leaving the patient defenseless against infection and other diseases. Cortisone-type drugs also interfere with the body's healing ability, and it is not uncommon for a person taking these drugs to have bone fractures or wounds that do not heal for long periods.

Some rheumatologists (doctors who treat arthritis patients) use gold injections. This method of treatment was abandoned years ago because it was considered too dangerous, but today gold treatments are finding their way back into medical practice. Another technique finding acceptance among arthritis doctors, despite its tragic consequences, is the use of chemotherapy drugs. The theory behind this drastic measure is that when a patient's immune system is knocked out, the patient's body is no longer able to form the antibodies that may be causing the inflammation in his or her joints. Other expensive and highly dangerous techniques include radiation therapy in the area of the inflammation, again with the intent of destroying the patient's immune response, and plasmapheresis, a procedure by which a patient's blood is drained, filtered to remove antibodies, and then reinjected into the patient.

While the traditional medical approach to arthritis is undeniably becoming more sophisticated, it also appears to be missing the mark. Not only do these treatments fail to get at the cause of the disease, they are becoming more expensive, invasive, and toxic and lead to the inevitable question, Do the ends justify the means? When traditional medicine begins to turn to anticancer therapies to treat arthritis—therapies that often are cancer-causing themselves and result in such radical side effects as nausea, hair and weight loss, and total devastation of the immune system—this question becomes even more pressing.

Dr. Warren Levin of Physicians for Complementary Medicine recalls that a couple of years ago the American Medical Association (AMA) put out a series of videotapes to teach physicians how to take care of and diagnose rheumatoid arthritis. The lecturer on the tape was adamant that nutrition has nothing to do with arthritis: "His whole face filled the screen, and he said, 'Nutrition has no place in the treatment of arthritis. We can use drugs.' That is the AMA way. They have not come to Physicians for Complementary Medicine to see what success we have with our methods and how the vast majority of our patients dramatically improve without the use of the toxic drugs that characterize American medicine's treatment of arthritis."

Alternative Treatments

"The way I treat arthritis is probably quite different from the approach of most physicians," says Dr. Peter D'Adano, a naturopathic physician. "As a naturopath, I was taught that we should not always think about treating a disease but about treating a person. Arthritis is a very good example of a disease which is highly individualized. Not only are there different types of arthritis, but people get it and express it in different manners."

It's a good idea to try to listen to the body and realize that it has an intelligence. In other words, if you are following a certain lifestyle and your problems are the result of that lifestyle, a change in lifestyle may change the illness.

People say that as the body gets older, the most natural thing in the world is for it to get decrepit. But give the body credit for the intelligence it has. When the body tells you something, if you listen and follow what it says, you will improve.

What is arthritis? It's pain. Why is it painful? Well, what have you been eating? Maybe you say, "I have a very good diet. I have pancakes in the morning with sausages. Then orange juice. I use saccharine." That is a diet loaded with substances that will bring complaints from the body. Instead, we must think of detoxification. Our air is noxious, our oceans are polluted, and so is the body. We have to help the body heal itself first by cleansing.

DIET AND NUTRITION

Dr. Peter Agho of the Healing Center says, "I do diet. Not just for arthritis. The thing about the whole diet is this. Change the diet, and the arthritis—along with obesity, high blood pressure, and other problems—will get better. The diet should include fresh fruit, including fresh fruit juice, and vegetables. You should eliminate animal fats and cut high-fat foods."

Dr. Howard Robins outlines his treatment: "We use a complete vegetarian diet, including a lot of green, leafy vegetables. These are important because of all the phytochemicals and phytoestrogens that help in all the chemical processes that are necessary to getting well again. We give them juices, six to eight fresh green juices a day—the best way to take in these chemicals."

Dr. Luke Bucci, author of *Pain Free: The Definitive Guide to Healing Arthritis,* notes that part of the reason people get arthritis is the lack of essential nutrients in a highly processed, refined diet. Sure, you get plenty of calories, protein, and fat—usually the wrong kind of fat. What you do not get is just as important—the minerals: magnesium, zinc, copper, manganese, boron. Many people are not aware of boron as a nutrient, but boron may turn out to be essential to our joints' health. These are what you do not get with the current, typical American diet. We look the substances that enable the joints tp repair themselves from the damage they sustain. That is why you want to start eating a whole-food diet that is rich in organic vegetables, fruits, and nuts.

Dr. Rich Ribner tells this story: "Recently, a woman came to the clinic with a terrible case of arthritis. She was in terrible pain and had been taking anti-inflammatory medication and tranquilizers. She was miserable. She said she thought about killing herself. I said, 'Stop this nonsense. I'm going to ask you to do something. You may not even want to do it.' She said, 'Anything.' I said, 'Between now and next week, I want you to drink six to eight glasses of water a day, but it has to be distilled or spring water. And eat nothing but brown rice, just brown rice.' 'But, but…' she began. 'Wait,' I said, 'You were talking about killing yourself. So listen, I'll add a few green vegetables to that.'

"You have to make sure there is a cleansing. Make sure they drink the water. Have a bowel movement daily.

"Well, this woman was so desperate that she stayed on the diet one week. When she came back, there was marked improvement. She still had a long way to go, but there was a change."

SUPPLEMENTS

Dr. Bucci believes that special nutrients can help prevent rheumatoid arthritis and that the most important substance for healing arthritis is glucosamine. There are several forms of it. With glucosamine sulfate, you should take 1,500 mg a day in divided doses; glucosamine hydrochlorides work quite well also. They "convince" your joint tissues to repair the damage. If the situation is not too far gone and you still have cartilage, you can rebuild it greatly, which may mean being pain-free.

Another very important nutrient is chondroitin sulfate. Chondroitin is synthesized to glucosamine in the joints. Chondroitin is one of the molecular "cements" or "glues" that hold together cartilage and let the collagen protein be laid down, forming the actual tissue.

Another interesting finding has been the value of vitamin C. This should be taken as 4,000 mg per day in two or three doses with meals. We have thought about using C for many other problems, but it is also a very important nutrient for the joints. Along with glucosamine, it is the only substance that can stimulate the cartilage to repair itself. Drugs have not been able to do this.

Another substance of value is vitamin E. Take 400 IU per day in one pill. It helps reduce pain, as has been shown in human clinical trials. Also useful is vitamin B_3 (niacinamide). This should be taken in a 150- to 200-mg dose three to four times a day. It will not kill pain right away—it takes time, maybe up to one or two years—but you'll see a gradual improvement in the range and function of the joint.

Magnesium and the obscure mineral boron are valuable. Areas of the world where there are low soil levels of boron show more osteoarthritis. Several human studies have been done that show that a very minor dose of boron, some 3 to 6 mg a day, can reverse the symptoms of osteoarthritis. This is very promising and exciting. I think boron is related to another mineral, magnesium, which has not had as many clinical trials. But we know it is extremely important for every healing process in the body. Therefore, there is a very definite link between boron and magnesium.

Interestingly, if you do not eat fruits and vegetables, it is almost impossible to get a dietary intake of boron, since it comes almost exclusively from vegetables and fruits.

"One of the questions I get as I go around the country," Dr. Luke Bucci continues, "trying to spread this message of the connection of nutrition and arthritis, is: 'Where is the evidence? No one's heard of glucosamine.'

"Well, I'm not the one who thought this up, though I may have rediscovered it. There is valid, strong scientific research and human clinical trials on this substance, millions of hours of use of glucosamine sulfate by doctors, mostly in Europe. Others in Europe are using substances they extracted from the cartilage itself, such as the chondroitin sulfate.

"There is a very large body of literature on the topic, with dozens of human studies and even more with animals. We know how and why these substances work because this is how the body heals itself. So I answer their question about where the studies are with my own question: 'Where's everybody been?' Why have people not read the prodigious literature available? Why don't people just open up their eyes and read?'"

AVOIDING CERTAIN FOODS AND CHEMICALS

Dr. Warren Levin points out that another important aspect to look at is allergies to foods and chemicals. After removing the offending substance from the patient's environment—whether internally with food or externally with chemicals—we see dramatic changes over and above what we see with just adding vitamins and minerals.

Some doctors believe that the most apparent cause of arthritis is common foods, what the patient eats all the time. Dr. Morton Teich stresses that the food the patient wants the most is the problem, such as milk. He cites a study by Richard Pettish (*Arthritis and Rheumatism,* February 1986, "Food Induced Arthritis: Inflammatory Arthritis Exacerbated by Milk") that shows that milk can cause severe allergies and arthritis.

Many studies indicate that food definitely causes problems; the nightshades, for instance, bring on allergies. They also cross react with ragweed.

Dr. Teich also warns us about the glycoproteins in milk, wheat, corn, and cinnamon, as well as inhalants such as dust, mold, and pollen. Chemicals are also vitally important in causing allergies, as are additives in foods.

HERBS

Letha Hadady, an herbalist, says that an important thing to remember about arthritis is that it is essential to eliminate the underlying problems that make it possible. Killing the pain is not enough; you need to eliminate the toxins that result from poor digestion and poor circulation.

She shares some of her herbal secrets for total health: using produce and herbal remedies, substances you can find in the grocery store, at the health food store, or through mail order.

In dealing with arthritis, one thing you must have every day is alfalfa. You could chew 10 tablets a day with a little water to eliminate much of the uric acid that can build up to create joint pain. Rhubarb also eliminates acid. It is a laxative, but it also breaks apart the crystals that form around your joints which give you pain.

Dandelion greens are full of vitamins and minerals. In fact, anything green is a rich source of calcium. Dandelions break down pain-giving acid, too.

Star fruit is a sweet, delicious fruit you can find in the grocery store or at the vegetable stand. Juice it. Add a cup and a half of cold water. Drunk three times a day, it will eliminate inflammatory joint pain, bleeding hemorrhoids, and burning urine. It it is cooling and cleansing.

It is important to realize that everyone's arthritic pain is not the same. Do you wake up in the morning with your joints feeling stiff and sore? Do they feel better after you move them around and after you exercise? If so, you need to take warming, tonic herbs that build vitality, increase circulation, and warm joints. Adding a pinch of turmeric to your stews will do this. Turmeric and cinnamon are a good combination for achy shoulders. If you have rheumatism that gets worse in cold weather, add a quarter of a teaspoon of turmeric and cinnamon to a little water and drink it as a tea.

Asafetida is a spice that is available in Indian stores. A little added to cooking beans or other hard-to-digest foods will help cleanse the body and warm the joints.

Another thing you can use is the resin myrrh; a few drops added to your tea will make your joints feel warm and your blood move, improving the circulation.

Hadady says that Asian medicine uses many herbs that can be added in cooking. For example, *tang kuei* increases circulation and warms joints. Another very safe and classic Chinese remedy, one that Chinese doctors have used for generations, is *du huo jisheng wan,* which makes arthritis in all parts of the body feel better.

Hadady's favorite—*guan jie yan wan*—is translated as "walk as smoothly as a tiger." This remedy brings the blood exactly where you need it: your hips, legs, and joints.

The wonder of Asian remedies is that a combination of herbs takes the painkiller where it needs to go. There are so many, including raw Tienchi ginseng, Efficacious Corydalis, *tien ma,* Three Snakes Formula, Mobility 3, Clematis 19, *du zhong, leigong ten pian,* and *rinchen dragjor-rilnag chenmo.*

GOOD PERSONAL AND INTERNAL HYGIENE

To understand the nature of the treatment, you have to understand that the first rule of health is good personal and internal hygiene.

What does that mean? Well, a lot of Americans eat fairly good diets some of the time but not all of the time. Whenever you eat something bad for yourself, you undo whatever a good diet has been accomplishing.

Not all diets are the same. I say get a good diet, but what does that mean? Does it mean eating hamburgers and cheeseburgers? No! It means a diet that is rich in live food. Does live food mean raw food? Not necessarily. It means nutrient-rich food loaded with life-supporting live enzymes. Give up meat, yes. Caffeine, absolutely. Sugar, yes. And give up chicken. Eat fish: the ones that are rich in the omega fatty acids that help lubricate joints and will help your heart. Mackerel, cod, salmon, and sardines are the most important fish for a good diet that helps prevent arthritis.

Take six glasses—and I'm talking about 12- to 14-oz glasses—of fresh organic juice. These juices should be aloe vera, cabbage, cucumber, celery, apple, and carrot. These are the mainstays, the primary beverages. (The aloe vera should be taken from the bottle, not as a plant, which has diarrheal properties.) Drink these juices unless you are hyperglycemic or diabetic, in which case you will have to stay away from carrot and apple because they raise your blood sugar level too high. Add such things as dandelions and a small amount of mint. Almost all the other vegetables can be juiced, and they are outrageously good, particularly for arthritis.

Make sure you are getting the right nutrients. To find out, you can check your blood. Make sure you get folic acid, niacinamide, pantothenic acid, vitamin D, and vitamin E (400 units/day). You can take from 2,000 to 20,000 mg per day of vitamin C, adjusting what you need each day, depending, for example, on how much stress you are under. If you are under stress, increase your dose. If you have a disease such as cancer or chronic fatigue syndrome, increase your dose even more. The necessary nutrients are vitamin B_{12} (1,000 mcg); vitamin B_6 (50 mg/day); vitamin B_2 (50 mg/day); vitamin B_1 (25 to 50 mg/day); vitamin A, a lot of which you'll get from the juices and fish oils (25,000 units/day); and MaxEPA (1,000 mg/day).

The minerals we need are calcium and magnesium (1,200 mg/day), iodine, and sea vegetables, which include wakame, kombu, nori, and hijiki. One 4-oz serving of these vegetables a day is good for the trace minerals. Also take phosphorous (700 mg); potassium (500 mg); sulfur, which can be found in garlic (2,000 mg); onions—an onion a day keeps the heart and blood circulation in good order—and manganese (25 mg). There are also more esoteric minerals such as evening primrose oil (200 mg/day), superoxide dismutase, coenzyme Q10 (100 to 200 mg/day), silicon extract, boron (5 mg), copper lysinate (2 mg), methionine, and selenium. Methionine is an amino acid found in soy. Selenium, by the way, is not in the soils. And if it is not in the soil, it is not in the plant, and so it will not get into our bodies.

Take enzymes. People with arthritis often have deficiencies in liver enzymes. Rebuild the intestine, the liver, and the pancreas. Take the plant-based enzymes, which are the primary nutrients.

Here is what it comes down to: You must eliminate milk, red meat, sugar products, green peppers, eggplant, tomato, tobacco, alcohol, salt, deep-fried foods, and preservatives. Then you will taken a major step toward rebalancing the body chemistry.

You are doing two things: detoxifying so that you do not have those triggers going off and damaging your body and fortifying your body with those green vegetables, supplements, minerals, and phytochemicals. You are exercising and doing other good things; in total, something has to work.

I know it sounds complex, but look at the benefits.

The average person with arthritis does none of the above. She will try simply to take a drug and hope for a miracle. But the miracle does not come. Who are you going to blame? The doctor? No. The pharmaceutical company? No. Blame your expectation that something outside yourself is better equipped to help you than is your own innate healing capacity.

CHIROPRACTIC

Many arthritis sufferers we interviewed for this chapter said that of all the things they tried to eliminate the pain, going to a chiropractor helped the most.

Dr. Mitchell Proffman, a chiropractor at the Healing Center, showed me two x-rays. The first showed bones that were nice and clean and square in shape; the second showed degeneration of the bones.

He showed what arthritis looks like in the human body: thinned disks and a little lip or spur, the body's defense mechanism to heal or shore up the area so that it does not totally disintegrate. He said a person might have a pinched nerve somewhere in her body, in the neck, for example, meaning it is out of alignment. He administers a gentle push with his hand, which is not painful, to move the bone back into position. The nerve energy comes through, and the joint can start to heal.

RECONSTRUCTIVE THERAPY

The noted physician Dr. Arnold Blank has used reconstructive therapy as an important means of treating arthritis. Reconstructive therapy, created in the 1920s by the osteopathic physicians Gedney and Schumann, works by stimulating the body's ability to heal itself. Their design was to help stimulate the body's ability to heal ligaments, tendons, and cartilage. The doctors found that by injecting substances that caused a slight irritation to these tissues, they could help the blood vessels grow into the region, thus bringing more oxygen, vitamins, and minerals, as well as fibroblast growth factor, into the cartilage, promoting tissue growth.

Dr. Blank introduced me to one of his patients: "George has had an injury to his shoulder due to chronic overuse. I have been injecting into the ligaments in and around his shoulder joint. This therapy works best when the patients are in an optimal nutritional state. Vitamin and mineral levels are important in our healing response and ability. The injection consists of a variety of different liquids. Primary liquids I use are calcium, lidocaine, and saline. They take a moment and really aren't painful. The majority of patients feel improvement after the first three or four treatments, developing some strength and feeling less pain, even increasing the range of movement.

"The nutrients we may use, natural ones, include substances that have an anti-inflammatory effect, such as vitamin C, shark cartilage, sea cucumber, glutathione, and glucosamine sulfate. All these substances are used once reconstructive therapy has begun because the new blood vessels going to the tissues will enhance healing. These nutrients may not work well when there are no blood vessels going into the area, and so they should be administered after the therapy has begun its work."

Another male patient recounts his experience: "I injured my back and didn't realize it until I started getting aches in the back of my leg. I had heard about reconstructive therapy, so I started on my back, had so many treatments, then I went to the hip, knee, and shoulder. They all feel great at present."

ACUPUNCTURE

Acupuncture has been used by countless people throughout the world to help alleviate the pain and suffering of arthritis. Dr. Yuan Yang of the Healing Center reminds us that arthritis around the joints causes much pain: "We put the needle around the joint to create circulation, taking the pain away. There may be cold, blocked blood and low energy, so I apply the needle for smooth blood. Moving blocked energy takes the pain out."

I asked her, "Are you saying that putting acupuncture needles around the joints where they are swollen will stimulate better blood flow and help relieve the symptoms?"

"Yes," she responded, "and then we have to do energy points. We must find the whole body energy points. Maybe we will work with the spleen point, the meridian and kidney points. These points will help circulation anywhere in the body and will make for better circulation and digestion."

PHYSICAL THERAPY

Shmuel Tatz works at Medical Arts at Carnegie Hall with an exercise physiologist, doing mostly hands-on treatment. He typically works with people who have arthritic problems from overuse syndromes or accidents. They work directly on the joints. For example, when working with a pianist who has problems with the hands, they will try to move the bones, separating the joints to make more space.

As Tatz explains, "Today in physical therapy we use many modalities. One of these is magnetic pulse therapy. We know of the positive effects of magnetism on the body. Scientists have developed a machine with different programs so that we can adjust for every different situation.

"We put electrodes on the body, for example, on the hip joint. Here it stays for 15 to 20 minutes. Usually patients report a very mild relaxing sensation, and the pain decreases.

"Many people with pain from osteoarthritis are afraid to be touched. People with a swollen knee, for instance, can do reflex therapy. For the knee we touch an acupuncture point on the ear, which gives relief."

Once this manipulation has had an effect, they start to exercise the knee by putting the legs in slings, relieving the pressure on the joint and making it easier for the patient to move the body. Trying to open the joint and make more space around the bones allows for better circulation.

The same can be done for every part of the body: the shoulder, neck, and so on. Movement is very important for people suffering with arthritis.

One patient, Lori, speaks about her improvement:

"Here at Medical Arts I was able to receive physical therapy, which has enabled me to avoid surgery and has greatly improved the quality of my life. I'm still dancing."

YOGA

Molly McBride, a yoga instructor, believes you do not have to stop working on your health simply because you may have some physical limitations. Even by working with something as simple as a chair, it is easy to stay fit and help yourself with the problems of arthritis.

The basis of yoga is breath and breathing practices, she says, which help circulation and also help flush the body out by collecting toxins so that they can be exhaled. Breath is the foundation of all the yoga stretches.

"We start with just taking a simple breath; the basic beginning exercise is a three-part breath. Let the air fill the abdomen, then the rib cage, then the upper chest. Exhale, letting the breath exit the upper chest, then the rib cage, and then abdomen. Inhale, exhale."

It is important to take time every day to do these breathing exercises. A really good time to do them is first thing in the morning, when your stomach is empty; if you have eaten, wait a few hours before you start. These breathing exercises can be combined with some simple joint lubrication exercises. To regenerate the body and increase the flow of oxygen through the system, to help release all the toxins that build up in the muscles and the protective cartilage around the joints, try simple yoga exercises.

Specific Treatment Approaches

In the following pages, we discuss some specific alternative approaches to treating arthritis. These include Dr. Jason Theodosakis's six-part program that works to optimize the body's own replacement of cartilage; Dr. Robert Liefman's balanced hormonal treatment; Dr. Marshall Mandell's allergy-related approach; Dana Ullman's homeopathic treatments for arthritis and fibromyalgia; the nutritional approaches of Betty Lee Morales, who has helped many people overcome arthritis and other degenerative diseases through the use of whole foods; and the special diet of Dr. Laurie Aesoph, a naturopathic physician, which helps both prevent and treat arthritis. Dr. David Steenblock's approach, which focuses on the correlation between arthritis and atherosclerosis, also is discussed. Although there are many other approaches, these have had a consistently high success rate, are not toxic or expensive, and in some cases may get to the cause of the disease rather than merely masking its symptoms.

DR. JASON THEODOSAKIS: MAXIMIZING THE ARTHRITIS CURE

Dr. Theodosakis is the author of *The Arthritis Cure* and a board-certified physician trained in exercise physiology and sports medicine, a lecturer on preventive medicine, a clinical professor at the University of Arizona College of Medicine, and the director of its Preventative Medicine Residency Training Program.

He begins on a personal note: "I've come up with my arthritis program out of necessity, both to treat patients and for personal use. I see a lot of patients mainly with osteoarthritis but also with the other types of arthritis. I developed my cure and published my book. I'm coming out with a new book, *Maximizing the Arthritis Cure,* which takes this treatment several steps further.

"My program is an integrated, comprehensive approach to creating a situation that optimizes the buildup of cartilage. I will basically use anything—diet, exercise, even medicine when it's called for. We hit it from all angles, including the psychological aspects.

"I'm very proud of this approach. We have changed the face of arthritis this year. The number of studies that have been done using elements that I've taken into my program has increased several fold. As many new studies were done this year with alternative treatments as were represented in the previous ten years."

He notes that his program addresses the causes of arthritis: "I believe that the hallmark of good medicine is not to just treat but to get an accurate diagnosis of where the problem originates and then try to reverse the reversible conditions whenever possible, in line with the knowledge of how the arthritis originated. If you have gout, for instance, with these crystals in your joint, you wouldn't want to just go through the standard treatment protocols for osteoarthritis, such as taking anti-inflammatory pills, because that won't eliminate the crystals."

NSAIDs, he remarked, are part of a $37 billion worldwide market that involvies such huge corporations as Whitehall-Robins, which makes Advil and Motrin; other NSAIDs are Aleve, which is naproxen sodium, and aspirin, which is considered an anti-inflammatory. According to Dr. Theodosakis, "They lead to thousands of deaths a year due to bleeding ulcers, kidney problems, and drug interactions. At a rheumatology conference I was at, it came out that none of these anti-inflammatories have been studied long term. Studies have suggested that they may even worsen the condition."

Dr. Theodosakis's program can be broken down into six components: diagnosis, supplementation with glucosamine and chondroitin, a change in biomechanics, exercise, and medical approaches.

DIAGNOSIS

"The very first step is getting an accurate diagnosis and working with the physician. Be up front with your doctor. In my book, I lay out what you should be telling your doctor and what your doctor should be asking you, the tests you should getting for a diagnosis, and so on. Even if you are in a managed-care setting where you get only five or ten minutes with your doctor, you have to know what information to get to use that time optimally. Getting an accurate diagnosis so you'll know what you are treating is step one."

GLUCOSAMINE AND CHONDROITIN

Use glucosamine and chondroitin as supplements. These are two natural supplements, taken from seashells and cow's cartilage, respectively. When taken orally, they actually improve the balance between breakdown and buildup of the cartilage. "These supplements are part of a treatment," he cautions. "Alone, these supplements are not the answer; they need to be part of a complete program. There is clear medical evidence to support their use. Several new studies are out this year, including two from the United States that have been completed but not yet published, using these supplements, one with Navy Seals and one with an orthopedic group in North Carolina. Both show positive results. The evidence on the value of this mounts."

Dr. Theodosakis has a website listing all these studies (www.drtheo.com). Further, he states, "I also set up a national reporting center for drug side effects related to glucosamine and chondroitin to see if any negative effects have been noted. So far, although millions of people are using these supplements, I'm not aware of any side effects. And I would be the first person to be aware of them if they were occurring."

The one problem with these supplements is that there are about 100 different brands on the market. In Dr. Theodosakis's opinion, "maybe as many as 30 percent do not meet the label claims. In other words, you are not getting what the bottle says. This is a very big concern of mine. It makes my treatment program look less effective if people are taking placebos. So, this is another thing you can get more information about on my website."

BIOMECHANICS

Biomechanics refers to the way the body absorbs shock from everyday movement. "You have different forces on your joint," he says, "and if you learn to dissipate these forces throughout your body, there is likely to be less damage to your cartilage. People can learn to improve their biomechanics. They certainly do in the sports arena, which you will see if you look at athletes as well as performers in such disciplines as ballet. They have wonderful biomechanics and can absorb and dissipate tremendous shock. So my patients are taught how to alter their biomechanics."

EXERCISE

Exercise is absolutely necessary for arthritis sufferers, but the wrong kind of exercise can worsen the condition. You need a specific program for whatever ails you, he says. If you have a hip problem, for example, you will need to do the appropriate exercises for that.

DIET

The fifth component is diet. In discussing a patient he cured, Dr. Theodosakis remarked, "The fasting in order to detoxify the body, the juicing, the vegetarian diet are all things I agree with 100 percent.

"Diet has a tremendous impact on arthritis for several reasons. One is weight control. A major risk factor for getting arthritis is being overweight. For example, women in the highest fifth of weight are eight times more likely to get arthritis of the knee than are women in the lowest fifth. Another factor is that different foods will either aggravate or alleviate arthritis. Some of the fish oils, omega-3 fatty acids, can help, while certain components of meat, such as arachidonic acid, can worsen the condition. You also need to eat a wide variety of fruits and vegetables, making sure you get a wide variety of nutrients and also taking supplements. With these nutritional elements, we are making sure your body has the optimal environment to win this cartilage battle."

MEDICAL APPROACHES

At this point Dr. Theodosakis's program moves into the medical approaches that are out there: the new prescription drugs, for example, as well as surgery for those who are too far gone, along with the psychological aspects, such as treating depression and looking at how the mind-body interaction affects arthritis.

RESULTS

Dr. Theodosakis describes what he calls "one of my most remarkable cases," that of one of his nurses. "She is about 40 years old. She had terrible arthritis, to the point where she was going to have her knee cartilage scraped off, she had so many crystals in it. She used my program for about four months and saw tremendous improvement. She was taking the supplements at that time, then she stopped taking the supplements—that was about two years ago. Now she's become a runner; she did a half marathon. But she would have been crippled if she had had the surgery.

"I have had a number of patients who were scheduled for joint replacement therapy and after going through this program were able to avoid the surgery. Many are pain-free. It won't reverse the bony changes that occurred in the joint, but it gives them the opportunity to exercise and do some of the things they want to do."

DR. ROBERT LIEFMAN: HOLISTIC BALANCED TREATMENT

Holistic balanced treatment (HBT) is derived from the work of the physician Dr. Robert Liefman (1920–1973). Dr. Liefman first used this treatment in 1961, after 20 years of research. Since that time more than 30,000 arthritis sufferers have received the treatment, and many of them are living pain-free, normal lives.

HBT is based on the results of Dr. Liefman's research, which showed that many arthritis sufferers, especially those with rheumatoid arthritis, have specific hormonal imbalances. Within the body there are naturally occurring hormones called glucocorticoids whose role is to reduce inflammation and raise the level of simple sugars in the blood. One of the ways these hormones raise blood sugar levels is by converting nonglucose molecules such as protein into glucose. If unchecked, these glucocorticoids can be responsible for the collagen breakdown of cartilage in joints, which may be a contributing factor in the development of arthritis. The glucocorticoids are balanced within the body by other hormones, such as testosterone and the feminizing hormones, which include estradiol; these hormones induce tissue building and hence balance the tissue-wasting effects of the glucocorticoids. If the body is not regulating these hormones, there are therapies to correct these imbalances. Dr. Liefman developed formulas consisting of varying amounts of three basic ingredients: (1) prednisone, an anti-inflammatory steroid, (2) estradiol, an estrogenic hormone, and (3) testosterone.

According to the proponents of HBT, the anti-inflammatory property of the steroid prednisone and the healing properties of sex hormones can be used to treat arthritic conditions with minimal side effects because of the balancing action between the different components. The anabolic, or building, quality of the sex hormones acts to control the catabolic, or destructive, effects of the steroidal drug therapy (these effects include infection, decreased immunity, improper healing, suppression of pituitary and adrenal function, and fluid retention). The feminizing and androgenic activities of sex hormones are kept in check both by the catabolic nature of the glucocorticoids and by careful adjustment of the concentration of the sex hormones in accordance with the specific requirements of the individual patient during treatment.

EARLY RESEARCH

Dr. Liefman, an American married to a Canadian, graduated from McGill Medical School in Montreal, Canada. During World War II he was drafted into the U.S. Army. A doctor in the medical corps, he was left relatively free to do research on endocrinology. After the war Dr. Liefman continued his research, focusing in particular on the hormones estrogen and progesterone. Around that time cortisone was being researched and developed at the Mayo Clinic by Dr. Philip Hench, who won the Nobel Prize in physiology and medicine in 1950 for his work on that drug. In the early stages of research cortisone was hailed as the miracle cure for arthritis for which scientists had been searching for many years. This fanfare caused many to begin funneling grant money into research on cortisone; accordingly, Dr. Liefman began to explore its potential uses and effects.

Early on, it became apparent that cortisone produces dangerous side effects when used alone. Dr. Hench and his associates continued their work to see how they could counteract the side effects of cortisone. As early as the 1950s Dr. Hench and his associates observed that there were fewer side effects when the drug was used concurrently with estrone (the estrogens include estradiol, estrone, and estriol) and that side effects were almost nonexistent when testosterone was used with the cortisone. It is unclear why Dr. Hench apparently discontinued his research into the benefits of combining hormones with cortisone to minimize the potential side effects. However, around this time both Dr. Liefman and another American physician, Dr. W. K. Ishmael, and his colleagues were conducting similar work which essentially confirmed the finding of Dr. Hench that the side effects of cortisone could be reduced greatly when it was administered in conjunction with the proper sex hormones.

Parenthetically, 30 years later, in November 1975, another group of researchers would confirm these results in a paper presented at the Southern Medical Association's 69th Annual Scientific Meeting in Miami Beach, which followed the direction of the work done earlier by Drs. Hench, Liefman, and Ishmael. In their study the researchers measured the responses of 14 women with severe rheumatoid arthritis who were given estrogen and progesterone in amounts similar to those present in pregnant women. (In 1948, Dr. Hench had observed the effect of pregnancies on 34 women. In 30 of the 34 pregnancies the women experienced substantial or total relief from arthritic symptoms during pregnancy. He also noted that the disease rarely began during pregnancy.) In the 1975 study researchers found that the response to the hormones was often very rapid and dramatic. Not only were decreases in pain and swelling noted, together with increases in mobility and strength, objective test results improved. The degree of inflammation decreased, and 6 of the 14 patients had normal sedimentation rates (which indicate the extent of inflammation) at the time the paper was presented. Before treatment, 12 patients had been moderately anemic; after the hormonal treatment, their blood tested normal. Also, x-rays indicated a lessening of soft tissue and bone softening (osteoporosis) and increased calcification of bones.

THE TREATMENT

When, in the 1950s, he received an offer from the Arthritis Hospital in Sweden to apply the results of his work, Dr. Liefman decided to leave Montreal. For a year he was given carte blanche to put to clinical use the research he had done on balancing the body's hormonal system. Much to his surprise, almost all the rheumatoid arthritis patients he treated showed great, if not total, improvement. A paper he wrote on his work was published in one of the leading medical journals in Sweden. Quite naively, Dr. Liefman expected that when he returned to North America, he would be acclaimed for the work he had done. He was sorely disappointed when his medical professors and colleagues were not interested in his findings. He attempted to sell his treatment to one pharmaceutical giant after another, but no one was interested because his hormone compounds could not be patented and thus could not generate the type of profits to which the drug companies were accustomed. These companies told Dr. Liefman that instead of bothering them he should give away his medication to the government. He went to the Veterans Administration (VA) and offered to treat veterans with his hormonally balanced formulas, but the VA rejected his offer because this medication had not been approved by the U.S. Food and Drug Administration.

Knowing the value of his treatment, Dr. Liefman began quietly treating patients in his home in Montreal. His first patient was a doctor who suffered from rheumatoid arthritis. After several days on the hormonally balanced treatment, all the doctor's crippling symptoms disappeared. The doctor in turn sent a child who was suffering from juvenile rheumatoid arthritis, and the same thing occurred. Word began to spread, and before long Montreal newspapers were running stories on this "miraculous" new treatment for arthritis discovered by a local resident.

The news of a miracle cure for an "incurable" disease was met with considerable skepticism in the United States. *Look* magazine even sent two investigative journalists to Montreal to "expose" this "quack" doctor who had bamboozled the Canadian press into believing that he could treat arthritis successfully. The journalists spent a week or so outside Dr. Liefman's home, where they observed people entering in wheelchairs and on crutches. After spending a few days there, many of those people left without their wheelchairs or crutches. Based on the personal observations of these journalists, *Look* presented a very favorable report on Dr. Liefman's work which explained his method of treatment and told about the high degree of success he was having. After the publication of that article, people from all over the United States and Canada flocked to Dr. Liefman for treatment. With this mass migration came the wrath of the medical establishment, which was outraged that an individual doctor could succeed where it had failed.

Over his lifetime and despite persistent harassment by the medical establishment, Dr. Liefman treated over 20,000 arthritis patients with a very high level of success. They were for the most part people who had tried orthodox medical treatment to no avail and had been essentially abandoned by the medical establishment as hopeless. Professor Henry Rothblatt, an attorney and a close friend of Dr. Liefman who defended him throughout the many legal battles waged against him, recounts how they met:

"I came to know about Dr. Liefman from a woman physician who learned about his treatment through *Look* magazine and went up to see him. She was literally left to die by her colleagues. She had been rheumatoid for 25 years. She had been in one of the leading hospitals in New York, and her colleagues said, 'Doctor, we have done everything that medical science can do for you. You are just going to have to suffer your last few years and make the best of it.' Well, she decided not to suffer. She went up to see Dr. Liefman, and within one week her crippling symptoms came to an end. She became one of his biggest fans and one of his most zealous disciples. It was through her that I met Dr. Liefman at a time when the Canadian bureaucracy finally decided to go to work on him."

The persecution of Dr. Liefman was unfortunate since his treatment has been so effective for an illness that affects so many people. The fact that it is innovative and unconventional is probably the main reason for its unpopularity within the medical establishment.

THE SUCCESS OF HBT

In contrast to the symptom-suppressing approach taken by the traditional medical establishment, HBT is designed to address the causes of arthritis. It does this first by restoring a positive protein-building balance within the body through the administration of the trihormonal formulas described above, which works to stop pain and inflammation. Second, according to Dr. Henry Rothblatt, "HBT is never administered without considering the particular need of the individual patient. The medication is adjusted for every patient so that the proper tissue-building and healing response can be obtained. Respect for the uniqueness and the unique need of the individual patient is one of the essential principles of the holistic approach to medicine."

Dr. Liefman developed four basic formulas to account for the different requirements of each individual using HBT: (1) White Cap, which contains prednisone, testosterone, and estradiol, (2) Black Cap, which has only prednisone and estradiol, (3) Red Cap, which contains prednisone and testosterone, and (4) Green Cap, which contains only prednisone and is used only to allow women to shed the endometrium proliferation caused by the intake of the estrogen-containing preparations. In turn, the proportions of these different compounds may vary from individual to individual and may be altered for the same person during the course of treatment. If, for example, a female patient begins to exhibit an adverse reaction to the treatment, such as the growth of excess body hair, the testosterone level in the medication will be reduced to eliminate those reactions. The same holds true for men who experience breast development or other sex-related changes as a result of the medication's estrogen content. Patients who exhibit some of the typical side effects of cortisone-type drugs will have the amounts of prednisone in their medication decreased, or appropriate increases in one of the sex hormones will be made to counterbalance the negative effects of the steroids. Generally, the adverse reactions to any of the elements in the compounds disappear within a short time once the proper balance among the hormones has been attained.

In addition to the importance of balancing the anti-inflammatory hormones with the sex hormones to establish a healthy protein-rebuilding environment, Dr. Liefman explored other biochemical interactions within the body which play important healing roles in arthritis. For example, he discovered that a growth hormone produced in the pituitary gland reacts synergistically with estradiol and testosterone to stimulate bone growth. He looked at the health of the pancreas to determine whether adequate insulin was being produced to ensure the efficient breakdown of sugar within the body, because without proper sugar metabolism, the body lacks sufficient energy to build and repair bones.

HBT also incorporates principles of nutrition and stresses the importance of regular exercise. The diet recommended in HBT eliminates junk foods such as sugar and sugar products and salty and processed foods such as luncheon meats and canned goods, fried foods, and refined foods. The diet is essentially moderate in protein and emphasizes high-fiber complex carbohydrates in the form of fresh fruits and vegetables, whole grains, and legumes. Vitamin and mineral supplements are used to bolster the patient's immune system and enhance the body's natural healing abilities. For instance, vitamin D is important for strong and healthy bones because it regulates the absorption of calcium from the stomach into the bloodstream, which carries it to bone tissue. Vitamins C and A are important for the maintenance and repair of collagen, the gluelike substance that holds the tissues together and is essential for joint and muscle stability. Vitamin E and B-complex vitamins are important for bone growth. Among the minerals, adequate supply and absorption of calcium, phosphorous, and magnesium are essential for the formation of healthy bones, while zinc and selenium are important immune system nutrients.

Exercise is also an important adjunct to HBT and is recommended to restore joint and muscle mobility and function as well as muscle mass lost during periods of inactivity. However, patients generally are told not to exercise until they are free of pain, swelling, and stiffness and feel confident enough to engage in it. Walking may be the first exercise; then, as patients improve, they can be given specialized exercises for the hands, knees, fingers, shoulders, and other areas which may have been affected by arthritis.

The medical establishment has basically ignored, attacked, or criticized HBT therapy even though its basis is drugs already widely used by physicians. All Dr. Liefman did was combine certain commonly prescribed drugs to maximize the benefits and minimize the side effects of each component drug. The balanced hormonal approach to arthritis did, however, do one unorthodox thing: It challenged the rigidly held position of the medical establishment that arthritis is an incurable disease. Was it for this reason alone that, before his death in October 1973, Dr. Liefman faced considerable opposition from the American arthritis community and was actively prosecuted by the FDA?

Here are some of the results arthritis patients have had over the years from using HBT:

PATIENT 1: MALCOLM

Malcolm had his first attack of arthritis when he was 21 years old. By the time he was 44, the pain had become constant. Deformities started to appear in the joints of his shoulders, hips, knees, upper and lower spine, and sternum. He was diagnosed with Strümpell-Marie disease (spondylitis), a form of arthritis which causes such severe deformities in the spine that the patient is literally doubled over.

Malcolm also had severe iritis, an inflammation of the eyes which is not uncommon in rheumatoid arthritis patients, and extensive retinal hemorrhages were found in both eyes. During the year before his treatment with HBT, he was taking 12 to 14 aspirin tablets daily, was receiving cortisone injections in his knee once a week, and had tried another medication which had no effect.

Malcolm began treatment with HBT in August 1962 after reading the *Look* magazine article in May. He experienced almost immediate relief. According to his physician, his arthritis had almost disappeared and his eyes were normal. When he was unable to get his medication in 1968, his symptoms began to return, but they subsided upon resumption of the HBT. About his treatment, Malcolm wrote years later:

"In August 1962, when I started the medication, I weighed 149 pounds and was using a cane. I could not turn my head and could do no physical work. Today I weigh 190 pounds (I am 5 feet 11 inches tall), show absolutely no sign of arthritis, and maintain an active schedule seven days a week. I have had my blood checked three times, and each time I have been pronounced to be in top physical condition.

"I would like to add that in 1961 I was in the hospital for tests and observation. X-rays showed that my hips were so clouded with calcium that the joints could not be seen, and five vertebrae in my back were fused. I was told that in about five years I would be so bent, I would not be able to sit in a wheelchair. About five years ago, for my own information, I had a set of x-rays taken and was told that my back and hips were in better condition than the average person's."

PATIENT 2: CYNTHIA

At age 19, Cynthia began to experience the symptoms of rheumatoid arthritis. Initially the arthritis was confined to her jaw and elbows, but over a period of 2 1/2 years, while she was undergoing treatment by a traditional physician, the arthritis spread to nearly every part of her body. Five years later Cynthia was so crippled with pain and stiffness that it took her a half hour to get out of bed in the morning. The morning after she started HBT, her pain had almost disappeared except for some stiffness and soreness, which also went away during the following three days. About her condition and her subsequent treatment at the Arthritis Medical Center in Fort Lauderdale, which administers HBT, Cynthia said:

"I was getting worse and worse. When I first went to my doctor, I had it just in my jaw and elbows. After 2 1/2 years, I had it in just about every place except my hips and knees. l couldn't turn my head at all.

"The doctor actually told me once that he felt really bad, that he had tried everything and didn't know what else to do, and that I had better go to the crippled children's center in Palm Beach. To tell a young woman that.... I just wanted to drive off a bridge. But I thank him for saying it because if he hadn't, I don't think I ever would have tried this place. I did it in desperation."

At the time Cynthia started HBT she was taking 30 aspirin tablets a day, which were causing headaches, ringing in her ears, and ulcers. She was spending approximately $1,000 a month on painkillers alone. While Cynthia found that she bruised and bled more easily after starting HBT, she notes that she had the same symptoms while taking large doses of aspirin. However, while the aspirin and other treatments did nothing to arrest the progression of Cynthia's arthritis, a day after she started treatment with HBT, her pain virtually disappeared, and it returned only when she forgot to take her medication. At present Cynthia is pain-free and works out three times a week at a health spa. She continues on her medication, but in much smaller doses than when she started treatment with HBT.

PATIENT 3: JUNE

June suffered from severe crippling arthritis for two years before starting treatment with HBT. Over that two-year period June received almost every form of traditional arthritis treatment available: gold injections, penicillamine, Butazolidin (phenylbutazone), small doses of prednisone, and 16 aspirins daily. June says that she was spending over $100 a week for medication alone. In the meantime she kept getting worse, and when she started HBT, she says, "I was immobile in my hands and shoulders. It was at that point that I thought, What's the use of living? I couldn't even turn my head." Additionally, her liver, stomach, and kidneys were damaged by the large doses of medication. She was forced to give up her business because she was too weak and in too much pain to work. Her medical bills were ruining her financially. The second day after June received HBT, her pain disappeared. June says about her progress with HBT:

"I woke up and I could move my ankles, I could move my hands and my feet. When I stood up, the pain wasn't there. I said to [my husband], 'My God, there's been a miracle.' It got better and better, and I guess within two months

I didn't even know I had rheumatoid arthritis. I got a bicycle, and I started dancing again and going to the beach again. It used to be if I lay on the sand, I couldn't get up again."

June continues to be pain-free, leading a normal life, and her medication has been reduced by more than half the initial amount.

DR. THERON RANDOLPH AND DR. MARSHALL MANDELL: ENVIRONMENTAL ALLERGIES

Environmental medicine, also called clinical ecology, was developed by Dr. Theron Randolph in the 1940s and 1950s when he observed early in his medical career that food allergies and sensitivities to environmental chemicals were a major contributing factor in a wide range of diseases, including arthritis. Dr. Randolph also noted that the causal relationship of allergy to disease was a very individualized phenomenon: One person could eat beef every day and never have an adverse reaction, while another person could develop a food allergy to beef even when consuming it only on rare occasions. Similarly, people with an allergy to the same product did not necessarily manifest the same symptoms. One might break out with hives, while another developed depression, and still another became arthritic. Dr. Randolph also found that seemingly innocuous chemicals found in the home, workplace, or school could in certain individuals trigger symptoms ranging from mental problems to aching joints to chronic fatigue.

The work of Dr. Randolph was applied to arthritis by Dr. Marshall Mandell, a board-certified physician from Connecticut and one of the country's leading environmental medical specialists. He has found that a considerable number of patients who come to him with arthritis or arthritislike symptoms are in fact suffering from a form of environmental allergy such as the ones outlined by Dr. Randolph. According to Dr. Mandell, "The basic process that underlies many cases of arthritis is a completely unrecognized or unsuspected allergy or allergylike sensitivity to substances that are part of daily life, including the food we eat, the liquids we drink, including the water supply, the chemicals that are deliberately or accidentally introduced into a diet, and the various forms of chemical pollutants in the indoor and outdoor air that get into our bodies." From his clinical experience, Dr. Mandell has found that more than half the patients he treats who would, by standard medical diagnostic techniques, be confirmed arthritics can be helped by means of simple dietary or environmental changes.

THE TREATMENT

"My approach and that of my colleagues in the field of environmental medicine and clinical ecology, supplemented by the benefits of nutritional therapy, begins by looking at the person who is predisposed to having arthritis to see if there are identifiable substances in the diet and environment which can trig ger or cause the episode of illness," says Dr. Mandell. "We deal with demonstrable cause-and-effect relationships. What we do is study the patient.

"First, we take a carefully formulated history which is designed to help identify people who have problems with foods, with various chemicals, with pollutants, and perhaps with seasonal airborne substances. From this, we are able to get a fairly good idea of what we're dealing with."

Before patients are tested for food or environmental allergies, Dr. Mandell often will have them fast or go on a restricted diet for four days to one week to rid the body of any residue of substances suspected to be responsible for the symptoms.

"Next," says Dr. Mandell, "we test these people using a technique known as 'provocative testing' to determine their response to extracts prepared from all the foods in their diet. The most commonly ingested foods are often the culprits, so it shouldn't come as any surprise that wheat, corn products, milk, beef, tomatoes, potatoes, and soy are leading offenders.

"The most common technique used for provocative testing is to place a few drops of the test substance under the tongue of the patient, where it is almost immediately absorbed. This is called 'sublingual' provocative testing. When we test in this manner, only small doses are used, so the effect is brief, but since the solution enters the bloodstream, the entire body is exposed. Symptoms can show up in the joints, muscles, brain, skin, or any other part of the body.

"If we are able to produce joint pain, stiffness or swelling, or redness within a few minutes after placing the solution under the tongue for absorption into the bloodstream, we know that we've found something that must be important, because we have flared up the patient's familiar symptoms—we have actually precipitated an attack of the patient's own illness.

"Many people will have what we call 'polysymptomatic illness,' meaning that many bodily structures, organs, or systems can be involved at the same time. The arthritic person's whole body may be sensitive, and this is why such patients may have a headache or fatigue or asthma or colitis, although they may not actually have any of the well-known allergies such as hay fever, eczema, or hives.

"We also find that many people react to chemicals. We have some people whose arthritis may be due in part or exclusively to the chlorine that is in the water supply, or perhaps to an artificial flavoring or coloring which is used very frequently, or perhaps to a preservative. We have people who have trouble because they are inhaling fumes such as tobacco smoke. We have people who in heavy traffic have trouble because the exhaust fumes will travel, along with the oxygen, through the walls of the lung into the circulation; once again, the whole body is exposed."

After Dr. Mandell determines the substances in the patient's overall environment which he suspects are responsible for arthritic symptoms, he double-checks with test meals of the specific substances.

"I confirm the results of our testing in the office with feeding tests," he says. "Three foods can be tested during the course of a day; however, for the test to be accurate, the food to be tested must be out of the person's system for at least five days. Sometimes we can get away with it for four days, but it is even better if that food has been completely omitted from the diet in all forms for five, six, or seven days. We give patients a single food as the test meal; since we want to test the food all by itself, we don't put any ketchup, pepper, mustard, sauce, or anything else on the food. Instead of a usual portion, we allow patients to consume as much of the single food as they can comfortably eat as an entire meal....

"Then we observe them for at least four hours. If we're able to reproduce that patient's specific symptoms, if we can actually turn the symptoms on and off like a switch, we know that we have nailed it down, because we have demonstrated a cause-and-effect relationship that can't be questioned. Should food be the primary causative factor, we will design a diet that eliminates all of those foods. Then, depending on how well they follow the diet, the patients will be either well or sick."

Dr. Mandell provides some examples of how allergic reactions can result in arthritis or arthritislike symptoms:

PATIENT 1: SARAH

Sarah was a rabbi's wife who began to have arthritis in her hands, but the flare-ups would take place only on Saturday mornings and then disappear during the course of the day. Using Saturday as a starting point, Dr. Mandell began to explore the possible sources of Sarah's "Saturday arthritis."

"Since she woke up with the arthritis in the morning," Dr. Mandell explains, "we knew it was not caused by something she was doing in the morning. So we went back 24 hours to explore Friday. What did she do on Friday? What did she eat? Drink? Breathe? What came into her system? Could it be, perhaps, the paraffin fumes from the candles on the table which were lit ceremonially every Friday night? Or could it be something they ate? Was it caused by something she was exposed to when she went to temple on Friday night, perhaps from clothing just taken out of the dry cleaner's? Or was it hair spray, perfume, cologne, or men with aftershave lotion? Was it that the temple had had the rug shampooed the day before the services or that the furniture was polished? I had no way of knowing, but I retraced all her activities, and then I tested her systematically.

"This actually turned out to be an easy one, and it was humorous, because the great 'Jewish penicillin,' chicken soup, was the thing that was undoing her. When I placed a few drops of chicken extract under her tongue, within minutes the knuckles that were affected by arthritis swelled up and became painful and red. I did this on a few occasions, and so we were able to demonstrate this. It is rare to find a patient in whom a single substance is the factor, but it does happen now and then. So here is a rabbi's wife with chicken and chicken soup arthritis—Friday night ingestion, Saturday morning appearance of arthritis."

PATIENT 2: A SURGEON

Dr. Randolph treated a surgeon who became so incapacitated by arthritis that he had to stop performing surgery and restrict his medical practice to office consultations. He had developed severe arthritis primarily in the hips, knees, shoulders, and hands and had received traditional treatment for 10 years. While he derived some relief from the treatment, he still was incapacitated. He had to walk downstairs backward, no longer had the strength or dexterity in his hands to perform surgery, and lacked the physical strength even to stand at the operating table.

The surgeon went to Chicago to see Dr. Randolph, who admitted him to the hospital and immediately put him on a pure spring water fast, free of chlorine and fluoride and without any of the contamination that affects city water supplies. Additionally, he was placed in a special room where the environment was controlled. There were no air fresheners or disinfectants and no bleaches, the floor was not waxed or polished, and the personnel were not permitted to smoke or wear perfume.

Within five days the surgeon was free of pain. He regained some dexterity in his hands and reported that if he was a little stronger, he felt he could return to the operating room and resume his normal work. Then he was given single-food feeding tests, and Dr. Randolph discovered that when he was tested with corn (cornmeal with some corn syrup), within a matter of hours he became miserably uncomfortable with severe pain in the shoulders and hips. He had so much pain that it felt as if he had been kicked by a mule. A few days later he was tested with chicken extract, and the effect was different. While he did not experience pain right away, the chicken affected his brain. He became so sleepy that he actually dozed off. When he awoke, he was in such severe pain that he was actually crying.

The surgeon found that as long as he avoided corn and chicken, he was virtually pain-free and could resume his regular daily life.

PATIENT 3: JANET

This example not only documents the dramatic effects which can be achieved by eliminating an offending food from an arthritic person's diet, it also shows the degree of resistance orthodox arthritis doctors have to accepting this even when it has been unequivocally demonstrated.

Back in the mid-1970s Dr. Mandell sent out a mailing to rheumatologists in the northeastern part of the country, indicating that he was studying the relationship between food allergies and arthritis and was interested in studying some of their patients free of charge. Out of 90 letters, he received six respons-es, of which three said yes and three said no. Through one of the doctors who agreed to send patients, Janet eventually saw Dr. Mandell. He discusses her testing and the results:

"I want to emphasize that we never tell the patient what the test material is, so we completely eliminate suggestion. When we tested her with pork, she had pain almost immediately in one finger on her right hand, and this was her arthritis joint. We caused the joint to swell up and become red and painful.

"This test was repeated three times, once a week, and after the last test I told her to stay off pork for at least a week and then have a large portion of it one morning as a feeding test. Once again the same thing happened. However, when she told her rheumatologist, the man who was willing to have her come to me, he said he didn't believe it because we didn't have any controls. This is … more than pathetic, it's almost a medical crime! Here the patient had her symp-tom reproduced … and the doctor says he doesn't believe what has happened to her."

The ironic thing about this skepticism on the part of the orthodox medical establishment is that many of the treatments it prescribes for arthritis have never been proved either safe or effective. Gold injections are a good example. This treatment is extremely costly, has very high toxicity, and is only rarely of benefit to arthritis sufferers. Furthermore, in cases where gold does provide some relief, rheumatologists are unable to offer a scientific explanation of how it operates within the body. Nevertheless, gold continues to be endorsed by the arthritis establishment while something as simple as eliminating a food from a patient's diet, even if that food has been demonstrated to cause the patient's symptoms, is ignored or criticized as being unscientific.

PATIENT 4: MRS. BULLOCK

Dr. Mandell has a friend, Dr. Bullock, whose wife suffered from arthritis. Dr. Bullock had noticed something strange about his wife's condition. When she went to the hospital for testing and treatment, her arthritis would improve, but the moment she returned home, the symptoms would flare up again. Her rheumatologist told Mrs. Bullock that he felt it was all psychological; the "pro-tective environment" of the hospital made her relax, and this had a beneficial effect on her arthritis. The rheumatologist concluded that something was "emotionally" wrong with Mrs. Bullock's home and that she should seek psy-chiatric help to discover what it was.

Her husband was skeptical about this, and after talking with Dr. Mandell, he began to look at possible environmental and dietary changes which could have been responsible for his wife's improvement in the hospital. Mrs. Bullock's problem, it turned out, was very simple. At home, she ate a very lim-ited southern diet which included certain favorite foods consumed daily or very frequently. When she was in the hospital, however, and was presented with a long list of foods from which to choose, it was like being in a hotel or a restaurant, and she ate an extremely varied diet. For Mrs. Bullock, varying her menu made all the difference in the world. Her husband created a diet that eliminated the major offending foods and rotated a wide variety of foods so that no one food had a chance to build up in her system. Her condition improved enormously.

DANA ULLMAN'S HOMEOPATHY FOR ARTHRITIS AND FIBROMYALGIA

Homeopathy is based on the idea that the cure for an illness is similar to its cause. As a result, treatment consists of administering small doses of a very diluted natural substance that would cause the symptoms of the condition being treated if it were taken in larger amounts.

Dana Ullman is the president of the Foundation for Homeopathic Education and Research and a board member of the National Center for Homeopathy. He is the author of five books on homeopathy, including *The Consumer's Guide to Homeopathy: The Definitive Resource for Understanding Homeopathic Medicine and Making It Work for You* (J. P. Tarcher, 1996), and *Discovering Homeopathy: Medicine for the 21st Century* (North Atlantic Books, 1991). Ullman describes the positive role homeopathy can play in treating arthritis, explaining how the homeopathic remedies are selected and what they're made up of:

TREATMENT FOR ARTHRITIS

"There are estimated to be 200 types of arthritis. I'm glad that [the medical establishment has] increased that number from before. [In the past], it's been … about 10 or 20. From the homeopathic point of view, every person with arthritis has his or her own species of arthritis. Homeopaths see disease as a syndrome. Just as a woman experiences premenstrual syndrome, which includes a certain degree of bloating and cramping as well as emotional changes, in homeopathy we consider that people with all diseases have a syndrome which involves a body-mind constellation of symptoms.

"Before rushing into the practical stuff, I want to comment about the research behind homeopathy, specifically in light of arthritis. The *British Journal of Clinical Pharmacology*, a major pharmacology journal, published a double-blind, placebo-controlled study on the homeopathic treatment of rheumatoid arthritis; this was way back in 1980. This study showed that 82 percent of the patients given an individualized homeopathic medicine got some degree of relief, whereas among those given a placebo, only 21 percent got that similar degree of relief.

"Rheumatoid arthritis, as many people out there know, is an autoimmune disease. It's not simply a disease of the joints. That's where it manifests in terms of pain and dysfunction, but the bottom line is that medicine today sees rheumatoid arthritis as a systemic disease. From a homeopathic point of view, conventional medicine is finally catching up with homeopathy [in recognizing that] all disease is systemic, that you cannot have just a disease in the joint. You cannot have just kidney or liver disease. Every manifestation of disease, that's only its most external source, and there's a complex of symptoms and syndromes that we all experience. All too often, in conventional medicine, they're unable to deal with the complexity and simply prescribe different treatments for different symptoms, not recognizing the unitary system that we are.

"There are several key approaches that homeopaths and the general public can use in order to make the best use of these homeopathic remedies to treat their own health problems of a musculoskeletal nature. One approach is the use of single remedies to treat the acute exacerbation of the problem. Acute exacerbation of the problem means an immediate problem of a short-term nature, like a flare-up of some sort. Homeopathy and homeopathic remedies can be used to allay and relieve some of the pain and discomfort that a person's having.

"A better approach, however, is using the single remedy prescribed by a professional homeopath. This provides what we call constitutional care. It's a more highly individualized remedy, not just for the acute flare-up but for the person's overall genetic health and entire health history. For the homeopath to do this, it requires a detailed interview, lasting at least one to sometimes two hours. And sometimes a homeopath doesn't prescribe on that first interview but needs more information. This type of care is probably, in my estimation, one of the more profound ways to augment the body's own immune defense system, to not just relieve a person's condition but to really initiate a healing and curative process.

"This is so important. We shouldn't just suppress our symptoms. Nor is it always adequate just to relieve them. Of course, relief is better than just living with it. We all have to be compassionate with everyone, including ourselves, who experiences pain and discomfort and look for ways—ideally, natural ways, first—to relieve our pain and discomfort. But ultimately, the real goal of a physician-healer has to be real cure ... not only temporary relief but getting underneath what's happening and initiating a curative process."

TREATMENT OF FIBROMYALGIA

To explain in specific terms how homeopathy can be effectively utilized, Ullman uses the treatment of fibromyalgia as an example:

"Fibromyalgia is also called fibrositis. For those who aren't familiar with it, it's a somewhat newly defined disease. At first, there was controversy as to whether it existed or not, but now there's basic acceptance that it is a condition. It's not officially arthritis, although it is thought to be a type of rheumatism where the person experiences pain and discomfort in the joints. But they can and will experience a variety—once again, a syndrome—of symptoms. And those symptoms can be extremely diverse. They can and will include fatigue and even emotional and mental changes such as poor concentration, anxiety, and irritability. There might also be an irritable bowel, headaches, and cramps. The syndrome comes on in exacerbations. The person may be fine at one point and then all of a sudden have all these symptoms.

"A study was published in the *British Medical Journal* on fibromyalgia. The researchers admitted into the study only those patients who fit the most popular homeopathic remedy used to treat the acute stages of fibromyalgia. It's a remedy called rhus tox [*Rhus toxicodendron*], which is poison ivy, believe it or not. [With] actual poison ivy, not only [does] an overdose cause skin eruptions, but if taken internally, and I don't recommend it, at least in a crude dose, it can and will have effects upon connective tissue that make the person feel extremely stiff, re-creating many of the symptoms that people experience when they have not only fibromyalgia but even many types of arthritis.

"They found that 42 percent of the people they interviewed fit this remedy. So they admitted these people into this study. In the first half of the study, half the people got a placebo and half the people got the real remedy. Then halfway through the study they switched, and the people who got the placebo now got the real remedy, and the people who began with the remedy got the placebo. The researchers found that when people began the real remedy, the homeopathic medicine, that's when relief began. And in this type of study, which is not only a double-blind placebo study—controlled and crossover is what it's called—the researcher is comparing patients with themselves. It's the most sophisticated type of research currently being done. It cannot always be done because these crossover effects, which we notice in homeopathy, are problematic since often homeopathic remedies have effects even after the person stops taking the remedy. So, when they begin taking the placebo, they're still feeling better. That sort of muddies the water. But this study did show, very clearly, that whenever people started to take rhus tox, they began experiencing relief. So, one thing I want to recommend to people out there is that maybe even before going to a professional homeopath, you can try rhus tox.

SPECIFIC REMEDIES

Rhus tox is also used in many, many musculoskeletal problems. For arthritis, it is one of the leading remedies. It is a leading remedy also for carpal tunnel syndrome. It's a leading remedy for lower back pain. Rhus tox is known for alleviating the type of pain syndrome in the joints which is worse on initial motion, in other words, when the person just begins moving that particular part of the body. But once they begin moving it more frequently, they loosen up and it doesn't hurt as much. Once they sit or lie down or sleep for any period of time, that's when they experience this rusty-gate syndrome again. So if you happen to have this type of rusty-gate syndrome, one of the remedies you need to think about is rhus tox. The people who need rhus tox also tend to have an exacerbation of their symptoms from cold and wet weather. Many people with various types of rheumatic conditions are hypersensitive to cold and wet weather.

"One of the nice things about homeopathy is that you can talk about this broad field of musculoskeletal problems. Although initially I was talking about fibromyalgia, these remedies can be used for many of these conditions. Another remedy that comes to mind is bryonia. Bryonia is an herb called wild hops. This is not the same hops that you drink in a beer. It's a different botanical substance entirely. This is for people with various types of musculoskeletal problems where any type of motion exacerbates the condition. By contrast, people who benefit from rhus tox have this rusty-gate syndrome where they feel worse only on initial motion and then loosen up and limber up. People who need bryonia, the more they move, the worse they are. Here is a really obvious difference. That's one of the unique and nice things about homeopathy. We can be quite precise in finding a remedy that fits each person because the bottom line is that we are all biologically individual. We don't have the same type of joint disease or headache or depression or fatigue. We all have our own unique constellation, our own pattern of symptoms, and homeopathy is an exclusively effective, individualized approach to using these substances from the plant, mineral, or animal kingdom to augment the body's own defenses."

Another remedy Dr. Ullman describes is honeybee (*Apis mellifera*) venom. "One of the other remedies that immediately comes to mind too [is] for various types of musculoskeletal problems, including fibromyalgia and arthritis, and also some carpal tunnel and repetitive strain disorder syndromes that are aggravated by heat or hot weather or hot applications. There is a medicine called … apis … which is [from] the honeybee. For those of us who have ever been stung by a honeybee, or at least we know what it's like, it's a burning and stinging type of pain, somewhat sharp. If you've ever had a bee sting, you also know that if you put ice on the bee sting, it provides some relief. But if you get near heat or you apply heat to it, it worsens the pain. Likewise, people who will benefit from homeopathic doses of apis will have joint pain with swelling, much like a bee might cause, because the bee not only causes that burning, stinging pain but also causes that inflammatory redness and heat. Thus, there will be swelling that will be increased by cold applications and aggravated by heat.

"One of the known parts of folklore is that beekeepers do not seem to get arthritis very often. Part of the reason for this is that they occasionally do get stung, though they don't react the way the rest of us do because they become more immune to it. Their body has developed more sophisticated histamine responses so that when there is any type of sting, the body just deals with it very rapidly and easily. And there's something about that sting that also provides protective effects. It's as if one were taking, if you will, a homeopathic medicine. You're taking something that will cause a similar syndrome to what the arthritis causes. I don't recommend bee venom therapy, usually. I don't recommend that a person with arthritis be stung multiple times by a bee. Not that I discourage it; I [just] think there are safer, easier ways, like taking homeopathic doses of bee venom, which is, once again, this medicine apis mellifica.

DOSAGES AND STRENGTHS OF HOMEOPATHIC MEDICINES

Dr. Ullman feels that it is important to understand some basics about the dosages in homeopathy and the strength of homeopathic medicines. "Don't be fooled by these extremely small doses. Don't think that just because we use small doses, you need to take more frequent repetitions of the remedy. During acute exacerbations, you do need to repeat them approximately every two hours in intense types of syndromes and every four hours in less intense syndromes. However, the idea of homeopathy is to take as few doses as possible but as much as necessary. It's a fine balance. In other words, at times you might take it more frequently, but then as pain and discomfort diminish, you reduce the frequency of taking the remedy.

"If you look in a health food store or pharmacy, it will list the name of the medicine, usually in Latin, because all homeopathic manufacturers have to be really precise on the source and species of the plant, mineral, animal, or chemical that we're using. But next to it will be a number such as 6x or 30c. Well, x refers to the number of times that particular substance has been diluted, 1 to 10. X is a roman numeral which stands for 10. So 6x means it was diluted 1 to 10 six times. C is the Roman numeral for 100. [If it says 30c], that means it was diluted 1 to 100 thirty times. Thus, the C potencies are a little more dilute because they're diluted 1 to 100. But both of these potencies are widely sold and widely effective, and generally we recommend that people who are not professionals in homeopathy should not use medicines higher than the thirtieth potency. The sixth potency, the twelfth, and the thirtieth are quite fine, quite effective. Although the two hundredth and the thousandth are even more effective, you have to be more knowledgeable about these remedies because the higher the potency used, the more precise the prescription must be.

"Another choice is not just the use of single remedies but various combination homeopathic remedies or formulas. These are mixtures of homeopathic medicines, usually two to eight of the most common remedies for a specific ailment, such as arthritic pain, back pain, PMS, allergies, sinusitis, and headaches. You see these in health food stores and pharmacies these days. Although these are not part of what would be called classical homeopathy and although they are not as precise as prescriptions, they are a user-friendly and quite effective means of providing help and relief to people, akin to using a single remedy for acute care.

"These formulas do not provide constitutional treatment. They do not really cure a person of their underlying problem. But they do provide wonderful relief. I do recommend that people consider using formulas when they cannot find the single remedy that they need or do not know how to find that remedy. Or they may know how to find the remedy but it is not immediately available, as is often the problem.

"There is a place for both single-remedy homeopathy, professional homeopathy, and formula homeopathy. In fact, in speaking of formula homeopathy, in terms of some injuries and trauma, I personally believe that people will experience—and I have observed this myself—even more rapid relief of an injury from using a formula of some sort. Because when you have an injury, you often need to give the person arnica [wolfsbane]. But at some other point, you need to give the person another remedy for the specific ailment. If it's a nerve injury, you give hypericum [St. John's wort]; if it's a connective tissue injury, you might give rhus tox or ruta [*Ruta graveolens*]. The bottom line here is that eventually anyone involved in homeopathy will need to give several remedies to the person. And I say, well, why not give several remedies together? A colleague of mine is a homeopath and a podiatrist. Every other day or so he conducts surgery on patients with various types of foot disorders, and he always gives a combination of homeopathic remedies, and he has systematically observed that people heal from the surgery better from a combination rather than just a single medicine given sequentially. I do want to acknowledge that there is some controversy over these formulas, but as far as I'm concerned, the controversy should be null and void."

BETTY LEE MORALES'S NUTRITIONAL APPROACH

Many practitioners of alternative health care who address degenerative diseases (e.g., cancer, diabetes, heart disease, atherosclerosis, and arthritis) in their practices agree that most of these diseases stem from a buildup of toxins in various parts of the body, which in turn results in metabolic dysfunction and eventually in the manifestation of the symptom typifying the particular disease. As to how these toxins begin to accumulate in the body, Betty Lee Morales, a longtime advocate of a natural approach to health and disease prevention, contributing editor of *Let's Live* magazine, and member of the National Health Federation, comments that this follows directly from modern lifestyles and circumstances.

"The pesticide sprays, the poisons that are getting into the air, soil, and water," she says, only worsen the conditions that she calls nutritional deficiencies. All these factors have a negative impact on what she describes as the weakest link: genetic inborn metabolic errors. "In short," she continues, "the proliferation of processed and refined foods, drugs, and man-made chemicals is really at the root of this rapid increase in all degenerative diseases.

"Although it is frightening, it is well to stop and think that there has been no advancement in the treatment or correction or prevention of degenerative diseases in the last 100 years."

EFFECTS OF PESTICIDES, FERTILIZERS, AND DEFICIENT SOIL ON FOOD

One of the specific sources of this problem is the manner in which food is produced and soil is treated in this country today. Dr. Max Gerson, one of the first physicians to take an environmental approach to the treatment of cancer and other degenerative diseases, referred to the soil as our "external metabolism." Even at the outset of his career as a medical doctor more than 60 years ago, long before the soil was depleted and stripped to the degree that it is today, Dr. Gerson was a strong proponent of organically grown, unprocessed foods.

According to Dr. Gerson, chemical pesticides and fertilizers essentially poison and denature fruits and vegetables by altering their chemical composition. For instance, he found that chemical fertilizers often cause the sodium content to rise in certain foods while decreasing their potassium levels. As chronically ill patients are very often chemically imbalanced, with excesses of sodium and deficiencies of potassium, the effects of the fertilizers are exactly opposite to what is required by these patients to begin to recuperate and serve to exacerbate their metabolic imbalances. In other words, even patients who have the willpower and determination to follow a strict regimen in which, among other things, salt and sodium are restricted and potassium is supplemented could find their efforts undermined simply by eating foods grown in chemically treated soil.

Additionally, says Morales, "When foods are grown in deficient soil, deficient plants result, and then the farmer poisons them with pesticides in order to bring them to harvest and to market. We must get back to taking care of the soil and regenerating it. It is not possible to keep taking from something without ever replacing it. It's just like a bank account; if you kept writing checks and didn't put more money into the bank, you would be bankrupt—and our soil is bankrupt. Through bankrupt raw materials and food, bankrupt animals and their by-products, we are producing nutritionally bankrupt people. The United States probably leads the world in excessive consumption of overly processed, overly refined carbohydrates and sugars."

Because of today's agricultural and manufacturing practices, foods once full of vitamins, minerals, protein, and fiber have indeed become bankrupt. Not only does refining wheat and other grains strip them of their fiber, the wheat grown on today's soils contains only a fraction of the protein content it once had. And this is not the only adverse consequence of modern-day food production. Even with thorough washing, many of these chemicals (pesticides, herbicides, etc.) are not removed. They penetrate the skin of fruits and vegetables and poison the body's systems.

If you eat meat, poultry, or dairy products, you are ingesting even higher amounts of toxic chemicals with your food. Meat production in the United States is big business, and the bottom line is maximizing profits, not consumers' health. American cattle are fed a myriad of drugs ranging from antibiotics to steroids, are given feed contaminated with feces and sprayed with pesticides, and are themselves sprayed with pesticides. All these chemicals remain as residues in the meat when it is consumed. As meat takes an especially long time to digest and is essentially fiberless, these chemicals are not easily eliminated and can accumulate to cause all sorts of toxic reactions within the body.

SUSCEPTIBILITY OF JOINTS TO TOXIC MATERIAL

Because of the specific physiology of the joints, they are especially susceptible to a buildup of toxic material which over time can result in arthritis.

Joints are surrounded by the synovial membrane, which is responsible for the production of synovial fluid. This fluid allows for smooth and efficient movement. Between the blood vessels and the inner portions of the joint, the only thing that keeps the blood from the inner surface of the joint is the synovial tissue; there is no structural barrier in this tissue which prevents toxic material from passing from the blood into the joint space. Usually the blood vessels have a surface called a basement membrane, a structural barrier that keeps the toxins in the blood and out of the tissues. In the synovial tissues, that structure is not present, and this allows any toxic material from the blood to pass into the joint space. Once it is in the joint space, this toxic material can scratch and irritate the joint.

According to Morales, "All these things ending in 'itis,' which simply means 'inflammation of,' such as arthritis, neuritis, and bursitis, are really just new and fancy terms for old-fashioned rheumatism. The new names make them appear to be different diseases when they really are not. Among 16 million osteoarthritics, the most common form of arthritis is called the 'wear and tear' disease of degeneration of the joint cartilage. There is much we can do to prevent that. If it has already taken us over, there is a great deal we can do to reverse it."

THE TREATMENT

Morales gives an example of how detoxification of the body and rebuilding of health with an improved diet can be used to prevent and treat arthritis.

"I work with people who are ready to do almost anything just to get a little relief," she says. "They don't even expect reversal, but sometimes they do experience it. One of my sisters was married to a professor at a leading university who was very skeptical of anything to do with diet and nutrition. When my sister developed rheumatoid arthritis, she also had five other diagnosed diseases, including high blood pressure, elevated cholesterol, and heart trouble. Her husband took her all over the world; they went everywhere looking for a magic cure. After they had spent over $40,000, she not only failed to get better, she was actually worse. They returned home and got a practical nurse to come in. She could not even wait on herself.

"Finally, when she reached the bottom of the barrel, she called me and said, 'Well, I would like to try the natural methods way to see if I can get some relief.' At that time she was on about five or six prescribed drugs and obviously had many problems from them: digestion, assimilation, constipation. I said that I would be very glad to help her. Then she said, 'I'll take these things, but I don't want my husband to know.' I said, 'Hey, back up a minute.' Although it broke my heart, I told her that I could not help her until she had suffered enough and was willing to do whatever she needed to do, especially since not all of it was going to be pleasant. I explained that she was going to have to examine her life closely and detoxify from years of faulty diet.

"Detoxification is a very important part of regaining health and maintaining it. I also told her that she could not do this on the sly without her husband knowing about it because it becomes a way of life. It begins with what you eat, the way you live, even the way you think, and you certainly cannot do it living in a house with another person and not have that person know what you are doing. 'In fact,' I said, 'he should be doing it too.' Then she got hysterical and said, 'Well, he's not open to it.' But I had to tell her that I couldn't help her by telling her to take these things, which are not drugs. The first thing you need to do is to start educating yourself. I sent her a few books, and I said, 'When you've read some of this and you are willing to say that you will really try anything, I'll give you three months. Then I will be happy to help.'

"She reached the point where she was in bed and could not go to the bathroom alone, could not hold a glass of water or a cup of tea. She called for me, and I went over. They live in a beautiful home and there is no problem with money, but when I outlined the things that were needed, both she and her husband said, 'Does it really cost that much?' I requested that they buy a juicer, the kind that grinds and presses, because it gives the maximum nutrition. I also wanted to bring in a practical nurse who was trained in this type of thing. I told them to think it over.

"They talked it over and decided that they would try it, so I sent over a juicer and 25 pounds of organically grown carrots. I gave instructions to the practical nurse to throw out everything in the cupboard that was opened and was refined or processed. Anything that was in cans or closed containers was to be given to Goodwill. I made it very clear that nothing was to go into that home that I didn't send in. I got rid of all the salt and sugar and all the easy-mix stuff—this was all a trauma to them because it costs money and nobody likes to throw away money. But I told her that she had to go the whole way or not at all.

"We put her on a seven-day detoxification to cleanse the small intestines and the bowel. She had coffee enemas every day for about a week. She had nothing but the juices, potassium broth, water and herb tea—no solid food for seven days. We broke the fast carefully. She had a massage every day, and I made sure she was taken outdoors at least once a day. I also had the nurse read different things to her every day so she would understand what her body was going through.

"Before she started the treatment, I sent her to a laboratory to have complete blood tests, and then after the cleansing, I had her do the same tests again…. Not that it was necessary in this case, but I knew that if she didn't see the results confirmed by a medical laboratory, she wouldn't believe them. Her cholesterol count was 535, which is incredibly high. Her doctor had told her that she was a walking time bomb. He was keeping her on drugs, but the cholesterol did not go down, although her liver problems increased.

"Three weeks later on this program—remember, this is a woman who could not get out of bed alone—she got up one day, went out to her own car, and drove down to the city to have her hair done. That's very typical of women and probably of men. As soon as they start to feel better, the first thing they want to do is look better. She wanted to have her hair done and get a facial and a manicure. It was a great morale booster. When her husband came home from the university, he did not know his own wife because she was up, was beginning to fix a juice cocktail, and they were so delighted that I never had more arguments or problems out of them. But she also felt so well that she decided not to wait the full six weeks to have the other tests done; it had only been three weeks. She went back to the medical lab and asked to have all the tests done over. She wanted to send her doctor a copy because she still was under the care of a medical doctor who had told her, 'These health food things won't hurt you, but they won't help you. It will only cost you some money, but you can afford it, so go ahead and do it.'

"When she had the second batch of lab tests [which showed substantial improvement] done and sent to him, he wrote her a letter in which he said, 'If you are going to pursue these quack remedies, I can no longer be responsible for your health, and I am dismissing you as a patient.' She called me up crying and said, 'I don't even have a doctor in case I need one.' She was still laboring under the horrible fear that this doctor had laid on her by saying that she could have a stroke or heart attack at any minute.

"We continued with the program. Within a total of three months, she was able to go on a South Pacific cruise with her husband. Today you won't meet two people who are better advocates of the nutritional way of living. They have gone 90 to 95 percent holistic and no longer feel that they have to be under the wing of a doctor who does not recognize nutrition.

"One of the positive offshoots of this is that my brother-in-law, who was a professor for 50 years at one of the most prestigious universities and a staunch opponent of the nutritional approach to healing, also turned 180 degrees around. He too had been taking quite a few medications for high blood pressure. He had what is called a Dupuytren's contracture, where the fingers curl down toward the palm and cannot be straightened—this is a classic vitamin E deficiency. After seeing what it had done for his wife, he said that he was ready to go on an intensive program and see what it could do for his fingers. His brother also had this condition and had had his tendons cut, so it obviously ran in the family. Fortunately, my brother-in-law was willing to try the nutritional program first. Today—he has just turned 80—he's in better health than he has ever been in his life. He is vital and virile and active and full of the joy of life, and the two of them are enjoying their life together so much when they could have been crippled and bedridden."

DR. LAURIE AESOPH'S SIX-STEP NUTRITIONAL APPROACH

Dr. Laurie Aesoph is a naturopathic physician as well as a medical writer. She has authored more than 200 articles on topics ranging from nutrition to herbs and homeopathy, and she also is a senior editor of the *Journal of Naturopathic Medicine.*

Dr. Aesoph describes what she sees as the relation between arthritis prevention and treatment and which foods may help treat this ailment and why:

"People with arthritis don't need to give up hope. Diet and nutrition are the foundation of good health anyway and can be used specifically to treat the more than 100 different types of arthritis that exist."

RESTORATIVE FOODS

"Many, many studies tell us that what I call restorative foods, which merely are the good foods we should be eating anyway, [such as] whole grains, fruits, and vegetables, are what we need to insert in our diet. The studies show not only that good diets help out with arthritis but that specific types of food seem to have healing qualities. For example, the oils from different fish have an anti-inflammatory and pain-relieving benefit for arthritis patients. Many fruits, vegetables, and even spices double as herbs. You can use those specifically for different arthritis symptoms.

"In an article printed in *The Lancet,* a British medical journal, in 1991, researchers put their patients on a cleansing diet. But eventually what they did is switch them over to a lacto-ovo-vegetarian diet in different stages, and they had a group that was their control, their placebo, which just ate as normal. They found that even on the lacto-ovo, where people are eating vegetarian diets but also eating eggs and dairy, the benefits continued throughout that year and at the end of the year. So here's evidence where we know that diet is helping.

"Even the Arthritis Foundation is admitting this. There are enough studies that they are taking notice. They have always said that of course, if you're overweight, there is stress on the joints, so if you have something like osteoarthritis or what we call degenerative joint disease, that's going to aggravate and wear out your joints. But they are also looking at studies involving food allergies and cleansing and fish oil, and of course the purines are involved with gout. And diet has always been a large part of treating gout."

STRESSOR FOODS

Dr. Aesoph asserts that it is equally important to minimize what she calls stressor foods from the diet: "Basically, the stressor foods are what set the stage for joint degeneration and breakdown to occur. And just to give you an example of what these foods are, look at the fat category. I want to remind [people] that fats per se are not bad. In fact they're essential, and there's something called essential fatty acids that we need to have—the fish oils fit into that category. But the trans-fatty acids—hydrogenated vegetable oils, for example, and margarine—[contain] too much saturated fat. Those are the sorts of things that are stressor foods and that we should be avoiding. Alcohol doesn't do us any good, nor does caffeine. Refined carbohydrates, such as sugars, flour, white rice, the different sweeteners, the artificial sweeteners such as aspartame and saccharine, processed foods, of course, and the additives and chemicals that are added to our foods are other things that we should also be avoiding.

"When you eat stressor foods, a lot of them really deplete the different nutrients: vitamins, minerals, and all the other phytochemicals and nutrients that we're discovering are in our foods. These, of course, are essential for general body function. Now, arthritis isn't just restricted to the joints. We've discovered that there is a link between the joints and different body systems, and so the immune system is involved. Rheumatoid arthritis is actually what we call an autoimmune disease, where the immune or defense system of your body is attacking yourself. So if you don't have the vitamins and minerals, your immune system isn't going to function as well as it can. Also, with regard to the intestinal tract, it's also vital that it function properly for all sorts of different conditions. When that isn't functioning right, it will aggravate an arthritic condition. I mentioned that if you are overweight, that will stress the joints. If you tend to eat stressor-type foods, that tends to play into or add to conditions of obesity. Also, we talk about stress in our lives, and I really believe that foods that are not complete in nutrition and aren't as whole as they should be are a stress on the body. So that doesn't help your body function any better.

"Also, if you are eating a lot of cooked or processed foods, they tend to be lower in the enzymes that help us digest our foods. There have been numerous studies done where when people eat a diet that is largely composed of cooked foods, their digestive systems, the pancreas, different organs that contribute digestive enzymes to the gut, have to work a little harder, which makes it harder to digest, and then that adds to your gut being a little thicker than it should be, and then that aggravates the arthritis down the road. So, you can see that there are direct and indirect effects that these stressor foods have.

"When you use natural medicine and conventional medicine, it doesn't need to be an either-or situation. You can also use nutrition to cut back on the medication that you're using. You can think of it as a compromise and perhaps gradually get away from the drugs. Also, if you happen to be on steroids, [such as] prednisone, if you plan to cut back and use nutrition, you need to work with your doctor on that. That's something you don't want to cut out cold turkey. The nonsteroidal anti-inflammatory drugs are not as much of a problem. But when going off any prescription drug or steroids, talk to your doctor first."

THE PROGRAM

Dr. Aesoph outlines her six-step nutritional program to overcome arthritis:

1. Cutting out all the stressor foods from your diet. You want to eliminate anything that is harming your body or undermining your body's functions and really setting the stage for joint problems to happen. These foods not only weaken the joints but impinge their ability to repair themselves as well. These are also the foods that add to excess weight, which can overburden the joints. Some of these foods are also high in purines, which tend to aggravate gout.

2. Cleansing the body with a real whole-foods diet and starting to add the restorative foods. This helps repair the gastrointestinal tract, which is an imperative part of healing arthritis. At this point you should be starting to learn how to incorporate healthy eating habits and what foods to choose.

3. Testing for and then beginning to cut out allergy foods.

4. Rebuilding the damaged joints and overall health again by starting to refine your choice of restorative foods. Sea cucumber at 1,000 mg may help, as can manganese at 25 mg and the bioflavonoid complex. Glucosamine sulfate and chondroital sulfate, both at 500 mg, can also produce phenomenal results. Flax at 1,000 mg from the omega-3 fatty acid group reestablishes normal fluid and osmotic pressure, the synovial fluid in those joints. Taking an alpha lypoic acid, the best all-around intracellular antioxidant, actually fights free radical damage inside the cell. Then you have a very powerful healing mechanism to get your joints circulating nutrients and oxygen and expelling carbon dioxide and waste products as they should. There are many supplements: minerals, vitamins, and herbs. Other ones that you can add are ginger, cumin, and cayenne. Cayenne cream can be rubbed on arthritic joints because it depletes substance p, which decreases pain.

5. Decreasing weight, if that's a problem, because it is a stress on the joints.

6. Eliminating any stress by learning to eat properly, such as by chewing your food properly and eating in a relaxed way.

DR. DAVID STEENBLOCK: ARTHRITIS AND ATHEROSCLEROSIS

Because of the susceptibility of the joints to the accumulation of toxic material which can scratch and irritate the inner linings, leading to the pain and inflammation that characterize arthritis, an analogy has been made between arthritis and atherosclerosis (degeneration of the arteries). In both diseases corrosive substances scratch the inner linings of the body part involved, causing irritation which can lead to degeneration. These substances can come from toxic material in the bowel which gets into the bloodstream. They can also come from food. In the case of atherosclerosis, these foods include cholesterol, fats, and fried foods, which, when they get into the blood, scratch and irritate the very sensitive inner linings of the blood vessels. The same substances can also pass from the blood into the joint space and irritate the inner linings of the joints.

According to Dr. David Steenblock, a physician specializing in the relationship of diet, nutrition, and arthritis, this correlation between arthritis and atherosclerosis is one of the reasons why a low-fat, low-cholesterol, high-fiber diet has been useful in treating arthritis. "Many patients on this type of diet," says Dr. Steenblock, "show substantial improvement because the fiber cleanses the colon and removes many of the toxic bacterial waste products, which frees up the blood system and makes it more pure. This in turn allows the toxic materials to be eliminated from the joints, and so the joints themselves can begin to heal."

HIGH-FIBER DIET

Dr. Steenblock also explains how a diet which eliminates processed foods and focuses on the consumption of high-fiber natural grains, fruits, and vegetables works specifically in the treatment of arthritis:

"We want to eliminate white sugar and white flour products and processed foods and foods which contain food additives because these processed foods cause abnormalities in the state of health of the intestine. When you eat processed foods with little fiber, the bacterial content of the colon changes from the so-called good bacteria, which are *Lactobacillus bifidus* and *L. acidophilus,* to organisms which are anaerobic such as anerococci and streptococci and organisms which generally are not healthy and produce many toxic substances themselves. When these toxic substances are present as a result of eating a diet high in refined food and lacking fiber, these toxins pass through the bowel into the blood. Also, refined foods, because they are so easily digestible and do not require work by the intestine, cause the muscle wall of the intestine to atrophy, or become thinner. This thinness of the wall allows more toxic material to pass through the bowel into the blood. Once it is in the blood, it can pass easily into the joints and cause more problems.

"The use of the high-fiber natural diet counteracts this trend because the fiber changes the bacterial content of the colon back to normal, and this eliminates many of the toxic materials, the carcinogens, and the mutagens which are formed otherwise, which are well-documented causes not only of osteoarthritis but also of cancer of the colon and atherosclerosis. The fiber also strengthens the bowel wall, making it thicker and healthier, and this creates more of a mucosal barrier between the colon's interior and the blood. Thus the diet should be more of a natural and raw foods diet if you want to get a good result."

Dr. Steenblock does warn, however, that people who have spent an entire lifetime eating refined, fiberless foods must approach a change to a raw, high-fiber diet with caution (excess dietary fiber can, for instance, cause calcium and zinc to be washed through the system so that calcium and zinc deficiencies result) in order to give their intestinal tract time to strengthen. A good physician with a solid background in nutritional therapy should be consulted before any drastic dietary changes are made.

CHELATION THERAPY

While atherosclerosis and arthritis often exacerbate each other, treatments other than diet which are directed at one condition often are beneficial in treating the other. For example, Dr. Steenblock discusses how chelation therapy, an intravenous chemical treatment (discussed more fully in Chapter 2) commonly used for atherosclerosis and heart disease, can also benefit arthritic patients:

"One of the problems with osteoarthritis is that the capillaries of the synovium have become rigidified, or more rigid than they should be, as a consequence of the aging process and of atherosclerosis. This limits the blood flow through these joints; therefore, the heat that is produced when the joint is put in motion cannot be taken away because the circulation is poor. As a result, pain occurs when you exercise, and conversely, when you are resting, the blood flow through that tissue is poor and toxic materials accumulate and can cause pain. Anything that increases the diameter and the blood flow through these capillaries will aid in the restoration process. This is where chelation therapy is very valuable because it actually gets into these small blood vessels and capillaries and removes the cross-linkage of the collagen and elastin. This makes these small blood vessels more pliable and elastic, gives them more diameter so that more blood can pass through them, and thus helps in the healing process."

SUPPLEMENTS

Different vitamins, minerals, and nutritive substances can play important roles in the treatment and prevention of arthritis. There is some evidence that the essential fatty acids furnished by substances such as cod liver oil, linoleic acid, and marine lipids, by replacing missing fatty substances in the synovial fluid, can be important in treating arthritis. The synovial fluid consists primarily of mucin with some albumin, fat, epithelium, and leukocytes. When the joint surfaces become irritated and undergo degeneration, some of the fat from the joint itself is lost. This fat acts as a lubricant and keeps the joint surfaces apart so that the cartilage-covered bone ends are protected and can move smoothly. When a person takes extra cod liver oil or other essential fatty acids, the oil goes to the joints and provides more lubrication.

Vitamin A, which is found in large quantities in cod liver oil, is also important for the maintenance of the mucous membranes of the body, which manufacture mucus to cleanse the body of infectious bacteria and toxins. Without adequate supplies of vitamin A, infection and accumulation of toxic materials can set in around the joints. Furthermore, a vitamin A deficiency can lead to insufficient production of synovial fluid; when this occurs, the joints lack proper lubrication, the cartilage becomes subject to drying and cracking, and movement becomes difficult and painful.

Because lubrication is vital to the smooth functioning of the joints, vitamin E, whose primary role is to protect against the destruction of the essential fatty acids by oxidation, is also an important antiarthritic nutrient. Both vitamins E and C, which generally act as free radical scavengers within the body, can be especially important in the treatment as they can "clinch" the free radicals present at the site of inflamed or irritated joints, thereby decreasing pain, swelling, and inflammation. According to Betty Lee Morales, university studies have also suggested that vitamin E can play an important role in neutralizing toxic substances in the air. Furthermore, Morales notes:

"Many women are stricken about the time of menopause, which suggests that arthritis has something to do with falling production of hormones within the body. Men go through menopause, but about 10 years later than women. If women would take extra vitamin E and make sure that they eat hormone precursor foods so that their bodies are fortified, then they would also be taking a step forward in preventing the diseases that are related to hormonal deficiency. Hormone precursor foods include the unrefined whole grains and pollen, which has all 22 free amino acids and is a great hormone precursor food for both sexes."

Many symptoms of arthritis are alleviated by establishing a proper balance of calcium and phosphorus in the body, since these are the two minerals most responsible for bone formation and healing. This can be one of the most confusing aspects of arthritis, because x-rays of arthritic joints often show excessive calcification. Afraid of further calcification, patients mistakenly believe that they must avoid calcium-rich foods. Actually, the calcification is due not to an excess of calcium but to malabsorption of existing supplies caused by an imbalance in the ratio of calcium to phosphorus. This imbalance is caused by two major factors. (1) excessive consumption of foods containing high levels of phosphorus such as meat, dairy products, and soft drinks and (2) the process of joint degeneration, which releases high levels of phosphates. This excess phosphorus at the joint site binds with calcium and results in calcification. Taking extra calcium orally does not contribute to this localized calcification. Rather, by increasing calcium levels in the blood, it draws the excess phosphorus away from the joints to bind with the blood calcium so that both are eliminated; this in turn inhibits calcification around the joints.

It should be noted here that soft drinks are the number one source of phosphorus in the American diet today. These drinks contain more phosphorus than most other foods or beverages, and the typical American consumes nearly 500 gallons of them a year. According to Dr. Steenblock, excess phosphorus is one of the major contributing factors to the development of osteoarthritis. He says, "We see this clinically in many people, who come with osteoarthritis in their early forties who are large consumers of soft drinks, who also consume excess quantities of meats and other high-phosphorus foods, and who do not eat enough of the green, leafy vegetables which contain calcium." The other problem associated with soft drinks is that most of them contain citric acids, which bind calcium and cause it to be excreted. "So," says Dr. Steenblock, "not only is there extra phosphorus in the soft drinks, they contain the material that takes calcium out of the body. If you want to develop osteoarthritis, that's a very good way of doing it."

PROTEOGLYCANS

Another therapy for arthritis entails the use of naturally occurring substances called proteoglycans, which are molecules made up of approximately 10 percent proteins and 90 percent carbohydrates. There has been very promising research in other countries on these substances, but to date little has been done in the United States. Dr. Steenblock explains this therapy:

"What we are talking about is a particular substance called chondroitin sulfate, which is a type of proteoglycan. In a person with osteoarthritis these substances gradually diminish in concentration in the joint as the joint becomes worn. If the chondroitin sulfate could be put back into the joint, this would inhibit the calcification process and also smooth out and seal the irregularities, the cracks, and the irritations which have occurred through time with wear and tear.

"Over the past 10 years or so, chondroitin sulfate has been used in both Europe and Japan for the treatment of osteoarthritis, rheumatoid arthritis, and also atherosclerosis. Again, there is a great similarity between osteoarthritis and atherosclerosis in the sense that both result from the wear and tear caused by irritative substances in the body. We need to protect these collagen surfaces from the irritative substances which circulate in the blood and ultimately get into the joint.

"Chondroitin sulfate appears to be one of the best treatments for both arthritis and vascular disease. When you take it orally, it actually enters into the body through the intestinal tract and will selectively go to the joints and all the areas of damage in the blood vessels. It not only acts preventively but also will help reverse the diseases that are present. This substance is now available in this country in health food stores.

"There are a few companies which are making it from an extract of the trachea called mucopolysaccharides. That is having very good results. Research in Europe and Japan is showing that this substance is probably the best form of therapy that there has been and probably will be for a long time in treating arthritis and vascular disease. The treatment is not, however, the sort of miracle drug type of treatment where you give the person one pill and get immediate results. What we are dealing with is a natural substance, and it takes time for these natural substances to create the result we are looking for, namely, healing of the injured areas. When you take these mucopolysaccharides, you have to take them for anywhere from two to four months in order to achieve results. Patients who stick with them are having very positive results and report upwards of 80 percent relief of pain and also a stoppage of the degeneration.

"There is another substance, which is derived from the New Zealand green lip mussel. There are a number of trade names for it. This substance is also a mucopolysaccharide, and it is effective in treating osteoarthritis as well as rheumatoid arthritis. This material is available in most health food stores.

"These mucopolysaccharides can also be used preventively to heal the small nicks and irritations that occur routinely in the blood vessels and joints. These substances immediately seal these little cracks and crevices so that they do not get larger. Our bodies are not really capable of doing that on their own, and we need to help them along with a little bit of these substances all the time so that our joints and arteries are protected."

Seeing the great variety of approaches out there, it behooves you, if you are suffering from arthritis, to stop watching fantasies of hard-bodied robomen or robowomen and begin a practical program which will ultimately involve both physical and spiritual growth.

Chapter 5

Birth Control

I n the United States today, few subjects are more volatile or politicized than birth control. My goal in this chapter is not to join the debate but to make sure that the information already available to some in the alternative health community is available to everyone.

No currently available form of birth control is 100 percent effective and risk-free, and no single method is right for everyone. A woman's fertility is a highly personal matter, and so the more you are able to feel in sync with your menstrual cycle and fertility, the better able you will be to make the right decisions about birth control for you and your partner.

Fertility Awareness

Fertility awareness, which also is called natural family planning, the Billings method (named after John and Evelyn Billings, two Australian researchers who helped popularize it), and mucus observation, among other names, is an underrated but extremely effective method of pregnancy prevention. This is not the old rhythm method promoted by the Catholic Church in the past, which was notoriously ineffective; each woman has her own "rhythm" that may change from time to time and may not fit into an established pattern.

Actually, fertility awareness can be characterized not as a method of birth control but as a way of life. That is, if you have a more accurate understanding of the dynamic physiological changes that occur during your menstrual cycles, you will be more aware of exactly when you are likely to get pregnant and will be better able to take preventive measures or, if you are trying to become pregnant, enhance your chances.

Some years ago, researchers at Princeton University reanalyzed a mountain of data that had been collected by the World Health Organization (WHO) on couples who used fertility awareness and found that this method was 97 percent effective in preventing pregnancy for those who understood its principles and used it as their sole method of contraception. This research puts to rest the widely held myth that fertility awareness isn't very effective.

Two myths that prevent many people from using fertility awareness as their main method of birth control are that it is difficult to learn and that women have to take their temperature every day and laboriously chart their menstrual cycles for the rest of their lives. This is definitely not the case. You can learn the basic principles of fertility awareness over a few months, and by knowing what to look for, you can learn to identify your fertile period intuitively with a high degree of accuracy without having to deal with charts and thermometers on a daily basis.

Essentially, a number of specific bodily changes signal the onset of a woman's fertile time. These include changes in cervical mucus, body temperature, sexual desire, and an ovulatory pain called mittelschmerz (middle pain).

Getting pregnant requires three factors: sperm, alkaline fertile mucus to nurture and transport the sperm, and a ripe egg in one of the egg (fallopian) tubes. The menstrual cycle begins on the first day of menstrual bleeding, and the average cycle lasts 27 to 30 days, although cycles as short as 21 days or as long as three to nine months are common). A viscous, "stretchy" mucous secretion manufactured in the glands of the cervical canal begins to ooze from the cervical opening at about day 10 of the average cycle and increases daily, peaking at days 14 to 16. Using a plastic speculum, you can actually see the clear mucus, which looks a lot like egg white, oozing from the cervical opening.

As production increases, the stretchy mucus seeps from the vagina and makes a sort of crusty secretion on your underpants or can be picked up by toilet paper.

At the same time that fertile mucus is beginning to develop, a ripe egg pops through the side of one of your ovaries and begins its trip of three to five days down the egg tube. As you approach ovulation, your temperature rises gradually and then, in most women, drops sharply on the day of actual ovulation. If fertile mucus is present and you have unprotected intercourse, the sperm slip easily along the liquid highway of mucus into the cervical canal, where they are kept alive for several days to regroup, as it were, and swim up through the uterus in search of an unfertilized egg.

The idea in using fertility awareness for contraception is to avoid having any sperm in the vagina at times when fertile mucus might be present. By carefully looking for the signs of ovulation (fertile mucus, a drop in temperature, mittelschmerz, and other signs), you can identify pretty specifically when that time is. The first part of the cycle (including menstruation) is considered the "unsafe" time because fertile mucus can appear early or at low levels, but any fertile mucus presents the possibility of pregnancy. Couples who use fertility awareness as a form of birth control avoid penis-in-vagina sex at this time but may enjoy other forms of sexual activity. Others use a barrier method of contraception until they are sure that ovulation has occurred. After ovulation, however, another egg will not appear, and so this is considered the "safe" time. After that time, according to researchers, it is perfectly safe to have vaginal intercourse without getting pregnant.

You can learn the tenets of fertility awareness from a number of excellent books, but many women and their partners find that taking a workshop with several sessions is the easiest and best way to learn. There are now a wide array of fertility detection devices that can be fun to use and are quite accurate. To find the nearest fertility awareness instructor, contact the Ovulation Method Teacher's Association, Box 14511, Portland, OR 97214. Many Catholic hospitals also teach this method.

RESOURCES FOR FERTILITY AWARENESS

Barbara Feldman, Director, Fertility Awareness Center and Birth Control the Natural Way, P.O. Box 2606, New York, N.Y. 10009; (212) 475-4490

Fertility Awareness Network, P.O. Box 1190, New York, N.Y. 10009. Send $4.00 and SASE for an eight-page introductory packet.

California Family Health Council, 3600 Wilshire Boulevard, #600, Los Angeles, Calif. 90010; (213) 386-5614

Diocesan Development Program for Natural Family Planning, 3211 Fourth Street, N.E., Washington, D.C. 20017; (202) 541-3240

National Family Planning Center of Washington, D.C., 8514 Bradmore Drive, Bethesda, Md. 20817; (301) 897-9323

The Male Condom

Condoms, which are latex rubber sheaths that unroll to cover the penis, are 90 to 98 percent effective in preventing pregnancy and provide the best protection from sexually transmitted diseases (STDs). The effectiveness of condoms can be raised to nearly 100 percent by combining them with the cervical cap, diaphragm, vaginal contraceptive film (VCF), or fertility awareness. Many people—both men and women—are reluctant to use condoms because direct skin-to-skin contact feels better. However, that thin rubber membrane may be all that stands between you and pregnancy or a variety of annoying or serious diseases. If you think of the entire body as being available for sexual stimulation, maybe covering up 1 percent of it isn't all that bad. Some people also worry that condoms cut down on sexual sensations and make it more difficult for a man to achieve orgasm. From a woman's perspective, many men ejaculate too readily anyway, and so delaying the man's orgasm may be an advantage.

Condoms are often thought of as a "male-controlled" method, but actually, the effective use of condoms requires the interest and willingness of both partners. Today both men and women buy condoms and keep them in their backpacks or at the bedside for ready use. Because of low cost and wide availability, condoms are the most commonly used barrier method in the world. Condoms come in a variety of styles, in different sizes, and with various aesthetic embellishments, with or without lubricants and/or spermicide.

To be effective, condoms must be used correctly. They should be unrolled along the shaft of the penis with a little space left at the tip to collect the ejaculate. Condoms may be lubricated or can be used with a variety of water-based lubricants (read the label), but they should not be used with petroleum-based lubricants such as Vaseline. When the penis is withdrawn after ejaculation, you or your partner should carefully hold the condom in place to ensure that no sperm are spilled into the vagina. For pregnancy protection, condoms should be used for all vaginal insertions. (For STD protection, you may want to use them in other types of sex play as well, such as anal insertions.)

Because of rumors about a high breakage rate, many people believe that condoms are not all that effective. To counter those fears, the U.S. Food and Drug Administration (FDA) has instituted more rigorous standards of testing, and so breakage rarely occurs. Condoms that are old or have been exposed to heat are more likely to break. If you are worried about breakage, use two condoms at a time. Also, try to buy them in small quantities and at places where turnover is high, such as large discount drug stores. If a break occurs and you are aware of it, insert spermicidal cream or jelly into the vagina as soon as possible.

If you have a variety of sexual partners and vaginal or anal intercourse is a part of your sexual activities, you should consider using condoms at each and every sexual session.

The Female Condom

The female condom somewhat resembles the standard male condom and can be bought over the counter, although it is more expensive than male condoms. It is a soft tube that is made of polyurethane, which is stronger and thinner than latex. It is inserted into the vagina like a lining. It has two rings. One is fitted around the cervix like a diaphragm, and the other remains outside the body and covers the labia. According to an article on the HealthWorld on-line website (www.healthy.net), the female condom has a failure rate of 5 percent when used under ideal conditions, but the average failure rate (since it is not always used in the most careful way) is 25 percent.

The female condom is said to provide effective protection against STDs, including AIDS, especially when it is used together with a male condom. It takes some learning to use properly, since it can get twisted if it is not inserted correctly. It may also reduce sexual sensation and the feeling of spontaneity.

The Cervical Cap

According to women's health and sexuality advocate Rebecca Chalker, "The existence of the cervical cap is one of the best-kept secrets of the twentieth century." This is an approach to birth control that is as safe and effective as the diaphragm but offers a good measure of spontaneity and the convenience of the pill. In Europe there are a handful of cervical cap designs, but in the United States there is only one; the Prentif cavity-rim cervical cap made by Lamberts Ltd. of London has been approved by the FDA for general use. The Prentif cervical cap looks like a large thimble made of soft latex rubber. As Chalker explains in *The Complete Cervical Cap Guide,* "a dollop of spermicide is placed in the dome. Then the cap rim is folded in half, tipped into the opening of the vagina, and guided with a finger to the back of the vaginal canal, where it readily slips over the cervix (the neck of the uterus). The cap stays firmly in place by gripping the cervix and forming a strong suction and provides a physical barrier to the sperm, while the spermicide affords an additional chemical barrier.

"Because it is smaller and more compact than the diaphragm, the Prentif has several distinct advantages. There is no large spring rim to press on sensitive vaginal walls, making it far more comfortable than the diaphragm. Thus, it can be left in place for longer than the diaphragm. The FDA recommends keeping the cap on for no more than 48 hours, but many women have reported keeping it in for three or four days with no problems. The cap stays snugly on the cervix, requiring no extra applications of spermicidal cream or jelly until it is removed. Consequently, it is not messy. Some women still prefer to use the cap more or less like a diaphragm, inserting it anywhere from a few minutes to a few hours before they anticipate having intercourse and removing it sometime the next day. Others keep it in for longer periods and especially like the convenience of being able to keep it in over the weekend."

Because of the cap's obvious advantages, many practitioners who fit the cervical cap now see it as the first choice among barrier methods and recommend the diaphragm only for those who cannot be fitted with a cap.

"Unlike the diaphragm," Chalker notes, "the cervical cap, with its greater freedom from spermicide applications and other inconveniences, can be associated with a greater enjoyment of sexuality. Of course, there is no perfect available birth control solution, and the cervical cap is no exception to that rule. The most vexing drawback associated with cervical cap use in the United States is that not everyone can be fitted with the four available sizes." According to Chalker, about 80 percent of women can be fitted: "If one of the four sizes fits you just right, then the cervical cap may be an excellent solution. In rare cases the cervical cap may develop an odor when left in place too long. Soaking for 20 minutes in water with 10 percent household bleach usually kills odor-causing bacteria. A well-fitting cap may occasionally dislodge. If you have repeated dislodgments, see your practitioner to reevaluate your fit."

About 200,000 women in the United States and Canada have been fitted with the cervical cap, and more than 2,000 medical practitioners who prescribe them are scattered across North America. Chalker notes that several new cap models are being studied and should be on the market before the end of the century. To find the nearest practitioner, call Cervical Caps, Ltd., at (408) 395-2100.

The Diaphragm

The diaphragm is considered a barrier method of birth control, but the spermicidal cream or jelly used with it is actually what kills the sperm and prevents them from entering the cervix. A diaphragm is a shallow cup made of soft latex rubber with a flexible rim that fits neatly into the palm of your hand. Once very popular, the diaphragm was overtaken in the early 1960 by the heavy promotion and the flood of research dollars behind the pill. The diaphragm is made in a variety of sizes, ranging from about two to four inches (50 to 100 mm) so that it may be fitted in accordance with the length of the vagina. When it is in place, one part of the rim is lodged behind the pubic bone, while the opposite part cups underneath the cervix in the back of the vagina.

A diaphragm with spermicide can be inserted up to six hours before vagina-penis contact. Between a teaspoonful and a tablespoonful of the spermicide is put into the shallow cup and then spread around, leaving a thin ribbon around the rim. Then, squatting, sitting on the toilet, standing with one foot raised, or lying down with your knees bent, you spread the lips of your vagina and insert the diaphragm into the upper vagina with the spermicide facing up. Then push the lower rim until the diaphragm locks into place. You should be able to feel the outline of your cervix with your finger through the rubber cup of the diaphragm.

The diaphragm should stay in place for at least six hours after intercourse to ensure that most of the sperm are killed. The maximum amount of time the diaphragm should be left in is 24 hours. If you have repeated intercourse while the diaphragm is in place, it is necessary to insert more spermicidal jelly or cream into your vagina with an applicator each time, leaving the diaphragm in place.

The standard for fitting the diaphragm is to use the largest size that is comfortable, but what is comfortable in the doctor's office or clinic may not be so comfortable after a few hours. If you are experiencing discomfort from a diaphragm, don't just put it in your drawer. Go back to your practitioner and ask for a smaller size. Then try using the smaller one, checking its placement both before and after intercourse for a month or so. If the diaphragm will not remain in place, you should consider another method.

The New Our Bodies, Ourselves recommends that when your doctor, nurse practitioner, or other women's health care provider fits you for a diaphragm, you want to make sure that you are correctly putting it in and taking it out by practicing before leaving the practitioner's office so that she or he can tell if you are doing it right. Alternatively, you can practice at home and then return to the practitioner's office with the diaphragm in place.

The diaphragm has few health risks. There is effectively no risk of it going farther inside than its correct position; if it pushes back against the rectum, it may be the wrong size. However, in addition to killing sperm, spermicide may kill off the lactobacilli in the vagina that keep yeast under control. To help counteract this, between diaphragm uses you can bathe the vagina with a solution of water and *Lactobacillus acidophilus* (available at most health food stores) by using a douche nozzle, a squirt bottle, or a plastic speculum. If a particular spermicide causes irritation either to your vagina or to your lover's penis, switching to a different brand may help.

About 20 percent of diaphragm users have occasional or recurrent bladder infections. This may occur because the rim bruises the urethra and makes it more susceptible to infection or because the spermicide alters the normal environment of the vagina and allows harmful bacteria to grow. If you are using the diaphragm and begin having recurrent bladder infections, you should look for a different method. If you have a prolapsed or otherwise displaced uterus, vaginal fistulas, or a protrusion of the bladder through the vaginal wall, the diaphragm is not an option for you.

As with other barrier methods, the diaphragm is effective only if you use it consistently and correctly. Studies have shown that the diaphragm is between 89 and 98 percent effective for women who use it during every session of intercourse (except during the menstrual period). However, the effectiveness of the diaphragm can be increased to nearly 100 percent by combining it with condoms or fertility awareness.

Your partner should not be able to feel the diaphragm, but if he does, it is usually only an awareness that something is there. Of course, using the diaphragm in no way compromises your fertility, and all you have to do if you choose to become pregnant is stop using it.

Vaginal Contraceptive Film

Another well-kept contraceptive secret is vaginal contraceptive film. This square inch of material that looks like plastic but turns into a viscous liquid after 5 to 15 minutes in the vagina is 28 percent nonoxynol-9, the sperm-killing ingredient in commercial spermicides. The film was designed to be used alone and seems to be about 85 to 90 percent effective when used that way, but most practitioners recommend that it be used with a cervical cap, diaphragm, or condom. Combining VCF with these barriers should increase their effectiveness to nearly 100 percent. Some people find the higher dose of nonoxynol-9—about three times as strong as regular spermicide—irritating. If this happens to you, you will probably have to stop using it. The other disadvantage of VCF is that it is somewhat expensive and not widely available in the United States. However, it is less messy than normal spermicidal cream or jelly and provides a stronger dose of spermicide. To find out where VCF is sold in your area, call Apothecus at (516) 624–8200.

The Pill

Birth control pills contain either a combination of synthetic estrogen and progesterone or progesterone only. In the first part of the menstrual cycle, higher-than-normal estrogen levels prevent the release of follicle-stimulating hormone (FSH). The absence of this hormone, which is manufactured in the pituitary gland, prevents an egg from developing inside the ovary. In the second part of the cycle, higher levels of progesterone thicken cervical mucus and inhibit the cyclic buildup of the uterine lining. If an egg were to be released or sperm were to get through the cervical mucus, the uterine lining would be too thin to support an implanted fertilized egg. The combination pills interfere with ovulation, thicken cervical mucus, and interfere with the buildup of the uterine lining. Progesterone-only pills, which are called minipills, only thicken cervical mucus and interfere with the buildup of the uterine lining.

In theory the pill is an elegant solution to the age-old problem of preventing unwanted pregnancies, and it has some positive aspects. Many women like the pill because its use can be completely separated from sex and there is no mechanical barrier to be aware of during sexual activity. Because the pill suppresses the menstrual cycle, its users often experience less painful menstrual cramps, fewer prementrual syndrome (PMS) symptoms, and a lowered risk of anemia. Women with endometriosis may experience a decrease in pain and other symptoms, and those who have a tendency to develop ovarian cysts are less likely to do so. Studies also show a lower incidence of pelvic inflammatory disease caused by gonorrhea as well as cancer of the uterine lining (endometrial cancer) and ovarian cancer (see Chapters 7 and 13).

However, the pill, even in its current low-dose formulation, has some significant drawbacks. Higher-than-normal levels of hormones not only have the desired effect of preventing pregnancy but also travel through the bloodstream and affect other organs that have nothing to do with contraception, often precipitating or exacerbating serious underlying conditions. In addition, synthetic hormones can affect mood or exacerbate a tendency toward depression. They may decrease the desire for sex or cause hair loss or fatigue, a bloated feeling, and weight gain over time. Some women don't experience any of these symptoms and enjoy the freedom from contraceptive jellies and devices, but others say that they simply don't feel like themselves.

The biggest problem that women have today with the pill is fear that it may promote the growth of cancer. Medical studies on this issue are conflicting, but too many studies show an increased cancer risk to dismiss this issue. Some doctors are begrudgingly acknowledging an increased risk among pill users in certain subgroups of women, especially women who have a mother or sister who developed cancer.

About 10 million women in the United States use the pill at any one time, but from 30 to 50 percent stop using it within a year because of undesirable side effects.

In the 1960s and 1970s high-dose pills caused serious problems for many women and are known to have caused a small number of deaths as well, but high doses equaled high effectiveness. The pill got a reputation for being 98 percent effective. Today most women take the progesterone-only minipill, which is only about 96 percent effective in normal use. This is still quite acceptable in terms of effectiveness, but it's not really much better than condoms, the cervical cap, or the diaphragm when those barrier methods are used consistently. Failures with minipills occur when women forget to take them or decide not to take them because they cease to be sexually active for a time. You can't just take one pill and be protected; it takes several weeks for the hormones to build up in your system.

Other failures occur because of normal fluctuations in women's hormone levels. You must take the minipill at the same time each day to get maximum protection. If you miss a day or two, double up on pills for at least two days. If you miss more than two days, you need to use another method, such as condoms or VCF.

There are numerous caveats you need to be aware of if you take birth control pills. You absolutely should not take the pill if you have heart disease, severe varicose veins, serious circulatory problems, liver disease, or breast cancer. You should seriously consider using another method if you have diabetes, hypertension, gallbladder disease, depression, epilepsy, migraines, irregular periods, or sickle cell anemia—the trait or the disease. A woman with these conditions may take the minipill safely but should do so only after a consultation with her doctor. You should stop taking the pill if you are planning surgery or must have your leg in a cast. The pill may interfere with the absorption of certain vitamins—including vitamins B_1, B_2, B_6, B_{12}, C, and E and folic acid—and may alter carbohydrate metabolism. If you smoke, the pill becomes far more risky for you.

Contraceptive Technology, a leading family planning handbook, has devised an easily remembered acronym, ACHES, to help make you aware of the danger signs of the pill:

A: abdominal pain (severe)

C: chest pain (severe), cough, shortness of breath

H: headache (severe), dizziness, weakness, numbness

E: eye problems (vision loss or blurring), speech problems

S: severe leg pain (calf or thigh)

If you experience any of these signs, call your doctor immediately.

In an article in *Alternative Medicine* magazine, Dr. Jeese Hanley reminds women that being in touch with the natural monthly cycle of hormones supports their intuition and creativity, yet women's lives today make it difficult for them to fully live out their female biological cycle. Taking birth control pills regulates their cycle to the point where they hardly notice that they're having a period. As Hanley puts it, "Many women become almost addicted to not being a woman, to not understanding the natural cycling of hormones and the feelings, increased sensitivity, intuition, and creativity this evokes." She sees this as a self-destructive tendency that will create health problems in the future. "Chinese medicine describes the uterus as the place where a woman's energy and essence reside, so we need to rethink our approach to uterine health," Hanley concludes.

Norplant

Norplant is a contraceptive that comes in the form of six silicone capsules about the size of matches that are implanted under the skin of the upper arm. The capsule releases a form of the hormone progestin (synthetic progesterone) that blocks ovulation and remains effective for as long as five years.

Dr. Hanley has noticed that the synthetic progesterone in Norplant interferes with women's hormonal balance and makes them upset and miserable: "Some patients tell me that using this form of contraception makes them feel as if a black cloud has settled over them." She adds that Norplant, like other synthetic progesterones, can cause irregular bleeding, weight gain, water retention, and depression. It disrupts thyroid function and has been linked to a greater risk of blood clots and cardiovascular disease.

In fact, about 200 lawsuits involving over 50,000 women have been filed against the manufacturer of Norplant, Wyeth-Ayerst Laboratories.

Sterilization

Many people are surprised to learn that surgical sterilization—tying, clipping, or cutting the fallopian tubes in women or cutting the vas deferens in men—is the most widely used form of contraception both in the United States and in the rest of the world. About 15 million women and men use this method.

Although it involves surgically altering parts of the body through snips and sutures, sterilization is the ultimate in "hands-off" birth control. Once the snips have healed, you never have to think about birth control again—unless, that is, you want to have a baby. Reversal rates for surgical sterilization are around 25 percent, depending on the type of procedure. This is a relatively low rate of success, and studies have found that regret is not uncommon among women and men who have had this procedure. Moreover, the surgery, which is not normally covered by insurance, may cost $15,000 or more. Once again, no available form of birth control is without its drawbacks.

In women the surgery is most often done through a small incision below the navel. The abdominal cavity is inflated with carbon or nitrous oxide, and a laparoscope is inserted through the incision to allow the surgeon to see and manipulate the egg tubes with various instruments. This surgery is usually done on an outpatient basis, and a light general anesthesia or spinal block is commonly used. Most women have some abdominal discomfort for one to three days and feel fully recovered within a week.

Chapter 6

Breast Cancer

Anyone who gets his or her ideas from the media will associate bra burning with the "wild-eyed" radical feminists of the 1960s. They seemed to be getting rid of their bras as a symbolic protest against women's being reined in by men. A deeper look back into the period, such as that provided by Alice Echols's brilliant *Daring to Be Bad: Radical Feminism in America,* will show that the idea of bra burning was both more thoughtful and part of a more provocative action than the stereotypical media presentations would indicate.

Although no bras were actually burned there, a protest against bras, high heels, girdles, and other "instruments of female torture" took place in Atlantic City in 1968 as part of a larger demonstration centered on the Miss America pageant. This show was castigated as nothing less than a cattle auction where women were paraded like meat on the hoof for the male gaze. In fact, it's often forgotten that the pageant stopped broadcasting temporarily when protests erupted in the audience and the protesters were ejected. That event was hidden from the television viewers, who were told that the station was experiencing "technical difficulties."

The critique these women offered was not a generalized protest but a targeted statement that the more women were paraded as objects of beauty, the less they were respected as individuals. The bras, they realized, were meant to enhance their image for men and thus to stress that they were to be looked at but not taken seriously. Ultimately, women's emphasis on appearance, which men promoted with their pageants, became a male rationale for discrimination in, for example, job promotions. Men claimed that women were so concerned with appearance that they had to wear bras to reshape their bodies and create an illusion. Such beings would be incapable of taking on weightier roles that involved objectivity and hard decisions, and so those positions in occupational hierarchies were reserved for males.

The feminist critique of this attitude seems as valid now as it ever was, but there was one weapon women didn't have in their arsenal of arguments against bras which is only now becoming available. This is the fact that bras, by constricting the flow of lymph in breast tissues, may play a large role in promoting cancer. Surprising as it may seem, bras distort the body as much as the ancient Chinese practice of foot binding distorted women's feet.

Breast cancer is the most frequently occurring cancer in women. We see 182,000 new cases a year, along with 46,000 fatalities. In 1950, 1 in 20 women was diagnosed with the disease; today, the number has risen to 1 in 8. Yet even the new conventional medical treatment for preventing breast cancer—the drug tamoxifen—is basically flawed.

Causes

Dr. Michael Schachter, a complementary physician from Rockland County, New York, describes some of the key factors in the development of the disease.

ESTROGEN

"Women whose menstrual periods start when they are relatively young have an increased risk for developing breast cancer, as do women who have a late menopause," explains Dr. Schachter. "This suggests that a woman who has a longer exposure to female sex hormones during her lifetime is at greater risk for developing breast cancer and that estrogen, the female sex hormone that stimulates cell growth, may play a role in its formation. Women who have no children and women who have children but do not breast-feed also have an increased risk. This suggests that the other female sex hormone, progesterone, may have a protective effect.

"Other known and accepted risk factors include an increased alcohol intake, a diet high in fat, being overweight, and a family history of breast cancer. This is because fat tissue can make estrogen and alcohol tends to stimulate its production. In summary, most risk factors seem to be associated with increased lifetime exposure to estrogen, decreased lifetime exposure to progesterone, or a combination of the two.

"Estrogen and progesterone tend to balance each other in the body. Excessive estrogen or reduced progesterone may lead to a condition known as estrogen dominance. The symptoms of estrogen dominance include water retention, breast swelling, fibrocystic breasts, premenstrual mood swings and depression, loss of sex drive, heavy or irregular periods, uterine fibroids, craving for sweets, and fat deposition in the hips and thighs.

"Estrogen tends to be transformed into two major metabolites in the body. They can be called the good and the bad estrogen, just as there are the so-called good and bad cholesterol. The bad estrogen, known as 16-alphahydroxyestrone, favors the development of breast cancer, whereas 2-hydroxyestrone seems to protect against it. Certain chemicals stimulate the formation of one or the other."

XENOESTROGENS

"Now that we've seen that the role of estrogen is very important," Dr. Schachter continues, "this leads to a discussion of something called xenoestrogens. *Xeno* means 'foreign,' and xenoestrogens are chemical substances that are foreign to the body but behave like estrogens. These substances mimic estrogen's actions. Some xenoestrogens can reduce estrogen's effects. These varieties, which are rapidly degraded in the body, usually occur in plant foods such as soy, cauliflower, and broccoli. They protect against the development of breast cancer. Other xenoestrogens, typically synthetic ones, appear to stimulate cancer growth.

"We are living in the petrochemical era. This period began in the 1940s as a result of technological advances in the procurement of oil and the manufacture of its products. In 1940 1 billion pounds of synthetic chemicals were manufactured; by 1950 the amount had increased to 50 billion pounds; and by the late 1980s 500 billion pounds of synthetic chemicals were being produced annually. Many of these compounds are toxic, mutagenic, and carcinogenic. The majority have not been adequately tested for toxicity, let alone for their environmental and ecological effects.

"Approximately 600 chemicals have been shown to be carcinogenic in well-designed, controlled, and validated animal experiments. And within the scientific community the overwhelming consensus is that chemicals carcinogenic to animals are also carcinogenic to humans. In large-scale epidemiological human studies, approximately 25 chemicals have been proved to be carcinogenic. For each of these 25 chemicals, animal research established carcinogenicity one to three decades earlier, making the animal studies all the more significant.

"Many synthetic chemicals behave as bad xenoestrogens, particularly pesticides, fuels, and plastics. They do so in various ways. Some enhance the production of the so-called bad estrogens that I mentioned earlier, and others bind to estrogen receptors, inducing them to issue unneeded signals to increase cellular growth. Xenoestrogens may enter the body through animal fat, since they tend to accumulate in fatty tissue and tend to concentrate as you go up in the food chain.

"Xenoestrogens tend to be synergistic so that a mixture of tiny amounts of many chemicals may have dire effects. As an example, at Mount Sinai in New

York City, Dr. Mary Wolf found that levels of DDE, a relative of DDT, were higher in 58 women who developed breast cancer than in those who had not. At Laval University, 41 women who had estrogen-responsive breast cancers had higher concentrations of DDE. And in a 1990 study of breast cancer and pesticides in Israel a strong relationship between the two was shown. In the 1970s Israeli women had one of the highest breast cancer mortality rates in the world, but in the 10 years that followed a 1976 ban on several organochlorine-type pesticides the incidence of breast cancer declined 20 percent, while it increased in all other industrial nations, strongly suggesting that the pesticides had a major causal effect on the development of breast cancer. Before the ban in Israel some dairy products there had pesticide residues as high as 500 percent above U.S. levels, and residues in human milk were 800 times that level."

POOR LYMPHATIC DRAINAGE

Another possible cause of breast cancer is poor lymphatic drainage, which may be caused by constrictions such as those caused by wearing a bra. Dr. Sidney Ross Singer, a medical anthropologist who did graduate work at Duke University, specializing in biochemistry, has championed this point in his book *Dressed to Kill: The Link between Bras and Breast Cancer.* He is also the founder of the Institute for the Study of Culturogenic Disease. He outlined what he sees as the solidly forged link between wearing a bra and the risk of breast cancer.

THE LYMPHATIC SYSTEM

I asked him to explain how the lymphatic system helps the body rid itself of debris. Although it's an essential body system, it has been little valued in traditional medicine. Historically, in fact, the role of oncologists and surgeons was to do damage to this system. If they found cancer in the lymph nodes, they believed it was necessary to get rid of them. Let's not forget that once they are lost, you do not grow new ones.

Singer explains: "The lymphatic system is so underemphasized by modern medicine. When I was in medical school, there was not even 10 minutes discussion of it. Yet it is a critical part of the body."

It's the circulatory part of the immune system. It consists of tiny vessels, like capillaries, microscopic in size and originating in all the tissues of the body. They drain the tissue of fluid, toxins, debris, cancer cells, bacteria, and so forth. The blood flowing through the blood vessels delivers oxygen and nutrition through capillaries under pressure. The fluid in the blood oozes out to bathe the tissues. This fluid is called lymph fluid. When you have a blister, the clear fluid that you see under the skin is the lymph fluid. It is the medium of exchange through which nutrients are delivered to the cells.

As the cells take in oxygen and food and give off their waste, some of the cell debris is flushed out through this other channel, the lymphatic system. Its tiny vessels have one-way valves to keep the fluid moving. They eventually take the debris to tiny organs called lymph nodes. The tonsils are examples of lymph nodes. For the breast, most of the lymph nodes are located in the armpits. These nodes are tiny factories for white blood cell production in response to infection. They filter out the lymph fluid, which then goes back to the bloodstream and through the heart.

HOW BRAS THREATEN THE LYMPHATIC SYSTEM

This pattern of flow is how the body works normally, Singer says. However, "when you wear a constrictive garment, the pressure of the garment, like the elastic of a bra, presses on these tiny vessels, shutting them off and preventing them from draining. They have no internal pressure; they are passive drains. They are not like the blood capillaries, which are under pressure from the heart. As soon as they are constricted because the bra lifts the breasts and gives them a different shape—which requires pressure—there is a backup of fluid in the breast, which is a condition called lymphedema, or edema for short." This pressure and backup can cause pain and tenderness in the breasts.

Before a woman has her period, her estrogen level is very high, and this causes generalized body fluid retention. This is what premenstrual syndrome is all about, a generalized, all-over-the-body edema. That goes away after the hormones drop and the woman starts having her period. But during that time of elevated fluids she has typically been wearing the same size bra she wore all month, yet her breasts have been a little bigger. As a result of the constriction from the bra, which has become like a tourniquet, the breast cannot drain the fluid, and it backs up, causing congestion in the breast tissue.

The end result, Singer explains, is that "the cells are sitting in their own waste and debris. The pressure builds, there's tenderness, and cysts form. That's why women get cysts in their breasts. These cysts, which are filled with lymph fluid, eventually become hard. This condition is called fibrocystic breast disease. Eighty percent of American women have it, and it's because of the bra."

If a woman gets rid of the bra, the constriction is gone, the cells can flush out the wastes, and the cysts go away. Singer has found that they are gone "within a matter of weeks, sometimes days. It may take a month to really to see the difference. For so many women, when their periods come, they have lost that tenderness. They don't even know when their period is coming. They used to say, 'Oh, my breasts are tender; my period must be near.' Now they cannot say that. That's gone. They stop wearing the bra, and the tenderness is eliminated."

HOW DOES THIS EVENTUALLY LEAD TO CANCER?

Why might this cause cancer? If you cannot flush toxins from the breast, which is what the lymph does, problems will arise. By toxins, Singer means those we find in our polluted world today, including carcinogenic herbicides and pesticides in food and water as well as plastic residues. All the foods we eat are wrapped in plastic. People should realize that the U.S. Food and Drug Administration (FDA) considers these residues an unintentional food additive.

"Once I bought a bottle of pure water," Singer recalls, "a plastic bottle. I drank it and left it on my shelf for about a month. I happened to open it and sniffed inside, and it reeked of plastic. So the plastic must have been leaching into this water. I called the FDA, and they said, 'Yes, we realize that plastic is getting in the food and water. We know these containers leak plastic, but we feel this is all within acceptable limits, so we don't mind.'"

We are eating these plastics that are known to cause cancer. Some medications also can cause cancer. We are filling our bodies with them. So, if they get stuck in the breasts due to constriction, the breasts become toxic. The toxic level builds up. There are also toxins that arise from the body itself, which, because of the constrictions, cannot be flushed out.

The cells all need oxygen to carry on their metabolism. If oxygen is low because of constriction, if you have edema, the cells aren't getting well oxygenated because they're sitting in fluid and cannot drain. Carbon dioxide and other waste products build up. Because the tissue is low in oxygen, the immune system begins to break down. Free radicals begin to develop, which can cause cancer.

Singer says, "Even without external toxins, I've been told by a toxicologist that the internal toxins the body creates could cause cancer. I think the reason we have such an epidemic is because we have such a toxic world these days."

By combining toxins with constriction, you have a formula for breast cancer and breast disease. This is a major link.

EVIDENCE FOR THE BRA-CANCER LINK

Singer went on: "We did a study on this, which is described in *Dressed to Kill*. We interviewed about 5,000 women in the United States in five major cities from New York to San Francisco. We felt if we were right, if there is this link between bras and breast cancer, then women who have breast cancer should exhibit different bra-wearing behavior than women who don't have breast cancer. We did our study and found that indeed that was the case. The incidence of breast cancer rises so dramatically with bra wearing. If you compare a woman who doesn't wear a bra with a woman who wears one 24 hours a day—and believe it or not, many women wear bras day and night, even when they are sleeping—there is a 125 times greater risk for the 24-hour wearers.

"Remember, they discovered that if you already have a history of breast cancer in your family, it increases your risk of getting the disease three to five times. That was considered major and led to women cutting off their breasts prophylactically to prevent cancer. This insane procedure is justified by doctors saying these women have a five times greater risk. But we found more than a 100 times greater risk. This is a causal link which explains the epidemic."

He challenges readers to compare bra-wearing cultures to those in which women do not wear bras. You'll find that breast cancer is confined largely to cultures where bras are worn. If there are no bras, there is very little breast disease. Men and women have about the same incidence of it. As soon as you bring bras into the picture, breast cancer rates soar.

X-RAYS

John Gofman, M.D., Ph.D., and professor emeritus of molecular and cell biology at the University of California, Berkeley, sounds the alarm on the harmful effects of x-rays in his book *Preventing Breast Cancer*.

The effects of x-rays take years, even decades, to manifest, which is why orthodox medicine does not pay attention to this danger. Indeed, x-rays are standard practice for medical diagnosis and treatment. "The incubation time is what has led organized medicine exactly in the wrong direction," says Dr. Gofman. "In the first half of the twentieth century medicine looked at treatments in this way: If you gave someone poison, the effects would be seen in weeks or months. They did not think in terms of years or decades. What we have learned about x-ray-induced cancer is that a very small proportion occurs in the first few years after the x-rays are administered. But most of them take 10, 20, even 50 years. Women with breast cancer who are 45, 50, or 60 are thinking, Why me? I haven't done anything wrong. What these women are not thinking about is what they were exposed to early in life. In the early 1940s, for example, pediatricians in New York City, Rochester, and the Pacific Northwest were giving children fluoroscopic examinations 12 times a year for the first two years of life as part of their well-baby examinations. Fluoroscopy is far worse than x-rays because the beam is left on for a long time. This laid the foundation for the development of breast cancer and other forms of cancer later in life. If you really want to know the story about breast cancer today, you have to ask yourself, What happened 30, 40, and 50 years ago?"

It is not the radiation itself that persists but chromosomal damage, Dr. Gofman says: "Inside the nucleus of every one of our cells is a string of DNA organized into 46 chromosomes. That's a treasure. Damage to your chromosomes is going to be there for the rest of your life."

Dr. Gofman bases his claims on well-documented research published in the 1960s and 1970s as well as his own work: "Ian Mackenzie, a great Nova Scotia physician, discovered the relationship between breast cancer and medical x-rays when he studied women who had been in tuberculosis sanitoriums and had received a treatment known as pneumothorax. This was a wonderful treatment that injected air into the chest cavity to rest the lung. It saved many lives. Unfortunately, during the course of treatment, these women were given 100, 200, or even more fluoroscopic exams to check whether the air had been placed in the lungs. Twenty to 30 years later, Mackenzie's work showed a 20-fold increase in breast cancer in these women. His results were published in 1965 in the *British Journal of Cancer*.

"Many people doubted his findings, saying that if he was correct, we would have seen breast cancer in Nagasaki and Hiroshima. Turns out nobody looked to see if this was the case. So one of the members of the Radiation Research Foundation looked and found exactly what Mackenzie had found.

"Arthur Tamplin and I raised a flag in *The Lancet* by saying that the Wanabo and Mackenzie studies suggest that breast cancer is one of the easiest cancers to induce by radiation. Today everybody who is anybody in medical science knows that breast cancer is related to ionizing radiation such as medical x-rays.

"A couple of years ago, I tried to answer this question—not whether x-rays cause breast cancer but what part of all breast cancers are being caused by x-rays? My estimate was about 75 percent. Everybody said, 'Oh, that's too high. It must be much lower.' Since that time I've done much more extensive work, and I have changed my numbers from 75 percent to more than 90 percent. Moreover, I now have enough data on a variety of other cancers to say that most cancers, not just breast cancer, are caused by medical x-rays."

Whether Dr. Gofman is 100 percent right or just partly right, whether medical x-rays are a primary cause of breast cancer and other types of cancer or merely an important secondary factor that until now has been ignored by our government and the medical establishment—in either case women need to recognize the seriousness of the problem and insist that radiation exposures be as minimal as possible.

"If you have a serious problem and you are told you need an x-ray, I don't want to stand in the way of your getting that x-ray," says Dr. Gofman. "But I want to be very sure that you are not getting a dose that is 2, 4, 8, or 20 times higher than is needed. I think there is room for at least a three- to fourfold reduction in dose, possibly even a 10-fold reduction. Every community should insist that its radiological facilities produce evidence that its doses are low. Mammography is a lesson in what you can do when you are pushed to the wall to do it. In the 1970s radiologists were giving 2, 5, and 10 rads per mammogram. When they were told that this would cause more cancers than it helped cure, they went to work and got the dose down to 0.3 a rad or less. That is a 20- to 50-fold reduction in the dose. Getting the dose down further should be a major national priority. If we do that, we are going to bring about the single most significant reduction in cancer incidence in this country. That's real prevention."

HIGH-FAT DIET

Earlier, Dr. Schachter gave one explanation of how fat can cause breast cancer. Here Dr. Charles Simone, director of the Protective Cancer Institute in Lawrenceville, New Jersey, gives another reason why fats generate disease: "We know that fatty foods actually convert normal cells into problematic cells.

Consuming high-fat foods, particularly unsaturated fats, increases free radical production, damaging the cell membrane. At this point the damaged cell has two choices. It can die. That's fine, because if it dies, you make another one. Or it can repair itself. In the repair process, a cell can go awry and metamorphose into a cancer cell. So fats cause free radicals, which damage cells, which in turn try to repair themselves and transform themselves into cancer cells."

Robin Keuneke, a natural food counselor with 13 years of experience, the editor of *Total Health* magazine, a lecturer, and the author of *Total Breast Health*, points to another factor: essential fatty acid deficiencies. These fatty acids are found in extra-virgin olive oil, she notes. Many studies have linked Italian diets, which contain lots of extra-virgin olive oil, to lower rates of breast cancer. Italian women do not have a low-fat diet, but neither do they have trans-fats in their diets. Trans-fats are unstable, highly reactive molecules that promote free radical oxidation and therefore can have mutagenic effects. They are found in margarines and other processed oils, shortenings, and confections such as cookies and candy. In Mediterranean cultures oils and fats in the diet come from monounsaturated fatty acids such as those found in olive oil or cold-pressed virgin flaxseed oil and in nuts, seeds, and grains. In these cultures it's common to dip vegetables and bread in a plate of olive oil on the table; you don't see margarine or, as a rule, butter there.

In America, by contrast, 95 percent of the population is deficient in the essential fatty acid alpha-linolenic acid. A study of the relation of trans-fats and breast cancer was done by Dr. Lenore Kohlmeier in 1997. She found that women with breast cancer have higher amounts of trans-fats in their body fats compared with women without the disease.

Other diet choices that seem connected to higher rates of cancer are cooked meat and fried foods. Keuneke notes: "One of the theses of my book is that burned meat and fried foods are linked to breast cancer. I found four studies linking burned meat, such as bacon, to cancer. Yet although the most recent study was published in November 1998, the so-called experts said there was not enough information to recommend changes in cooking. They went on to claim there was only one study out making the connection between fried foods and cancer."

This is not true. The first study was published in 1972. It was a population study looking at Seventh-Day Adventist women, who have a relatively clean diet. It found that women who ate the greatest amount of fried potatoes had the highest rate of breast cancer.

Her conclusion: "I warn you that when you read an Associated Press report that says there is only one study out there, look a little further before you believe it. Unfortunately, so much information we receive is commercially driven." Keuneke wondered what would happen if experts came out and told women that eating fried foods was linked to breast cancer: "Imagine how many fast food restaurants would be closed down."

OTHER FACTORS

Dr. Simone cites two other factors as leading contributors: "We know that tobacco is the number two cause of cancer in our country and the number two cause of breast cancer as well. Regarding alcohol, we know that two to three drinks per week is enough to confer a two- to threefold risk of getting cancer of the breast independently of everything else. So the number one, two, and three causes of breast cancer—a high-fat diet, smoking, and alcohol consumption—are totally within our control."

Symptoms

The initial symptoms of breast cancer include thickening, a lump in the breast, and dimpled skin. Later on there may be nipple discharge, pain, ulcers, and swollen lymph glands under the arms.

Once breast cancer is diagnosed, the prognosis depends on the course of the disease. Dr. Schachter explains: "The staging of breast cancer involves the size of the cancer in the breast, whether it has spread or metastasized to regional lymph nodes, and whether it has metastasized to distant organs. The more lymph nodes involved and the greater the size of the tumor, the worse the prognosis. Stage zero is limited to the topmost layer, and the five-year survival rate is about 90 percent. In stage 4, in which cancer has metastasized to lymph nodes above the collarbone or has distant metastases to organs such as the liver, lungs, and brain, the five-year survival rate drops to 10 percent."

Clinical Experience

Before we outline the steps you can take to prevent breast cancer, let's look at one step that is highly touted by conventional medicine, but which I would not recommend. This is the use of tamoxifen. We saw earlier that excessive estrogen production is held responsible by some for breast cancer. This is the rationale for prescribing tamoxifen. However, asserts Sherrill Sellman, psychotherapist and author of the best-selling book *Hormone Heresy*, this treatment is far from the panacea it is claimed to be.

WHAT IS TAMOXIFEN?

Tamoxifen, Sellman explains, "is the leading drug being given to women with breast cancer. Millions of women are on it."

Tamoxifen is in a class of drugs collectively known as SERMs, serum estrogen receptor modulators. Although the way these drugs work is not totally understood, it is believed that SERMs block the action of estrogen on the breast tissue, which in turn inhibits the growth of tumors.

So how does tamoxifen prevent breast cancer? Sellman says, "The theory is that it works like a weaker estrogen." Estrogen is a major factor in the growth of breast tumors. Many but not all breast cancers require estrogen to grow. These types of tumors have a site on the cell called an estrogen receptor. Tamoxifen competes with estrogen to reach these receptors, where it creates a barrier that prevents estrogen from binding to the cell.

In theory, then, tamoxifen acts like a phytoestrogen, although it has contradictory effects. In the breast it seems to reduce the effects of estrogen on tumor growth, yet in other parts of the body it acts like one of these estrogens, stimulating growth, for example in the uterus, where it can cause endometrial cancer. "It's unpredictable," Sellman stresses, "in the sense that we don't really know what are going to be the consequences in a woman's body."

THE HISTORY OF TAMOXIFEN

Tamoxifen has been used for over 20 years as a treatment to prevent a recurrence of breast cancer. It has been only moderately successful in preventing new tumors, but even this moderate success has come at a cost. While tamoxifen may benefit some women with breast cancer, it is also a highly toxic drug with serious side effects.

In the early 1980s American researchers began to speculate about whether tamoxifen might actually prevent breast cancer in women who had never had the disease. So in 1992 the National Cancer Institute initiated a $60 million clinical trial to test tamoxifen as a cancer preventative. Thirteen thousand healthy women who were at higher than average risk for breast cancer were enrolled in the trial. Half the women took tamoxifen (20 mg a day); the other half received a placebo.

From the beginning, the Breast Cancer Prevention Trial was controversial. Critics of the trial were outraged that healthy women would be exposed to the health risks associated with tamoxifen.

Results of the trial were made public in April 1998. At first glance, the trial results seem impressive. Women in the trial who took tamoxifen had a 44 percent reduction in breast cancers compared with the placebo group. But these results are misleading; tamoxifen also caused uterine cancer, blood clots, and cataracts. In fact, women who got tamoxifen had almost 3 times the rate of endometrial cancers and blood clots. Two prominent health groups, the National Women's Health Network and Public Citizen, have calculated that for every 1,000 women who take tamoxifen, there will be 2.9 fewer cases of breast cancer, but 2.8 more cases of extremely serious health problems. Even more important, results of the trial show there is no difference in overall survival rates or in the number of women who died of breast cancer.

In addition to cancers, blood clots, and cataracts, tamoxifen also caused strokes, hot flashes, vaginal discharge, mood changes, menstrual irregularites, and skin rashes.

In October 1998, the FDA approved the use of tamoxifen to reduce the risk of breast cancer in healthy women. But even members of the FDA's own advisory committee voiced concerns about giving tamoxifen to healthy women. One committee member noted that every woman who took tamoxifen was exposed to the health risks, but only a few women would benefit from the drug. Dr. Samuel Epstein, one of the world's leading cancer experts, has said that prescribing tamoxifen to healthy women as a cancer preventative is "disease substitution, not disease prevention." In fact, the FDA was unwilling to approve tamoxifen for prevention, and reworded the recommendation to approve it only for "risk reduction."

Critics of the FDA say that approval of tamoxifen as an anticancer drug is premature. Two European studies found tamoxifen provided no benefit as a preventive measure. Still other criticism focuses on the statistical model (known as the Gail model) used to assess breast cancer risk for women considering taking tamoxifen as a cancer preventative. Opponents say this model greatly overstates risk, putting large numbers of women into a high-risk category and therefore eligible to take the drug. Finally, the short-term nature of the NCI study—only 25 percent of women enrolled in the trial were followed for more than four years—means that possible long-term effects of tamoxifen could not be determined. In addition, because breast cancers can take 10 to 15 years to develop, the short follow-up of women in the clinical trial means that nobody really knows if tamoxifen prevented breast cancers or merely delayed them.

Remember, above all, that tamoxifen is a carcinogen. "What really seems insane about this," in Sellman's opinion, "is that they are giving women who are dealing with breast cancer a known carcinogenic substance as treatment. This never made sense."

Sellman makes a further point about the drug's manufacturer. The company that manufactures tamoxifen, sold under the brand name Novaldex, is Zeneca Pharmacuticals, whose parent company, ICI, makes many herbicides and chlorine-based chemicals, which are known cancer-causing agents. She notes, "On the one hand, this company is causing breast cancer by making these products and, on the other hand, it is making breast cancer treatments using chemicals that supposedly prevent breast cancer from occurring."

TAMOXIFEN'S ADVERSE EFFECTS

The health risks associated with tamoxifen are the same for women who have breast cancer as for those who take it as a treatment to prevent a recurrence. Sellman says, "One woman who was diagnosed with breast cancer was given tamoxifen and started to lose sight in one of her eyes. She was going blind. When she started to lose sight in her second eye, she got really terrified and stopped taking tamoxifen. After that her sight returned."

Tamoxifen may also cause liver damage and liver cancer. Animal studies found a link between tamoxifen and liver cancer in rats, but the results of human studies have been less conclusive.

But Sellman believes that many doctors simply don't make the connection. "This is often overlooked, because it is thought that when women are diagnosed with breast cancer, when they find liver cancer also, it is a secondary cancer assumed to be caused by the same source. What is not understood is that liver cancer is often directly caused by the tamoxifen treatment. In fact, one researcher called tamoxifen 'a rip-roaring liver carcinogen.'"

A Swedish study looked at 1,327 breast cancer patients who took 40 mg of tamoxifen each day for two to five years. Comparing this group to one of the same size that didn't take the drug, it was found the tamoxifen users upped their chances for getting uterine cancer sixfold.

Sellman notes the further irony that, while in general it is recognized that cancer is partly caused by people's exposure to the vast sea of pollution we now live in, the only solution proposed is to try another chemical. She quotes Dr. Susan Love: "It is a sad state of affairs when we have to add yet more chemicals to counteract the effects of other chemicals."

WHY DO WOMEN STILL TAKE TAMOXIFEN?

Strangely enough, many women's groups are supporting and advocating this treatment. Most of the time, however, these are groups that take money from the pharmaceutical industry. But other women's groups have been the primary activists opposing tamoxifen, the lead group being the National Women's Health Network. And there have been so many false reports and so much misinformation that unless you really investigate the issue thoroughly, you will very seldom get access to truthful data. As Sellman says, "It's very easy to play with results, stats, and studies to make it look like something wonderful is occurring when in fact it is a scam. This drug has the potential to be such a big money spinner. It is already the number one drug given to women with breast cancer. The industry will stop at nothing to get its drug out there. Health is not their primary concern."

Prevention

While the possibility of a positive diagnosis for breast cancer is terrifying, it is empowering to know that there are steps that can be taken to prevent the condition, that minimally invasive treatments are often beneficial, and that it is possible to avoid a recurrence.

Dr. Tori Hudson, a naturopathic physician in Portland, Oregon, says, "I believe that breast cancer is a preventable disease. Just look around the world. Women in our culture have one of the highest—if not the highest—incidences of breast cancer, while women in Asia have the lowest.

"The reason is diet. To make a big story simple to understand, cultures that have a vegetarian diet or are closest to a vegetarian diet have the least breast cancer. That's how it all pans out no matter how you look at it. This implies that cultures that eat less fat, especially less animal fat, have the least breast cancer.

So the big picture is really clear. Eat a lot of vegetables, fruits, and whole grains and beans. Those foods provide protection."

Letha Hadady, an herbalist and educator in New York City, visited China to learn why Chinese women haved such a low incidence of breast cancer compared with American women and those in other western nations. While diet was a big part of the picture, she learned that other factors came into play as well. To prevent breast cancer, Asians build immunity through diet, cleansing herbs, and the avoidance of pollution, stress, negative emotions, smoking, alcohol, and radiation: "They have much cleaner habits than we do." In addition, Hadady made this important discovery: "I found it quite interesting that breast cancer is considered a disease of melancholy in China. That feeling of heaviness in the chest leads to poor circulation and excess phlegm. This leads to two conclusions: Increase circulation and you have a better chance of prevention, and reduce phlegm. The easiest way to reduce phlegm is to stay away from foods such as cheese, chocolate, fried foods, and milk. You will not find dairy in the diet in China. Their diet tends to consist of grains and greens."

Of course the easiest of all preventive strategies is to follow the protesters mentioned at the beginning of the chapter and simply chuck your bra. Going braless is certainly wise, and not just in terms of breast cancer. If you think about how men and women look at women's breasts in our society, you will see that we have made them more significant than they should be as an isolated object. We should be looking at the whole person.

If a woman's breasts begin to sag or if one of them is not quite the same size as the other, often she'll say to herself, "My God, I'm not perfect," or think, I'm not as interesting to my mate. Women go through absolutely destructive surgical procedures such as inserting implants. They don't consider that if they didn't have the bra, they could have stronger upper chest muscle activity, which would actually keep the breast firm for much longer.

Look at women who are braless in Africa. In their sixties and seventies they have still have firm breasts, while here a woman's breasts sag in her late twenties or early thirties.

We need to reconceptualize the muscular system so that we see having a stronger chest as part of having a healthy overall musculoskeletal condition. Instead of having stooped shoulders and a craned neck with arthritis, we should be doing exercises to strengthen the shoulders, deltoids, pectorals, and all those muscles in the upper chest—the ones that don't get exercised—so that they can support the breasts without a bra. Wearing a bra is a foolish and stupid social idea, about as useful as wearing a necktie. It's a dumb thing to do.

In his book *Breast Health: A Ten Point Prevention Program* Dr. Simone outlines the following plan for optimal breast health:

Optimize nutrition.
Take antioxidant supplements.
Avoid tobacco.

Avoid alcohol.

Avoid estrogens.

Exercise.

Minimize stress.

Become spiritually involved.

Increase your awareness of sexuality.

Get a good regular physical examination starting at age 35.

Reexamining Conventional Assumptions

When a diagnosis of breast cancer is made, minimally invasive therapy may be just as effective as more intrusive standard medical approaches, according to Dr. Robert Atkins, a well-known advocate of holistic medicine: "Women develop a lump in their breast and appropriately have a mammogram or biopsy which leads to the diagnosis. At this point the trouble begins. The doctor gives the patient two choices: a mastectomy or a lumpectomy with radiation. A paper just published on this reported a third option that was every bit as good regarding survival rate and life expectancy. That was simply to do a lumpectomy without the radiation."

Dr. Atkins goes on to say that women don't realize that after the diagnosis and treatment there is much they can do to regain total health: "The biggest fallacy of all is when doctors tell patients after therapy that they've done all they can do and there is nothing left to do. This ignores the whole concept that people can get healthier by enhancing all their internal systems to make sure that the neoplasia, the process of forming cancer, no longer takes place. In other words, cancer is not the tumor itself; cancer is a process.

"Once you know that, you can ask, 'What can nutrition do?' You will learn that it can help in multiple ways. First and foremost, free radicals trigger the formation of cancer and the recurrence of cancer. Nutritional antioxidants can help slow down the formation of free radicals. Additionally, plant foods have antioxidant and immune-enhancing properties."

YOUR DIET AND OTHER NUTRITION-BASED APPROACHES

ANTIOXIDANTS

To prevent and reverse free radical damage to breast tissue, Dr. Steven Rachlin, an internist in Syosset, Long Island, New York, has his cancer patients follow this daily protocol:

Emulsified vitamin A (up to 50,000 IU)

Beta carotene (up to 100 mg)

Vitamin B_1 (400 mg)

Vitamin B_6 (500 mg)

Folic acid (3,200 mcg)

Vitamin C (up to 5 g)

Coenzyme Q10 (270 mg)
Flaxseed oil (1 tbsp)
Cat's claw (1,800 mg)
Melatonin (up to 10 mg)
Shark cartilage (1 mg/kg of patient's weight)
Pycnogenol (150 mg)
Essiac tea (several ounces)
Pancreatic digestive enzymes (up to 40 g)
Aloe vera juice (9–12 oz)

MINERALS

Dr. Schachter states that trace minerals play a vital role in the prevention of free radical damage: "The body contains certain antioxidant proteins, such as SOD (superoxide dismutase), which help neutralize oxidatively induced free radicals. SOD requires three minerals—zinc, copper, and manganese—to function properly. Deficiencies of any one of these minerals may predispose to oxidation damage, with a resulting increase of susceptibility to breast cancer.

"Adequate amounts of calcium and magnesium are also important. Considerable evidence exists supporting the role of selenium in preventing and treating cancer. A dose of 200 mcg daily is safe, and large amounts may be given with monitoring. Chromium and molybdenum may be supplemented as well, and these are also important.

"Recently I have begun to use the whole range of trace minerals in colloidal form as a supplement. That's a liquid form where the minerals are bound to organic chemicals. We use about 70 different minerals. Many of these minerals are in trace amounts, have already been shown to be essential, and are probably lacking in our synthetically fertilized soil. I believe these colloidal trace minerals will play an important role in bolstering the immune system."

DIET

As was mentioned earlier, a diet that is largely vegetarian and low in fat, mainly consisting of whole fresh foods such as vegetables, fruits, whole grains, nuts, and seeds, protects against breast cancer.

Hot, spicy foods, oily foods, and stimulants such as coffee, black tea, drugs, and alcohol should be avoided. Water should be pure, free from fluoride, chlorine, pesticides, and other synthetic chemicals. Many urban and suburban water supplies cannot be trusted and need filtering. Since some filters remove chemicals and chlorine but not fluoride, a reverse-osmosis type of water purifier is recommended.

Certain foods are medicinal in their ability to protect against breast cancer. They include soybeans, soy products, and lima beans. Isoflavones and phyto estrogens found in soybeans, soy products, and lima beans protect against cancer. The low incidence of breast cancer among Japanese women is largely attributed to the widespread eating of soybeans. Other cancer-fighting foods include:

FLAX. The omega-3 fatty acids in flaxseeds and flax oil protects against breast cancer.

FISH. Fish high in omega-3 fatty acids include salmon, tuna, sardines, mackerel, and herring.

CRUCIFEROUS VEGETABLES. Vegetables such as broccoli, cauliflower, and Brussels sprouts contain cancer-fighting substances.

MUSHROOMS. Reiki, shiitake, and maitake mushrooms have strong anticancer properties.

ONIONS. Robin Keuneke considers onions vital: "If we look at the Thai diet, we notice that the Thai people eat a great amount of onions. People may say it's a smelly food to eat, but in the Mediterranean countries, where rates of breast cancer are low, they eat raw onions as well. A tip is to slice them thin and sprinkle a little bit of sea salt on them. This takes the bite out. In India they also eat a lot of raw onions, sprinkle salt on them, and add a dash of vinegar. It's a terrific thing to add to a salad."

HERBS

Natural herbal substances are a veritable gold mine for protecting women against breast cancer. Some herbs to know about are listed below:

CARNIVORA (VENUS FLYTRAP). This powerful herb is popular in Europe but less known in the United States. In Germany it is even used to wipe out cancer that already exists.

ESSIAC. Essiac is a Native American herbal combination that has a synergistic effect in putting an end to cancer and aiding in its prevention.

CAT'S CLAW. A cat's claw formula is used by the Peruvian Indians for the prevention and treatment of cancer.

EVENING PRIMROSE, BORAGE, AND BLACK CURRANT SEED OILS. All these herbs supply gamma-linolenic acid, which is known for its strong anticancer activity.

XIAO YAO WAN. This combination of digestive herbs increases circulation, builds blood, and breaks apart fibroids. The Chinese say it prevents breast cancer caused by phlegm and feelings of melancholy, which impede circulation to the chest. *Xiao yao wan* is available in Chinatowns throughout America.

DANDELION. Dandelion helps prevents cancer by breaking up phlegm and eliminating it from the system. Excess phlegm can turn into tumors.

ASTRAGALUS. Astragalus is a wonderful immune-system-strengthening herb that can be used in cancer prevention or as an adjunct to cancer treatments. Letha Hadady says, "It has worked wonders for my friends on chemotherapy who take this between sessions for strength." Add a teaspoon of astragalus powder to some pure water and drink once or twice a day. Or try Astra-8, a combination of astragalus and other immune-system-strengthening remedies in capsule form that is found in health food stores.

ROSEMARY. Rosemary has been highly researched and is recommended even more than soy for its breast-protecting qualities. According to Keuneke, "Use rosemary in a vinegarette or to marinate fish. Try to buy rosemary on a regular basis. Perhaps make a salad dressing with rosemary and garlic, fresh lemon, and extravirgin olive oil. All those ingredients are wonderful foods that are eaten throughout the Mediterranean."

MINT. Include mint in your diet on a regular basis. Mint has a phytochemical in it called limonene, which is effective in fighting breast cancer. In one study, it was found to reduce mammary tumors in animals up to 80 percent. The foods containing limonene are mint, dill, sage, celery seed, caraway, and organic citrus peel. The last item is also found in the Thai diet, which uses a lot of lime peels.

TURMERIC. Turmeric also contains a vital phytochemical that has been found to prevent mammary tumors in animals.

ENZYMES

Keuneke says, "I had the pleasure of interviewing Dr. Keith Singletary from the Functional Foods for Health program at the University of Illinois. He's done a lot of research with herbs and spices. I brought up a thesis I'm exploring about breast cancer rates in Asia. Women from Thailand have the lowest rate of breast cancer in Asia. We've always heard about low rates of breast cancer in China, but why, I wondered, do the women in Thailand have this extremely low incidence?

"Dr. Singletary thought we should note that so many herbs are consumed raw there, as well as other foods, such as fruits. Thai women eat more raw foods, herbs, and spices than any other women in Asia. Thus they ingest a lot of enzymes."

Enzymes are organic substances that help create reactions in the body, such as breaking down fats. They are linked to breathing and all the bodily functions we need to live and stay well. There are 3,000 enzymes in the body. A healthy person can produce enough enzymes to fight off cancer cells, but things such as free radicals from smoke, pollutants, junk foods, and medications interfere with enzyme production.

"So, as you can imagine," Keuneke says, "there are many people who are low on enzymes. To combat this people can increase the amount of raw foods in their diet and increase fresh juice—juice all kinds of fruits and vegetables."

Numerous studies, she recounts, link enzymes and breast health. Over 90 were conducted by universities throughout the world regarding the beneficial effects of enzymes. Much of this work has been done in Germany.

ESSENTIAL FATTY ACIDS

In Keuneke's opinion, "We need to use linoleic acid. It has a bad rap because some feel it is linked to cancer. However, we have to distinguish between different sources of this oil. It's available in safflower oil, corn oil, and processed oils, but these are not the healthiest sources. Healthy, nonprocessed forms have been consumed for hundreds of years by people in areas with low incidences of cancer."

We can't generalize here, she cautions. "Sesame seeds, for example, contain linoleic acid. People in the Far East and Middle East eat sesame seeds, and that's where they have lower rates of cancer." They also eat almonds, which contain anticancer phytochemicals and are a rich source of calcium. Sunflower seeds contain linoleic acid and are also an abundant source of zinc. Organic, unrefined sunflower and sesame seed oils in small amounts are fine to use in vinaigrettes and are healthy sources of omega-6 fatty acids.

PROTECTING OUR DAUGHTERS THROUGH NUTRITION

"We can really help protect our daughters from getting breast cancer as adults—and also protect our sons from prostate cancer—by taking positive steps at an early age, when the young cells in their bodies are being formed," notes Keuneke. "We can get rid of the processed food consumption and set a healthy example.

"Many people I know are interested in nutrition and practice what they preach. Their children love fruits and vegetables because they see that their parents enjoy eating them, and these parents know how to prepare them in a way that makes them taste delicious. It is sometimes hard because kids do tend to eat junk food in high school. But parents should do the best they can and try to set an example."

The studies are there, by the way. For example, increased yogurt consumption in young people has been linked to decreased breast cancer in adults. So be sure to have a nice yogurt with acidophilus available. That is a protective food. Other studies show that consuming soy at a young age is linked to breast health in adulthood. Exercise, making sure there are enough nutrients in the diet, and getting a really great vitamin for children are important.

OTHER DETOXIFICATION THERAPIES

EXERCISE

Dr. Schachter notes, "Any activity that removes accumulated toxins in the breast reduces the chance of women developing breast cancer. Studies show that aerobic exercise is associated with decreased cancer risk, as exercise promotes lymphatic drainage and sweating helps remove toxins from the tissues.

"Although I am not aware of any direct studies showing reduction of breast cancer with a detoxification program using saunas and certain nutrients as is done with the Hubbard method of detoxification," says Dr. Schachter, "I do know that this procedure has been clearly shown to reduce pesticides and other toxic chemicals in the bloodstream and in fat tissues. Since high levels of these substances increase the risk of breast cancer in women, reducing them with this detoxification method should help reduce the risk of breast cancer to women."

MASSAGE

Lymphatic detoxification is aided by manual lymphatic drainage (MLD), a simple method of massage that uses light, slow rhythmic movements to stimulate the flow of lymph in the body. Massage therapist James Kresse notes that this is especially important for women suffering from lymphedema, a condition that often occurs after a mastectomy: "When our lymph nodes are not functioning properly or have been irradiated or removed, an excessive accumulation of stagnant waste occurs. The lymph system becomes overloaded, thus forming lymphedema.

"MLD should be applied directly after surgery rather than when a massive edema has formed. This will guard against any possibility of a blockage in the system or alleviate any that exists. Studies in Europe show that severed lymph vessels regenerate with constant MLD therapy. The therapy makes the scars from the mastectomy more subtle, which increases the mobility of the arm. It also lessens pain from surgery and the uncomfortable sensitivity that occurs." (For more on MLD see the subsection "Lymphedema," below.)

IMMUNOAUGMENTIVE THERAPY

In the 1950s Dr. Burton and a team of researchers discovered immunoaugmentive therapy (IAT), a nontoxic, noninvasive method of controlling cancer by restoring the patient's own immune system. Although the therapy was successful, Burton left the United States after medical politics prohibited him from practicing here. In 1977 he opened the Immunology Research Center in Freeport in the Grand Bahama Islands, where thousands receive treatment for the disease.

Since Dr. Burton's death, Dr. John Clement, an internationally respected cancer specialist who studied with Dr. Burton, heads the center. Dr. Clement gives an overview of the treatment: "The intellectual basis of the treatment is that many cancers can be controlled by restoring the competence of the patient's immune system, as the body's complex immune-fighting system may well be the first, best, and last line of defense against many cancers.

"The method we use is similar in any type of cancer we treat, although each patient has her treatment tailored to the results of her own blood test. We do not deal with toxic chemicals in any way. We assay the blood for the factors we believe are aiding the patient's cancer. By identifying these factors, we are able to control them, put them back into balance, and hopefully destroy the patient's cancer."

Regarding breast cancer, Dr. Clement says: "We have had patients with breast cancer who have had no other treatment but IAT for upward of 20 years who have no recurrence of disease. While we are still claiming only to control their cancer, you will see that to all intents and purposes, by any kind of medical description, they have been cured."

Dr. Clement reports less success with patients who come to him after extremely arduous chemotherapy and those with advanced cancer where there is a loss of bone marrow and fluid collection in the abdomen or pleural effusions in the lungs.

Addressing other forms of cancer that affect women, Dr. Clement states that IAT is often successful with cancer of the cervix if it is caught early, even after surgery. Additionally, lung cancer, which is becoming more widespread among women and generally is not treatable by conventional methods, can be more successfully treated with IAT: "We have a good measure of control with adenocarcinoma of the lung and with squamous cell carcinoma. If fluid is present, however, which indicates a more severe type of disease, very often we do not have much control. Nor do we have much luck with the type of cancer that is associated with smoking, small cell lung cancer. This is because small cell lung cancer grows rapidly. Tumors will double in size in just 30 days. Our treatment does not work quickly enough to do these patients much good." As for ovarian cancer, Dr. Clement states, "We have been lucky. We have been able to control this cancer in people even after metastases and recurrences of the cancer after operations and chemotherapy."

THE MIND-BODY CONNECTION

Exploration of the effects of outlooks and emotions on health and disease processes has opened up an exciting area of science known as psychoneuroimmunology. Researchers have discovered that the mind, nervous system, and immune system interact with one another at the cellular level. When we feel joy, we enhance our healing mechanisms. Conversely, when we feel fear or hopelessness, we generate disease.

Dr. Carl Simonton, medical director of the Simonton Cancer Center in California and coauthor of *Getting Well Again* and *The Healing Journey,* is one of the early pioneers in this field. In the late 1960s, as a radiation oncologist, he noticed that emotional factors and patient attitudes influenced the course of treatment. His research led him to an extensive body of literature, where he learned that the three biggest mental influences on cancer are a tendency to respond to stressful situations with hopelessness, the bottling up of emotions, and a perceived lack of closeness to one's parents. This understanding prompted Dr. Simonton to look at the influence of counseling on the course of treatment. He discovered that survival times doubled, quality of life improved, and there was a better quality of death as a result of counseling efforts.

Dr. Simonton firmly believes that emotions drive healing systems and that the imagination and standard counseling can be used to increase a patient's will to live: "The emphasis of our approach is to focus on what is right with the individual. We ask, What are the person's goals and aspirations? What are the person's main sources of inspiration and creativity? What is the person's sense of purpose and destiny? As people become clearer and more connected to these concepts, they rediscover a strong desire to live. That in turn enhances their inherent healing mechanisms.

"As we explore these areas, we begin to address those things that interfere with achieving these very important aims. One primary culprit is unhealthy beliefs. To demonstrate this, I would like to give an example of a patient I have worked with for over 20 years. This 36-year-old woman came to me in 1976 with metastatic breast cancer that had spread to her ribs and spine. Her father was a physician, and her husband's family had run a retail store for three generations. She was involved in helping her husband run the family business.

"Her religious and spiritual life was important to her. It was a great source of strength. She wanted more time to be involved in religious administration and spiritual counseling. As she began to pursue these areas, her beliefs about how she should be the good daughter, the good wife, and the good mother came into play. These beliefs were all quite rigid, allowing virtually no freedom for her own creativity. Over time we helped her make a shift in these beliefs and behaviors that was central to her recovery.

"She has been free of disease for 15 years. Currently, she is weller than well and runs marathons. The family store burned down about 10 years ago. Now she works primarily in church administration, doing religious and spiritual counseling, which is what she always wanted to do."

Dr. Simonton emphasizes that there is a relationship between all types of cancer and rigid thinking: "Here we tend to be controlled by beliefs about how we should be or have to be. That allows very little room for the expression of the spirit. Becoming aware of the direction in which our life force wants to go is essential for renewing vitality and healing power. It becomes important to listen to the voice within and to develop ways of enhancing that. This takes practice."

Dr. Simonton says that the way we use the imagination can mean the difference between success and failure in treatment: "In our imagination, we must think about the things we do for ourselves that are helpful. There are three areas that we need to look at: our beliefs about treatment, our beliefs about the body's ability to heal itself, and our beliefs about the disease itself.

When a person is first diagnosed with cancer, if she shares the common cultural perspective, she believes that cancer is strong, that the body is weak, and that treatment is harsh. In keeping with these beliefs, a person is going to experience much in the way of undesirable side effects and less benefit. As we look at those beliefs, we find that they are not at all compatible with reality; cancer is a weak disease composed of weak cells. It is important to remind ourselves that our bodies have always been able to recognize and destroy cancer cells since before we were born. Shifting those images helps healing occur."

THE SOURCES OF RESISTANCE TO ALTERNATIVE THERAPIES

When we see dreadful practices such as cutting away healthy women's breasts and giving women drugs that cause one kind of cancer while preventing another kind, the question arises as to why alternative therapies are resisted.

INDUSTRY

Many people believe that industry in general has a vested interest in disputing the findings of alternative medicine. For example, one might imagine that Dr. Singer's book would wound the bra industry, since it told women to stop wearing those halters. But he was surprised that it was not from the bra business that most of the opposition to his book came. In fact, the bra industry is beginning to *support* his findings. He acknowledges: "When we came out with our book in 1995, we got complaints from the Apparel Council, which is based in New York and is the trade association for the multi-billion-dollar bra industry. They called my publisher and threatened him with a lawsuit if he published the book because they were so worried. Now they are admitting that 80 to 90 percent of the public is wearing bras that are too tight." The industry claimed that women were wearing the wrong sizes. Singer says that is like "blaming the victim . . . I don't know how you can wear a push-up bra and not have it too tight. Its purpose is to be too tight."

What happened was that the industry began promoting bra fittings, which all the department stores now offer. "That's the answer the bra industry is coming up with. They're saying that if you wear a well-fitted bra, it will not cause damage. Of course, they are not being any more specific about what they mean by damage. If you look on the Internet under bras nowadays, you will see advertised bras that claim to be looser, that won't affect the lymphatics. They are even citing our book."

MEDICINE

The bra industry may have been able to cope with Dr. Singer's message, but the medical profession has refused even to acknowledge that it exists. Singer says: "I have a press kit now that is an inch thick. I have been around the world, on television, I've done hundreds of radio shows, been in dozen of magazines, done untold interviews. This has been all over the place, yet nowhere is it ever mentioned in the mainstream medical literature. It's been censored."

A number of problems arise from the paradigms and orientation of modern medicine. A central difficulty with the medical establishment's treatment of cancer is its close connection to the cash nexus: "When you look at the numbers on breast cancer and the money that is being made on working with those who have the disease, you'll see that the medical industry is profiting in the billions from this disease every year. There are 200,000 women who are going to be diagnosed with breast cancer this year. Each woman's treatment will amount to $50,000 on the average. That's $10 billion just this year. That doesn't include all the mammograms."

Sherrill Sellman's experience with the tamoxifen lobby has taught her the same lesson. As she sees it, "Researching my book was a real eye-opener, for I found that women are an industry and cancer is an industry. There is really only one motive driving it. The central focus is that money is to be made, and if women's lives have to be sacrificed in pursuit of profits, they will gladly be sacrificed by the companies. That's the sorry state of affairs."

Aside from their fiscal interest, doctors are locked into restricted paradigms, Singer says: "Doctors have a tremendous interest in career development. When their careers are focused on treatment, they will have little interest in prevention. The prevention of disease should not be given to the treatment industry, which is exactly what has happened in this country."

The lack of interest in treatment was corroborated by Dr. Georgi, director of the National Cancer Institute's nutrition division. He said that less than 5 percent of the NCI's budget for breast cancer was earmarked for prevention.

In Sellman's words, "The fact that there are options that are safe and nontoxic will never see the light of day in the medical model. That's because we know that in the medical model drugs are foremost. Doctors are really impotent because all they have are drugs and procedures. Anything outside those two options is not in their world. This spells disaster for women, yet in the medical profession nothing else is offered."

This doesn't mean there will not be treatments, but that they will be limited to those which bring in large fees and follow the medical paradigm, which, as we have seen, involves solely surgery and drugs. I believe the day will come when all these cancer treatment centers will be seen differently. People in the future will be looking at them and saying incredulously, "You really were doing preventive mastectomies because of this foolish gene notion?"

As Singer puts it, "I'd take off a bra before I'd take off a breast." But the medical establishment doesn't see it that way.

Another of Singer's criticisms of the medical establishment asserts that its research agendas are often set by ignoring the difference between humans and animals. "Remember, the difference between a human and a rat is that we have created a culture, institutions, and other stuff. Rats don't wear bras, for example. Now, most research is done on animals. A doctor doing this research will be thinking simply, 'A mammary gland is a mammary gland,' assuming it can be studied equally well in a rat, a monkey, a cat, or a woman. This is so ridiculous when you deal with a lifestyle-caused disease, which cancer is known to be. You have to look at people and how they live."

WOMEN THEMSELVES

If doctors have the excuse of a distorted worldview and a desire for money to explain their fear of innovation, how do we explain why women are so often bamboozled by physicians and the media when the facts are out there? Why, for example, do they keep eating toxic foods? We have a tendency to follow our early conditioning and stick to the foods we learned to love. We go for soft, crunchy, salty, and sweet foods. It's like smoking and drinking and doing drugs. People are not so stupid that they don't know these substances are harmful, yet look at how many millions of people are using them and doing other abusive things to their bodies.

If you ask someone drinking vodka, "Do you think this is doing you good?" she'll know that it's not beneficial in any way. Certainly she won't say, "I'm going to drink some vodka today because it's good for me." We know these substances are bad for us. But there's a difference between knowing what is bad for us and being willing to be responsible for the consequences.

When a disease happens, people face a gray area in their life and find that they have not been raised to be fully responsible for seeking out as many ways of looking at a problem as possible. They have been given black and white, and they get confused when they discover that what a favorite authority figure said to do actually causes disease. If you are in that type of position at this point, you don't know what to believe because you were not allowed to do relative thinking. You were taught absolute thinking and learned that authority figures cannot be wrong. So even when they are wrong, you have a hard time disengaging your trust factor and overcoming these prejudices. All the experts I spoke to had their own recipes for moving people beyond their prejudices and unhealthy worldviews. Krupka says, "I like to tell women when I lecture that each woman should think for herself. She should be willing to take a look at cultures that have lower rates of cancers and see what they're eating. Ask about them. Do they eat trans-fats? Do they eat junk food?"

Singer has tried innovative ways of getting his message across beyond simply lecturing and making appearances. For example, he has used art to make the public aware of the link between bras and breast cancer. He contacted a conceptual artist named Nicolino, who had previously done a project called Bras across the Grand Canyon, which, says Singer, is "all about body image and body politics and Barbie and things of this sort. It focuses on these cultural messages that women get that are so destructive.

"We collected 40,000 donated bras from across America. These bras were woven into a 40-foot-wide by 100-foot-tall (that's four stories) tapestry called the National Bra Tapestry that is in the image of the Statue of Liberty. It traveled across the country in fall 1998 and was presented to President Clinton."

This has been a way to alert the public, because, as Sellman also believes, the only way the breast cancer epidemic is going to end is through grassroots efforts.

Patient Stories

MARYLOU

I have always been interested in holistic medicine, and I was a great fan of Carlton Fredericks. In 1989, when I discovered a lump in my breast, I sought help directly from a holistic doctor, Dr. Robert Atkins. I went to him before any diagnosis because I knew that if I had to have surgery, I wanted to see someone who was open-minded about alternative therapies.

The lump was malignant, and I had a modified radical mastectomy. Fortunately, my lymph nodes were clean, but the tumor was not a hormonal tumor and it was a very aggressive one.

I started therapy with Dr. Atkins that consisted of a low-carbohydrate diet. That meant absolutely no caffeine and no sugar of any kind. I was also on a program of vitamins and nutrients targeted to my specific problem. Once a week I was given an intravenous drip of an anticancer formula developed by Dr. Atkins that was largely vitamin C.

Soon after surgery I had a problem. The tumor grew back into the incision. Both the surgeon and Dr. Atkins advised radiation, which I was given for five weeks. While I was undergoing radiation, I did the IV weekly, and it alleviated any side effects of the radiation. I wasn't tired, and I was able to work half days.

A month or so after the radiation, the tumor came back again in the area of the incision, and again it was removed. I continued Dr. Atkins's therapy. That was almost seven years ago, and I haven't had a problem since. I am still on the diet and the vitamin program. The intervals between the IVs have been extended to two months.

There is no question in my mind that Dr. Atkins saved my life.

RITA

I got breast cancer 10 years ago, when I was 39. I had conventional surgery but would not undergo chemotherapy or radiation. Since I had no positive node involvement and no metastases after surgery, I was told that I was fine and that there was nothing else to do. But because it was a very large tumor and an aggressive one, I was concerned about it. Since I had been involved with natural medicine for a long time and was pretty well educated in it, I started to search for ways to prevent the return of the cancer.

I discovered a lot of things. I went on a one-year program of injections of a formula that was mostly mistletoe. I had to get the prescription for the vials and send away to Switzerland for the formula. I injected myself with the herbal formula.

I did a lot of reading, and I took courses in Chinese herbology. I learned about several herbalists and studied with Letha Hadady over the years. I took several workshops with her where I learned about Chinese herbs and the whole philosophy of Asian medicine as well as the ayurvedic and Tibetan systems. Over the years, I have taken formulas of Chinese and western herbs.

The results are difficult to show concretely. All I can tell you is that I don't have cancer and that ten years later, after having had a very aggressive kind of tumor, I am still fine.

I believe in natural medicine. I also believe very firmly that it is important to have a practitioner, to not use the local health food store as your medical adviser. Everybody has to be examined individually.

SUSAN

When I was 46 my doctor found tumors in my breasts and my uterus. He screamed at me to see a surgeon, but I refused. The reason I said no is because of what happened to one of my best girlfriends, Kimberly. Kimberly was 34, beautiful, and very sensitive, with a wonderful husband and three stepchildren. She found a lump on her breast and went to the doctor. Her mammogram was negative, but they did a biopsy anyway and found that it was cancerous. Three days later she had her breast lopped off. That was followed up with lots of chemotherapy. Her hair fell out ,and she vomited 24 hours a day. She couldn't keep any food down. Then they did radiation, and her skin burned up and two of her ribs broke. Most people don't know how dangerous radiation is. I had seen enough. I wouldn't touch any of that medicine with a 10-foot pole.

I decided that I was going to try to heal myself using entirely natural means. By the way, I was already in a stage IV situation, and my doctor had given me two months to live. So I had this deadline. I had to get well by February 15.

Norman Cousins, who wrote a best-selling book about healing through laughter, says that a doctor shouldn't tell a patient that he or she is terminally ill. When you tell people they are going to be dead in 18 months, they will die in exactly 18 months. To counter that, I gave my immune system the opposite message. I had to get well in two months. Otherwise, I would lose my breasts, my uterus, and probably my house and my studio too because I don't have health insurance. I believe in giving yourself a deadline in a positive way rather than in a negative way. Giving your body a positive deadline sets a healing situation in motion. And of course, the brain is the main master of the immune system, so what you tell yourself will influence what happens to your body.

I got a lot of books out of the library. One said to eat brown rice. Another said to visualize. Still another said to do psychological work on yourself. I decided that I needed a whole program covering every single aspect of my life. I called my program MOTEP: the Marathon Olympic Tumor Eradication Program. It's a funny title, but it shows how hard I worked on it.

First of all, I joined a Y and swam a mile per day. While I was swimming, I would incorporate Dr. Carl Simonton's visualization technique. I had used it before to get rid of a lump in my neck that I got from using acrylic paint. So I did have some experience at "self-lumpectomy," and this is what I was attempting to do.

I started to talk to myself in a very positive way, visualizing the tumors as shrinking and going away. This occurred during the Gulf War, so I would visualize a Scud missile actually hitting my breasts and little white particles of the tumor floating into the water. I would actually see this. Then, when I would take a sauna after the swim, I would visualize the tumor as actually melting.

All day I would invent these very aggressive visualizations. When you visualize, you don't want passive imagery such as snowflakes or Tinkerbell sprinkles. Those are ineffective. You want to use very aggressive imagery: sharks eating your cancer, or Pacman, or Scud missiles hitting your tumor. It helps to believe that you can conquer this disease. So I believed 100 percent in my program.

My program also consisted of special foods based on the macrobiotic diet. I ate whole grains and fresh juices, vegetables and fruits, and some fish. No meat and no dairy products were included. I had lots of carrot juice because the beta carotene is very healing. I also meditated and chanted to get rid of stress.

There are two major points in my program. One is to detoxify the body, and the other is to destress because your body cannot heal if you are full of heavy-duty anxiety. You want to calm your body down with meditation, chanting, and other spiritual activities, such as white-light meditation, in which you visualize a white light cleaning out your body.

I also got myself into group therapy because this has been shown to extend the lives of cancer patients. Furthermore, I healed my relationships. People in good relationships with social support are the ones who live the longest. So you want to mend your relationships or get out of them. If a relationship is destructive, you don't want to be in it. A woman in my group is going through a terrible divorce, and she has breast cancer. She decided to go away to Puerto Rico to Ann Wigmore's healing place for a while. I think that's the best thing she can do. She needs to get away from her stressful situation so that her body can heal.

I broke up with a boyfriend and turned him into a friend because he was causing me a lot of distress. He was going out with other women and bringing out feelings of jealousy and anger in me. I cleaned out all those negative emotions from my body.

One month later my body went through a horrible healing reaction called inflammatory breast cancer. My breasts turned bright red and hard as a rock, and my left arm was totally paralyzed. Unfortunately, inflammatory breast cancer is not recognized as a healing reaction. If a surgeon cuts the body at that time, the patient dies immediately from the trauma. Women need to support their bodies at this time. Then they have a great chance of living through it.

I continued with my program throughout my healing crisis. Three weeks later—this is one week before my appointment—I knew I had won the battle. My yellow-green hue disappeared, and natural color came back to my cheeks. Two days later both tumors were gone. This was five days before my appointment. My body responded to my deadline.

My doctor was shocked not to find any lumps. He examined my breasts three times to be sure. He looked for my uterine tumor, but that was gone too. He finally said that I should make a video about my experience. That's when I decided to write my book, *Keep Your Breasts: Preventing Breast Cancer the Natural Way.*

Women around the country are using this program to get well without subjecting themselves to surgery or drugs, and we have had outstanding results. One woman changed her mammogram results in only 10 days from the time she told them to clear, and she was high-risk. Another woman dissolved a lump in only two weeks. Once you have the information, it's easier to utilize than it is when you have to look here and there and try to piece it together as I did.

Fibrocystic Breast Disease

CAUSES

Fibrocystic breast disease is caused by overcongestion from foods that clog the system, such as wheat, dairy products, refined foods, and fats. Caffeinated products such as coffee, tea, chocolate, and soft drinks are hard on the body and add to the problem, as does a sluggish thyroid gland, which makes metabolism more difficult and leads to constipation, causing a buildup of toxins. Toxic accumulations worsen congestion and can manifest as breast lumps (cysts). Stress worsens the condition.

SYMPTOMS

Fibrocystic breast disease shows up as single or multiple breast lumps. Cysts are usually harmless but are related to a higher than normal chance of contracting breast cancer later. Mammograms determine whether breast lumps are benign.

Drs. Ruth Bar-Shalom and John Soileau, naturopaths from Fairbanks, Alaska, add that the symptoms may also include tenderness and pain in the breast. In an article on the American Association of Naturopathic Physicians website (www.naturopathic.org) they stress the importance of learning breast self-examination and performing it every month, a week to 10 days after the menstrual period starts. This enables you to recognize the cystic areas. If you are not sure whether a lump is a cyst or something else or if there is a discharge from the nipples, consult a physician.

CLINICAL EXPERIENCE

DIET AND NUTRITION

A diet high in complex carbohydrates can make a difference; fruits, vegetables, grains, beans, and some fish are recommended. Red-hot peppers, cayenne pepper, and regular or daikon radishes cut through mucus and help eliminate breast lumps.

According to Drs. Bar-Shalom and Soileau, the most important dietary measure for reducing cysts is to eliminate from the diet all forms of caffeine, including coffee, tea, chocolate, and soda. Meat, especially the hormone-containing commercial type, should be avoided as much as possible. Finally, since constipation can aggravate fibrocystic breast disease, it is important to eat more vegetables, fruits, and whole grains and drink 8 to 10 glasses of water a day.

SUPPLEMENTS

These nutrients offer extra help when combined with a cleansing diet.

ANTIOXIDANTS. Among the antioxidants, use selenium and vitamins A, C, and E.

MAGNESIUM. Magnesium cleanses the tissues by entering cells and forcing out excess calcium and other minerals.

IODINE DROPS. Iodine speeds the metabolism of the thyroid gland. As the metabolism perks up, breast lumps tend to disappear. Iodine drops from seaweed can be obtained in the drugstore in a saturated solution of potassium iodide or Lugol's solution. There is also an Edgar Cayce remedy called Atomodine. In addition, health food stores sell iodine drops in the form of liquid kelp. Before you use iodine, a thyroid blood test should be done to check for thyroid antibodies. This ensures that there is no thyroiditis, an inflammation of the thyroid gland.

Drs. Bar-Shalom and Soileau suggest the following supplements:

MULTIVITAMIN.

VITAMIN B COMPLEX. 50 mg twice a day.

VITAMIN B$_6$. 100 mg twice a day.

VITAMIN E. 600 IU per day.

FLAXSEED OIL. 2 capsules or 1 tablespoon a day.

BETA CAROTENE. 150,000 IU per day. If you are pregnant or of childbearing age, take no more than 15,000 IU a day.

AMINO ACIDS. Take 1,000 mg each of choline and methionine a day to remedy the hormonal imbalance which is said to result in formation of cysts.

HERBS

Herbalist Letha Hadady recommends the following plant remedies to break up congestion in the chest and release phlegm and mucus from the system before they lead to more serious problems:

XIAO YAO WAN. This formula is a combination of digestive herbs that increase circulation, build blood, and break apart fibroids. *Xiao yao wan* is available in Chinatowns throughout America.

DANDELION. Dandelion tea or capsules can be taken every day to break apart fibroids.

Bar-Shalom and Soileau recommend in addition poke root and iris versicolor taken as tinctures. Take 5 drops of each three times daily for up to three months. Do not take these herbs if you are pregnant.

EXTERNAL TREATMENTS

CASTOR OIL PACKS. According to the medical psychic Edgar Cayce, stimulating liver circulation ends constipation. Substances that clog the body and form breast lumps are then eliminated. To do this, rub castor oil on the skin over the liver. Cover this area with a towel and place a heating pad over it. Do this for 20 minutes each day.

PEPPERMINT OIL. Rubbing peppermint oil on breast lumps diminishes them by stimulating the circulation.

PHYTOLACCA OIL AND HYDROTHERAPY. Joseph Pizzorno has found success with this combination treatment: "We have a woman put a hot compress on her breast so that it gets real warm. She then covers the area with phytolacca oil. After the application, she covers it with a cold pack. We combine herbal medicine with hydrotherapy to help the cysts drain out of the breasts. I use that treatment with a lot of women and have had quite a good response."

HOMEOPATHY

Drs. Bar-Shalom and Soileau suggest the following homeopathic remedies. Choose one based on how well it matches your symptoms and then take it under the tongue three times a day, stopping when the symptoms are relieved.

PHYTOLACCA. Use phytolacca, 6c potency, for hard, sensitive breasts or when you have multiple nodules.

CONIUM MACULATUM. For sharp pain in the nipples and for breast swelling, take conium, 12c potency.

SEPIA. When irritability accompanies breast swelling, take *Sepia*, 6c potency.

COLON CLEANSING

See the section "Colon Cleansing" in Chapter 2.

YOGA

Gary Ross, M.D., a family physician and certified yoga instructor from San Francisco, recommends yoga poses, meditation, and breathing exercises to alleviate fibrocystic breast disease brought on by stress and a sluggish thyroid. These three postures increase blood flow to the thyroid and chest area:

SHOULDER STAND. On a mat or thick blanket, lie flat on your back. You may place a rolled towel under your neck. Raise your legs over your head so that your body is in a U formation. Rest the elbows firmly on the floor and support the back with both hands. Adjust your body so that it is completely vertical. Then press the chin against the chest. Hold still as you breathe slowly, concentrating on the thyroid gland. You may be able to do this for only several seconds at first, but then you will be able to work up to one minute. To come down, lower the legs slowly toward the head. Then lower the back to the floor one vertebra at a time. When the back is on the floor, continue to lower the legs gradually until you are once again flat on your back. Do this once in the morning and once in the evening. To get the full benefit, follow with the fish pose.

FISH POSE. Lie on your back with the legs straight or folded. If the legs are straight, place the hands under the buttocks with the palms down. Otherwise, hold on to the crossed feet. Resting on the elbow, arch the chest and neck back. The head should be on the floor, but do not apply pressure there. Support should come from the elbows. Do not bend the neck too far back as that can impede circulation. Focusing on the thyroid, breathe deeply in this position, holding for 30 seconds.

COBRA. Lie facedown with the elbows and palms down on the floor or mat and the palms beneath the shoulders. With a smooth, gradual motion, raise the eyes upward and then the head, neck, and spine, one vertebra at a time. Allow the area below the hips to remain on the blanket. Hold the pose and then come out of it using reverse motions that are equally slow and gradual. Breathe in as you come into the posture, hold the breath while in the cobra, and breathe out when coming down.

In addition to these yoga asanas, Dr. Ross advocates deep-breathing exercises to bring more energy into the chest area. Visualization creates a mind-set that helps make lumps disappear. Further, meditation creates spiritual and mental tranquillity that is conducive to healing.

PATIENT STORIES: DOCTOR ROSS

A 24-year-old woman came to me with benign lumps on one breast. She had had a lifelong history of severe constipation, requiring laxatives and enemas. On top of that, she basically lived on muffins, breads, and coffee.

The first thing we did was take her off all caffeine. That included coffee, tea, chocolate, and soft drinks. To eliminate the congestion, we asked her to stop eating muffins and bread.

This was a start, but it didn't address her constipation. I investigated that further and found that she had a mild case of subclinical hypothyroidism. This means that her blood tests for thyroid function were normal, but clinically she felt sluggish and constipated with slightly dry skin and a low body temperature. This condition is crucial to correct; when thyroid function is low, the body is unable to metabolize excessive amounts of congesting foods. I put her on a low dose of natural thyroid. That, coupled with dietary changes, antioxidants, magnesium shots, and castor oil packs, absolutely changed her life. The breast cysts and constipation went away. Her energy picked up. It was absolutely amazing.

Another excellent case involves a 29-year-old woman who also had breast lumps. In her case, this related to stress, heavy caffeine intake, and smoking. Of course, I advised her to cut out the caffeine and smoking right away, which she did. I had her rub peppermint oil onto the breast lumps to stimulate the circulation. As circulation increases, the body decongests and the lumps tend to go away, as they did in this case.

A third case is a 33-year-old woman who was under a lot of stress. In her case, what seemed to work best was a combination of yoga, meditation, and breathing exercises.

LYMPHEDEMA

Lymphedema, a swelling of the limbs caused by an accumulation of lymph fluid, affects 1 percent of the U.S. population. Health practitioner James Kresse explains, "There are two types of lymphedema. The first is *primary lymphostatic lymphedema,* an inherent condition that predominantly affects women in their midthirties but can manifest at birth or during adolescence. The second is more common and frequently occurs in patients who have had mastectomies or the removal of malignant tumors. The large increase in the incidence of breast cancer and subsequent mastectomy operations is one of the major reasons for the rise in lymphedema today. Secondary lymphostatic lymphedema can occur from six months to three years after the initial surgery."

SYMPTOMS

Lymphedema appears as a swelling or skin thickening in a limb. It is important to detect the condition early, and this can be done in several ways. Kresse advises, "Notice any jewelry becoming tighter on the affected limb over a short period of time. Or squeeze the affected limb for 10 seconds. If an indentation is noticed, notify your surgeon immediately or measure your arm with a cloth tape measure around your wrist and forearm. If you notice an increase in the circumference of your arm, call your surgeon right away."

CLINICAL EXPERIENCE

MANUAL LYMPHATIC DRAINAGE

Lymphatic detoxification is aided by manual lymphatic drainage (MLD), a simple method of massage that uses light, slow rhythmic movements to stimulate the flow of lymph in the body. "This type of therapy is very, very light," says Kresse. "It's almost featherlike. We're working on the parasympathetic nervous system. A regular massage stimulates the sympathetic nervous system. That is our fight-or-flight nerve. The parasympathetic nervous system is our night nerve, our rest and relax nerve. This is the nerve that lymph drainage affects in order to calm the patient down."

COMPRESSION BANDAGING

In addition to MLD, compression bandaging is used to apply pressure around the affected limb. Exercises performed with the bandage enhance muscular contractions that help with lymph flow.

LIFESTYLE CHANGES

Kresse states, "If lymphedema is not brought under control with a combination of MLD, specific exercises, and a no-protein, no-sodium diet, along with decongestive therapy or the use of a pneumatic pump, the affected limb can swell to an unsightly size and become life-threatening.

"There are dos and don'ts that a person should be aware of. Just to mention a couple, as far as the dos are concerned, the person needs to practice meticulous skin care with the use of pH-balanced lotions and creams to protect the skin. Following a good nutritional program consisting of lots of fruits and vegetables is helpful. Salt and fatty foods should be eliminated, and protein intake should be limited. It is important to maintain an optimum weight, as obesity contributes to lymphedema. Exercise such as swimming, walking, and stretching is excellent. Incorporating deep diaphragmatic breathing techniques, along with specific exercises taught by an MLD therapist, is good. While sleeping, the patient can elevate the limb by tilting the mattress or by placing pillows under the arm. Antibiotic solutions should be carried at all times for incidental cuts, scratches, or bites. Infection should be treated at the first sign.

"Precautions to take include not subjecting oneself to extreme temperature changes such as hot tubs, saunas, steam baths, and other thermal treatments. Care must be taken when using instruments on the affected limb, such as the instruments used in manicures and pedicures. Pets must be watched to see that they don't scratch or bite. Blood pressure readings, injections, vaccinations, and acupuncture should be avoided on the infected arm. Constrictive clothing and jewelry should not be worn. Heavy prostheses can cause excess pressure on the affected limb. Care must be taken when cooking, gardening, and doing daily chores. Finally, heavy objects must not be lifted. This can cause a lymphedema right away or somewhere down the line."

Other therapies that help lymphatic conditions include rebound exercise, ozone therapy, enzyme therapy, colon hydrotherapy, deep breathing exercises, and a good vitamin and herbal program.

PATIENT STORY: SUSAN

I had been overexposed to the sun and wound up with a severe toxic reaction. It was sun poisoning that went one step further and became lymphedema. Instead of just having blisters on the surface of the skin with lymphatic fluid in them, my lymphatic fluid was backed up. The lymph nodes weren't clearing up the blisters, and the fluid wasn't coming to the surface the way it should. So I wound up with a severe case of lymphedema. My ankles were the size of my knees, and I couldn't really walk. I let myself get dehydrated because I couldn't even take going to the bathroom. It was the most horrible thing I ever encountered.

I finally dragged myself to the Healing Center after three or four days of agony. That's when I began alternative treatments. I had a vitamin infusion using 75,000 mg of vitamin C. I had lymphatic massage and was prescribed homeopathic remedies. I was also prescribed huge amounts of bioflavinoids as well as quercetin, essential fatty acids, and lecithin.

I also used magnets, which were great. Not only did they help the lymphatic drainage, they freed me from pain. I applied those to my legs: first ceramic magnets and then electromagnets. These really helped with circulation and healing.

I had great relief and was once again able to walk normally instead of dragging my feet.

Chapter 7

Cervical Dysplasia, Fibroids and Reproductive System Cancers

Cervical Dysplasia

Cervical dysplasia is an abnormal growth of cervical tissue caused by the sexually transmitted human papillomavirus (HPV), the same virus that is responsible for cervicitis, genital warts, and cervical cancer. These conditions can be detected with a Pap smear.

CAUSES

The likelihood of a woman contracting cervical dysplasia increases with intercourse at an early age, unprotected sex with several male partners, smoking, birth control pills, and weak immunity. Dr. Tori Hudson explains, "Women who have intercourse at an early age are more vulnerable to getting genital warts and cervical dysplasia because the cells of the cervix at that age are more susceptible to being infected by the virus.

"Smoking is the biggest factor in acquiring cervical dysplasia and cervical cancer. If you smoke, and you are exposed to the virus, you are much more likely to develop dysplasia, and you are much more likely to develop cervical cancer from your dysplasia. We know that nicotine actually lodges in the glands of the cells of the cervix. When exposed to the virus, the DNA can change to take on more abnormal features. If you have genital warts and you smoke, it is much more likely that they will turn cancerous as well.

"Oral contraceptives are known for creating a folic acid deficiency, and folic acid deficiency is associated with acquiring cervical dysplasia and having the disease progress to cancer."

SYMPTOMS

Dr. Hudson describes cervical dysplasia as a progressive syndrome that develops over time: "After initial exposure to the virus, there is no indication that anything has changed. Later, immune changes may occur. Warty tissue may develop, then mild dysplasia, moderate dysplasia, severe dysplasia, carcinoma in situ, and then invasive cancer." Since these symptoms are not evident upon physical examination, Pap smears are necessary.

CLINICAL EXPERIENCE

PREVENTION

Since HPV is sexually transmitted, the conditions associated with it are preventable. Notes Dr. Hudson, "Cervical dysplasia, genital warts, and cervical cancer are all sexually transmitted diseases. That should make an impression on all of us, because it really dictates how we should protect ourselves.

"Obviously, we shouldn't smoke. We should protect ourselves by having safe sex and a healthy immune system. If you take birth control pills, it is advisable to take folic acid. A good maintenance dose would be 800 mcg daily. Those are the main ways to protect against cervical dysplasia and genital warts." Additional preventive daily supplementation may include 1,000 mg of vitamin C and 25,000 IU of beta carotene.

To catch the condition early, Dr. Hudson stresses yearly Pap smear exams. Statistics show that the longer women wait between Pap smears, the higher the incidence of cervical dysplasia and cervical cancer.

DIAGNOSIS

Before treatment, it is essential to get fully diagnosed to determine the stage of the illness. If a woman has an abnormal Pap smear, her partner needs to be examined by a urologist for warty tissue. Otherwise, they will pass the virus back and forth, reinfecting each other. Diagnosis by a licensed, well-trained alternative practitioner will determine whether a woman is a candidate for natural treatments only or needs to integrate these approaches with conventional methods.

CONVENTIONAL TREATMENTS

Conventional medicine usually does nothing to treat mild dysplasias and genital warts. "Basically, they wait to see if it gets worse," says Dr. Hudson. "Often the body can reverse mildly abnormal states to normal on its own, as the body has an extraordinary ability to heal itself. But when it can't , then the disease progresses, and the downside of waiting becomes apparent."

In the later stages, aggressive measures may be taken. The preferred conventional treatment is known as LEEP (loop excisional electrosurgical procedure), which uses an electrical wire to cut out abnormal tissue. This is less expensive and less traumatic than the method of treatment previously used, called cone biopsy or conization. In advanced disease states, a hysterectomy may be needed to save a woman's life.

NATUROPATHIC TREATMENTS

Women with cervical dysplasia often have excellent results using naturopathic approaches. Dr. Hudson notes, "In the results of a research study that I conducted at the College of Naturopathic Medicine in Portland, we treated 43 women with varying degrees of cervical dysplasia. Through my treatment protocol, 38 of the 43 reverted to normal, three partially improved, and two had no change, meaning that they didn't get better and they didn't get worse."

Dr. Hudson's protocol consists of three parts: systemic, local, and constitutional treatment. She stresses that after a woman follows the protocol for three months, it is important for her to once again be examined by a health practitioner and to obtain another Pap smear. Sometimes a biopsy is also needed.

SYSTEMIC TREATMENT
Beta carotene, 150,000 IU daily.
Vitamin C, 3,000–6,000 mg daily.
Folic acid, 2.5–10 mg daily. Note: High doses of folic acid must be prescribed by a naturopathic physician. After three months, the amount of folic acid is decreased.
Immune herbal formulation

LOCAL TREATMENT
Vitamin A suppositories
Herbal suppositories

CONSTITUTIONAL TREATMENT
Dietary changes. An optimal immunity diet is low in fat and high in whole grains, vegetables, and fruits. Immune system inhibitors such as coffee, sugar, alcohol, and fat are omitted.
Use of condoms
Avoidance of smoking

HERBAL TREATMENT

Amanda McQuade Crawford, a medical herbalist, uses herbal infusions to treat cervical dysplasia. In her book *Herbal Remedies for Women*, Crawford recommends the following infusion, made by steeping the herbs in water that has been boiled:

Take 1 teaspoon in water or herbal tea three times a day for two to four months.

Crawford also recommends herbal douches. Her favorite douche uses 1 oz of wheatgrass juice for every 6 oz of sterile water. If wheatgrass is not available, she recommends the following douche solutions:

1 oz marshmallow root

4 oz periwinkle leaf

1 oz goldenseal root

1 oz *gotu kola* herb

Grind the herbs and mix with 4 oz of boiling water. Strain, and allow the mixture to cool to room temperature before using.

1 cup warm, but not hot, sterilized water

15 drops of thuja essential oil

1 oz calendula oil

15 drops vitamin E oil

You can also add:

4–6 drops of blue chamomile essential oil

4–6 drops of geranium essential oil

Dilute the oils in water and mix together well.

IMMUNOAUGMENTIVE THERAPY (IAT)

Treating cervical cancer by restoring the patient's own immune system has also proved successful at John Clement's Immunology Research Center in Freeport in the Bahamas. Dr. Clement specifies that success can occur if the treatment is begun early, even after surgery. (See Chapter 6, Breast Cancer.)

Fibroids and Uterine Bleeding

Fibroids are growths composed of muscle tissue that are usually benign. They attach themselves to the inner or outer wall of the uterus. One in five women over 35 has them; the majority of these women are African-American. These tumors grow in response to estrogen levels. Medically, they are also referred to as fibromyoma uteri and leiomyoma uteri.

CAUSES

Complementary physician Dr. Robert Sorge says that fibroids are nature's way of encapsulating toxins that result from an unhealthy diet and lifestyle: "Most of our patients with this condition consume tremendous amounts of coffee. As far as I'm concerned, this is something that every person concerned about their health must stop drinking. Diet sodas, greasy fries, pizza, potato chips, doughnuts and danishes, and other devitalized foods add to the problem."

Registered nurse and licensed acupuncturist Abigail Rist-Podrecca, of New York City and Kingston, New York, adds that Asian medicine sees fibroids as the result of blockage to the uterine area: "This can be caused by anger, emotional upset, or a history of problems with menstruation, where it is either late or prolonged. Sometimes, after an abortion, the endometrial wall will still have some cells from that particular pregnancy. Further down the line, that can develop into fibroids."

SYMPTOMS

Small fibroids are symptomless, but when they grow, they may result in painful periods, bladder infections, and infertility. Uterine bleeding is another common symptom, explains Rist-Podrecca: "If the fibroid is located on the inside of the uterus lining, then you will have this uterine bleeding, which usually sends women to the gynecologist, where she opts for hysterectomy. If the fibroid is located on the muscle wall, there is not so much bleeding but the fibroid will continue to grow."

Dr. Sorge adds that bleeding is the body's attempt to restore balance, according to naturopathic medicine: "Circulation and oxygenation of the uterine muscles and blood vessels are diminished, and metabolic waste products begin to build up. Bleeding is the sign of a highly toxic condition attempting to correct itself."

CLINICAL EXPERIENCE

CONVENTIONAL APPROACH

Small fibroids that do not cause problems are sometimes removed by a procedure known as a myomectomy. This procedure removes the fibroid only and does not interfere with a woman's ability to have children.

For larger tumors or fibroids that cause heavy bleeding, hysterectomies are the standard treatment. Dr. Herbert Goldfarb, a gynecologist and assistant clinical professor at New York University's School of Medicine, reports that the majority of these operations are unnecessary, as well as dangerous: "Each year 750,000 hysterectomies are performed, and 2,500 women die during the operation. These are not sick women, but healthy women who go into the hospital and do not come out. Surgical procedures have morbidity, which means complications, and they have mortality, which means death."

In addition, hysterectomy can be psychologically destructive. As Goldfarb explains, "Some women want the operation and are all right about it, but most women feel like lambs being led to slaughter. They really don't want to have this procedure done, but their physicians give them no alternative.

"A new laser procedure, called myoma coagulation, has the potential to end the use of hysterectomy for fibroids once and for all, but most people don't know about it. My book *The No Hysterectomy Option* was written in response to my frustration at having a technology to help women avoid hysterectomies, but women not knowing about it. Sometimes women need hysterectomies, but often they are told they need them for frivolous reasons. My book is designed to help women understand when a hysteroctomy is needed and when other options are available. I always like to say that a hysterectomy may be indicated, but may not be *necessary.* Our best customer is an informed consumer.

"We could avoid hysterectomies in well over 50 percent of the patients now having them. Breaking it down, somewhere between 10 and 20 percent are done for cancer. At this point, I am not going to say that these can be avoided, although some of the ones done for precancerous conditions of the cervix can. But hysterectomies for conditions like endometriosis are not needed. Endoscopic procedures, laparoscopic procedures, and the judicious use of alternative medications will control these conditions. Regarding fibroids and bleeding, we can take care of this with myoma coagulation if the condition is caught early enough."

According to Dr. Tori Hudson in a column in *Prevention* magazine, one alternative to hysterectomy is hysteroscopic surgery, which is used when a fibroid is protruding into the uterus. The surgeon inserts a hysteroscope (a tubular instrument that allows the surgeon to visualize the interior of the uterus) through the cervix and shaves away the fibroid with instruments passed through the hysteroscope. The hysteroscope is also used to shrink larger fibroids with lasers or electric currents.

An alternative for relatively small fibroids on the outside of the uterus is laparoscopic surgery. The laparoscope, an instrument used to visualize the interior of the abdomen, is inserted through an incision in the abdomen, and the fibroid is vaporized by an electric current or removed surgically, using instruments passed through the tube.

Dr. Vicki Hufnagel, using the new technique of female reconstructive surgery (FRS), has been successful in removing uterine fibroids regardless of the size or number of tumors, limiting both blood loss and surgical complications.

MYOMA COAGULATION

Dr. Goldfarb lectures extensively to doctors on this new technology, which has enabled him to successfully prevent hysterectomies in hundreds of women with fibroids and uterine bleeding. Here he describes how he discovered the technique and why it works: "Approximately five years ago, on a trip to Europe, I observed a technique where a fibroid was being pierced with a special type of laser which destroyed the fibroid tissue and subsequently shrunk the tumor.

"When I returned to the United States, I performed the first myoma coagulation. (Other physicians call it myolysis.) A young woman with a fibroid tumor was undergoing a tubal sterilization. I pierced the fibroid with a laser fiber, and lo and behold, the fibroid disappeared. Five years later, this woman is functioning perfectly well. The fibroid is gone, and she has absolutely no symptoms.

"Subsequent to that, I performed this technique in well over 300 patients. A number of my colleagues also perform the procedure. I travel from coast to coast, north to south, lecturing and teaching. Physicians are uniformly performing it."

The typical candidate for this procedure is a woman uninterested in reproduction, since the uterine wall may become too weak to support a pregnancy. Also, the size of the tumor must be 10 cm or less (approximately 6 in). If the fibroid exceeds this size, it can be reduced with the medication Lupron: "Lupron reduces estrogen levels in the body, and temporarily reduces the size of fibroids. With Lupron, we get a 30 to 50 percent reduction in size."

Once the tumor has become smaller, coagulation can be performed, which shrinks it another 50 to 75 percent and puts an end to the problem: "When we do this procedure, we literally undermine the tumor by destroying its blood supply. As we put needles around the fibroid, it turns blue, showing that the blood supply has been interrupted. Fluid and blood go out, and the tumor shrinks. It becomes stringy tissue and just sits there, becoming very small, eliminating the need for removal. The patient has no symptoms and can go about her life without the need for further surgery."

The cost of myoma coagulation is equal to that of other operations, but this treatment is cost-effective in the long run: "The good news is that patients come into the hospital in the morning, have the procedure done, and go home in the afternoon. That saves the insurance company significant amounts of money. Also, these patients go back to work within a week so that there is very little cost in terms of disability."

DIET AND EXERCISE

Fibroids grow in response to estrogen, and so nutritionist Gracia Perlstein advocates the natural lowering of estrogen through diet and exercise as a first-line defense against fibroid growth.

As Perlstein explains, "Research shows that an over-fatty diet increases estrogen in the diet, and we know overweight women produce more estrogen. So the first approach would be dietary.

"The best diet for a woman attempting to decrease the size of her fibroids, or at the very least keep them from getting any larger, consists of whole foods and is semivegetarian or vegetarian. The best protein sources are from vegetables and include whole grains, especially millet, amaranth, quinoa, buckwheat, whole-grain oats, and brown rice. A wonderful way to cook whole grains is to put one part grain to four parts water in a slow cooker. Before going to sleep, turn the cooker on low or automatic shift, which starts high and goes lower. When you wake up in the morning, you have a creamy, delicious whole-grain cereal. That's a wonderful way to eat whole grains every day.

"Eat small quantities of legumes daily. Soybeans and foods made from soy, in particular, contain isoflavones that discourage tumor growth. Foods made from soy include tofu, fortified soy milk, miso, and tempeh. A variety of other beans can be used to make wonderful ethnic dishes: black beans, adzukis, pinto beans, chickpeas, mung beans, lentils, and lima beans. Grains and beans are your best source of proteins.

"If you eat meat, I recommend eating only small quantities of it, no more than 3 oz per day, an amount that fits into the palm of your hand. It should be only from animals that are free-range and grass-fed, with no hormones or antibiotics. A good way to get animal protein is to make soup stock with chicken or fish bones. Simply put them in pure water and simmer with a little organic cider vinegar for a couple of hours or overnight. Red meat, poultry, and conventional dairy products, which come from animals that are fed hormones, should be avoided entirely.

"The liver detoxifies excess estrogen, so you want to support liver function by avoiding all recreational drugs, alcohol, fried foods, coffee, and any processed or refined foods. Be sure to drink at least two quarts of pure water a day to help your bowels and kidneys. You are trying to remove excess estrogen from the system, and this is supported when your organs of elimination work properly."

Exercise is also very important, says Perlstein. "Regular exercise will reduce excessive estrogen levels. Most people are familiar with the fact that hard-training women athletes sometimes reduce their estrogen levels to the point where they stop menstruating. We are not after that kind of effect, but regular exercise is very beneficial and helps the body remove excess estrogen."

For further uterine support, Perlstein recommends the following supplements and herbs:

Balanced oil supplement (a mixture of flax, borage, and other unrefined, natural, organic oils), 1 tablespoon daily

Multiple vitamin/mineral supplement

Iron and herb supplement. This should be taken if there is anemia from heavy bleeding. Avoid high doses of iron as they are implicated in cancer and heart disease

Vitamin E, 400 units, twice daily

Silica supplement

Vitamin C with bioflavonoids, 1,000 mg five times daily, divided over the course of the day

Evening primrose oil, 100 mg, three times daily

False unicorn root tincture, 15 drops in a small amount of water, taken every hour, for acute uterine problems

Shepherd's purse tincture, 15 drops in a small amount of water three times a day, may stop excessive bleeding

White ash may reduce size of fibroids

Perlstein asserts that such a comprehensive program of diet and lifestyle changes, geared toward reducing excess estrogen, gives the body the tools it needs to shrink fibroids or keep them from growing any larger. In addition, the side effects of such a program are wonderful: "You will be slimmer and have more energy than you would using conventional methods, which have harmful effects."

WESTERN NATUROPATHIC TREATMENTS

Complementary physician Dr. Anthony Penepent recommends fasting for excessive uterine bleeding, excluding life-threatening situations where a woman needs hospitalization: "This condition signals liver poisoning. During the course of the month, a little fasting might be in order, in addition to a very strict hygienic regimen, to straighten out the condition. I have had patients with all forms of dysfunctional uterine bleeding, and I cannot remember any woman who followed my instructions who did not have a good result."

OIL-SOLUBLE LIQUID CHLOROPHYLL. Dr. Joseph Pizzorno, N.D., president of John Bastyr College of Naturopathic Medicine, says this old natural therapy can quite effectively put an end to abnormal uterine bleeding. Oil-soluble liquid chlorophyll is available in capsules. Two to three are usually taken two to three times a day. Dr. Pizzorno says that for some unknown reason, the chlorophyll seems to relieve this condition: "Many people think this works because it improves clotting, but it turns out that women with abnormal uterine bleeding do not have clotting abnormalities. So why it works is not clear, but the bottom line is, it works quite well."

WESTERN HERBS. According to Judy Griffin, Ph.D., an herbalist from Texas and author of *The Woman's Herbal,* as quoted in *Positive Health* magazine, treating fibroids involves decongesting the liver by using safe herbs that can be taken over an extended period of time, including dandelion and vitex berries. Vitex is particularly beneficial for fibrocystic disease because it lowers estrogen levels.

CHINESE HERBAL MEDICINE

Rist-Podrecca says the following herbs are good for stopping dysfunctional uterine bleeding when taken under the supervision of a Chinese herbal practitioner:

Poo wha. Made from bee pollen.

Er jow. From the hide of an animal.

Chuan xiong (*Ligusticum wallichi*). Regulates bleeding by the amount taken. Too much causes uterine bleeding, and too little stops it.

Han lian cao (warrior's grass). Helps tone the spleen and uterus and stops intense uterine bleeding.

ACUPUNCTURE

Acupuncture points that relate to the uterus are found on the ankle. Rist-Podrecca explains how electrical acupuncture to this area helps reduce fibroids: "We use a small electrical current. This makes the uterus contract and expand. It palpates the area slightly to get the body to recognize that the fibroids are there, increase circulation, and start vibrating the fibroids so that they are released."

HOMEOPATHY

Beth MacEoin, a homeopath and the author of *Homeopathy for Women,* as quoted in *Positive Health* magazine, says that since fibroids are a chronic condition, they are best treated by a practitioner. For acute symptoms, however, a number of remedies may be effective; these must be chosen based on whatever specific symptoms a woman is experiencing at a given moment. "The idea is that for a remedy to be active, the remedy chosen must match the symptoms as closely as possible. So it would be very important to select that remedy with the help of either a practitioner's support or a very good, solid self-help manual."

With that in mind, consider the following remedies for uterine bleeding and fibroids:

IPECAC. Dr. Marjorie Ordene, of Brooklyn, New York, recommends this remedy to stop acute hemorrhaging with bright red blood. "When given in the 200 potency, every 15 minutes, ipecac slows down the bleeding. That's two pellets under the tongue, until the bleeding actually stops. I have had success with a number of patients, and other physicians have reported this as well."

SHINA AND SABINA. Dr. Ken Korins says the two remedies to think of first for heavy bleeding are shina and sabina. Shina is for heavy, dark blood that forms clots and leads to debility and exhaustion. Sabina is also for clots, but here the blood is bright red. When large clots are being expelled, there is a laborlike pain that radiates from the sacrum to the pubis.

SECALE. Women who need secale have dark blood that is almost black. Periods are profuse and prolonged.

PHOSPHORUS. Phosphorus is indicated when there is bright red blood with no clots.

TRILLIUM. Trillium is indicated when bleeding is very heavy and bright red. The person characteristically feels faint and dizzy after bleeding. Periods occur biweekly, and the woman feels worse with even slight movement.

AURUM MURIATICUM. This remedy may reduce the size of fibroids. It should be used when there are no other symptoms, such as heavy bleeding, and there is no particular discomfort.

HYDRASTINUM MURIATICUM. This remedy has been known to cure large fibroids, especially when they seem to be on the anterior wall of the uterus, pushing on the bladder and causing symptoms of urinary frequency and pain.

Reproductive System Cancers

Women are susceptible to ovarian cancer, uterine or endometrial cancer, and carcinomas of the uterine cervix. Of the three, ovarian cancer occurs most often and is increasing in frequency. Uterine cancers are easier to detect in the beginning stages and tend to be more treatable, whereas ovarian cancers are rarely discovered early on, and are terribly damaging to the woman's quality of life.

OVARIAN CANCER

Women who are sedentary and don't exercise have an increased risk of ovarian cancer, explains Dr. Susanna Reid, a naturopathic physician at the Center of Natural Medicine at the Center for Women's Health in Darien, Connecticut. Dr. Reid also believes that being overweight, smoking—especially if you are postmenopausal—consuming alcohol and milk, eating meat (especially fried meat), and eating a diet lacking in fruits, vegetables, and fiber also increase the risk of ovarian cancer. The drug tamoxifen is associated with ovarian cancer, and hormone replacement therapy may also increase the risk of this cancer.

Ovarian cancer usually manifests after menopause, especially in women who have few or no children, were unable to conceive, or gave birth later than the average age. Other factors that place women at risk include a past history of spontaneous abortions, endometriosis, type A blood, radiation to the pelvic region, and exposure to cancer-causing chemicals, such as asbestos.

Women should look for the following early indications of ovarian carcinomas: abnormal vaginal bleeding, weight loss, and changes in patterns of urination and bowel movements. While a Pap smear will not detect ovarian cancer in the beginning stages, ovarian cancer can be diagnosed through annual pelvic exams.

Dr. Reid emphasizes therapies to help prevent reproductive cancers. Once reproductive cancer has appeared, she believes the role of natural medicine is to help heal the body after any surgery, for, she says, most reproductive cancers are not curable with natural remedies.

"I focus a lot on lifestyle. Fruits and vegetables have been shown in epidemiologic studies to protect against ovarian cancer, so I suggest that people put a lot of fruit and vegetables in their diet. Carotenoid-containing foods appear to specifically protect against ovarian cancer, carrot consumption in particular. Vegetable fiber is also important. Green vegetables and carrots seems to have a particular affinity for the ovaries and help protect them from reproductive cancers. Cruciferous vegetables in particular are very important in increasing natural killer cell toxicity. Whole grains also provide protection."

One of Dr. Reid's guiding principles is to have people return to natural or raw foods as much as possible. She says that animal products have a strong association with ovarian cancer and recommends eliminating animal products from the diet. "That even includes yogurt, which many people think is one of the best dairy products to eat. I don't think a person can be too careful. Ovarian cancer doesn't have a very positive prognosis, so if anything, a person should do too many things rather than not enough.

"Legumes seem to help as well and also help eliminate alcohol; wine consumption is associated with an increased risk of ovarian cancer. Although green tea isn't specific for ovarian cancer, it does act specifically on breast cancer, so that might be something a woman would want to add to her diet. Also, moderate exercise increases immune function and is an important aspect of treatment."

Dr. Reid says that women with ovarian cancer seem to have a problem with the antioxidative mechanism in their bodies, and suggests using antioxidants like vitamin E and selenium to help deal with oxidative conditions in the body. Indole-3-carbonyl may also be useful. "There is a new herb called *Camptotheca acuminata* that the National Cancer Institute is studying that seems to show some promise in the treatment of ovarian cancer."

CERVICAL CANCER

Cervical cancer is associated with cervical dysplasia. Although not all cervical dysplasia results in cancer, it can be the first stage of a malignancy.

Oral contraceptives and DES (diethylstilbestrol), reduced physical activity, multiple sexual partners or having the first intercourse at a young age, smoking, frequent douching, genital herpes, and multiple pregnancies are all associated with cervical cancer.

In the early stages of cervical cancer symptoms are usually absent, although there may be a watery vaginal discharge or spotty bleeding. Signs of advanced cervical cancer include dark, odorous vaginal discharges, fistulas, weight loss, and back and leg pain. One's chance of survival increases with early discovery through yearly Pap tests.

Dr. Reid warns that cervical cancer can begin as a chronic inflammation that, if not treated, becomes cervical dysplasia and eventually becomes cervical cancer. She says that cervical conditions may be related to a virus. "Natural medicine has a really good track record in treating cervical dysplasia before it gets to cancer. I would not treat cervical cancer with natural remedies. A woman would normally have the cervix removed surgically.

"To treat cervical dysplasia, we use a diet high in fiber as well as flax seeds, olives, and avocados. There is some recent research that shows that olives contain immune-enhancing substances. And of course, I recommend a lot of fruits and vegetables."

Dr. Reid also recommends using supplements and botanicals. These include folic acid, beta carotene, and vitamins E and C with bioflavonoids. She also has a six-week set protocol that utilizes suppositories. It begins with mild herbal suppositories, which she alternates with more intense herbal suppositories followed by a healing herbal suppository. In one study, 38 of 43 patients with cervical dysplasia using this treatment had their Pap smears revert to normal.

ENDOMETRIAL CANCER

Endometrial cancer is associated with hormones, including hormone replacement therapy with or without progesterone, a history of infertility, failure to ovulate, the use of drugs containing estrogen, and uterine growths. Tamoxifen is one drug that significantly increases the risk for endometrial cancer.

According to Dr. Reid, other risks include not having given birth to any children, beginning menopause after age 55, being overweight, using alcohol, and eating a diet high in calories, especially when you are postmenopausal. Eating meat and saturated fats—even fat from fish, especially processed fish—and low consumption of vegetables, fruit, fiber, and legumes, are also risk factors. Other poor dietary habits that increase risk are drinking soft drinks and consuming sugar. Oral contraceptives seem to decrease the risk of endometrial cancer.

The symptoms of endometrial cancer are abnormal bleeding in the vaginal area, especially after menopause, and pain in the lower abdomen or back. A Pap smear does not always catch endometrial cancer early, but the cancer can be detected with a surgical examination of the uterus.

As with other reproductive cancers, Dr. Reid believes that endometrial cancer has to be surgically treated. "It's not something that we would ever treat in natural medicine."

Dr. Reid says that natural treatment is focused on helping the patient heal from surgery. She uses therapies that facilitate healing, such as zinc and antioxidants and anti-inflammatories such as bioflavonoids and quercetin and bromelain. The specific therapy depends on how the surgery was done. "If it was done vaginally you can use hydrotherapy treatments on the abdomen. There is a time in during which you have to be quiescent because clots are setting, so you don't want to encourage bleeding. Patients should drink lots of fluids and eat very light foods, so their bowels are minimally taxed and their digestive systems can rest as the abdomen is healing."

COMBINATION TREATMENTS

Gar Hildebrand, president of the Gerson Research Organization in San Diego, California, says that more patients would triumph over reproductive system cancers if a combination of approaches was employed. This is the case because contemporary treatments for ovarian cancer are disappointing. While they can make cancers disappear for weeks or months at a time, they fail in the end as the cancer returns with a vengeance to finish the job. In fact, orthodox survival rates for ovarian cancer patients are only between 5 and 10 percent. Cancers of the uterine cervix initially exhibit higher success rates with surgery, which may involve the removal of the uterus (hysterectomy), as well as both ovaries and the fallopian tubes (salpingo-oophorectomy), in addition to x-ray and hormone therapies. But there is no guarantee that the cancer will not return. He states, "No one should be treated by a single specialty, and then watched in hopes that the cancer will not come back. It's not scientifically justifiable, nor is it acceptable to the patient. Sitting and waiting just causes horrible, immune-suppressing anxiety." Here Gar Hildebrand informs us about multiple modalities that work best for patients with ovarian and uterine cancers:

NUTRITION

"Let's say a woman with an ovarian cancer has just been admitted to Memorial Sloan Kettering Cancer Center. The first thing the doctors will do is a laparotomy. She will be opened up, and a surgeon will get the bulk of the tumor out. I have no problem with that.

"But the second step would definitely not be to use drugs that kill tumors. Tissue damage always accompanies cancer; unless it is addressed, the cancer is sure to reappear. In other words, throughout the body tumor toxins cause cells to lose potassium and swell with extra salt and water. This state is worse around the tumor itself. Often a treatment that goes into the bloodstream fails to penetrate to a tumor effectively because the tissue next to the tumor has no immunity. What's really needed, then, is for the patient to be stabilized physiologically. The ideal treatment would be for the person to receive nutritional salt and water management, a diet that nourishes and corrects the water retention in the cells. We're going to feed the whole body to try to get the tissues back to normal functioning."

Hildebrand recommends a diet that detoxifies and stimulates cells back to health. "Doctors have long been aware that most cancer patients have an aversion to meat. They'll smell it and gag; that's a self-defense mechanism. It's absolutely essential for these people to stop taking in heavy proteins—animal proteins and sometimes even heavy vegetable proteins like legumes—for a while, just to clear up. The tumor is converting that stuff into caustic chemicals, related to the ammonia we use in our laundry machines. It's those chemicals that create damage systemwide.

"We can also detoxify the body by supplying oodles of plant chemicals, called phytochemicals. These foods can be eaten cooked or raw, and should include vegetables of all sorts, fruits, and a few whole grains. Fruit and vegetable juices are especially important. You have to flood the system with nutritious fluids such as carrot and green leaf juices. Apple juice should always be added because apples contain a material that is very good for cellular energy. If you put those juiced phytochemicals into the body every hour, these cancer patients will have their cellular enzyme systems speeded up so that the individual cells can spit up toxins.

"Eating an excess of empty calories and proteins creates toxicity that causes the immune system to overproduce white blood cells that aren't very adept at what they do. Once you restrict protein and calories and get the nutrient level up, these patients' immune systems become intelligent again. They stop making excess stupid white cells and create more lymphocytes that are interested in more types of challenges. In other words, you get a very lean, mean immune system."

In addition to changes in diet, most patients need additional weapons in their fight for survival. Hildebrand explains why the following therapies are so important:

COFFEE ENEMAS

"These enemas have been used by thousands of cancer patients, outside the realm of traditional medical care, because they work. Boiled coffee in retention enemas stimulates the liver's enzyme system, which in turn causes great relief from pain in cancer patients. The liver has more than a thousand documented medical functions. When we help it work better and faster, a cancer patient's overall physiological condition changes, sometimes within hours and certainly within the first several weeks of treatment. You have a whole different person. People come off gurneys and out of beds, excruciating chronic pain is eased, and addiction to morphine is broken.

"Every three minutes, all the blood in our bodies goes through the liver. Our livers and small intestine walls have an enzyme system with a fancy name that we will call GST for short [GST refers to the glutathione S-transferases]. This enzyme system naturally responds to cancer in the body by going up, and coffee enemas have been shown in laboratory experiments with rats, and in later experiments with humans, to produce increased liver bile flow and to stimulate the GST enzyme system. In fact, it's raised to 700 percent of normal levels of activity. When the GST system is running that fast, it can effectively remove tumor toxins from the bloodstream. And it doesn't take very long. The effects of these coffee enemas will last for sometimes four, six, or eight hours before a feeling of discomfort and pain around the tumor returns. They're that effective.

"You have to know how much coffee to use: a quart of water with three tablespoons of coffee boiled in it. That's cooled and strained, not filtered, because a filter would remove some of the molecules that stimulate the GST enzyme system. The coffee is safely taken into the colon, while the person is lying on his or her right side, retained for 10 to 15 minutes, and then released.

Patients doing this without the supervision of a physician should know that anything cooler than 100 degrees is going to cause cramping in the intestines."

HYPERBARIC OXYGEN

Hildebrand states, "We're also going to try to increase circulation with full-body-immersion oxygen therapy. Hyperbaric oxygen treatment is given in a diving chamber that used to be used to treat the bends. There's been a lot of fascination with ozone in cancer treatment in the alternative field. But what we found is that ozone applications raise tissue oxygen only by 25 to 50 percent, whereas hyperbaric oxygen can predictably raise oxygenation by 800 to 1000 percent. This means that tissue around the tumor, which doesn't have enough oxygen to function, can get sufficient oxygen for energy production. This will also allow the tissue to repair itself by producing a high-potassium, low-sodium environment, so that this edema can come out of the tissue."

COLEY'S TOXINS

Hildebrand states that this treatment has the most glorious record of any treatment in the cancer literature, especially when combined with the Gerson diet program, consisting of hourly glasses of fresh juice and coffee enemas: "I am hopeful that much interest will be sparked in this therapy because right now the only reports I've seen of long-term survival for ovarian cancer patients have been from a combination of these approaches.

"The word 'toxin' is a little confusing, because Coley's toxin is not really a poison. It refers to a bacterial endotoxin that is an immune stimulant. I would put that directly into the abdominal cavity once the tissue around the tumor has been stabilized.

"Coley was a physician who searched the literature for cancer treatments after a heartbreaking experience of losing a child patient to the disease. Much to his surprise, he found a skin infection called erysipelas. Erysipelas is caused by a streptococcus that causes a skin fever of 105 to 106 degrees Fahrenheit. This fever causes an inflammatory infection which interferes with tumor action.

"Coley constructed a live erysipelas vaccine, which was too toxic at first. Some patients died, but others experienced a tumor regression. He went through a lot of trial and error and eventually settled on something which we now call *Serratia marsecens.* He mixed the *Serratia* and the strep in a ratio of 1,500 cells to one, and then crushed the mixture through a microfilter to liberate the internal toxins of the bacteria. This liberated antigens, which in turn caused the immune system of the patient to think that there was a chronic infection that had to be fought.

"The effectiveness of Coley's toxins seems to be due to the fact that the immune system, when turned on, can cause a lot of dust to rise. These patients need to be put into an intensive care unit and hooked up to monitors in case there is a problem, although there have never been any heart attacks or kidney failures reported in the 900 cases that have been thoroughly studied. Then a tiny amount of toxins is administered intravenously for four hours through a drip. About two hours into the process, the immune response begins. The patient will develop chills and shaking that last for about half an hour to 90 minutes, followed by a rise in temperature of about a degree every 10 minutes. Once that temperature hits 105 or 106, the ICU staff lies the patient down or puts in a suppository of Tylenol to stop it.

"The reaction is the immune system's response. This is not a poison. This is not a toxin. It's not like chemotherapy making your hair fall out or causing bone marrow suppression. The Coley's toxins are much more like what happens when your immune system decides to cure you of an infection. So the symptoms are more flulike, without the nausea and vomiting. After the second or third IV application, patients usually get sleepy and actually nod off. The fever lessens progressively. In other words, there's a honeymoon period.

"Coley himself said that if you don't keep these up for at least three or four months, in booster dosages, you won't get a permanent response. The literature reveals that gains are lost when Coley's toxins are given in lower concentrations or for shorter durations. But when they are properly used, there is an extraordinary 50 percent cure rate in advanced, inoperable uterine and ovarian cancers."

THE BENEFITS OF AN OVERALL APPROACH

Gar Hildebrand reemphasizes the importance of utilizing any and every cancer protocol that works: "We believe that it's time we stopped living in an either/or world where orthodoxy is over on one side and the marginalized alternative professions are in the trenches and foxholes, and nobody talks. We believe it's time to get the doors and windows of communication open so that we can find the context for each of these treatments and the way they fit together. Our own experience reveals that using the nutritional approach takes a toxic load off the immune system and speeds up intracellular enzymes so that they can repel toxins and pull them from the blood rapidly. Calorie and protein restrictions and a diet high in nutrients can lead to the sensitization of a tumor. Years of experience show that diet therapy alone can produce monthly fevers, and tumors may or may not regress through those fevers. But if you stimulate the immune system when those fevers are hitting, you have a much greater chance of tumor reduction. That's why we suggest the marriage of these disciplines and the respectful recognition of the role of every aspect of anticancer medicine that's ever been developed."

Patient Stories

MORGAN: CERVICAL CANCER

I still have cervical cancer, but I am working on overcoming it through a number of approaches. I watch my diet very carefully. I feel that my condition is in an early enough stage where I can handle it nutritionally. But it's not just nutrition that I have to deal with. I have to deal with all the emotions that help to create disease in the body. It's also a matter of detoxing. I do colonics and a lot of juicing. I take supplements. And I do meditation, and exercise.

The major reason I started to see a nutritionist was, of course, the wake-up call, the cervical cancer, which was just diagnosed three months ago. But I had also had ulcerative colitis for almost 20 years.

I feel like I now have energy again. I exercise at least several times a week, which was literally impossible before. I even had trouble getting up a flight of subway steps without feeling exhausted at the top. So I have several different things that I am working with: nutrition, meditation, and detoxification. I'm working on it.

"Now I have to find a gynecologist who is holistically oriented because my primary care physician dropped me after I refused to have a hysterectomy. I feel very lucky. I feel that someone else trying to deal with this would have followed the recommended course of action and would have given up her reproductive rights, allowing herself to be mutilated, and always being fearful of having the cancer reappear.

Also, I feel that the cancer is nothing more than a wake-up call. Your body is saying, "Hey, something is wrong here. You're out of balance. You need to address this, this and this." If you don't, disease is the end result. Now I am vegetarian and doing a lot of things differently. If I didn't, I might not be alive now. I might be at a higher risk for the cancer to spread throughout more of the body. This doesn't mean that I am 100 percent there. I still have a lot of work to do. But I feel very hopeful.

A PATIENT OF GAR HILDEBRAND'S: OVARIAN CANCER

The ability of diet therapy to produce tumor regression in ovarian cancer is best illustrated by the experience of a woman named Leslie. This woman had an omentectomy, a bilateral salpingo-oophorectomy, and a complete hysterectomy. She had tumors all over the inside of the back wall of the abdomen, on the pelvis, and on other organ structures, which were left for chemotherapy. But she declined the chemo and tried dietary therapy.

Several weeks later, this woman had a sudden fever response. It hit fast and was so debilitating that she could not even move. This is a classic reaction to diet therapy that patients sometimes have. Her husband put her to bed; he stopped measuring her temperature and started icing her down at 105 degrees. Leslie had this fever for 24 hours. When it was gone she said, "I know I'm going to be okay. I know I'm going to be fine." Today, Leslie is alive and well, and living in Florida with her husband.

Chapter 8

Chronic Fatigue Syndrome

Some of you may remember the preface to Charles Baudelaire's *Fleurs du Mal* (Flowers of Evil). Baudelaire was a premier poet of modernism, one of the first to put his hand on the pulse of what we now consider the contemporary condition, at least for urban dwellers: continual agitation, distraction, and resentment and a life lived under a bombardment of toxins and media inanity so fierce that it can wreck one's health and sanity. Baudelaire begins by saying that he intended to pick up his pen to write a long essay, but when his eye fell on the front-page headlines of a tabloid on his café table, he was overcome by such lassitude that he couldn't lift a finger. Such unbearable fatigue is often a product of modern society's overstimulating environment and soup of pollutants. One disease related to this situation, whose roots reach back to the mid-nineteenth century when Baudelaire was writing, is chronic fatigue syndrome.

This chapter will look at the current understanding of ths disease, whose origin and definition are a matter of controversy, and then at some of the treatments that have proved useful.

Chronic fatigue syndrome poses a major problem for traditional medicine. The medical establishment has fumbled in its treatment to the point of sometimes claiming that the illness does not exist, but chronic fatigue is a major problem in the United States. Millions lack the energy they once had, ranging from people who have just a little bit of energy to those who are maximally depleted, in bed and unable to function.

In 1988 the Centers for Disease Control (CDC) in Atlanta, Georgia, devised the term "chronic fatigue syndrome" to describe a state of constant exhaustion. Chronic fatigue syndrome—a syndrome is a disorder that includes a collection of symptoms but is not necessarily a disease entity—is quite similar to certain other disorders that have been known for centuries. In the nineteenth century, for example, a common complaint of middle-class women was neurasthenia, which was characterized by chronic exhaustion and a variety of other physical symptoms.

Dr. Neenyah Ostrom, author of *America's Biggest Cover-Up,* emphasizes that chronic fatigue syndrome is very difficult for the average doctor to diagnose, especially because the CDC's definition of it is so misleading that nobody can figure out what the illness is supposed to be. In late November 1995 there was a meeting at the CDC to discuss changing this definition. It turned out that researchers wanted to define it out of existence so that anyone who was tired could be said to have chronic fatigue syndrome.

Ostrom argues, "If you speak to any clinicians who see people with this condition, they will tell you it is very easy to diagnose. They can tell within moments of talking to a patient whether the patient has it, since the symptom complex is unique."

Why is it that for years Americans with a debilitating illness were not recognized as having a disease? They were simply told that chronic fatigue syndrome does not exist. Dr. Dean Black says, "If you go back to the last century, you can read about women suffering from nervous disorders—so many of them that clinics had to be set up to care for them. There was always the search for a cause, but one couldn't be found, and so, without a cause, doctors wouldn't say it was a disease. It had to be in the patient's mind. This is not a new way of sweeping things under the carpet."

Dr. Ostrom comments, "Since there are debates in the government on whether chronic fatigue syndrome exists, very few therapies have been tested for chronic fatigue patients."

Dr. Black brings up another historical example to explain traditional medicine's current difficulties in coming to grips with chronic fatigue syndrome. He says we need to go back to the origin of the current paradigm in the seventeenth century, when René Descartes promulgated his doctrine of universal doubt, which held that one could know nothing without using the scientific method: "People would say things to Descartes, but he would explain them away, saying, 'I can see this, this, or this equally plausible alternative.' He felt we could know things for certain only if we had a scientific method whereby we could define truth in a rational cause-and-effect manner. Now, that method had a certain number of rules, one being that there had to be a straight line between a single cause and a single effect. Deviate from that and you introduce so much complexity that the idea of certainty is lost.

"Medicine's power base is the idea of its basis in certainty, which hinges on the concept of a single linear cause-and-effect relationship. That's why medicine is always looking for a single causal factor. This is called the theory of specific etiology."

Dr. Black compares the situation of chronic fatigue syndrome to that of the Epstein-Barr (EB) virus, which was initially thought to cause chronic fatigue syndrome, although later this theory was challenged. "That is why they were so happy to discover this EB virus," he explains. "It seemed marvelous to them because it served to justify the single-cause idea. Yet, as has been frequently pointed out, everyone may have Epstein-Barr [it is so widely distributed]. Chronic fatigue syndrome is caused by many factors operating together. But this idea has been excluded by traditional medicine, which refuses to come to grips with multifactorially generated disease. Medicine is reluctant to accept this multifactorial explanation because it holds to this idea of absolute truth, which requires simplicity and must have one cause and one effect."

Dr. Andrew Gentile stresses that we need to be able to differentiate between chronic fatigue syndrome and other health problems: "Since chronic fatigue syndrome has no known cause, we need to rule out other disorders whose cause we do know. The working definition provided by the government for this disease says there is no other illness at the root of it. Differentiating it calls for great care, since fatigue is ubiquitous as a symptom of many diseases, such as anemia, low thyroid, hypoglycemia, and a variety of other illnesses. These other illnesses must be clearly ruled out."

Symptoms

Dr. Gentile calls chronic fatigue syndrome a degenerative disorder that causes fatigue and usually begins after the onset of flulike symptoms. The fatigue is not a simple tiredness; it is an exhaustion accompanied by feelings of unwellness. Many people have difficulty getting out of bed and may become weakened to the point of needing to lie down all the time. Often patients are bedridden for months; extreme tiredness can last for years.

Chronic fatigue syndrome may be accompanied by depression, irritability, headaches, low-grade fever, infection, confusion, focusing difficulties, spaciness, diarrhea, sharp muscle pain and weakness, swollen glands, and sleep disorders. The patient is not able to fall asleep or stay asleep and does not feel refreshed or restored even after much sleep.

As Dr. Gentile describes them, "Patients will go from one room to another, and when they get to the new space, they cannot remember why they are there. They cannot remember the name of a colleague they worked with for years. There are difficulties with concentration and an inability to read complex texts. So there are cognitive symptoms, sleep disorder, flulike symptoms, frequent sore throats, tender lymph nodes, and often fevers and chills."

Causes

VIRAL POSSIBILITIES

Although many resist the multicausal explanation for chronic fatigue, as Dr. Gentile notes, some healers have been able to develop such an explanation: "There is now the feeling that a single cause is not sufficient, and moreover, in the world of treatment it is now much more productive to work on caring for the symptoms than on continuing a quixotic search for a single cause. Healing is really the charge of medical research."

Dr. Martin Feldman tells us that chronic fatigue syndrome involves severe fatigue with a 50 percent reduction in capacity. There is a continuum of fatigue problems, and chronic fatigue is on the low end. "One will find two factors involved," he states. "First, there is a flulike infection, either a new or a renewed one, and often, though not necessarily, a history of such infections, whereby the viral mix—for there may well be more than one virus involved—weakens the immune system. The second point is that this immune system difficulty somehow pulls down hormonal function. Almost all patients with this syndrome have low adrenal function, and many have low thyroid function. So we have a hormonal mix-up causing fatigue, but behind this is the viral disease pulling down the immune system."

According to Ostrom, what is probably behind the chronic fatigue disorder is a virus that was first found in AIDS patients. It is called human herpes virus 6 (HHV-6): "What is interesting is that there are two types of this virus. One form is found very widely in the general population, and the other is found in people with cancer, AIDS, chronic fatigue syndrome, and other immunological problems. That virus can attack the immune system very effectively, and I believe it will eventually be found to be instrumental in causing chronic fatigue syndrome, AIDS, and some forms of cancer."

Dr. Gentile adds that a plethora of studies have looked at viruses in connection with this syndrome. One theory posits a single viral agent. In fact, he states, "I have heard chronic fatigue syndrome being called a number of things from Epstein-Barr to mononucleosis.

"Epstein-Barr was brought into the discussion by way of a lab in Philadelphia that exclusively studies this virus. One of the lab assistants was negative for current and acute Epstein-Barr virus, but during the course of the study the assistant developed the symptoms of chronic fatigue syndrome. He was treated and found to be positive for Epstein-Barr virus. So we had the first studied case in which a person went from Epstein-Barr-negative to Epstein-Barr-positive at the same time that he had all the symptomatology for chronic fatigue syndrome. That began a flurry of studies investigating the Epstein-Barr connection. We now know there is not a high degree of correlation between the symptoms of chronic fatigue syndrome and Epstein-Barr serological titers. So Epstein-Barr is probably not the cause of chronic fatigue syndrome."

Dr. Gentile goes on to note that the EB virus is widely distributed in the populace. Most people have it by age 8. Thus, there is no clear distinction between those who have it and those who do not. We would expect many more people to be ill with chronic fatigue if it were indeed Epstein-Barr that was causing it. As a result, this candidate for being the cause of chronic fatigue syndrome has fallen into disfavor.

"However," he persists, "several other candidates have presented themselves, including HHV-6 (formerly called HBLT), a B-lymphocyte virus that was studied by the National Institutes of Health. But again, studies showed that this virus is very widely distributed and thus could not be the distinguishing agent responsible for the syndrome. Other studies are proceeding. Wistar, a renowned laboratory in Philadelphia, is looking at a retrovirus, HTLV-2,[human T-cell lymphotropic virus] as a possible cause."

Dr. Neil Block reminds us that quite a few viruses have been implicated in some forms of fatigue syndrome. These viruses include, along with EB, herpes virus, Coxsackie virus, adenovirus, and enterovirus as well as a number of lesser known ones. He echoes Dr. Gentile in saying, "The one that has received the most attention, Epstein-Barr, has not panned out as an answer, and indeed, in some sufferers it plays either a very minor role or no role at all. But it can't be dismissed. And most cases deserve to be tested with an Epstein-Barr viral titer to determine the antibody status, whether there is or has been current or past infection with the Epstein-Barr virus."

Other viruses that have been implicated are the hepatitis virus and the influenza virus, which have been known to cause fatigue two or three months after the original virus has disappeared.

Dr. Majid Ali says, "It's very enlightening to look at Epstein-Barr. I come from Pakistan, and for us Epstein-Barr was not a kissing disease. Because of poor sanitation, all of us were exposed to the virus as children. But we came through the exposure with intact immune systems. Our immune systems fought off the Epstein-Barr, and we acquired a certain resistance. In this country people will get infectious mono or Epstein-Barr (those are the same thing) later. They get it in college or high school. It's the so-called kissing disease. They will be sick for four or five weeks and lose some weight. They'll be tired for some months and then snap back."

However, he states, there is a different possible scenario. "Think of people in their thirties and forties with good jobs. They are not fit and are under tremendous stress. Their nutrition is awful, and now along comes Epstein-Barr, and it floors them. The problem," Dr. Ali states, "is not that Epstein-Barr is more virulent; the problem is that their molecular defenses are shattered. Their bodily ecosystems are destroyed, and so they have no ability to fight back. So whether

Epstein-Barr is a devastating terminal attack on their immune system or a garden-variety illness they can easily get over depends on the state of their previous health. You give Epstein-Barr to little children, and they generally survive very well. In fact, they generally don't even know they have this disease. So the issue is not the power of the virus but that of our defenses."

Dr. Gentile states, "The consensus among practitioners is that a single virus probably does not cause this illness. We have to carefully distinguish between cause and trigger. Clearly, a virus may trigger a cascading set of events in various body systems: neural, endocrine, cognitive, hormonal. A variety of abnormalities may be found in these systems, but if viruses do trigger these imbalances, then they quickly hide within the normal cells—which is usually how viruses behave—while their effects wreak havoc in the body system."

It is as if the virus triggered something in the immune system that makes the system unable to self-regulate and find its way back to homeostasis. Thus, each time the immune system is stressed by a toxic load from the environment or food allergies or when infections are reactivated, there is a breakdown. The flare-ups and relapses occur and recur frequently, reproducing all the symptoms. These relapses then compound themselves. If a patient is not sleeping every night, symptoms such as exhaustion and a deranged immune system crop up.

"We know, by the way," Dr. Gentile adds, "that the rhythms of this illness dovetail nicely with 90-minute circadian rhythms. In sleep, we have a REM [rapid eye movement] cycle that occurs every 90 minutes, and this is the cycle by which our immune system is synthesizing proteins. The immune system works lock and key with this cycle. But if one has a sleep disturbance caused by a virus or a set of viruses from this disorder, one's sleep will be off and so the immune system will be off."

ENVIRONMENTAL FACTORS AND ALLERGIES

As we saw, Dr. Ali sees the surrounding environment and lifestyle as playing causal roles. He says that the immune system becomes injured by environmental pollutants such as mold, formaldehyde, and pesticides as well as by allergenic foods or by poor nutrition, stress, and a lack of physical fitness. He gives equal emphasis to all four areas.

Dr. Shari Lieberman, a professor at the University of Bridgeport School of Nutrition, expands on this point. She has published articles and several books, including *The Real Vitamin and Mineral Book.*

She begins bluntly: "We as a country are not healthy. We have all these discussions, lectures, books, and so on, concerning a healthy lifestyle. We have the information, but we are not actualizing it. I don't think people understand how all of the body's circumstances are impacted by the immune system."

She goes on to specify why weak immune systems are so prevalent: "Number one is that we have all this technology and all this food, but we are really starving ourselves, because we are eating food that is nutritionally poor," that is, doesn't have enough antioxidants. This includes the well-known ones, such as vitamin E and C, selenium, and beta carotene. People should also be getting the antioxidants that are less well known, such as lycopene, quercetin, bromelain, and catachin. She says, "We have a plethora of plant compounds in our available foods that we are simply not eating. What does your average American eat today? Fast foods and other foods that don't contain much nutrition. So the foundation for repair is pretty lousy. We don't have the functioning mechanisms in place because we don't have the nutrients to fuel those mechanisms.

"I'm sure," she goes on, "that people have heard about antioxidants and oxidative stress and free radicals many times, but they don't understand that free radicals and oxidative stress can damage any of our cells. If we think of macular disorders, we see that these radicals can damage your eyes. They will damage your arteries and cause coronary artery disease and so on. However, the other crucial thing is that they can actually damage immune cells. They can oxidize white blood cells; they can oxidize killer cells."

Antioxidants can stop oxidative stress from destroying our immune cells: "Oxidative stress will actually form like a rust on the cells. These cells will die. They'll be obliterated. The antioxidants, by contrast, can augment our existing immune functions. They will stop these free radicals from damaging the components of the immune system such as the T cells, the macrophages, the lymphocytes, and the other white blood cells."

Dr. Michele Galante also believes that allergies are important: "The patients I have seen have been very allergic not only to pollens and airborne agents but especially to foods and chemicals. These people are so sensitive and so debilitated that a short exposure to perfume, nail polish, gas fumes, carbon monoxide, or even just paint, such as from a freshly painted room, will give them headaches, make them weak, even make them emotionally upset. Chronic fatigue syndrome is closely connected to allergy."

Ostrom seconds this notion. People with chronic fatigue syndrome often develop allergies they never had before. For instance, they will exhibit violent allergic reactions to medicines and show new food sensitivities: "In patients with chronic fatigue syndrome (and AIDS as well), a portion of the immune system shuts down, while another portion, which causes immune reactions, is revved up almost 100 percent. These people respond immunologically to things that their immune system would not have recognized before they got sick.

"Some of these allergy-causing substances are unavoidable. Chemicals in our environment, aside from those in our foods (coloring, preservatives, and so on), are everywhere. There is chlorine in our water; the air is filled with pollutants—things that were not in our ecological system 50 or 60 years ago. Recent phenomena that accompany technological advances, such as the mercury in silver amalgam dental work, are weakening our systems. Each of these chemicals in itself does not necessarily have so strong an impact, but exposure to all of them together, day after day, for many years, overloads the liver and immune system. Electromagnetic influences, previously ignored, are now also under discussion. Many believe the cathode rays from computers affect the electromagnetic fields of the body, for instance, as does the electromagnetism of cellular phones, radio waves, and television waves—things relatively new to our environment."

FOODS AND YEAST INFECTIONS

Dr. Ali sees children with fatigue and attention deficit disorders: "Tests will show that the child is allergic to wheat, dairy, peanuts, sugar. The doctor tells the mom she has to change everything she feeds him, and she is ready to collapse. But talk to her six or nine months later, once she knows all the other wonderful food options she has, and she is happy. The child resisted at first, but then his problems began to clear up. Halloween came, and he nose-dived. He began to clear up again. Thanksgiving, he nose-dived. Christmas, he nose-dived."

Dr. Galante also focuses on food, pointing to processed foods, white sugar, white flour, hydrogenated products, and chemicalized food as lacking vitality. People are eating these foods in far too great a quantity. Through food therapies which remove these foods, he has seen relief from hypoglycemic reactions such as mood swings and manic depressive symptoms, at least in the less severe cases.

Another problem in chronic fatigue syndrome is *Candida*, both external and internal. But Dr. Ali reminds us not to go looking for a doctor to cure us of yeast since it is always present in our bodies: "You do not want to get rid of it but instead achieve 'gut balance' and restore the gut ecosystem." *Candida* is just one possible problem; he tests for the nine different kinds of yeast.

METABOLIC REGULATION

Chronic fatigue syndrome can also be explained in terms of immune system depression related to a failure in metabolic regulation. When glucose production is up, it brings on hypoglycemia, with a high degree of glucose in the blood causing an increased level of insulin, which lowers the glucose level excessively. Because of poor utilization of glucose, fatty acids increase in the blood to provide a sufficient level of energy. A high level of triglycerides will occur, and the immune system will be depressed because it needs a new army of T lymphocytes, which are not being produced because of derangement in lipid metabolism.

VITAMIN AND HORMONAL DEFICIENCY

Dr. Neil Block connects these problems to lifestyle. Those who do not have the best lifestyle, such as smokers and drinkers, and those who do not breathe the best air often lack B nutrients, and this affects the immune system. Even if you are taking a number of vitamin B pills, make sure you are on a multi-B regimen so that none of the B vitamins become scarce in the body.

Lack of vitamins C and E and beta carotene can also affect your immune system, as can a lack of minerals, particularly calcium, vanadium, copper, magnesium, potassium, molybdenum, boron, iodine, selenium, and chromium. The trace minerals are especially important for organ function.

Dr. Block also points to hormonal imbalances, particularly thyroid imbalance (especially hypothyroidism), which is found in females in a prevalence of 6 to 1 over males. It tends to develop spontaneously between the ages of 20 and 50, although it can come at any time, often from unknown causes. The rare causes, which are the ones known for this disease, involve either a superabundance or a deficiency of iodine in the body, although the latter is unlikely in our society, where we have iodized salt and other sources. Another rare cause is consuming too many of certain vegetables, such as cauliflower, broccoli, and Brussels sprouts, which tend to bind the active ingredient and inhibit thyroxin production.

Other hormones frequently out of the normal range include the adrenal hormones. "There are a number of tests we can run for this, none of which is perfect," Dr. Block continues, "for we have to remember that the adrenal gland is really two glands in one. On the inside, the adrenal medulla is making adrenaline and noradrenaline, and the outer coating, the adrenal cortex, is making cortisonelike substances that are related to our immune system and blood sugar control as well as corticoid steroids. The last thing the adrenal cortex is important for is modulating the male and female hormones that are in conversation with the pituitary gland and primary sexual organs. And, lastly, some chronic fatigue syndrome patients have imbalances in gender hormones. It is not unusual to have imbalances in the estrogen that governs the ovarian function or in other governors, such as LH [luteinizing hormone] from the pituitary gland or progesterone." In fact, women frequently come to Dr. Block with lack of menstruation, milky discharge from the breast, breast tenderness, or more menstrual cramps than usual. And every month one or two men come who are low in blood testosterone.

DRUG USE

Dr. Galante remarks, "The allopathic drugs, conventional drugs, antibiotics, and steroid usage are major influences. The use and abuse of hese drugs in childhood, for example, sets up chronically weakened conditions that will extend into adulthood and contribute to a predisposition for chronic fatigue. These drugs are suppressive in nature, not curative. They themselves impose an illness on the system. This may be one of the largest of the causal factors."

Dr. Ali talks about a young person suffering from chronic fatigue syndrome who went to a medical clinic and was given a prescription for steroids. We know steroids suppress the immune system, so why would anyone give these drugs to someone with this disorder? Steroids can create a sense of well-being and euphoria for a couple of days, but it is false. An unenlightened patient will take the steroids; an enlightened one will reject them.

PSYCHOLOGICAL FACTORS

Dr. Gentile tells us that chronic fatigue seems to reduce stress tolerance. Sufferers cannot exert themselves or they will relapse into fatigue if they try to walk or swim. He has had patients who were marathoners before contracting the illness. They report that they had been working hard and then got sick with fever and chills. The illness waxed and waned. They would feel better at times and go back to running but then quickly relapse. These patients cannot tolerate stress in either thephysical or the psychological form. Stress will exacerbate the illness again and again.

Dr. Block adds that these stresses that affect chronic fatigue syndrome patients are the same ones that affect us in everyday life. They cause faltering in many bodily systems, such as the neurotransmitters, which are missed in examinations by many doctors who are not aware of gamma-aminobutyric acid (GABA), dopamine, serotonin, and other neurotransmitter chemical levels.

According to Dr. Paul Epstein, a key tenet of naturopathic medicine is to treat the underlying cause: "A person diagnosed with chronic fatigue syndrome has a suppressed immune system, which can be documented by blood tests and other measures. But what caused this? It may be improper diet; then the patient will need to eat properly. But we also need to ask why he adopted that diet in the first place. If the answer is stress, we can then ask what caused the person to follow certain patterns of reaction to stress. As we treat the patient, going through all the different problems layered one on top of the other, we eventually get in contact with the person's core self.

"One way to make this contact is through the inner child. Many people have been influenced by John Bradshaw's work on recovering and healing the inner child and on seeing how the wounds and scars of childhood may have led us to create lifestyles that are addictive. Thus, even as I help the person medically by giving advise on diet, stress reduction, and so on, I remember this. If we do not touch deeper problems, healing may not occur."

Clinical Experience

DIAGNOSIS

Dr. Michael Vesselago, former chief medical resident at the Virginia Mason Medical Center in Seattle, Washington, uses laboratory tests to diagnose his patients and then treats them accordingly. He looks for viruses and for excess *Candida* as well as for allergies and stress: "I test the person for allergies with an IgE RAST [radioallergosorbent test] and get back a report showing how the body responds to over 100 tested foods. We adjust the diet so that the person is no longer eating allergy-causing foods, and that alone brings about a significant improvement in over 70 percent of individuals.

"If someone collapses unduly fast or wakes up tired and requires several cups of coffee to get going, then I will focus on the adrenals first. I do a test for adrenal function that involves checking cortisol, which is one of the main adrenal hormones. From that I get a picture of how well the adrenal glands are coping with stress during the day."

Dr. Martin Feldman says that the first step in the analysis of any patient who comes to him with fatigue, whether mild, moderate, or severe, is to profile the patient to see how she or he fits with the five major problems associated with the syndrome. Almost all people with chronic fatigue syndrome have at least one of these problems, and so they are a good place to begin tests. These five indicators are as follows:

1. An immune viral breakdown, leading to low adrenal function: "You'll find that almost all chronic fatigue syndrome people have low adrenal function once you test the adrenals properly."
2. Thyroid imbalance: "A large proportion, though a little less than half, have these issues."
3. Vitamin B deficiency.
4. Hypoglycemia.
5. Cerebral allergies.

After doing these tests Dr. Feldman tests the thymus, spleen, and lymphatic system. "It's very easy, yet very hard, to test the thymus because you have to use electrical energy," he says. "You could test the T- and B-cell counts. That's easy to do, but it's very expensive, so in daily practice it's easier to test thymus electrical energy. You can also do this for the spleen. When we find a weak thymus circuit, we can try any aspect of therapy within the weakened circuit to obtain a resonance that will help strengthen that circuit."

Dr. Gentile is more concerned with self diagnosis: "If you feel you have chronic fatigue syndrome, ask yourself these questions:

➤ Do I not just feel tired but have had debilitating fatigue for six months?
➤ Do I have flulike symptoms?
➤ Have I not found any physiological cause?
➤ Do I have pronounced sleeplessness?
➤ Do I have low stress tolerance so that if I take a short walk or try any sport, I feel vaguely ill and tired?

If you answer yes, you may want to consider a fuller assessment of yourself by a physician."

Dr. Majid Ali states that most physicians have a tendency to focus narrowly on one or two aspects of a problem. But, he says, "I don't think trying to find a diagnosis for one or two symptoms is terribly important. What is important is how the patient describes his or her suffering. We need to think of what we can do at a molecular and energetic level to relieve his or her suffering and restore his or her health.

"I've seen patients whose lives have been devastated by chronic fatigue syndrome. They've gone through all these drugs, antivirals, steroids. With each drug, they get better initially and then nose-dive. What do we do?

"Think of chess. In chess, the queen is the most powerful and the pawn is the weakest piece. But as a good chess player knows, there are many games in which the lowliest piece, the pawn, can take that all-powerful queen. This can be done by a player who is able to 'read the board.' And I think what a good holistic physician has to be able to do is read the board , that is, look at the patient's whole situation and then, as a doctor, ask yourself: 'Should I first work on the kitchen, what the patient eats, or should I first work on self-regulation, control of breathing, and so on, or must I first create some hope, make the patient talk to other recovering patients and take a workshop?'" Making the correct choice of initial therapies should take precedence over minutely analyzing the symptoms.

FINDING THE RIGHT TREATMENT

The key to finding treatment for chronic fatigue syndrome, according to Dr. Gentile, is choosing an empathetic expert who believes the disease exists: "It has reached the level of scientific respectability, and most practitioners and medical examiners believe it exists. It is important to have someone who is up to date on the literature and who has seen at a minimum 50 to100 patients, someone who understands the ups and downs of the disease and is aware of the number of different treatments that have developed."

He points out several ways to locate a credible expert. For one thing, there are chronic fatigue syndrome support groups in every major town in our country and now worldwide that have lists of physicians who have tended to specialize in the disorder. There are national groups such as the Chronic Fatigue Syndrome Association. They maintain a list of doctors who understand the disease and have treated it and are sympathetic and believing.

"This last trait is so important," Dr. Galante explains, "because many sufferers have gone through scores of doctors. We're treating a woman now who has already seen 75 physicians all over the world. She was ready to give up because she feels people do not believe her. So a critical part of treating this illness is belief. A second thing to bear in mind is that because this is a chronic illness with a wide range of symptoms, it will tend to fall between the cracks of all the medical subspecializations. With this disease, it will not be adequate to go to a single physician. It would be worth considering putting together a team, which would include a GP/internist, one who works both with traditional and alternative therapies; an allergist/infectious disease specialist; and a psychologist/psychiatrist. This team could coordinate to work out a treatment plan, working so that the client understands what is coming next. And if these treatments don't work, they could determine why that might be and what would be worth trying next."

THE SPIRITUAL ELEMENT

Dr. Ali tells us that in dealing with a chronic, devastating illness like this, hope and the spiritual element are essential for long-term success. He has had case histories that truly stretch the bounds of credulity: "Creating hope is very easy to do; sustaining hope is difficult, but it is central to healing. Before I see a patient, he or she has seen at least seven specialists. They've had biopsies, CAT [computed tomography] scans. When they come to me, it's not that easy to simply reassure them that they'll get better after they've seen the previous failures. But fortunately, by the time they get to me, they've listened to some of our tapes, read our books, and, most important, talked to some of the other patients who have gotten better. So when they come in, and they've seen our nursing staff, our ancillary staff, they see we are all serious. If they ask how my program differs, we say this: They do not have the option to remain sick."

SUPPLEMENTS

Another significant treatment mode uses supplements. The hope, according to Dr. Lieberman, is not only to repair damage and stabilize the weakened immune system of a chronic fatigue sufferer but to overboost the system:

"Consider the fact that we have all these pollutants in our environment and are exposed to all these viruses. Can we do anything not just to repair but to augment our immune systems? This is going beyond just stopping the damage and trying to superfortify the system. A decade ago to talk about this was heresy, and it was considered a ridiculous direction to try to go. Now we have hundreds of scientific studies that have shown that higher levels of specific nutrients can boost immune function."

One of the most famous studies looked at vitamins E and C: "They didn't do it with older folks, since there are so many studies showing that if we give nutrients to the elderly population, we clearly get improvement and immune-enhancing benefits. But what about younger people from their twenties to forties whose immune systems are under siege? Those younger people were the subjects of this study, which was published in the *American Journal of Clinical Nutrition*.

"It looks at the effects of giving 400 IU of vitamin E and 1,000 mg of vitamin C over the course of a year," she explains. "What they did was very interesting. They gave vitamin E alone to some subjects and saw that it boosted immune function beyond its normal level. Then they gave vitamin C alone and found that it too boosted immune function. But when they gave them together, the resulting immune boosting far exceeded what happened when either one of the nutrients was given alone."

Lots of studies have looked at the synergy between different antioxidants: "So if you really want to do this and achieve an improved immune system, take the supplements together. Bear in mind that if you just take one antioxidant, if you just take vitamin C or just vitamin E, you are not going to get the benefit you would from taking these things together."

At Dr. Ali's clinic I watched a nurse making up an intravenous (IV) chronic fatigue syndrome protocol with vitamin C, magnesium sulfate, pantethine, calcium, pyridoxine, and a multivitamin formula. She says that patients who come in are very tired and have joint pains, headaches, and memory loss. These IVs help repair cell membranes and boost the immune system, which will then hopefully function better. About 90 percent of her patients have responded well. Dr. Ali will usually order a set of five to begin with, she says, and after that he can measure the patient's response, see how deep the problem is and whether she requires further drugs.

"I see these drips as jump-starting the cellular enzymes," Ali says. "The enzymes, which are detoxification enzymes, are dependent on minerals and vitamins. If I feel there is enough time, when the patient is not acutely ill or has been chronically ill for a number of years, I will try to use a more conservative approach. But when I see people with severe, incapacitating fatigue, I use the IV. In fact, in one of our studies where we compared one group that had the IV and one group that didn't, we saw that the IV speeds up the recovery process."

Dr. Ali continues, "We have 14 different formulations or protocols to manage different clinical problems in our IV drips. For chronic fatigue syndrome, we use vitamin C, magnesium, calcium, pyridoxine, pantethine, zinc, B vitamins, molybdenum, potassium, copper, and selenium. Most of our protocols have 15 to 18 items, and we change their quantities depending on the individual's state."

Ostrom notes that the antioxidants with vitamins C, E, and A are efficacious in treating chronic fatigue syndrome, as they are with AIDS, since both conditions involve the same immunological battle. In these cases the systems are under fierce attack from free radicals, viruses, and in some cases bacteria. The supplements help reequilibrate and repair damage done by the molecules and help boost the immune system.

"First, we have to get the vitamins really right," Dr. Feldman says, "since they are the building blocks of the immune system. People suffering from chronic fatigue syndrome are deficient in such things as vitamins A, B5, B_{12}, and E; bioflavonoids; the essential fatty acids; zinc; selenium; and GLA (gamma-linoleic acid). All those must be put into order before we can proceed further."

Dr. Lieberman gives additional recommendations: "First, for immune boosting, I would say take vitamin E, making sure it's the natural alpha form. A preventive range would be between 400 and 1,200 IU per day."

Next is beta carotene: "With the fat-soluble vitamins, make sure they are natural. The natural ones do work differently, and their biological activity is much higher. There are many natural beta-carotene supplements available that also mix in some of the other natural carotenoids. An optimal amount would be from 25,000 to maybe even as high as 100,000 IU. I take 100,000 IU a day of natural beta carotene."

For vitamin A recommendations, let's turn to Patrick Holford. For 15 years he has been a researcher and clinical nutritionist. He has written over 10 books, including *The Optimum Nutrition Bible,* and is the founder of the Institute for Optimum Nutrition, a nonprofit center in London devoted to research on and the practice of correct nutrition.

He emphasizes that vitamin A is very important for the immune system because "it helps strengthen cell walls. The amount we should be taking as an ideal amount to strengthen the immune system is on the order of 30,000 to 40,000 units of vitamin A each day. That dosage is achievable, or at least three-quarters of that is achievable, from diet alone as long as we eat on a regular basis those orange, red, and yellow foods: fruits and vegetables. The organic carrot is a good example. A single carrot can give you 10,000 or even 15,000 units of vitamin A.

"I would recommend supplementing your dietary intake with an additional 15,000 or 20,000 units of vitamin A, of which up to 10,000 is in the animal form known as retinyl. Retinyl is also available in vegetable form in a supplement called retinyl palmitate. Basically, one takes 10,000 units of some kind of retinyl and the remaining 10,000 units in the form of beta carotene, which is the vegetable precursor of vitamin A. You can get the remaining amount in the diet. That helps strengthen the cell walls."

Lieberman also reminds us of the importance of C. "For vitamin C," she says, "if you are really living in a very polluted environment as we are in New York, you should take 2,000 to 6,000 mg a day (or 2 to 6 g). Divide that dosage throughout the day. You wouldn't want to take 6,000 mg at one time, but maybe 2,000 mg two to three times a day. That is a great place to start in boosting immune function."

For selenium, you'll need 100 to 200 mcg each day. Lieberman thinks 50 mcg really isn't enough. You have to go to 100 to 200 mcg a day to really get the benefits.

Holford mentions that zinc is also important. "What actually helps get the immune system fighting well?" he asks. "Principally, I'm speaking here about the lymphocytes, which the body produces in giant quantities. In a half hour, for example, the body will make a million of these immune cells." A key nutrient that helps support this process is zinc, yet the average person is getting only about half the amount of zinc she needs. You need about 15 to 20 mg a day, which you can get from seeds or nuts, sweet corn, and peas and also from fish and meat. Nothing can grow without zinc, Holford notes: "It's so vital for growth. If you plant it and it can grow, then it's got zinc in it." You can probably obtain up to 10 mg of zinc from your diet, which leaves to 5 to 10 mg more that you need. He recommends supplementing with 10 mg in a good multivitamin.

With respect to B vitamins, Holford says, "B_6, B_{12}, folic acid, and pantothenic acid (called vitamin B5) are important for improving the strength of your immune cells. The ideal level of those varies somewhat, but I would recommend 50 mg of B_6, 50 mg of pantotheic acid, a bit more folic acid, such as 400 mcg, and of B_{12}, 10 or 20 mcg. You should be able to obtain all of this by taking a good high-strength multivitamin."

Liberman reminds us that supplementation is not sufficient on its own: "It's not enough to just take these supplements. You also have to clean up your diet, making sure you are eating a balance of raw foods such as salads, fruits, and vegetables, things that you can eat raw and really retain the active enzymes. A lot of the plant-based antioxidants are destroyed or rendered inactive during the cooking process, although other nutrients are rendered more absorbable by the same process."

Balance is the key. To achieve it, make sure you eat a lot of salads, raw fruits, and vegetables and drink a lot of fresh juices. Try to take these immediately after they are juiced. Don't leave them in the refrigerator for any length of time. Also, eat whole-grain foods like lentils and beans and quinoa. If you eat in this way, you'll get a wide range of plant compounds.

You won't want to swallow a capsule for each of these nutrients, because you'd end up taking thousands of capsules a day. You don't want to take a capsule of lignins or isoflavones, for these can be obtained from soy or chickpeas. Quercetin and a lot of the phenolic antioxidants are obtained from berries and fruits that have a lot of pigments in them.

Dr. Neil Block discusses his treatment: "If proteins or amino acids are low, we can try to individually supplement the amino acids. If minerals are lacking, they can be given individually or in tandem, trying to operate by an economy of scale so that a patient doesn't have to take from more than 10 to 15 bottles at a time.

"As for hormonal imbalance, I have 20 to 25 percent of my chronic fatigue syndrome patients on thyroid hormone. I prefer to use the more natural brands of thyroid hormone. Again, I believe in giving both the male and female hormones. We also have to try to adjust the pancreas and adrenals. For the pancreas I use chromium or chromium picolinate. For adrenals, the glandulars or homeopathics, and sometimes things such as licorice tend to help multiple hormones. If we are working on the pituitary, we use glandulars, the homeopathics, and on rare occasions I use a lot of the amino acids to try to build neurotransmitter activity. The amino acids to be used are arginine, tyrosine, and phenylalanine. Tryptophan was also once useful to me until they took it off the market. I'm also not afraid to use, correctly and in small doses, items obtained from the pharmacy. What I tend to shy away from are the tranquilizers, such as Valium and Librium. I do make use of antidepressants on occasion."

Often his patients have seen other physicians and holistic healers and may need only one or two things to turn the body around on multiple levels:. "With neurotransmitters being easily adjusted nowadays, with items like the newer antidepressants such as Paxil and Zoloft, which lack drastic side effects and have a response beginning in two to four weeks, they're worthwhile. It's nice for a patient who has suffered two, four, or six years to take these new agents and within two to four weeks get at least some indication of the direction in which he or she is going."

The following daily supplementation requirements are recommended for boosting immune strength. Large doses of vitamins should not be taken without supervision by your health practitioner.

A (as pure A)—15,000 to 20,000 IU divided into 10,000 IU of retinyl and 10,000 IU of beta carotene

Beta carotene—25,000 up to 100,000 IU

B_6—50 mg (test for your reaction first)

pantotheic acid—50 mg

folic acid —400 mcg

B_{12}—10 or 20 mcg (all the B vitamins can be obtained in a good, high-strength multivitamin)

C (buffered)—To bowel tolerance. Try sago palm, not a corn source. Buffering neutralizes acid.

E—2,000 mg two to three times a day

Quercetin—250 to 1,000 mg

Pycnogenol—150 to 300 mg

Essential fatty acids—100 to 350 mg (obtainable from sunflower, sesame, safflower, evening primrose, or soybean oils and black currant, a tablespoon a day)

Zinc—5 to 10 mg

Selenium—100 to 200 mcg (oceanic)

Coenzyme Q10—100 to 300 mg

ENZYMES

Another area of supplementation that has only recently come into focus is enzymes. Dr. Steven Whiting, the author of *The Complete Guide to Optimal Wellness,* has spent a long time looking at the value of enzymes in improving the immune system. He has 20 years of experience in the field of clinical nutrition, holds a doctorate in biochemistry, and has worked in a number of hospitals, offering alternative perspectives.

It's one thing, he explains, to take in nutrients, but it's quite another to absorb them at the cellular level, which is the only place where they can be of any value. Enzyme formation in the body starts with the saliva, with the enzyme ptyalin. Enzymes are also present in the stomach, intestines, and so on, to help with food absorption.

There are two forms of supplementation, and it is important to understand the difference between them. One type of product you can get at health food stores consists of whole enzymes and actually contains such things as pepsin, rennin, and trypsin, the real enzymes. They have their place, and they have their drawbacks. Their primary use is for chronic disease and for people who are very debilitated. The big problem with using them is that the body can grow to be dependent on them quite rapidly. When they are taken orally in the form of supplements, the body is not always encouraged to make them on its own.

"The second group of supplements," Whiting says, "is called enzyme precursors. These are substances that not only contain the raw materials for the body to build its own enzymes but frequently contain the vital stomach acid hydrochloric acid, which helps the body build many of the protein digestants. Remember, proteins are digested in the stomach, and carbohydrates and starches are digested in the intestinal tract. This is why a very unique enzyme system has been created and needs to be maintained."

He continues: "For the average person looking for a good enzyme product, I recommend one that would contain at least the following things. First, hydrochloric acid. After years of eating junk foods and dead, lifeless foods, we need it to help with stomach digestion. According to a recent survey by the University of California at Berkeley, only 9 percent of the population eats the recommended number of fresh fruits and vegetables per day. This product should also contain protein digestants, which should include papain and pepsin. There should be fat digestants, ox bile and pancreatin. Also a starch digestant, which would be bromelain."

"The bulk of the five years of research I have done for my book is about what I call whole-spectrum nutrition. We have been able to isolate about 102 nutrients that the body needs every day. These include the 16 vitamins, the three fatty acids, 8 to 12 amino acids, and about 72 minerals.

"What we found out in working with patients, such as those with chronic fatigue syndrome, in a clinical environment is that the concept that has developed in the last 20 years of using potency to address chronic diseases may have been only part of the picture. In reality, we are finding that the ratio of nutrients to each other is as important as if not more important than potency alone."

He illustrates by talking about calcium absorption. Calcium is one of the more difficult minerals for most people to absorb. As they age, people's overall pH increases, and they lose the natural acids in the body, making calcium absorption even less efficient. Dr. Whiting describes a study he conducted with Paul Saltman, head chemist at the University of California at San Diego, in 1991 on the use of calcium. They divided 59 postmenopausal women into several groups: "One got a placebo, one got calcium, one got a mixture of trace minerals, and the fourth group got calcium with the trace minerals. Essentially, at the end of two years all the women had experienced substantial bone loss, which would be expected because of osteoporosis in that time period—all, that is, except the last group, who got the calcium and the trace minerals together. They actually had a 2 percent increase in bone density.

"This is very indicative of what has been found in many recent studies, which is that it is the combination of nutrients that is extremely important." Thus, when Dr. Whiting sees a patient with chronic fatigue syndrome, "The first thing I recommend is that she take a full spectrum of supplements that provide all the needed vitamins and minerals. Once they are on a full program, we will be in a much better position to address various health challenges."

CHINESE HERBAL THERAPIES

The herbologist Letha Hadady says that the tradition of herbology is very rich in China, with many herbs to choose from for healing the immune system. These strengthening agents are Chinese ginseng, dandelion, false ginseng, *Andrographis, Eclipta alba,* and honeysuckle.

After using these herbs, we should act to kill germs and viral infection with such herbs as honeysuckle flower, *Andrographis,* and dandelion. Having built strength and killed germs, we must build blood using Chinese blood tonics, such as *han lien tsao,* which is called *Eclipta alba* in Latin and grows wild in the American southwest. It builds blood without any side effects, such as inflammation. You can take it every day in powdered form.

She also mentions *fo ti,* which builds blood while it keeps us cool: "One part of herbal treatment for viral infection is taking antibiotic and anti-inflammatory herbs such as dandelion, a cleansing agent that keeps us cool. It can be put in salads and soups and may be found in health food stores as capsules."

Honeysuckle flower grows outside in the garden. Boiled as tea, it will eliminate a sore throat and fever as well as kill pneumonia, staph, and strep germs.

There are three types of ginseng: American, Chinese, and false. The American type provides more moisture and more saliva and is good after a fever. Chinese ginseng, called *ren shen,* gives us energy. *Dang shen,* or false ginseng, makes us feel stronger without feeling hotter. All can be used in soups. When *dang shen* and astragalus are used together, the first lifts our energy and the second sends our defenses to the surface.

Cayenne pepper increases circulation and makes us feel stronger. It can be used by those who do not find it irritating.

There are also herbs for relaxing the nervous system. Siberian ginseng can be taken as an extract or in capsule form. Valerian, taken in capsules, can quiet the nervous system: "For people who are depressed," Hadady says, "we need to bring them to their center as a way to be grounded and to feel more whole. Use ginger and mint. Mint helps bring the worries out of the head, and ginger helps burn them away, because it is digestive and heating and so it brings us warmly to our centers. They make a good combination."

High Energy preparation is an herb mixture that uses western and Oriental ingredients: *gotu kola,* American ginseng, damiana, red clover, peppermint, and cloves. It strengthens the adrenals and lungs.

Hadady adds that cloves and hot water will increase your energy and make you breathe more deeply.

OTHER HERBAL FORTIFIERS

Dr. Lieberman has looked at American plants to find ones that can strengthen the debilitated immune system that accompanies chronic fatigue syndrome.

"I'd say hands down that about the most important herb in this area is licorice root," she says. "A specific valuable compound found in this root is glycyrrhizin, available at health food stores as a supplement. It's not the easiest thing to find, but a few companies make it. Glycyrrhizin is just remarkable at boosting the lymphatic and immune systems, the white blood cells, and the thymus gland."

Glycyrrhizin can actually be therapeutic in relation to some of the viruses implicated in chronic fatigue syndrome. For condyloma, Lieberman reports "unbelievable results giving glycyrrhizin both orally and intravaginally for women. So glycyrrhizin is a nutrient that I think is key if you are dealing with some sort of viral syndrome."

There is one caveat. If you are prone to high blood pressure, take your blood pressure from time to time while taking glycyrrhizin. "I haven't seen many patients' blood pressure go up when taking this, but it will occasionally happen," Dr. Lieberman notes. Perversely enough, conventional medicine treats people with chronic fatigue syndrome by recommending that they take loads of salt. "This is the most ridiculous thing I've ever heard," Lieberman notes. "This won't help. What will help is glycyrrhizin, which may also play a role in ameliorating the postural hypotension that these patients are facing." Glycyrrhizin stimulates the production of interferon naturally. It supports the thyroid gland and boosts natural killer cells and other aspects of immune functioning. A therapeutic dose ranges from 75 to 300 mg per day. Take your blood pressure from time to time to make sure it is in check.

Another antiviral is echinacea. Dr. Lieberman believes that it is not used nearly enough for viruses such as condyloma and cytomegalovirus or for chronic disease and immune dysfunction. Many people use it for influenza, which is also a virus, but they don't think of echinacea as useful for these other viruses, which it is. Echinacea has a remarkable ability to naturally stimulate interferon, natural killer cells, and phagocytes. Anyone who has ever played Pacman will understand the action of phagocytes, which search for and destroy viral cells and bacterial cells.

The liquid extracts of echinacea work best. Most of the research on it was done by Madaus AG in Germany, whose extract is known as EchinaGuard. Use 50 drops once or twice a day, depending on the severity of your symptoms. It's been recommended that you use echinacea four days on, four days off. There is some concern that if you use it all the time, you may adapt to it and it may stop boosting certain aspects of immune function. We don't know that for sure, but to be on the safe side, that's my recommendation. But I keep my patients on glycyrrhizin long term, though I gradually cut the dose down and maybe eventually have them on 75 mg per day as a prophylactic.

DIETARY CHANGES

Dr. Majid Ali sees eating right as a way to prevent or combat chronic fatigue syndrome. Corn and wheat are big culprits. Better grains are wild and brown rice, amaranth, quinoa, teff, and spelt. Soy products are also very good. The other good sources of carbohydrates are lentils and different types of beans. Tomatoes, potatoes, and yams are okay, but only in moderation. Foods containing white flour are a no-no, as is white rice.

"Lentils and beans are good sources of protein. Egg is excellent, but many people are allergic to it." Dr. Ali also recommends protein drinks in the morning because their amino acids give sustained energy. Sugar and carbohydrates, by contrast, provide a roller coaster effect; they are useful only when you are doing an endurance type of physical activity, in which case you need carbohydrates. But most people do much better without sugar and carbohydrates.

Dr. Ali does not insist that his patients follow a vegetarian diet but recommends little beef. Unusual meats such as venison and pheasant are better, he says. "We provide a list to patients of places where they can order such meat. Cornish hen and turkey are fine. Hunted fish (deep sea fish) are good. Cultured fish are not recommended. They're beginning to put fungicides into fish raised in fisheries. If you want fish, eat the deep sea ones. (Unless you have serious mercury sensitivity—then you should avoid fish.)"

He feels that eating certain fats is essential but that one should avoid oxidized, processed, denatured fats and animal shortening as well as corn oil, palm oil, and coconut oil. If you do not have milk sensitivity, butter is possible. You can make ghee by warming butter and skimming the white part off. It is delicious, and those who cannot tolerate butter can still tolerate ghee. Use virgin olive oil, the type you find in Italian stores.

Avocado oil is an excellent source of monounsaturates, but not if it is processed. For supplemental oils, flaxseed is excellent. People should make a habit of using flaxseed in salad dressing.

Dr. Galante advocates using many live foods that can be eaten right from nature without cooking, such as raw fruits, vegetables, and sprouts. They can provide tremendous energy, with a lot of enzymes and nutrition. They take little energy to digest and give much energy back.

Turnips and parsnips, both root vegetables, are very high in calcium. Green leafy vegetables give needed chlorophyll and oxygenate the blood. Radishes, red and green peppers, and eggplant are excellent, and ginger can be used to flavor any juice. Celery is a good diuretic, and cabbage is high in beta carotene, as are all the green leafy vegetables. Sprouts are the best source of protein. An ounce of wheatgrass, which is high in chlorophyll, is equal to 22 ounces of the choicest vegetable you can imagine.

Dr. Lieberman, who has written a book called *Shiitake, King of the Mushrooms,* recommends this vegetable highly. "Let me go into some detail on the shiitake mushroom," she says. "First and foremost, remember that this is a food. You can put it in a salad or cook it in soup. It's considered a delicacy in Japan. Back in the feudal period there, it was traded for its weight in silver, it was so rare and highly regarded.

"Some studies done on shiitake use the whole mushroom, but others use an extract from it known as D fraction. Most studies on this are specifically looking at cancer, both animal and human studies. D fraction is a highly concentrated extract of part of the mushroom known as beta-1,3-glucan and beta-1,6-glucan.

"What these plant compounds are able to do is really quite remarkable. They can preserve immune function during chemotherapy. It also works a little differently from chemotherapy. Chemo will kill cancer cells, but it also unfortunately kills healthy cells." Here is the significant point: "What D fraction does is kill cancer cells indirectly by boosting part of the immune system that will then kill the cancer cells." So D fraction has a phenomenal effect in helping immune function, which could be valuable in aiding the immune system of those suffering from chronic fatigue.

Lieberman adds that garlic is a wonderful nutrient that, like other plant compounds, can be eaten; it doesn't have to be taken as a supplement. "However, if you can munch garlic and still maintain a good social life, you are very lucky. Otherwise, there are nice capsules, some of which have been odor-modified. That's for people like myself—if I eat garlic, people will know about it." Over 500 scientific references describe garlic's benefits. "Let's compare that to aspirin," she says angrily. "After one positive study—one—every physician on the planet, nearly, was recommending it to his or her patients. If you recommended a dietary supplement after one study, you normally would be nailed to the cross."

In these 500 references one finds that garlic preserves immune function as well as playing a role in other areas, such as protecting against cancer and cardiovascular disease.

HOMEOPATHY

Homeopathy is Dr. Galante's specialty; it has been very effective against chronic fatigue syndrome. Homeopathic remedies, all made from natural substances, are given in microdoses.

To talk about one particular remedy, though, is not appropriate, Dr. Galante explains, since the essence of homeopathy is to select for each individual a remedy based on her or his unique physical constitution and manifestation of symptoms.

ACUPUNCTURE

Registered nurse and acupuncturist Abigail Rist-Podrecca points out that the *chi,* or bioelectrical energy, flows through pathways called meridians in the body. Disease, she says, is associated with an energy blockage. Acupuncture needles inserted in some of the 365 points that can be used open the blockages so that the energy can flow smoothly through the meridians. In addition, the needles dilate the blood vessels so that more blood flows through the area, bringing more oxygen and nutrients, which aid all aspects of health.

TAI CHI

A benefit of tai chi is that it increases one's awareness both internally and environmentally. "Then you can choose which to work on, whether there is something physically wrong or something in the environment that needs to be corrected," says Eric Schneider of the Northeastern Tai Chi Chuan Association.

According to Schneider, you have to cultivate a part of your body that can observe phenomena dispassionately without having to grab on to every experience and run with it, so that when you find yourself in in stressful situations you can say quietly, "Oh, so this is what is happening now. What can I do about it? What are my options, and how am I feeling?"

However, it takes 10 years to achieve what is called the *gung chi,* which means that the body is able to contain energy. This is not a quick fix.

IMAGERY AND HEALING

Dr. Paul Epstein says imagery is a therapeutic technique that helps people explore through words and symbols so they can understand the language of the subconscious.

According to Dr. Epstein, "Usually what comes up is the issue that is at the core of what will be the healing. People may get in touch with childhood wounds or abuse from the past that needs healing. Perhaps they'll get in touch with the fact that the work they are doing is not real work.

"In one such case, with a person suffering from chronic fatigue syndrome, we found that the illness was a case of a person trying to get love. She had not let go of trying to get love from her mom and dad. She was still stuck at that place. And the pain and the grief of not having that love were not only weakening her immune system but keeping her stuck in the unhealthy way she was living her life."

Dr. Majid Ali reiterates some of Dr. Epstein's message: "What I demonstrate to my patients is that the way you look at the world around you determines the biology under your skin. If you can be in a self-regulatory, healing mode, your brain activity, heart activity, muscle energy, skin energy will all be functioning positively. Or you can be trying to figure things out, think everything through in an overly intellectual way, and your biology will be as up and down as the

New York skyline. This is the stress mode, and it causes disease. Another mode is an even, steady-state mode, a resting mode.

"Our goal is to perceive the energy in these modes and understand how the energy profoundly affects the electrophysiological profile. Can we allow this energy to guide us into the healing mode? We want a transition from an ordinary, thinking, nervous stressful mode that causes disease to a nonthinking, meditative, deep-breathing mode that makes us well. That is our goal."

AYURVEDA

Dr. Nancy Lonsdorf, medical director of the Maharishi Ayurveda Health Center in Washington, D.C., and coauthor of *A Woman's Best Medicine,* defines fatigue as an imbalance in the body's rest-activity cycle. According to ayurvedic principles, the natural structures of rest cycles allow the body to recover from activity cycles: "A state of chronic fatigue means that the body has not fully rejuvenated itself."

Dr. Lonsdorf reports that many of her clients overcome fatigue by adhering to the basic rules of Maharishi Ayurveda, which address rest, activity, digestion, cleansing, and meditation:

REST

Lonsdorf says: "One of the simplest things we can do is pay attention to our sleep cycles. Many Americans just don't get enough sleep. They think they should be able to get by with five, six, or seven hours when most of them need eight or more.

"When we sleep and awaken is also important. This has to do with an understanding of the three doshas, or fundamental principles, that operate in nature. Doshas are expressions of nature's intelligence that guide all activity in our bodies and in nature. These three fundamental principles are called vata, pitta, and kapha. Vata governs movement, everything that flows in the body, all digestive action down to elimination, and all circulation. Pitta is the energy cycle, the fire and transformation. Last is kapha, the structural dosha, the muscles, bones, and connective tissue that give substance to the body. It includes everything that holds the body together as one piece of matter.

"Vata, pitta, and kapha govern our rest-activity cycles. For best sleep, Ayurveda tells us that we should start our rest during the cycle that is organized for calming down. This is the kapha time, between six and ten in the evening. Most people naturally start to feel sleepy then. If we go to sleep at this time, we will fall asleep quickly and our sleep will be the most rejuvenating.

"The other side of the coin is getting up. Benjamin Franklin had the right idea when he said, 'Early to bed, early to rise makes a [wo]man healthy, wealthy, and wise.' Ayurveda agrees with this and says that getting up early gives us more energy throughout the day. If we get up during vata time, between two and six in the morning, we will be the most active and energetic.

"It is very important for a woman to rest more during menstruation. This is a time for the body to rejuvenate, clear out, and purify. Limiting activity and resting more at this time give women more energy for the entire month."

ACTIVITY

"We also need more physical activity to rejuvenate the body. Ayurveda teaches that different body types are suited for different types of exercise and that we should exercise according to the dominant dosha in our system.

"Let's start with the vata type. The vata-dominant person is light in build with a small bone structure and tends to be high-strung and energetic. These people should exercise but not overexercise. Walking or bicycling 30 to 60 minutes at a comfortable, easy pace or doing a light exercise such as yoga is best for this body type. Too much exercise causes this type of individual to become overly anxious, not sleep well, and become weak.

"The kapha body type is the opposite. This person has a heavy bone structure and tends to put on weight and keep it on. Too little exercise results in lethargy and a sluggish type of fatigue. The best exercise for overcoming this type of fatigue is a vigorous workout. Joining an aerobics class or scheduling time regularly to walk with a friend helps keep this type of person motivated, since kapha-dominant people tend to procrastinate.

"Pitta, the middle body type, has a medium bone structure and lots of natural energy. These people tend to be athletic and to enjoy sports. The only problem is that they are workaholics who can forget to take the time to exercise. The pitta type is dominated by heat, so cooling types of activities such as skiing in the winter and hiking on a mountain trail in the summertime are more balancing and tend to make these people feel better.

"A couple of other points on exercise. It is very good to exercise in the morning, during the sluggish kapha time from 6 to 10 a.m. That will keep us going the whole day. It will improve metabolism, increase appetite, and help the digestion. Altogether, that will give us more energy."

DIGESTION

"The third area of treatment for fatigue is digestion- and diet-related. According to the ayurvedic system, how we digest food and how the cells of the body get nourished by that food are related to how energetic or how fatigued we feel. In fact, Ayurveda has a precise word for lack of good digestion: *ama*. *Ama* refers to residues, or improperly digested food molecules, that get deposited in the arteries, bones, or joints. *Ama* can be as simple as excess cholesterol, gallstones, or uric acid which can create gout, or it can be glucose-related end products that get stuck in the tissues and cause stiffness and aging. Good nutrition creates less *ama* and gives us more energy.

"I would like to add that it is best not to eat late at night, since this can interfere with good sleep. Eating after eight o'clock is to be avoided. Less food in the evening gives us better, more rejuvenating sleep."

CLEANSING

"One other ayurvedic treatment for fatigue cleanses the body of accumulated impurities or *ama*. It is known as *pancha karma*. *Pancha* means "five," and *karma* means "action"; this therapy consists of five actions or treatments. It is basically a physical treatment involving several days' work with a trained technician. During this time special herbal oils are applied to the body to soften impurities. Then some mild cleansing therapies, such as herbalized steam, are used to open the channels of circulation. A mild herbal enema follows, which helps eliminate contaminants. A study published in the *Journal of Social Behavior and Personality* reported that this therapy resulted in 40 percent less fatigue."

MEDITATION

"The imbalance between rest and activity also includes our perceptions about life. Basically, every waking moment, we have our attention on the field of activity. We experience through the senses, we think, we emote, and we relate to other people. We are always active. When we take that awareness to the field of silence, we greatly energize the mind and nervous system. This has a tremendously rejuvenating effect. We do this through meditation. In Maharishi Ayurveda, we use TM, the transcendental meditation technique, because that has been scientifically shown to give excellent results in terms of improving health and reducing anxiety and other stress-related conditions."

NATUROPATHY

Gracia Perlstein, an alternative health care practitioner with a private practice in Belle Terre, New York, says that for chronic fatigue, food is the best medicine: "We really don't have any existing drugs on the market to help this condition. In fact, most drugs will weaken immunity and delay recovery further. It is best to approach this with natural supports to inherent healing processes." While there are no quick cure-alls, Perlstein makes the following recommendations to speed up recovery.

DIET

A diet of pure, dense, nutrient-rich whole foods is imperative for this condition: "You want to include plenty of fresh organic vegetables. Cruciferous vegetables such as broccoli, cauliflower, and Brussels sprouts are very important for their immune-enhancing properties. You want onions and garlic, the poor man's cure all: "Choose from a wide assortment of whole foods. Don't eat the same few over and over again. In this weakened state you can develop allergic responses to foods consumed repeatedly in large amounts. Eating different foods will ensure that you get a variety of nutrients and will keep you from developing allergic responses. Amaranth, quinoa, and other grains not commonly eaten by Americans are good to include.

"Really emphasize the green foods. Have a dark green salad daily. Super green powders are very helpful as well. Add them to juices, but do not emphasize sweet fruit and carrot juice.

"Eat an adequate amount of high-quality proteins. The best sources are vegetarian because of the low toxicity and ease of digestion. Good vegetarian proteins are tofu, tempeh, fortified soy milk, and legumes. You can benefit from small amounts of fresh fish because fish is high in omega-3 fatty acids. But there are some precautions you must take. Be sure to find a market that gets fish from clean, unpolluted waters and make sure they do not dip it in chlorine, which is a common practice. If you eat farm-raised fish, it should be organically raised. If you eat poultry, it should be naturally raised as well, free of hormones and pesticide residues. Consume only small amounts of animal protein, no more than 3 to 4 oz a day.

"The best way to have protein is in a soup. An excellent old Chinese recipe for an immune-enhancing soup combines a whole astragalus root with onions, garlic, ginger, and free-range chicken, fish, tofu, or tempeh. Some fresh green vegetables and a handful of brown rice are added to that. The soup is brought to a boil and then simmered. Some miso is added for flavor. This is highly nourishing, easy to digest, and excellent for helping a weakened individual regain strength.

"Drink plenty of pure water daily. In colder seasons unsweetened herb tea, such as immune-supportive echinacea tea, is a very good source of liquid. Cold water is a little shocking to the digestive system for people with chronic fatigue syndrome, so you want warm liquids and plenty of them."

SUPPLEMENTS

To enhance energy further, try the following immune-enhancing supplements.

Multivitamin and mineral complex. This should be a good-quality hypoallergenic supplement. Be sure it includes magnesium, chromium, and zinc. Many people with chronic fatigue are low in these.

Vitamin C at 5,000 to 10,000 mg should be taken throughout the day. Every two hours take 1,000 to 2,000 mg. Much higher doses can be taken with an intravenous vitamin C drip. This method has proved highly beneficial for overcoming chronic fatigue.

Coenzyme Q10 at least 75 mg

Lactobacillus acidophilus + *Bifidobacterium bifidum.* Take as directed on label

Vitamin E at 400 to 800 units

Garlic capsules: 2 or more with meals

Vitamin B complex at100 mg three times per day
Vitamin B$_{12}$ at 100 mcg
Essential fatty acid supplement:. 1 to 2 tablespoonfuls
Geranium at 100 mg

HERBS

Herbs are nature's medicines. The ones listed here concentrate on building and strengthening the immune system:
Echinacea
Pau d'arco
Cat's claw
Siberian ginseng
Astragalus

In addition, Perlstein reports excellent results with lomatium complex: "It is one of the best things I have found for overcoming chronic fatigue syndrome. If you were to use one herbal complex, that would be it."

EXERCISE

The little strength a person has can be improved through gentle exercise. Perlstein says, "Being outdoors is best. Try walking, even in cold weather. If you bundle up, you can do it. Getting fresh air is very, very important.

"In terms of physical disciplines, yoga and tai chi have wonderful balancing effects on the endocrine and immune systems. Some kind of physical discipline is imperative for regaining health."

MIND-SET

Perlstein concludes by pointing out the strong mind-body connection in both getting and overcoming chronic fatigue syndrome: "Studies show that chronic fatigue syndrome generally manifests itself in people who feel they have overwhelming life circumstances. They do not feel empowered to make positive changes in their lives. This has a damaging effect on their immune systems. "When you have chronic fatigue, you want to do your best to be optimistic. You want to be grateful for your life experiences. Try to focus on the positive. That will help keep the body more balanced. When you do have emotional issues, try to resolve them completely. Do not repress negative emotions. Do not tell yourself that they are unimportant or inconsequential. It is very important to resolve your emotional conflicts completely.

"Creative movement is very helpful for that—dance in particular, with beautiful music. If you feel you cannot confront an individual or a situation, at least put on music and somehow work out the emotions with your body. Creative dance can help with this."

OTHER LIFESTYLE CHANGES

If adrenal function is depressed, Dr. Michael Vesselago treats it specifically with glandulars, vitamins, magnesium, and calcium:. "Sometimes I also have people take vitamin B_{12} injections to support adrenal function. Sometimes, just with adrenal treatment, people get 30 percent, 40 percent, 50 percent better inside a few weeks."

However, Dr. Vesselago looks at medical treatments as short-term help for making patients more comfortable and better able to function. He stresses that changes must be made on a deeper level if they are to be lasting: "When we talk about wishing for the good old days, part of that wish is for a slower pace and a more humane way of life. So part of what I do is talk to people about their lives. I make them aware of how their motors are racing all the time. I encourage them to start an aerobic exercise program because rhythmic, sustained, repetitive, total body activity supports the adrenals and dissipates much stress. Look at how you feel after you have been out for even a half hour's walk.

"I also recommend meditation. People are always racing around in heavy traffic or are surrounded by phones that ring all day long. Even television has their minds racing a mile a minute. Turning inward for 20 minutes once or twice a day with the eyes closed allows the system to take time out.

"One technique for decreasing the stress response is called breath awareness. A person can become aware of her or his breathing any time of day, during any activity. It really grounds you in the here and now. It brings your focus back to the body and decreases stress. So there are little things you can do just in the course of the day that make a difference."

DRUGS

Ostrom mentions a new drug which may yet be helpful: Amplygin, which is currently in U.S. Food and Drug Administration (FDA) trials, appears to fix a very important immune system antiviral pathway. Found to work for AIDS, it has yet to be proved against chronic fatigue syndrome.

Dr. Galante opines that antibiotics can certainly be called for when all else fails, in cases where the system has been debilitated, perhaps by too much previous drug use. However, the state we are aiming for is one in which the energy in the body will overcome all problems.

THE SELF-HEALING PROCESS

Dr. Epstein elaborates on his earlier position: "What is needed in treating chronic fatigue syndrome or AIDS and similar problems is a new approach. We should be looking not for the quick fix or what will work for everybody but for an approach that is individualized and holistic and empowers the patient to get involved in the cure and gives that patient belief and hope that healing is possible.

"There are two points in my treatment that I've been told by patients have helped them most: that I have given them hope and belief that healing is possible and that I have shown them that there are things they could do to help themselves. I don't heal anybody. Doctors don't heal anybody. They support people as they heal themselves."

Dr. Epstein wants to help patients listen, explore, and understand the message of their disease, which is the key that unlocks the door to recovery: "After the diagnosis and medications, natural or other, there still has to be an exploration of healing for this person. We might have conditioned immune-suppressant responses built into our attitudes, beliefs, the way we live our life, the way we think, and the way we eat. An illness cannot be fixed from the outside; there is no magic bullet for chronic fatigue syndrome.

"People heal themselves by engaging in a self-healing process, by looking at their life and its meaning. It may seem rather complicated, but it is not. It is based on the knowledge that we do not get sick overnight. The condition may manifest suddenly in certain symptoms, but it took years and years to arrive. And it was not from one virus, not just from Epstein-Barr or herpes or parasites, low blood sugar, or electromagnetic pulsations. It was a combination of all of them."

Detoxification takes time. It might take you a year to really cleanse. You need a rational diet so that you can get rid of the food polluting your system. Bring in the healthy foods, exercise, meditation, and acupuncture. If you are what you eat, eat what you appreciate becoming. Remember that the mind is a powerful healer and also a powerful slayer. Surround yourself with positive thoughts and people who will support your endeavor to live a natural lifestyle. Chronic fatigue syndrome can be cured. Every day you can be processing health and overcoming disease.

Chapter 9

Cosmetic Surgery

When the book *Subliminal Seduction* by Wilson Bryan Key appeared in the 1960s, it caused quite a stir by laying bare some of the seamier activities of the advertising industry. Exposed, for example, was a technique used in movie theaters that was so outrageous that it was eventually outlawed. Unscrupulous owners would insert one or two frames with such messages as "Buy Popcorn" into films they were showing. These messages flashed by so quickly the audience was not consciously aware of them, yet later during the film many people would go to the lobby to—you guessed it—buy popcorn.

Another equally suprising phenomenon described in the book concerns the average, unenlightened American male, the "breast man" who prefers women with noticeable chests, the bigger the better. I'm not talking about mature men who in choosing a female friend or companion look for spiritual and mental qualities first, but the so-called machos who love the pinups TV and Hollywood provide.

In examining this phenomenon, Key studied sample covers of *Playboy* magazine, which commonly features busty women. He carefully studied the models' poses, the relation between the models and the viewers, and the facial expressions displayed, and found that these cover girls, though on the surface they were sex objects, latently appeared to the readers as mother figures. Thus, he argues, the machos who are attracted by these large breasts are driven not so much by lust as, subconciously, by the desire to throw them-selves on Mama's bosom.

Whatever the truth of Key's argument, he calls attention to many American males' preference for large breasts. Many women, influenced by this male per-spective but not having breasts considered big enough, have their breasts enlarged through plastic surgery,.

Let's pause right here to puncture one myth. This is the idea that all women who get implants to enlarge or reshape their breasts do it out of vanity. Very often, in fact, women get implants because they need a breast reconstruction after an illness or accident or because of a physical malformation.

This chapter explores how the breast implant procedure works and then turn to the risks associated with implants. You may be surprised to learn that these risks extend not only to the women who have the surgery, but to the chil-dren they give birth to afterward. We will meet some people who are trying to raise awareness of the problems associated with these implants, and will exam-ine the safest ways to surgically remove implants as well as how to detoxify the body to lessen the effects these procedures are bound to have on one's health.

Since women—and men—are lining up every day for cosmetic surgery, let us first look at the pros and cons of cosmetic surgery in general.

Sometimes cosmetic surgery may benefit a person who has physical fea-tures she feels are hampering her; she believes there's no other way to deal with this problem. In that case she should have the surgery, of course. But I also often see cases in which people have had procedures done and an observ-er is tempted to ask "Why?" In others, the observer might ask not just "Why?" but "How did they select the person who performed the surgery, which wasn't done very well?"

Let me tell an anecdote here that might amuse you, if you have a taste for the grotesque. I was in Hollywood on a tour in Beverly Hills. It was after 1 a.m., and I and a friend went to a restaurant that he told me was a good late-night place to eat. In one of the sections a party was going on.

I couldn't believe what I saw. I felt I had entered a Todd Browning movie, because every single person at the party looked like a freak. Nobody looked natural. Their cheeks, noses, lips, necks, breasts—nothing looked real. Some of the faces looked like someone had put a plastic bag over the person's face and pulled it from behind.

I was thinking, All this money, all these connections, what didn't they see, what questions didn't they ask, how many times have they had surgery done? I'm not talking about older people. Most of these people were probably in their forties and fifties. What was going on? Hadn't *any* of them thought to ask, "Is this the best procedure?" For instance, could a laser do better than a surgical procedure in which the surgeon has to cut and tuck and pull?

That got me thinking about the new laser technolgy which is being increas-ingly used for cosmetic surgery. To find out more about it, I talked to Dr. Debra

Sarnoff, a graduate of Cornell University and George Washington University's School of Medicine. She is one of the premier laser surgery experts in North America, specializing in cosmetic dermatology and dermatological surgery. She's written numerous articles and is certified by the American College of Physicians. Currently she is an assistant professor of dermatology at New York University. Her latest publication is a complete guide to laser cosmetic surgery entitled *Beauty and the Beam.*

Laser Surgery: A New Development

Dr. Sarnoff sees lasers as a great new tool. "New methods and uses for laser surgery are emerging almost every month. Lasers can't do everything, but they have truly made a difference in cosmetic surgery, particularly in relation to what may seem minor problems, such as broken blood vessels on the face and around the nose, brown spots, age spots, liver spots, whatever you'd like to call them, on the tops of the hands or in the chest area."

Lasers have proved helpful with problems such as removing a now-unwanted tattoo. They are also useful for spider veins on the legs. Women may shy away from wearing skirts when they have nice legs but a map of spider veins makes them very self-conscious. Or perhaps they have scars from teenage acne, before we had effective treatments for acne and people were left with pockmarks on the face. Maybe it's just wrinkles. A woman may feel young on the outside, but when she looks in the mirror she sees these wrinkles, and she wants to stay looking young, vibrant, and healthy. "Things like this," says Dr. Sarnoff, "are often correctible with laser surgery."

There is a big difference between what a laser can accomplish and what typical plastic surgery can accomplish. Dr. Sarnoff mentions that plastic surgery can be done with care and dignity, so that it doesn't create specimens like the ones I saw in Beverly Hills. Those people might have been overpulled or pulled too tight, or perhaps they had more than one procedure. Sometimes in L.A. people will start early, maybe in their thirties, which means that in their fifties, they may be having a third face-lift. "There's just so much pulling and so much tucking one can do. You are eventually going to develop the 'wind tunnel look,' where you look as if you'd gone through a wind tunnel."

However, Dr. Sarnoff insists, this is not good plastic surgery. "That is not the kind of thing that anyone would be proud to have as their patient walking around. That's not the result you want to see. When everyone can clearly tell that you had something done, that's the antithesis of what we are trying to achieve, because good plastic surgery should be surgery that is natural-appearing, " Dr. Sarnoff stresses. The goal is to look like a healthier, more vibrant, more youthful version of yourself, not to have an artificial look.

Laser surgery does not involve the same kind of pulling, Sarnoff explains. It uses light beams; lasers are essentially beams of light applied to the skin.

Unlike a scalpel, which actually cuts the skin and causes some bleeding, a laser beam will pass through the skin without causing any bleeding. It has a particular target that it is trying to eradicate, and it can do this because it has a particular color. In the early twentieth century Albert Einstein eloborated the principles of radiant energy that were later developed by other physicists into laser (light amplification by stimulated emission of radiation) technology.

An example of what laser surgery can do well is provided by a person with broken blood vessels on her face and a ruddy complexion that leads people to believe she's an alcoholic, even though she doesn't drink at all. What she has is a genetic tendency to be very red in the face and to have many broken blood vessels.

If you seek out a dermatologist or a plastic surgeon, look for someone who is experienced and trained in lasers and who has the right laser with the correct light beams to use on the overlying skin. Dilated blood vessels are a problem lasers can correct with little downtime and little discomfort in a very simple procedure that can be done during a lunch hour, in 20 minutes or so. So for something like that a laser is a major breakthrough.

There are certain problems that only lasers are capable of solving, just as there are certain problems only scalpel surgery can solve. For example, Dr. Sarnoff says, "There's no way that pulling and stretching and tightening the skin, through surgery, can change the quality of the skin. If your problem is that something is wrong with the quality of the skin, very often a laser can help that."

RESURFACING THE SKIN

One cosmetic surgery procedure that can be done well with lasers is what is called resurfacing the skin. We all develop wrinkles as we get older. After smiling, laughing, and expressing ourselves with our faces for all these years, most of us develop lines around the eyes—crow's feet—as well as lines on the upper lip. Lip lines are particularly frustrating to women because they have more of them, since their skin is different than men's.

Dr. Sarnoff says that even the best face-lift in the world will not eradicate those lines. Something has to be done to resurface the skin. "In the old days, we used a machine called a dermabrader, which was like a little sanding machine that people used to try and peel off the top layers of the skin. In other cases, doctors used acid as a chemical peel. The theory was that when the skin healed, it would be much smoother and the wrinkles would not be as apparent.

Then, says Dr. Sarnoff, "Along came this generation of lasers. The laser can be used to peel off the top layers of skin as opposed to using a chemical or a dermabrading machine."

This procedure involves going to a reputable physician, preferably a dermatologist or plastic surgeon who is experienced in this technique, and having the top layers of skin removed in a controlled way with a laser. Healing will take at least 10 days, during which the recovering patient has to lie low. She will look like she had the worst sunburn ever. The skin will be red, moist, and chapped. She won't be able to put on makeup for at least 10 days.

The cost of resurfacing the entire face can be between $4,000 and $5,000. There may be some added costs for the operating room, as well as charges for anesthesia.

AGE SPOTS

Many women have sunspots or age spots, what is called photodamage, from all those years of baking in the sun before we knew that ultraviolet rays are potentially harmful. Sarnoff explains, "A lot of that sun damage will be entirely reversible if the beam of light can be used to strip off those top layers of skin. That type of laser resurfacing is a fairly involved procedure that really takes a commitment and a healing time. It's not the kind of thing you just pop in to have as if you were going to the deli and do a little laser over your lunch break. That laser resurfacing is a bigger deal."

BROKEN BLOOD VESSELS, HAIR REMOVAL, TATTOO REMOVAL

Dr. Sarnoff adds, "We are also using lasers now to help lighten stretch marks and to deal with birthmarks. The costs for these procedures are usually more in the hundreds of dollars. It depends on how large the discoloration or the tattoo is and how much time is required. For something like a tattoo, usually several visits are needed. They would be spaced about six to eight weeks apart, and it would not be unusual to need up to eight treatments to clear a tattoo completely."

Procedures such as zapping broken blood vessels and removing little brown spots are simpler; the side effects are usually no more than a little bruising, crusting, or scabbing, something you might want to wear a small bandage over or apply a little antibiotic ointment to, but nothing that would keep you out of work or prevent you from functioning. Many times people have these procedures and go right back to work.

Lasers can also be an an alternative to electrolysis for hair removal. There are many benefits to laser hair removal as compared with electrolysis. The procedure can be done very rapidly, and the patient can immediately return to what she was doing before.

KNOW WHAT TO ASK

Dr. Sarnoff warns that a savvy consumer must ask the right questions. She must learn whether a procedure is a one-shot deal or wil have to be repeated. And you should ask how long the improvement will last. Certainly you want something that is going to be cost-effective. Some laser treatments are really long-lasting. Laser removal wrinkles has been around for about five years, and people who had the treatment when it was first introduced still look good. With hair removal, by contrast, very often the hair will grow back in a few months. Dr. Sarnoff stresses that you have to know that before you commit. "I think it is very important to ascertain ahead of time approximately how many treatments are needed and what you should expect."

KNOW THE RISKS

There are risks, Sarnoff cautions. One is that you will pay good money and be disappointed because your underlying problem will still be there. "Something else that consumers have to be aware of is scarring. It's usually not the case that scars occur, and with a doctor who is well trained and experienced, I think that the technique is very safe. Nonetheless, it is a topic that definitely needs to be addressed before the procedure is done."

Sometimes there are some temporary changes in pigment. As the skin is healing, it can become a little darker or lighter than the surrounding skin. You must be aware how often this happens and know whether it is in fact only temporary or could be permanent.

There are very different types of lasers. Each beam of light accomplishes a different purpose, and the potential hazard from each is different. Still, there are some universal precautions that all competent laser providers follow. You need the correct eyewear, for example. Each laser is set at a very specific wavelength, and the protective eyewear needs to be specific to that wavelength.

Postoperative instructions make a difference, too. If you're removing tattoos or broken blood vessels, there is usually nothing else to do. However, with skin resurfacing, Dr. Sarnoff cautions that it is extremely important that patients follow the protocol afterward so that they do not get any kind of infection and heal properly.

LASERS AND RADIATION

The number one fear people have about lasers is that they involve harmful radiation. But, as Dr. Sarnoff explains, the word "radiation" in the spelled-out version of laser actually refers to the verb 'radiate,' meaning 'to give off light.' Most of the beams of light used in lasers are in the visible light range. That is, they are part of normal light. The only unique thing about lasers is that they are monochromatic. You might have a red beam or a yellow or green one, as opposed to natural light, which is a blend of all the colors of the rainbow. Laser light is non-ionizing; it's basically safe, as opposed to x-rays or ultraviolet light from the sun, which are ionizing. Ionizing radiation may change our cells and damage our chromosomes. We can get in real trouble with that type of radiation; but most lasers are not in that part of the electromagnetic spectrum.

FINDING THE RIGHT PERSON TO DO THE PROCEDURE

Another fear that people express to Dr. Sarnoff involves whether the specialist they are seeing is qualified. Physicians don't need any board certification to perform laser surgery and, in fact, one doesn't even have to have a medical degree to use lasers. Lasers are relatively new; many have been around only about 15 years. There are many wonderful doctors who trained at reputable universities and passed their boards in their respective fields, but the advent of lasers came after they graduated. Not every doctor has kept up with the technology and really understands it. A doctor might be board-certified in one particular field but know relatively little about laser techniques, but could get a laser this afternoon and start to do any of the procedures. Consumers have the right to know about the doctor's actual experience in laser surgery.

In Dr. Sarnoff's opinion, if you are considering cosmetic laser surgery, "The best thing to do is to ask around in your community. Start by asking your regular doctor, your neighbors, your friends, and anyone you know who might have had a laser procedure done similar to the type you are interested in. You can also call groups for a recommendation, such as the American Academy of Dermatology, the American Society of Plastic and Reconstructive Surgeons, or the American Society of Laser Medicine and Surgery."

She suggests that you make more than one consulting appointment. You want to meet the doctor and ask how many procedures like yours he or she has performed. Ask if you can see photos of the doctor's work. This may not be necessary for some of the minor procedures, but if you are thinking about resurfacing your face, it is very important to know that the doctor is experienced and is going to do it correctly.

As long as it is in the right hands this type of cosmetic surgery can be practical and safe. I cannot say that for the next cosmetic surgery procedure we will look at: breast implants.

Breast Implants

Dr. Susan Kolb described to me why in her experience women have breast implants and how the implants are put in. Dr. Kolb has been a board-certified plastic surgeon for 17 years and is a founder of and senior surgeon at the Plastikos Surgery Center in Atlanta. She's a fellow of the American College of Surgeons and the American Society of Plastic and Reconstructive Surgeons.

Since 1962, she says, 2 million American women have had silicone breast implants to increase the volume of their breasts. A woman with small breasts may want them to be larger. However, there are also other reasons. "Sometimes, after nursing, the breast tissue involutes. Women who have had this happen want to obtain the fullness of the breasts they had before they nursed." She adds that the most prevalent reason for this surgery is not a matter of aesthetics so much as "because of reconstruction after cancer or because of traumatic or congenital deformities. Sometimes women are born with breasts of different sizes."

She describes what happens in breast implanting. "The nature of the procedure as we do it now is to make an incision either below the breast, around the nipple, or in the axillary [the armpit]." Usually, the surgeon makes a pocket underneath the chest wall muscles. It is possible to put the implant above these muscles, but if that is done, the skin may stretch out and leave the breast drooping. So, if at all possible, you put the implants under these muscles.

"Right now," she continues, "we are using saline implants." Saline implants are made of a silicone shell filled with salt water. The shell is either smooth or textured, and depending on the procedure, sizers are placed underneath the chest muscles and inflated with water to determine the size that is to be fitted. Then the sizers are removed, and the implants inserted.

WHAT ARE THE RISKS?

The biggest risk of implants has to do with placing a foreign object in the body. Dr. Kolb points out that as we learn more about placing such materials in the body, it is clear that some people's bodies are less tolerant of these substances than are others'.

One problem is that a woman can get bacteria and infections around the implant. Moreover, both bacteria and fungi can live inside the saline in implants. "I have taken implants out where the water is kind of brackish or grayish, and fungus has been in the implant itself," Kulb states. "Since we know that implants can leak, we have to worry about what will happen if the fungus or bacteria leak out into the body. Plastic surgeons as a group are very concerned about this, and there has been a lot of discussion in our journal about what the true risk of this is."

Studies have shown that implants serve as a breeding ground for infections, such as tuberculosis. Kolb says that at her practice, they do cultures of the capsules inside the implants, and they have found a positive culture rate for infectious bacteria of somewhere between 40 and 50 percent. The rate is almost 100 percent for women who are having a lot of pain in the area. She says that if a woman is feeling pain around an implant, "we have to assume that there is a subclinical infection there."

The second risk is deflation. It's a silicone envelope and, like most manufactured containers, will eventually leak. According to Kolb, the engineering data show that timplants begin to leak between 8 and 15 years after the procedure. "This is the silicone gel implants, and now that we are putting saline in, I think we should assume that they will leak as well. When the saline implants leak, you tend to go flat, while with the silicon gel it was difficult to tell if they were leaking. Even the MRIs that are done to determine if they are leaking are not 100 percent accurate. They have about a 15 percent mistake rate." She also notes that some implants leak right after women get mammograms. The textured implants don't seem to tolerate that procedure as well as smooth implants do.

Dr. Douglas Shenklin elaborated on why implants leak. He is a board-certified pathologist who has taught about the effects of implants on the body at the University of Tennessee since 1983 and has published over 270 papers and reviews on this subject. He says that he has had patients who have had implants in for 20 years without a rupture, but the consensus is that about 50 percent rupture in around 10 years and about 70 percent do so in 17 years. After 20 years, you are living on borrowed time. "The longest one we had that didn't rupture lasted around 26 or 27 years and then it was removed," he says. "It fell apart shortly after the surgeon took it out."

Dr. Shenklin explained that the outer layer of the implant is is a very thin shell, about the thickness of an ordinary sheet of photocopying paper. It can fold back on itself like an accordion. When it is put into the body, it is subject to the normal motions. An implant that has been placed behind a muscle distorts the muscle and puts pressure on it. Once it becomes a little bit redundant in the space that is created by the scar tissue that forms around it in the body, the possibility that the implant will crease and fold is very high. That crease is one of the areas where it will rupture.

Some of the very early implants had what were called fixation patches. They were made of Dacron on the back side and were meant to be sewn to the tissues. They represented points of stress in the design. Many implants that are inflatable, either by adding saline to a special compartment or expanding the central compartment, have a valve in them, and those valves represent a defect in the wall. Just like a valve on the inner tube of a tire, the valve creates a stress point. Sometimes those valves are not well designed either and breakage will start right there. So there are many places where rupture and deflation can occur.

The diseases associated with silicone implant leakage include siliconosis, which creates a series of symptoms that may resemble those of other diseases. A number of patients suffering from siliconosis have been diagnosed with fibromyalgia, for example. There is also good clinical evidence, both laboratory and research, that so-called connective tissue diseases occur in relation to the implants.

Not only do these implants leak, but the outer walls may flake off. Kolb notes, "I use smooth wall implants, which are less likely to flake off, get into the scar capsule around the implant and into the lymph nodes, and leak out into the body, causing an immune response." Even so, some silica particles get out of the shell and into the scar tissue, and they can eventually make their way into the lymph nodes, even from smooth wall implants. In some people this can cause an immune response. There is some evidence that the likelihood of this happening can be related to a woman's particular HLA (human leukocyte antigen) type or genetic makeup. It's widely accepted that anyone with a family history or any personal history of autoimmune or connective tissue disease should not get these implants."

Although these problems of implant leaks and flaking are well known, what is less well documented are their ultimate health effects. This is because few studies have been commisioned on the subject. Dr. Shenklin draws a contrast between breast implants and implants made of substances other than silicone that are implanted in parts of the body other than the breast. Both types of implants break down and cause health problems, but only the latter have been sufficiently studied. He states, "All implants wear down." Devices such as metal hip joints and other implantations have similar problems. The surface does break down over time. The joint is in constant use as you walk and sit and get up.

He states, "It's a balance between the objective of getting this implant and the risks involved. For example, take a person whose hip is more or less frozen and basically inactive because of severe arthritis whose health can degenerate and even lead to death due to the immobility. It's a good idea to replace that person's hip joint. But you do it with the understanding that sometimes the implant does not perform correctly."

Breast implants are different from other implants in that the other implants were thoroughly studied before they were put on the market. Dr. Shenklin comments that if you consider orthopedic implants in general, the risks of certain adverse effects are fairly well known because these things were investigated relatively carefully before the procedures began to be done on a large scale.

He gives the example of Swanson implants for finger and toe joints, which are made of hard silicone. Alfred Swanson of Michigan, an orthopedic surgeon, designed these devices in cooperation with the Dow company in the 1950s and early 1960s. He was extremely careful with the research he did to try to understand the long-term consequences. "This is in stark contrast," Shinklin says, "to what has been done with so-called aesthetic devices. Comparable research was not done before these devices were put on the market. So we are now learning from the large-scale experimentation that has been done on the women themselves who have silicone in their bodies."

Since we lack thorough scientific evidence on the health risks associated with implants (though as we will see later much more work is now being done on this subject), we should note some stories of women who have become sick from the implants.

Dr. Kolb herself had silicone implants. "I had silicone gel implants from Dow Corning that were put in in 1985. In 1994, I started having chest wall pains, pains down my arms. My immune system seemed weakened. I got sinus disease, periodontal disease, and fungus that I had never had before. I experienced muscle aches along with neurological symptoms such as dizziness. My hair was falling out. I knew, since I was treating so many women who had leaking or ruptured breast implants, that this was probably what was causing my problems. So in January of 1997 I had my implants removed. Sure enough, I found the implants had been leaking very badly."

Although she may regret it, she decided to get new implants with saline, because at that time she didn't realize that these implants also had problems. She says that she also wanted to gain experience with those implants and that many of her patients had questions about what they were like and what the risks were.

In her experience, the saline implants feel very different in the body than the silicone gel implants do. The specific gravity of silicone gel implants is closer to that of natural breast tissue, so they feel more natural, unless you get a hardening of the capsule of scar tissue that forms around the implant—known as a capsular contracture—which was very prevalent when they were putting them above the muscle. Saline implants are put below the muscles to mask some of the problems, but they are sloshy. She says to imagine bags of water under your chest wall muscles: "It's not real natural."

Equally drastic consequences of having breast implants followed for Kathy Johnston, a registered nurse, who worked for 16 years as a clinical specialist before she became physically disabled due to the rupture of her 10-year-old silicone breast implants. She founded the United Silicone Survivors of Missouri and now serves as president and medical director of that organization. She also works with the Toxic Discovery Network, which publishes *The Toxic Journal*.

This is how she tells her story: "I had my implants removed in 1994 after there had been a rupture. At the time of my rupture, I was standing in my office—I was an oncology nurse—and it literally felt as if a snake had slithered across my body in the upper torso. It was as if a bubble had transported itself across my chest wall.

"I had been having a plethora of symptoms. There I was, a cancer nurse. I was having immune system problems, had been diagnosed with Epstein-Barr, had headaches. The doctors I was working for had no idea what was wrong with me. There were days I was working and I was sicker than my cancer patients. I would have to go lie down because of my terrible headaches. I had flulike symptoms daily.

"This went on for years. The doctors said, 'You're over 40. You have a small child at home. You're tired. You have hormonal depletion. These are symptoms of life.' That is what I was being told. It's time women stood up and said no! I was 40 years old, but I was a healthy individual. "This is not correct," I said. Then I was diagnosed, eventually, as being in the late stages of connective tissue disease."

HOW DO IMPLANTS AFFECT CHILDREN?

Joann Mersano describes the biological effects on the children of parents who have implants, including not only mothers with breast implants but also fathers with penile implants, cheek implants, and other types of implants. This is perhaps the most neglected area of study in the already neglected field devoted to understanding the health hazards of implants.

Mersano was born with a tumor on her right breast, and, after it was removed, her breast never developed properly. She had a breast implant, and 19 years later she became sick. The children she had during that time developed symptoms similar to her own. In 1992, after realizing there were no formal studies establishing a link between parents with implants and high levels of toxicity in their children, she began to gather evidence. Eight years ago she founded the Children Afflicted with Toxic Substances Foundation, a nonprofit foundation that alerts parents to the dangers of implants.

According to her data, women are not the only ones who can be endangered by implants; they can also affect the safety of the fetus. "First of all," she says, "we know that these implants are not expected to last a lifetime. Moreover, the silicone in such things as cheek implants—at least the hard silicone device used in some of them, as well as the gel in TMJ [temporomandibular joint] implants and the harder rubber type of silicone used for chin or pectoral implants—all of these can degrade and leach into the body." The degradation of each type of silicone is a little different. There can be a variety of problems.

In her research, she has come across a number of significant questions: "One question that has been raised in terms of fetal health is that with breast implants, the silicone may not be that much of a danger—though it is a danger—in comparison to the secondary chemicals like benzene and toluene, as well as formaldehyde, all of which are also used in these implants."

Other questions are: Do these substances cross the placental barrier? And, if the substances have gotten into the mother's blood, does the baby get a double dose, first across the placental barrier and later in the breast milk?

Mersano has gathered information about children born to mothers with these implants, children implanted with devices themselves, and mothers who breast-fed their children and then showed various problems. A study of children born to women with reconstructions and implants showed that a small number of them had developed a very rare disorder, esophageal motility disorder (EMD), in which the esophagus doesn't function properly; it is a symptom of scleroderma. Dr. Jeremiah Levine at Shriners Children's Hospital conducted this preliminary study in 1994. He says, "If you picture your esophagus as an inchworm, as you swallow, it moves whatever you are swallowing down to the lower part of your stomach. With this disorder, it basically just sits like a stovepipe. It doesn't function right." The gastric juices and acids can come back up from the stomach, creating problems with bad teeth and throat, constant stomachaches, and various other problems. Dr. Levine went on to publish other studies of children born to mothers with implants, documenting problems with blood and urination, and the esophageal motility disorder kept appearing in later studies.

Because of these studies and others she has been collecting, Mersano has become convinced of the significantly deleterious effects of implants on children. She warns mothers with implants to pay attention if their children complain of headaches or have rashes or are fatigued. "In my study of these children, I find that many kids complain that their knees hurt and their legs cramp. A 3-year-old said she didn't want to ride her tricycle because her legs hurt." She also notes that as an effect of these implants, "You'll find cases where the kid is vomiting all the time or complaining of stomachaches. I mean more than just your normal, occasional stomachache."

She warns that even more serious disorders in children are associated with the implants, such as attention deficit disorder. "We've seen abnormal bone growth where children's legs are bowed and they have lordosis. We've seen muscle weakness and we've gotten reports from doctors of rare renal problems where boys have frequent bladder infections and stenosis (narrowing) of the urethra. That's just a few of the problems we are looking at."

In her opinion, if you had implants at the time you were pregnant and your child has any of these complaints, you need to go to your pediatrician and have a serious talk. Say, "Look, I know that information is being gathered on the relationship between implants and the kind of health problems my child is having." Help him or her learn about this issue.

ROLE OF THE IMPLANT MANUFACTURERS

Mersano is an extraordinary woman who decided that because scientists had never considered this problem, even though hundreds of cases had been reported anecdotally, she would conduct her own study of this situation through correspondence with doctors and sufferers. "I'm just a mom, let me say, but over the years I've worked with many researchers and have read all the studies on the subject. If we go back, we find the manufacturers knew that silicone migrated. It traveled to the ovaries and uterus and crossed the placental barrier. But they never conducted any long-term rigorous studies on the substances they were providing."

As she sees it, the implant manufacturers followed the strategy of the tobacco industry, thinking, If we are caught, we can just say there's no study. That'll be our spiel.

When studies are done, especially those paid for by manufacturers, they tend to be whitewashes. Mersano comments, "Just recently the manufacturers published two studies, one out of Canada and one out of Denmark, stating that it was okay to breast-feed" if you have implants. All these studies did was look at records of children who were hospitalized, yet many of the children who have these symptoms are not hospitalized. She believes there are no existing studies on which you can base a decision on whether it is safe to breast-feed or not.

She notes they've had 40 years to conduct studies on this, but the manufacturers have decided not to do the studies. "We know that there are adverse effects. Just the chemicals alone that are used in these implants, such as formaldehyde, we know are of great concern."

Kathy Johnston has also noticed the weakness of many studies of implants. "Recently, so-called scientific panels have come out saying the danger of these implants has not been established. I was shocked to hear this. Not only as a woman who has been injured by breast implants, but as a medical profession-al. I see the discrepancy between what has happened to women and what these experts talk about. I see where the PR is going and it's absolutely absurd. Nowhere in this report [from June 1998] did they talk about the the known ill effects of the implants. Nowhere did they talk about the migration of silicone in human beings. We have silicone migration recorded in the blood, brain, lymph nodes, liver, and ovaries. This is all documented histology and patholo-gy. For this panel not to take a look at this is, for me, absolutely absurd."

As I've often said on my radio show, we need to investigate a panel's asso-ciations and previous work in the field to see what makes them experts. When the U.S. Food and Drug Administration (FDA) said Prozac was safe and had a panel give it a clean bill of health, I looked into the background of that panel and found all kinds of gross conflicts of interest.

As an indication of the accuracy of such panels, note a *New York Times* report of April 14, 1999, which mentioned a group of lawyers representing a women's group suing a panel of "experts" who released a report exonerating breast implants from causing harm. The lawyers said they had discovered that one of the experts, Dr. Peter Tugwell of the University of Ottawa, had not only received money but was soliciting more from Bristol-Meyers, a breast implant maker. One certainly wonders how unbiased a student of the health risks of the implants will be when he is on the payroll of the very company he is investigating.

Johnston notes that the National Institutes of Health (NIH) are doing a metastudy of breast implant studies. They are looking at what these studies concluded and how accurate their findings are. The NIH did a study about two years ago commenting on the research done so far on breast implants. They said that the studies that have been done were flawed; they were not large enough to be statistically significant.

Dr. Louise Britton of the National Cancer Institute was scheduled to release her findings in 1999, addressing these discrepancies in earlier studies. She points out that all the studies that have exonerated the makers of the implants have looked at women who had implants for less than five years. As Johnson notes sardonically, again seeing the parallel to the tobacco industry, "That's tantamount to looking at smokers who have smoked for five years or less and concluding that cigarettes have no relationship to lung cancer."

PUBLIC ACTION

Earlier we mentioned that Kathy Johnston works with the Toxic Discovery Network, which has done yeoman service in publicizing and fighting to get this health issue studied. One thing her group has done is help sponsor national legislation: the Silicone Breast Implant Research and Information Act, referred to as the Boxer-Green Bill, introduced by Senator Barbara Boxer of California and Representative Gene Green of Texas on June 10, 1998. It is designed to help coordinate breast implant research and ensure that adverse effects of implants on women and their children will be uncovered. It will also try to establish the best treatment options.

The legislation consists of three parts. It establishes a federal coordinating committee; it will help support research on breast implant recipients; and it will identify and correct problems related to FDA regulation of breast implants, specifically the inaccurate information the agency has given out about all breast implants.

According to Johnston, "The Toxic Discovery Network certainly thinks it is past due for Congress to take meaningful action to ensure that women and their doctors have adequate information regarding breast implants. What we need is unbiased scientific research and proper medical treatment. We in the Toxic Discovery Network and women in other organizations across the country will keep reintroducing this legislation in each Congress and keep fighting for it until it is passed. I encourage women to write their senators and representatives about this important bill."

In mid-1999, both the Senate and House versions of the bill were in committee.

Meanwhile, doctors in the U.K. have recognized the problems with these implants. They have been trying to define the disease or diseases that these implants cause. Siliconosis was the name given to these conditions by the British Society of Allergy, Environmental and Nutritional Medicine on September 9, 1998. They defined it as a condition caused by having silicone in one's body, which is not a substance existing in nature. Siliconosis involves local, regional, and systemic problems.

The American doctors who took part in that debate were phenomenal physicians who have backgrounds in studying how breast implants impair the health. These participants included Dr. Henry Jenny, author of the book *Silicone-Gate,* a plastic surgeon and inventor of the saline breast implant; Dr. David Smalley, a consulting pathologist from Memphis, Tennessee; and Dr. Robert Garry, an immunologist from Tulane University. These physicians voted 90 to 0, with four abstentions, to describe this deleterious condition stemming from the implants as a new malady: siliconosis.

REMOVING IMPLANTS

A woman who has implants should seriously consider removing them. Dr. Shenklin says, "The primary therapy for helping a person detoxify from silicone poisoning is to start with getting the implant out. It doesn't matter what type of implant it is, since if it is saline, it still has a silicone coating on the outside, which is what the body is reacting to. Get it out and do not replace it, since doing so often leads to a worsening of the condition."

In fact, as Dr. Kolb points out, Shenklin has done research on women who have had their silicone implants removed and had saline ones inserted. There is an immune system memory of the silicone, which may cause health problems. Kolb says, "I've removed over 300 implants and I've noticed that if we put the saline back in, then the women tend not to get better as quickly from the health problems caused by the orginal implants as they would if we took everything out. What I tell women is: If you're really ill in any way, whether neurologically, metabolically, or whatever, and are getting toxic from the silicone, get the implants out. Rest a while and get better.' They need to go through a detoxification program, which helps them get rid of not only the silicone but also some of the heavy metals that are causing the problems they have."

Women may be reluctant to remove these implants, however. Dr. Vicki Hufnagel, a gynecological surgeon, talks about the worries women have and her own procedures for dealing with the removal. "I have seen plenty of women with breast implants who are dancers, actresses, or models, and I have seen terrible, terrible results. I have seen deformed breasts, and I have seen women who are fatigued, depressed, and in pain. Where their skin was once soft and supple, it is now hard and wrinkled. They look like they have aged 20 years.

"We did blood studies of women with implants and found antigens to the silicone. All their immunological studies were abnormal. To my mind, many of these women are experiencing a silicone reaction. It is real, not a figment of crazy women's imaginations."

Dr. Hufnagel adds that all implants cause damage from silicone, even those with saline: "A lot of women say, 'I'm going to have a saline implant and it is going to be safe.' That's a myth. All implants made are made of silicone. Saline is put in a silicone holding capsule."

Fragments of silicone react with tissue even when the capsule remains intact. Dr. Hufnagel learned this after operating on a patient to remove saline implants and sending tissue to a pathologist for an analysis: "This was big news, and I flew to Washington with it. Here a woman with a saline implant, without a rupture, without a leak, with silicone only being used to hold her saline, gets silicone in all of her chest wall tissue. I reported it to the FDA and they took no action."

Removing implants to reverse the problem has never been a simple option. Women who consider this choice are often talked out of it by surgeons who tell them that their breasts are too stretched out and that they will look terrible afterward. "Women are too scared to do anything about it," Dr. Hufnagel says. "They are afraid that they are going to look worse than they did before the implants were put in, which probably was fine to begin with. A lot of this image issue about having breast implants is probably due to social problems that we have in our society."

Indeed, once implants are removed, women's breasts cave in and become grossly deformed. This sad state of affairs prompted Dr. Hufnagel to devise new surgical methods for restoring breast appearance during breast implant removal.

Dr. Hufnagel's challenge was to figure out how to take implants out without having the breasts cave in. She reports success using an argon beam: "I asked myself, 'How do we shrink the dead space that has been created in a woman's body from tissue being pushed out?' I use the argon gas to send a heat-fiber type of electricity in a spraylike manner. This will not burn the body, but it will shrink tissue. We take the whole chest wall, where this envelope is, and we shrink it. That prevents massive deformity.

"We operated on two small, thin women who had large implants in very small chests. Normally, they would have been deformed once we had removed their implants. But we have had good outcomes. We really think we've hit on something.

"Also, by using the argon beam, we are ablating the reactive tissue and allowing new healthy tissue to grow in its place. This is breakthrough surgery." Dr. Hufnagel adds that ending the need for such operations depends on psychological and sociological factors. "The silicone problem is going to be with us as long as women don't like themselves."

Before surgery, Dr. Hufnagel advises women to learn as much about silicone as they can, to get a complete diagnostic workup, including a silicone antibody test, and to follow a good vitamin program. "Surgery is stressful to go through, so build up your body," she advises. "Not too much vitamin C for the first two weeks, as it will increase scar formation. You want higher amounts of vitamins A and E. Avoid vitamin C until two weeks after surgery.

"Learn everything. Ask questions. Ask to look at pictures of women who have had their implants removed. If they don't remove the capsule, be sure that they at least biopsy it and submit it for tissue analysis to look for silicone.

"Finally, report your case to the FDA. Every case should be reported. That doesn't mean that the government is going to take action. But if we have enough people, someone someday may stick their nose in the file and find out, 'My goodness, after the FDA retracted their announcement on silicone, they got all of these reports and still did nothing.'"

DETOXIFICATION

Once the implants are out, the body has to be detoxified. Dr. Shenklin has developed one protocol for this. "What we do is treat the immune system to try and quiet it down. I've been using a drug called Plakenol on my female patients. We give a moderate dose over a 10-day period and stop and see what the effect has been. Sometimes we have to give a second round later. We use anacytal, which helps to detoxify the body.

"My protocol for detoxification is holistic. It has to do with diet, trying to eat more fresh foods, exercise, and stress reduction techniques." For supplementation, he recommends inositol, a B vitamin that helps hydroxylate the crystallized silicate in the tissues. For more severe problems, he give an IV formula containing vitamin C and minerals. For the fibromyalgia, magnesium is very helpful.

He doesn't believe that the health problems women with implants have all stem from one thing unless, of course, the silicone is leaking very badly. These patients, for example, have mercury fillings and they have heavy metal toxins from living in the city and breathing lead all of the time. The effects are cumulative, as with any toxic disorder. Part of the real challenge is therefore to try to figure out all the different components and then treat all of those things together in detoxifying.

To continue with Dr. Shenklin's detoxification protocol, "We put our patients on immune supplements. We have a mixture of minerals and herbs that are good for the immune system; we also have superantioxidant vitamins. Many of the women who take this mixture get a boost of energy just from the nutritional supplement involved. It's something their bodies were lacking. So we start them off with this before we remove the implants, because we don't want them to have an adverse reaction. Their immune systems are always in poor condition, as you can tell from looking at their T-cell counts and other indications."

With such programs, the ill health associated with implants can be reversed.

Chapter 10

Diabetes

D iabetes mellitus is a serious condition that in the late 1990s affected nearly 16 million Americans a year. Today diabetes is the third leading cause of death in the United States and a primary cause of new cases of blindness, renal disease, and nontraumatic amputations. Dr. Robert Atkins, a complementary physician from New York City, says, "In 1960, 1 percent of the American population was diabetic, but now it is 3 percent. Diabetes has tripled in the last 35 years. In addition, certain subsegments of the population are more often affected; African-Americans, for example, are disproportionately affected." Women who take oral contraceptives may be increasing their risk of getting diabetes, since oral contraceptives have been associated with lower vitamin B levels, which can lead to glucose intolerance.

Causes

Diabetes is closely associated with heart disease, and the incidence of both conditions increased when Americans began to change their dietary patterns. "There is a wonderful book written about 25 years ago," Dr. Atkins continues, "called *The Saccharine Disease,* by Dr. Cleave. He made observations, one of which was "the law of 20 years," which says that after you introduce refined carbohydrates into a culture, two illnesses emerge two decades later, diabetes and heart disease. We know that a Third World diet without refined carbohydrates leads to no heart disease and no diabetes. When one illness emerges, so does the other. Studies of this sort have linked diabetes with heart disease. We know that a woman who is diabetic is three times more likely than women in the general population to get heart disease."

Under normal circumstances, insulin is released by the pancreas in response to elevated levels of sugar in the blood. It promotes the transport and entry of glucose to muscle cells and various tissues, thus lowering blood sugar levels. In a diabetic, part of the process is interrupted as a result of a deficiency in, resistance to, or insensitivity to insulin.

INSULIN DEFICIENCY

For many years, it was thought that diabetes is purely and simply a deficiency syndrome in which the body does not produce sufficient quantities of insulin for proper glucose metabolism and assimilation. More recently, it has been learned that many diabetics do produce enough insulin, but their cells do not take it in. The problem is, then, due to insulin insensitivity or resistance.

INSULIN INSENSITIVITY

Insulin enters cells at points known as receptor sites. When the receptor sites are plugged because of fat, cholesterol, inactivity, and obesity, insulin cannot enter. As a result, glucose stays in the blood and creates hyperglycemia, or high blood sugar. This excess sugar is diagnosed as diabetes. In such cases, there is no need to increase insulin production but rather a need to enhance insulin sensitivity. A person with diabetes needs to work at making his or her own insulin more efficient, and simply increasing the amount of insulin will not do that.

INSULIN RESISTANCE

Insulin resistance is a phenomenon that is closely related to insulin insensitivity. With insulin resistance, there is also a sufficient or even overabundant supply of insulin, but allergic responses prevent insulin from doing its job. Usually allergies to specific foods suppress the activity and efficiency of insulin. Different factors may be responsible for a disordered carbohydrate metabolism in different people. Wheat, for instance, may create symptoms of high blood sugar in one woman and corn may affect another. Offending substances can be determined on an individual basis with food allergy tests.

Different factors are responsible for the two main types of diabetes.

Type I diabetes is the most serious form of the disease. Type I diabetes used to be called juvenile diabetes, because for many years it was believed that this type of diabetes only occurred in the childhood or teenage years. This form of diabetes is characterized by a true insulin deficiency. It results when the pancreas is damaged from some exotic viral infection or even a highly toxic state. The disease may also be a genetic condition. In type I diabetes the beta cells in the pancreas that produce insulin are destroyed. Since type I diabetics have an insulin deficiency, they have to take insulin by injection daily, and generally for life.

Maturity-onset or type II diabetes is more of an acquired disease. It is often precipitated by chronic excess weight from poor diet and/or lack of exercise. It may also be brought on by overconsumption of stressor foods or other allergens that are insulin resistors.

Type II diabetes accounts for some 90% of all diabetes in the U.S. It occurs most frequently in adults over age 40. In type II diabetes, the beta cells in the pancreas still produce insulin, but for a variety of reasons there may be insufficient insulin production or the body may not be adequately using the insulin that is produced. Thus this form of the disease is characterized by complications of insulin resistance and insulin sensitivity rather than, in most cases, a true deficiency of insulin. For this reason, maturity onset diabetes can frequently be non-insulin-dependent.

Symptoms

Often there are no symptoms present, especially in the beginning stages of type II diabetes. Obesity is sometimes a sign of a prediabetic state, especially when the excess weight is concentrated at the waistline and just above the waistline. Classic diabetic symptoms are more often experienced by type I diabetics and include frequent urination, especially at night, great thirst and hunger, fatigue, weight loss, irritability, and restlessness. Progressively, the eyes, kidneys, nervous system, and skin become affected. Infections and hardening of the arteries commonly develop. In type I diabetes, coma from a lack of insulin is a constant danger.

Clinical Experience

TRADITIONAL APPROACHES

INSULIN

Before the development of insulin in the 1920s, diabetic patients had a bleak prognosis. Sufferers saw the condition rapidly go from bad to worse as complications such as blindness, gout, and gangrene developed. Overall life span was drastically shortened.

In the beginning, insulin appeared to be a miraculous drug, and it probably was. The life span of diabetic children was extended from months to decades. Today, many of these children live normal, productive lives.

Insulin is still the primary therapy for type I diabetes. Type I diabetics generally take insulin at least once a day, frequently several times a day. While some type II diabetics require injections of insulin, many are given oral hypoglycemic medications. Many type II diabetics incorrectly believe that these pills are simply a form of insulin, but that is not the case. None of the oral medications used to treat type II diabetes contain insulin. They are designed to help your body use the insulin that is in your pancreas more effectively, or to stimulate better insulin production. Consequently, oral medications can only be used by diabetics whose pancreas still makes some insulin. In addition, some type II diabetics can control their diabetes entirely through diet and exercise.

COMPLICATIONS AND BLOOD SUGAR CONTROL

Although diabetes can cause a wide variety of complications, from kidney and eye problems to nerve damage, some of these complications can be reduced considerably by carefully controlling blood sugar. For many years doctors assumed that diabetics whose blood glucose levels were as close to normal ranges as possible reduced their risk of serious complications. In 1993, the results of a nationwide trial, the Diabetes Control and Complications Trial (DCCT), one of the largest studies ever conducted, confirmed that diabetics in the intensive control group, with glycohumaglobin rates that averaged 7.1, reduced their risk of eye disease by 76 percent compared with the less aggressively managed group, with glycohumaglobin rates of 8.9 percent. Across the board, diabetics in the intensive control group had a 50 percent reduction in all serious diabetic complications. Although the trial was conducted only on type I diabetics, experts believe that the findings of the study apply to all diabetics.

CURRENT DIETARY RECOMMENDATIONS

The findings of the DCCT study make diet and eating habits even more important for diabetics than previously. Eating the right foods can help maintain proper blood sugar levels, as well as helping to boost your immune system. In 1994 the American Diabetes Association changed the dietary guidelines for diabetics.

In the past there was one standard diabetic diet, prescribed for all diabetics. Now the ADA recommends that diabetics work with experts in diet and nutrition to individualize their diets. In the past, complex carbohydrates, like potatoes and bread, were restricted because it was believed that they caused moderate increases in blood sugar. The new dietary recommendations recognize that complex carbohydrates are not the problem they were once thought to be. Emphasis is now put on the total amount of carbohydrates in a meal, rather than the source. Diabetics are frequently taught to count carbohydrates, and match medication requirements to carbohydrate intake. This is especially true for insulin-dependent diabetics.

Unlike simple sugars, complex carbohydrates are beneficial. Although both are broken down into glucose, the latter do not go directly into the bloodstream. While simple sugars immediately enter the blood, complex carbohydrates go through a long process of digestion and only very gradually release sugar into the blood. Therefore, they do not then contribute to the high blood sugar levels, as do simple carbohydrates. Instead, they stabilize and improve health.

In addition, fat and protein are more carefully monitored than in the past. Diabetics who are overweight are told to keep fat intake to no more than 20 to

25 percent of total calories. Large amounts of protein may be related to accelerated kidney damage. This is because protein must be immediately processed by the body; it cannot be stored. This puts a great stress on the nephron cells, which filter the body's toxins. Many diabetics suffer from kidney deterioration as a result and must receive dialysis or a kidney transplant. Studies show that the elimination of meat from the diet is often enough to reverse kidney damage.

THE NATURAL APPROACH

Despite its severity, diabetes need not be as debilitating as it usually is. While there is currently no cure, there are ways of enhancing the body's natural defenses through nutrition, avoidance of allergy-producing substances, and exercise. A healthy lifestyle and alternative approaches to treatment can decrease the amount of insulin or oral medications needed by some persons, although type I diabetics will need to continue taking insulin for life.

The goal of treatment can and should be to build up the body's ability to function as independently as possible. When changing to a more holistic approach to treatment, it is important not to immediately discontinue any of your diabetic medication. Instead, a preventive medicine physician should assist in the gradual transition. With a doctor's guidance, medication may be reduced or completely eliminated with time. Complete elimination, however, is not always possible.

Physicians who practice alternative approaches to treating diabetes for the most part employ a program combining exercise and dietary modification aimed both at better nutrition and at weight loss, where indicated. Medications are used only as second- and third-line approaches. This sort of program usually controls the disease and its ancillary complications in a less invasive, more efficacious manner, in a short period of time.

While type II diabetics respond most dramatically, even type I diabetics may be able to reduce their insulin dependency. More importantly, they are able to alleviate many of the insidious complications that have come to be thought of as intrinsic to diabetes.

DIET

Since diabetes and heart disease are so closely related, Dr. Atkins recommends that some people with diabetes follow a Dean Ornish program, in which they drastically cut down on dietary fats. The best diet consists of organic vegetarian foods, eaten raw, sprouted, steamed, baked, or stir-fried with little or no oil. Those who have a true insulin disorder will not fare well on a high-carbohydrate diet, since diabetes is a carbohydrate metabolism disorder. "It is important to know who needs carbohydrate restriction versus who needs fat restriction," Dr. Atkins says. "To determine that, there are a variety of tests, including a cholesterol profile in which we look at the ratio between the triglycerides and the HDL [high-density lipoprotein]. When a person has a blood sugar disorder leading to a lipid disorder, the ratio is extremely high. To be really safe, the number should be approximately the same or the HDL should be higher than the triglycerides. It is perfectly appropriate to spend five or six weeks on one diet and then get all of your parameters checked again, and then spend five or six weeks on the other diet and get them checked again. In that way, you can make an intelligent decision."

EXERCISE

An exercise regimen is crucial for burning calories and normalizing metabolism, and is especially important for overweight adults, who are often inactive.

Exercise also heightens the body's sensitivity to insulin. By lowering cholesterol, it lowers triglyceride levels in the blood, making cells more available for glucose assimilation. This is why the insulin requirements of diabetic athletes always drop while they're engaged in swimming, soccer, and other sports. Athletes also notice an increase in their insulin requirements when they cease doing their physical activities for an extended period of time.

Athletes are not the only ones who benefit from exercise. Ten to twenty minutes of light exercise after each meal helps reduce the amount of insulin necessary to keep blood sugar levels under control. A brisk walk gets the body's metabolism working a little faster so that food is more easily absorbed. That prevents blood sugar from rising too high.

An exception to the rule involves diabetics with heart disease. In these patients, exercising after eating may precipitate an angina attack because of the transfer of blood from the intestines to the legs and other parts of the body.

ALLERGY TESTING

Testing for food allergies can determine which foods are responsible for insulin resistance. Clinical experience has shown that this approach to treatment is the most useful way to get to the root of adult-onset diabetes and reverse the condition. Patients can usually be weaned from insulin, since an insulin deficiency is not the cause of the problem. Eliminating allergy-producing foods may also foster weight loss. This occurs because people crave foods when they are allergic to them. When these foods are taken out of the diet, the desire for them eventually stops.

To determine whether a specific food is causing hyperglycemia, a doctor can monitor a patient's blood sugar before and after that food is eaten. Foods that raise the blood sugar cause allergic reactions and should be eliminated.

SUPPLEMENTS

In addition to diet and exercise, the following supplements are important to know about:

CHROMIUM PICOLINATE. Chromium helps normalize glucose levels in insulin-dependent diabetics.

MAGNESIUM AND POTASSIUM. These minerals also help to maintain a glucose tolerance level.

ZINC. Zinc is essential for normal insulin production.

ENZYMES. Enzymes useful in controlling insulin-dependent diabetes are digestive protylase, amylase, and lipase.

VANADYL SULFATE. Vanadyl sulfate may be the most important mineral for diabetes. It was discovered in France in the late 1800s and used to help diabetics before insulin appeared on the market. It works at the cellular level and is most effective when taken three times a day.

TOPICAL TREATMENT FOR DIABETIC ULCERS

Ulceration at various locations plagues many patients with diabetes and cause a condition that is often serious enough to warrant amputation. This tragedy can be averted with a simple solution. According to clinical studies, raw, unprocessed honey is an ideal dressing agent for almost every type of wound or ulcer. It sterilizes the ulcerated area, and often works even after antibiotics fail.

OTHER APPROACHES

Mucokehl (made from the fungus *Mucor recemosus*), which was originally developed in Germany, may actually reverse diabetic neuropathy. People using this remedy get feeling back in their extremities, and their eyesight improves. Many practitioners also recommend chelation therapy for reducing diabetic retinopathy and healing foot ulcers.

MONITORING AND PREVENTING DIABETES

Diabetics and those who wish to prevent diabetes can do a great deal to monitor themselves. It's important to look for the presence of antibodies that attack some of the body to defend against an ingested allergen. This is easy to see if the symptoms are blatant, but not if they are subtle. The thing to look for is a general lowering of the body's immune response. The best way to see this is to go five days without eating the food (or any of its relatives) you wish to test. If you want to test milk, abstain from cheese, ice cream, and all other dairy items or processed foods that contain milk as an ingredient. After five days, eat a meal consisting of just milk and eat generous amounts of it. Then tune in to your body's response. If you experience headaches, stomachaches, pulse rate changes, increased heartbeat or blood sugar, depression, lethargy, dizziness, or even delusions, you can see that your body has reacted negatively to this substance. In other words, you have an allergic response to it. You will have to back off from it. Leave it alone for 12 weeks initially. When it is reintroduced into the diet, it must be rotated with other foods. Eat it in modest amount no more often than once every four days.

"Of course, there are a lot of good things about that four-day basis," says Dr. William Philpott, a prominent diabetes researcher and clinician. "You will eat... 30 or 40 kinds of foods instead of the half dozen you've been eating. This is a very wholesome thing. To have the necessary nutrition you will have a wide range of foods." It is a good idea to try introducing new foods into your diet, ones that you have never thought to eat. Try not to eat any foods more frequently than twice a week.

Dr. Philpott recommends that you invest in some diabetic equipment so that you can monitor your blood sugar an hour after each meal. "At least 110 is optimum," he says, "and 160 or beyond is high blood sugar. Before the next meal, test your blood sugar again to make sure it is at least 120 before starting your next meal. If it is not, wait and exercise. Get it down before your next meal. Monitor your pH from saliva; it should be 6.4. If it is below 6.4, you are having a reaction to the food. Measure your pulse; if it varies drastically, you are reacting to the food. Blood pressure is more significant. Physical symptoms, mental symptoms, and blood sugar are the most important. They are absolutely essential. It will take about 30 days to do this."

Gestational Diabetes

About 3 percent of nondiabetic women develop a type of diabetes called gestational diabetes during pregnancy, usually in the last trimester. Gestational diabetes is diagnosed with an oral glucose tolerance test. In many cases this type of diabetes can be controlled with diet and exercise. Although gestational diabetes disappears after delivery, as many as 50 percent of women with gestational diabetes will develop diabetes later.

Dr. Susanna Reid, a naturopathic physician at the Center for Natural Medicine at the Center for Women's Health in Darien, Connecticut, says that diet and exercise are the key to controlling gestational diabetes.

Dr. Reid advises women with gestational diabetes to learn how to eat on the low end of the glycemic index. The glycemic index was developed around 1982 by Dr. Sullivan, who gave people glucose and then measured how high the sugar level in their blood rose. He then established that level as 100 percent of the glycemic index. He repeated the experiment by giving people various foods and measuring how high their blood sugar would go just as he had with glucose, and assigned then each food a percentage.

Dr. Reid says that foods we don't normally associate with sugar may still be high on the glycemic index. "A baked potato and puffed rice are both 100 percent on the glycemic index, which means that they raise your blood sugar significantly. This is bad for your body; it goes into a state of alarm when your blood sugar rises so quickly and significantly, and it produces more insulin. Since the rate of rise is so rapid, the body tends to overproduce insulin and people get what is called reactive hypoglycemia (low blood sugar). Then they have to eat sugar to get their blood sugars back up again. Therefore you need to eat foods low on the glycemic index to avoid either hypoglycemia or reactive hypoglycemia."

She explains that the position of some on the glycemic index may seem counterintuitive. These include fruits, nuts, and legumes. For example, peaches, plums, grapefruit, and cherries are between 20 and 29 percent on the glycemic index. But potatoes and even carrots and parsnips and rice are at the top level. She says, "When you eat foods that are high on the glycemic index, you need to have a healthy fat with them. Doing this seems to prevent the rapid rise in blood sugar. If you had a baked potato, for example, you'd want to have olive oil in it."

Foods that you may think would be low on the glycemic index, such as vegetables, are often among the highest. "Peas are between 50 and 59 percent on the index and corn is between 60 and 69 percent. Yams are very high, but sweet potatoes are much lower on the index than yams. Brown rice and all the grains tend to be very high."

EXERCISE

Dr. Reid also tells her patients about the importance of exercise for gestational diabetics. She says that by exercising regularly, we can often keep our blood sugar levels within the normal range. "When a person exercises, it improves insulin's ability to remove glucose from the blood and also decreases insulin resistance. If you exercise 60 minutes a day at 60 to 70 percent of the maximum heart rate, then usually after just one week of exercise you'll see an improvement in the glucose tolerance test. But be careful not to overdo it and cause your blood sugars to drop too low."

Reid warns that a woman should not attempt to become a world-class athlete while pregnant. "But she should continue and enhance her current exercise program. There are some things that she needs to be careful about. She should not lie supine and attempt to lift weights, she shouldn't get too warm, she should maintain adequate hydration, and she probably shouldn't take up a new sport in which balance is a main requirement because she is having to adjust daily to changes in the shape of her body and her orientation in space. She wouldn't want to do anything where she might fall, such as inline skating at top speed."

Reid's favored exercises are running and walking. "Women need to feel free to move when they are pregnant. It is not a pathological state. They are not ill."

NUTRITIONAL SUPPLEMENTS

Reid cautions against using some herbal supplements during pregnancy. "Most of the herbs are contraindicated in pregnancy, so one has to be cautious in treating gestational diabetes. For example, traditional herbs we would use to treat non-insulin-dependent diabetes, which gestational diabetes usually is, are bitter melon (*Mamordica charantia*), fenugreek, elecampane (*Inula helenium*), and garlic and onion supplements. All those are contraindicated in a pregnant woman. Ginkgo and jerusalem artichoke are not contraindicated, and in all of the research that I've done I can't find a contraindication for *Gymnema sylvestre*, which is an herb that seems to increase the pancreas's ability to produce insulin, which would be advantageous in patients with gestational diabetes."

Patient Stories

DR JULIAN WHITAKER

Dr. Julian Whitaker, who has worked with many diabetic patients, has had considerable success with a program that emphasizes diet, vitamin and mineral supplements, exercise, and practical education. Here he describes two cases. The first was a 27-year-old patient who was taught to use these essential tools.

"He was on insulin for about six months and was also having hypoglycemic reactions. When we saw him, he was taking only 10 to 12 units of insulin per day and his blood sugar levels were very low. Whenever you have a situation like this, you can cut down on the insulin and then eventually get off it completely. We measured in his blood a protein called C peptide which measures the body's production of insulin. If his pancreas was not producing insulin, his C peptide would be about zero. This patient had a close to normal C-peptide, meaning that his pancreas was producing insulin. We put him on a program to sensitize his body to the lower levels of insulin his pancreas was producing. This included exercise, a low-fat diet, and vitamin and mineral supplements…. It has now been about nine months, and he has been without insulin. His blood sugar level would go to about 140 or so after breakfast, but then he was told to exercise, and when he keeps up his program, his blood sugar level stays under control. I think this indicates that you have a very powerful tool in diet, exercise, and minerals which is patently ignored by most physicians treating diabetes as they systematically utilize insulin and oral drugs for their diabetic patients."

Another case of Dr. Whitaker's illustrates the shortcomings and even abuses of traditional diabetic treatment and at the same time shows how an alternative approach may be more appropriate and efficacious.

"Five years before I first saw this patient, he had had mild high blood pressure for which he was started on diuretics. He used hydrochlorothiazide, a thiazide diuretic. This drug has a tendency to lower potassium and elevate blood sugar, findings that are well known and are listed in *The Physicians' Desk Reference*, but it is still the most commonly used prescription medication worldwide. The patient's potassium level dropped, he developed some cardiac arrhythmias, his blood sugar level began to go up, and his problem was diagnosed as high blood pressure plus diabetes. He was placed on oral medications that failed to lower his blood sugar, so he was placed on insulin. When a patient like this gentleman, who did not have any diabetes to speak of but had a drug-induced form of diabetes, is placed on insulin, his blood sugar drops to a very low level. The body responds to this low level by generating glucose from the liver and shooting the blood glucose up very high so that when the highs and lows are checked, the physician feels the patient is out of control and increases the insulin level; this, of course, only increases the rebound, or the up and down characteristics, of the blood sugar. This is what happened. Not only was he having much higher and much lower blood sugar levels, he was having one or two hypoglycemic attacks a day. He kept going back to the hospital with this problem, and when he arrived there, his blood sugar would be high, so they increased his insulin. He was taking 130 units of insulin daily and was also taking additional medication for cardiac arrhythmias and high blood pressure, which he didn't have, and 17 prescription pills daily.

"When we saw him, we realized that he had not had any dietary advice at all. This, I think, is in some way systematic malpractice. We very rapidly took him off of all of his medications. When we instituted a low-fat, high-carbohydrate diet plus an exercise program under close monitoring, we were able to test his blood sugars two to three times a day. We cut his insulin in half in two days and then eliminated it after another two days. For nine days he went without insulin, and his blood sugar never went back up again. We stopped the diuretics and gave him additional potassium. His blood sugar never went back up again, and he was able to lose some weight in the short time he was with us. When he went home and continued the low-fat, high-carbohydrate diet plus exercise, his weight continued to drop; he lost, I think, an additional 20 pounds. Over this period of time, he never required medications again. Here he had been treated by two board-certified, highly specialized, highly respected physicians in his community, who had been doing—and I went over his chart very carefully—everything appropriately, according to standard methods of practice. In other words, it is currently acceptable that some kind of drug is given for mild elevations of blood sugar. The practice isn't even frowned upon. It's also currently acceptable to prescribe a diuretic for mild blood pressure elevations, even though the diuretic may cause problems down the line.

"As a result of following these currently acceptable methods of therapy, the patient was rapidly deteriorating not from any diseases he had but from the treatments he was given. We were able to use diet and exercise to cut through the requirement for medications, and he is still, a year and a half later, not taking any medications. Now he's quite a bit healthier. I think a diabetic patient is prone to excessive drug use not only in the treatment of the initial condition but also in the treatment of conditions associated with diabetes. But when you use a diet and exercise program to cut through that, you can eliminate a tremendous amount of prescription medication, as was done in this patient."

DR. WILLIAM PHILPOTT

Dr. William Philpott's treatment is based on the detection of insulin resistance factors in specific food and chemical allergies as they affect the individual patient's ability to utilize available insulin supplies efficiently. He describes what happened in his treatment of a 60-year-old man who was a diagnosed type II (maturity-onset) diabetic:

"He was placed on an oral medication which he took twice a day. However, I saw him 11 years after that diagnosis at his present age. His fasting blood sugar was usually around 300. The doctors said, 'We are going to have to go to insulin.' He was very weak—just terribly fatigued—and depressed too. He had read my book *Victory over Diabetes* and wanted to give it a try before he went on insulin. When he came to me he was not on insulin yet; he was just ready to be put on insulin. I simply put him on foods that he just never would be addicted or allergic to and put him on intravenous vitamin C, B$_6$, calcium, and magnesium for about four days in a row.

"By the time we reached the fourth day his fasting blood sugar was normal. On the sixth day, we started feeding him foods that he more commonly used. One of those foods was wheat, and within an hour his blood sugar was 270. At about three or four hours it had normalized and we were able to give him another meal. With rye it was 275. On garbanzo beans it was 206, millet was 189, and even milk was 176. Oatmeal was 206. So we had at least a dozen foods that gave him high blood sugar. Actually the most important was the wheat, which he ate religiously every day.

"We find the cereal grains containing gluten—wheat, rye, oats, barley, buckwheat—to be the most serious reactors. Through the years, only sugar and glucose have been used as the criteria for response, but we found much higher reaction to wheat.

"As we studied him, we grew a fungus from his mouth and from his stool and rectal area called *Candida albicans*. He also had rather high antibodies. A lot of diabetics are made toxic by this organism.

"We spotted that and found that he was deficient in magnesium and folic acid. We found that he was taking in 400 mg of caffeine, in coffee, every day. This was an important factor that was helping to disorder his functions. Now, knowing the foods he reacted to and leaving them out of the diet for at least 12 weeks while treating his infection and making his nutrition optimum, we were able to very quickly leave him with good energy, good control, and no high blood sugar at all.

"Instead of going on insulin, here we have him strong with no high blood sugar at all and without infections. If we had just given him insulin and paid no attention to this fungus infection, he'd still be toxic. If you monitor him from any standpoint you wish, this man doesn't have diabetes. That's the difference between the types of symptom management: just giving insulin to cover this insulin resistance that he had. We measured his insulin, and actually he had a normal amount of insulin.

"His problem was insulin resistance. Now he knows that the disease process is not deteriorating him any more. The consequences of this deterioration are depression, weakness, infection by fungi and viruses, and soon the whole degenerating disease process. Now we have him on a high-fiber diet, which will feed the right kind of bacteria. There will be good bowel function, moving the toxins out of the body, which is necessary.

"But this is a very small part of what you need to do. People should lose weight and should use this kind of diet, but there is something much more central to this disease process, which is the insulin resistance to the food and your ability to isolate which foods prevent your body from using insulin properly."

Herbal Pharmacy

Plants containing phytochemicals with antidiabetic properties, in order of potency, are as follows:

Cichorium intybus (chicory)
Rauwolfia serpentina (Indian snakeroot)
Thymus vulgaris (common thyme)
Arctium lappa (gobo)
Carthamus tinctorius (safflower)
Passiflora edulis (maracuya)
Opuntia ficus-indica (Indian fig)
Taraxacum officinale (dandelion)
Tetrapanax papyriferus (rice paper plant)
Canavalia ensiformis (jack bean)
Linum usitatissimum (flax)
Pueraria lobata (kudzu)
Hordeum vulgare (barley)
Inula helenium (elecampane)
Althaea officinalis (marsh mallow)
Oenothera biennis (evening primrose)
Avena sativa (oats)
Triticum aestivum (wheat)
Medicago sativa (alfalfa)
Panicum maximum (guinea grass)

Plants containing phytochemicals with insulin-sparing properties, in order of potency, are as follows:

Cocos nucifera (coconut)
Plantago major (common plantain)

Chapter 11

Eating Disorders

P aul Goodman, a radical social theorist of the 1950s and 1960s, wrote one of the most interesting analyses of *On the Road* by Jack Kerouac. That 1957 novel was about dissatisfied youth, dubbed "beatniks" by the press, who restlessly moved about the United States, dissatisfied with the anti-intellectual culture and conformism of the Eisenhower years. Most critics either decried or fulsomely praised the book, depending on their reaction to its literary and political message. In his review Goodman looked at what the novel's protagonists, who had become role models for disaffected youth, ate for dinner, noting that their favorite foods were hamburgers and French fries. In a time before fast-food restaurants, this was an avant-garde cuisine. Goodman argued, though, that this soft type of food, which does not have to be chewed, symbolically represents a desire to avoid conflict. Not only were the beatniks dropouts who didn't want to get involved in the success-oriented rat race of American society, they didn't even want to commit to masticating their food. For Goodman this indicated a lamentable withdrawal from life's struggles.

Whatever the merits of Goodman's analysis, his basic point—that what people eat says a lot about who they are—is repeatedly illustrated in this chapter as we look at various eating disorders and fad diets.

Food Cravings and Emotional States

Dr. Doreen Virtue, former director of a clinic and inpatient psychiatric unit specializing in eating disorders, has a Ph.D. in counseling psychiatry and is the author of several books on dieting and health, including *Constant Craving from A to Z.*

The first thing to do in approaching the topic of food cravings is to distinguish between a craving and a desire to compensate for nutritional deficiencies. "Most nutritionists would have you believe that nutritional deficiencies are at the heart of all food cravings," she says. "The problem with that approach is that it still leaves many food cravings unexplained. Food cravings tend to be so specific. For example, a person may crave a hard-boiled egg but not a soft-boiled egg. Or a person may want a chocolate candy bar but not chocolate pudding. It sounds bizarre and a little childish, but anyone who has experienced food cravings will understand how intense and specific they can be.

"Another reason why nutrient deficiencies may not be the only possible cause of these cravings is that not everyone satisfies his or her craving for food before the craving passes. Just as mysteriously as the food craving appears, it may vanish. A food craving can change as easily as a person's state of mind." Virtue has been researching food cravings for 12 years and has found patterns that correlate with people's personalities and emotional issues. Again and again, for instance, she found that someone who craved, say, bread was very different from someone who craved ice cream. It's similar to drug-taking behavior. Someone addicted to marijuana, say, has a very different personality and style than someone addicted to another drug.

Noting this correlation, she says, "I investigated further to look at the correlation between personality, emotional and spiritual issues, and how they are connected to food cravings. I did a great deal of research in university libraries, looking at the psychoactive, that is, mood-altering, chemicals found in different foods. I'm not talking about chemicals such as pesticides. I mean the inherent properties, such as vitamins, minerals, amino acids, and so on, that actually can increase or decrease our blood pressure and trigger the pleasure centers of the brain and other areas, chemicals that really affect our moods and energy. What I found is that we all tend to act as intuitive pharmacists. We tend to crave foods that will bring us to a state of homeostasis, which means balance or peace of mind. Whenever we are upset, it is normal for us to do something to fix that. If we don't want to take direct action, for instance, by making changes overtly in our lives, a more covert way of dealing with the upset is food cravings, which are cravings for a chemical that will make the body feel at peace."

From this point of view, Virtue believes that food cravings should be dealt with by trying to understand their underlying emotional sources. Instead of getting angry at yourself for having food cravings, thinking, Oh, I'm so weak. I should have more willpower, it's better and healthier to listen to those cravings, which are a form of intuition. As Virtue puts it, "Deciphering them is almost like dream interpretation. They can give us guidance in our lives and help us in many ways."

We noted earlier that a food craving is not due to a nutritional deficiency. Nor is it due to physical hunger. Virtue explains, "Let's think about the difference between emotional hunger and physical hunger. They can feel identical, and actually, this is one of the most important points in managing the appetite: to know the difference between emotional cravings and physical cravings."

She notes several underlying differences. For one thing, emotional hunger comes all of a sudden, out of the blue. As she puts it, "You feel like you are starving. Whereas physical hunger is gradual, at one moment you might just feel a little pang in your stomach, then over the course of the next hour or so it grows into a voracious hunger."

The second difference is that emotional hunger is usually for a very specific food. It has to be rocky road ice cream or it must be a pepperoni pizza. Physical hunger, while it may have preferences, is open to different types of food. It doesn't require an exact type of food to be satisfied.

Third, Virtue says, "Emotional hunger is always above the neck, whereas physical hunger is based in the stomach. Emotional hunger is a kind of 'mouth hunger' where in your mouth you get a taste for a certain thing. It's a very cerebral type of hunger. It is also very urgent. It has to be satisfied now, whereas physical hunger says, 'I am hungry, but I could wait 15 minutes or a half hour if I needed to.'"

The demanding nature of emotional food cravings is due to the urge's misguided attempt to fill an emotional hole: "One of the reasons emotional hunger is urgent is that it really is uncomfortable with the feeling and wants to make that feeling go away. Emotional hunger also is usually paired with some upsetting emotion. And if we stop for a moment when we are experiencing this emotion and ask, 'Could there possibly be something that upset me that I wasn't acknowledging?' as we go into introspection, we usually see that a clerk was rude or a driver cut us off on the road. We are upset, not really hungry."

Physical hunger arises from a real physical need, not from emotional needs. Emotional hunger, since it is not related to actual physical need, has a strong psychic component: "When we do try to satisfy it, we almost go into a trance where we are eating without realizing we are eating. It's as if someone else's hand were holding the fork or the spoon. It can be designated as 'automatic' or 'absentminded' eating. With physical hunger, you are more aware of, more tuned in to what you are eating: you are satisfying it."

This is why many holidays involve overeating and eating foods we normally would not touch: "One reason that, for instance, most people can think of a Thanksgiving when they overate is that a lot of intense emotions take place around that holiday. Maybe you are with your family and someone overdrinks and gets into an argument, or it may be all these emotions in a happy way. So one of the reasons we overeat at Thanksgiving is because of these intense feelings we may not know what to do with. Even after we are stuffed, we keep going. Of course, the food is delicious, but this goes beyond that, because true physical hunger stops when you are full."

SPECIFIC TRIGGER FOODS

Usually, if you really look at it, Virtue notes, there are a few trigger foods that cause a voracious appetite. If you want to find out what your triggers are, you can ask a friend or someone who eats with you, "What kind of food do I seem to binge on?" If you are aware of your own food cravings, you can ask yourself, What's going on and how do I feel?, the same way you would about stress.

Virtue says, "What I've found is that several factors are involved that correlate the particular trigger food to the emotions. One is the texture. Is the food crunchy or soft or chewy? The next is the actual physical components and the underlying chemical properties that either increase or decrease blood pressure, elevate or lower mood, and create neurochemicals that alter mood. The last thing is the flavor or the taste, whether it's spicy, salty, sugary. All these things have to do with who we are as a personality."

Again, identifying your trigger foods is a way to understand what your underlying fears and other emotions are expressing. "Instead of getting mad at ourselves for craving these things," she counsels, "we need to see our cravings as a blessing in disguise. It's the body's way of talking to us. It's just like when a person puts his or her hand on a hot plate. Then the body talks back and says, 'Get that hand off that heat.' Our appetite is trying to do the same sort of thing and give us a message."

THE FIVE CORE EATING STYLES

Food cravings, Virtue observes, are paired with specific ways of eating, or what she calls core emotional eating styles: "There are five core emotional eating styles. Although most people center on one style, it is possible to be more than one. Some people are all five, although that is very uncommon."

"The first one is the binge eater. This is a very black-and-white eating style. You are a binge eater or you are not. It's a person who, in response to a certain trigger food, as if she or he had an allergy, goes on an eating binge when she or he tastes this food. Refined white flour and sugar are very common binge foods. Such people actually need to abstain, as if they were alcoholics staying away from alcohol, in order to manage their appetites."

The second style of overeater is the mood eater: "This is a person who overeats in response to very strong emotions. It's usually someone who is very sensitive. She may not overtly express her feelings, but deep within she feels emotions very strongly. This is often an intuitive person. Sometimes she will overeat because of other people's emotions which have upset her. This is a person who can heal very easily from overeating by keeping a food journal every time she has a craving and then writing down what she ate and the accompanying emotion. She can then identify what emotion will send her into mood eating and plan other ways to cope when this emotion appears.

The third type is the self-esteem eater: "This is the person who, often because of life events, has low self-esteem and issues about worthiness. Such a person will feel she doesn't deserve success. She often tends to berate herself or even criticize herself in front of others. Whenever she starts to lose weight, she gets frightened because she might be getting some attention from the opposite sex, which can scare her, especially if she has had a history of any kind of sexual abuse. She may feel that she does not deserve happiness and will sabotage herself. This type of woman will often benefit from talking to a skilled eating-disorder therapist."

The fourth type is the stress overeater: "This person will overeat when there is a lot of tension in the air. She'll go home from work and head right to the refrigerator." According to Virtue, a stress eater does really well by exercising. She should also schedule some fun and relaxation into the week. Spending time outdoors is good, as is any kind of spiritual practice. It doesn't have to be religion. Meditation and yoga are helpful for stress eaters.

The fifth type of overeater is the snowball-effect eater: "This is the kind of person who, just like a snowball rolling down a mountain, will gain speed and momentum in her eating after going on a strict diet. She will say, 'I'm not going to eat anything except for three little things at each meal.' This is unrealistic. Every day she begins adding more and more to the diet without realizing what is going on. As her plate gets fuller, her weight goes up, like a snowball."

Dealing with these types of unregulated eating, then, means following the Socratic injunction "Know yourself." Once you understand which emotions and situations are driving you into these unwanted patterns, you can take steps to satisfy your emotional cravings in less destructive ways.

Insulin Reaction and Overeating

Having examined the emotional basis for overeating, let's look at its biological basis in the body's glucose cycle. Colette Heimowitz has a master's degree in nutrition from Hunter College, is certified in health and nutrition by Pratt University, and has 20 years of clinical experience in weight management.

The number one biological cause of obesity in our sedentary population, she maintains, must be understood in terms of insulin resistance: "In a normal homeostasis, an individual ingests a carbohydrate and it raises the glucose levels in the blood. When someone eats protein or fat, by contrast, this doesn't happen. Once the glucose level rises in the blood, it sparks an insulin response from the pancreas. What the insulin does is take the glucose to the peripheral tissues, either to the fat cells, the liver, or to muscle as storage. When we age, as a result of years of eating refined carbohydrates, maintaining high-sugar diets, and living a sedentary life, the insulin is no longer efficient at taking the glucose to the peripheral tissue.

"One of two things happens. Either the glucose levels remain high or the insulin is constantly being produced—overproduced in a prediabetic state—and fat is constantly being stored. When we are sedentary, the process of burning glucose for energy is not happening. It will even provoke the reaction more."

Among the factors that contribute to insulin resistance, "one, of the utmost importance, is lifestyle, a sedentary lifestyle. Some research was done with retired master athletes. Glucose tolerance tests with insulin levels were studied before putting them on bed rest for only one day. The glucose tolerance factors were normal, and the glucose in the blood was normal, because they were still leading an active life, not an elite athlete life, but still one that was active. After one day of bed rest, the glucose tolerance test was repeated and the glucose levels were much higher."

Equally important, Heimowitz says, was a history of eating refined foods, which "the American public is known for—taking the bran out of food, taking the fiber out of food, and replacing the essential fatty acids with hydrogenated fats. This causes a complete stress on the insulin level. The glycemic index of foods [a measurement of the amount of glucose found in the blood as a result of eating a specific food] is much higher, provoking more of an insulin response. The pancreas eventually gets trigger-happy."

There is also a genetic component. It has been shown that people whose parents have a history of diabetes or cardiovascular disease have a weak gene that makes them susceptible to this particular condition. She says, "They especially have to be careful and have an active lifestyle and a low-saturated-fat, higher-protein, lower-carbohydrate diet."

TREATMENT: FOOD AND SUPPLEMENTS

To alter this continuous fat and flabby syndrome, a lower-carbohydrate diet is needed to give the pancreas a rest. Heimowitz recommends eating "low-glycemic-index-type foods, that is, complex whole foods such as fruits and vegetables." She also recommends specific supplements for the insulin-resistant individual.

Alpha lypoic acid is the biological spark plug in converting glucose to energy. She states, "It can lower and stabilize glucose levels and stimulate insulin activity. Some research was done with diabetics being given 600 mg daily, and it stabilized their glucose levels without any medication. A nondiabetic or hypoglycemic person could probably use 200 to 300 mg a day."

The mineral vanadium, found in vanadyl sulfate, also reduces insulin resistance; 15 to 30 mg a day is appropriate.

Chromium is a component of the glucose tolerance factor, a molecule essential for normal insulin function in glucose metabolism. Usually 200 to 1,000 mcg daily is the range for a beneficial effect.

Heimowitz also emphasizes "essential fatty acids, which are grossly lacking in the American diet and also improve insulin sensitivity and reduce insulin resistance. So supplementing the diet with 3,000 to 6,000 mg of the omega-3 fatty acids is appropriate."

Vitamin E is also important. It relieves some of the oxidative stress caused by excessive glucose, which results in free radicals. It will also reduce the risk of cardiovascular disease. Heimowitz adds, "Excessive insulin also causes a lipidation of the triglycerides, and that causes free radical pathology. The excessive insulin also thickens the aortic valve. You are at a higher risk of cardiovascular disease. The vitamin E should be anywhere between 400 and 800 IU daily."

Zinc also influences carbohydrate metabolism, increases the insulin response, improves glucose tolerance, influences the basal metabolism rate, and supports thyroid function; 50 to 100 mg of zinc a day is important.

Magnesium helps maintain tissue sensitivity so that insulin is more effective at taking that glucose to the peripheral tissues. Magnesium helps control glucose metabolism and also decreases sugar cravings; 500 to 1,000 mg a day is recommended. "Sometimes," she cautions, "when you go as high as 1,000 mg, it may cause diarrhea, so the dose should be determined individually. People should start at 500 and work up slowly."

Heimowitz notes that manganese has been shown in studies to be important for insulin activity: "Manganese-deficient rats showed reduced insulin activity and impaired glucose tolerance. This lack also lowered glucose oxidation and the conversion of triglycerides in the rats' adipose tissues. However, the manganese should be dosed in relation to zinc and copper because they will compete at the cell site. So as little as 35 mg of manganese is all you need. The proportionate amount of zinc would be 100 mg."

She notes further, "If someone has hypotension because of the insulin resistance, the amino acid tyrosine could also help control the hypotension; 1,500 mg to 3,000 mg daily is appropriate. Hawthorn berry, an herb, can also help control hypotension; 240 to 480 mg is a good range.

"When there is cardiovascular involvement, with a high risk, especially with low HDL [high-density lipoprotein] and elevated triglycerides in individuals with insulin resistance, coenzyme Q10 is also appropriate. I suggest 100 to 200 mg a day."

TREATMENT: EXERCISE

As we saw in the experiment where retired athletes were forced to remain in bed, lack of exercise also causes blood sugar problems. Thus, exercise is key. Heimowitz recommends that "for exercise, we look at the fitness level of the individual. I wouldn't tell someone who has been a couch potato to go out and exercise an hour a day. The fitness level needs to be increased slowly so the body can adjust to the different mechanisms that are going on.

"Someone might want to start with a brisk walk in the morning for 30 minutes every day. That's a good start. If they have foot or knee problems, a good swim or stationary bicycle—anything that results in some kind of sweat or heating up of the body to help burn some of that glucose in the blood, which will allow the body not to produce so much insulin because you are burning the glucose for energy.

"Then, as the fitness level increases and the person feels more comfortable, I usually recommend that she take her pulse, using the equation for finding the optimal pulse rate that is described in exercise books. As the person's pulse becomes more normal as she exercises, she may increase the level of exercise. The walk goes into a jog and then into a run. I think an hour a day, especially if you are sitting behind a desk all day, is appropriate, at least six times a week. Some kind of activity is needed every day."

Why Popular Diets Don't' Work: The High-Protein, Low-Carbohydrate Scam

The multifaceted approach to combating eating disorders presented so far combines assessing your emotional state, exercising, eating right, and taking supplements. This is in contrast to the faddish, highly touted wonder diets that appear in the media every season. These diets are more often feel-good panders to eaters' worst cravings than scientifically sound practices.

Dr. Joel Furman is a board-certified physician in private practice in Belle Mead, New Jersey, who specializes in preventing and reversing diseases through nutritional methods. He is the author of *Fasting and Eating for Health*.

"High-protein, low-carbohydrate diets have become increasingly popular over the past few years," he notes, "and doctors who promote these diets list a number of reasons why people with weight problems need to get onto this type of diet. One reason they give is that these people's bodies do not metabolize carbohydrates properly, a condition popularly referred to as insulin resistance."

"In fact," Furman cautions, "such diets, promoted in some of the most heavily promoted, best-selling diet books, are among the most dangerous. Among these books are *Enter the Zone* by Barry Sears, the Atkins books, and *Protein Power* by Michael Eades."

The problem is not the connection between the insulin reaction and bad eating habits but how these books recommend breaking the habits: "All these people who read these books, wanting to lose weight by eating a high-protein, low-carbohydrate diet, remind me of people who want to lose weight by snorting cocaine and smoking cigarettes. In other words, there are lots of ways that may work to help you lose weight, but we are interested in more than just having a person temporarily lose weight. We want a diet that is going to enable us to lose weight and protect our health simultaneously, not something that will end up making us look thin in a coffin or increase our cancer risk."

These diets, he goes on, counsel replacing one bad food, refined carbohydrates, with another, animal fats: "You know, some of these high-protein-diet gurus claim that they have the truth [about the value of eating meat and animal products] and that there's a conspiracy among the 1,500 scientific studies that continue to point to the association between the consumption of meat, eggs, and dairy products and cancer, heart disease, kidney failure, constipation, gallstones, and hemorrhoids, just to name a few. They are overlooking the fact that you must pay a price with your health for eating increased animal proteins as a way to lose weight."

"Of course, there is one good point in what these people say," he adds. "It's true that refined carbohydrates such as pasta, bread, sugar, sweets, candies, bagels, croissants, potato chips, and all the junk food that Americans eat are not doing us any good. This junk now constitutes about 50 percent of the American diet. We know that this food is linked to heart attacks, cancer, obesity, and diabetes. That is absolutely true."

However, the gurus "are taking the fact that these highly refined, low-fiber carbohydrates can cause increased insulin levels, obesity, and insulin resistance, showing that those are dangerous foods and then saying that therefore the diet should be low in carbohydrates and high in animal protein.

"But that's a jump that the nutritional and scientific literature doesn't make. As a matter of fact, there are no data showing that a person on a high-carbohydrate diet rich in unrefined carbohydrates, such as mangoes, cabbage, beans, legumes, and squash, is in any danger. In fact, many studies show that a diet centered on unrefined carbohydrates—vegetables, whole grains, legumes—will not raise blood sugar or insulin levels."

What people don't realize, Furman goes on, "is the value of plant protein. Compare a steak to broccoli, for example. Let's look at the protein comparison for 100 calories of steak and 100 calories of broccoli. Sirloin steak has 5.4 grams of protein for 100 calories, and broccoli has 11.2 grams. In other words, green vegetables are very rich in protein. Beans are very rich in protein. We can devise a diet that is very low in animal fat or totally vegetarian, but with a good, satisfactory amount of healthy protein.

"People have to realize that there is a big biochemical difference between animal and plant protein. Plant protein lowers cholesterol; animal protein raises cholesterol. Plant protein is a protector against cancer; animal protein is a cancer promoter. Plant protein promotes bone strength; animal protein promotes bone loss. Plant protein has no effect on aging or kidney disease, and animal protein accelerates both of them. In other words, plant protein is packaged along with fiber, phytochemicals, vitamin E, and omega-3 fatty acids. Animal protein is packaged with saturated fat, cholesterol and arachidonic acid."

Therefore, "if you are on a diet such as the Atkins diet or another high-protein diet in order to lose weight, you are paying a price with, for example, the risk of increased cancer."

In Dr. Furman's opinion, after studying the food recommendations of these diets, "I suspect that a person really following one of these high-protein diets that restrict fruit and carotenoid-rich starches—found in foods such as sweet potatoes, corn, and squash—could be more than doubling her risk of colon cancer.

"There are studies that show a clear and dose-responsive relationship between increased cancers of the digestive tract and low fruit consumption. High fruit consumption has a powerful dose-response relationship to reduction of mortality from all causes of death. The only other food that even approaches this powerful effect of reducing cancer is raw vegetable consumption. So I suggest that if you are going to average 60 to 70 percent of your caloroes from fat and animal products with no fruit, you have to consider that diet exceedingly dangerous."

Dr. Furman describes his own experience of the difference between patients on a plant-protein-rich diet and those on an animal-protein-heavy diet: "Now, I am a physician in practice, so I can watch what happens. In 10 years I may have seen 20,000 patients and treated them with aggressive nutritional interventions that emphasize plant protein. I have a good success rate. I get about 95 percent of my diabetic patients off insulin in two or three months, and this is with a primarily vegetarian diet. Their sugars go down. The long-term effect is that their health improves; their cholesterol drops, and their triglyceride levels drop. It's a diet that is rich in natural foods and unrefined foods."

By contrast, patients who had been trying to control their sugars on high-protein diets did not do as well: "They've gotten some improvement in their glucose responses, but they come in with higher creatinine, and they've hurt their kidneys.

"These are patients who came to me after following the diets recommended by these high-protein proponents. Some came with kidney failure after having damaged their kidneys by eating a high-protein diet. Diabetes itself damages your kidneys enough. You don't have to add to this a diet that accelerates kidney damage." What happens is that the high-protein diet leads to ketosis, a toxic condition in which brain is fed the wrong type of fuel, instead of glucose.

"They used to use ketogenic diets to treat children with seizure disorders when they were unresponsive to medication. Medical studies showed that these diets resulted in very serious metabolic consequences over time. Investigators report that they caused hemolytic anemia, abnormal liver function, renal tubular acidosis, and spontaneous bone fractures. In other words, it's a dangerous way of eating that will age us prematurely and slowly accelerate the calcification of our kidneys and the destruction of the kidneys with time."

Another danger of these diets is that they promote growth. To the uninformed, it might seem that growth-promoting foods are good, but Furman warns, "If we eat foods that accelerate growth, we speed up aging. Growth is very similar to aging. Laboratory animals that grow the fastest die the youngest. If we feed them foods that maximize growth—especially when they are young—it's almost like we are causing their bodies to age rapidly.

"On a cellular level, the body has to remove wastes and has to repair DNA damage. Eating a diet that activates the cell and activates the DNA and makes the cell replicate and grow is in a sense overworking or overtaxing the body's mechanisms of detoxification and DNA replication. From one perspective, you are prematurely aging the species. With breast cancer, for example, the more slowly a woman grows and the later is her age of puberty, as marked by the first menstrual period, the lower is her chance of developing breast cancer. The object should not be to make our kids weigh 150 pounds by the time they are 12. The object is not to grow as rapidly as possible."

Nutritionists 30 years ago believed it was good to feed kids in a way that maximized growth. But, Furman suggests, "Now we have learned that the opposite is true. The less we feed an animal, the longer it lives. We want to choose a diet that is rich in nutrients, sure, but low in fats and calories. The only way you can devise a diet that is rich in nutrients and includes an assortment of fibers, phytochemicals, antioxidants, and trace minerals is to eat a large quantity of vegetation in your diet, which has to include green vegetables and things like that. In other words, if we were to analyze the nutrient density of all foods, we would find that vegetables such as salad, broccoli, and string beans would always come out as having the highest nutrient density."

Why Popular Diets Don't Work: The Blood-Type Diet

Other popular diets advocate eating according to a person's blood type. These diets have sold many books, and the authors have appeared on all the shows. The authors say, "It's your blood type. You have to eat this for your blood type." I've seen a ton of scientific evidence that could disprove that and show its lack of validity. So why is that approach not being challenged by the American public or the media?

According to Furman, these diets are popular because they give free rein to people's ingrained bad habits: "I think it reinforces what people want to believe. People are addicted to their rich diets. They are looking to hang on to any reason, however irrational it may be, to not have to change.

"If you talk to smokers, you'll see the same thing. You'll hear how irrational are the reasons they give for why they must still smoke and how they have diminished in their own minds the strong reasons against smoking. The same is true with eating. People want to rationalize why it is okay to do whatever they are addicted to doing. "The American addiction to such things as junk foods is such that when you stop doing it, you get uncomfortable. The problem is that the American diet is so toxic and so unhealthy that when people try to go off it, when they skip a meal and start eating fruits and vegetables, they feel sick. They get headaches and abdominal cramps. They get shakes and confusion. Then they think that it must be this new diet. It must be that eating healthily is making them sick. They must need this rich animal-fat protein and the junk food. In other words, they don't see that this is a temporary phase that lasts a week or two, when they are withdrawing from caffeine and the rich nitrogenous waste. You might feel a little ill when you change your diet. That slight resistance to change is one basis of people's addiction to harmful foods, and it makes them turn to these quack diets."

THE THREE (CRIPPLED) LEGS OF BLOOD-TYPE DIET THEORY

Referring to James D'Adamo's book *The Blood Type Diet*, Furman maintains that "D'Adamo's whole theory of blood types is based on three legs. If we look at these legs in detail, we see that they fall down and the whole thing collapses."

LEG 1: AGGLUTINATION

D'Adamo's first claim is that eating certain foods for certain blood types will cause agglutination as a result of lectins in the food. "He really shows a very poor understanding of human physiology," according to Furman, "because he is looking at agglutination on a lab slide, not in the body. The body has various mechanisms to prevent agglutination with the immune system and through the production of various enzymes in the gastrointestinal tract. In other words, looking on a slide at a person's blood is not the same thing as what goes on in the body. If people were having agglutination from lectins, all the type O's who agglutinate with beans and wheat would be dead by now because agglutination would cause infarction of the brain and organs. In other words, the whole thing is so ridiculous that it's almost silly to have to discuss it."

LEG 2: POISONOUS CHEMICALS

Leg 2 of the theory is that the indocyanine test has shown that some chemicals are more poisonous for certain people. Furman argues, "This is also a hypothesis which is not supported by one article in the scientific literature. The author completely ignores enzymes such as intestinal transglutaminases, which are secreted in response to lectin-induced damage. He ignores the transmission of peptides to the gut and the intestinal tract that inhibits the absorption of these things. In other words, these things do occur, there are lectins in various foods, but the body knows about it, we've been brought up with this for millions of years as our genetics have evolved and the body has evolved mechanisms to handle it."

LEG 3: HYPERSECRETION OF ACID

Leg 3 of the theory holds that type O's hypersecrete hydrochloric acid so that they can digest animal protein better. To Furman's mind, "that also falls on its face.

"First of all, this diet guru says that type O's have more ulcers. Ulcers are not caused by hypersecretion of acid, so he's wrong on that point. The other thing is that type O's have been found to include all different types: hypersecreters, undersecreters, and normal secreters of acid. Moreover, hypersecretion of acid does not give you the ability to digest protein in the first place. Protein is digested by pepsin, and the acid in the stomach makes the right type of environment to activate the pepsinogen in the pepsin. If you hypersecrete acid, the higher acid will decrease the activity of the pepsin and interfere with protein digestion. So theoretically if this idea were correct and not part of some one-size-fits-all diet theory of lumping all the type-O people into one secretion state, it wouldn't make sense even in relation to hypersecretion's relation to digestion.

"Another aspect of the third leg of this theory is the idea that a type O has the ability to break down cholesterol easier than other people can. That also is not true. We thought in the 1960s that alkaline phosphatase was involved in lipid absorption, but in recent years we have discovered that it has a different function altogether."

Furman's resounding conclusion is that "every leg of his theory, all the scientific reasons that are given by this author for the rationale behind his diet, fall flat on their face when you scrutinize them. His diet doesn't have a leg to stand on."

Anorexia, Bulimia, and Obesity

Anorexia involves compulsive dieting to the point where the anorectic eats so little that she becomes malnourished and may actually starve herself to death. It is signaled by muscle wasting, loss of menstrual periods, body image problems, and an exaggerated fear of becoming fat. Bulimia is characterized by compulsive eating and forced vomiting or the use of laxatives or diuretics to eliminate many of the calories that are consumed during binge episodes. Obesity is seen as an enormous increase in the ratio of fat to muscle, the result of eating to excess, far beyond what the body needs.

Carolyn Costin is the director of the Eating Disorder Center and the author of *The Dieting Daughter* and other books. She came to the study of eating disorders through her own experience: "I had anorexia nervosa myself when I was about 16 years old. I had a pretty severe case, was 79 pounds for a few years."

CAUSES

In Costin's opinion, a number of seemingly benign factors, such as the emphasis on exercising and dieting in our culture, as well as interpersonal family pressures may cause a woman or adolescent to fall into any of these negative eating practices.

The problem with diets is that they often disappoint their users. "The main thing I say to people about any kind of diet program is, 'Don't do anything to lose weight that you're not prepared to do for the rest of your life, because going on a diet certainly implies that you'll ultimately go off it.'"

So what happens when you go off it? This will lead to disillusionment and weight disorders, such as constantly going on and off trendy diets, unless a person realizes that a healthy lifestyle, not a temporary eating change, is the only answer to maintaining proper weight: "So really, what it always comes down to, always—and everyone ultimately finds this out in the end—is that it's a balanced way of eating and having a lifestyle that is, I think, one that lets you be not just physically healthy but emotionally healthy too."

Another problem is that a healthy desire to exercise can be developed in the wrong way. This, Costin says, is "a little bit like an activity disorder. They can't not do it. There's an addictive component that makes them have to do more and more. Things in their life get put on hold in order to do the activity. They will continue to do it even if they've been injured or are in pain or it's snowing outside. And the way the eating disorders correlate with activity disorders, there are certainly a lot of anorectics and bulimics who also have activity disorder."

In Costin's view, eating disorders are also caused by the way people obsessively codify rules of eating, what she calls "the Thin Commandments." She notes, "Over the years I started to come up with these rules that people with eating disorders have, such as 'If I eat anything, then I have to exercise and burn it off' or 'I have to wear clothes to make myself look thinner. I have to punish myself if I've eaten anything fattening.'"

Delving deeper, one finds that eating disorders are often rooted in relationships girls form with their parents, particularly their mothers, though not the type of relationship that's commonly assumed to be at fault. "In the beginning," Costin explains, "anorexia nervosa was often blamed on overcontrolling mothers. But that's way too simplistic." Rather, the problem is the type of role models that mothers sometimes provide for their daughters. Costin asks, "What are little girls learning from these role models about their bodies and about weight and about food?"

Not only those who actually end up with eating disorders but almost all young women and girls are influenced by these role models. Costin says, "When you have statistics that 80 percent of fourth-grade girls report that they're dieting and 10 or 11 percent of those girls report that they're vomiting on these diets, you've got to look at what's happening with their role models."

Costin describes a 6-year-old girl in her waiting room who said she was really excited at having chickenpox. Asked why, she said it meant going to bed without any dinner. "I said, 'Well, what's so good about that?' And she said, 'Because it means I didn't have any calories.' The thing is, she's 6. Her mother was a binge eater seeing me for treatment. But kids are little sponges. And she hears her mother talking about calories are bad and calories are in food, so she just learns that part of being female is trying not to have too many calories."

Fathers also can have a negative influence. "I talk to fathers a lot," Costin comments, "about being conscious about what they say about female bodies when they're reading magazines or watching television or things like that. I talk to them about not just praising their daughters for the way they look, which is a very common thing that fathers do with their little girls. A lot of praise and attention focus on appearance as opposed to internal validation. And also just a lot of paying attention to who their daughter is, doing things with their daughter."

Finally, there is mounting evidence that eating disorders have some basis in genetics. Costin states, "It's pretty clear from twin studies that we're going to learn more and more in the next few years about genes that predispose people to inherit this. It's probably going to turn out that there's a biological predisposition. And then maybe a cultural trigger sets it off. Thus, there's a swing back to a more biological basis of these illnesses and not as much of a focus on the big, bad culture. But I think there's no doubt that the culture plays a big role in it, which is why we see over the years an increasing incidence of anorexia and bulimia. But I think it's a combination of someone who has a predisposition and dieting, which is certainly a risk factor. So if more of the population is dieting, more people who have the biological predisposition are exposed to this trigger."

TREATMENT: NUTRITION

Costin outlined some of the basic approaches to nutritional therapy. "There are many ways to do nutritional therapy with eating disorder patients," she notes. "One is educational. A dietitian will do some educational sessions. The patients have a lot of myths about food such as 'If I eat anything with sugar, it's going to turn into fat' or 'If I eat anything at night, it's going to turn into fat.' So you send them just to be educated."

More complex is "another model that's education combined with therapy." This is needed because "patients' food fears are related to some very deeply rooted psychological stuff. So you combine nutrition therapy and nutrition education."

There are various ways to do this. "For example," Costin explains, "I can send someone to a dietitian, and they get a food plan set up. They get some help, and they go for a few weeks, and then they continue with their therapy, but they don't go back for more nutritional sessions until they're ready to take the next step."

TREATMENT: PSYCHOLOGICAL COUNSELING

The first step in counseling a woman with an eating disorder is to help her analyze why she has this problem, Costin explains: "We start off asking her, 'Why do you have this disorder? What's good about it? How has it helped you? Let's talk about the advantages of it.' The woman may look at us sideways. But it's important because she needs to understand how it's come to serve a purpose. And that's the whole psychological aspect of it.

"A woman will have some desire to maintain her disorder because it helps her feel in control; it helps her feel unique and special; it's a way she deals with anger. Getting to the emotional aspect is really, really important, and if you don't deal with that, I think you don't really deal with the illness."

TREATMENT: SUPPLEMENTS

Costin finds supplements helpful in treating eating disorders: "We're using amino acids in some cases with patients instead of medication, and it's working. It's pretty interesting. We use tyrosine and tryptophan and glutamine."

More specifically, she recommends "the use of tryptophan, particularly with bulimia nervosa. We use it for people who have trouble sleeping as well. Phenylalanine also, for depression. Tyrosine for depression. For people who are often given medications such as Ritalin, we use a combination of tyrosine, glutamine, and phenylalanine together."

REFEEDING

In working with recovering bulimics and anorectics, it is necessary to begin returning to normal eating patterns gradually. Costin explains, "In fact, a lot of the deaths that happened early on with anorexia occurred during the refeeding process, because the heart just can't take the volume that you start giving it if you do the refeeding too fast."

In her practice, "We slowly raise the patients' calories. We get lab tests two to three times a week. We take their pulse in the morning and sometimes even during the day and after meals just to make sure their bodies are handling the stress that comes from refeeding. You can't just take someone who's emaciated and say okay, start eating."

TREATMENT: COGNITIVE THERAPY

Dr. José Yaryura-Tobias, an orthomolecular psychiatrist, also finds that because of the life-threatening severity of a condition such as anorexia nervosa, any nutritional approach must be preceded by a program of cognitive therapy: "Anorexia nervosa, from our perspective, is an obsessive-compulsive disorder that is related to self-image, the way that we perceive ourselves. Basically, anorexia nervosa is the process by which a human being self-starves. Thirty percent of the population who self-starve eventually die.

"In the vast majority of cases, when patients come for a consultation, they are already very emaciated. The chemistry we can measure is very altered. From the biochemical viewpoint, we know that there is a groove related to an area of the brain called the limbic system. This is the hypothalamic area, which regulates sugar, thirst, appetite, and so forth. This information can help us classify some of these patients but does not tell us how to manage and eventually cure the problem. The rest of the problem, we feel, has to do with body-image perception, the way that these patients see their own bodies. They feel too fat. They have different perspectives than the rest of us do.

"How do we treat this condition? Basically, we use a nutritional approach after the patient has undertaken a behavioral program with cognitive therapy. Cognitive therapy is important because the idea is to educate the person about her problems and to discuss with her how many false beliefs she has have about who she is, why she thinks this way, why her body looks the way it does for her, and so forth. So false-belief modification is an important part of treatment."

Breaking the Cycle of Food Addiction

As I have said and written for many years, food cravings and food addictions often mask food allergies to the very foods we crave.

Dr. Hyla Cass, a holistic psychiatrist who integrates psychotherapy and nutritional medicine, describes her experience treating patients suffering from food addiction as follows: "Some time ago, a psychologist who specializes in eating disorders began to send her clients to me because she had heard that antidepressant medications work for these patients. I had shifted to a more holistic way of looking at things, so I told the psychologist that before I did anything with antidepressants I would try some other things. With certain eating disorders, such as food cravings, the underlying problem is a food allergy. We often crave the very foods to which we are allergic. Typically, it's the very things we want to eat that are the most damaging, that create the symptoms. In fact, it's like an addiction to alcohol: As you abstain from the foods you're addicted to, you begin to have withdrawal symptoms and crave those foods even more.

"In order to break the cycle in cases of food addiction, just as in breaking the cycle with drinking (alcoholics are actually allergic to alcohol), you need to supply the body with the appropriate nutrients. When we correct the deficiencies and restore body balance, the food cravings and allergy symptoms will often be relieved. Rather than having to rely strictly on 'willpower,' it is possible for individuals to break addictive cycles by achieving metabolic balance through avoiding the offending foods and supporting the body with a balanced nutritional program of vitamins, minerals, and amino acids. Often the cravings will then simply go away. It's quite remarkable: With a good vitamin and mineral product, you can often put a stop to the food allergy and its accompanying symptoms.

"I may order a plasma amino acid analysis, a blood test to determine which amino acids—-especially among the essential ones which the body cannot synthesize by itself—-are low. The amino acid glutamine, in a dose of 500 to 1,000 mg, is particularly useful for reducing cravings, including alcohol cravings.

"There are other things to do for food allergies as well," Dr. Cass adds. "Addictions and allergies are often related to magnesium deficiency and can be corrected by supplementation. There are also techniques that can actually eliminate food allergies through the use of acupuncture and acupressure."

"As we can see," Dr. Cass concludes, "there are many ways, other than psychotherapy and medication, to approach what at first seems like a psychological problem."

Dr. Doris Rapp, a pediatric allergist and environmental medicine specialist, gives us more details concerning the connection between food cravings and allergies: "In my experience, eating disorders and alcoholism can be related to allergies. Frequently, eating disorders are food addictions. When you have a food sensitivity, there is a certain phase of it that makes you really crave that food. And if you happen to be addicted to wheat or baked goods, for example, you can never get enough of them, with the result that you may become obese. To give another example, men who are addicted to corn may drink a lot of beer and can become alcoholics. They're sensitive to and addicted to the beer, but it's the corn—-or sometimes some other component—-in the beer that is causing the problem. Sometimes, for those with an allergy to grains, they may feel 'drunk' after eating cereal or certain types of baked goods."

You Can Recover from Eating Disorders

Carolyn Costin, however, disagrees with those who say that eating disorders such as bulimia are an addiction like alcoholism: "It's really, really important that you can be recovered from conditions such as anorexia and bulimia. With alcoholism, you have it and your body responds to alcohol differently. For your whole life you can't have a drink because you are then going to be off the wagon and compulsively drink." This is distinct from eating disorders: "For example, the approach to bulimia shouldn't be, well, okay, if you eat chocolate you binge on it, and therefore you can't eat chocolate. I think that instead we have to learn how to teach you that you can absolutely be in control of this. You have to learn how to have it without binging and purging it.

"The bottom line is that the new studies show that people become fully recovered from these illnesses. It takes a long time. The new research shows approximately five to eight years, but the recovery rates are high, much higher than originally was thought. It's like 76 percent full recovery with anorexia nervosa. There's fewer studies on bulimia, but it's pretty good."

More on Physiological Causes

Research shows that anorexia nervosa, bulimia, and obesity may be the result of a zinc deficiency. Dr. Alexander Schauss, Ph.D., C.E.D.S., a clinical psychologist and eating disorders specialist from Tacoma, Washington, reports that science has long been aware of this connection: "We've known since at least the 1930s that when animals were experimentally placed on diets deficient in zinc, those animals would develop anorexia. Our interest in eating disorders in relationship to zinc has to do with the observation that when humans are placed on zinc-deficient diets, they too develop eating disorders."

"By characterizing three of the most common eating disorders," Dr. Schauss continues, "you can see how vital zinc is. In morbid obesity, when people are significantly overweight in such a way that it could shorten their life span or increase their risk of disease, we know that there is an inverse relationship between the level of obesity and the level of zinc, meaning that the more obese they are, the less zinc they have in the body. We don't know yet whether this is cause or effect, but it is a very important observation because at the other end of the continuum, with anorexia nervosa, self-induced starvation, we also have individuals who are generally always zinc-deficient. We believe there is strong evidence today, from studies done at the University of Kentucky School of Medicine, Stanford University, and the University of California at Davis, in addition to our research institute's work, that the lower the zinc status is, the more likely it is that the patient will not recover from any treatment plan to resolve the anorexia."

Stress is commonly associated with the onset and continuation of eating disorders and can also be understood in terms of zinc loss, since constant mental stress results in the depletion of this mineral. In 1975 it was reported that between ages 15 and 20 zinc loss caused by stress is at its lifetime peak. Women are more prone to stress-related zinc loss than men are and therefore more likely to have eating disorders. Dr. Schauss explains, "The answer may lie in the fact that males have prostate glands and women do not. Zinc is highly concentrated in the prostate in males; it provides a mineral that is essential for the development, motility, viability, and quantity of sperm. If a male is under psychological stress, he can catabolize or seek out stores of zinc in the prostate. Since women don't have a prostate, they will catabolize the zinc from other tissue.

"In women, the richest source of zinc is found in muscle tissue and bone. A common feature of anorexia is muscle wasting and an increased risk of osteoporosis. Anorectics actually catabolize or eat their own tissue as a way of releasing nutrients that they are not getting in the diet. The last muscle, and one that contains only about 1 percent zinc, is the heart muscle. When the body starts to scavenge zinc out of heart muscle tissue, it can interfere with the heart's function, which contributes to bradycardia, tachycardia, arrhythmia, and eventual heart failure. It is particularly dangerous when patients with damaged hearts are in recovery. As they put on weight, they add extra pressure to the heart. That is what killed the singer Karen Carpenter, for example."

TREATMENT: LIQUID ZINC

Liquid zinc has a positive effect in the treatment of eating disorders, as it is directly absorbed into the blood. Powders, tablets, and capsules, which must first be broken down by the stomach and absorbed by the small intestine, do not work as well because many eating disorder patients are unable to digest nutrients properly. Dr. Schauss has found only one brand available in the United States, Zinc Status (supplied by Ethical Nutrients of San Clemente, California), to be effective in clinical trials. Other liquid zincs are not autoclaved (sterile); although they are cheaper, they have not proved effective. Once the patient shows marked improvement, a good zinc supplement will do unless deterioration occurs, in which case the more expensive Zinc Status is needed again.

While results are not usually immediate, taking from several days to weeks, once liquid zinc takes effect, its benefits are long-lasting. According to Dr. Schauss, "In 15 years I worked with hundreds of eating disorder patients. Until I saw this treatment, my colleagues and I felt that the best we could expect in long-term outcome in treating patients with either bulimia or anorexia was maybe a 20 to 30 percent recovery. In our five-year study, we found that bulemics had a 64.1 percent success rate after recovery on the liquid zinc treatment. In anorexic patients, our five-year follow-up study found an 85 percent recovery rate. These are extraordinarily high recovery rates for a condition that is considered difficult to treat and insidious."

Besides being highly effective, liquid zinc is inexpensive, costing between $12 and $15 a day. This makes it a first-choice treatment for eating disorders, especially when you consider the options. "Within twenty years of initial diagnosis, a British study found, 38 percent of patients with severe eating disorders are dead," says Dr. Schauss. "Many times the families have spent enormous amounts of money keeping their children alive, as the average institutional cost is about $650 a day."

Another favorable finding is that liquid zinc can lift the depression that is usually associated with eating disorders. Dr. Schauss reports, "In our eating disorder studies, we used a multidimensional design and evaluated the mood state of our patients. One of the first things to improve in patients was the degree of depression that they were experiencing based on psychometric instruments such as the Beck Depression Scale and the Profile of Mood Scales, among other depressive indexes. The fact that we have discovered this antidepressive effect and could document it in patients under blind conditions is of great value."

Patient Story

Dr. Schauss gives the following account of one patient's recovery:

"We were doing blind studies, which means that neither I nor the patients were aware of whether they were receiving a placebo or liquid zinc. One of the women in the study was 47 years old. She was a psychotherapist who had been treating patients with eating disorders for the last 15 years and who herself had bulimia involving about five binge-purge episodes per day for the last 34 years. She could hardly recount a single day in the last 34 years when she did not engage in bulemic activity. We have a protocol in which we give a small amount of liquid zinc, about 5 or 10 ml, which is less than a tablespoon. We ask a person to swirl it around in his or her mouth for a few seconds and to tell us what he or she tastes. Zinc has a strong metallic taste. If the person can't taste the solution, it's evidence of a systemic zinc deficiency. This has to do with a zinc-dependent polypeptide known as gustin that helps us distinguish metallic tastes.

"The zinc tasted like water to this woman. Since she couldn't taste anything, she thought that she was receiving a placebo. She followed the protocol, taking about 120 ml of the zinc solution spaced out through the day, about 30 or 40 ml each time on an empty stomach.

"Four days later she called back saying that she couldn't explain why, but she had no desire to binge or purge that day. That was the first day she could recall feeling that way in 34 years. This is very similar to the experience that we have had with hundreds of bulimics we've studied.

"We were intrigued about how a simple nutrient such as zinc could cause a major change in the way the brain functions and in the perceptions of the individual. When you've done something for 34 years, whether it's cigarette smoking, nail biting, or engaging in bulimia, you have to wonder how it is possible for that obsessive-compulsive type of behavior to disappear in just four or five days.

"It has now been five years since that day, and she has never gone back to bingeing and purging. More important in terms of the study, she received no psychotherapy, nor did she have any contact with me personally. The protocol was given to her by a staff member. So we're quite convinced, in this case and in hundreds of others, that it was the liquid zinc that was effective rather than some tangential treatment."

As Goodman noted, eating patterns are rooted in styles of life while being entwined with the country's culture and the body's physical system, The alternative approach tries to work on all these levels flexibly to make your eating patterns saner and your health more positively inflected.

Chapter 12

Endometriosis

E ndometriosis is a condition in which the glands and tissues that line
the inside of the uterus (the endometrium) grow outside the uterine
wall. Normally, cells build up in the uterus each month in preparation
for pregnancy, serving as a nest for an incoming embryo. When pregnancy does not occur, the lining is shed and appears as menstrual flow. In
endometriosis, endometrial-type cells may attach themselves to the fallopian
tubes, ovaries, urinary bladder, intestinal surfaces, rectum, part of the colon,
and other structures in the area.

Between 7 and 15 percent of American women have endometriosis. One of
the goals of the medical treatment of endometriosis is to reduce the stimulating
effect of estrogen on these cell "implants." Since there is no cure for this illness,
the most that natural care can do at present is to work on relieving the pain.

Dian Shepperson Mills, a nutritionist and tutor at the Institute for Optimal
Nutrition in London, has been a trustee of the National Endometrial Society
for number of years and is the author of *Endometriosis: A Key to Healing
through Nutrition.* She explains that the implants cause a problem "because
the endometrium is designed to shed blood at the end of every month if a
pregnancy has not been achieved. So these endrometric implants which are
scattered around on the bowel and the bladder and so on do likewise; they
shed blood. When you are having a normal period, the blood comes out of the
body down the vagina. However, with endometriosis, the implants bleed into
the abdominal cavity, and the blood is trapped in there because it has no exit.
Thus, people with endometriosis get considerable amounts of pain."

However, Mills explains, women with the tiniest spots of endrometriosis often have far more pain than women who have large lumps of endrometriosis. There seems to be no rhyme or reason as to why all this pain occurs mainly in women who have small amounts of endrometric implants.

She adds that there is a problem with this illness beyond the pain: "We also think that the reaction going on in the body, which is trying to remove the implants, which the body's immune system knows should not be there, may affect people's fertility in some way, although we don't know how. It's believed that it is mainly the chemical secretions by the immune cells which are trying to remove the endometrium that are affecting the sperm or the ova."

Women may experience menstrual pain, pain on ovulation, pain on intercourse, and problems with fertility. As Mills says, "It affects 1 in 10 women, so it's almost like looking at asthma or diabetes in that it is experienced by a lot of people. Yet it's not very well known, for it's very difficult for some women to talk about this, as it's such a personal thing."

Causes

The exact cause of the condition remains a mystery, though several theories exist as to why it happens. These are some possible explanations.

RETROGRADE MENSTRUATION. Blood flows backward instead of downward through the cervix and out of the body. It is thought to go out the fallopian tubes and into the pelvic and abdominal cavity. Once it is there, cells from the exiting blood implant themselves outside the uterus onto other tissues.

LYMPHATIC CHANNELS. Cells of the endometrium lining pass through lymphatic channels or migrate via blood and then implant themselves outside the uterine cavity.

GENETIC PREDISPOSITION. Certain families are predisposed to the condition.

IMMUNOLOGIC DISORDER. The immune system is deficient in some way, causing tissue to proliferate in abnormal areas. The idea is that through some type of immune deficiency, hormonal and chemical influences cause endometrial tissue to become activated at different times in the cycle.

CHILDBEARING. Childbearing in combination with methods of contraception may be responsible.

Symptoms

About 70 percent of women with endometriosis have severe, chronic symptoms. Endometriosis can produce slight or severe pain, ranging from mild cramps to agony and dysfunction. Endometrial implants produce chemicals, including prostaglandins, which cause the uterus to contract, resulting in cramping. Pain also results from swelling, inflammation, and scarring of affected tissues. It is usually cyclical and most commonly occurs just before menstruation. Some women have pain during sexual intercourse any time in the month.

Where and to what degree pain is felt depend on the location of the endometrial tissue and the degree to which it has spread outside the uterus. Some women have pain during urination as a result of implants on the bladder. Some have pain during bowel movements because of colon and rectal implants. There can be ovarian pain or pain radiating to the back or buttocks or down the legs. Upon a manual gynecological examination, there may be pelvic pain.

Internal bleeding may occur as well as nose bleeding or bleeding from another orifice at certain times of the month. Any cyclic bleeding is suspect for endometriosis. Other symptoms that sometimes appear include aggravated premenstrual syndrome (PMS), bladder infections, fatigue, and lower back pain. Endometriosis may result in infertility when it interferes with ovarian function.

Clinical Experience

DIAGNOSIS

Endometriosis can be suspected in the presence of one or more of the symptoms listed above, but the only real way to confirm a diagnosis is with a surgical procedure known as a laparoscopy, which allows the doctor to actually see and biopsy tissue. Sonograms and magnetic resonance imaging (MRI) scans may be helpful, but they are not definitive in making the diagnosis.

The proper diagnosis is important, notes Dr. Anthony Aurigemma, because while endometriosis is considered benign, it can become malignant.

CONVENTIONAL THERAPY

Treatment usually consists of medical prescriptions for pain control and reduction of endometrial growth. Antiprostaglandin medicines such as indomethacin, ibuprofen, and naproxen are often given to reduce pain.

Another popular pharmaceutical, danazol, is also used for this purpose, but in some women it does not provide total or lasting relief. Studies show that danazol has a good effect after surgery to remove adhesions. After some of the adhesions have been removed, it may help an infertile woman become pregnant. A side effect of the drug is that it may increase cholesterol, especially the low-density lipoprotein (LDL) variety, which is implicated in accelerated arteriosclerosis. The adverse effects of all these drugs can include weight gain, edema, decreased or increased breast size, acne, excess hair growth on the face and perhaps even in a developing fetus, and deepening of the voice.

Hormones are sometimes given to fool the body into believing it is pregnant, since pregnancy seems to retard or prevent the development of endometriosis. This method appears to have some benefit, but the side effects include depression, painful breasts, nausea, weight gain, bloating, swelling, and migraine headaches. Since the side effects can be fairly severe, this is not a popular method.

Newer drugs, called gonadotropin-releasing hormone compounds, are sometimes given by injection. These agents suppress pituitary gland release of the female hormones follicle-stimulating hormone (FSH) and luteinizing hormone (LH), causing what is called a clinical pseudomenopause. They help reduce pain in many women and decrease the size and volume of endometrial tissue after surgery.

Through the advanced surgical technique of female reconstructive surgery (FRS) developed by Dr. Vicki Hufnagel, the uterus and ovaries can be repositioned, thus reducing the deep pelvic pain that is associated with endometreosis.

DIAN MILLS ON NUTRITION

"Pain is very different for every woman, but endrometriosis pain is unlike any other pain," notes Mills. "It's just so overwhelming when it's severe. Some of the women I have talked to say that it is worse than giving birth. The muscle cramps that you get in the uterus and in the intestines are just excruciating. I might add that I have this problem, so I do know that it is absolutely awful. Some women don't get much pain. It's a very personal situation. Some women get pain on the left side, some on the right, some in the center. It's very difficult for doctors, because every patient presents with pain in a different place.

"Orthodox painkillers can dull it but never take it away. When I started looking at nutrition for the endocrine system, I came across lot of research which suggests that if you are deficient in various nutrients, it may affect the way your body deals with pain. These nutrients would be the essential fatty acids, such as evening primrose oil, fish oil, linseed oil, safflower oil, and vitamins C, E, and K. All these are important in the body's control of pain. The B vitamins, particularly B_1, seem to be important in building up the endorphins, which are the body's natural painkillers. Also, there is an amino acid called DLPA, which is DL-phenylalanine, which seems to help in dulling pain. Also, there are zinc, selenium, and magnesium."

If you are deficient in many of these nutrients, your body may not be able to cope well with pain. Mills says, "If we look at, say, magnesium, we see that it is very important in allowing muscles to relax. Calcium and magnesium balance one another. Calcium causes muscles to contract, and magnesium allows them to relax. Seeing that the uterus is one of the largest muscles in the body, it would be quite important to make sure you are getting enough magnesium-rich foods, such as green leafy vegetables, nuts, and seeds. The same is true of

B vitamins. There are lots of those in vegetables and fruits. That's also where you'll get vitamin C. Zinc will be found in nuts and seeds. Selenium would be in seafood."

In general, she advises that a woman make sure she eats a well-balanced diet. "That's not the only thing," she adds. "You also have to make sure that your digestion is working. If you're not digesting properly, then the nutrients don't get to where they are supposed to go, however well you eat."

DIGESTION AND THE REPRODUCTIVE SYSTEM

"We know that with this disease, the endometric implants require estrogen in order to proliferate, that is, to grow, produce blood, and excrete," Mills continues. "We know that the body deals with estrogen in several ways. Every cell in a woman's body produces estrogen. The ovaries and the adrenal glands also produce it. It is used sensibly by your body as a messenger to trigger the ovaries and reproductive system to work."

For this process to function properly, "you need to have your liver enzymes working effectively, because all estrogen is sent to the liver to be degraded, and then it's bound to fiber from the food you eat in order to be excreted. It's very important that your liver be working effectively and that your diet be rich in fiber from cereals, fruits, vegetables, nuts, and seeds in order for your body to deal with the estrogen. The liver enzymes which deal with estrogen need B vitamins in order to work. Again, it's important to make sure you are eating foods rich in B vitamins.

"At the same time, you need various enzymes in the gut that will deal with the estrogen. They also depend on your having good gut flora. Don't forget that we all have 4 pounds of bacteria in our gut, good bacteria, friendly bacteria. Most of it, the bifida bacteria, is very important in helping your body work. Now, if you've taken a lot of antibiotics or have been on hormones or the pill and hormone replacement therapy (HRT) and feel very stressed from the pain of endometriosis, it is more difficult for your gut flora to work effectively. So you need to take something like a digestive enzyme and an acidophilus tablet as well as make sure you have good fiber in your diet. Note, though, that sometimes wheat fiber is not the best; oat fiber may be better. You should also have lots of fruits and vegetables. That can help your liver and digestion deal with the estrogen as well as help your reproductive system."

REBUILDING HEALTH

Consuming the right nutrients and digesting those nutrients properly form the basis of Mills's treatment for endometriosis:

"Once I have a patient who has a major endometriosis problem, the first thing I look at is her digestion. If she doesn't get the nutrients from food or any supplements she takes, nothing will work. So, you have to heal the digestion first. If she has constipation or diarrhea or heartburn indigestion, I will give her digestive enzymes, acidophilus, and possibly slippery elm. Then, once we've got that healed, you can try a digestive supplement, such as a multivitamin, and some magnesium, zinc, and vitamin C.

"You have to analyze what is wrong with each individual person and tailor the treatment specifically to her needs. Generally, for endometriosis, I try to ensure that the woman is taking evening primrose and fish oil. The supplements also must be wheat-, yeast-, sugar-, and dairy-free. By taking magnesium, zinc, the probiotics, and the digestive enzymes, you are working through the body system from different angles to try to relieve the pain while supporting the endocrine and immune systems."

NATUROPATHY

Dr. Tori Hudson, a naturopath from Portland, Oregon, believes there is most support for the immunological weakness theory of endometriosis because women with this condition have altered immune cells and fewer T lymphocytes. By improving immune function with supplements, diet, and botanicals, she claims to help many patients: "I've seen women with severe pelvic pain who were scheduled for surgery one month from the date I saw them. My treatment helped them recover completely without the surgery." She adds that most, but not all, women respond to her protocol, which is designed to stimulate a maximal immune response. The basic program consists of the following.

Antioxidants

Vitamin C: to bowel tolerance, up to 10,000 mg

Beta carotene: 150,000 to 200,000 IU

Selenium: 400 mcg

Vitamin E: 800 to 1200 IU

DIET

Changes in the diet are made to further stimulate the immune system. This is accomplished by lowering fat; adding whole grains, vegetables, and fruits; and eliminating immune system inhibitors such as coffee, sugar, alcohol, and high-fat foods. Foods such as cheese and meat have high amounts of estrogen and are omitted, because estrogen aggravates the disease. A mostly vegetarian diet is best for lowering estrogen and stimulating the immune system.

BOTANICALS

Two botanical formulas are included. One contains chaste tree berry, dandelion root, motherwort, and prickly ash in equal amounts. A half teaspoon is taken three times daily. The other formula contains small doses of toxic herbs that must be carefully prescribed by a naturopathic physician.

In addition, Dr. Hudson sometimes prescribes natural progesterone made from wild yam. The wild yam extract is converted in the laboratory to natural progesterone.

OTHER SUPPLEMENTS

Dr. Susan M. Lark, a physician in Los Altos, California, who is the author of *The Women's Health Companion: Self-Help Nutrition Guide & Cookbook* (1995), recommends vitamins, herbs, and minerals that will decrease estrogen stimulation of the endometrial cells.

VITAMIN A in the form of beta carotene: a maximum daily dose of 5,000 IU to help decrease the excess menstrual bleeding that may occur with endometriosis.

VITAMIN B complex: 50 to100 mg with an additional dose of up to 300 mg daily of vitamin B$_6$. These vitamins help the liver convert excess estrogen into less stimulating forms.

VITAMIN C: 1000 to 4000 mg of bioflavonoids daily. Vitamin C not only regulates estrogen levels but reduces cramps and bleeding by strengthening capillaries. You can get bioflavonoids by eating citrus fruits (including the inner peel), berries, the skins of grapes, alfalfa, buckwheat, and soybeans and taking 800 mg a day of vitamin C as a supplement.

VITAMIN E: 400 to 2,000 IU a day. If you have high blood pressure, begin with 100 IU and work up to the higher levels gradually. Vitamin E helps even out the effects of high levels of estrogen.

ESSENTIAL FATTY ACIDS. Essential fatty acids (EFAs), including linoleic and linolenic acids, are the source for the manufacture of prostaglandins, which prevent cramping of muscles and blood vessels. Good sources of EFAs are raw seeds, especially flax seed, nuts, salmon, mackerel, and trout. They can also be taken as dietary supplements.

HERBS. 100 mg per day maximum dose of fennel, anise, blessed thistle, black cohosh, and false unicorn root works to restore hormonal balance. You can also use white willow bark and meadowsweet to reduce pain, fever, cramps, and inflammation of the endometrial implants. Be sure to follow the directions on the label, since these herbs can cause an upset stomach and diarrhea.

ASIAN MEDICINE

Dr. Roger Hirsch, a naturopathic doctor in Santa Monica, California, who specializes in Asian medicine, says that the Chinese approach to gynecological imbalance is holistic: "What do I mean by holistic? It treats the mind and body as an integral unit like a gloved hand. If you move the hand, what is moving, the glove or the hand? The body or the mind? They move in concert. If there is a psychological, emotional, or spiritual imbalance, it may show up on the physical plane and cause a 'stuckness' or endometrial situation."

The Chinese diagnose endometriosis by looking at the way the blood flows in the body, specifically in the pelvic cavity. This is determined by the appearance of the root of the tongue, which represents the pelvic cavity. "If a woman has endometriosis, there will be raised bumps and papillae in the back of the tongue and perhaps a greasy yellow coating," Hirsch says. "If you look at the back of your tongue in the mirror and see raised bumps that are red and fiery, especially during the time of menstruation, you may well have endometriosis." (For an explanation of how Asian medicine treats endometriosis as it relates to infertility, see Chapter 17.)

HELLERWORK

Hellerwork is a bodywork technique derived from Rolfing. Both modalities use deep tissue work to improve body structure, but Hellerwork is different in that it is not painful. Certified Hellerwork practitioner Sarah Suatoni of the Pelvic Floor Rehabilitation Laboratory for Women with Endometriosis at St. Luke's Hospital in New York City gives an overview of the process: "There are three components to Hellerwork. There is a hands-on part, which feels much like a massage; a movement educational aspect; and a mind-body dialogue aspect.

"In the hands-on process, we analyze the body much as a chiropractor would, looking at the posture, or the structure, as we call it, to determine which parts of the body are out of balance. We look to see which myofascial tissue connections are creating this misalignment. Then we work with our hands to release it. That in a sense is also the beginning of movement education, because this isn't done to the client but with the client. In other words, I put my hands on a spot, and we work closely together with visual images or deep breathing to help the person identify the misalignment, feel it, and then release it.

"The second part of the work is movement education, in which we do very simple everyday movements. We look at how a person sits or stands. In the case of computer programmers, we look at how they sit at the computer and use their arms. We look at whatever it is that may be contributing to the dysfunction in the body, and then we begin to look at how we can have the person move in a way that will not create the same problem.

"Last but certainly not least is mind-body dialogue. We work under the belief that our emotional patterns, memories, and attitudes are reflected in our bodies. In the same way one needs to look at a movement pattern in order to shift some sort of physical dysfunction, one needs to look at emotional patterns or beliefs in order to shift those as well. We dialogue with clients in order to identify underlying emotions or memories. Then we look at how clients might better facilitate emotions or memories so that they are not manifesting them through physical dysfunctions.

"This work is a process where people come in for 11 sessions. Once a week for an hour and a half is ideal, although other time frames are possible. Each session touches upon a different part of the body and different aspects of the being."

Suatoni tells how she began using Hellerwork to treat endometriosis and similar chronic conditions: "I met Dr. David Kauffman, a urologist, who determined that women with interstitial cystitis had severe spasm of the pelvic muscles. He has since started working with patients with endometriosis, vulvodynia, vestibulitis, and a number of other conditions that show the same symptoms of severe spasm or contraction. Dr. Kauffman was using biofeedback and felt that he needed someone who did hands-on work to accompany the biofeedback treatments. That's how I began.

"I determined that he was indeed right. When I put my hands on the deep pelvic muscles, they were in severe contraction. We do not know why this is so. Whether it is a cause or effect of the disease is still a question. We do know, however, that teaching women to feel those muscles and to learn to relax them releases a great deal of pain.

"I do a normal series of Hellerwork on these patients because each part of the body is connected to every other part. It's the hip-bone-connected-to-the-thigh-bone thing. If the pelvis is in contraction, it has been affected by all the other related areas. So I work on the whole body as well as the pelvic area.

"I find that most of my patients do not know how to relax. Education is extremely useful. I place my hands into the deep pelvic muscles and teach women how to feel them. The beginning of the process is just to help them locate the muscles, feel the muscles, and then learn that they have control over them. They can, in fact, relax and release the contractions.

"The second part of the process involves movement. We look at the way women walk, sit, and breathe. Slowly they begin to realize that they have been holding on to these muscles all their lives. This insight is the beginning of their awareness of what is happening.

"Then we look at different situations in their lives that tend to exacerbate their condition. Issues of control are often involved. For example, when they are having a big fight with somebody or having a difficult day at work, they tend to grip these muscles tighter. Once women make this connection, their awareness is further enhanced. They realize that on a really bad day they grip those muscles tightly. Hopefully, once they identify what is happening, they can begin to release. Then their pain is greatly alleviated.

"So this is really an educational process about the whole body. Specifically, it is a process of learning about how not to grip and grab those muscles so that they do not spasm and create pain.

"The last part looks at emotional patterns that may be creating some of the physical problems. Endometriosis in particular has been called the working woman's disease. On an emotional level, the disease is speaking to masculine and feminine aspects being out of balance. Most of these women lead very ambitious, fast-paced lives. They are doers and achievers who are often magnificently bright, aggressive, and successful. However, they are not really in touch with their feminine aspect. I am using feminine in the Jungian sense, which refers to receptivity and surrender and applies to men and women. These aspects of being are less present in their lives. In a sense, the disease is a voice saying, 'It is time to bring life into better balance.' Certainly, the disease forces them to do that because most women must slow down, receive help, and do things they have never done before. Ideally, women begin to replace the receiving they get through medical care with receptivity in other aspects of their lives, and disease symptoms lessen.

"Although this process deals with mind-body relationships, this does not imply that these diseases are imaginary. Some women have been told for years that their disease is all in their head, when there are all kinds of physical evidence for the disease. Rather, the disease is the result of a set of relationships between the mind and body. Hellerwork and other forms of bodywork help because they are process-oriented and look at relationships. Once women start understanding these relationships, they find that they have a whole lot of power to overcome disease and regain health."

HOMEOPATHY

Homeopathy is another holistic therapy that addresses underlying emotional causes. Dr. Aurigemma has been treating his patients homeopathically for 10 years and claims that the therapy is completely safe and highly effective. "There is no doubt in my mind that something actually happens and that it helps people," he says. "I utilize the remedies because I see them work. What spurs me on is the continuous improvement of most of the patients I see."

Patient Stories

LINDA

Dr. Aurigemma outlines one patient's progress with homeopathy. "A 35-year-old woman who was diagnosed with endometriosis via laparoscopy in 1981 came to my office. She had a history of migraine headaches; vaginal yeast infections; pain beginning in her hips and going down to her knees as well as midmonth pain in the uterine area; shooting, throbbing ovarian pain; pain while running; and pain after overeating. Premenstrually, she experienced headaches, anger, bloating, crankiness, and sensitivity. She had headaches the last day of her menstrual cycle and the day after the cycle ended.

"In homeopathy, part of the diagnostic process includes an assessment of how people appear. These were some of her personality characteristics. She was bright, lively, and pleasant. Even though she seemed to be in pain, she was not irritable. She said she alternated between being warm and feeling chilly and that she easily got overheated. In addition, she claimed to be spontaneous and very quick to act. Also, she was an animal rights activist who took in strays. She said that she did not harbor anger. Instead, she tried to get things out in the open. In terms of her eating habits, she was not a very thirsty person. She liked to drink cold water and herb teas, and she would occasionally have a glass of wine with a steak dinner. She said that she liked salads, spicy foods, and borscht but that creamy foods were too rich. She smoked one to two cigarettes per day two or three times per week.

"Her fears included claustrophobia: not liking to be in tunnels, elevators, or crowds. Thunderstorms bothered her. She was somewhat weepy at sentimental movies.

"I studied her symptoms, personality characteristics, foods, likes and dislikes, and fears. Based on this information, I came up with a particular homeopathic remedy which I asked her to take twice a day four or five days a week.

"Approximately three months later, she reported feeling 70 to 80 percent better. Her uterine pain and headaches had decreased, premenstrual symptoms were less severe, and there was an almost total disappearance of her yeast infection. At that point she was given another single dose of the same remedy, but in a higher potency. I gave this to her in the office, and it was not repeated.

"A month later she returned and said that she was improving further. There were no headaches at all with her period and very little pain. The yeast flared up but then got better. On that visit I gave her no remedy at all and told her to come back in three months or if the symptoms started to return.

"Three months later, in September, she came back with some return of headaches when the period was ending. Even so, the headaches were still about 50 percent better than they had been in the first place. The yeast infection was 90 percent improved, and the monthly pain was about 75 percent better overall. This was without any further remedy. At this point, I gave her another dose of the same remedy to take daily five days per week. That was three months ago. Since that time, I have not seen her.

"The subjective estimates of health were given to me by the patient, since there is no physical way to measure improvement. She is more functional, better able to do things, happier, and pleased with the treatment. She plans to continue. Her symptoms are fewer and certainly less intense. In seven months her periods became easier, and between periods she feels more comfortable. There were no side effects from the remedy other than an aggravation of her yeast infection for a few days, which then subsided. That was due to a higher potency of the remedy. Homeopathic remedies can aggravate symptoms. Very often that aggravation is a sign that the remedy is correct and is bringing things to a head, getting the body to focus on the problem and then getting rid of it.

"She is functioning better and is less uncomfortable, but we do not know whether the endometrial tissue has shrunk or gone away. The only way to really know that is by doing another laparoscopy, but a person is unlikely to undergo surgery when feeling better."

Linda describes her experience treating endometriosis with Ayurvedic medicine. "I had constant abdominal pain from the endometriosis for 21days out of every month. For many years, I took 8 to 10 aspirin a day and sometimes stronger painkillers. In four years, I had been to three gynecologists, two internists, and a gastroenterologist. I had laparoscopic surgery and then was given Lupron injections. Lupron [a gonadotropin-releasing hormone compound] is a drug that blocks estrogen and causes the endometrial tissue to shrink. After three months on Lupron, the pain from the endometriosis was gone, but there were some terrific side effects. Hot flashes interfered with my sleeping. I also had a lot of trouble with joint pain. But by far the worst side effect was loss of bone density. This is the reason why you are not supposed to take drugs like Lupron for more than six months in your lifetime. After I stopped taking Lupron, the endometriosis came back within a month or two. At that point, my gynecologist said my best option was another drug that could also affect bone density or a complete hysterectomy. It seemed as if I didn't have any acceptable options left.

"At that point, I found Dr. Lonsdorf, an Ayurvedic doctor, who recommended certain herbal mixtures for me. She also suggested other measures that are simple to follow and of benefit to everyone: sipping hot water throughout the day to aid digestion, eating the main meal in the middle of the day and eating less toward the end, cutting down on meat and working toward a more vegetarian diet, getting to bed by ten and up by six—that is, trying to get more in touch with the circadian rhythms—using massage to stimulate circulation, and practicing meditation to calm the mind.

"I incorporated as many of these suggestions into my life as I comfortably could. Within a few weeks the pain from the endometriosis was almost completely gone. I have been under Dr. Lonsdorf's care for almost a year and a half and almost never have any discomfort anymore. I have much more energy and am much calmer. Some other problems I had, such as low blood sugar, have also cleared up. In fact, the Ayurvedic medicine helped me so much that my husband and both of our daughters see Dr. Lonsdorf now."

A NATURAL HYGIENE SUCCESS STORY

Dr. Anthony Penepent describes one patient's success treating her endometriosis with natural hygiene.

"One woman came to see me who was on prescription narcotic medication for the pain. The medicine gave her no relief, and she was at the point of wanting a hysterectomy to get relief from the pain. I put this woman on a natural hygienic regimen for a couple of weeks. First she fasted for five days. Then she followed up with a nutritional plan.

"Let me briefly describe a typical hygienic regimen. The patient has a breakfast consisting of a vegetable juice or a vegetable and fruit juice combination, a blended salad, a piece of fruit, perhaps some hot cereal, and a couple of soft-boiled egg yolks. Lunch is a vegetable juice or vegetable and fruit juice combination, a blended salad, a cup or a little more than that, a piece of fruit, and then some raw nuts or unsalted raw-milk cheese. For the evening meal the patient starts with juice again, blended salad, tossed salad, and steamed vegetables such as string beans, broccoli, or escarole. Then she goes on with the main course, which includes a steamed potato or yam, natural brown rice or another whole grain, and a legume. I also might supplement the meal with egg or cheese, depending on the protein needs of the woman. Of course, there are variations for individual patients.

"After following this general plan, this patient was pain-free at the end of one month. That was 10 years ago. Right now she is pregnant with her second child, whereas before she was infertile. Natural hygiene has tremendous implications for endometriosis. There is absolutely no reason why a woman should have pain or be infertile because of such a simple condition.

"From my perusal of the literature I can see that endometriosis is plainly a condition of liver toxicity, where the liver is failing to completely break down the estrogen hormones that the body is manufacturing. These breakdown products wreak havoc in the form of endometrial tissue in the pelvic cavity."

Chapter 13

Environmental Illness

Technological advances in our society have been accompanied by unprecedented challenges to our bodies and our health. The ability to change our looks and our bodily processes with a pill or an implant, along with a variety of other changes, combined with a multitude of potentially carcinogenic types of microscopic pollution in our air, water, homes, and workplaces, have caused an overload on our immune systems that can produce a condition called environmental illness.

In the 1970s environmental medical specialists—allergists who view a person's whole environment as having the potential to create an immune system response—realized that many allergies were a major factor contributing to illnesses and diseases that traditionally had been left out of discussions of allergic responses. Migraine headaches, depression, and arthritis are just a few of the conditions that were found to be allergy-related. While clinical data have supported this work, many traditional allergists and immunologists believe that there is insufficient theoretical explanation of these phenomena to accept them as scientifically valid.

Women tend to be more prone to environmental illness than are men, in part because a number of chemical toxins actually mimic estrogen in the body, causing an insufficiency of that hormone. Also, both birth control pills and silicone breast implants can compromise women's immune systems.

Causes

Dr. Stephen M. Silverman of Port Washington, New York, says that thousands of poisons in our food, water, and surroundings are responsible for environmental illness: "The first thing you must realize is that what you eat can have a tremendous effect on your immune system. One of the most toxic foods that people expose themselves to unknowingly, for example, is hydrogenated oil. People don't realize how widespread that ingredient is. It's in crackers, all commercial breads, potato chips, pretzels, and cookies, and it has a very strong damaging effect on the immune system.

"Along with what you eat, you must consider what you drink. Most people are being exposed to tap water, whether directly from the sink or outside when they buy a cup of coffee or tea. Probably one of the highest exposures to carcinogens comes from this source. In 1989 Ralph Nader's group identified over 2,000 chemicals commonly found in people's drinking water. When water is tested over the course of the year, it is tested for approximately 120 chemicals. When you are told that the water is safe to drink, it means that it is safe with respect to what it was tested for. You have no idea about the other 1,900 chemicals. Insecticides and pesticides in the water have been associated with Long Island's high rate of breast cancer. Certainly, if they can create cancer, they can cause immune system damage.

"Among the other factors that can set you up for illness are the things you put on your body. I am talking about cosmetics, moisturizers, and hair sprays. We know through medical applications of the nicotine and estrogen patches that what you put on your skin will be absorbed into the bloodstream. If you were to take a look at the ingredients in your cosmetics, hair sprays, and underarm deodorants, you would see that they are loaded with chemicals. You have to realize that when you use these chemicals every day, they eventually get into the bloodstream. When you think about it, is it possible that these chemicals have no effect on your immune system? It's almost impossible.

"In addition, there are environmental factors. One of the most important rooms to be safe in is the bedroom. If you happen to have a carpet that is outgassing, by which I mean releasing chemicals at a very low level, and some of those chemicals are suspected carcinogens, despite how well you may be eating, you are going to get sick from that carpet. When we sleep at night, we are supposed to detoxify. Your body attempts to purify itself at night of any additives or toxins in foods that you may have eaten. If you have a toxic bedroom where the carpet, the paint on the wall, or a mattress loaded with formaldehyde is releasing gas, and if you're reacting to these chemicals, then eight hours a night, instead of restoring your immune system, you may be causing it severe damage."

According to the environmental medicine specialist Dr. Marshall Mandell, "There is absolutely no question that environmental factors play a major role in many diseases; where they do not actually start the disease, they can complicate it. Anything that makes your illness worse is important for you to know about."

In the same way that cocaine goes right from the nose of the user to the nervous system in a matter of seconds, producing a wide variety of effects, toxins in food or air produce a range of effects in the systems of highly sensitive individuals. Conventional physicians and traditional allergists simply miss this phenomenon by recognizing only a very limited range of symptoms. If their patients aren't sneezing or itching, they will not recognize the possibility that an allergy may be present. But logically, once a doctor recognizes that minute flecks of animal dander or pollen in the air can produce marked symptoms, is it so difficult to see that chemical toxins in meat or milk or air pollution, among a host of other possible causes, might also have an adverse effect? Simply put, the human race has evolved over millions of years and has adapted to most of the conditions on this planet. But many of the pollutants and toxins we are dealing with have arisen over the last 30 to 50 years. Our bodies just haven't had time to evolve in response to these changes in our environment. Unless we act sensibly by at least recognizing this discrepancy, we may cause great damage to ourselves and our environment.

Whatever you breathe in enters your body along with the oxygen. If your home, work, or school environment is polluted, the pollutants will travel through the walls of the lungs, go into the blood vessels of the lungs, and ultimately reach the heart through the pulmonary circulation. Similarly, chemicals, additives, and contaminants in our food and beverages will pass through the digestive system and reach the heart. Once there, they will be pumped through the bloodstream. Every tissue in your body is exposed to what you eat, drink, and breathe. That is why so many people are sick today.

"Research shows that women are more prone to environmental illnesses," says Heather Millar, author of *The Toxic Labyrinth*. "The reason is that many chemicals, such as formaldehyde, benzene, phenols, and chlorine, have estrogen-mimicking properties. These chemicals take the place of estrogen in the body. The body thinks that it has enough estrogen and doesn't make enough. Estrogen is responsible for reproduction as well as many other vital functions in the body. Problems occur when the body calls upon the estrogen it thinks it has but doesn't.

"Silicone breast implants are making women terribly ill. They have a tendency to grow fungus inside the implant, which adds a problem to an already existing one. Fungus is extremely hard to get rid of once it starts to grow. After breast implants are removed, women do not feel better. This indicates that their immune systems have been damaged. It will probably take a very long time for them to recover, and we do not know the long-term effects."

Symptoms

Symptoms vary with a woman's constitution and may include fatigue, aching muscles, a flulike feeling, ringing in the ears, burning eyes, headaches, migraines, disturbed sleep, shortness of breath, food allergies, a heightened sense of smell, loss of balance, inability to concentrate, memory loss, anxiety, panic attacks, depression, and irritable bowel syndrome. There is a marked progressive debilitating reaction to consumer products such as perfumes, soap, tobacco smoke, and plastics.

Clinical Experience

CONVENTIONAL APPROACH

Environmental illness was first recognized in the 1980s, but mainstream medicine still generally disregards this syndrome. When patients come in with the symptoms of sensitivity to a toxic environment, doctors often do not know the correct protocol. Standardized blood tests appear normal, leading doctors to assume that no problem exists.

Another problem is that most doctors today are not trained to work with a disease that affects the whole body. Millar, who suffered from the condition, notes, "In the medical community we have created a world of specialists. Physicians are now neurologists, cardiologists, rheumatologists, and so on. We have gotten away from the old-fashioned approach. We no longer have general practitioners. Before, you would go to a doctor's office and tell him your history from start to finish. He would look at you as a whole individual, checking the psychological as well as the physical aspect of the body. Only then would he make an assessment.

"Now technology has compartmentalized the body. The neurologist looks only at the symptoms of numbness, tingling, and headaches. The rheumatologist looks only at arthritis, joint pain, and aches. The infectious disease doctor looks only for infection. What happened to me was, I would go in and give a detailed history of what was happening. The doctor, according to his specialty, would look only at one specific area. He or she did not want to hear about the other symptoms I had.

"What we are failing to realize with all this supertechnology in medicine is that the body works in harmony. You do not have one body system that works separately from something else. They all work together. So if you are having symptoms in one system, you are probably having symptoms elsewhere."

DIAGNOSIS

In her book, Heather Millar has a checklist to help people determine whether they may be suffering from environmental illness. These are some questions she asks people to consider:

Do I have a toxic lifestyle?

Have I had breast implants?

Does my environment contain chemicals that could be making me sick?

Do I feel ill at work?

Do I feel ill at home?

Do I live in a new home?

Have I recently painted or installed a new carpet?

How much plastic do I have in the home?

Does my neighborhood contain chemicals that could be making me sick?

"Discovering the cause of the problem is a detective process," Millar says. "It involves taking a close look at your home, workplace, and neighborhood.

"Start with your home. You may ask, 'Why didn't we have these problems before? We always painted our house and put new carpet in.' What I'd like to suggest is that technology has changed a lot of chemicals and manufacturing processes. Since the 1980s we have added more synthetics and are now seeing their effects. A lot of these products emit gas. The newness smell is a gas that is coming off. Basically, it's a chemical soup that is very hazardous to our health. Also, since we live in energy-efficient buildings, we do not have the ventilation needed to lessen the concentration or these gases.

"Plastics present further problems. They have a lot of these estrogen-mimicking properties. Softer plastics have more toxicity. We used to live with metal, wood, and glass. These are far safer alternatives. When replacing plastic with wood, consider the type of finish on it. Does it smell?

"Then look at the workplace. Ask yourself, what are you doing as an occupation? Are you working with chemicals on an ongoing basis? Or are you working in an energy-efficient office building that was recently renovated? Is it currently being renovated? Does it have no open windows? Do other people in the office frequently get colds and flu or feel unwell?

"Finally, examine your neighborhood. Where do you live? Do you have chemical manufacturing in your backyard? Is there some kind of toxic incinerator nearby? What is in your water supply? What kinds of pesticide regulations does your neighborhood have?

"You may react differently to toxins in your environment than your coworkers do. For example, in my workplace, which was extremely toxic, my symptoms were mainly neurological. Other colleagues were diagnosed with chronic fatigue. Still others experienced asthma or fibromyalgia, which is an aching of the muscles. We react differently depending on our genetic predispositions."

Fortunately, there are physicians who do recognize the illness, and there are tests available to pinpoint the condition. Occupational health doctors and environmental physicians prescribe tests that look at solvent levels in the blood. They look at pesticide levels in the blood and check mineral levels, which are usually low in people who suffer from chemical exposures.

FOUR CLUES TO PROPER TREATMENT

Dr. Michael Schachter, a clinical ecologist, or environmental medicine specialist, identifies four contributing factors which he considers key in his examination and in determining a course of therapy:

> The quality of nutrition generally and the identification
>   of any nutritional deficiencies
> Infections
> Psychological stresses
> Toxicity

According to Dr. Schachter, the course of therapy should be determined by the condition of the patient in regard to these four criteria.

Dr. Schachter is also concerned with improving the oxygenation and energy utilization of the body at the cellular level. Anything we can do to improve that process is going to strengthen the immune system and thereby help reduce a person's tendency toward sensitivity and reactions. Thus, Dr. Schachter encourages the use of oxidant therapies, but only up to a point, since oxygen in too great quantities can have a damaging effect. The key here, as in virtually every area of health, is balance.

The first and foremost oxidant therapy must be aerobic exercise. Keeping in mind that oxygen is the main nutrient of the body, it is easy to understand that as we improve oxygenation, we improve the body's ability to detoxify and enhance the immune system. Beyond exercise, a number of new nutrients are available to enhance oxygenation, such as germanium and ubiquinone, as well as a variety of traditional oxygenation techniques.

Vitamins and minerals are another key component in Dr. Schachter's approach. He sees vitamin A as a major protective factor that guards against both chemical sensitivities and infections. Thus, cod liver oil, which parents once gave automatically to children, is indeed an excellent preventive medicine with its high concentrations of vitamins A and D. In treating children with recurrent ear infections, Dr. Schachter has found that by simply enhancing their diet, removing most of the sugar and refined foods, and adding a spoonful of cod liver oil, the ear infections can be controlled and prevented in many cases. Other useful vitamins include vitamin C, vitamin B_{12}, and vitamin E, which is an antioxidant. Selenium and beta carotene are also important antioxidants. Vitamin B_{12} can help counteract the adverse effects in the body of pesticides in the environment. Moreover, while conventional physicians may test for vitamin B_{12} levels in the bloodstream, normal levels may be present in the blood while there are deficiencies at the cellular level.

According to Dr. Schachter, infections are a key factor in going from troubled to good health. Frequently, infections will yield to nontoxic treatments.

Take *Candida,* for example. Patients who have repeatedly used antibiotics, include a lot of refined carbohydrates in their diet, and may have been exposed to steroids or birth control pills tend to develop a chronic overgrowth of *Candida,* a yeastlike, funguslike organism which we all have in our bodies. In certain cases the infection will give off toxins which may impair the immune system and produce a variety of symptoms. Some of these symptoms will be the result of food and chemical sensitivities which have been aggravated by the infection.

Dr. Schachter has found that starting the patient on special diets which exclude refined carbohydrates, especially sugars and alcohol, and include various nutrients, especially certain fatty acids which inhibit *Candida* growth, will go a long way toward controlling the infection in many cases. He also notes that garlic has strong anticandidal properties.

Chronic viral syndromes are another key problem. A previously healthy individual suddenly gets a flu and instead of recovering completely experiences frequent fatigue, exhaustion, swollen glands, sore throat, night sweats, anxiety, and loss of appetite. However, conventional testing shows nothing definite. More sophisticated testing may show exposure to various viruses, but the main problem here may be that the person's immune system just isn't responding as it should. Dr. Schachter has obtained excellent results in patients with this profile by using nutrients to bolster the immune system. Intravenous vitamin C may be used, along with germanium and a variety of other vitamins and minerals given orally. In cases of herpes virus, for example, he may use high doses of the amino acid lysine, which has antiviral effects for the herpes virus and certain other viruses. For short treatment periods, he may administer as much as 10 to 15 g of lysine per day.

Psychological stress is another key factor, according to Dr. Schachter. Environmental medicine specialists, he warns, must be careful that in emphasizing the importance of the physical environment they do not underestimate the importance of psychological factors in determining the strength of an individual's immune system.

As for toxicity, Dr. Schachter feels that hydrocarbons and other chemicals are already playing a major role by damaging our immune systems, as are heavy metals. He sees chelation therapy as a valid treatment to detoxify our systems of the effects of heavy metals. Chelation therapy has also shown impressive results in patients with cardiovascular disease.

In summary, in treating an allergic or chemically sensitive patient, Dr. Schachter believes it is important to look at the specific kinds of food allergens and chemical sensitivities that may be involved, employing rotation diets and neutralization diets, but also to go beyond these issues to seek any underlying factors which could be important, such as infections, chemical pesticide poisoning, heavy metal poisoning, and stress. It is important to deal with each aspect independently, and it is equally important that the program be synergistic and able to make the patient less sensitive to her or his environment.

DETOXIFYING THE BODY

Without detoxifying the system, all other steps to repair the body will be of no avail, says Dr. Silverman: "When people are ill, they're frequently thinking, What should I take to repair my system? But usually half the battle is figuring out what is hurting the immune system, and more often than not that means figuring out what can be taken away. People are under the impression that they can take B vitamins, minerals, and immune stimulants while continuing to drink toxic water with insecticides, pesticides, and metals and eat foods that they react to and still get better. They don't get better, because although they are taking good nutrients, they are still poisoning their bodies."

Dr. Zane Gard, an expert in toxicology, reports methods of detoxification that have impressive results in the reversal of environmental illness: "Heat stress detoxification includes wood saunas, hot sand packing, steam baths, and sweat lodges. The history of these approaches goes back several thousand years. Careful supervision is required. Heat stress detoxification can be effective but requires knowledge of toxins and their potential effects on the body. If it is not administered properly, there can be a lot of complications, and the patient can actually end up worse.

"The biotoxic reduction program was designed with the toxic-chemical-syndrome patient in mind. It is a comprehensive, medically managed program that addresses toxicology, psychology, neurology, pathology, and immunology. The program must be followed seven days a week, three to five hours a day, for a minimum of two weeks. It would be nice to have off on Saturday and Sunday, but patients actually regress one or two days every time they take a day off during the first two weeks. So it has to be every day during that initial period.

"The program consists of increasing niacin, aerobic exercise, sauna therapy, and other therapies as necessary. With those who have neurological damage, other therapies will be needed, including a therapy that stimulates the myelin sheaths of the nerves to regenerate. As a result, many peripheral neuropathies completely reverse. In over 80 peripheral neuropathies, including multiple sclerosis (MS), we have only two patients who did not fully recover.

"In a study of patients in our program, the average blood toxin levels after 21 days of therapy are as follows: toluene drops from 19.3 to an average of 0.34, ethyl benzine drops from 14.7 to 0.1, xylene drops from 72.9 to 0.94, 1:1-trichloroethylene goes from 7.7 to 0.92, and DDE goes from 5.7 to 1.8. We know that DDT, which is the parent compound of DDE, will be 97 percent removed within four months. You continue to detoxify for a good four months."

DETOXIFYING THE ENVIRONMENT

It is no longer enough to watch what we eat or the medicines we take; in the twentieth century environmental toxins have become an unavoidable reality, especially for those living in densely populated urban areas. The very air that we breathe on the streets or in our homes and offices can attack our health;

noise pollution and artificial lighting add to the physical and mental stress of urban life.

The myth is that you should look for the big toxin. But it's the chronic, day-in, day-out exposure to small toxins that does you in. It may take decades—none of these environmental toxins, even asbestos, will knock you out right away—but you may pay for your lack of awareness with lung cancer, leukemia, arthritis, or heart disease down the line. Perhaps worst are the subtle symptoms of fatigue, anxiety, and minor nagging physical problems which you come to accept as a normal part of life.

Elimination of the unseen substances that attack your system stealthily, over time, is half of achieving good health. If you never use any supplementary vitamin, mineral, or herb but simply eliminate those factors which depreciate your health, you should be able to live to 100 years of age in a healthy way. One group of people, nearly 70,000 in number, in the north of Pakistan at the base of the Himalayas, often live to 90 or 105, putting in full days of work daily until they die. It may not be possible for all of us to live in the pure atmosphere of the Himalayas—not to mention emulating the diet, activities, and social structure of these people—but we can alter our environment realistically and functionally. A good place to start is where we live.

Dr. Alfred Zann, a fellow of the American College of Allergists and the American College of Physicians, has written a book, *Why Your House May Endanger Your Health*, which explores the relationship between our homes and our well-being more thoroughly than we can here; much of the following discussion is indebted to information he shared on my radio show as well as to Dr. Richard Podell.

THE SICK BUILDING SYNDROME

The "sick house" is a relatively new development. Materials and methods used to construct houses have changed considerably since World War II; an extreme example is the energy-efficient office buildings built during the energy crisis of the 1970s, about which we'll have more to say later in this chapter. But not only are houses built with more emphasis on energy efficiency—which means heavy insulation and minimum ventilation to the outside—the construction materials themselves, as well as the furnishings—carpeting, fabrics, furniture—are new, often more convenient, cheaper, lighter synthetic compounds unheard of in prewar houses. The particleboard which is so useful in modern house and furniture construction exacts a price for this convenience; it is a silent time bomb, giving off invisible, odorless—but no less dangerous—vapors years after it is installed.

Formaldehyde is a major culprit in the modern house or office building. Particleboard, new synthetic carpets, insulation, many interior paints, and even permanent-press fabrics can give off formaldehyde. It is invisible and odorless except in high concentrations, but even quite low chronic levels can cause symptoms ranging from burning eyes and headaches to asthma and depression. New houses may be built largely of materials which vaporize formaldehyde for years; the worst culprits are mobile homes, which also are often poorly ventilated.

Another important factor in a house's potential toxicity is its source of heat. Combustion-heating appliances using natural gas, oil, coal, kerosene, or wood can all create afterburn by-products even if you can't see or smell them. Good ventilation can help but makes it harder to keep a house warm. Electrical heat, though expensive, is the safest source.

What can be done about a toxic house? Some changes can be made in the furnishings, floor coverings, and ventilation and heating systems, but often much of the problem lies in structural components which would be expensive and difficult, if not impossible, to alter. Building your own house or having it built with attention to all the materials used is one solution if you can afford it or have the time and skill. If you are looking for a place to live, consider an older home. Prewar houses were often constructed of bricks, plaster, and hardwood, not the chemically treated plywood, composite board, and other synthetic materials used almost universally now. If synthetic materials were used in an older house, they will have had years to emit their toxins. Often a house built before the energy crisis will allow more air circulation. Ceilings are often higher, allowing fumes to rise away from the inhabitants.

There may be disadvantages in an old house, however; molds and mildews may have accumulated over the years. Old carpet is a fertile ground for mold as well as accumulated dust, animal hair, and whatever toxins have been tracked in or sprayed over the years, but it can often be pulled up to reveal a hardwood floor. Outdated heating systems can usually be replaced without too much trouble.

If moving or rebuilding your house is not an option, you can still do a lot to detoxify your home. We'll identify the weak spots room by room.

THE GARAGE AND GARDEN

An attached garage is like a toxic waste dump stuck to the side of your house. Many garages have heating and cooling systems which lead directly into the house; anything that can be absorbed through any crack or ventilation system will end up in the house. What's in the garage? The car, of course, and gasoline. Gasoline vaporizes. The afterburn fumes caused by inefficient burning of gasoline are mostly carbon dioxide, which has no odor and is invisible. Breathing these fumes results in headache, dizziness, and mood swings. (Think of people stuck in traffic jams, breathing the afterburn of all the cars around them for hours at a time.) When you park a hot car in the garage and close the door behind it, the hot oil in the engine is volatile and gets into the air. Park the car outside and wait for it to cool off before you bring it into the garage.

Other things you may keep in the garage—paint thinners and removers and turpentine—also vaporize easily and stay in the air for months at a time. If you smell a rag that was used for paint thinner three months ago, you will see that it is still giving off these fumes. Try to minimize the number of these substances in your garage. If you must keep them, use a small shed or garbage can outside the garage to store them. And the garage should be ventilated out, not into the house, with a suction fan. There should be no ducts from the garage into the house.

Your garage is probably where you keep chemicals you use on your lawn and garden: pesticides, fungicides, or herbicides, for instance. In the first place, do you really need them? Look at it this way. If it's going to kill an insect, a plant, or a mouse, it's a toxin and it can affect you, your pets, and your children. If you spray a weed killer on your lawn and then walk around on the lawn, you will repeatedly be bringing it inside on your feet. It doesn't just go away. Think of all the things you bring in on your feet and think, for instance, of your kids playing on the carpet, perhaps putting things into their mouths that have been on it.

Taken individually, none of these things is going to kill you, but be aware that everything you spray outside is likely to be in the air you breathe or will make its way back into your house and settle there. There's no real need to run this risk: We can use diatomaceous earth and natural biological controls or just weed without spraying.

THE BASEMENT

A typical basement in a private home is often damp. People like their lawns unencumbered by debris that might wash down from the gutters of the roof through the downspout, and so the downspout is kept close to the house. Thus the water runs off the roof, down the downspout, and into the ground directly by the foundation of the house. You might just as well run this water directly into the basement, since its walls are rarely waterproof. A little dampness in the basement is enough to support a healthy growth of mold, which can then permeate the house. A forced-air system of ventilation, which has ducts running to the basement, will create a vacuumlike effect that will suck particles of mold into the system, to be dispersed around the house.

Many people react to mold whether it is eaten or inhaled, a point that is obvious to anyone who begins to sneeze as soon as she or he walks into a damp basement. More insidiously, though, mold which is inhaled even in small quantities cross-reacts with mold which is ingested in food. This effect, known as concomitancy, means that a small quantity of inhaled mold which in itself would hardly cause a noticeable reaction will enhance sensitivity to foods which contain mold.

Any food made by fermentation can induce this reaction. Wine and vinegar are fermented fruit juice, cheese is fermented milk, yeast in bread fer-ments, and even mushrooms are in the mold family. Thus, it is easy to ingest mold three times a day, exacerbating our inability to tolerate the mold which has circulated upward from a damp basement. Obvious symptoms are sneezing and watering eyes, but allergic symptoms can also be systemic, making them harder to pin down to a specific source. Fatigue, headaches, depression, and even arthritis can have a basis in chronic allergic irritation.

In addition to water coming into the basement from the downspout, groundwater can roll down a hill toward the house, which then serves as a dam. You can raise the earth around the house to divert its flow away from the house. If a high water table is the problem, a sump pump is needed. Thoroseal, a dense cementitious material, can be applied to the outside block foundation as caulking to keep water out.

If the basement is still damp, a dehumidifier can help, but these work well only above a temperature of 50 to 60 degrees Fahrenheit. Chemicals such as baking soda are only temporary measures. The best way to remove the mold is to scrub the area with sulfur water. The basement can be hosed down and the water removed with an industrial vacuum.

THE KITCHEN

What's the most dangerous toxin in most kitchens? Gas. You should always have a vent in the kitchen; it has been shown that cerebral allergies are often directly attributable to the gas burnoff of pilot lights on stoves, which leak constantly. If you often have headaches and suspect that they are more common when you're spending time in the kitchen, try disconnecting your stove when you're not using it. If this makes a difference, you should consider replacing the gas stove with an electric one. Not only gas ovens are a health risk, though. Microwave ovens can leak; a defective microwave creates a very unhealthy environment within about eight feet around it.

The freon in the condenser of the refrigerator is a highly volatile, dangerous chemical. It is a very good idea to replace refrigerators that are more than 10 years old.

The refrigerator contributes to another seldom considered form of pollution found especially in the kitchen: noise pollution. You should be able to tolerate background noise of about 30 to 35 decibels. Noise higher than 50 decibels becomes uncomfortable. Above 80 decibels, you become substantially irritated, and noise above 100 may cause ear damage or central nervous system overstimulation. The compressor in most refrigerators is up to 60 decibels. You don't appreciate this until you turn on a refrigerator when everything else is totally quiet. But think of a kitchen with a television or a radio on, things cooking, telephone conversations—you can't even hear the refrigerator, and the noise level may be up around 100 decibels. The kitchen is one of the most stressful places because of this level of background noise. Even if you are unable to replace appliances such as refrigerators and air conditioners with less noisy ones, you can cut down on the number of noisemakers you are using at the same time.

Street noise can be irritating in any room. Noise-buffering double-fold drapes can keep noise down as well as insulate.

Mold and mildew are common invisible toxins in a kitchen. When was the last time you changed the water tray in your refrigerator? Under the condenser coil is a tray to collect water, but it can also collect all kinds of mold. Mold spores are in the air all the time, and you're inhaling them. If you're sensitive and your immune system is low, you'll feel it: Your eyes will get puffy, your nose will clog, and your throat will get sore. Keeping this area clean and dry could make a big difference.

Look under your kitchen sink; you'll be amazed at the range of toxic chemicals you keep there, so close to your food. Cleansers, for instance, especially ammonia-based products, often vaporize easily. Ammonia is very toxic and will stay in your blood for hours after you've smelled it. When you wax the kitchen floor, the floor wax will evaporate and you will breathe it in. Try to install floors that will not need waxing, but if you don't want to tear up your current floors, you might want to settle for a matte finish rather than a high sheen if you have to constantly apply volatile chemicals to get that sheen. As with the weed killers and insecticides in your garage, there are alternatives to chemical cleaners in the kitchen. Apple cider vinegar and hydrogen peroxide mixed half and half in cold water do the same job as ammonia. This preparation will clean windows and glassware perfectly, too.

Roach sprays are very stable. They can last for months and vaporize constantly. A dog or cat licking the floor can pick them up directly. A safer alternative is to use boric acid. You can mix it with sugar as a bait, but be sure pets and children can't reach it; line all the counters and fittings underneath with a strip of this no thicker than a pencil. This mixture is not volatile and is safe as long as it's put only in inaccessible places. Diatomaceous earth is safe and works well too. Or use the roach motels which use resin that roaches get stuck on instead of poisons.

Aluminum-based cookware in which the aluminum can come into contact with food should not be used. Aluminum has been implicated in Alzheimer's disease. It is a heavy metal that lodges in the blood, brain tissue, and central nervous system, where it can cause motor problems. Aluminum foil is all right to store cooked food but should not be used in cooking, where it can oxidize in microscopic amounts. You can't see this, but it can get into your food and your body. Teflon and all other nonstick coatings should also be avoided. They easily scratch or flake off with age, getting into food as well as exposing it to the often inferior metal underneath.

Next time you fill up a glass with water from the kitchen tap, consider that it may contain over a thousand chemicals, including those which the government puts in, such as fluoride; traces of herbicides and pesticides that have leached down into the water supply from fields; and traces of metal, rust, and molds from the inside of your pipes. Most water filtration systems can remove only a portion of these; the finer particles, including toxic chemicals such as pesticides, come through. If you live in a polluted area and your water supply is from underground streams, buy bottled water. I would buy plain distilled water. You get minerals from food; you don't need them from water. Since 72 to 74 percent of our bodies consists of water, we should be sure it is the purest water possible.

THE BATHROOM

One of the most common causes of allergy is what we put on our bodies: soaps, deodorants, and cosmetics. We use these things day in and day out, rarely thinking about their effect on us. For example, women who wear lipstick every day and lick their lips are absorbing chemicals never meant to be eaten. Perfumes vaporize and get breathed in. Read the ingredients of your antiperspirant; most likely it contains an aluminum-based compound which can be absorbed through the skin and carries the risks of aluminum outlined above. You can minimize these sources of toxins by using natural soaps and shampoos made out of vegetable ingredients, a nonfluoride toothpaste such as Dr. Bronner's or Tom's, mouthwash which you can make yourself with a little ascorbic acid in water, and natural loofah pads to scrub yourself.

The bathroom is one of the wettest rooms in the house and is a likely site for mold. It's important to air out the bathroom after a shower or bath and let it dry out. A window fan to evacuate the moist air is a good idea. Bathrooms are too often closed up most of the time and can be like little poison chambers that trap the perfume, deodorant, and cleaning fluid fumes in a small space. Odor disguisers such as pine- or lemon-scented aerosol sprays are worse than useless; the odor is a molecule floating around in the air that can be removed only by letting the air escape. Products that claim to take away odors only cover them up with a chemical which probably smells worse and is certainly worse for you.

The "disinfectant" cleaners so popular for bathroom tiles and tubs are virtually useless. To disinfect something, you have to boil it for 20 minutes, but within 1 minute it will be covered with germs again. Those germs are not going to kill anyone despite the fear tactics used to market these cleaners. Their heavy aromatic odors are often more of a problem than the germs; pine, for example, is a resinous material that is quite troublesome to allergic or sensitive people.

Never store medications in the medicine chest; it's hot and humid in the bathroom, and this can cause them to go bad. Store medicine and vitamins in the refrigerator.

As in the kitchen, look around the bathroom and think about potential toxins: cleaners for the tiles and sink, toilet fresheners, and so on. Do you need all those things? Can you substitute natural, nontoxic products?

THE BEDROOM

We spend a third of our lives in the bedroom; if you live 72 years, that means 24 years in bed. An ecologically ideal, safe place to spend all this time should be as free of dust as possible. Many bedrooms have wall-to-wall carpeting, which is an ecological disaster. Carpeting is toxic in several ways. Whereas new synthetic-fiber carpeting contains chemicals, such as formaldehyde, which will vaporize for a year or more, old carpets collect dirt, yeast, fungus, and mold. Dust mites live in rugs. Through an electron microscope these mites look like tiny dinosaurs; their diet is chiefly composed of the shed human skin cells which are another large component of dust. House dust mites can be wafted into the air by currents and breathed into the lungs. People who are allergic to them react as they do to cat or dog dander. Like dander, they can get into your eyes and make them red and puffy.

Think about ripping up your old carpet and putting in nice hardwood floors. They're easy to maintain and nontoxic. The Japanese have never had polyvinyl fluoride or no-wax floors; they use natural resins on wood, and some of these floors are 500 years old. If you feel you must have carpets, buy wool or natural fiber rugs with natural dyes. Stay away from synthetic carpets. And learn to vacuum efficiently. Most people just zip the vacuum over the carpet; by the time the dust has had a chance to get up through the nap into the air, the vacuum has moved on and has only raised the dust. You've actually increased the pollution in the air. Run the vacuum very slowly over the carpet, giving the dust you raise time to get into the vacuum.

You may be sleeping on foam-filled synthetic pillows and using synthetic-fiber pillowcases and sheets. Replace them with down-filled pillows and comforters and pure cotton sheets. Be aware of what you're putting in your sheets when you wash them; bleaches and fabric softeners are potential irritants. Many manufacturers of bedding use chemicals to which many people are allergic to fireproof the material. The way to test for this is to sleep on bedding which is not treated to be fireproof and see if your symptoms disappear. Again, if you feel better when you are sleeping away from your house on vacation, it should alert you to the fact that something in the bedroom is causing trouble.

Sleeping on clean sheets that are changed frequently reduces possible reactions to dust and dust mites. When you wash bedding, it's best to avoid perfumed detergents, antistatics, and softeners and look for biodegradable brands. Bleach should be oxygen bleach, not chlorine, which leaves an irritating residue. Miracle White, made by Beatrice Food Company, works well. If you suspect that a pillowcase, for example, is bothering you, wash it with a simple unscented detergent, rinse it three or four times, and try it again to see if the problem goes away.

Electric blankets can affect the electromagnetic field around the body and should be avoided. It's also best not to sleep near a digital clock, which can affect the body's electromagnetic system from three feet away.

Even your closets can affect your health; mothballs emit a poisonous gas. Try a mixture of rosemary, mint, thyme, ginseng, and cloves that has the additional advantage of smelling good.

AIR QUALITY

If you ever see the sun slant into a room at a certain angle, you know how much dust and smoke are in what you thought was clear air. It's there all the time. An air purifier with a negative ionizer is the best way to eliminate airborne toxins: spores, dust, cigarette smoke, hydrocarbons and pollutants from the street, cat hairs, and positive ions. The ionizer bombards the room with negative ions which attach themselves to the positive ions of pollutants, which then drop to the ground and can be filtered out by the filtration system.

Humidifiers are fine for improving air quality as long as you use distilled water in them. Otherwise mineral deposits from the water will end up all over your carpet, floor, and furniture.

PLANTS

One efficient and natural air-quality improver is living greenery in your house. The more plants in your environment, the better. A large number and variety of houseplants will increase the oxygen level in the air. Green, nonflowering varieties are best, since they will not give off pollen. Plants are also a great natural air pollution filtration system. They help maintain humidity levels and a proper electricity balance in the air. They also create a living energy field which we can share and be invigorated and calmed by.

LIGHT

Your visual environment is more important than you might realize. If you feel tired, ill, or depressed inside in the winter, especially if you live at a high latitude where the days are very short, and if you spend most of your day indoors, you may be suffering from seasonal affective disorder. In this condition the hypothalamus of the brain is deprived of full-spectrum natural sunlight—most artificial lights use only a part of the spectrum. The best solution is to allow plenty of natural light into your house; use double-glazing rather than small windows or heavy drapes if insulation is a concern. Try to spend time outdoors or arrange your activities so that you're near a window. If getting more daylight is beyond your control—the days are short, your house is dark, and you must stay indoors—the situation can be improved with full-spectrum lightbulbs. Full-spectrum incandescent lighting works on a completely different principle from that of fluorescent lighting (discussed in the section on the workplace below) and is more natural for the eyes. These bulbs are available in health stores in all sizes; using them in your office as well as in your home can make a big difference in your energy level and mental state.

HEAT

In cold areas we shut down for the winter, closing and sealing the windows to avoid ventilation from the outside. These practices contribute to the toxic state of the air inside.

Oil heaters often burn inefficiently and release unburned oil fumes into the house. An afterburn catalyst that is available on the market now can recycle these fumes, creating a clean air burn. Electric stoves are not a problem. Gas or oil space heaters are one of the worst offenders. Dry radiated heat can dry up your nose and skin. Wood-burning stoves may seem rustic and natural but can be one of the worst sources of indoor pollution.

In forced-air combustion heating systems that use gas or oil, a little pinhole not infrequently develops between the heat exchanger, which is next to the combustion chamber, and the air going past it to be heated. As the air that you're going to breathe goes around that heated chamber, it sucks in the partially combusted gases. You may not even perceive this in the air, because it's at a very low level, but over a six-month period this air can produce severe illness. Therefore, you must have your forced-air system checked out electronically for these pinholes every year. The smell test is not satisfactory. If you don't do this, you're at risk.

THE WORKPLACE

The energy crisis of the 1970s led to a generation of very well insulated but poorly ventilated office buildings. People who work in these buildings often complain of fatigue, nasal congestion, dizziness, and a host of other mysterious symptoms, yet there has been clear-cut documentation of toxic levels of pollutants in very few cases. The levels of toxins in these buildings are rarely high enough to provoke official alarm, but they are high enough to cause fatigue and illness through long-term, chronic exposure. Even low levels of organic chemicals, pesticides, formaldehyde, carpet cleaners, and tobacco smoke can affect those exposed to them for a long enough period.

The individual pollutants can be located and reduced, but the single most important factor is ventilation. Monday is the worst day for headaches and stress, at least partly because the ventilation systems have often been shut down over the weekend; you're breathing old, stale air. The ducts of your office air venting system probably haven't been cleaned in years. Dust and molds have built up inside them and are coming out into the air you breathe when the system is restarted. Ask the maintenance people to clean them; if they won't, get a heavy-duty charcoal filter and put it in the vent with a thick white insulation pad over it. These filters can be bought inexpensively at any hardware store. In one week the insulation pad will be covered with black particles large enough to see.

If it's noisy where you work, wear earplugs. You can also make your desk more pleasant with a small portable ionizer. The ionizer can actually fit in your pocket and is also useful in airplanes or on the dashboard of your car.

The fluorescent lighting often used in offices flashes on and off rapidly and constantly, placing great stress on your central nervous system. Although you are not consciously aware of this very rapid flickering, your eye and nervous system are overstimulated by it; two or three hours of work under fluorescent light can have the effect of three or four cups of coffee. At a certain level of overstimulation the central nervous system will shut down, and you will find yourself deeply fatigued. Replace the fluorescent lighting at your desk with a lamp which uses incandescent bulbs and use the natural full-spectrum light-bulbs described earlier. It's best to have an office with a window or skylight for true natural lighting; if you don't have one and can't arrange it, it's especially important to have natural—and sufficiently bright—lighting.

Stay away from the photocopier at the office as much as possible; it uses very volatile chemicals. Don't leave typewriter ink or correction ribbons lying around open; put them in a sealed plastic bag when they are not in use. An exhaust fan on the ceiling will help draw away vaporizing fluids.

Patient Stories

HEATHER MILLAR

I started becoming ill a year before I realized what was happening. At first I just thought I was tired. I was having trouble getting out of bed. I was drag-ging myself to work. I would come home feeling exhausted. Sometimes I had asthmalike symptoms and couldn't quite catch my breath. I wondered why this started all of a sudden when I was 30 years old, because my understand-ing was that most people develop asthma as children. I attributed these symptoms to working and living a fast-paced lifestyle, and I ignored them. One day my wrist started to ache for no apparent reason, which made me wonder if I was getting arthritis. But I ignored that as well and thought it would go away. I had these warning signs for a year before collapsing at work in September 1993.

I had woken up feeling as if I had the flu but thought I was well enough to go to work. I had gone shopping with my mom that morning and had had dif-ficulty walking up stairs. When I arrived at work, I realized that I was feeling quite unwell and that I would be able to work only part of my nursing shift. At the end of the first hour, I needed to go home because I was too ill to walk down the corridor and deliver medications to my patients. It was then that I returned to the nursing station and collapsed. I could hear, but I couldn't move. I felt as if I were paralyzed. I couldn't communicate with the other nurs-es who came to attend to me.

They took me to the emergency room, but I started to feel better and went home. I decided that I had the flu and that I would be better in three days.

Three days of flu evolved into a year and a half. During this time, I experienced many difficulties. The problem with environmental illness or chemical sensitivity is that you have a wide array of symptoms that come and go. You don't really know where to start and what connections to make. These are some of the symptoms I experienced.

Flu symptoms plagued me every day and became worse with time. As time passed, I was having more difficulty getting out of bed and walking around the house. I was extremely tired. No matter how much I slept, I just could not seem to get enough sleep. Even small tasks that shouldn't take much energy overwhelmed me. Cooking a meal was too much to even think about.

I also started having disturbed sleep. Despite my fatigue, I would wake up between two and four each night with numb hands. Sometimes I would have an incredible thirst. And sometimes I would wake up shaking as if I had a very high fever.

At one point I lost sight in my right eye. This happened for a short time but was extremely frightening nonetheless. All of a sudden, the vision in my right eye became completely silver, as if I were trying to look through a piece of tinfoil.

I had headaches with stabbing pains in my temples and a burning sensation in the back of my neck that made it difficult to turn my head. If you try to drive a car or move to do something, you realize how important it is to have range of motion in your neck.

The next month, I started to experience food allergies. It started with a few things. First I wasn't tolerating wheat very well and stopped eating it. Then I noticed that I did not feel well after drinking coffee and milk, so I eliminated them also. As the months progressed, I was unable to tolerate more and more foods. By January, I was virtually down to two foods: lamb and yams. By February, I lost my tolerance for everything. I was caught in a vicious cycle. I knew I needed to get nutrition in order to turn my health around, but eating these foods would make me even sicker.

As I became increasingly ill, my sense of smell became more and more acute. All of a sudden perfumes were a problem. I absolutely hated going to the department store and passing the perfume counter. I couldn't stand the smell of car exhaust either. I even avoided the hardware store because of the strong smell in there. Going to public places became difficult, as many people wear scented products such as clothes washed in scented laundry detergents, perfumes, and aftershaves. I would walk into a room, and if someone had perfume on, I would suddenly feel like I had the worst flu. My shoulders and muscles would start to ache. I would feel short of breath. I would get a headache.

A heightened sense of smell is part of the illness. People who are not affected need to understand what is happening when individuals with environmental illness ask, "Please do not wear that fragrance because it makes me feel sick."

I also started to have ringing in my ears. That would come and go, so I never could associate it with any particular event. Sometimes it would affect one ear, sometimes both. It was bothersome trying to have a conversation with somebody and trying to hear that person over the ringing in my ears.

Additionally, I felt dizzy. I had days when it was even difficult for me to stand up and navigate my way to the bathroom. Several times I fell over.

One of the most disturbing symptoms that I had was difficulty concentrating. I could no longer read something from start to finish. It would take me three to four tries to read material I should have comprehended in the first reading.

I also noticed that I was forgetful. Previously I had had an exceptional memory. All of a sudden I noticed that I couldn't remember things that were extremely important. At age 30 I was wondering if I was getting the beginning stages of Alzheimer's disease, the loss of memory was so apparent. Some days my memory was better than others, and some days my ability to concentrate was better than others.

Then there were the panic attacks. My heart would race while I was driving my car on the interstate. I did not understand why I felt better on residential streets. Later, I realized that I had difficulty on the interstate because the exhaust was so much more prevalent there. Every time I was exposed to exhaust, my heart raced; I felt anxious and had difficulty concentrating.

I also felt extremely anxious in shopping malls. I have since learned that there are extremely high levels of chemicals in shopping malls, such as formaldehyde, emitted by new building materials. These synthetics are highly toxic. What I couldn't understand was why I felt anxious at some times and not others. The reason was that some shopping malls are less toxic than others, and some stores, because of the types of merchandise they carry, are also better than others.

The day I collapsed at work was the last day I worked as a nurse. I kept assuming that within a month I would feel better and go back to my job. One month rolled into two, two months into three, and three months into a year and a half.

Being a nurse, I felt that I would receive the support I needed. After all, I was a medical person myself. What I experienced instead was how a patient feels when he or she is told that nothing is wrong. I had always been on the other side of things. I found this new perspective extremely alarming.

The medical community has become technologically based. Everything relies on a diagnostic test. I would go in, and they would run a gamut of tests. As with most people with environmental illness, the standard tests would come back negative. The doctors would then tell me that there was nothing wrong. This was disturbing because I was extremely ill. I was so sick that I could hardly get up off the couch. Nor could I make myself a meal. Going to the bathroom was an effort. How, on a diagnostic test, could I look perfectly normal?

When the doctors could not diagnose me, they said that I was suffering from stress. But this was not the case. Before I got sick, my life was wonderful.

I had one of the least pressured jobs I had ever had, and I was enjoying what I was doing. At the end of a contract I would go on vacation to Europe for a month. I was about to get married. My life couldn't have been better.

Stress is becoming the catchall diagnosis in the medical community. We must ask why so many people in our society are being told that they have stress, panic disorder, anxiety, and depression. That category is growing larger and larger. People have to ask, Why is this happening in our society? Is something chemical bringing this on? Do we need to make changes in the environment?

If you are feeling some symptoms of toxicity, it is time to take action now. Don't wait until you end up, as I did, in a wheelchair, bedridden, and completely intolerant to food.

DR. GARD ON ONE PATIENT'S EXPERIENCE:

A 56-year-old white female came to us with swollen, painful joints, especially the right knee. She was scheduled for a knee replacement. Her history indicated that she worked in a closed building as a counselor to students. Nine of the 12 teachers in this building had similar problems. Most of the complaints began after a new carpet installation.

A biotoxic reduction was started. Within the first hour of the program she was able to bend her right knee. By the second day she was able to move with less difficulty and ride the stationary bike. Upon completion, she was pain-free and had full range of motion in all joints. This was over four years ago, and the patient is still well.

Her laboratory work revealed toluene, 24.9 before the program and 1.4 after; ethyl benzine, 12.3 before and none after; xylene, 83.2 before and none after; styrene, 123.6 before and none after; chloroform, 5.4 before and none after; 1:1-trichlor, 1.4 before and 0.5 after; tetrachloroethylene, 1.5 before and none after; dichlorobenzene, 11.1 before and 4.3 after.

Chapter 14

Heart Disease

Heart disease among women is a much greater threat than many people believe; twice as many women die from heart disease as from all forms of cancer combined. A major reason for this is the loss of estrogen that accompanies menopause, for estrogen protects the cardiovascular system.

Causes

Lowered estrogen is just one of many factors that contribute to heart disease in women. "Overall, there are 247 risk factors that can damage the heart," states Dr. David Steenblock, a complementary physician from California. "A risk factor is anything that injures the inner lining of the blood vessels that supply the heart with oxygen and nutrition. Any agent that injures this inner lining, such as tobacco, air pollution, food additives, high blood pressure, and gasoline fumes, can initiate atherosclerosis, the so-called hardening of the arteries. Then the accumulation of such things as cholesterol, calcium, scar tissue, and fat causes atherosclerotic lesions, which gradually go on to occlude, or block, the arteries to the brain and the heart. When the arteries to the brain [the carotid arteries] are blocked you have a stroke, and when the arteries to the heart [the coronary arteries] are blocked, you have a heart attack."

Dr. Michael Janson, president of the American Preventive Medical Association and author of *Vitamin Revolution in Health Care*, describes other common heart ailments, some of which are precipitated by atherosclerosis.

ANGINA PECTORIS

Janson says, "Clogged arteries leave the heart muscle with inadequate oxygen. As everyone knows, muscles hurt when exercised beyond their oxygen capacity. When not enough blood flows from the coronary arteries to the heart muscle, people experience pain in the chest. Sometimes they feel pain in the jaw, the shoulder, or even the wrist. Often they do not realize that this is referred pain coming from the heart itself."

CONGESTIVE HEART FAILURE

"Hardening of the coronary arteries can lead to a number of other problems," Janson explains. "When heart muscle tissue functions inefficiently, more blood comes in than is pumped out. In other words, with each beat the amount of blood being returned to the heart is more than the heart muscle can handle. Fluid backs up, and other tissues, such as the lungs and legs, can get congested. Congestive heart failure leads to shortness of breath, water in the lungs, and swelling of the ankles."

HIGH BLOOD PRESSURE

Janson says, "High blood pressure can be the result of dietary habits; lack of exercise; high stress; being overweight; having too much caffeine, sugar, alcohol, or, in particular, salt in the diet. In the past few years, some reports have said that salt does not make much of a difference for most people. The fact is, that's not true. Even a slight elevation in blood pressure is enough to increase the risk of heart disease."

Symptoms

Heart disease is a gradual process that takes years to develop into a serious condition. At first there are no warning signs. If the coronary arteries become severely blocked, a person may experience shortness of breath or chest pains (angina pectoris) that are relieved by rest.

Clinical Experience

CONVENTIONAL TREATMENTS

MEDICATIONS FOR HIGH BLOOD PRESSURE

Dr. Janson believes the general public is being misled into believing that medications for high blood pressure are safe and always necessary: "We all hear advertisements on the radio telling us to stay on these medications for life. They say that no symptoms tell you whether or not your blood pressure is high. Therefore, if you are taking medication for high blood pressure, you must stay on your medication and never, ever stop. That so-called public service announcement is really a sales pitch from the drug companies that make the medications. We know that these medications actually cause more heart disease and that they create side effects in addition to the high blood pressure."

Dr. Steenblock warns, however, that patients who depend on medication to control high blood pressure should not self-discontinue: "Many people have this idea that since the doctor is not getting at the cause of their high blood pressure, it is somewhat illogical for them to take their blood pressure medicine. True, doctors often do not have the answer. Still, if you fail to take your medicine and your blood pressure gets out of control, you can develop heart disease and go on to have a stroke."

The solution here is to work with a complementary medical physician until your heart health is restored. In some cases, medication may be needed long term, even for a lifetime, but no one can fail to benefit from improving lifestyle and diet. The following sections can serve as guidelines.

RISK ASSESSMENT

Diagnosis is an important first step. Before any one begins a cardiovascular health program, a doctor should take the following factors into account: family history, blood pressure, cholesterol level, weight, and stress electrocardiogram (ECG) tests. After assessment of the person's risk factors, the program can begin.

DIET

The power of a vegetarian diet in a cardiovascular health program was recognized in a now-famous study by Dr. Dean Ornish. The Ornish study placed heart patients on a protocol of healthy vegetarian foods, daily aerobic exercise, and relaxation. At the end of a year, a significant number of patients showed improvement in their heart condition, and in some the disease was even reversed.

Dr. Paul Cutler, a complementary physician from Niagara Falls, New York, says, "Medicine in general owes Ornish a great deal of gratitude. He showed that a drastic reduction of fats was most important. I believe that the total dietary fats should be well below the typical average of 40 percent. Modern nutritionists are saying 30 percent. I try to get fat content down to 10 percent of the total calories. I see improvement in angina just by reducing the fats to that degree."

There is not much controversy about what is wrong with the standard American diet with its high amounts of animal proteins, saturated animal fats, dairy products, deep-fried foods, and refined carbohydrates. The average American diet consists of 43 percent fats and 14 percent proteins and the rest is mainly carbohydrates. The average daily intake of cholesterol is 450 to 500 mg. But there is controversy over the proper foods for those with heart disease. There are over 60,000 dietitians in the United States, and they have been a primary source of information on what a sick person should eat. After all, physicians graduate from medical school with only an hour or two of learning about nutrition. However, even though dietitians are well-trained, there is a split in the field. Only a very small percentage of dietitians believe the standard American diet plays a large role in causing the diseases we are beset with, including heart disease.

The American Heart Association recommends that we cut fat intake to 30 percent, with only 10 percent of this in the form of saturated fats (fats found particularly in land animals, palm and coconut oils, and hydrogenated vegetable oils). We have been told that margarine, made from "polyunsaturated fats," is good for the heart and will lower cholesterol. That is simply not true; margarine is loaded with the fatty acids that contribute to heart disease. Instead of margarine, use olive oil, canola oil, or flaxseed, almond, safflower, sunflower, or soy oil. Of these, olive oil would be at the top of my list. But don't have margarine.

No more than 10 percent of the oils you eat should be polyunsaturated fats, such as those found in some vegetable oils, including corn and cottonseed oils. According to the American Heart Association, we should get the rest from monounsaturated fats such as olive oil and take in less than 300 mg of cholesterol each day.

While the dangers of saturated fats to heart health are well known, Dr. Ray Peat, a distinguished scientific researcher in Eugene, Oregon, says unsaturated fats can be just as damaging: "Many people have been soaking their bodies in unsaturated vegetable oil diets for years. As a result, every time they get hungry or face stress, their blood sugar falls, their adrenaline rises, and these unsaturated fats are drawn out of storage. Once released, they immediately start poisoning the lining of the blood vessels and all the cellular energy-producing systems. In 1960, this effect was demonstrated by a group in England which saw that adrenaline, either natural or synthetic, caused damage to the circulatory system. It turns out that this occurs after unsaturated fats become mobilized. They hit the lining of the blood vessels, where they cause lipid peroxidative damage."

Dr. Janson adds that people should avoid foods such as sugar, salt, white flour, white rice, and particularly any shortening or hydrogenated vegetable oils found in products like margarine and vegetable shortening: "Whenever you see vegetable shortening, hydrogenated vegetable oil, or partially hydrogenated vegetable oil on a label, avoid that product. These are not foods. In fact, I consider margarine an industrial waste product that is fashioned to resemble food."

He recommends a low-fat, whole-foods diet: "The diet should be high in complex carbohydrates, including whole grains, beans, vegetables, and fruits. Remember, flavonoids, which are plant pigments, are present in fruits and vegetables and in some beans and grains. These are very protective, and most of them are not available as supplements.

"I think the diet should be largely vegetarian, although a number of studies show that fish also reduces levels of heart disease and cancer. Fish may or may not be the reason for this. It may be that eating more fish means eating less chicken and meat. Cutting those foods out of the diet helps cut down on heart disease."

Broccoli and other vegetables are the first foods to turn to. We eat broccoli and all kinds of produce, seeds, legumes, and grains to get our beta carotenes and maybe vitamin C, but they also contain important phytochemicals. These phytochemicals include beta carotene, alpha carotene, ascorbic acid, ash, boron, caffeic acid, calcium, chlorophyll, chromium, citric acid, copper, glycine, iron, linoleic acid, lysine, magnesium, niacin, oleic acid, phosphorus, potassium, riboflavin, selenium, thiamin, tryptophan, and zinc, among others. There are 1,000 different phytochemicals that are important in protecting us from cancer. Among them are the phytoestrogens, which guard against prostate, breast, and lung cancer. These chemicals have all kinds of healing properties. Chlorophyll, for instance, helps purify the blood and acts as a detoxifier.

You can lower your blood pressure by eating vegetables such as garlic, broccoli, and asparagus. You should have at least five servings of vegetables and three of fruits each day, raw, steamed, or juiced. Once you start, you will notice a world of difference in your overall vitality. Other invaluable heart foods are rice and beans, which are complete proteins rich in fiber and B-complex vitamins.

We grow up with the pernicious myth that if it is not an animal protein, it is not a complete protein and so is not really nutritious. I did studies at the Institute of Applied Biology that proved conclusively that beans, legumes, and all grains contain complete proteins just like animal proteins, without the saturated fats. They are not high in calories and are rich in vitamins, minerals, and essential oils.

Hence, people in cultures that have rice and beans as a dietary staple have, historically, been quite healthy. There are thousands of ways to prepare these foods. Go into a health food store and look at the different preparations along with all the other foods sold. When you see the variety, you will not feel deprived by not having steak and potatoes.

EXERCISE

"Aerobic exercise and an improved diet should go hand in hand," notes Dr. Cutler. "Aerobics help the good cholesterol go up significantly, which in turn helps remove cholesterol from arterial walls after the cells are through with it so it is less likely to form plaque." Exercising aerobically means getting the heart rate up three or four times a week. A doctor can help determine how much exercise is needed.

Dr. Janson adds that people should stretch before and after an aerobic workout: "The stretching has another benefit in that it relaxes the body and keeps people limber and more flexible. That makes it easier to continue an aerobic exercise program."

Exercise is, however, not a panacea. Some people mistakenly assume that cholesterol can be burned off by exercise and activity and that as a result, people who engage in athletics and body building can eat more meat and eggs without suffering ill effects. There is no scientific basis for this notion. To the contrary, studies have shown that good conditioning and muscle tone do not necessarily put a person in good cardiovascular condition.

Dr. Julian Whitaker refers to "studies done on marathon runners in South Africa in which five of them died of heart attacks. These were conditioned long-distance runners. They all had cholesterol levels of 270, 290, etc. They were very fit but not very well."

SUPPLEMENTS

Supplements provide wonderful support for the heart and sometimes help eliminate or reduce dosages of medication. The following are nutrients you should know about. In addition, two other beneficial supplements are chondroitin sulfate A and evening primrose oil (1,500 mg/day).

ANTIOXIDANTS Antioxidants help protect the heart from free radical damage, also known as oxidation. Antioxidant nutrients include vitamin E, beta carotene, vitamin C, and selenium. Free radicals damage the tissues lining the arteries, which leads to atherosclerosis and plaque deposits. Antioxidants, particularly vitamin C, can prevent this from happening by protecting the lining of the arteries. Vitamin E has several functions. Aside from being a protective antioxidant, it reduces the stickiness of the platelets, little blood fragments that initiate blood clots. This effect is helped by the addition of essential fatty acids and garlic to the diet. Minimizing free radical damage and keeping platelets from clogging the arteries give arteries a chance to heal and recover. There is more room for oxygen to flow through the arteries to reach tissues. It is estimated that between 400 and 800 units are useful in preventing stroke. You may go higher, up to 1,200 or 1,600 units, unless other medical conditions preclude a higher level. I believe we would cut the incidence of stroke by 20 percent, saving 50,000 to 100,000 people a year, just by having everyone take this little, inexpensive supplement.

L-ARGININE. L-arginine is an amino acid that has been receiving well-deserved attention in the medical literature for its ability to produce nitric oxide. Nitric oxide benefits the arterial walls in several ways. It helps the smooth muscles in the arterial walls relax, promoting an antianginal, antihypertensive, and antistress effect. Additionally, research shows that L-arginine reduces the activation of platelets, the small bodies that can initiate arterial spasm and plaque development. Other studies show that L-arginine slows plaque development and even reverses small amounts of plaque buildup. "I've seen it work," says

ALTERNATIVE TREATMENT SOLUTIONS **281**

Dr. Cutler. "Taking 2 to 3 grams of L-arginine per day has quite a marked antianginal effect. L-arginine now is a must in my protocol for nutrients. Usually I start with about 1,000 mg per day, and raise the levels if that amount isn't helping."

L-CARNITINE. The heart muscle needs to burn fat for energy, and L-carnitine allows this to happen. Dr. Janson explains, "L-carnitine gets fat into the little engines inside the cells called mitochondria. These little mitochondrial engines are where fat is burned for energy. Your heart muscle needs to burn fat for energy, and the only way it can get the fat into that little engine is with the amino acid L-carnitine. At the same time, that inner mitochondrial membrane requires another nutrient to burn the fat: coenzyme Q10." Dr. Janson recommends that people take 500 mg L-carnitine two to three times a day. You should take L-carnitine along with vitamin E, because they work together synergistically.

CHROMIUM PICOLINATE. Chromium picolinate has been shown to be beneficial both for the heart and for blood sugar levels..

COENZYME Q10. Coenzyme Q10 is a nutrient that should be taken by anyone who has heart problems or who wants to avoid getting them. Along with L-carnitine, it helps prevent angina and protects the heart muscle by letting it burn fat for energy more easily. It also improves heart health by reducing blood pressure and arrhythmias. As an antioxidant, it prevents the damage to blood vessels that leads to hardening of the arteries. Therapeutic levels are between 50 and 150 mg for mild heart disease. More severe heart disease may respond to 200 mg.

LECITHIN. Lecithin is made from soy. Not only does it keep the arteries strong and healthy, but it helps emulsify fats, helps the brain, and is good for memory as well as the heart.

MAGNESIUM. Magnesium increases blood flow by allowing muscles in the arterial wall to relax. Usually 500 to 1,000 mg is needed.

MAXEPA. MaxEPA, a combination of EPA (eicosapentaenoic acid) and DHA (docosohexaenoic acid), also known as fish oil, is part of the omega-3 and omega-6 fatty acids found in salmon, sardines, and mackerel. Since many people do not eat these fish, they should be getting these fatty acids in fish oil. The recommended daily dose is 500 to 1,000 mg. Clinical and epidemiological experience as well as scientific studies have found that people who eat a lot of fish have less heart disease than people who do not.

NIACIN (VITAMIN B3). A 15-year study on the effects of niacin published by the American Heart Association in the mid-1980s connected the use of niacin to a significant reduction in heart attacks and death from heart disease. Long-term niacin use has also been associated with decreased rates of cancer. Niacin should be taken under medical supervision, since it can affect liver function.

Dr. Janson adds, "Other B vitamins, such as folic acid and B_{12}, can help lower blood levels of homocystine, a risk factor for heart disease."

TAURINE. Taurine, an amino acid, is another important antioxidant that helps prevent atherosclerosis. Additionally, it can avert heart failure by improving the strength of the heart's contraction. That increases the outflow of blood from the heart and reduces congestive heart failure. Generally, 500 mg is taken twice a day.

THYROID SUPPLEMENTS. Thyroid supplementation may normalize high cholesterol, according to Dr. Ray Peat: "High cholesterol indicates a thyroid hormone deficiency. A clear demonstration of this was seen in the 1930s in patients whose thyroid glands were surgically removed. After the operation, cholesterol levels became abnormally high, but they returned to normal with thyroid supplementation." He adds that thyroid extract is linked to fewer heart attacks: "One of the foremost American researchers in the field, Broda Barnes, wrote *Solved: The Riddle of Heart Attacks* after finding that patients in one group had far fewer heart attacks than did patients in another group. All the low-heart-attack group did differently was take thyroid when they needed it."

VITAMIN B_1. Among the B vitamins, vitamin B_1 is the most important for the heart: 25 to 50 mg daily.

VITAMIN C. If there is one vitamin everyone needs to take every day, it is vitamin C. If you have a cold or flu, you may require 50,000 mg for quick recovery; for heart disease, you may require substantially more. Get over that old-fashioned idea that all you need is one glass of orange juice to get the necessary vitamin C. That idea went out with the horse and buggy. Now we have thousands of studies of the valuable properties of vitamin C, which can help with everything from cancer to heart disease and diabetes. I would take 500 to 1,000 mg, five times a day. Vitamin C washes out of the system, so you need to take it throughout the day. Two well-known specialists in coronary heart disease recommend that their patients take vitamin C before going to bed at night because they find it helps prevent heart attacks during sleep and in the morning, which is when the majority of heart attacks occur.

HERBS

In addition to the herbs listed below, consider taking barberry, black cohosh, and butcher's broom.

BUGLEWEED. Bugleweed is a remedy for heart palpitations and elevated blood pressure. It may also alleviate anxiety, since elevated blood pressure is frequently associated with a rapid pulse rate, anxiety, and agitation.

CAYENNE. Capsaicin, the active ingredient in cayenne, helps the heart in many ways. It stimulates circulatory function, lowers cholesterol, reduces blood pressure, and lessens the chance of heart attacks and strokes. By decreasing blood levels of fibrin, it also reduces the risk of forming blood clots that cause heart attacks and strokes.

GARLIC. Among its many benefits, garlic helps lower blood pressure and decrease cholesterol. When combined with vitamin E, it lessens the frequency of blood clots in arterial walls, which in turn helps prevent heart attacks and strokes. The recommended amount is 500 mg or more of deodorized garlic taken twice a day.

GINKGO BILOBA. *Ginkgo biloba* helps improve small blood vessel circulation.

HAWTHORN BERRY. Hawthorn is an overall heart tonic that works against arrhythmia, angina, high blood pressure, and hardening of the arteries. It aids circulation and ameliorates valvular insufficiency and an irregular pulse. Hawthorn berry can also correct acid conditions of the blood. It can be safely taken every day.

MISTLETOE. Mistletoe is a cardiac tonic that stimulates circulation. Fifteen drops of tincture taken three times a day or three cups of tea daily can help lower blood pressure and alleviate heart strain. Mistletoe should not be overused, nor should the berries be eaten.

MOTHERWORT. Motherwort helps stabilize the electrical rhythm of the heart. The amount taken should be monitored by a doctor.

WILD YAM. Wild yam stimulates production of DHEA. Low levels of this hormone have been related to higher incidences of heart disease. Wild yam can provide added protection and is completely safe.

CHINESE HERBAL THERAPY

Letha Hadady, one of the leading herbalists in the United States, says most Americans do not go to the doctor when they are a little sick; they wait until they are really suffering. They may have chest pains or difficulty breathing, but they generally don't go to the doctor nor, of course, to the herbalist. They say, "I'm tired; I'm under stress," and ignore it. That is a terrible approach because some of the underlying problems of heart disease are the ones they are complaining of: fatigue, stress, and poor digestion. Poor digestion and fatigue lead to cholesterol buildup, which leads to pain and heart congestion. People try to breathe more deeply and reduce stress when they experience these early symptoms, but that does not help. But changing your diet, taking herbs and foods that reduce cholesterol, will definitely help.

Hadady's clients often have conditions that they believe are unrelated to heart disease; but her special training as an herbalist enables her to see a connection to the heart. Mind, body, and spirit are interconnected, and the heart is affected by all of these things. Depression, for example, is related to a weak heart. Insomnia, poor concentration and palpitations are all signs that poor circulation could be affecting the heart.

Many Western doctors will say that herbs, especially Oriental ones, have not been tested. This is a prejudiced position. When you go to a public library or consult an on-line medical search and reference service such as Medline, which is available free, to any interested person, you find 3,500 studies on Chinese herbs alone. The majority of the research is done in Asia, and for Americans to say this research does not count is racist.

Quite a number of these remedies are available in health food stores, by mail order, or in your local Chinatown. The ingredients are always in English or Latin on the back.

Hadady points out that one of the major underlying problems associated with heart disease is fatigue. Chinese doctors link the heart's health to the strength of the adrenal glands—not an obvious connection. Hadady states, "If I had a patient complaining of fatigue and being overweight, I would suspect heart problems—if not then, somewhere down the line, so I would work on the adrenals. To strengthen the adrenals, you can get the herbal preparation from Chinatown called Goldenbook. It adds to immune energy and will help with kidney and heart problems. We strengthen what is weak so the heart will not falter."

Hadady explains that clove, a spice we have at home, is a strong stimulant. A pinch in the late afternoon will act like coffee. Coffee is a major problem because it increases painful, sluggish circulation in the gastrointestinal tract that affects the whole circulation, meaning that the heart will not run smoothly. A pinch of clove will replace coffee better than anything else can.

Siberian ginseng, a blend of various ginsengs, is beneficial. The ginsengs are adaptogens; that is, they help us maintain energy as well as aid us in living under a high level of stress. They support the nervous system. Raw tienchi ginseng, one that Americans are less familiar with, comes in powdered form. A half teaspoon in cool water, taken every day, will reduce cholesterol and pain around the heart.

One Chinese remedy that is especially valuable in relation to heart pain and blood vessel congestion is *dan shen wan*, which combines salvia and camphor. The camphor dilates the blood vessels while the salvia increases the heart's action. Another valuable remedy is *guan xin su he wan*, which contains frankincense. Both frankincense and myrrh improve circulation. Frankincense increases blood flow around the heart. You can take it once a day to prevent heart attack. It can be chewed and swallowed. Hadady recommends it even if you have no heart symptoms. It has healthy ingredients such as liquid amber and sandalwood, which keeps the esophagus and chest cool.

Yans shen jia jiao wan is a combination of ginseng and other herbs that free the circulation of the blood in the brain. This is not just for victims of heart attack but also for those with stroke and hemiplegia (paralysis of one side of the body). People with high cholesterol and those at high risk of heart trouble can take one dose a day as a preventive measure.

Baoxin wan is a remedy for heart attacks. If you feel faint and experience pain and weakness, you sniff it like a smelling salt. If the pain is great and you feel the onset of an attack, take it orally. It includes ginseng and liquid amber. It treats the congestion of the blood vessels around the heart and opens up the blood vessels.

Some of the underlying problems leading to a heart attack, such as excess weight and cholesterol, are well countered by herbal remedies. One preparation whose name is self-explanatory is Keep Fit, Reduce Fat. The ingredients are ginseng, hawthorn, and other herbs that are good for the heart. Hawthorn, a slightly bitter, slightly sour berry, works as a digestive. You can take a capsule of Keep Fit after meals. Cholesterol is reduced, and the muscle of the heart is made stronger.

Evening primrose oil is another useful herb for reducing cholesterol. Chinatown is an excellent place to purchase this remedy since the prices are apt to be considerably lower than those for comparable items in health food stores.

Another popular remedy in Asia is green tea, which has even been reported in the *New York Times* as being very good for reducing cholesterol. "This is a good alternative to other caffeine teas," Hadady notes, "because the caffeine in it is very low. It gives the satisfaction of a bitter tea while reducing cholesterol."

Bojemni slimming tea protects the heart. It includes hawthorn. *Xiao yao wan,* a digestive remedy that boosts circulation and combats depression, contains ginger, mint, and other herbs; it eases the flow of bile, eases the digestive process, and reduces chest congestion.

Digestive Harmony is an American-made product that contains Chinese herbs, one of many such products that are now on the market and sold door to door or through mail order. "This is part of a trend now," Hadady explains, "a very important trend in herbalism, of using Asian herbs manufactured with American standards. Digestive Harmony can be ordered from Oakland, California. It will ease the underlying troubles related to heart disease.

"Remember that depression is in part a heart problem," Hadady goes on. "The heart is not just a digestive center, but is related to our emotions. Depression is rightly associated with heart disease since it affects the heartbeat. When we are not happy and our emotions are not smooth, we feel it in the heart.

"Some remedies that combat depression come to us from China. Coschisandra strengthens the energy level and keeps us from losing the energy we have. It is good for both the adrenals and the heart. It fights against poor memory, poor concentration and depression. Also try *anshen bu nao pien,* available in all the Chinatowns in the United States. It is for depression, blood deficiencies and heart-related problems such as panic and anxiety.

"Also useful is *mao dong qing,* which is the Chinese name for holly, and it comes in capsule form. It is for chest pain and prevention of heart trouble. You can take several of these capsules each day as a preventive. If you already have heart problems, it reduces cholesterol, congestion, and pains.

"In general," Hadady concludes, "Chinese remedies for the heart also treat not just pain, but also emotional problems: sadness, anxieties ,and other mental suffering."

CHELATION THERAPY

Chelation therapy is especially popular since coronary bypass surgery has been pronounced ineffective for up to 65 percent of the people receiving it. Coronary bypass surgery and cardiovascular drugs and medications do offer slight, though highly invasive, relief of the acute complications of heart disease. However, chelation therapy, which is being administered to hundreds of thousands of heart disease patients, is proving quite successful and is considerably safer and substantially less expensive than bypass surgery. It is not new, having been in use for over 40 years.

The EDTA used in chelation therapy bonds with toxic metals and calcium and carries them out of the bloodstream through the kidneys, slowing or reversing some plaque formation in the arteries and thus retarding the degenerative process. EDTA enhances blood flow, permitting more essential oxygen and nutrients to circulate and be absorbed by the body. As chelation therapy is more commonly used, chelation specialists feel that it will become the most important heart disease therapy offered in the future.

As Dr. Steenblock describes it, "EDTA binds with calcium that has deposited in artery walls and is excreted from the body through the kidneys. In addition, it breaks down scar tissue and allows the arteries to become softer. In other words, it takes the hard out of hardening of the arteries."

When deciding whether or not to administer chelation therapy, Dr. Cutler tests patients for heavy metal buildup. "I look for elevated iron and copper levels in the blood. I also measure something called the serum ferritin, which reflects artery tissue levels of iron. If I start chelation, as the iron levels come down in the blood, there are also clinical improvements in angina and exercise tests. And there are angiogram and treadmill test improvements as well

"If I do not find any abnormality in these metals, I do what is called a challenge, which means I give one chelation treatment, collect urine for 24 hours afterward, and observe the metals that come out. Based on these results, I make the decision as to whether I want to chelate the person."

Dr. Steenblock, who has administered chelation therapy for almost 20 years, uses the treatment more extensively. He explains why it is so valuable for most individuals: "In their forties most people develop some degree of atherosclerosis due to cholesterol, scar tissue, fat, and calcium, which accumulate in the artery walls.

"You have to try to prevent all these risk factors by keeping your diet low in fat and cholesterol and by exercising, thinking properly, avoiding chemicals, and taking antioxidants to protect the inner lining of the blood vessels. In addition, you can break down scar tissue and remove calcium with chelation.

"Studies show that if you start chelating in your forties, you can actually reverse all the atherosclerosis as soon as it starts to develop. If you have done things that have not been perfect in your life—you haven't eaten right, you have been under too much stress, you have smoked—by the time you are 40, you will have some degree of atherosclerosis. Chelation can reverse this process and keep those arteries more pristine.

"By the time you are 60, the amount of calcium that has been deposited in your arteries is 10 times what you had in your arteries at 10 years of age. Al Fleckenstein, a leading cardiovascular drug researcher, said in one of his books that the amount of calcium present in the walls of the arteries is the single most important risk factor in the development of atherosclerosis. In other words, as calcium accumulates in the arterial walls, it promotes the development of atherosclerosis; atherosclerosis develops because you are gradually accumulating this calcium. If you can remove the calcium somewhere between the ages of 40 and 60, you can change that ratio, reverse the whole process, and put off the development of atherosclerosis for a number of years. That's for prevention.

"Of course, if you have outright disease, you can be helped as well. I have been doing chelation since 1977, so I have treated thousands of patients, and most do not come for prevention. They come for treatment of disease. They come in with angina or claudication [lameness due to leg pain]. With chelation, most of the time these symptoms disappear. If they do not, it is usually because the person has advanced disease and needs more than the standard 30 treatments. When people who are 75 or 80 years old come in with advanced disease, I tell them that they need to start out with 30 treatments—that's one treatment twice or three times a week. They wait a month or two, and then come back and do another 30. This process continues until we clean out these arteries because it takes time to reverse all of the terribly occluded blocked arteries that develop over many, many years of bad living."

STRESS MANAGEMENT

Virtually all the authorities agree that if you want to get a handle on heart disease, you have to deal with stress. Stress or distress is a major problem for the American psyche.

For a long while we have known that stress is a contributor to heart disease, but only recently have we begun to understand the physiological basis of the connection.

Richard Friedman, Ph.D., of Harvard Medical School, remarks that when we are confronted with stressful situations, most of us try to oversolve the problem. We constantly try to fit square pegs into round holes, and when we find that is not going to work, we turn inward, brood, and look for ways to dissipate stress, frequently by acting inappropriately, such as overeating, drinking or taking inappropriate drugs or medications. This contributes to the disease process.

Dr. Friedman says there is a link between stress and cardiovascular disease. When we are stressed by a fear of physical or psychological danger, the body exhibits a fight-or-flight response as it prepares to deal with an enemy. Very recent research indicates that the body readies itself not to bleed if it is cut or injured, which makes a lot of sense from a biological and evolutionary perspective. However, if the threats are psychological and you have a bad diet, you may be going through stressful incidents 20 or 30 times a day, triggering the fight-or-flight response. Each time this happens, the body prepares not to bleed by making the blood platelets stickier. This internal clotting takes place every time you get angry, whether on a supermarket line or in a traffic jam. Over time this continual clotting can contribute to plaque buildup in the arteries. A heart attack that may occur when you are 50 years old would not have occurred until you were 80 if you had undergone less of the buildup induced by platelet stickiness.

Stress also contributes to heart disease by increasing free radical damage to tissues and increasing spasms in the arterial walls.

When you are exposed to a biochemical or psychological stress, a host of changes take place in addition to platelet stickiness. The body's ability to fight off viral and bacterial infection is be lessened by the weaknesses induced by stress. Stress compromises the immune system's ability to fight off opportunistic diseases.

There is some good news, though, about our ability to fight off the debilitating conditions that lead to a heart attack. Dr. Friedman notes that just as continued stress leads to a weakening of the system, there is an opposite effect, one that has been labeled by his colleague at Harvard Dr. Herbert Benson as the "relaxation response." Eliciting this calming response on a daily basis makes it less likely that you will have high blood pressure or arteriosclerotic plaque buildup or a heart attack down the road.

The relaxation response should be combined with other behavior modifications to create a healthier response to stress, and all these tecniques should be combined with the best medical care. That is the way to optimize your health.

Dr. Friedman tells us how the relaxation response is induced: Use whatever strategy you have available to let go of any muscle tension you may be experiencing. Make sure your muscles are loose and your jaw lets go. After you feel a bit more comfortable, focus your attention on your breathing. If you find yourself having any distracting thoughts, do not let them bother you or take you away from the process. As soon as you have a distracting thought, simply say to yourself, "Oh well," and return to a concentration on your breathing and to a thought or image that allows you to stay calm, peaceful, and relaxed. Become aware of the cool air coming in your nostrils and the warm air going out. Keep this up till you are deeply relaxed.

Other ways to overcome stress are exercise, deep breathing, visualization, tai chi, yoga, meditation, *qi gong,* mantras, massage, Reiki, biofeedback, and aromatherapy. An essential oil blend of *ylang ylang,* lavender or peppermint, and marjoram added to oil and applied during massage helps calm the system and may even lower blood pressure.

TREATMENT OF HELICOBACTER PYLORI

Dr. Paul Cutler says that recent research links the *Helicobacter pylori*bacterium to high incidences of heart attacks and strokes. "*Helicobacter pylori* causes ulcers and chronic gastritis. Most practitioners are well aware of the higher incidence of stomach complaints in patients with heart disease. Apparently, this little bacterium, which comes from contaminated foods, burrows its way into the stomach wall. In its attempt to fight off the body's defenses, it produces toxins that initiate plaque development and thickening of the blood. This points to a strong correlation between stomach ulcer disease and coronary artery disease."

Fortunately, this problem is simple to cure, says Dr. Cutler: "You can use one particular type of honey that is high in hydrogen peroxide or cider vinegar, bismuth, and extracts from licorice. Or you can take a one-week course of three antibiotics to kill this bacteria, probably 97 percent of the time. It is very gratifying as a physician to see not only stomach symptoms but angina improve, sometimes dramatically, with the treatment of this common bacterial parasite."

HOMEOPATHY

Dr. Ken Korins explains how his specialty, homeopathy, seems to get results with heart disease: "Homeopathy works by giving very small doses that are extremely individualized to the person's symptoms and physical state. These doses work by means of a type of vibration or energy that stimulates the body much as acupuncture does."

Many traditional practitioners dismiss homeopathy due to a colossal ignorance of the evidence. These physicians say this therapy has never been proved by randomized, double-blind studies in the way more scientific procedures have been. Dr. Korins argues that is absolutely incorrect. He tells us that a 1991 *British Medical Journal* article by Kleijnen reviewed 107 clinical studies of homeopathy. About 80 percent of them found that homeopathy had positive effects. Many of these were extremely rigorous studies. A double-blind study in the *Journal of Pediatrics,* for example, showed extraordinary results from homeopathy.

What kinds of heart problems improve with homeopathy? Hypertension is one. Homeopathy can also help people recovering from congestive heart failure, cerebrovascular accidents, arteriosclerotic heart disease and a very wide range of other conditions.

In classical homeopathy, the specialist selects a single remedy. Korins elaborates: "We don't rely on a lot of tests and the high technology that goes with them. We prefer to look at what symptoms a person has and how they present themselves. For example, if a person is having angina, tightness, a squeezing sensation, a remedy such as songea or cactus, which is extremely effective in treating angina, is called for. Sometimes there is a congestion in the head, a hot feeling when the blood pressure goes up. The prescription there might be gloline.

QI (CHI) MANIPULATION

An Asian treatment that has some success with heart patients is the manipulation of *qi (chi)* energy. This term refers to all the nonliquid, biological energy that circulates through the body. Dr. Jeie Atacama, D.D.M., LaC., uses *qi* to accomplish healing. He estimates that in 20 years of practice he has helped between 3,000 and 5,000 people. Rebalancing *qi* energy can help greatly with heart disease by rebuilding the body's health and restoring its self-healing powers.

This practice works exactly like acupuncture. It does not use needles, but it shares with acupuncture a focus on the meridians of the body. In a technique he learned from his father, Dr. Atacama uses his fingers directly on the patient's skin. U points are found on either side near the base of the spine. One point is connected to the large intestine, which is part of the body system particularly in touch with the *qi* energy. The treatment session should be done three times a week for as many weeks as are called for by the condition. If the problem is cramps in the leg due to poor circulation, 10 sessions will get rid of the problem.

As Bill Moyers showed on his television reports on Asian philosophy, healing practices such as *tai chi* and *qi gong* depend on channeling internal *qi* energies to rebalance the body.

PSYCHOLOGICAL, SOCIAL, AND SPIRITUAL FACTORS

Most healing programs focus on physical modalities. We look at diet, exercise, supplements, and substances to avoid, but people are beginning to understand that more subtle factors have a powerful influence as well. Dr. Ron Scolastico, a spiritual counselor and author of *Healing the Heart, Healing the Body,* believes that the process of remaining healthy involves four important elements: "The first element is our physical life, which most people know a great deal about. The second element looks at our mental life. It is becoming clearer and clearer that our thoughts promote or hinder health and in some cases actually cause disease. The third element addresses our emotional lives. Feelings, particularly love, have a profound effect. The fourth element addresses spiritual factors. I believe those energies come from ther soul, which is an incredible source of power, love, and wisdom inside each of us."

Dr. Scolastico says we must draw on each of these factors as needed. Sometimes we must take physical steps such as seeing a doctor and taking medications or herbs, but sometimes that is not enough: "For example, one of my clients developed congestive heart failure after a painful divorce, along with pericarditis, which is an inflammation of the membrane surrounding the heart. She failed to respond to medical treatment, and her condition began to worsen. As I worked with her, she realized that she had lost touch with her soul. The divorce had wreaked such havoc in her emotional life that she could no longer feel love.

"Every day for six months she took an hour to connect with her soul. By doing this, she was able to regain a feeling of deep love for her body and herself. Today she is symptom-free and believes that without inner work she might be dead. So, many times, we need not only physical treatment but mental, emotional, or spiritual work to augment that process."

To promote health at every level, Dr. Scolastico advises the following:

Connect with your spiritual nature. Religious or not, we need to accept the existence of some benevolent, healing force larger than our personality and physical being. Once we realize we are never alone or abandoned, amazing changes can happen.

Be mindful of your thoughts. We all have negative thoughts, but this alone does not cause illness. Swallowing them and engaging them does. We must learn to release negative ideas. This work takes time, and we should not be hard on ourselves when our thoughts are less than perfect.

Follow the physical principles of health. Living in a healthy way includes eating the right foods, exercising, and getting enough rest, play, and social activity. Giving to others has a beneficial impact on health.

Create love in your life every day. This is perhaps the most important principle of all. Research shows that love affects every aspect of our beings, including the physical. When we feel love, all body systems work better. The endocrine system produces beneficial hormones. Muscles relax, so that the flow of oxygen to the cells increases. Immune system function is enhanced.

When we are filled with self-love, our health is strongest and our lives improve all around. Recent studies show that teaching self-esteem improves academic performance and promotes emotional stability and greater health.

"A powerful way to enhance self-love," advises Dr. Scolastico, "is to notice when you are creating negative thoughts and feelings about yourself. Then consciously create an experience of love for yourself right at that moment, using the power of the word to augment the process. You can say, 'I just noticed I'm creating these negative thoughts and feelings about myself. I now choose to use my imagination, my creativity, and my will to create an inner experience of love for myself right now, in this minute.'"

Another way to build love into our lives is to set aside time each day for building loving energy. Dr. Scolastico says, "For at least five minutes, use your mind, open your heart, and create love in your feelings. You can do that by imagining a person you love. Let your feelings for that person fill you as you bring that loved one fully into your thoughts and feelings. Let the corners of your mouth lift up in a smile. Just let your heart swell with love. You won't need a scientific test to prove the benefits."

Equal in importance to self-love is the love we share with others. Connecting with family, friends, and community gives us a sense of belonging that is invaluable to our well-being. Recently, a link between social bonds and heart health was reported in *Natural Health*. The magazine summarized 30 years of research on the town of Rosetto, Pennsylvania, and concluded that the most important risk factor for heart disease is a lack of community and intimate relationships. In this town, people lived in three-generation households with grandparents, parents, and children. There was a lot of interaction among families and much participation in community organizations. The incidence of heart disease was virtually nil even though residents ate high-fat diets and did not go out of their way to exercise. In fact, there was less coronary heart disease in Rosetto than in any other population in the United States.

HERBAL PHARMACY

Plants containing phytochemicals with antihypertensive properties, in order of potency, include the following:

Viola tricolor hortensis (pansy)
Sophora japonica (Japanese pagoda tree), bud/flower
Oenothera biennis (evening primrose)
Lactuca sativa (lettuce)
Cichorium endivia (endive)
Vigna mungo (blackgram)
Chenopodium album (lamb's-quarters)
Raphanus sativus (radish)
Portulaca oleracea (purslane)
Brassica pekinensis (Chinese cabbage)
Avena sativa (oats)
Amaranthus sp. (pigweed)
Chrysanthemum coronarium (garland chrysanthemum)
Anethum graveolens (dill)
Taraxacum officinale (dandelion)
Spinacia oleracea (spinach)
Cucumis sativus (cucumber)
Brassica chinensis (Chinese cabbage)
Allium cepa (onion)

Plants containing phytochemicals with antiarteriosclerotic properties, in order of potency, include the following:

Cucumis melo (cantaloupe), cotyledon
Juglans regia (English walnut)
Persea americana (avocado)
Cucumis sativus (cucumber)
Carthamus tinctorius (safflower)
Prunus armeniaca (apricot)
Papaver bracteatum (great scarlet poppy)
Helianthus annuus (sunflower)
Juglans cinerea (butternut)
Lagenaria siceraria (calabash gourd)
Bertholletia excelsa (Brazil nut)
Papaver somniferum (opium poppy)
Sesamum indicum (sesame)
Pinus edulis (pinyon pine)
Cannabis sativa (marijuana)
Cucumis melo (cantaloupe), seed
Cucurbita foetidissima (buffalo gourd)
Nigella sativa (black cumin)
Oenothera biennis (evening primrose)
Pinus gerardiana (chilgoza pine)

Plants containing phytochemicals with anticardiospasmic properties, in order of potency, include the following:

Theobroma bicolor (Nicaraguan cacao)
Cimicifuga racemosa (black cohosh)
Spirulina pratensis (spirulina)
Gentiana lutea (yellow gentian)
Ephedra sinica (ma huang)
Phaseolus vulgaris (black bean)
Vigna unguiculata (cowpea)
Aegle marmelos (bael de India)
Asparagus officinalis (asparagus)
Theombroma speciosum (macambo)
Helianthus annuus (sunflower)
Capsella bursa-pastoris (shepherd's purse)
Abelmoschus esculentus (okra)
Malva sylvestris (high mallow)
Agathosma betulina (buchu)
Sonchus oleraceus (cerraja)
Nasturtium officinale (berro)

Durio zibethinus (durian)
Arachis hypogaea (peanut)

Plants containing phytochemicals with antiarrhythmic properties, in order of potency, include the following:

Lactuca sativa (lettuce)
Portulaca oleracea (purslane)
Coptis chinensis (Chinese goldthread)
Cichorium endivia (endive)
Avena sativa (oats)
Vigna mungo (black gram)
Raphanus sativus (radish)
Chenopodium album (lamb's-quarters)
Brassica pekinensis (Chinese cabbage)
Anethum graveolens (dill)
Amaranthus sp. (pigweed)
Spinacia oleracea (spinach)
Cucumis sativus (cucumber)
Coptis japonica (huang lia)
Chrysanthemum coronarium (garland chrysanthemum)
Taraxacum officinale (dandelion)
Phaseolus vulgaris (black bean)
Strophathus gratus (quabain)
Brassica chinensis (Chinese cabbage)

Plants containing phytochemicals with antianginal properties, in order of potency, include the following:

Catharanthus lanceus (lanceleaf periwinkle)
Carya glabra (pignut hickory)
Carya ovata (shagbark hickory)
Chondrus crispus (Irish moss)
Portulaca oleracea (purslane)
Phaseolus vulgaris (black bean)
Papaver somniferum (opium poppy)
Avena sativa (oats)
Vigna unguiculata (cowpea)
Spinacia oleracea (spinach)
Tephrosia purpurea (purple tephrosia)
Ammi visnaga (visnaga)
Trichosanthus anguina (snakegourd)
Glycyrrhiza glabra (licorice)

Prunus serotina (black cherry)
Nyssa sylvatica (black gum)
Juniperus virginiana (red cedar)
Rhizophora mangle (red mangrove)
Symphoricarpos orbiculatus (buckbush)

Plants containing phytochemicals with anti-ischemic properties, in order of potency, include the following:

Portulaca oleracea (purslane)
Ipomoea aquatica (swamp cabbage)
Panicum maximum (guinea grass)
Viola tricolor hortensis (pansy)
Moringa oleifera (ben nut)
Asparagus officinalis (asparagus)
Elaeagnus angustifolia (Russian olive)
Frangula alnus (buckthorn)
Ipomoea batatas (sweet potato leaf)
Bertholletia excelsa (Brazil nut)
Ribes uva-crispa (gooseberry)
Linum usitatissimum (flax)
Fagopyrum esculentum (buckwheat)
Ipomoea batatas (sweet potato root)
Capsicum annuum (bell pepper)
Capsicum frutescens (cayenne)
Pisum sativum (pea)
Lens culinaris (lentil)

Plant containing anti-infarctal phytochemicals include *Jateorhiza palmata* (calumba), root.

Full Alternative Therapy Programs

DEAN ORNISH'S PROGRAM FOR REVERSING HEART DISEASE

The Ornish Program at Beth Israel, which opened in 1993, has four components:
1. Moderate, supervised exercise.
2. Stress management, involving stretching exercises, some yoga poses, and the teaching of relaxation and meditation techniques.
3. Low-fat, vegetarian diet with no animal products and no added fats.
4. Group support sessions where patients meet to learn more about their problems and act to express themselves.

The main focus of the program is to modify risk factors known to increase the dangers of coronary disease. It is not that different from a general medical program. The goals are to reduce weight, lower cholesterol and blood pressure, control diabetes, stop smoking, and control stress.

In a 1989 study reported in the British medical journal *Lancet,* two groups of heart patients were followed. One group adhered to the Ornish guidelines, and the other took the regular medical treatment for coronary disease. One year after starting the Ornish program, there was a reversal (improvement) of the coronary artery disorder as measured by an angiogram. In a follow-up study of the same group five years into the program, a PET (positron emission tomography) scan (then a state-of-the-art procedure) demonstrated that there was still a significant improvement in blood flow to the heart. This follow-up study was published in September 1995 in the *Journal of the American Medical Association* (JAMA).

"One thing we emphasize to patients who enter this program," Deborah Matra, R.N., says, "is that they need to regard what is required as a prescription from their doctor. They need to stick with the diet and exercise, do the stress management routine daily, stay with it as they would honor a doctor's prescription."

THE HEALING CENTER:
INTRAVENOUS VITAMIN AND OZONE THERAPY

We have been led to believe that genetics plays a primary role in all diseases, and it probably does in many. We must see, however, the connected symptoms. We must see that diet and lifestyle play an enormous role, far more than genetics, though genetics is a contributing factor. The Healing Center, in New York City, takes a holistic approach to healing. They use state-of-the-art, even avant-garde, techniques—vitamin C drips, dietary counseling, acupuncture, massage therapies, chelation, and body therapy—and they have had magnificent results.

One patient, John, talks about his experience: "I'd say that I'm 95 percent responsible for my ill condition, out of sheer laziness and neglect. I weigh about 600 pounds, and I realize I am apt to get various diseases because of my weight. I have already suffered some: high blood pressure, fatigue, severe viral and bacterial problems, and edema of the right leg that causes cramps. I have trouble flexing the joints."

In the African-American community to which John belongs, there is, unfortunately, a high incidence of death from coronary heart disease and far too many cases of high blood pressure. John notes that much of his disease arose from faulty lifestyle habits: growing up eating too much fat and a lot of meat and drinking alcoholic beverages, all of which undermine health.

Dr. Howard Robins described his work when he was at the Healing Center. "We try," he said, "to let the body heal itself from all its injuries and weaknesses. We do not focus on one illness, but on the body as a whole. This is how holistic medicine was originally formulated

"We have a medical doctor who assumes charge of the patient's medical condition, a homeopathic practitioner; a nutritionist who does extensive nutritional counseling with each patient on vitamins, herbs, and minerals; an acupuncturist who also prescribes Chinese herbal remedies to strengthen a weak organ system; and a dentist who removes mercury amalgam fillings, which cause fatigue and weaken the immune system. We also have a chiropractor who rebalances the back structure to create better innervations so the nervous system won't misfire and damage the organ system. Since all the body's systems are interconnected, we need to put everything back in order."

Dr. Robins's particular specialty was intravenous vitamin C and ozone therapy. He explained that in vitamin C therapy a person is built up very rapidly to large doses, to the 100,000-mg range and eventually to the 200,000-mg range. High levels of vitamin C cleanse the artery walls of calcified fatty plaques. The program also added EDTA in the drip, which melts the calcium bonds to the walls so the plaque is freed and the EDTA and vitaminC can wash it out of the body. Then the solution cleanses and heals the scars left by the low-density lipoproteins, healing the walls so that plaque will no longer adhere to them.

In ozone therapy—called major autohemotherapy—about 300 cc, or 10 oz, of blood is drawn and an oxygen-ozone combination is mixed into it. The blood is then infused right back in, which takes about 30 minutes. The ozone helps oxidize fatty plaques, in a sense liquefying them and removing them from the walls, while making the red blood cells more flexible so that they can slip through the clogged arteries. This last measure is very important in preventing the need for bypass surgery and getting rid of angina pain.

Dr. Robins traced ozone therapy back to World War I. It was found that men who had been burned by mustard gas, injured, or shot and were kept in the back of the hospital tent, where the electric generators for the field lights were, were getting well. Eventually, doctors realized that the cause of the improvement was the ozone gas created by leakage from the generators. That began the work on ozone as a means to heal and prevent the amputation of limbs that had developed gangrene. "We've seen some miraculous results of ozone therapy at the Healing Center, for it's one thing that really does work."

DR. JULIAN WHITAKER: NUTRITION AND EDUCATION ARE KEY

Dr. Julian Whitaker was on the medical staff at the Pritikin Center. Nathan Pritikin helped millions of people by prescribing a diet that eliminates refined carbohydrates and animal fats and putting patients on a strict but moderate exercise regimen. In 1979, Dr. Whitaker went on to found the Whitaker Wellness Center in Newport Beach, California. He has expanded the Pritikin program, adding special vitamin supplements and eliminating most, if not all, animal protein from the prescribed diet.

Dr. Whitaker runs an intensive five-day nutritional and educational clinic designed to teach people dietary and exercise guidelines that can help them prevent or overcome heart disease. Many patients attend the clinic as an alternative to major surgical procedures and/or drug therapy. They are frequently able to avoid these invasive and toxic treatments; more important, in the long run they establish or regain a healthful lifestyle and vitality that they had assumed was beyond their grasp.

Dr. Whitaker's treatment is as much a matter of education as of actual therapeutic intervention. Patients learn what they can do about their conditions so that the responsibility becomes theirs. Once patients understand how nutrition, vitamin supplementation, and exercise can help stop and even reverse most heart conditions and cardiovascular diseases, they must be resolute in applying this knowledge to their own lifestyles. They make these changes a routine part of each day.

"Heart disease," Dr. Whitaker states, "is not really as much a disease of the heart as it is a disease of the artery." The arteries carry blood to the heart at a uniform rate of flow, and if that flow is interfered with—speeded up or slowed down—the heart must adjust its activity to compensate for the change. If the arteries become clogged, the blood supply to the heart may be insufficient to the point where "the heart muscle begins to die in sections. These are what we call heart attacks, when a section of the heart muscle does not receive enough oxygen and simply dies."

It is important to understand that the heart itself usually remains healthy until the arteries are damaged. If the arteries become too rigid or are obstructed by clots and occlusions, they are not able to get the blood supply to and from the heart at a steady, healthy rate. "Heart disease" patients must be taught first and foremost how to repair and maintain the cardiovascular system in general rather than the heart specifically.

THE PROGRAM

Dr. Whitaker considers the three major risk factors to be elevated cholesterol levels, elevated blood pressure, and cigarette smoking. Other high-risk factors he looks for are obesity, diabetes, and lack of exercise. These too are important but are not as strong or as predictive as the other three."

Once patients understand the basic causes of their problems, the Newport Beach Program is geared to teach them how to deal constructively with the situation. Naturally, patients who smoke must give up the habit. Then they learn how to structure a diet that will attack the root causes of the disease as well as the symptoms. While surgical and drug remedies may relieve symptoms temporarily, they do not deal directly with the underlying causes of disease and rarely effect an actual cure or reversal of the dysfunction. Dealing effectively with the actual disorders leads ultimately to the disappearance of symptoms. This can be very exciting if you are one of the millions of people who have long suffered from cardiovascular problems that traditional physicians consider insurmountable without radical and invasive intervention.

ELIMINATING ANIMAL PROTEINS

Early on, Dr. Whitaker's patients are taught about reducing fats in their diets. Dairy products and processed meat are the chief culprits here. Eggs especially should be avoided by those with heart and cardiovascular diseases. Just like meat, eggs are directly related to elevated cholesterol levels, leading to damage and corrosion of the epithelial tissue lining the arterial walls.

"In the blood," Dr. Whitaker explains, "fat tends to coat the red blood cells with a fatty layer. "This causes a reduction in the electromagnetic charge of the blood cell. All our blood cells have to carry oxygen through the capillaries. To get through the capillaries, these blood cells have to go single file, because the capillary is about 7 microns—about 1/10,000 of an inch—in diameter, and the red blood cell is about the same size. You cannot force four or five blood cells through the capillary at the same time; that would be like trying to get seven people to go through a single doorway. When you eat fat, it causes these blood cells to clump together. When they get to the doorway of the capillary system, they can't go through. Many researchers have measured the actual oxygen uptake of heart muscle before and after a fatty meal. They have documented that there is a 15 to 30 percent drop in oxygen utilization and oxygen availability to normal heart muscle after a fatty meal."

People who continue to consume meats, cheeses, eggs, and other animal proteins, says Dr. Whitaker, cannot seriously reduce their overall body fat. Strangely enough, even animal products such as yogurt that may have no fat or cholesterol trigger an internal reaction that treats them as if they did simply because they are animal products. Dr. Whitaker describes a patient who could not lower his cholesterol level even though he had eliminated all meat and dairy products from his diet for four years. It was determined than his daily nonfat, cholesterol-free yogurt was the culprit. The reason for this phenomenon is unclear, but when you are suffering from heart disease, you are not as concerned about reasons as you are about results.

Dr. Whitaker estimates that by getting away from animal proteins, "you shift from 49 percent fat down to around 15 percent fat, and you shift your carbohydrates from 40 percent on the American diet up to maybe 65 to 75 percent. This will dramatically lower blood cholesterol if the shift is made accurately. The drop in the cholesterol level should be anywhere between 15 and 30 percent. It will also aid in weight loss, triglyceride control, and blood pressure control."

One can effectively reduce the intake of animal proteins by adding more carbohydrates to the diet. Dr. Whitaker explains that with animal proteins, which have only two sources of calories—fats and proteins—it is still necessary to add carbohydrates for a balanced diet. However, carbohydrates contain all three caloric sources—fats, proteins, and carbohydrates—and therefore can replace animal proteins. Instead of bacon and eggs, you might have a whole-grain cereal or bread with fruit. Pasta and rice and bean dishes such as bean tacos and burritos along with vegetables and a high-fiber salad with plenty of calcium-rich dark greens constitute a fine substitute for the standard meat and potatoes. There's nothing wrong with potatoes in and of themselves, but by the time they are smothered with butter, sour cream, and ketchup, they become fatty and high in cholesterol.

By turning away from meat and dairy products while increasing the proportion of fruits, vegetables, legumes, grains, breads, cereals, and pastas, heart disease patients replace high-fat, high-cholesterol foods with high-fiber, powerhouse-type foods. This switch lowers the patient's blood cholesterol levels, while the additional fiber will help clean out whatever fat and cholesterol are already clogging the system. Even foods containing significant amounts of fat, such as nuts and oils, can be used in moderation.

Olive oil, a monosaturated fat, "seems to be less deleterious to the system," Dr. Whitaker states, "than some of the polyunsaturated fats, such as corn oil and sunflower oil, which are common in our food processing. Greeks and Italians, who eat substantial amounts of olive oil, have been found to be in better health than, for example, Israelis, who eat a substantial amount of corn oil and sunflower oil."

In the case of nuts, some are better to consume than others. Walnuts, for example, have substantial amounts of omega-3 fatty acids, which are very beneficial for cardiovascular health. Peanuts, however, may contribute to sluggish blood flow related to serum cholesterol levels; they can be more harmful than even butter, a well-known villain. This information comes from rabbit studies conducted by Dr. Julian Whistler at the University of Chicago.

ESTABLISHING HEALTHY HABITS

Besides the quality of the fats heart patients consume, it is crucial for them to reduce the overall quantity of fats. Dr. Whitaker insists that "you need to reduce the fat intake by about 50 percent of what the American population is eating now to be at what I consider to be the upper limit of fat intake."

One reason why many people do not change their lifestyles sufficiently to establish good health is that they are encouraged by their doctors to maintain the average range of white blood cells, cholesterol, and triglycerides. Dr. Whitaker believes that his patients deserve better than this. He tries to get them to stablish healthy, not just average, levels of these heart disease culprits. They do this through exercise and socializing, proper vitamin and mineral regimens, and the reduction of animal fats in the diet, replacing them with complex carbohydrates.

CARBOHYDRATES

Carbohydrates are preferred to fats because they do not have the high cholesterol levels that fats have and do not deposit sludge in the arteries, interfere with normal blood flow, or damage the inner arterial walls. Carbohydrates are high in fiber, vitamins, and minerals, all of which promote overall cardiovascular health. They also do not convert into fat very readily, although many people believe, partly because of misinformation from the scientific community, that carbohydrates are fattening.

Dr. Whitaker explains: "It is very difficult for carbohydrates to actually put fat weight into your system; some studies have shown that carbohydrates are not converted into fat nearly as rapidly or as efficiently as many scientists used to think. The conversion of carbohydrates into fat takes more energy than is actually present in the carbohydrate molecule trying to be converted, so the body just doesn't do it. The primary thing that really deposits fat into fat is fat itself. Often, when people add carbohydrates to their diet, they add them to an already increased fat diet. Generally, when I put people on an increased carbohydrate diet, they will almost always lose weight, and they will call begging me to give them something to stop the weight loss if they are truly following a 70 to 75 percent carbohydrate diet. Believe it or not, the high-carbohydrate diet we use causes a weight loss that creates a problem."

It should be made clear that Dr. Whitaker does not recommend an increased intake of all carbohydrates. A lot of carbohydrates, particularly simple and processed carbohydrates, are nothing but junk food. Processing breaks down their fibrous cellular structures and robs them of much or most of their vitamin and mineral content. Cakes, jams, sugared fruit juices, baked goods, highly processed breads, and bleached flours and flour products are examples. Often the only thing left in these foods is sugar. The carbohydrates espoused in Dr. Whitaker's program are unprocessed, unrefined, and wholesome complex carbohydrates such as whole grains and fresh fruits.

VITAMIN AND MINERAL SUPPLEMENTS

Vitamin and mineral supplementation is another significant part of Dr. Whitaker's program. Vitamins A, B_6, C, and E are especially important, along with the minerals selenium, calcium, magnesium, and chromium.

Between 25 and 50 mg of vitamin B_6 may be used. Some B vitamins, such as niacin, are used in large doses much as a drug is used. "If there is an elevated cholesterol and triglyceride level which doesn't respond adequately to our diet," Dr. Whitaker explains, "we will use niacin at a rate of 500 to 700 mg per meal." This is strictly a therapeutic dose and should be used only in conjunction with a physician's prescribed treatment.

Vitamin C is of particular significance in maintaining the sound structure of arterial walls since it promotes strong, healthy connective tissues. Dr. Whitaker cites a Canadian study in which guinea pigs (which were used because they, like humans, do not manufacture vitamin C) were deprived of vitamin C: "Their arteries began to corrode because the connective tissue inside the artery gave way, allowing cholesterol to go into the system."

When vitamin C was restored to the guinea pigs' diet, arterial damage not only slowed but began to reverse. Evidence such as this has convinced Dr. Whitaker that vitamin C plays a critical role in cardiovascular health. "In my opinion," he says, "early on the most important vitamin, if there is a single one, would be vitamin C."

It is especially important that the patient's blood remain thin and free-flowing, and this is where vitamin E plays a role in Dr. Whitaker's treatment. Vitamin E is an anticoagulant that keeps blood platelets from clumping together so that they can pass easily through narrow openings and small cap-illaries. It is also an antioxidant, protecting the arterial cells from damage from free radicals.

Dr. Whitaker also uses MaxEPA, a blood thinner and anticoagulant that acts somewhat like vitamin E. MaxEPA, he says, "is beneficial to a patient who has an elevated level of triglycerides plus elevated cholesterol. We use large doses of it at that stage. We will use large amounts per meal to drop the triglyc-eride and cholesterol level." He goes on to note that MaxEPA is ineffective in lowering cholesterol levels when very low levels of triglycerides are present. Dr. Whitaker warns that MaxEPA alone is not a "panacea for lowering the choles-terol," as some sponsors have made it out to be, but is very effective when inte-grated with an overall treatment program.

Mineral supplementation is equally important. Magnesium has been found to be deficient among heart patients, up to 50 percent lower than in noncardiac patients studied recently at the University of California. To restore the mineral to acceptable levels, Dr. Whitaker uses injectable magnesium for angina patients. Diuretics, which are commonly prescribed to lower blood pressure in patients with cardiovascular disorders, deplete magnesium as well as potassi-um. While most physicians are careful to replace the potassium lost during diuretic treatment, few replace the magnesium. This can cause further compli-cations, especially since the loss of magnesium affects serum calcium levels. This is part of the reason Dr. Whitaker believes that "diuretics, and the way they are currently used, are making a lot of people worse instead of better."

WHY CONVENTIONAL THERAPIES ARE NOT THE ANSWER

Dr. Whitaker believes that technology has been confused with science. Just because it is possible to do a coronary bypass or angioplasty does not neces-sarily mean that it always makes sense to undertake it. Bypass surgery involves severing the artery before the blockage and rerouting the blood flow through an unblocked blood vessel taken from the leg. "It has been conclusively demonstrated," he states, "that bypass surgery fails to reduce mortality rates for 75 percent of heart patients who undergo the procedure." While failing to cure many heart disease victims, such surgery frequently puts the patient at needless risk, with 0.3 to 6.6 percent of such patients dying after the surgery. Still, Americans spend between $2 billion and $3 billion a year on coronary bypasses.

Similarly, catheterization has an insufficient scientific basis in Dr. Whitaker's opinion, yet thousands of catheterizations are done almost routinely. Catheterizations are used to detect arterial blockages and open them up, often in conjunction with a balloon angioplasty or a bypass. Angioplasty, a procedure in which a catheter is snaked through the arteries to open up blockages, has been hailed as a great technological feat. However, it has a death rate of 3.5 percent and a conversion to bypass rate of 15 percent, and the whole procedure must be repeated in more than one in three cases because it does not work the first time.

An obvious problem with this routine approach to dealing with heart disease is that the catheterization itself—sticking a catheter inside the heart—can cause harm. To perform this exploration without good reason is dangerous, yet it is commonly done to patients who do not have life-threatening conditions and frequently don't even suffer from chest pain.

Moreover, the results of catheterization are not dependable. Dr. Whitaker explains: "Studies were done comparing the blockages found in patients who had been recently catheterized and had died from some other cause, and they did an autopsy within 30 days of the catheterization. When they looked at the arteries at the autopsy and looked at the angiogram picture and the way it was read, they found very little correlation. Even more alarming is the fact that different doctors viewing the same catheterization had different opinions concerning the exact location of the blockage. Studies at the University of Iowa showed that blood flow measurements taken during surgery were quite different from what had been indicated by the angiogram."

WHY DR. WHITAKER'S PROGRAM WORKS

The success of Dr. Whitaker's lifestyle approach indicates that the healing power that comes from rebalancing one's mind and body has been vastly underestimated. Surgery and medication cannot slow the progression of arteriosclerosis, for instance, but basic lifestyle changes can accomplish this quickly and dramatically. Lifestyle changes address the cause of heart disease and allow the body to heal itself when given the proper tools and directed by a disciplined, discriminating, and essentially positive attitude.

DR. JOHN MCDOUGAL: FOOD IS THE BEST MEDICINE

Dr. John McDougall, unlike many physicians in the preventive health care field, practices what he preaches: vegetarianism. He feels that food is the best medicine; traditional therapies may be introduced in crisis situations, but the body benefits most from the restoration of normal biochemical balance. The standard American diet, he feels, has lost its ability to maintain that balance. A natural diet, free of animal protein and consisting of small amounts of food eaten many times a day, can help restore it. His vegetarian diet helps not only people with heart disease but those who suffer from cancer, arthritis, and obesity.

Today, the American Heart Association, the National Institutes of Health, and other well-established organizations are recommending moderate changes in the way people eat. Unfortunately, this so-called prudent diet does not fully address the underlying issue. If people are consuming foods or engaging in lifestyles that cause disease, suggesting that moderation be exercised is like suggesting that they try to get moderately better. To achieve more than "moderate" health, people must do something more pronounced than making token gestures: They must make drastic changes in diet and lifestyle.

DRASTIC CHANGES IN DIET AND LIFESTYLE

Dr. McDougall, author of *The McDougall Program: Twelve Days to Dynamic Health,* believes that the American public needs to be informed about the best diet available, not just a moderate or prudent one. The reasons many physicians suggest only minimal changes in the diets of heart disease patients is that they, like their patients, do not know what the best diet is. Since nutrition has been given so little attention in medical school curricula, few doctors know how to prescribe diets appropriate for specific conditions. They tell their patients to cut down a little on fat, add a bit of fiber, and so forth, but patients with heart disease have their lives on the line and need much more informed direction.

DIETARY HISTORIES

Dr. McDougall began taking dietary histories of his patients to see if he could get some clues to helping patients who were not being healed by the traditional treatments. He took dietary histories of every one of his patients for the next three years and was amazed by what he found.

Practicing in rural Hawaii, he had a unique opportunity to study an isolated group of sugarcane plantation workers through several generations. The first, older generation was made up of Japanese, Chinese, and Filipinos who had come to Hawaii in their teens or early childhood. Their children, grandchildren, and great-grandchildren were natives of Hawaii and had a very different background in terms of lifestyle and diet.

The members of the older generation possessed far superior health to that of the second, third, and fourth generations despite all having been in the same location and the same industry for years. The members of the first generation were trim and hardy, still vital and vigorous even in old age. The younger generations, by contrast, were commonly obese or at least overweight, plagued with diseases that Dr. McDougall had been taught were primarily genetic: diabetes, colon cancer, heart disease, and high blood pressure.

Clearly, genetics was not the issue here. The only variable Dr. McDougall could clearly establish was dietary history. The members of the older generation were primarily vegetarians, consuming very few high-fat, high-cholesterol animal products such as eggs, cheese, and milk and instead eating most-ly rice and vegetables. The younger generations, raised in Hawaii instead of Asia, had become accustomed to the American diet of animal products and meats, highly refined and processed foods rather than whole foods, and sugar- and salt-laden snacks. Dr. McDougall came to realize that diet is a far greater factor in the incidence of degenerative disease than he and others in his field had been led to believe.

He also noted that, in a broader perspective, throughout history it has always been those in the upper, rich, privileged classes who have been plagued by the degenerative diseases. The royalty of past centuries were the people who had the means to enjoy rich diets replete with fats, including dairy and meat products. The feast was a routine part of their privileged life, and glutto-nous eating was a major source of socialization and entertainment. The poor peasants who tilled the earth from sunup to sunset could afford to eat only what they themselves grew—grains, vegetables and potatoes—a simple diet high in starch, complex carbohydrates, and fiber. This "poor man's diet" was largely responsible for the fact that the peasantry rarely suffered the degener-ative diseases so common among the elite: heart disease, diabetes, gout, and the like. The diet rich in saturated fats, cholesterol, and salt might have been fit for a king, but it certainly did not keep the king fit.

Dr. McDougall also pondered the fact that for hundreds and even thou-sands of years the general populace had not depended on high-protein foods such as meat and dairy products for their daily nutritional needs. In New Guinea and South America whole civilizations revolved around sweet pota-toes; the Indians of North America were hunters for whom meat was only an occasional treat, the main diet being primarily corn-based. For Asians, to this day, rice has been central. Europeans originally ate high concentrations of grains, breads, and, later, potatoes. Africans consumed mostly grains and beans. In Mexico and Central America, rice, corn, and beans provided the main sustenance. In the Middle East, wheat, sesame seeds, and chickpeas have been the traditional mainstays of the diet. Even today in many of these parts of the world meat is consumed infrequently.

We find almost invariably that among cultures and civilizations in which starch forms the basis of the diet, there is a very low incidence of obesity, high blood pressure, and heart disease. Dr. McDougall recalls that one of his professors could remember a time when heart failure—that is, a heart attack—was a "curious disease" in Hong Kong. People would gather around the victim to witness this rare affliction. That was 33 years ago, and since the diet in Hong Kong has been westernized, the occurrence of heart attacks has risen sharply.

Wherever the traditional high-starch, high-carbohydrate diet is main-tained, one finds stronger, trimmer, healthier people. On mainland China, for instance, where the traditional rice and soybean diet is still very much a part of the culture, there is little degenerative disease. One seldom sees an over-weight Chinese person. That same trim person with a strong heart and healthy cardiovascular system would quickly become obese, atherosclerotic, and hypertense if he or she came to the United States and adopted western ways of eating. Heart disease is not the only disorder resulting from the Western diet. In Japan, following World War I, there were only 78 cases of prostate cancer among the entire population. In the United States today, there are thousands of prostate cancer cases every year. The incidence of breast cancer is far high-er in the United States than it is in places that still adhere to starch-based diets, such as China and Japan.

WHAT IS THE BEST DIET?

As Dr. McDougall discovered in his research, the best diet is one based on high-starch, complex carbohydrate foods with a high fiber content. This includes whole grains, legumes, fruits, and vegetables. The worst diet consists of high-fat "delicacies," or what Dr. McDougall calls the feast foods, basically animal protein: milk, eggs, cheese, beef, pork, poultry, and even chocolate. Americans' declining health is directly correlated with the rising consumption of these foods.

FOCUS ON COMPLEX CARBOHYDRATES

Dr. McDougall works at getting his patients off diets high in cholesterol, fat, and salt and onto diets high in fiber and starch. His complex carbohydrate diet is preferable for several reasons. For one thing, it fills the stomach with much less food more quickly. Although people eat partly to fill the stomach—to feel satisfied and relieve the pangs of hunger—for many people this is the sole con-sideration in establishing eating patterns. However, it is important to realize that all foods are not equal in the way they fill people up.

Carbohydrates provide what are called low-density foods. Fats are high-density foods. The higher the density of a food is, the less bulk it has. The less bulk there is, the more that must be consumed to fill the stomach. If you eat a small portion of low-density, high-bulk foods, you will feel just as sat-isfied as you would after consuming the same size portion of high-density, low-bulk foods, usually from the meat and dairy groups. Thus, you eat fewer calories to feel just as full as you would from eating far more eggs, meat, and cheese.

It is easy to see why people who eat primarily meat and dairy items are more likely to become obese. Consequently, Dr. McDougall's patients will lose 6 to 15 pounds a month eating as often as they want to by eating only the low-density starches and none of the high-density fats. They are encouraged to enjoy eating and not be afraid of it, as are so many overweight and obese people. The patients' top priority is to choose the proper types of foods.

THE PROBLEM WITH FATS

Another reason Dr. McDougall's patients are taken off fats is that fats are a chief cause of coronary artery problems. This is because fats are a fuel; they are stored energy. The body can synthesize fats; they are part of the cellular structure and are found in people's hormones, enzymes, and brains.

Essential fats are those which must be obtained through diet because the body does not produce them. The primary source of these essential fats is plants. They also come from meat, but meat is only a secondary source. The animal from which the meat or dairy product is obtained has the essential fats because it ate plants containing them. People can choose to bypass the animal altogether and go directly to fat sources in the form of vegetables, grains, and legumes to fulfill the essential fat requirements. If you choose to eat meat, however, you are getting a highly saturated fat that is far rougher on the cardiovascular system than are the polyunsaturated plant fats.

One of the first effects of fat in the system is to make people obese. This is why half the people in the United States are overweight and the other half are on diets and exercise programs to avoid becoming overweight. This obsession with obesity would be entirely unnecessary if people restructured their eating habits and lifestyles. People living in central New Guinea, Japan, and other places where the inhabitants primarily eat plant foods and wholesome, unprocessed carbohydrates are not concerned about their weight even though eating plays a key role in their cultures. They don't need to be, because the cause of obesity does not exist for them.

Fat makes people obese because it is easily transported to body fat tissue once it has been consumed. Carbohydrates, in contrast, become stored energy in the form of glycogen in the muscles and liver. Only with great difficulty does the body convert carbohydrates into fat. In victims of heart and artery disease, fat, especially animal fat, plays a sinister role by causing a sharp rise in cholesterol. The presence of excess amounts of cholesterol in the blood damages the inner walls of the arteries. The high level of cholesterol in the American diet is directly related to the epidemic of heart disease that people in this country now face.

Many cardiologists tell their patients to eat white meat instead of red meat, but Dr. McDougall points out that this will not reduce fat and cholesterol levels significantly. Beef may be 70 percent fat, but chicken is 40 to 50 percent fat. While eating chicken is an improvement, it will not reverse arterial blockage and heart conditions. If a patient is suffering from too much fat intake, why should that patient be told that it is all right to eat food that is one-third fat? Why not instead consume foods that range from 1 to 10 percent fat at the most? To get an idea of the relative fat contents of various foods, consider chocolate, a food with a 55 percent fat content, whole milk at 50 percent at solid matter, eggs at 65 percent, cheese between 70 and 90 percent, a "good steak" at 82 percent, and luncheon meats—cold cuts—up to 90 percent. Compare these high-density saturated fats with low-density, polyunsaturated vegetable fats such as the potato, with a meager 1 percent fat, rice at 5 percent, and fruits ranging from 2 to 10 percent fat. Realizing that these fruits and vegetables also contain high-quality fiber, which is essential to free-flowing blood and arterial health—something that is altogether lacking in meat and dairy items—it becomes clear that choosing complex carbohydrates over animal fats lays a solid foundation for recovery from heart disease. After all, the causes of the heart disease are being eliminated almost entirely from the diet.

While the fat content of white meat may be less than that of red meat, the cholesterol levels may actually be higher. While 3-oz servings of beef and pork have 85 mg and 90 mg of cholesterol, respectively, turkey has 83 mg and skinned white chicken has 85 mg. Patients told by their cardiologists to switch to fish may also be victims of misinformation, since some types of fish have as much cholesterol as meat and poultry do. Many people with coronary and/or vascular problems are deceived by inaccurate information into thinking they are choosing the best possible therapeutic diet when in fact they are not.

HOW THE PROGRAM WORKS

Dr. McDougall found the earliest recorded reference to this sort of healing approach in the Bible, in the book of Daniel. Daniel's men had become sick from eating rich foods, and rather than offer them a magical cure or secret medicinal concoction, he had them ingest only vegetables and water. This high-starch, high-fiber diet helped them regain their normal health in only 10 days. At Dr. McDougall's hospital, practically everyone in the program is able to get off drugs and experience drastically reduced cholesterol, triglyceride, and blood sugar levels in a mere 12 days, the duration of the program. Their diet is similar to the one Daniel's men were given over 2,500 years ago.

There is no quick cure, however. The disorders plaguing these patients have been arrested, but true reversal and restoration of coronary and arterial health take months to accomplish. The special diet used in the program is not a temporary one but must be continued for as long as the patient wishes to avoid reestablishing heart disease and vascular dysfunction. In other words, the new eating habits are not really a diet but, along with a structured and progressive exercise program, constitute a whole new lifestyle.

During Dr. McDougall's 12-day live-in program, people with heart disease are taught how to let go of their high-fat diets and how to choose and prepare high-quality complex carbohydrate meals that are high in starch and fiber. At breakfast, coffee, ham and eggs, and white buttered toast with sugar jam might be replaced by oatmeal with strawberries. A whole-grain bread without the fat-laden butter, maybe topped with a real fruit jam instead of sugary jam or jelly, might be paired with herbal tea or a hot beverage derived from grains rather than coffee beans.

Patients are taught to distinguish simple from complex carbohydrates. The simple sugars may be called glucose, fructose, maltose, or lactose: they are found in honey, corn syrup, milk, molasses, maple syrup, and fruit juices. They provide the body with quick-burning fuel which does little to sustain energy levels evenly or over an extended period of time. In a processed state, they do not even retain their fiber and nutrient values and become little more than highly concentrated sugars full of calories with little nutritional value. These types of carbohydrates should be avoided, but not as much as the fats and animal products.

Complex carbohydrates, in contrast, provide a very slow burning fuel that is stored in the muscles and provides a steady energy supply throughout the day. Potatoes, rice, and vegetables such as peas, corn, and asparagus contain ideal forms of carbohydrates.

Dr. McDougall offers a variety of suggestions regarding starch-based meal planning, preparation, and variation using a carbohydrate-centered diet: "The foods we suggest are corn, pasta, rice, most vegetables, grains, and all fiber-rich foods. For breakfast, you can have oatmeal or other hot whole-cereal meals, grains, waffles, and pancakes. For lunch, you can have all kinds of soups, such as lentil soup, bean soup, tomato soup, onion soup, or pea soup, as long as you make the soup yourself. Main entrees for dinner can be spaghetti with marinara sauce, curry vegetable stew, brown rice casseroles, baked potatoes, bean burritos without lard or oil, Indian curry dishes, and all kinds of Chinese and Japanese dishes. You can have all these foods as long as they are not processed in any way and are made fresh."

All the foods Dr. McDougall recommends are high in starch and fiber and have naturally balanced amounts of minerals, vitamins, and other nutrients. When these foods are eaten in the whole, natural state, they provide a highly nutritious source of calories and essential nutrients. They contribute to overall good health and optimal, easily maintained low body weight. People who adhere to these dietary changes have experienced great and rapid success. According to Dr. McDougall, during his patients' brief stay at the clinic, their "blood cholesterol drops an average of 28 points. Their triglycerides drop and blood sugars drop in a matter of four or five days. These people change from cardiac cripples who can't walk 15 or 30 feet to people who are walking three or four miles and exercising."

TREATING HIGH BLOOD PRESSURE

Besides the symptoms of their diseases, many people suffer greatly from the medications they take to treat those diseases. Dr. McDougall relates, "We take people who come in on medications for high blood pressure, and they just want to get off those medications because the side effects are so horrendous. They may even be on 10, 12, or 15 medications. It's rare that we can't get them off."

Here is an example of such a patient: "I had an accountant come into my office and state that he was on 20 drugs and wanted off them. Actually, he was on 12 high-blood-pressure pills, one diabetes pill, and several heart pills. After four days on a healthy diet consisting of no salt, low-fat, and no cholesterol, he was off all his medication; his blood sugar, which was 235, fell to 168; and his blood pressure, which started at 190/110, became 150/70."

High blood pressure is not in itself a disease. It is a condition or symptom which may accompany a more generalized disease state, specifically, heart and arterial disease. Blood pressure rises when arteries damaged by excessive dietary fat, oil, and cholesterol begin to close. Decreasing the area the blood can flow through is like putting your thumb over part of the opening of a garden hose: The pressure increases, and the water squirts farther. If you increase the amount of water flow at the same time—say, by turning the faucet on higher—the pressure becomes even greater and the water squirts farther still.

High blood pressure may also be caused by a combination of too much salt and too little potassium. Sodium attracts water, so the presence of salt draws even more fluid into the bloodstream and the pressure gets even greater. Processed foods usually have been stripped of potassium and have excess sodium as well. People eating these foods will therefore have low potassium levels.

To treat high blood pressure, the most obvious step is to clean out the arteries by eliminating fat, oil, and cholesterol ingestion. In other words, you take your thumb away from the hose nozzle and the pressure is reduced. Can you imagine leaving your thumb there while trying to reduce the pressure? You would be overlooking the obvious cause of the pressure buildup. Dr. McDougall says that this is exactly what happens in traditional treatments of high blood pressure: "We treat blood pressure," he says, "by lowering it, which makes as much sense as giving aspirin to someone with an infected toe. We've lowered the fever but have not cured the infection. When there is a sign that the blood vessel system is diseased, we use blood pressure pills to eliminate the sign, but the disease stays. What we should do is deal with the cause. So far only a half dozen people in our program have not been able to eliminate blood pressure medications. Over the last 10 years, I have treated over 7,000 people.

"Let me tell you about a minister at the church I've gone to for several years. This young man, who is only 32 years old, had blood pressure problems for 10 years and had been taking blood pressure pills for two years before I saw him. He was recently married and was having problems with sexual function. He was being treated by a doctor who gave him the standard line: 'You're on pills for high blood pressure; we don't know what causes the problem, and you'll be on them for the rest of your life with no chance of getting off them.' He finally decided to see me, and when he asked what could be done for him, I told him to stop taking the blood pressure pills and told him how to do this (he was taking the kind that can't be stopped immediately). He changed his diet. This was over a year ago, and his blood pressure went down from the high level of 160/95 to 110/70 in two to three weeks. He lost 30 extra pounds he'd been carrying around since his teenage years, and he's absolutely drug-free and feels wonderful. He still sees the doctor who told him he'd never get off blood pressure pills and gloats a bit as the doctor takes his blood pressure and finds it perfectly normal. The doctor's response to all of this is, 'It was a coincidence.'"

Dr. McDougall says that this sort of "coincidence" occurs in more than 90 percent of cases where patients have changed their diet dramatically. This occurs because his patients all make the required dietary changes. Frequently, people are not willing to make these changes. Probably the greatest obstacle to improving people's heart conditions once they have been taught how critical diet and exercise are is their reluctance to make such vast changes in their lifestyles.

DR. ERIC BRAVERMAN'S APPROACH TO HYPERTENSION

Dr. Eric Braverman has published over 60 papers in peer review journals and is the author of numerous books, including *Hypertension and Nutrition: The Amazing Way to Reverse Heart Disease Naturally*. Like Dr. McDougall, Dr. Braverman believes that a general wellness program that combines a proper diet, supplementation, and exercise is the best way to treat hypertension. The diet he recommends combines these elements with a special nutrient formula designed to lower high blood pressure and then help maintain good cardiovascular health.

Dr. Braverman believes that the primary cause of hypertension and heart disease is the accumulation of heavy metals such as lead, aluminum, and cadmium that produce arterial hardening as people age. With that hardening comes an increase in blood pressure because an aging body is no longer as flexible as it once was. This problem is compounded by the loss of estrogen, progesterone, testosterone and DHEA, depending on a person's sex, and the loss of growth hormone. According to Dr. Braverman, the danger of hypertension and heart disease begins at a blood pressure level that exceeds 120/80, and in some cases, the risk level may be 110/70.

Not surprisingly, the first step in Dr. Braverman's approach to treating high blood pressure is a diet that adds potassium and restricts sodium and cholesterol intake. Regarding the ongoing debate about the cholesterol content of eggs, Dr. Braverman asserts that high cholesterol usually has more to do with the other elements in the average person's diet than with eggs being the central culprit. As he puts it, "The average person is still eating white flour, junk food, and garbage essentially. So cholesterol intake will throw off cholesterol levels. But as a rule you're making 90 percent or more of the cholesterol in your body, and it's triggered by the diet. So, if you're eating a Null diet or a Braverman style diet, then the eggs are going to be a good food for you as long as you're not allergic."

SPECIAL NUTRIENT FORMULA

Dr. Braverman also advocates the following nutrient formula to lower hypertension: 200 mg of garlic, 200 mg of taurine, 50 mg of magnesium, 10 mg of potassium, 20 mcg of selenium, 4 mcg of zinc, 20 mcg of chromium, 50 mcg of niacinimide, 50 mg of vitamin C, 50 mcg of molybdenum, 50 mg of vitamin B_6, and 1,000 units of beta carotene. "Then," he says, "you just multiply that from about 5 to 10 to get a balance of those. Those are what I call the poor hypertensive nutrients.

"We've worked hard on a supplement called the heart or hypertensive supplement. On the basis of the research I did, we put all these nutrients in one pill, so you could lower your blood pressure naturally with one vitamin that you could take a lot of. However, one doesn't have to do that. There are many ways to take these supplements, but it's clear now that supplementation is one aspect of lowering your blood pressure."

OTHER PARTS OF THE PROGRAM

Despite the fact that supplementation is a useful tool in lowering high blood pressure, Dr. Braverman stresses, "The defeat of high blood pressure is a transformation of being and lifestyle." A person who exercises, keeps his or her weight down, generally maintains a low-fat, low-salt diet, and gets useful supplementation preferably through diet, but alternatively in pill form, will be better off for it in the fight against heart disease."

Other possible ways that Dr. Braverman suggests to lower hypertension include the use of borage and fish oil; relaxation; meditation; an electrical stimulator that has been FDA-approved for anxiety; melatonin; and last but not least the revolutionary role that retreats to healing centers and wellness programs can play in people's lives when they are trying to precipitate a long-term lifestyle change. Dr. Braverman explains: "Many, many individuals can go to health retreats, go on juice fasts, go on new dietary regimes, start cleansing techniques, and exercise, and they reverse their blood pressure, their weight, their blood sugar. Even I continue to underestimate the revolutionary nature of the wellness movement which says to the drug company and the drug managed care hospital network, no." He cites a recent example of a patient who had hypertension, diabetes, and a weight problem. After she went through a wellness program, all her health problems took a dramatic turn for the better.

Choosing a Therapy

Five years ago, I suggested to a leading cardiologist that the use of vitamin E, stress management, exercise, dietary changes, power walking, and proper supplementation would make a vast difference in the prevention and treatment of heart disease. He looked at me and responded, "No way. It's not scientific. It won't work." Today *JAMA, New England Journal of Medicine, Medical Tribune, Lancet,* and many other major medical journals recommend the same treatments that doctor disparaged five years ago. Thanks to the pioneering work of Dr. Dean Ornish and others, the concept of alternative treatment is less controversial and people are now willing to accept these treatments if they seem to offer the best possibility of health. Hopefully, in the future we will not have to reject any form of treatment, but accept the best features from each as they lead to better health.

Having reviewed the material in this chapter, you should know enough about the available alternatives to radical surgery and drug treatment to decide whether you prefer to seek traditional or alternative care for cardiovascular distress. Whatever sort of care you seek, you should monitor the progress you are or are not making to determine whether it may be feasible to abandon one course and embark on another. If you seek alternative treatments, you can find references in this book. In either case, select a competent physician and weigh his or her advice carefully, remembering to give serious consideration to your own observations of your response to the treatment. Don't be afraid to demand the best and most appropriate care available. When you are dealing with heart disease, your decision could be a matter of your own life or death.

Patient Stories

SYLVIA

An ultrasound test disclosed that my carotid arteries were 95 percent closed. I didn't want an operation, and while sitting in the doctor's waiting room, I discovered an alternative. While waiting to be examined, I overheard patients discussing chelation therapy.

After 28 chelation treatments, my carotid arteries are only 70 percent closed. I plan to continue with this therapy. It has made a difference in my life. I also have osteoporosis. Since the chelation, I can walk more freely and without too much pain.

KAREN

I was looking for stress management because I have a pretty stressful job. When I was down in Port Jefferson I saw a sign that read "Long Island Reflexology." I took the number and made an appointment to see Gerri Brill. That was three years ago. Since then, I've been diagnosed with moderate hypertension.

One evening, just out of the blue, I decided to take my pressure before I had a session and then afterward. I found that whereas before the session, my pressure was 150/100, it fell afterward to 120/80, which is the ideal number. This convinced me that reflexology had some of the health benefits that had I read about.

I find reflexology immensely energizing and relaxing, and go for a session every two weeks. It's an hour and a half of complete relaxation. You're away in a different place, and when you come back, you feel more energized and able to do your normal routine.

Chapter 15

Herpes

S ome viral infections, such as a cold or the flu, are like bad party guests you can't persuade to go home. They seem to hang around forever, although you know they will eventually leave. After a few weeks of misery, the cold and flu depart. But there are other viruses, notably herpes, that come to the party with a bedroll and tablecloth, planning to take up permanent residence. Perhaps this behavior will remind some readers of the classic film *The Man Who Came to Dinner.* A nasty, crotchety, but influential writer comes for a weekend visit to a couple seeking his favors, then breaks his leg and ends up staying in (and ruling) the house for months.

There are a number of types of herpes. One is the common cold sore, which usually occurs before another, more aggressive virus, such as a cold, is going to take hold in the body. That's why it is called a cold sore. Cold sores on the lips are usually referred to as fever blisters. A cold sore is classified as herpes simplex virus 1 (HSV-1). A more serious kind of herpes is genital, sexually transmitted herpes, called herpes simplex virus 2 (HSV-2). There is also herpes zoster, which used to be called shingles. Finally, Epstein-Barr virus is the form of herpes that causes mononucleosis.

Michele Picozzi, a health writer who specializes in natural medicine and the author of *Controlling Herpes Naturally,* points out that there is some controversy about the relationship between the two HSVs. There is no agreement on the status of "herpes simplex 1, which occurs, technically, above the waist, most often on the face or the lips, and simplex 2, which occurs below the waist. There is a body of evidence that they are actually different viruses, and they are classified as such. However, some researchers think they are both the same virus, which acts differently in different parts of the body. This would indicate that there is merely a herpes simplex 1 that is appearing at different sites."

In 1997, the *New England Journal of Medicine* reported that one in five Americans over age 12 is infected with genital herpes. This represents a fivefold increase, particularly among white teenagers and whites in their twenties, since the late 1970s. The figures for both HSV-1 and HSV-2 infection combined range from 50 to 60 million persons in this country alone.

Herpes can be pervasive, persistent, painful, and embarrassing. It also represents a fairly serious health risk both to the individual and to the community because many people who have herpes, particularly genital herpes—that is, anywhere from 20 to 25 percent—don't know they have the disease, since they don't experience symptoms. Even without symptoms, they can transmit the disease. Herpes is very contagious, and it has no cure.

As Picozzi notes, "Herpes has remarkable staying power. Once you contract herpes, you have it for life. It never leaves the body. It lies dormant in the nerve endings at the base of the spine. Thus the possibility of infecting people over a lifetime is considerable if there are recurrent outbreaks.

"An epidemiologist at the Centers for Disease Control in Atlanta, Georgia, has published a figure indicating that most people who have genital herpes will have another episode within 12 months. Other research indicates that HSV-1 has a recurrence rate of 14 percent, while genital herpes has a return rate of up to 60 percent or more."

Aside from the facial and genital areas, herpes can affect the eyes and the brain, with more serious health consequences. Herpes sores can also increase a person's risk of contracting AIDS, as the *New England Journal of Medicine* reported in 1997. In addition, for the numerous people who already have a diminished or compromised immune system, recurrent outbreaks of herpes can put a further strain on their immune reserves.

There is, however, some evidence that contracting facial herpes as a child lowers the risk of contracting genital herpes or even AIDS as an adult.

Causes

Some factors involving both food and emotional and physical states can cause herpes to recur, although the exact mechanism by which this happens remains a medical mystery.

According to Picozzi, "Stress is considered to be the number one precursor to a herpes outbreak, and this applies to all types of stress: emotional, mental. or physical. Physical stress would includee such things as overexertion, exercising too long, exercising in the sun, and doing a type of exercise which your body is not ready for. For example, you may be lifting weights and trying to increase your weight load. That may put a strain on the body. Stress inhibits the production of interferon, the body's antiviral agent. That's important, because herpes is a virus. Stress also inhibits the body from creating antibodies to fight off infection."

Certain foods have been found to cause herpes recurrences. These are primarily foods high in the amino acid arginine, including chocolate, peanuts, sunflower seeds, soy, and coconut. There are also some foods that raise the acidity of the blood. A high blood acicity level can irritate soft tissues, which is usually where herpes appears. These foods are sugar—that is, processed sugar—white flour, and red meats.

Exposure to strong sunlight—ultraviolet B (UVB)—has been shown to be a major factor in causing facial herpes, that which occurs on the lips, around the nose, or on other parts of the face.

Some people have a recurrence of facial herpes because there has been a trauma to the skin, for example, when they have dental work. Some people have a sensitive mouth, and so just the friction of the dentist working in that area can cause the virus to recur.

Also implicated are seasonal changes, particularly the transitions from winter to spring and summer to fall, when the body goes through certain adjustments and detoxifying periods. This can also cause herpes to recur, depending on how well you are taking care of yourself at that particular time.

Genital herpes can be sexually transmitted, and pregnant wpmen can transmit the virus to their unborn children. Moreover, prescription drugs that lower immunity, such as antibiotics, steroids, and antidepressants, can set off an attack

Warning Signs

About 50 percent of people who have recurrent infections of herpes virus experience warning signs. Medically, these signs are known as a prodrome. These sensations are usually experienced in the area where a previous infection has occurred.

Picozzi explains, "The most common of these is a tingling or an itching, twitching sensation. Some people feel heat or a crawling beneath the skin, or "pins and needles." Some feel as if they are coming down with the flu. They feel fatigued. Their lymph glands are swollen, and they have other muscular aches and pains throughout the body. These signals from the brain can last anywhere from a few seconds to a few days."

She describes some recent work on the emotional triggers of an outbreak: "The most interesting thing I have found in researching herpes is the mind-body connection. Most people with genital herpes will tell you that for them, stress is the biggest precursor for an outbreak. I have found that this connection goes even deeper. I call it the overlooked psychological connection.

"A naturopath and psychologist in the Philadelphia area, Dr. Wayne Diamond, as far as I know has been the only health practitioner to study this phenomenon in any depth, and he has come up with some very interesting conclusions.

"He conducted a series of clinical research projects that involved patients with both viral and bacterial skin conditions. He concluded that there are two sets of emotional conditions that almost always precede an outbreak in people who are prone to recurrent herpes infections. The emotions he specifically zeroed in on are, first, unexpressed feelings of anger or anxiety and, second, ambivalence or fear of loss. He believes that these emotions diminish the power of the human glandular system, which has a large effect on the body's immune system. Stress and anxiety take a toll on the body by increasing its temperature, which can affect how nutrients are absorbed, and they can also create more stomach acid, which eventually gets into the bloodstream."

Symptoms

Genital herpes causes surface sores on the skin and the lining of the genital area. In women, sores can appear on the cervix, vagina, or perineum and may be accompanied by a discharge or vaginal blisters. There is often a burning sensation, especially at the onset of an outbreak. Other symptoms may include urinary problems, fever, and lymphatic swelling. Intercourse is painful and should be avoided during an outbreak to prevent transmission. HSV-2 occurs intermittently and usually lasts five to seven days.

As the name implies, facial or oral herpes tends to attack the skin and mucous membranes on the face, particularly around the mouth and nose. These cold sores tend to appear as pearl-like blisters. Although they don't last very long, they can be irritating and painful. Herpes zoster, the result of the varicella zoster virus, causes agonizing blisters on one side of the body, usually on the chest or abdomen. Pain is usually felt before effects are seen, the result of overly sensitive skin covering the affected nerve. The symptoms may last from a few days to several weeks.

Conventional Treatment

There is no conventional medical cure for herpes, although drugs are commonly given to lessen symptoms. The most often prescribed of these is drugs acyclovir (Zovirax), which supposedly reduces the rate of growth of the herpes virus. Herpes medications have many potential side effects, including dizziness, headaches, diarrhea, nausea, vomiting, general weakness, fatigue, ill health, sore throat, fever, insomnia, swelling, tenderness, and bleeding of the gums. In addition, acyclovir ointment can cause allergic skin reactions.

Natural Remedies

Herpes sufferers will be glad to learn that natural remedies are often highly effective in shortening the length of outbreaks and diminishing their frequency. Here are some of the important ones to know about.

NUTRITION AND LIFESTYLE CHANGES

When herpes strikes, it is always a good idea to rest and eat lightly. Short fruit fasts, with plenty of pure water and cleansing herbal teas, can be very helpful. Good herbs to include are sage, rosemary, cayenne, echinacea, goldenseal, red clover, astragalus, and burdock root. Beneficial bacteria, such as those found in nondairy yogurt and in supplements containing lactobacillus and acidophilus, support the digestive processes necessary for the maintenance of the immune system. Other nutrients that directly enhance the immune system include garlic, quercetin, zinc gluconate, buffered vitamin C, and beta carotene (vitamin A). In addition, 500 mg of the amino acid L-lysine, taken two to four times a day, can produce excellent results. Bee propolis is anti-inflammatory, while B vitamins combat stress. Also good are bee pollen, blue-green algae, and pycnogenol.

Nervous system stressors, such as caffeine, alcohol, and hard-to-digest foods such as meat, should be avoided, especially at the onset of an attack. Foods high in the amino acid arginine, such as chocolate, peanut butter, nuts, and onions, are also associated with higher incidences of outbreaks.

Since stress promotes outbreaks, it is important to make time for activities that alleviate tension. Among the many possibilities are biofeedback, yoga, meditation, deep breathing, and exercise.

Toothbrushes should be changed frequently and completely dried before reuse to prevent reinfection. Soaking them in baking soda also fights germs.

MORE ON SUPPLEMENTS

Picozzi takes a holistic approach to fortifying the system to prevent a herpes outbreak, beginning with supplements. She says, "Antioxidants and B vitamins are the supplements that are important to people with herpes since they both support immune function. On the antioxidant side are vitamins A, C, and E. On the B vitamin side, B_6 and B_{12} are very important. I would recommend, though, that the B vitamins be taken in a combination or complex as they work synergistically. Minerals such as selenium and zinc are particularly helpful in supporting the immune system."

Most important, she says, is L-lysine. "For people with herpes, lysine should be the first line of defense. This is found in both alternative and traditional fields of medicine."

Dr. Steven Whiting, author of *The Complete Guide to Optimal Wellness*, has 20 years of experience in the field of clinical nutrition, holds a doctorate in biochemistry, and has worked in a number of hospitals that offer alternative perspectives. He has spent a great deal of time looking at the value of lysine.

"Lysine is an isolated form of an amino acid. Herpes, like so many viruses, requires complete protein in which to replicate. The lysine molecule mimics the virus's favorite protein structure, yet it is missing several bonds that are vitally important to the virus's lifestyle. When you increase lysine in the blood, the herpes virus attaches itself quite quickly to the molecule, and then it is too late. It is unable to replicate. You can shorten the outbreak of herpes down to a matter of a few hours with this treatment. In fact, if you catch it soon enough, you can keep the outbreak from occurring."

He recommends a full-spectrum program for the management of herpes.

"First take vitamin C, which is a powerful antioxidant and should be used in the presence of all viral infections. Take 2,000 mg as a minimum per day. Vitamin E used topically, for example, on the lips, will relieve pressure and irritation quite rapidly. It also is a powerful antioxidant and helps prevent cross-linkage at the outbreak. Take zinc, 100 mg per day, and copper, 2 mg per day. Acidophilus is certainly very important in any viral condition because of the die-off of the viral material, which eventually has to be processed in the colon. Take four to six capsules once or twice a day. Finally, and most important, is L-lysine, which can be purchased at your health food store in isolated form. In order to achieve saturation at the cellular level, you'll need 1 to 3 g a day, but take that only for an actual outbreak."

Dr. Whiting says that if you suffer from cold sores around the lips and you begin to feel itching in that area, that's the time to start the treatment. If you are in a period of excessive stress, or you feel a cold or flu coming on, these are also also classic times when you are liable to experience an outbreak, so you want to begin taking lysine before the blisters start to form. Take 1 g, three times a day. That is the basic recommendation for herpes.

Dr. Whiting notes, "We have had tremendous success with this treatment at our institute using that formulation as long as we use it with a full-spectrum approach."

However, as Picozzi notes, lysine is not useful for everyone. "Some people don't do as well as others using lysine alone to control herpes. Some dietary supplement manufacturers have come out with formulas containing lysine with some supporting herbs and vitamins that some people may find more effective. Lysine also helps the body form antibodies, helping the immune system fend off challenges like the herpes virus. It also nourishes the blood."

She has also found that "another supplement, a glandular thymus extract, can be very important for people with chronic infections because it helps boost the production of white blood cells. There are also two new types of food-based supplements—olive leaf extract and red marine algae—which are showing promise in inhibiting the growth of the herpes."

HERBS

Picozzi also see herbs as an important part of the treatment."Some herbs are very good for building and maintaining immunity. They include echinacea and licorice root, both of which have been shown to have interferon-like properties. Echinacea also has some antiseptic qualities. It helps the body regulate the glandular system."

Also recommended is goldenseal, which is very important because it regulates liver function and in addition is reported to cleanse and dry the mucous membranes, the site where herpes often appears.

Siberian and American ginseng are invaluable in helping the body boost its resistance to stress and infection because they support the adrenal glands and the nervous system.

Tarragon is good because it contains caffeic acid, which has been found to prevent herpes. Tarragon has been shown to be beneficial for fatigue, particularly when taken in combination with lemon balm, also called melissa. Lemon balm has become very popular for both internal and topical use. It's best taken as a tea, two to four cups a day.

Herbs should only be taken for short periods, say one or two weeks, and under the supervision of a health care practitioner.

Plants containing phytochemicals with antiherpes properties, in order of potency, are as follows:

Myrciaria dubia (camu-camu)
Glycyrrhiza glabra (licorice), plant or root
Viola tricolor hortensis (pansy)
Sophora japonica (Japanese pagoda tree), bud or root
Oenothera biennis (evening primrose)
Malpighia glabra (acerola)
Coffea arabica (coffee)
Aesculus hippocastanum (horse chestnut)
Rhizophora mangle (red mangrove)
Citrus limon (lemon)
Camellia sinensis (tea)
Abrus precatorius (crab's eyes)
Podophyllum hexandrum (Himalayan mayapple)
Mangifera indica (mango)
Origanum vulgare (wild oregano)
Phyllanthus emblica (emblic)
Allium cepa(onion)

HOMEOPATHY

According to Dr. Erika Price, a practitioner of classical homeopathy and holistic healing, classical homeopathy is the most effective form of treatment for people with the herpes virus: "The properly chosen remedy will motivate and empower the individual's own defense systems to fight back against anything harmful to it," she claims. Unlike orthodox medicine, homeopathy does not suppress ailments. This is very important because when you suppress a disease, it doesn't go away but goes somewhere else deeper inside you. That is, it goes into an organ that is more important than the skin. Homeopathy has no adverse effects and can only be of benefit. When the patient's physical, mental, and spiritual nature is taken into account, a cure can be found. The following remedies may prove extremely helpful for cold sores.

NATRUM MURIATICUM. When sores are on the lips, especially in the middle of the lips, the 30c potency of this remedy should be taken twice a day.

PHOSPHORUS. Cold sores that manifest above the lips, accompanied by itching, cutting, and sharp pain, should be treated with the 30c potency of phosphorus twice a day.

PETROLEUM. For cold sores that erupt in patches and become crusty and loose around the lips and mouth, petroleum is indicated. A 9c potency is needed three times a day.

APIS. Apis helps cold sores around the mouth and lips that are accompanied by stinging; it also helps painful blisters that itch and burn. A 6c potency is needed three to four times daily.

The following remedies may be helpful for female genital herpes.

NATRUM MURIATICUM. This remdy is indicated when the herpetic lesions are pearl-like blisters and the genital area feels puffy, hot, and very dry. A 6c potency, four times a day, may be beneficial.

DULCAMARA (BITTERSWEET). Women who tend to get a herpes outbreak in clusters on the vulva or the hair follicles around the labia and vulva every time they catch a cold or get their period probably need dulcamara in a 12c potency two to three times a day.

PETROLEUM. Petroleum may be beneficial if herpes eruptions form in patches and the sores become deep red and feel tender and moist. Outbreaks usually occur during menstrual periods, and most often affect the perineum, anus, labia, or vulva. A 9c potency should be taken three times a day.

The following remedies may be helpful for shingles.

ARSENICUM ALBUM. This remedy benefits most cases of shingles, especially when the individual feels worse in the cold, worse after midnight, and better with warmth. If taken at the onset of an attack, it is best in a 30c potency twice a day for two to three days. After the first three days, *Arsenicum album* is indicated if there is a burning sensation in the areas that were affected by the zoster eruptions (typically the chest and abdomen). At this point 12c, taken two to three times a day, is best. This remedy is excellent for the getting rid of the burning sensation that is often present.

HYPERICUM PERFORATUM (ST. JOHN'S WORT). This is a wonderful remedy for any kind of nerve pain. It is indicated whenever there is intense neuritis and neuralgia with burning, tingling, and numbness along the course of the affected nerves. Take this remedy in a 30c potency, two to three times a day, as needed.

When taking homeopathic remedies, Dr. Price reminds patients not to touch them directly, since that may disturb the vibration of the medicine. Instead, shake them into the bottle or tube cap and from there place them under the tongue until dissolved. Avoid coffee, mint, camphor, and chamomile, which work against the remedies. It is also important to note symptoms; as they change, so must the remedy.

AROMATHERAPY

The use of essential oils has gained popularity in the United States, where they are used widely in skin and body care products. However, the medicinal value of certain oils has long been accepted in other countries, particularly France, where in many instances, their antimicrobial properties make them an acceptable replacement for drug therapy. Aromatherapist Valerie Cooksley, author of *Aromatherapy: A Lifetime Guide to Healing with Essential Oils,* says that pure essential oils, properly used, can heal cold and canker sores. One mouthwash she recommends combines five drops each of peppermint, bergamot, and tea tree oil with raw honey, which is used as a carrier. This is important, as oils do not mix with water. The mixture is then added to a strong sage or rosemary tea. Rinsing with the formula several times a day balances the pH of the mouth and helps heal infections. Using this daily may even prevent outbreaks.

Additional spot treatments alleviate pain and restore health. One that Cooksley recommends involves dabbing a cotton swab with myrrh oil and applying it directly onto cold and canker sores. Another aromatherapist, Sharon Olson, dabs a cotton swab with diluted tea tree oil and places it on the cold sore to kill the virus. She follows this up later with lavender, which soothes the sore and stimulates the growth of new skin. The addition of fresh aloe vera gel further promotes healing. A side benefit of the therapy is its ability to lift the spirits. "When I get a cold sore, I get depressed," reveals Olson, "so I usually inhale some rosemary or basil to lift my spirits and clear my mind."

As this book emphasizes throughout, you shouldn't become fixated on one alternative approach, but be willing to experiment with different methods in order to build up a well-rounded, eclectic program. Dr. Whiting makes this point in relation to nutrition: "Too often, we as nutritionists have looked at isolated supplements as ways to deal with these ongoing health problems. When we do that, we ofttimes forget that the body is the greatest state of equilibrium ever developed biologically. Without maintaining that equilibrium, we have a big problem. The body runs on balance and not on extremes. Most of us enjoy the extremes. We go from one to the other, and that alone provides an endless amount of stress on the biochemistry."

Once you have developed a mix of healthy practices as part of your lifestyle, you can eliminate or minimize the outbreaks of the bug who came to dinner.

Chapter 16

Hormonal Imbalance

D isturbance of a woman's hormonal cycle can play a major role in the development of various medical conditions. Women are affected both by their monthly hormonal cycle and by the hormonal phases associated with the life cycle of adolescence, maturity, pregnancy and childbirth, and menopause, so an understanding of these natural cycles is invaluable in understanding and treating a multitude of symptoms.

Causes

Sherrill Sellman, a psychotherapist and writer on women's health, author of the best-selling book *Hormone Heresy,* tells us that for the body to function properly, estrogen and progesterone have to be in balance. Progesterone and estrogen stimulate each other and help balance each other. One function of estrogen is to stimulate estrogen-sensitive tissues, which include cells in the breast, ovaries, and uterus. Estrogen helps develop the curviness of women. It produces their secondary sex characteristics. It is a very powerful stimulant of these tissues. Progesterone, on the other hand, helps slow down the growth of cells and stabilizes mature cells so their growth doesn't get out of hand. The proper relationship, as Nature designed it, is one of checks and balances.

"We are seeing a predominance of estrogen in relation to just a little progesterone," Sellman says. "That's caused by the drugs and food we eat and the disharmony in our own bodies. It's been noted that 50 percent of women over the age of 35 are not ovulating each month. Now only if women are ovulating, releasing an egg, can a little endocrine gland called the corpus luteum, which is the primary source of progesterone, be formed on the surface of the ovary. If a woman doesn't ovulate due to stress or bad diet, she can go a whole month without producing the progesterone to balance the estrogen. As a result, women are progesterone-deficient."

DIET AND LIFESTYLE FACTORS

Dolores Perri, a nutritionist from New York City, lists factors that can interfere with normal hormonal production and balance:

ALCOHOL. Alcohol blocks the body's gammalinolenic acid (GLA) production, preventing the manufacture of natural hormones. This quickens the aging process. Alcohol creates deficiencies in B vitamins, magnesium, and calcium, which upsets hormone balance. Further, alcohol damages the liver, which in turn interferes with hormone metabolism.

ANIMAL PROTEINS. Animal proteins are loaded with hormones and synthetic antibiotics that throw our own hormone levels out of balance.

BIRTH CONTROL PILLS. Birth control pills deplete the body's B vitamins, which are needed for natural hormone production; increases susceptibility to allergies, and may cause liver damage, which can affect hormonal balance.

CAFFEINE. Caffeine is found in coffee, tea, chocolate, soft drinks, and certain medications. Like alcohol, it blocks GLA production. In addition, chocolate inhibits the liver's breakdown of hormones, and tea interferes with the absorption of iron and zinc, particularly if drunk with meals. Caffeine also raises adrenaline levels and increases stress.

EXERCISE. Professional athletes and women who train vigorously may use up so many vitamins and minerals that the body has insufficient means to maintain normal hormonal production. This can lead to an abnormal menstrual cycle and even the absence of menstruation altogether

PHOSPHATES AND POLYPHOSPHATES. The phosphates and polyphosphates found in many food products–such as soft drinks, processed meats, and cheese–can interfere with the absorption of nutrients.

SMOKING. Cigarettes contribute to hormonal problems by increasing the need for vitamins and minerals to detoxify the poisons in tobacco smoke. This reduces the amount of nutrients available for hormone production.

STRESS. Stress is a major contributor to hormonal imbalance. Any type of adverse stimulus that requires the body to change and adapt, such as day-to-day hassles, psychological trauma, financial problems, and environmental pollution, can cause stress. External stress can cause hormones to decline, which puts stress on internal body systems, further diminishing hormonal production and possibly interfering with immune function, which can lead to the development of allergies and autoimmune illnesses such as thyroiditis or lupus. Conversely, stress can create problems by causing the body to secrete too many hormones.

SUGAR. Sugar interferes with nutrient absorption, particularly B vitamins. It also interferes with the circulation of hormones throughout the body.

WEIGHT PROBLEMS. Excess weight adversely affects hormonal balance. The ratio of fat to lean body mass is critical in the initiation and continuation of the ovarian cycle. Being too thin is equally undesirable. If you fall below a certain weight, the pituitary hormone stops sending messages to the ovaries, and ovulation and menstruation stop.

OTHER FACTORS. Other conditions that contribute to hormonal imbalance include food sensitivity, allergy, chronic illness, candidiasis, menstrual and gynecological problems, drugs taken over long periods of time, and low levels of thyroid hormone.

Symptoms

Dr. Elizabeth Vleit, founder and medical director of the Women's Center for Health Enhancement and Renewal at All Saints' Hospital in Fort Worth, Texas, and author of *Screaming to Be Heard: Hormonal Connections Women Suspect and Doctors Ignore,* describes some of the conditions that hormonal imbalance can trigger and tells when they are likely to occur: "Women's bodies are cyclic in their response to hormones. They have a monthly rhythm of hormonal changes from puberty to menopause, which have a critical bearing on many dimensions of health. Men's bodies, on the other hand, have a tonic pattern of secretion, which means that the same amounts of key hormones are produced every day. They vary within 24 hours in terms of their hormone production. But basically each day is similar to the day before and the day after.

"For women, the first half of the menstrual cycle is dominated by a rise in ovarian estradiol. This is the primary estrogen that is active at receptor sites on all the cells in the brain and body, from puberty to menopause. This rise in estrogen allows the ovary to prepare the follicle that will become the egg released at ovulation.

"At ovulation, when the egg is released, the estradiol level drops briefly. The egg then takes over and produces progesterone for the second half of the cycle. Progesterone levels rise, and estrogen levels rise again, though not as high as in the first half of the menstrual cycle. Progesterone and estrogen drop prior to bleeding, when the egg is not fertilized. The body sheds the lining of the uterus and starts over.

"When hormones fall, right before bleeding, a drop in certain critical brain neurotransmitters, such as serotonin and endorphins, is triggered. This is associated with mood changes women describe—feelings of irritability, insomnia, depression, or anxiety. This may be a time in the cycle when women get migraines. The drop in estrogen that triggers changes in serotonin, norepinephrine, and endorphins sets off a cascade of blood vessel spasms that are involved in migraine headaches. That also affects chemical messengers involved in regulating the immune system, the gastrointestinal tract, the heart, heart rate, blood vessels, and as many as 400 other functions.

"We also see hormonal connections in women who have the diffuse muscle aches of fibromyalgia. These women often develop aches and pains and tender points after some type of hormonal change, such as postpartum or post–tubal ligation, or following a hysterectomy, even if the ovaries are left in place. We see this in menopause too. If we look at the patterns of this type of pain in women, we see that 80 percent of fibromyalgia patients are female, and that the average age when fibromyalgia appears is about 44 or 45."

Sherrill Sellman notes that infertility and miscarriage are both directly related to hormonal imbalance: an excess of estrogen and a deficiency of progesterone.

Clinical Experience

TESTS

Dr. Vleit says women need to be aware of the relationship between hormonal cycles and medical conditions: "One of the ways to do that is to track patterns relative to cycles, and to test the blood for various hormones that women's bodies produce. I've developed an approach to doing that by measuring the hormonal levels at the right time of the menstrual cycle. This helps women know what is happening to their hormone levels at the time that they are having symptoms. I become frustrated when doctors tell me that we don't need to measure the female hormones because they vary. I respond that that's the whole point. They do vary, and how they vary, relative to women experiencing problems, is what we must find out in order to offer them the most constructive options."

It is also important to check thyroid function. Thyroid hormone controls progesterone, cholesterol, and the ovaries. It acts as a cascading system. When not functioning properly, other hormones get out of balance.

NUTRITION

The typical American diet is high in fat, protein, caffeine, simple sugars, and salt, ingredients that interfere with optimal hormonal balance. These foods create a vicious cycle. They fuel premenstrual cravings for sweets and chocolate, and giving in to them worsens the cravings.

Perri advises us not to reach for a prescription drug for hormonal problems. It is better to eat high-quality organic foods and avoid foods that throw the system off balance. Beans and legumes are better sources of protein than meats, which are loaded with hormones. In addition, Perri recommends cold-processed oils, nuts, seeds, fatty fish, and beans. "These foods are all very high in GLAs," she notes. "The GLAs help us make natural estrogen in our own bodies."

SUPPLEMENTS

Wild yam and DHEA promote production of natural estrogens in the body, if the body needs them. If estrogen is not needed, these supplements are eliminated by the body, making them completely safe to use. Magnesium and calcium may also be beneficial, since most women do not get enough of these nutrients.

HERBS

Blue cohosh, black cohosh, yarrow, and chaste tree help balance hormone production. Other balance-promoting herbs include raspberry leaf, *dong quai,* wild yam, and passion flower.

Janet Zand, a naturopath, doctor of Oriental medicine, and acupuncturist, uses programs that rotate the herbs being used in accordance with the four weeks of the menstrual cycle. Herbs used during the first two weeks nourish blood and balance hormones; those used during the second two weeks clear the liver, which tends to become congested during these last two weeks.

In an article on the HealthWorld Online website (www.healthy.net), Zand recommends the following general herbal program for balancing the hormonal system and building general resistance. If you have severe PMS, check out Chapter 28, which discusses her programs for PMS.

First two weeks: combination of red raspberry leaf and *dong quai,* as a tablet, capsule, tea, or tincture, three times a day.

Third week: astragalus, American ginseng, or Chinese ginseng. These adaptogenic herbs tone the deep immune system. Take as a tablet, capsule, tea, or tincture, three times a day.

Fourth week: combination of goldenseal and echinacea. These herbs have antiviral, antibacterial, and anti-inflammatory properties. Take as a tablet, capsule, tincture, or tea, three times a day.

Chapter 17

Infertility

pproximately 2.5 million American couples are unable to conceive. The question of what can and should be done to conquer infertility is not only a complex medical issue but, with the advent of more and more advanced techniques for getting around nature's roadblocks to conception, at times a thorny ethical dilemma as well, with high emotional stakes.

After 10 years of fertility tests and treatments, Carla Harkness, frustrated by the lack of consumer-oriented literature on the subject, consulted over a hundred medical specialists and put together *The Fertility Book*. Harkness sees infertility as an emotional life crisis that is largely unacknowledged by society: "Reactions include grief and mourning, loss of self-esteem, and impaired self-image. Couples often have difficulties communicating with one another. Their sexual relationship is tested and damaged. All in all, it is a traumatic experience."

She adds that an early end to pregnancy, due to miscarriage, produces the same frustrations: "The failure of a fertilized egg to implant is amazingly common. Often up to 50 percent of fertilized eggs do not make it past the initial two-week period to implantation. Up to 20 percent of confirmed pregnancies are miscarried in the first trimester in women under 35 years old. As a woman approaches 40, that number can exceed 25 percent, and by the age of 45, the miscarriage rate is almost 50 percent. The emotional impact of miscarriage is similar to the emotional impact of infertility. There is often grief and mourning that are not accepted as genuine mourning in our society. Couples often hear things like, 'I guess it was meant to be,' 'Something was wrong,' or 'You'll have another.' That is often of little solace to someone feeling this kind of loss."

Causes

Reasons for infertility include endometriosis (a condition in which the glands and tissues that line the inside of the uterus grow outside the uterine wall; see Chapter 12, Endometriosis); poor diet; deficiencies in folic acid, vitamin B_6, vitamin B_{12}, and iron; heavy metal toxicity; obesity; immature sex organs; abnormalities of the reproductive system; hormonal imbalances; and genetic damage from electromagnetic radiation. In men, saunas and excessive vigorous exercise can diminish sperm production.

It may surprise you to learn that the birth control pill and other sources of estrogen can add to the problem. Barbara Seaman, an advocate for women's health issues and author of *The Doctors' Case Against the Pill*, whose publication led to detailed product warnings being included in birth control pill prescriptions, concludes that the chemicals in the pill may increase infertility in three ways: by suppressing the natural productions of hormones; increasing the risk of sexually transmitted diseases (STDs), especially chlamydia; and upsetting the assimilation of nutrients.

ABNORMAL MENSTRUAL CYCLES

As Seaman reports, "Fertility experts confirm that many women who have been on the pill for a long time have problems reestablishing their monthly cycles. In Switzerland, Fabio Bertarelli, the billionaire owner of the largest company to manufacture fertility drugs, publicly states that he owes his fortune to the birth control pill. In 1993, Bertarelli told the *Wall Street Journal* that his typical customer is a women over 30, who has been taking birth control pills since she was a teenager or since her early twenties. When she got off the pill, her normal cycles did not come back."

Seaman adds: "Fact is, there are a lot of nutritional issues involved. If a woman has been on the pill for a long time, she may be very low in folic acid; vitamins B_1, B_2, B_6, B_{12}, C, and E; and trace minerals zinc and magnesium, all essential to normal fertility. Sometimes just getting on a really good diet with really good supplements can get her back into a fertile cycle without needing heavy-duty drugs. It should be noted, however, that any dietary supplements used should be low in vitamin A, niacin, copper, and iron, the levels of which tend to be elevated in pill users."

Robin Wald, a nutritionist and health-care writer who specializes in infertility, explains further how birth control pills can cause hormonal imbalances that affect fertility.

"The hypothalamus is the gland that produces gonadotropin-releasing hormone, the hormone that triggers the pituitary gland to secrete other hormones that are important for fertility. These hormones, follicle-stimulating hormone, which tells the ovaries to start producing and maturing an egg each month, and luteinizing hormone, which ripens the egg and allows it to be released, signal the ovaries to produce estrogen and progesterone so that you can have a normal menstrual cycle. It's a very complicated and complex system and must be in a very particular balance to function properly; for the egg to ripen and mature; for the egg to be released and travel through the fallopian tubes; and for progesterone to be there to build up the endometrial lining to nourish an egg, so that if it's fertilized it can be implanted and nourished and grow so that it doesn't miscarry. When you have too much estrogen that suppresses pituitary gland function, you disrupt the normal hormone balance."

CHLAMYDIA

"Another reason the pill is bad for female infertility," notes Barbara Seaman, "is that it promotes the growth of chlamydia. This condition has reached epidemic proportions in the United States, with over half a million new cases yearly. Chlamydia causes pelvic inflammatory disease, which can then cause sterility. Usually, the first time it strikes, chlamydia does not render a woman sterile. Women who get the condition once should give up the pill right away."

TOXIC SUBSTANCES

Wald also cautions women trying to conceive to avoid exposure to toxic substances that not only may interfere with conception but have also been linked to miscarriage and birth defects.

"The first thing I tell people to avoid is tobacco smoke. If you're a cigarette smoker and you plan on getting pregnant, quit smoking. Tobacco is very high in chemicals, including cadmium, which is a toxic heavy metal that accumulates in the reproductive organs of both men and women. It interferes with sperm production in men and hormone production in women. Secondhand smoke can cause similar problems.

"I also encourage people to stop drinking, even if they only drink moderately. Alcohol interferes with fertility by causing liver toxicity. The liver is the primary organ for building up cholesterol to form the steroid hormones which are important to reproductive health. Marijuana and other drugs can also cause liver toxicity and should be avoided.

"In addition, I suggest that people eliminate caffeine, both in coffee and sodas; switch to decaf coffee or herbal teas, and increase your water intake. Although the subject of caffeine and fertility is controversial, studies have shown that as few as two cups of coffee a day or two cans of caffeinated soda can increase your chance of a miscarriage by four times and your infertility by 50 percent.

Wald further cautions women to avoid taking some over-the-counter medications. "A lot of women who experience menstrual discomfort think nothing of taking an aspirin or ibuprofen. But nonsteroidal anti-inflammatory drugs are also harmful to the reproductive system.

"One thing to avoid that cannot be overemphasized is pesticides—both pesticides that have been sprayed in your garden and pesticide residue from food that you buy. Pesticides are very toxic to the reproductive system. This is because pesticides are in a class of chemicals called *xenoestrogens,* synthetic chemicals that act like estrogen on the body. Overexposure to xenoestrogens can result in a condition called estrogen dominance. In estrogen dominance there is too much estrogen circulating in the body, which throws off the balance and production of other hormones that are essential for fertility."

Other sources of xenoestrogens are food additives, preservatives, and meat from animals that have been fed hormones. Dairy products also contain xenoestrogens, both from the cows' own hormones and from hormones given to them to promote milk production.

Clinical Experience

ASSISTED REPRODUCTIVE TECHNOLOGY

"The laboratory options have just exploded in the past decade for infertile couples," Carla Harkness reports. "In 1978, the first 'test-tube' baby was born in England through a process called in vitro fertilization. Since then, the process has been instituted worldwide. There are now over 260 clinics practicing some form of that kind of laboratory fertilization, which is now called Assisted Reproductive Technology or ART.

"Now the boundaries have even exceeded menopause. Before, you had the practice of donor sperm for artificial insemination. Now there is the ability to fertilize donor eggs from younger women with the husband's sperm and to implant those eggs in an infertile woman who is over 45 or 50. She is able to carry a child to term that is not genetically related to her. These kinds of options have all become available, and they offer a great deal of hope to many couples."

ETHICAL ISSUES

While modern advances in fertility treatments offer a wealth of new possibilities, they also raise new ethical concerns. "A number of religious groups have raised questions about the intervention of technology in the natural process of reproduction," Harkness explains. "There is also a theme of pronatalism at any cost here, emphasizing that to be complete as couples or as women, people absolutely must birth a biological child. Another big issue revolves around extending maternal age past nature's deadline of menopause. Before, women in their mid-40s probably weren't able to get pregnant because their bodies would stop that function. Now, it is possible for women in their 50s and 60s to become pregnant. This raises a number of questions: Is that putting too much demand on their bodies? What about the age difference between them and their children? What about obligations to aging parents while having little ones in your midlife? Additionally, there is a legal and moral question revolving around the status of unused, frozen embryos in the event of death and divorce.

"There are further questions surrounding the availability of this expensive technology to those without the means or the medical insurance. Unfortunately, these treatments are quite expensive. From the moment you walk into a specialist's office asking for an evaluation, you start incurring costs in the hundreds of dollars for examinations and tests, all the way to thousands of dollars for the in vitro techniques. It's about $10,000 per cycle for a straight in vitro lab procedure, all the way up to $15,000 if egg donor in vitro fertilization is utilized."

Many women distrust scientific intervention in general. Problems with IUDs have caused pelvic inflammatory disease resulting in infertility. Diethystilbestrol (DES), an estrogen replacement often used as a "morning-after" pill in the United States even after it was linked to cancer and anomalies of the vagina and cervix, has been another big problem, as has thalidomide. Now there is a concern about using female hormones to stimulate ovulation. With most infertility treatments, whether the problem is due to the man or woman, it is mainly the women who undergo the drug treatments, the surgeries, and so forth. What are the long-term effects of exposing women to these drugs?

NATURAL OPTIONS

Dr. Marjorie Ordene, a gynecologist from Brooklyn, New York, believes that while there is a place for technology in fertility, women are too quick to seek out these methods, and she suggests trying various natural options first.

PINPOINTING TIME OF OVULATION

Women should learn to recognize their time of ovulation by taking their temperature first thing in the morning, before getting out of bed: Says Ordene: "Usually, temperature rises in the second half of the cycle, two weeks before menstruation. The mucus that is produced around the time of ovulation has a clear and slippery quality. This is the kind of mucus that is needed for the sperm to penetrate the cervix." (See Chapter 5, Birth Control.)

LIFESTYLE

Women should maintain a healthy diet and follow a basic exercise program. Fertility specialists Talha Sawaf, M.D., Yehudi Gordon, M.D., and Marilyn Glenville, writing in *Positive Health* magazine, recommend eating organic foods as much as possible and avoiding food additives, coffee, and tea. They advise eliminating nonessential medications and avoiding exposure to radiation, hazardous substances in the workplace, pesticides, and pollutants such as toxic metals. They point out that becoming as healthy as possible before conception improves the quality of the egg and sperm, thereby maximizing fertility and reducing the risk of miscarriage. Conversely, fertility is decreased by poor nutrition, vitamin or mineral deficiencies, and too much alcohol, cigarettes, and stimulants.

DIET

Robin Wald, who suggests that the very first step in optimizing fertility is to examine your diet, says that the standard American diet does not promote either health or fertility. She recommends an organic, whole, live foods diet. "A potato chip is a good example of what I mean. A potato grows from the earth as a potato. When you turn it into chips and fry it, that's not a whole, live food any more. That's a very refined, dead food.

"The advantage of eating live food is that the nutritional value and the quality are that much higher. Good nutrition is vital when you're trying to get pregnant. Vitamins, minerals, fats, amino acids, and other nutritional components from our foods are essential for keeping the reproductive system healthy. Eat fresh fruit and vegetables, especially leafy green vegetables like collard greens, kale, Swiss chard, red chard, and beet greens, which are very high in folic acids and loaded with calcium. Folic acid is essential for preventing birth defects like spina bifida, and calcium will aid in building your baby's skeleton as well as keeping your own bones healthy."

She suggests minimizing your intake of processed flour, bread, baked goods, and pasta, and incorporating more whole grains into your diet. She recommends brown rice, millet, quinoa, oats, and buckwheat. "Whole grains are loaded with fiber and have very high nutritional quality. Raw nuts and seeds are also good, as are chickpeas, lentils, black beans, and pinto beans, which are both high in fiber and a good source of nonanimal protein.

"Fiber is important in promoting the excretion of toxins and bound-up estrogens from the gut. If you have insufficient fiber to move things through your intestines in a timely way, these estrogens sit in the gut and get reabsorbed into the body. So instead of having environmental estrogens or estrogens your body has created circulating through your body once, they're now going through a second, third, or fourth time, which contributes to estrogen dominance."

Wald advises eating soy products, like tempeh and miso. "Soy is a good source of phytoestrogens, which have a chemical structure similar to estrogen. Phytoestrogen tricks your body into thinking that it's getting estrogen, but the advantage of phytoestrogens is that they tell your body to lower its own estrogen production, which helps balance your estrogen levels. As well, phytoestrogens block the absorption of xenoestrogens."

EMOTIONAL AND SPIRITUAL ISSUES

Often, a woman has apprehensions about becoming pregnant that need to be addressed. It may be reassuring to talk to the inner child and let her know that even though there will be another child, the little girl in her will still get the attention she needs. This kind of spiritual work is often important in achieving pregnancy.

Sawaf, Gordon, and Glenville note that feelings of blame, guilt, anger, and frustration that infertile couples often experience will have a negative effect on their fertility. Discussing such issues, perhaps with a counselor, can resolve these negative feelings and improve the chances of conception.

Infertility is a very stressful, major life event, and stress can itself adversely affect fertility. Robin Wald describes how stress affects reproductive function. "Every time there is a stress response in your body, the adrenal glands secrete a group of hormones that have an inhibitory affect on the hypothalamus, which is the master gland that signals the production of the hormones needed for reproduction. When you have excessive stress, the hypothalamus does not function properly.

"Stress can also cause a condition called hypoprolactin anemia. Prolactin is another hormone that prepares the breasts for milk production. If a non-pregnant woman has high levels of prolactin, it will make conception difficult because it can shut down ovulation.

"If you're under a lot of stress, do whatever you can to reduce it," Wald suggests. She recommends yoga, meditation, breathing exercises, spiritual work and prayer, visualization and imagery, bodywork, and massage as ways to lower stress levels.

Nutritional supplements can also help. Wald recommends vitamins C and E, beta carotene, alpha carotene, coenzyme Q10, and antioxidants to protect against stress-induced free radical damage.

ASIAN NATUROPATHIC APPROACH

The traditional Eastern approach to fertility depends less on modern technology and more on time-tested knowledge. Dr. Roger Hirsch, a naturopathic physician from Santa Monica, California, explains Chinese philosophy and infertility treatments based on this point of view: "We look at making the abdomen happy. This is an aphorism for correcting the digestion, menstruation, and hormones, so that women can conceive. Of course, raising the man's sperm count and sperm motility is important as well, because it is not just the woman who is infertile in an infertility situation. A key to this is the way the blood flows in the pelvic cavity."

According to Sawaf, Gordon, and Glenville, Chinese medicine uses acupuncture, massage, heat, or crystals applied at points along the energy pathways, or meridians, to balance the flow of energy in the body. Changing the diet, decreasing emotional tension, and balancing heat and cold will increase the effectiveness of the basic treatment. Thus acupuncture is more effective when used together with herbs to regulate the menstrual cycle, promote ovulation, and increase general vitality, all of which enhance fertility. Chinese medicine can be combined with assisted reproductive technology to minimize stress and help women tolerate drugs and surgery.

INCREASING PELVIC BLOOD FLOW

A study of endometriosis-induced infertility was performed in China and published in the *Shanghai Journal of Traditional Chinese Medicine and Medicinals* in 1994. Forty patients were treated with neon laser acupuncture, retention enemas, and injection into the endometrial nodes with common sage root, which is a blood-vitalizing or blood-moving herb. Of the 40 patients treated, the size of lumps diminished and symptoms disappeared in 17, and 13 women conceived. Among the women who conceived, six had suffered from fallopian tube blockage and seven from ovulatory dysfunction. There was a total amelioration rate of 97.5 percent.

SEXUAL HYGIENE

Avoiding sexual intercourse during menstruation is another important consideration in reversing endometriosis and infertility. It has been demonstrated that Israeli women as a group have a low percentage of endometriosis. This is related to laws in the orthodox Jewish religion which say that you can't be with a man during menstruation. Chinese medicine agrees. Having intercourse during menstruation causes an imbalance of energy and results in the migration of endometrial tissue into the pelvic cavity.

HERBS

HERBA EPIMETI. "In Chinese medicine," says Dr. Hirsch, "herbs are used to tone renal/adrenal function because reproductive function is related to the kidney and to functions related to the kidney. The actual viability of the eggs for a woman over 40 is related to kidney yang function." One herb that is very good for kidney yang is an aphrodisiac called *herba epimeti*, which translates in English to "horny goat weed." The Chinese noticed that goats become sexually active after eating this particular plant. They put the plant into the herbal formula for women who are kidney yang–deficient, and they noted that it increased sexual desire.

LUTAIGOU. *Lutaigou*, the gelatin that comes from boiling the antlers of deer, is used by the Chinese to help women over 40 who are trying to extend their egg-producing years. It helps slow down the biological clock.

WORMWOOD. In the European system, we have wormwood, which creates more circulation in the pelvic cavity. The Chinese use this along with daughter seed and fructose litchi, a little red berry.

DONG-QUAI AND CORTEX CINNAMOMI. Both of these help the circulation in the pelvic cavity. *Cortex cinnamomi* is not the cinnamon you put in your mulled cider, but a cinnamon with a very thick bark.

ACUPUNCTURE

In China, acupuncture has been used in the treatment of infertility for centuries. The first published account of this is seen in medical literature dating back to 11 A.D. The Chinese look at five principal organs—the liver, spleen, heart, lung, and kidney—and use acupuncture to release blockages from these systems so that energy, or chi, can move freely. This helps the body return to good health. Promoting fertility is one benefit that can be obtained.

Acupuncture to kidney points releases psychological blocks that interfere with reproduction. Dr. Hirsch uses the treatment to help patients overcome deep-rooted fears connected to sexual abuse: "If there has been early abuse, rape, or incest, there sometimes is a problem with hormone maturation. In other words, fear causes the hormones to become dormant. This is related to the kidney, as this organ controls reproductive function, endocrine function, and hormonal function. I needle points along the kidney meridian to help establish a connection between the heart and the uterus. I also use the Bach flower remedies walnut and crab apple. Walnut breaks links, and crab apple cleanses."

Dr. Hirsch connects another psychological issue—low self-esteem—to endometriosis and infertility: "In treating self-esteem issues, I work on the heart and kidney points. The acupuncture points that seem extremely valuable for this are pericardium 5 and 6. If a practitioner is having a problem with understanding whether or not a psychological issue is involved in the infertility, and the patient does not know what the issue is, pericardium 5 can be needled. If something is holding the person back, that will bring an event or dream to memory, and the patient will understand why she is stuck. In treating self-esteem issues, we may also release stress by needling the heart 7 point, heart 9, and sometimes heart 7 to heart 5.

"We also address conception vessel 17, which is between the breasts. This is a very important place for women because it opens their energy. It also helps relieve liver chi congestion or stuckness. Remember, the liver and the liver hormones, both in Chinese and Western medicine, govern the flow of blood in the pelvic cavity."

WESTERN NATUROPATHIC APPROACH

Dr. Joseph Pizzorno says that as a naturopath and midwife he saw numerous infertile couples and discovered two causes of the condition that were not generally recognized by the orthodox medical profession: "The first was pituitary insufficiency. The pituitary gland was not secreting enough of the hormones needed to stimulate the ovaries to mature, ripen, and produce a viable ovum.

Most of these women had been on birth control pills for long periods of time. Even though they had been off the pills for several years, their pituitary never functioned fully again.

"With these women I did two things. I gave them a herbal concoction using herbs that are commonly used for women's health problems, which are supposed to stimulate proper pituitary functioning. I also gave them raw pituitary gland from an animal. There were surprisingly good results with this treatment. A urine test beforehand measured the level of hormones from the pituitary. If a patient had low hormone levels, I would then use this protocol with them. A surprising number became pregnant once their urinary hormone levels returned to normal.

"The second major cause was pelvic inflammatory disease, where there were infections in the fallopian tubes, the little tubes that go from the uterus to the ovaries. Infections leave scars. Then the ovum cannot penetrate the tube and get into the uterus for fertilization.

"An age-old hydrotherapy procedure, called sitz bath, helps end this problem. A woman gets two big pots of water. (We use washtubs that are about 3 feet in diameter.) One tub gets filled with hot water (as hot as she can stand it). When a woman sits in it with her arms and legs out of the tub, the water level reaches her umbilicus. The other tub gets filled with ice cold water. That tub is filled to the point just below the umbilicus. In other words, there is more hot water than cold water. The woman sits in the hot water for five minutes, and then in the cold water for one minute. She alternates back and forth three times.

"The first time a woman does this, she will find it startling. But after a while she will actually start to like it. She does this every day. After a few treatments, she starts getting a discharge. As near as we can make out, this discharge is the body throwing off scar tissue and toxic material in the ovaries. This is a particularly dangerous time for a woman to have intercourse. The ovaries are starting to open up, and there is a high probability of an ectopic pregnancy. The egg will only be able to go partway down the tube since the tube is not yet open enough for it to get all the way into the uterus. We therefore tell women no unprotected intercourse for at least three months while doing these treatments every day. Again, a surprising number of them become pregnant."

RESTORING THYROID BALANCE

Even as far back as the 1930s, alleviating low thyroid conditions was found effective against infertility. Dr. Ray Peat says, "Over the last 15 years, I have worked with quite a few women, some who have tried for as long as 10 years to get pregnant. Several had spent as much as $100,000 on other treatments. Consistently, within a few weeks of correcting their thyroid, they get pregnant."

To keep thyroid levels up, women should snack frequently and eliminate unsaturated fats. Although unsaturated fats are often touted as beneficial, recent studies show them to inhibit thyroid secretion. More high-quality protein may be needed, especially by women following a weight-loss program or a vegetarian diet. A daily minimum of 40 g is recommended. Taking a thyroid supplement for a short period of time can greatly help. "People whose thyroid function is suppressed can benefit from a week or two of thyroid supplementation," Dr. Peat advises. "They don't need to take this indefinitely."

NATURAL HYGIENE

Anthony John Penepent, M.D., practices natural hygiene, which he has known about his whole life. In fact, he says that it made his own birth possible: "Members of my family were natural hygienists before I was born. Back in the forties, my mother fasted for 30 days at Dr. Christopher John Cursio's hospital in Rochester, New York, the Castle of Health, so that she could conceive and retain pregnancy."

Today, Dr. Penepent follows the principles of natural hygiene when treating any medical condition: "Over the years, I have seen many wonderful things happen with natural hygiene which would not have been possible with allopathic medicine." Explaining infertility, Dr. Penepent says there are many causes, but that all of them can be treated similarly: "There are many mechanisms that can come into play. You can have basic amenorrhea or failure to ovulate. You can have any variety of hormonal imbalances or fallopian tube obstruction. In 40 percent of the cases it is not the woman's fault, although she may take the blame to save her husband's ego. The man may have a low sperm count, depressed sperm motility, or abnormal sperm morphology. These are all possibilities. Then again, conception may occur but the egg or ovum may not have sufficient nutrients for the embryo to develop. What happens then is you have unrecognized spontaneous abortions that make it appear as if the woman is infertile, when in actuality she just has a nutritional deficiency.

"In many cases, an infertile woman can conceive and go on to have a successful pregnancy with a minor amount of dietary change. In the case of the fallopian tube obstruction, it may be necessary for her to fast for several days. I remember one patient, a rabbi's wife, who was childless. Because of their religious beliefs, it was absolutely essential for her to bear children. In her particular case, I put her on a fast for several days and followed that up with a nutritional regimen. She was able to conceive within six months."

SUPPLEMENTS.

The right nutrients can make a difference in whether or not pregnancy is possible:

COLLOIDAL SILVER. When chlamydia is causing infertility, colloidal silver helps to clean up the system.

VITAMIN E. High doses of vitamin E balance hormone production. Under the guidance of a health-care professional, an individual should start slowly and gradually increase dosage.

ZINC. Zinc is particularly important for helping men to fertilize and mobilize sperm. Generally 50 mg per day is needed.

CONSUMER ADVOCACY GROUPS

Carla Harkness recommends becoming a part of a consumer advocacy group that can provide individuals and couples with support and information. One group, called Resolve, has its national office in Somerville, Massachusetts, and a string of chapters across the country: "Resolve is a great ally that provides literature, referrals, and legal advocacy to the infertile. Chances are, wherever you live, there's a chapter by you."

Herbal Pharmacy

Plants containing fertility-promoting phytochemicals, in order of potency:
Myrciaria dubia (camu-camu)
Malpighia glabra (acerola)
Cucurbita foetidissima (buffalo gourd)
Rehmannia glutinosa (Chinese foxglove)
Aloe vera (bitter aloes)
Helianthus annuus (sunflower)
Pinus pinea (Italian stone pine)
Ceratonia siliqua (carob)
Nigella sativa (black cumin)
Juglans cinerea (butternut)
Cnidoscolus chayamansa (chaya)
Citrullus vulgaris (watermelon)
Lupinus albus (white lupine)
Nasturtium officinale (berro)
Cucurbita pepo (pumpkin)
Cinamomum cassia (cassia)
Arachis hypogaea (peanut)
Momordica charantia (bitter melon)
Allium schoenoprasum (chives)
Sesamum indicum (sesame)

Chapter 18

Lupus

L upus, or systemic lupus erythematosis, is an autoimmune disorder of the connective tissues that affects eight times more women than men. *Lupus* is the Latin word for "wolf," and *erythema* means "redness"; the typical red skin sores caused by the disorder are said to resemble a wolf's bite. Lupus can be mild or life-threatening; it affects 1 out of 130 women between the ages of 20 and 40. Females of African, Native American, and Asian descent develop the condition more frequently than those of European ancestry.

Causes

Lupus occurs when antigen-antibody cell complexes circulating through the body are deposited in various body tissues such as the kidney and skin, causing inflammation. Symptoms may be exacerbated by infections, extreme stress, antibiotics, and certain other drugs. Although the exact cause of this disease is unknown, hormones are believed to aggravate it, particularly estrogen, which is why so many women are affected. According to an article by Anthony di Fabio, of the Arthritis Trust of America, which is posted on my website (www.garynull.com), lupus seems to be related to the use of estrogen therapy, indicating that it may be to some extent hormone-dependent.

Symptoms

Initial signs include arthritis, a red "butterfly" rash across the bridge of the nose and on the cheeks, weakness, prolonged and extreme fatigue, and weight loss. There may also be fever over 100 degrees, light sensitivity, skin sores on the neck, hair loss, chest pain, Raynaud's disease (a constriction of circulation in the extremities that causes fingers to turn white or blue in the cold), joint pain, muscle inflammation, anger, depression, and anemia. If the central nervous system is involved, seizures may occur.

Additional symptoms include mouth or nose ulcers and a nail fungus, which is an outgrowth of infection by *Candida albicans.* Often lupus sufferers have headaches. The characteristic skin sores are raised reddish patches that become scaly and crusted. When they fall off, they leave white scars. If these sores spread to other tissues in the body, tissue wasting may occur.

Lupus may begin abruptly with a fever, or slowly, with infrequent flare-ups. Those whose symptoms appear only in the skin have a better prognosis, while those whose kidneys and brains are affected have a poorer prognosis. In some patients, many different organs—lungs, heart, kidneys—are affected.

Clinical Experience

TRADITIONAL WESTERN TREATMENT

Mild cases of lupus are treated with nonsteroidal anti-inflammatory and analgesic drugs such as aspirin, ibuprofen, indomethacin, and sometimes phenylbutazone. Prednisone, a form of cortisone, may be given for arthritis and muscle aches. In severe cases of lupus, steroidal drugs are prescribed for internal and external use. However, long-term use of these medications can damage the liver and weaken the bones. Steroids depress the immune system, leaving the body vulnerable to infection.

For both mild and severe forms of lupus, says Anthony di Fabio, traditional treatments only relieve symptoms; they do not get at its causes.

NATURAL THERAPIES

Alternative practioners have successfully treated lupus with a variety of therapies, generally based on changes in diet and appropriate supplementation.

HERBS AND SUPPLEMENTS

To lessen inflammation, use pycnogenol, cat's claw, black walnut, omega-3 fatty acids, and flaxseed oil. Pau d'arco and aloe vera juice act as blood cleansers. A good nervous system tonic is *gota kola*. Colloidal silver is antibacterial, antifungal, and antiarthritic.

According to Johnathan Wright, M.D., a nutritionist from Kent, Washington, writing in the December 1995 issue of *Nutrition and Healing,* vitamin B_6, up to 500 mg three times a day, will help relieve symptoms. People with lupus also need supplementation with hydrochloric acid. He adds, "All lupus patients have food allergies, and will improve when this condition is handled." In addition, over half of women have low levels of DHEA and testosterone and need to take these hormones as supplements. (His article can be found at www.garynull.com)

Other practitioners recommend vitamin B complex, vitamin B5, vitamin B_{12} as an injection, vitamin C with bioflavonoids, vitamin A, vitamin E, proteolytic enzymes, digestive enzymes, zinc, calcium and magnesium, essential fatty acids, amino acids such as L-cysteine, L-methionine, and L-cystine, beta carotene, garlic capsules, and selenium.

INTRAVENOUS THERAPIES

According to di Fabio, Ronald M. Davis, M.D., of Seabrook, Texas, reports success treating lupus patients using EDTA (edetate calcium disodium) chelation therapy with DMSO (dimethyl sulfoxide, an antioxidant), and intravenous hydrogen peroxide. Dr. Davis initiates treatment of lupus and other autoimmune diseases by giving antifungal drugs such as metronidazole, since it appears that some antibodies related to autoimmune disease are produced in response to fungal microorganisms found to be present in such diseases.

ACUPUNCTURE

Acupuncturist and massage therapist Gina Michaels, of New York City, explains that she individualizes her acupuncture treatments according to each patient's unique profile: "The Chinese recognize that there are different kinds of arthritis. One type is from heat and wind, another from cold and damp. Western pharmacopeia treat them all the same, but we make a differentiation according to the symptoms that the client is displaying. Then a strategy is formed.

"Each decision an acupuncturist makes looks at the large picture. For example, if the person has a headache, along which meridian is that headache located? Is it the gallbladder channel? The stomach channel? Are they having other symptoms, such as fever or sweat? Is the central nervous system affected? All of this is very, very important in deciding what treatment protocol to choose.

"There are eight meridians formed during conception that go to a very deep constitutional level. Treating these is very useful for illnesses that are systemic or of a much deeper nature."

DIET

The Arthritis Trust of America recommends that people with lupus avoid overeating; minimize intake of cow's milk and beef; eat more green, yellow, and orange vegetables; eat nonfarmed cold-water fish several times a week; avoid alfalfa sprouts and tablets containing L-canavanine sulfate, a substance that can worsen lupus; and avoid taking L-tryptophan, which can exacerbate the autoimmune reaction.

The diet should be high in vegetables and low in grains. Wheat grass is excellent for reducing inflammation. Foods detrimental to healing include peanuts, bread, corn, soybeans, and other foods that can produce fungi and molds. In addition, alcohol, spinach, and carrots may aggravate the condition. Acid-producing foods, such as orange juice, meat, and dairy products, can also be harmful.

Fasting. Di Fabio quotes Joel Fuhrman, M.D., who says, "Having fasted over a thousand patients with various diseases I can say without hesitation that fasting is very often the only avenue that a patient can use to establish a complete remission.

"This is especially true with autoimmune illnesses like lupus, where it is almost impossible to shut off the hyperactive immune system with nutritional modifications alone, without total fasting." Fasting, he explains, is not merely a method of detoxifying. "The body clearly has the mechanism to adequately handle the removal of endogenous wastes generated in the fasting state. In fact, fasting has been shown to improve or normalize abnormal liver function." No drugs of any sort should be taken while fasting.

EXERCISE

Regular exercise is important, because it helps to keep the joints moving.

STRESS MANAGEMENT

Lupus can flare up during times of extreme stress. Working at a job one dislikes can be a contributing factor, for example. It is important for people to examine their lives and to create circumstances that promote health and happiness.

AROMATHERAPY

Essential oils can help calm the emotions and eliminate flare-ups. Rubbing tree oils such as pine and cedar directly onto the joints can diminish swelling. A drop of chamomile, lavender, lilac, or neroli can be placed on the palms and breathed in for relaxation. When there is chest congestion, eucalyptus is excellent for clearing the nasal passages and lungs.

HERBAL PHARMACY

Plants containing phytochemicals with antilupus properties, in order of potency:

Portulaca oleracea (purslane)
Triticum aestivum (wheat)
Ipomoea aquatica (swamp cabbage)
Morinda citrifolia (Indian mulberry)
Chrysanthemum coronarium (garland chrysanthemum)

Rumex acetosa (garden sorrel)
Luffa aegyptiaca (luffa)
Mimosa pudica (sensitive plant)
Peperomia pereskiifola (perejil)
Hibiscus rosa-sinensis (Chinese hibiscus)
Zizyphus jujuba (black date)
Basella alba (vinespinach)
Daucas carota (carrot)
Tropaeolum majus (nasturtium)
Hordeum vulgare (barley)
Symphytum offinale (comfrey)
Cinnamomum cassia (cassia)
Centella asiatica (*gota kola*)

Chapter 19

Menopause

Menopause marks the end of the female reproductive cycle, which typically occurs between the ages of 45 and 50 but can happen anywhere from 40 to 60, or even earlier as a result of surgery or illness. Menopause is said to begin when a woman goes through one complete year without a period. The stage before menopause, called perimenopause, may last as long as 10 years. Many women harbor misconceptions about the nature and effects of menopause. Yet in cultures where menopause is less feared, symptoms are virtually nonexistent, and in fact menopause is anticipated as a rite of passage into a stronger, wiser time of life.

Causes

"It is a myth to imagine that the ovaries fail at menopause," says Sherrill Sellman, international seminar leader, psychotherapist, and author of numerous articles on women's health and of the best-selling book *Hormone Heresy*. "During perimenopause, the ovaries go through a last hurrah. The body is making very high levels of estrogen, trying to kick-start the ovaries so they can keep going. There is no winding down, but rather very high levels at this time, though they tend to fluctuate quite erratically, causing hot flashes.

"Nature produced the ovaries, which are endocrine glands, to keep working throughout a woman's life. There will be a reduction in hormone levels because during this period she is shifting out of her reproductive nature into a new stage of life. She does not need to be producing the hormones required for ovulation. At menopause her body shifts just enough so she is no longer able to produce eggs, but she is still producing adequate levels of estrogen to maintain the functions of her body. The two main estrogens are estradiol and estrone. The estradiol drops only about 15 percent from what it would be during perimenopause, and the estrone drops about 40 to 50 percent. But the body does continue to produce hormones.

"At menopause the outer part of the ovaries, which has been more responsible for producing eggs, begins to shrink because eggs are no longer being created, but the inner part, called the inner stroma, actually gets switched on for the first time. It produces hormones that look after the heart, blood vessels, skin, and libido, protecting the woman's body and her well being.

"Furthermore, when estrogen production by the ovaries declines, other parts of the body are switched on, such as the adrenals, which help turn body fat into estrogen. So even women who have hysterectomies, if they are healthy, are able to create enough estrogen to keep themselves vital without needing supplementation."

Sellman adds that progesterone levels do seem to be low at perimenopause and low progesterone affects a woman more at this stage than does low estrogen. These levels can be assessed through saliva assay tests—which, she asserts, should be the gold standard for assessing hormone levels, not blood assay tests, which are now widely used. "Saliva tests are widely available in the United States and give accurate readings. Blood tests generally show only 1 percent to 9 percent of the hormones circulating in a woman's body, which will lead doctors to think women are deficient. It's this type of misdiagnosis that leads to mistreatment."

Symptoms

One of the first changes perimenopausal women experience is in the frequency of their menstrual cycle. The time between cycles may increase or decrease, or they may skip a month. Usually blood flow is reduced, but women may also experience heavy, irregular bleeding. Other common symptoms associated with menopause are hot flashes, dry skin, mood swings, depression, irritability, vaginal dryness, night sweats, bladder infection, fatigue, and sleep disturbances.

"Many changes appear in perimenopausal women, but the negative ones usually arise from stress, bad diet, pharmaceutical drugs, exhausted adrenal glands, and other things—not from lowered estrogen levels," says Sellman. "I believe, based on my own experience, that the symptoms of menopause—and also those of PMS, which are produced by the same imbalances—are really the result of poor health. When we can correct these imbalances, our hormones automatically go back into balance and we receive all the benefits. Women need to understand that a healthy liver, a healthy digestive system, a healthy adrenal system, and getting the colon working are the factors that contribute to healthy hormone production."

Sellman says that it is well known that there are cultures that do not associate the cessation of menstruation with negative consequences. "The Japanese, for example, don't have a word for menopause or hot flashes. They look at it just as a transition period, but not one with a significant effect on a woman's life. So the symptoms we are told are inevitable, that all women must endure, are actually symptoms of imbalance. I've found that to be true in my own case. When I notice symptoms appearing, such as night sweats or cramp or fatigue, I get immediate relief when I work with natural healing methods."

Clinical Experience

MISCONCEPTIONS ABOUT MENOPAUSE

MENOPAUSE CAUSES A LOSS OF SEX DRIVE

According to clinical psychologist Dr. Janice Stefanacci, society expects menopausal women to lose their sex drive, but this does not have to happen. "Many women fear that they are going to lose their passion and sexuality. Really, only a small portion of women who go through menopause have their sex drive adversely affected. For these women who lose their sexual desire or have difficulty becoming and staying aroused, help is available. But most women do not experience sexual arousal problems, and many report feeling more sexual because the risk of pregnancy is gone."

MENOPAUSE CREATES PSYCHOLOGICAL PROBLEMS

Dr. Linda Ojeda, author of *Menopause Without Medicine,* says many women see menopause as the beginning of the end. "They believe that life is going to be downhill from this point on. They no longer think of themselves as youthful, as able to contribute to society. They fear that their behavior will become erratic, hysterical, and out of control. This is not true. When we reach fifty, we do not turn into raging maniacs, and we are not more susceptible to clinical depression. In some women, however, lowered levels of estrogen, endorphins, and serotonin, substances that affect mood, can create mood swings. Levels can be raised naturally in these women.

"We know that beliefs and attitudes affect the transition. In Asian countries, symptoms are virtually nonexistent. In these countries, menopause is looked at as an important event in a woman's life. She now has more prestige and is viewed as a wise, older woman. Women anticipate this time of life with relish. If you are approaching menopause with fear and trepidation, you need to examine your attitude."

MENOPAUSE IS A DISEASE

The medical community has created this belief by stressing the need for hormone replacement therapy. In reality, menopause is not a disease but a natural transition that should be dealt with naturally.

DANGERS OF HORMONE REPLACEMENT THERAPY

"Hormone replacement therapy is based on deceit," asserts Sherrill Sellman. In the 1970s, women turned their backs on supplementation with estrogen alone because it had been found to cause endometrial cancer. So the drug companies came up with hormone replacement therapy (HRT), which used a combination of estrogen and a synthetic progestin like Provera. They used a synthetic because natural progesterone, which has no toxic side effects, cannot be patented. To sell HRT to women, who were scared of hormones after the revelations of the 1970s, the companies claimed that HRT reduced the risk of a condition most women were unaware of: osteoporosis.

Sellman says, "Osteoporosis was intentionally made to appear as specifically a woman's disease, which it never was. And the image of the dowager's hump which it could lead to was a terror that overrode women's fears of cancer. The image was that this new disease would lead their bones to crumble and leave them aged and handicapped."

In the early 1990s, a new reason for healthy women to take this powerful carcinogenic steroid was introduced. HRT was said to be a way to protect the heart. A Harvard study of about 46,000 female nurses found that those who had taken HRT had a lower incidence of heart disease by up to 50 percent. However, when that study was more fully investigated, it turned out that the women with lower rates of heart disease were actually women who were healthier in general. Compared to the group who were supposed to have a greater incidence of heart disease, they were wealthier, more likely to exercise, and had better diets; fewer of them had diabetes; and they smoked less. The women who didn't take HRT were more likely to have diabetes, smoked, were poorer, and didn't visit their doctors. Also not reported in the study was the fact that the women who took HRT had a 50 percent increase in strokes. This, then, was a flawed, biased study.

By now HRT, originally supposed to be only a short-term treatment for relief of menopausal symptoms, had become a long-term treatment given to prevent other conditions, conditions which only *might* occur. But giving it to healthy women with no history of heart disease, to perhaps prevent them from one day getting it, is dangerous. In truth, according to Sellman, the use of hormone replacement therapy is actually killing women because it is increasing their risk of cardiovascular disease.

"It's important to understand that the way these drugs are pushed creates the fear that menopause itself is a risk factor in heart disease. The rationale for giving HRT to postmenopausal women is that when you arrive at menopause your risk of getting heart disease or stroke will skyrocket and, therefore, you need protection. But studies from reputable researchers show that this is a myth. There is no rapid increase of heart disease in postmenopausal women. There is simply a rise in heart disease as women move on in life in general. The doctors who push HRT as a preventive for women's heart disease seem not to take into account the fact that men also have a higher incidence of heart disease as they age.

"Some thought that women overtake men and develop a higher incidence of heart disease later in life, but that also is not true. Many things contribute to increased risk of heart disease, but menopause is not one of them. Women are being given this false information, and so are doctors, because their main education comes from the pharmaceutical industry.

"The final myth on which hormone replacement therapy is based is that women become estrogen-deficient as they age. But, in fact, very few women have this estrogen deficiency. It's important to understand this point, so that women can claim power over their bodies and their health.

"Recent studies have challenged the theory that hormone replacement therapy is beneficial to the heart. A study that came out in August 1998—sponsored by Ayerst, the company that manufactures the number-one replacement estrogen, Premarin—used estrogen and progesterone in an attempt to show the benefits of HRT as a secondary treatment for the women in the study who already had some sort of heart disease. They gave half the women hormone replacement therapy and the other half a placebo. After five years, they discovered that in the first year of treatment, the women taking the HRT had a 50 percent increase in heart attacks. Over the five years, the risk decreased. The conclusion was that women who already had heart conditions got no overall benefit from HRT. But this glossed over the horrible fact that HRT increased heart problems the first year. What was more, women taking it had three times as many blood clots in the legs than women taking the placebo. There was also an increase in gallbladder disease.

"The estrogen and synthetic progestin used in HRT are not natural substances, but powerful steroid drugs. About 120 risks and side effects are associated with this combination, some of which are life-threatening, including not just heart problems but cancers of the reproductive organs, breast cancer, increased risk of diabetes, asthma, thyroid imbalance, and immune dysfunction.

The manufacturers' own package inserts warn that these drugs should not be taken by women who have current problems with or a past history of clotting, thrombosis, stroke, cardiovascular disorders, high lipoproteins (a specific type of blood fats), severe hypertension, or lipid metabolism disorders. Estrogen and progestin will increase the possibility of strokes and clotting, since they thicken the blood and raise blood pressure. And these factors all contribute to the possibility of heart disease."

Dr. Kent Hermsmeyer, a professor of medicine and cell developmental biology at Oregon Health Sciences University, put rhesus monkeys whose uterus and ovaries were removed on a regimen of estrogen and progesterin. Another group got estrogen and natural progesterone. The monkeys on the synthetic formula developed vascular spasms; their coronary arteries shut down. He only saved them by injecting them with a drug that reversed the condition. But with estrogen and natural progesterone, there were few effects, hardly noticeable. These results indicate that not only is estrogen a factor in increasing risk of heart disease but so is progestin, since it constricts the arteries.

In another study, Dr. Peter Collins at the National Heart and Lung Institute in London gave one group of women natural progesterone and estrogen and another group the synthetic combination. Put on a treadmill, those taking the synthetic mixture had a remarkably decreased ability to work out. They became exhausted. Those using the natural progesterone showed no ill effect.

"So it seems perverse to give women either estrogen alone or the HRT combination when it is known that these synthetic hormones cause strokes and blood clots," Sellman concludes. "In fact, there is a class action suit underway in Britain by women who claim they have gotten strokes and clots directly from the HRT. I've known women who have had strokes due to HRT."

Progestin also contributes to birth deformities. That is why women on the pill are told not to get pregnant. It also impairs the liver and the gallbladder, and may contribute to depression and headaches. It promotes increased facial hair, fluid retention, infertility, and miscarriage. A large number of women now have endrometriosis, which is at least exacerbated, if not caused, by synthetic estrogens and progestins. Progestin interferes with blood sugar, increasing the risk of diabetes. Progestins are just as dangerous as estrogens in causing a range of serious health problems.

Another important point is that estrogen and progesterone are not just sex hormones. They regulate and influence all the systems of a woman's body, including the digestive, immune, circulatory, and nervous systems. Because tampering with these hormones has grave consequences for a woman's physiological and psychological health, it must be done with great awareness and concern. Instead, what happens is that HRT plays havoc with her physiology.

First off, she gains weight, since taking estrogen leads the body to convert food into fat and store it. This is Nature's way of helping women survive famine. Furthermore, dieting and exercising alone will not take HRT-caused weight off.

Other consequences of estrogen dominance are fibrocystic breasts, depression, mood swings, anger, fluid retention and bloating, fatigue, migraines, and headaches. Estrogen lowers the libido—it does not increase it. There is foggy thinking and memory loss. Fibroids, which are the number one reason women have hysterectomies, are fed by excess estrogen. There are also aches and pains (fibromyalgia), infertility, miscarriage. Too much estrogen can block the uptake of thyroid hormones, so women develop thyroid problems. Estrogen excess also weakens muscle tone and makes the skin sag.

One of the more serious consequences of a prolonged excess of estrogen, as mentioned, is an increase in breast cancer. The latest finding from the Boston nurses study, which has been going on for 18 years, is that women on HRT who have been taking synthetic estrogens and progestins for 10 years or more have a 100 percent increased risk of breast cancer. The combination of progestin with estrogen was even more deadly than taking estrogen alone, for progestin, as mentioned, is also carcinogenic, associated with a higher incidence of reproductive cancers: breast, endometrial, and ovarian.

"The level of propaganda from doctors and the drug companies is so great that, for the average woman, the myth that without HRT they will deteriorate starting at menopause, become useless, decrepit, and powerless is enshrined as truth," Sellman declares. "But Nature didn't make a mistake. It did not program women to decline. If we are going downhill, it's our own doing, because we don't understand how to help the body regenerate."

With respect to osteoporosis, Dr. Bruce Hedendal of Boca Raton, Florida, comments, "Most people are told that estrogen prevents osteoporosis. This is true to some degree. Around menopause, synthetic estrogen replacement therapy is effective for five to seven years only. It slows down the bone loss, but it does not reverse it in any way, shape, or form. The studies have shown that eight to ten years after menopause is finished, there are no benefits to estrogen replacement therapy on bone loss."

Dr. Robert Atkins, director of the Atkins Centers for Complementary Medicine, confirms that one side effect of estrogen therapy is insulin resistance. "This syndrome is characterized by low blood sugar, high blood pressure, or high insulin levels. But the most frightening one of all to most women has to do with upper body obesity."

NATURAL THERAPIES THAT WORK

Natural therapies can make HRT unnecessary. I completed a year and a half study of people who went on a strict program of cleansing and detoxifying, eating no animal proteins, no meat, no sugar, no caffeine, no processed food. They exercised six days a week for an hour. They drank lots of fresh organic juices, sometimes as much as a gallon a day, and certain herbs.

Three women in that group who had been postmenopausal—one who had been so for 18 years and had had a hysterectomy—returned to a premenopausal state of health. Skin wrinkles were gone, energy restored, human growth hormone was back, and hormones were balanced. The gray, thinning hair of one 71-year-old woman grew back brown and thick. Another woman had a low libido, and her mucus membranes were dry, as was her skin. Her skin and mucus membranes regained moisture, and she enjoyed a level of health and energy that she hadn't experienced for years. Her toenails and fingernails, which had been brittle, yellow, and cracked, became pink and fresh. This was all without medication or any hormone replacement therapy. We just gave her body a chance to rebalance itself; we honored it by not giving it anything that would have led to an imbalance.

DIET

Jane Guiltinan, a naturopathic physician from Seattle, Washington, says, "A lot of women don't know that there may be alternatives to estrogen replacement therapy. There are some very good plant sources of estrogens in some of our foods. In fact, you can get significant amounts of plant estrogens. They have been shown in several research studies to improve menopausal symptoms. "The food that has the highest content of estrogen is soy. Soybeans, tofu, tempeh—anything made with soy—will contain plant estrogens. Oats, cashews, almonds, alfalfa, apples, and flaxseeds contain smaller amounts of estrogen. A woman emphasizing those foods in the diet can experience significant decreases in her hot flashes." Studies suggest that too little magnesium in the diet is one cause of hot flashes. Magnesium can be found in whole grains, beans, and soy products.

Sugar, which can cause hot flashes and other menopausal symptoms, should be avoided. Sugar, coffee, and alcohol adversely affect the blood sugar and can disturb the emotions.

Ann Louise Gittelman, author of *Before the Change: Take Charge of Your Perimenopause,* notes that weight gain, a common problem in peri-menopausal and menopausal women, can be minimized by eating the right kinds of foods. These foods are incorporated in Gittelman's Changing diet plan. "Low-glycemic, or slow-acting, carbohydrates will supply lots of energy for their calories. My favorites are those that are lower on the glycemic index, which is a list of carbohydrates ranked as to how they develop into blood sugar in your system. I like yams rather than white potatoes, and I like whole rye meal rather than wheat. I choose unprocessed carbohydrates that are moderate to low on the index, which also provide high-quality fiber to help eliminate excess estrogen from the system by lowering blood levels of this hormone.

"In addition, a number of fruits and vegetables are particularly high in phytochemicals and phytohormones. These include apples, grapefruits, lemons, pears, peaches, and a wide variety of vegetables that are high in fiber and loaded with phytochemicals.

"I have found that a diet with the right amount of proteins, fats, and low-glycemic carbohydrates not only helps regulate sexual hormone production, but also helps to balance the hormonal response to food, which I think is critical in keeping blood sugar levels stable. A level blood sugar helps to prevent perimenopausal symptoms like depression, mood swings, and hot flashes, and it leads to weight loss without any effort.

"Fats are important on the Changing diet plan. We need to add essential and beneficial fats, not take them away. These come in the form of the high-lignan flaxseed oil, olive oil, toasted nut seeds, and avocado. These fats stabilize blood sugar levels.

"So we're getting our blood sugar stable, we're assisting in long-term energy, and more importantly, we're providing the raw material for hormones, particularly progesterone, which is the key hormone in perimenopause."

Another natural source of phytohormones is the natural thickening agent kuzu. Several natural foods recipes incorporate kuzu in sauces in place of flour, making this a way to both enjoy healthy foods and alleviate symptoms.

VITAMINS AND MINERALS

The following nutrients provide an additional boost to good health in the menopausal years:

MULTIVITAMINS. Women need a natural multivitamin/mineral supplement containing higher amounts of magnesium than calcium and high amounts of B and C vitamins. A good multiple vitamin helps build the adrenal glands, which lessens emotional symptoms.

VITAMIN E. This vitamin is known for its ability to rejuvenate the reproductive system and alleviate hot flashes. Low amounts of FSH (follicle-stimulating hormone) and LH (luteinizing hormone) are related to hot flashes, and vitamin E helps increase levels of these brain hormones. It also helps lessen vaginal thinning and dryness. Mixed (beta-, delta-, and gamma-) tocopherols are best as they are found together in nature. D-alphatocopherol is also preferred over synthetic vitamin E. Generally, 400 IU per day should be taken in the beginning. The dosage can be gradually increased to 600 IU, although some women may need up to 800 IU.

ZINC. This mineral supports ovarian function. A good source is zinc picolinate. It can also be taken as an amino acid chelate or as zinc methionine. The recommended dosage is 25 to 30 mg per day.

B COMPLEX. B-complex vitamins are important throughout life, but there is an extra need for these during menopause. They can be obtained from whole grains and green vegetables. B_5 (300–400 mg/day) and B_6 (150 mg/day) are especially helpful during menopause. Folic acid, in prescription doses, is a valuable replacement for female hormones, according to Dr. Carlton Fredericks.

ESSENTIAL FATTY ACIDS (EFAS). EFAs, which are precursors to the natural hormones in the body, are very important for both men and women. People on low-fat diets should pay special attention to this. A diet too low in fats can lead to an increased risk of cancer and aging. Omega-6 fatty acids can be found in flaxseed, sesame, pumpkin, and safflower oils. Omega-3 fatty acids are found in fish oil capsules or fish. Both are needed. EFAs help prevent or treat vaginal dryness.

VITAMIN D. The best source of vitamin D is sunlight. It can also be taken in supplementation (400–600 IU/day), although caution should be taken not to get too much of this vitamin. Another source of vitamin D is salmon oil. People living in polluted environments need more vitamin D.

CALCIUM. Calcium is essential to prevent osteoporosis; supplementation should begin before the onset of menopause. There are many forms to choose from. Dairy is a poor source because many people have an intolerance to it. Calcium citrate is easy to digest, as it is already in an acidic medium. Calcium carbonates are alkaline and therefore more difficult to digest. Amino acid chelate is an excellent source of calcium. Calcium lactate is another good source. Calcium gluconate can be made into a powder and mixed into drinks; 1300 mg per day, from food and supplemental sources, is the recommended dosage. If it is not being absorbed well, more may be required. Each person should be analyzed to see the amount needed.

GAMMALINOLENIC ACID (GLA). This is available as evening primrose oil, borage oil, or blackcurrant seed oil; 200 mg per day is recommended.

BORON. Research shows boron to be a precursor of both female and male hormones.

SUPPLEMENTS THAT HELP CREATE HORMONES

Sherrill Sellman advocates natural progesterone, which is an identical match to what the body makes, as opposed to the synthetic progestins, like Provera, which are molecularly altered and thus don't fit exactly with the body's hormone receptors. Instead, these synthetics give instructions that are out of harmony with a woman's physiology. By increasing progesterone levels with natural progesterone, women can eliminate and reverse many of the conditions resulting from estrogen dominance, such as hot flashes, depression, low libido, breast tenderness, fluid retention, and digestive problems. Progesterone helps normalize thyroid function and blood clotting. Progesterone is the hormone that is predominant right after ovulation, and it increases women's libido. Finally, progesterone oxygenates the cells.

PREGNENOLONE. Taking 25 to 30 mg a day helps the body create female hormones.

DHEA. Natural DHEA, found in wild yam extract preparations, rejuvenates the body.

PROGESTERONE CREAM OR SERUM. Progesterone is a woman's rejuvenating hormone; it protects against cancer and fibrocystic cysts and increases the beneficial effects of thyroid hormone. In addition, it guards against osteoporosis by putting calcium back in the bones. After menopause, progesterone can be taken three or four weeks out of the month. Wild yam cream contains progesterone and can be purchased over the counter. Natural progesterone can also be taken orally.

ESTRIOL. This natural, friendly estrogen has been shown to inhibit breast tumors in animals. Some gynecologists are beginning to recommend estriol for menopausal women because it is safer and more effective than synthetics.

TRIPLE ESTROGEN. This formula is 80 percent estriol and 20 percent estrone plus estradiol. Estriol affords protection against breast tumors. Together, estrone and estradiol help reduce the risk of osteoporosis and cardiovascular problems. There are no negative side-effects.

HERBS

A number of herbs on the market help relieve perimenopausal and menopausal symptoms by restoring the progesterone-estrogen balance. They include alfalfa, black cohosh, blue cohosh, Chinese ginseng, damiana, fennel, licorice root, motherwort, red clover, red raspberry leaves, sarsparilla, and certain forms of wild yam. Flaxseed contains lignan, a phytohormone fiber that removes excess estrogen from the system. This is particularly important, since too much estrogen is believed to fuel breast cancer. Whole flaxseeds can be ground up or can be taken as flaxseed oil.

CHINESE HERBAL THERAPY

The Chinese have been using herbs to treat women's problems for 5,000 years. Roberta Certner, President of the New York State Association of Professional Acupuncturists, says that Chinese medicine sees a woman as giving birth to herself at menopause, since she no longer has an obligation to her children. This philosophy thinks in terms of cycles of seven years. When a woman is 49—often the age when menopause begins—it sees her lifespan as half-finished. "The next half of the lifespan is for self-growth."

Certner explains that "Chinese medicine is adamant that women shouldn't be suffering from night sweats, insomnia, mood changes, and other symptoms, and herbal formulas are good for this purpose. They help to rebalance the energies of the body so that a woman doesn't feel at the mercy of these tremendous moods and powerless over bodily changes."

According to Certner, one virtue of Chinese medicine is gentleness: "People aren't forced to take medications which reduce libido function, which set up terrain for heart conditions. It really addresses the mechanism itself and not just the symptoms. The reason Chinese medicine works is that it goes to the root of the problem. If progesterone is low, you enhance the progesterone, using something like dioscorea or leonorus, whose name itself means 'mother root.'" Many different herbs are available to the practitioner, who chooses the ones to use in a given case according to the nature of the particular person involved. As Certner says, "Chinese medicine doesn't really treat conditions— it treats people."

Chinese medicine classifies herbs into three categories: tonic, medicinal, and poisonous. You can safely take tonic herbs for long periods; you can take medicinal herbs for short periods when you need them; and you should never take poisonous herbs, which can cause harm. Abigail Rist-Podrecca, an acupuncturist knowledgeable in Chinese herbology, explains that tonic herbs are of two types: yin and yang. Everyone contains both yin and yang, which are opposite types of energies: yin is, as Rist-Podrecca says, "the female, the recessive, the deeper organs," and yang is male and includes more active and superficial organs. The cooler yin herbs will tone the yin organs, while the hotter, yang herbs affect the yang organs. (Additional information from my interviews with Certner and Rist-Podrecca can be found on my website, www.garynull.com.

Important tonic herbs in Chinese medicine include:

ASTRAGALUS. Known as the poor person's ginseng, astragalus fortifies the immune system.

DONG QUAI. *Dong quai* tones the uterus and stimulates production of female hormones. It is helpful for anemia since it builds the blood.

GINSENG. Ginseng contains a natural steroid that tones the adrenals and pituitary, regulating the endocrine system. It is good for all major organs, and therefore is known as the king of the tonics. It regenerates, retards aging, and promotes sexual functioning. To diminish hot flashes, cook until it is soft and cut into small pieces. As a rule women should avoid the stronger red types of ginseng; these are better for men.

HER SHOU WU. This herb promotes longevity. It is good for the kidneys, liver, and nervous system, and for clearing the eyes. Although it gives a tremendous amount of life energy (chi), it does not stimulate but rather acts as a mild sedative. It is said to promote the three vital treasures: spiritual bliss, sexual energy and radiant health. It also promotes hair growth and darkens the hair. It can be cooked along with an equal amount of ginseng.

LICORICE ROOT. This phytoestrogen-containing herb detoxifies, regulates, and stimulates glands, and is good for the stomach. Combined with other herbs, it is used for ulcers.

WU-WEI. *Wu-wei,* or schisandra fruit, was used by royal women and emperors to promote sexual potency and prevent aging. Other uses include relieving neck and shoulder tension, protecting and enhancing the skin, and, when used over long periods, purifying the blood, helping the kidneys, and sharpening the mind. Because it has both yin and yang aspects, *wu-wei* promotes balance.

OTHER USEFUL HERBS

CHASTE BERRY. Vitex, or chaste berry, is commonly referred to as the menopausal herb because it alleviates many symptoms, including hot flashes, vaginal dryness, and mood swings. It works by raising the progesterone level.

GINKGO BILOBA. Studies demonstrate ginkgo's effectiveness in leveling mood swings.

WILD YAM contains benefcial progestrone, the precursor of estrogen. This gives a woman the building blocks to create more hormones.

HOMEOPATHY

The homeopathic remedy chosen should correspond to the symptoms described. According to Ken Korins, a classically trained homeopathic physician in New York City, only one should be used for best results. Sometimes it's a matter of trial and error; if one does not work, another can be tried. These are some of the remedies Dr. Korins recommends for menopause:

REMEDIES FOR HOT FLASHES

The following herbal remedies are used for specific types of hot flashes.:

LACHESIS. Heat is felt all day long, while cold flashes may be experienced at night. Once the menstrual flow begins, all the symptoms disappear. Symptoms are worse with pressure and heat, and better with the onset of discharges or flows. Increased sexual desire is also associated with a need for lachesis.

BELLADONNA. There are many hot flashes. The face looks red and feels hot, and there is hot perspiration coming from the face and a pounding, throbbing, congested feeling in the head. Often there is dryness. Condition improves with resting quietly in the dark. Symptoms worsen with light, cold air, and sudden jolts. The emotional state can border on hysteria with rages.

GLONINE. Hot flashes are focused, with pressure in the head and feelings of congestion. There may be an associated rise in blood pressure at the time of the flashes. Symptoms are worse with heat and better with cold air. Emotionally, there is a fear of death; there is mental agitation.

AMYL NITRATE. Flashes of heat are accompanied by headaches. Often they are associated with anxiety and heart palpitations.

MANGANUM. Hot flashes are associated with nervous system depression. The body does not want to move. Symptoms improve when patient is lying down. Emotional state is peevish and fretful. There is a loss of pleasure in joyful music, but a profound reaction to sad music.

REMEDIES FOR FLOODING

The term "flooding" refers to irregular periods which stop for a while but are very heavy when they return. The following remedies may also help younger women with extremely heavy periods:

CHINA. There is heavy bleeding, with dark, clotted blood, leading to debilitating fatigue. Symptoms get worse with drafts and light pressure, but better with strong pressure and heat. Emotional symptoms are apathy with a strong disposition toward hurting other people's feelings (not the normal state).

SABINA. The period is characterized by heavy, bright red, clotted blood. Expelling the clots is painful, and pain radiates from the sacrum to the pubis. Emotional symptoms are irritability and a dislike for music.

SECALE. Periods are profuse and prolonged. Blood is almost black. Symptoms worsen with heat and improve with cold.

PHOSPHORUS. There is easy, frequent bleeding of bright red blood, often with no clots. The patient is low-spirited, with multiple fears. Also, memory may decrease. Another symptom is constant chilliness.

REMEDIES FOR VAGINAL DRYNESS AND THINNING:

SEPIA. The vaginal area is itchy and dry. There is a sense that the uterus is falling out of the vagina. There is also a loss of libido. Symptoms tend to be worse with standing, cold and rest, anything that causes venous congestion. Symptoms are improved with anything that increases venous flow, such as motion. Emotionally, there is an indifference to loved ones, sadness, and a tendency to weep easily.

NATRUM MURIATICUM. Vaginal dryness makes sexual intercourse very painful. Discharges tend to be acrid and burning. There is often a loss of pubic hair. Emotional state is one of depression and irritability, which is worse with consolation. Symptoms also tend to worsen around 10 o'clock in the morning.

BRYONIA. Vaginal dryness is accompanied by severe headaches. Any motion is painful and distressing. Condition improves with rest.

NITRIC ACID. Vaginal dryness reaches the point where the mucosa fissures, causing splinterlike sensations in the vaginal area.

EXERCISE

Regular exercise can reduce the frequency and severity of hot flashes. This is because it decreases FSH. For best results, it is a good idea to begin exercising before menopause begins. Otherwise, exercise may trigger hot flashes. Exercise also alleviates mood swings and depression by naturally raising serotonin and endorphin levels in the brain. The best exercises to engage in are dancing, brisk walking, running, swimming, biking, and tai chi. Additional benefit is derived from cross-training, doing different exercises on different days. This prevents any one part of the body from becoming overdeveloped or overstressed.

AROMATHERAPY

"Aromatherapy is truly holistic because it is a mind and body treatment," states Ann Berwick, author of *Holistic Aromatherapy and Women's Health.* "I think this is part of the secret of its power." Berwick uses essential oils to help alleviate a number of conditions, including hormonal imbalance in women going through menopause. "Cyprus, fennel, and clary sage are believed to have estrogenlike effects. For overall balancing, I recommend to my clients that they use these oils in a lotion or body oil, and apply it to their body two or three times a day. When women are experiencing hot flashes, I also suggest that they breathe in peppermint or basil on a tissue throughout the day. I find that a great help for most of my clients."

AYURVEDIC MEDICINE

Menopausal women report relief and rejuvenation from ayurvedic formulas using herbal phytoestrogens and phytoprogesterones. Ayurveda believes that balance is the key to perfect health. It basically determines which body/mind type a person is and helps people choose the type of foods they should eat and the type of exercise that is best for them. Chapter 8, "Chronic Fatigue Syndrome," discusses some ayurvedic principles in detail. You can also read *Perfect Health* and *Ageless Body, Timeless Mind* by Deepak Chopra.

REFLEXOLOGY

In Chapter 28, "Premenstrual Syndrome," Laura Norman outlines reproductive system reflex points. Here she gives additional information on specific ways to relieve menopausal symptoms: "For menopause, in addition to working the reproductive organs, I also would encourage you to work your thyroid gland, as this will help take over when the ovaries produce less estrogen. This is how to find this point: the base of the toes reflects the neck area where the thyroid is located. Press your thumbs into the base of your toes and thumb-walk across that ridge, particularly in the base of the big toe.

"Another area to massage is the adrenal gland reflex point. You are on the big toe side of the foot. Go about a third of the way down your foot. You are under the ball of the foot, in line with the big toe. If you press your thumb into that area, it will provide energy when you feel fatigued.

"Also, the pituitary gland, which helps all the other glands to work, is located in the center of the big toe. Pressure applied there helps stimulate that area. Both feet should be massaged equally."

HERBAL PHARMACY

Plants that are helpful during menopause, in order of potency:

Oenothera biennis (evening primrose)
Helianthus annuus (sunflower)
Psophorcarpus tetragonolobus (asparagus pea)
Lablab purureus (bonavist bean)
Moringa oleifera (ben nut)
Nasturtium officinale (berro)
Sinapis alba (white mustard seed)
Cucurbita foetidissima (buffalo gourd)
Cicer arietinum (chickpea)
Sesamum indicum (sesame)
Phaseolus vulgaris (black bean)
Spinacia oleracea (spinach)
Cucurbita pepo (pumpkin)
Trigonella foenum-graecum (fenugreek)
Basella alba (vinespinach)
Corchorus olitorius (Jew's mallow)
Brassica nigra (black mustard)
Vigna radiata (green gram)

Chapter 20

Menstrual Cramps and Irregular Menstruation

Painful and difficult periods are so commonplace in our society that some women have come to think of them as normal. However, they are not normal at all. Many experts feel that the symptoms of menstrual cramps (dysmenorrhea) are related to dietary practices as well as to unresolved emotional difficulties.

Causes

"What causes menstrual cramps?" asks Dr. Pat Gorman. "In addition to toxins found in foods with preservatives, additives, and caffeine, they are due to putrid proteins found in dairy and red meat. These foods contain a lot of hormones that upset the system. In addition, foods fried in heavy oils cause problems and should be cut out immediately by any woman interested in getting rid of dysmenorrhea."

Dr. Gorman adds that the Chinese attribute this condition in part to pent-up anger and frustration: "If you are not happy with your life, if you are angry with people, you must work this out. The liver, which stores blood and prepares it for the period, is also responsible for anger. That's not a Western concept, but with my patients I find that working out anger helps the liver relax. As a result, there is far less of a problem with dysmenorrhea."

Dr. Marjorie Ordene, a gynecologist in Brooklyn, New York, agrees that hormonal and psychological factors cause painful periods and explains the underlying factors: "What causes dysmenorrhea is exaggerated uterine contractions. These contractions are mediated by receptors in the uterine lining that are stimulated by hormonal and psychological factors. Hormonal factors that stimulate the uterine receptors have actually been isolated. They are chemical messengers called prostaglandins. Two things are clear: People with menstrual cramps have an excess of prostaglandins, and there is an imbalance in the types of prostaglandins they produce."

She adds that eating foods we are allergic to can increase prostaglandin production: "For example, many women are sensitive to yeast, and eating baked foods, breads, pastries, and processed fruit juices can cause an increase in prostaglandin production."

Symptoms

There are different types of menstrual pain. Usually it is experienced as a spasmodic cramp, but there can also be an achiness, a feeling of heaviness in the lower abdomen, or discomfort in the lower back or thighs. Other symptoms may include nausea, vomiting, loss of appetite, diarrhea, headache, dizziness, tiredness, anxiety, and depression.

Dysmenorrhea usually begins at the onset of menstruation and lasts a few hours, but it can begin premenstrually and remain for several days. According to traditional Asian medicine, if the tongue has a thick white coating, the problem is the result of too many of the wrong types of proteins, while a thick yellow covering signals toxicity from protein.

Clinical Experience

CONVENTIONAL TREATMENT

Medical doctors often prescribe medications such as ibuprofen to inhibit prostaglandins. While these agents work to relieve menstrual cramps and the accompanying symptoms, problems occur when drugs are taken month after month. The side effects can include gastrointestinal bleeding, decreased blood flow to the kidneys, and leaky gut syndrome, a condition that allows undigested food particles to enter the blood.

NATUROPATHIC TREATMENT

DIET

Changes in diet can decrease overproduction of prostaglandins and restore normal balance. Cool green foods help reduce hot stabbing pains and inflammation. It is good to eat foods such as organic grains, legumes, oatmeal, and steamed green vegetables. Deep-sea fish such as salmon, tuna, and mackerel can be included, as well as flaxseed oil. Hot spices should be avoided, along with fried greasy foods, sugar, salt, alcohol, and stimulating foods such as garlic and onions. Foods that produce allergies should be eliminated as well.

Women who have nerve-related menstrual pain can benefit from tofu but should stay away from too many cold raw salads, hot spicy foods, and even white potatoes. The herbalist Letha Hadady suggests this soothing recipe: warm tofu cooked with sweet spices such as pumpkin pie spices and nutmeg. This quiets the nerves and helps a woman feel nurtured and relaxed.

FASTING

Dr. Anthony Penepent, a physician who practices natural hygiene, helps patients with painful menses by placing them on a strict hygienic regimen: "I put them on a fast one day before the onset of their period. In serious conditions, I might have them fast one day and then prescribe juices or juice blended with salad and fruit for the following days until they complete their menses." (For a description of a typical hygienic regimen, see his patient's experience in Chapter 12, Endometriosis.)

SUPPLEMENTS

EVENING PRIMROSE OIL. Taken throughout the month as a daily supplement, evening primrose oil prevents headaches and blemishes that occur just before the period.

MAGNESIUM CITRATE. Magnesium deficiencies are common and result in the release of prostaglandins that cause spasm and pain. Magnesium is antispasmodic and helps relieve the problem. Take 300 to 500 mg daily and work up to bowel tolerance.

HERBS

The following herbs help alleviate menstrual problems.

GARDENIA AND PHILODENDRON. These are popular in Chinese medicine and can be obtained by prescription from an herbalist.

CORN SILK TEA. This tea helps get rid of the bloating that comes from too many hormones stored in the blood. Women's Rhythm also eliminates bloating. This Ted Kapchuk formula can be found in certain health food stores or ordered from Kahn Herbs.

XIAO YAO WAN. This a wonderful remedy that can be purchased at pharmacies in Chinatowns in major cities, such as Pearl River Pharmacy in New York City.

It helps digestive processes. Not only does this formula relieve painful periods, it also alleviates anger.

GREEN TEA. Green tea is cooling and satisfying and has very little caffeine. A pinch of tea can be added to a pot of boiled water, steeped for five minutes, and sipped throughout the day. People experience an energy pickup from the digestion being activated, not from the nerves being stimulated. Green tea helps soothe sharp, stabbing pains.

ALOE VERA JUICE OR GEL. Aloe can eliminate headache, irritability, fever, stabbing pain, blemishes, and bad breath associated with menstrual cramps. Aloe also reduces acid from the stomach and liver and is slightly laxative. Just add to juice, tea, or water.

DANDELION. Dandelion helps break apart impurities in the system. It can be bought as capsules or tea.

SARSAPARILLA. Sarsaparilla helps hot, stabbing pains brought on by inflammation. It is anti-inflammatory, antiseptic, diuretic, and soothing.

VALERIAN. Valerian is a sedative herb that makes a woman feel quieter, more relaxed, and grounded. It is especially good for nervous women who experience insomnia, anxiety, crying jags and emotional upsets, and other nervous problems. Valerian quiets the nerves that go to the uterus.

YUNNAN PAI YAO. This combination of herbs helps reduce heavy bleeding and stabbing pain. Because it increases the circulation, internal bleeding is healed and swelling and pain are reduced.

HOMEOPATHIC REMEDIES

Homeopathy was developed in Germany over 200 years ago by Dr. Samuel Hahnemann. The word "homeopathy" means "like cures like." The same substances that cause a disease in a healthy individual can heal an ailment in a sick person when they are diluted and given in minute proportions.

Homeopathic physician Ken Korins, M.D., explains that the dilution process is what makes homeopathic remedies so safe: "Homeopathy is a vibrational medicine. We are dealing with very subtle energies. Substances are given in extremely small dilutions that cannot possibly have any toxic effects. In fact, if you were to analyze these substances, you would not find a trace of the original material in the final dilution."

The correct homeopathic remedy is the one that most closely matches the symptoms that manifest themselves. Dr. Korins recommends that dysmenorrhea sufferers choose among the following:

COLOCYNTHIS. Colocynthis is a frequently indicated remedy that is useful when you have a severe onset of sudden cramps, particularly on the first day of menstruation. Emotionally, intense irritability and anger are associated with the menstrual cramps. A key indication is that you feel better when your knees are pulled up toward the stomach and held with firm pressure.

MAGNESIA PHOSPHORICA. Magnesium phoshorica helps spasmodic cramps with bloating. The key indication for this remedy is that you feel better from warmth. Magnesia phosphorica and colocynthis help alleviate the symptoms in 85 percent of cases.

PULSATILLA. A key indication for pulsatilla is variation; the cramps and the flow of bleeding are changeable. The pains themselves are typically cutting and tearing and may be felt in the lower back or kidney region. Generally, you feel worse in warm stuffy rooms and better in the open fresh air. Emotionally, you tend to be mild, gentle, and weepy when entering the menstrual state and prefer the company of other people to being alone.

VIBURNUM. Viburnum is indicated when the menses are very scanty and often late. In fact, they may last only a few hours. When you get cramps, the flow of blood stops. Cramps tend to radiate to the sacrum and the thighs. You may feel faint or feel like passing out.

CIMICIFUGA. Cimicifuga is indicated for spasmodic, cramping pains. The pain radiates across the pelvis from one thigh to the other. It is often associated with a premenstrual headache. Increased flow results in more pain. Emotionally, you may feel nervous to the point of being scattered and often are somewhat depressed.

CHAMOMILLA. Chamomilla is helpful if you are either hypersensitive or insensitive to any pain. Emotionally, you tend to be irritable and contrary. Someone brings you something that you ask for, and then you don't want it. During intense periods, you may become dependent on coffee and other stimulants and sedatives. Another symptom is anger. When you become angry, your symptoms become worse.

AROMATHERAPY

Marjoram, clary sage, and lavender are wonderful analgesics. Eighteen to 20 drops of oil added to a lotion or oil and massaged into the abdomen and lower back will help relieve menstrual pain. Breathing in the cooling fragrances of rose, lavender, or sandalwood can alleviate sharp, stabbing pain.

STRESS MANAGEMENT

Deep abdominal breathing, meditation, tai chi, and other mind-body disciplines eliminate frustrations and anger that bring on pain. Additionally, it is helpful to slow down the pace of life from the time of ovulation to the period.

Amenorrhea and Menorrhagia

Amenorrhea and menorrhagia are medical terms for abnormal blood flow. "Amenorrhea" refers to the cessation of bleeding or very light and infrequent periods, most often caused by an abnormally functioning hypothalamus, pituitary gland, ovary, or uterus as a result of drugs or surgery that removes the ovaries or uterus. "Bulemics and anorectics also exhibit this pattern," notes Dr. Pat Gorman, an acupuncturist and educator from New York City. "Sometimes this is caused by excessive dieting and overexercise driven by self-hatred. Not accepting who she is, a woman thinks, I've got to make myself thin, beautiful, and perfect. If this is going on at the end of the cycle, when toxins are being released into the system, the woman is aggravating her body to the point of saying, We're not going to give up this blood. We desperately need it. Forget ovulation, forget periods."

Dr. Ruth Bar-Shalom and Dr. John Soileau, naturopaths from Alaska, in an article on the website of the American Association of Naturopathic Physicians (www.naturopathic.org), list several other causes of amenorrhea. First, it happens normally after a woman stops using birth control pills, during pregnancy, and during all or most of the breast-feeding period. It is important to establish that pregnancy is not the reason for amenorrhea, since some of the remedies for this condition may harm the woman and her child while she is pregnant or nursing.

Malnutrition, crash diets, obesity, stress, intensive exercising, extreme obesity, abuse of antidepressants and amphetamines, and mental illness are other causes of amenorrhea, say Drs. Bar-Shalom and Soileau. When a young woman of 16 has not yet begun to develop sexually, when weight fluctuates dramatically, and when amenorrhea is accompanied by severe depression, drug use, or pain, consult a qualified health-care professional.

With menorrhagia the opposite scenario occurs, and there is profuse bleeding. The condition can be debilitating, sometimes bad enough to warrant immediate attention in a hospital's emergency ward. "The Chinese say menorrhagia is caused by excess toxins and heat in the blood from foods containing preservatives, additives, and caffeine, especially coffee. It's like water in your car radiator becoming low," Dr. Gorman says. "The engine will overheat and explode. Alcohol adds more toxicity because it constantly removes water from the blood. As water diminishes, it heats up the blood. When the blood is what we call 'hot,' or fast-moving, it's very hard for the body to hold it in. It can't stop the bleeding."

The emotional profile of a menorrhagic individual is someone who sees herself as a victim. Dr. Gorman explains: "This person feels the need to serve everybody. She does not know how to set boundaries. Whatever anybody wants, they get. She keeps pouring out her energy and pouring out her blood."

Dr. Vicki Hufnagel, a gynecological surgeon and activist for women's health rights, adds that heavy bleeding is often a sign of an underlying problem in the female system, especially when it is accompanied by pain. The problem frequently is due to a hormonal imbalance. "Anything can throw off a cycle," says Dr. Hufnagel, "including emotional stress, insomnia, too much estrogen in the system, or too little light, as in the winter. Other physical problems that can cause menorrhagia are fibroids, polyps, and a malfunctioning thyroid gland."

Before you can restore the blood flow in patients with amenorrhea or menorrhagia, you must discover the reason for the problem. Once the cause is addressed, periods should return to normal.

SYMPTOMS

Oriental medicine can diagnose amenorrhea and menorrhagia by examining the skin. Amenorrhea manifests as pale, sallow, slightly yellowish skin from a deep lack of blood and nutrients. Often this is accompanied by a great deal of emotional anxiety. With menorrhagia, the tongue has a red tip and tiny red dots. When the condition is long term, a woman can become anemic.

HORMONAL BALANCING FOR MENORRHAGIA

Dr. Hufnagel says that hormonal dysfunctions in women with menorrhagia can be corrected with oral doses of natural progesterone. "Often the creams women use are not adequate because they don't cause a rise in the blood level. We often have to give what we call oral physiological levels of progesterone. I give women natural hormones in a cyclic manner, the way the body should be getting them."

Hormone balancing also can be accomplished through the diet. Fatty diets cause higher levels of estrogen in the system, which in turn can cause menorrhagia. Lean diets and exercising with weights produce more testosterone, which in turn helps balance hormones and put an end to menorrhagia.

NATURAL HYGIENE APPROACH TO AMENORRHEA

Anthony Penepent, M.D., a natural hygienist from New York, says amenorrhea is one of the easiest conditions to correct. Mostly it stems from undernourishment and can be corrected with a diet that includes two green salads daily, using romaine lettuce, fresh lemon juice, olive oil, and some brewer's yeast. You should also include two pieces of fresh fruit and two soft-boiled eggs in the daily menu. When amenorrhea is caused by a thyroid condition, a thyroid supplement is needed. Additionally, if stress is in the picture, the stressful situation must be remedied. For more serious cases, additional dietary intervention is necessary. Usually, small changes in diet are all that are needed. Dr. Penepent says, "Even if the woman doesn't follow a completely natural hygienic regimen and is not vegetarian, she still can get tremendous results simply by increasing the amount of green leafy vegetables in the diet and providing concentrated nutritional sources, such as eggs and unsalted raw-milk cheese."

CHINESE HERBS.

The following Chinese herbs have specific effects on the blood and are needed at different times of the monthly cycle. Dr. Gorman recommends working with a health practitioner to create an individual protocol and monitor progress but offers these general guidelines.

AT THE BEGINNING OF THE CYCLE:

DONG QUAI. High in vitamins A, E, and B$_{12}$, this bloodbuilder can be taken most days of the month, up to the point of menstruation, or just before it begins if there are strong premenstrual symptoms. "You don't want to be building blood if you are having trouble moving that blood," Dr. Gorman warns.

WOMEN'S PRECIOUS. This formula is a tremendous blood builder that is taken for about three weeks after the period ends. Women's Rhythm is then used the following week.

AT THE END OF THE CYCLE:

GARDENIA. Gardenia is taken when the symptoms of premenstrual syndrome (PMS) arise. By moving blood that is stuck, gardenia helps relieve that heavy, bloated feeling. (See also Chapter 28, "Premenstrual Syndrome.")

WOMEN'S RHYTHM. Women's Rhythm helps release a woman's blood. It is usually taken a week before the period to help move toxins out of the organs. (Women's Precious and Women's Rhythm are Ted Kapchik formulas that can be found in some health food stores and ordered directly from Kahn Herbs.)

CAN BE TAKEN EVERY DAY:

FLORADIX WITH IRON. This wonderful product is available in most health care stores. Liquid Floradix is superior to the dry form because it contains more live nutrients.

NATUROPATHIC APPROACH

DIET

Doctors Bar-Shalom and Soileau state that women with amenorrhea need adequate protein, which means eating a number of grams per day equal to half your weight in pounds. They advocate fish and chicken instead of red meat, as well as nuts, seeds, and beans. Second, they advocate eating seaweed of all kinds.

SUPPLEMENTS

Those doctors recommend the following supplements: 400 IU of vitamin E a day; 25 mg of B-complex vitamins a day, 1,000 mg of vitamin C twice a day, and 1,200 mg of calcium a day.

HERBS

Several herbs are good for amenorrhea, say Drs. Bar-Shalom and Soileau.

GINGER TEA. Drink one to four cups of ginger tea each day (made from powder or grated fresh ginger).

BLAZING STAR, FALSE UNICORN, BLUE COHOSH, CHASTE TREE, AND ANGELICA. Mix together equal parts of these herbs and steep 1 tablespoon of the mixture in a cup of boiling water for 20 minutes. Drink three cups a day. You can also combine tinctures of these herbs. Drink 1 teaspoon of the mixed tinctures added to 1/4 c of water three times a day.

TANSY AND PENNYROYAL TINCTURES. These tinctures are used for persistent amenorrhea. Add 15 drops of each to a cup of hot water and take up to three cups a day for no longer than five days.

PHYSICAL MEASURES

Doctors Bar-Shalom and Soileau stress the importance of focusing on deep breathing, consciously giving yourself periods of relaxation, and getting sufficient exercise to reduce stress as much as possible. Thye also suggest types of physical therapy that will help alleviate amenorrhea.

SITZ BATH. Make an infusion of a pound of oatstraw boiled for a half hour in 2 quarts of water and add it to warm bathwater. Sit in the water, which should reach your navel, with your feet propped on a chair outside the tub. Cover your top so that you stay warm. Soak like this for 10 to15 minutes once or twice a week.

CLAY COMPRESS. Sterilize clay by heating it in a low oven for an hour and then grind it and make a paste with water. Apply the paste to your abdomen, cover with a cloth, and leave until the paste dries.

CASTOR OIL PACK. Put a cloth soaked in castor oil on your abdomen and then cover with plastic and then a dry cloth. Rest for an hour.

HOMEOPATHY

Two homeopathic remedies are good for amenorrhea, according to Drs. Bar-Shalom and Soileau.

NATRUM MURIATICUM is for amenorrhea that occurs after extreme mental strain in women who have trouble expressing emotion. Use the 12c potency.

PULSATILLA is for a woman who misses her periods after stressful and emotional situations. Take it in the 6c potency three times a day for three weeks or until the period begins.

Toxic Shock Syndrome

Toxic shock syndrome (TSS) is a rare but serious and sometimes fatal disease. The victims tend to be tampon users under the age of 30, especially those between 15 and 19. This sudden and serious disease affects persons with severely compromised immune systems who are poisoned by a strain of bacteria called *Staphylococcus aureus,* phage group I. This type of staph produces a substance called enterotoxin F, which can overpower and destroy a weak body.

Toxic shock syndrome is linked to the introduction of tampons with four new ingredients in the early 1980s. Before then tampons were made primarily of cotton. In the 1980s, though, highly absorbent polyester cellulose, carboxymethyl cellulose, polyacrylate rayon, and viscose rayon came into use. Three of these new ingredients were soon taken off the market; today only one of the new ingredients, viscose rayon, is in use. Today's tampons are either entirely viscose rayon or a blend of cotton and viscose rayon. In addition, the tampons on the market today may contain an assortment of chemicals, including pesticides used in growing cotton, chemicals used in the manufacture of viscose rayon (lye, sodium sulfate, and sodium hydroxide), and dyes (some of which have been considered carcinogenic since the 1950s).

One theory about the cause of TSS is that the vagina is normally an oxygen-free environment that limits the growth of dangerous bacteria. However, air is trapped between the fibers that make up tampons. When that air is inserted in the vagina along with the tampon, the possibility of toxin production increases. Even after the tampon is removed, some of its fibers may remain.

TSS was originally thought to affect only women who wore high-absorbency tampons, but now it is known to affect newborns, children, and men as well. The initial indications can include a high fever, headache, sore throat, diarrhea, nausea, and red skin blotches. These signs can be followed by confusion, low blood pressure, acute kidney failure, abnormal liver function, and even death.

A severe case of TSS is a medical emergency that may necessitate hospitalization. However, there are many natural ways to support the system once a crisis is over for quick recovery and prevention of recurrence.

NATUROPATHY

Dr. Linda Page, the author of *Healthy Healing: An Alternative Healing Reference,* developed a protocol for healing from TSS out of necessity: "I actually came close to death on an operating table from TSS. I had to bring my body back, and I did it herbally. It took a couple of years, and now I can speak from experience."

HERBS

Dr. Page's personal ordeal gave her a great deal of confidence in the power of natural remedies. The following herbs helped her overcome toxicity, restore immunity, and return to health.

GINSENG. Both *Panax ginseng* and *Panax quinquefolius* (American ginseng) varieties are general tonics that balance and tone all body systems as well as improving the circulation. Ginseng should not be used when there is a high fever.

CAYENNE AND GINGER. These nervous system stimulants can help the body recover from shock. They can be taken internally or applied to the skin in compresses.

HAWTHORN EXTRACT. Hawthorn speeds up and normalizes the circulation and restores a sense of well-being.

DIET

In addition to herbs, Dr. Page ate supernutritious foods that could be easily digested and quickly utilized by her failing system. These foods included high-potency royal jelly, bee pollen, wheat germ, brewer's yeast, and unsulfured molasses. The addition of green drinks, including chlorella, barley grass, spirulina, and wheatgrass, supplied her with high potencies of vital minerals. "All these go into the body very quickly and help it recover even from a death situation," explains Dr. Page. "By going on a program of concentrated nutrients, I was eventually able to create a state of health that was better than before."

PREVENTION

Alternatives to tampons have included sea sponges. However, sea sponges are no longer sold as menstrual products. A 1981 report alleged risks from embedded sand, chemical pollutants, bacteria, and fungi. No additional studies were done, but the U.S. Food and Drug Administration (FDA) halted menstrual sponge sales. Another alternative is called the Keeper, a rubber cup that sits in the lower vagina. The Keeper may hold an ounce of menstrual blood and should be emptied several times a day. This device does not promote the growth of bacteria in the vagina. However, the Keeper is not widely available. Tampons that are 100 percent cotton and thus present less risk than do modern superabsorbent tampons that may also contain added chemicals are available in many health food and natural goods stores.

PATIENT STORIES

CLAUDIA

I had two basic areas of concerns. Number one, I had a very troublesome menstrual cycle. Number two, I have certain characteristics that place me at a slightly higher risk for breast cancer than other women. Because of these two factors, I wanted to go beyond the traditional Western medical approach. Certainly, I wanted to use what Western medicine had to offer, such as getting regular examinations, but I also wanted to take an additional step. That's why I sought herbal remedies and holistic health care.

Back in November 1993 I went to a health care seminar given by Letha Hadady on breast health. I was very impressed by the information that was given. I made an appointment with Letha after that, and the remedies she gave me were very helpful.

Before I had the herbal remedies, my menstrual cycles were extremely heavy, I had mood swings, and I was very prone to exhaustion. I was extremely irregular. When I started taking the herbal remedies, the menstrual cycle became very regular again, approximately every 30 days. The flow was more regular, and the cramping was easier to deal with. The mood swings disappeared, and I became balanced. My own body told me that this was certainly working for me. The herbs have made a fundamental difference in my life.

Chinese herbs are different from American herbs because they are given in combination. They address a number of symptoms at one time, and they are also cost-effective, which I think is important for many people today.

This is something that a woman can choose to use in conjunction with regular health care approaches: self-exams, medical care, proper nutrition, and addressing emotional health.

SUSAN

I had a job I loved, but it was very stressful. I wound up with amenorrhea for a few weeks. Since I am not yet premenopausal or even perimenopausal, I was upset by that.

A friend told me about a product called Eternal, a herbal tincture that contains damiana leaf, saw palmetto, and a lot of other wonder substances that help with hormonal rejuvenation. My friend had been on Premarin for almost 20 years because of hot flashes after a hysterectomy and found great relief from Eternal. I tried it, and to my relief, it counteracted the effect the stress was having and brought my periods back. Everything is back to normal, and I no longer have a problem.

Chapter 21

Mental Health Problems

A s you read this chapter, it may be useful to remember one of the central insights of Jean-Jacques Rousseau, one of the founders of modern thought. Drawing on the findings of the crude anthropology of his day, he greatly idealized primitive life and wrote about "noble savages" who, unlike their civilized counterparts, lived in unrestricted freedom, where they could play as they worked, and where each woman and man moved among equals. Although this picture was a distortion of reality, what still seems accurate in Rousseau's comparison is the idea that civilization brings with it a host of neuroses, anxieties, and psychological distresses that would be totally unknown to the members of earlier social systems.

Anxiety

The most common type of anxiety is called neurotic anxiety, or anxiety neurosis.

CAUSES

Anxiety can have many different causes. Psychiatrist Helen Derosis, associate clinical professor of psychiatry at the New York University School of Medicine and author of *Women and Anxiety,* points to external pressures on women who lead busy lives and have never learned to plan properly and set priorities:

"Practically everyone I encounter in this country is anxious to some extent. One can be slightly anxious or very anxious, anxious occasionally or continuously. The most devastating type involves being anxious all the time over the little things we have to do everyday. People worry that somehow things will not turn out right for them.

"If we compare today's women to those of the 1970s and 1980s, the earlier period had a lot of very young women who were delighted with the women's movement, although they might not have taken full advantage of the opportunities life seemed to offer. Many of them would say, 'Well, I have a college degree so I can do anything I want.' This is not true. You have to work for anything you get. Eventually, they would come to me distracted and anxious because things were not working out well.

"A woman about 25 years old came to me who was very bright and educated and was working for a large TV company. She wanted to be a producer, but was only a gofer, though at a very good salary. She was very upset, disappointed, and angry. She would cry to her husband every night when he got home. Yet as soon as she realized it wasn't possible to achieve that goal so quickly and saw that life was not as easy as she thought, she calmed down.

"Earlier, a doctor or psychiatrist would have treated her with Valium and said her problems were not real, all in her head. Remembering those older treatments, a patient will come in today asking for medication, which is not a solution. Getting over anxiety involves growing. If you can keep growing, you will have problems, but the constant activity of being alive, thinking about what you want to do next, and planning how to achieve it will keep you from being bogged down in anxiety.

"In fact, if we look at women suffering from anxiety, we see there is not much planning in their lives. Women in their fifties and sixties, especially those who are married, expect their partners to make all the decisions and do all the planning. If the partner tells his wife in a reasonable way what to do, she may accomplish quite a lot, but she would not have taken the initiative and gone out and done it on her own. These older women have been constantly dependent on their husbands. Some of them, after being prodded by their husbands, may after a while be able to go out and begin acting independently.

"Today's women are under unique pressures. A large number of women work outside the home, but often have children and household chores as well. They have gotten themselves into the habit of rushing, overworking, tolerating employers who are not very kind. They think they should be doing two or three things simultaneously. But since that is impossible, they develop a helpless fear.

"Furthermore, they hear the cry, 'Compete, compete, compete.' This causes a great deal of anxiety and tremendous distraction if a woman has to keep looking over her shoulder to see if any competitors are gaining on her. Competition is constantly touted in this country as wonderful, but it isn't. The only place it is wonderful is on the basketball court or the football field. It is not healthy in everyday life. These women are not only competing at work; they are often competing with their partners.

"Anxiety often arises when a woman is in a situation of conflict. She is trying to go in two directions simultaneously and so can't go either way.

"An anxious woman will complain, cry, appear distracted, want help, feel helpless and not know what to do with herself. Once a woman told me she couldn't sleep so she got up and scrubbed the kitchen floor and then she felt better. Often as soon as you use your body, you reduce anxiety. I tell women they must do simple physical fitness exercise; they don't have to run miles.

"A woman who faces multiple tasks has to take the responsibility for planning. If a woman has too many things to do, she has to begin by deciding what her priorities are and get things done in order of importance. We all know women who have jobs and families and are working as if they had double or even triple jobs. These women push ahead, but they are exhausted most of the time. Year after year, they don't give themselves time to go on a trip, get their hair done, or take time for the simplest enjoyment."

HOW METABOLISM AFFECTS ANXIETY

From the perspective of orthomolecular psychiatry, practically any nutritional deficiency that affects the mind (and almost all do in one way or another) can cause anxiety as a symptom.

A glucose tolerance test is important in determining whether sugar is being properly metabolized. Anxiety attacks can occur when sugar levels get too low, as in hypoglycemia. Hypoglycemia can also cause a rebound effect when adrenaline is secreted to raise blood sugar levels. This adrenaline rush also causes anxiety. Orthomolecular psychiatrist Dr. Michael Lesser checks out sugar tolerance "rather than getting involved immediately in looking for Oedipal or pre-Oedipal fantasies," because in a recent review of his cases he found that 92 percent of people with neuroses had abnormalities in the glucose tolerance test.

Dietary recommendations based on the results of a glucose tolerance test may help a patient far more effectively, quickly, and safely than either psychotherapy or drug treatment will. The main objective is to create stability so that sugar levels neither drop nor rise too sharply or rapidly. For a hypoglycemic, a high-protein diet is recommended by Dr. Lesser because it digests very slowly, sending just a small trickle of sugar into the bloodstream so that the blood sugar is kept stable for a long period of time. Then, when the patient eats frequently, the blood sugar remains stable. "I have these patients eat six or seven times a day, small snacks so as not to put on weight," he reports. "Actually, they can handle more calories than they could if they were eating one, two, or three large meals a day because the body is set up to metabolize the small meals frequently. When you have a large meal, you cannot metabolize all that nutrition, and the body turns a portion of that into fat."

THE ROLE OF DIGESTION

Dr. Walt Stoll, a board-certified family practitioner who combines his traditional Western (allopathic) training with holistic healing practices, has found that anxiety disorders are often linked to an inability to completely break down proteins during the digestive process into their amino acids.

"Just three or four amino acids still hooked together (peptides), if they get through the intestinal lining, can stimulate the immune system to make antibodies against them. Since the body is also made up of peptides hooked together to make proteins these antibodies can attack us. To an antibody, a peptide is a peptide. It frequently doesn't matter whether the peptide came from outside the body or is a part of the body. It is now being found that many of the chronic diseases that are so baffling to the allopathic disease philosophy of conventional Western medicine are related to autoimmune processes.

"In addition, "some of these peptides have been found to be identical to certain brain hormones (endorphins) that are associated with panic attacks, depression, manic depression, schizophrenia, and other conditions. In these cases—with more certain to be discovered-—there is no need for the immune system to be involved; the effect is direct. The two first examples to be discovered were peptides from imperfectly digested casein (milk protein) and gluten (wheat protein). Of course, these are the two most commonly eaten foods in our culture."

Dr. Stoll usually sees patients after they have tried a number of different therapies. "These patients come with stacks and stacks of records documenting that nothing seems to have worked in spite of every imaginable test having been done and every imaginable treatment having been tried. Psychoactive drugs have either worked poorly or have even caused the problem to worsen because the side effects exceeded the benefits.

"Since every other conceivable cause has been ruled out by the time I get to see them, I am free to look for the things that have not been evaluated. One of the first things I look for is how well the lining of their intestinal tract protects them from their environment. I frequently find that either they don't have the normal bacterial balance in the colon or that they have gone beyond that stage to having candidiasis. *Candida* can escape from our control only if the normal bacteria are not under control. If *Candida* has converted from the yeast form, which is a normal part of the intestinal flora, into the disease-causing fungal form, it further damages the lining so that the leakage of peptides is much greater.

"The greater the amount of peptide leakage, the more likely it is that the brain will interpret these protein particles as being identical to the endorphins it produces during panic attacks, depression, and the like. This leakage is responsible for the increasing sensitivities we see in patients who are sensitive to environmental substances other than foods. In most cases, it is much simpler to correct the leakage than it is to eliminate the substance. But why not do both?"

According to Dr. Stoll, dramatic improvement is often seen once the reason for the leakage is corrected. "The antibodies involved last only for 72 hours. Once the leakage is stopped completely, symptoms lessen substantially in just a few days; even a reduction of the leakage helps. There are many patients today who have had that kind of experience. Not everyone's mental symptoms are caused by poorly digested food playing tricks on the brain. However, in my experience it is the most commonly missed diagnosis and one that is relatively easy to resolve."

CLINICAL EXPERIENCE

20-STEP PLAN

Dr. Helen Derosis has a 20-step plan for reducing anxiety. The first step is to identify one thing that causes anxiety or creates tension, guilt, anger, and so on. "Don't forget that one of the main problems in anxiety is that the person cannot discriminate between distracting and anxiety-producing components of her life. So, I ask her to put her finger on one item.

"For example, one of my patients had a teenage son who was troubling her a great deal. She said her son was coming to the dinner table that summer without any shoes, in his underwear, and with dirty, unkempt hair. She would yell at him, then they would argue, and he would get up and stomp out. Then she'd feel bad because she was kicking him out. In other words, those little details of life. So I asked, 'What is it that bothers you the most?'

"She responded, 'It's his wearing underwear to the dinner table.' Then she added, 'But he does so many things to get me mad.'

"I stopped her and said I wanted only one thing. Then I asked, 'What could you do about that one thing?' This was the second step. Once you have isolated a problem, you have to plan what you are going to do about it.

"I also suggested that she behave in a low-key way, for she had been carrying on just as her son did, and it never got her anywhere. In fact, it made things worse.

"She was able to keep quiet for quite a while and then she thought, 'What if I got him some summer shorts. Maybe he might wear them.'

"So she asked him if he might like them and he said, 'Yes.' She did that, and he wore them all summer. Every once in a while, she would grab them and put them in the washing machine. As a result, their whole relationship changed. But this change involved one of the little details that can make life easy or anxiety-filled.

"I believe that any woman who is willing to grow can benefit from this program. I give my patient an outline. I tell her to start with this and tell her there's no hurry. I ask her to get a notebook and make some notes on the outline. Then she starts my 20 steps. She doesn't have to do every step or follow exactly the order I have given. But as she chooses and works on a step, she should jot down what she is doing, noting the plan she is working out.

"The third step, once a plan has been made, is to follow it. Sometimes it takes a woman a while to get to this third step. She may like the plan but sit around weeks before going through with it. Finally, when she has carried out the plan, she needs to evaluate it. Did it succeed? Did it fail? Did it succeed to some extent or fail to some extent? And why? If it failed dismally, she should choose another plan, and make sure it is doable—that is, possible for someone with her background and experience. If she selects her plan that way, she won't be likely to fail easily. And once she has succeeded, she will be happy with that step.

"A woman can experience the benefits by following up on even one step. It's amazing how quickly she can feel the blanket of anxiety she may have been living under start to lift."

DIET AND NUTRITIONAL REMEDIES

Orthomolecular treatment of anxiety involves approaches that would rarely be thought of in traditional psychiatry. These include metabolic studies, digestive analyses, diet modifications, and stress-reduction techniques.

Dr. Michael Lesser stresses the fact that good nutrition is also important, since junk foods can spur anxiety. Simple, processed carbohydrates such as white sugar and white flour products may give a quick lift to the a person with hypoglycemia, but this is followed by excessive insulin secretion that drives the blood sugar down again, only to be pumped up once again by an adrenaline rush. This episode leaves a person with cold hands, jitters, anxiety, and panic.

Special nutrients can help alleviate this problem, especially chromium—also called the glucose tolerance factor- which helps normalize blood sugar. Zinc and the B vitamins, especially thiamine and vitamin B_1, are also beneficial. Vitamin B3, or niacin, has also been identified as an antistress factor. It lowers cholesterol and triglyceride levels, which are increased by anxiety, and affects the brain in ways that are similar to the effects of tranquilizers. Dr. Lesser is convinced of the efficacy of this nutritional approach, but emphasizes the need to be patient when looking for results.

It may take months for the condition to begin to clear because "the body has been often run-down for a number of months or years, and you have to gradually repair all the cells in the body. The old cells have to die off and be replaced by new ones that are better nourished. The natural life span of cells varies throughout the body. Some, such as blood cells, live 120 days, so you cannot really expect sudden dramatic improvement unless the condition has come on suddenly and you have caught it early."

According to Dr. Allan Spreen, a specialist in nutrition-based medicine, anxiety disorders respond to treatment with certain natural substances. The advantages of treatment with natural substances can be numerous and substantial: by freeing people from having to take more toxic medication, the holistic approach can spare the patient the medication's side effects as well as the extra expense.

"Some amino acids, when given individually," says Dr. Spreen, "can be very effective in calming down the symptoms of anxiety disorders and panic attacks." For example, tryptophan, which has been banned from public sale as a nutritional supplement, "was used as a sleeping agent until there was a problem with some batches of it being contaminated, which caused a syndrome that was related not to the tryptophan but to the contaminant. Some doctors use tyrosine for depression and anxiety. The 'DL' form of phenylalanine is often used on a short-term basis for depression and can be very effective if given correctly. It can lessen anxiety and depression in people by giving them more of an 'up' mood. Phenylalanine is also an appetite suppressant for many people. If they're given correctly, there seems to be no toxicity associated with amino acids, and they're much cheaper than antidepressants or antianxiety prescription medications."

Another nutritional approach is advocated by Dr. Steven Whiting, author of *The Complete Guide to Optimal Wellness.* He argues, "Once we have addressed the question of whether you are eating the proper foods, then you need to take certain supplements."

For Dr. Whiting, key supplements are calcium and magnesium. "We have been told that the B complex is centrally important. Although this is true, the importance of calcium and magnesium should not be underestimated. Remember, at periods of high stress, calcium and magnesium as well as vitamins C, B_1, B_{12}, and pantothenic acid are consumed by the body at a phenomenal rate. One recent clinical study showed that up to 1,200 mg of pantothenic acid can be consumed in a 24-hour period of severe anxiety. With the recommended dietary intake of those nutrients well below that, we can see it is not sufficient for high-stress periods.

"So in addition to these supplements that are commonly given for stress, calcium and magnesium are probably the best weapons we have because of their action on the central nervous system. I would recommend 800 mg of calcium and 400 mg of magnesium every four to six hours, as well as at bedtime. By accelerating that, you can create what I designate 'a natural tranquilizer replacement.' While it should be used only for short periods of time, it certainly can be used for three to five days with no side effects whatsoever."

Dr. Whiting also believes in using vitamin and mineral supplementation to replace tranquilzers. He notes, "A combination which I have used successfully to replace such harmful drugs as Valium and Librium goes as follows: calcium at 600 mg, magnesium at 400 mg, vitamin B_6 at 200 mg, potassium at 1,600 mg, and vitamin B_{12}, 500 mcg every four hours under the tongue. This is used every four to six hours. We have had a phenomenal response with this, in terms of removing people's need for these highly habit-forming drugs."

STRESS REDUCTION

In addition to dietary modifications and nutritional supplements, anxiety may be ameliorated by relaxation techniques, yoga, massage, exercise, and stress management. An orthomolecular psychiatrist will often suggest these approaches before turning to drugs. Drugs, unlike nutrients or stress-reduction techniques, often become addictive. If you suffer from anxiety and then develop an addiction to drugs that were intended to help that problem, you will only have augmented the agony you were trying to eliminate. In addition, the direct side effects that drugs often have may leave you less capable of living a normal, healthy life than you were when you first underwent treatment.

Orthomolecular psychiatry also puts psychotherapy on the back burner. The shortcoming of psychotherapy, according to Dr. Michael Lesser, "is that most people who suffer from anxiety have only a limited capacity to deal with it through insight psychotherapy. There is a real risk and danger that an individual, by concentrating on her pathology—phobias and anxiety—and by delving deep into her childhood and looking for trauma, will become 'fixed' on the idea of her pathology. Rather than becoming more able and competent, she will become fixed in her neurosis and in some cases will become even more anxious as a result of exploring the so-called unconscious. I have seen many cases—I am not saying this occurs in every case; perhaps I am seeing only the failed cases—of individuals who have been in psychotherapy for 4, 6, 8 or even 12 years with no apparent improvement. It seems to me that when a case goes on that long, someone should think about the possibility of using another approach."

Obsessive-Compulsive Disorders

Obsessive-compulsive disorders affect an estimated 6 million Americans. They are characterized by repetitive thinking and the inability to control or put a stop to this thinking process. As Dr. José Yaryura-Tobias explains, these thoughts become urges that are so demanding that it appears to the person who has them that they *must* be carried out. Two of the main compulsions are double-checking and hand washing.

CAUSES

According to Dr. Yaryura-Tobias, "As to why this condition exists at all, we don't have a sure answer to that question. The behavior may result from a learning process that takes hold during childhood… It may relate to changes in neurotransmitters—the chemical substances in the brain that build bridges between nerve cells so that they can transmit signals from the outside into our system or, in the reverse direction, direct us to act to affect the outside world. The key neurotransmitter that is being studied in this regard is serotonin."

SYMPTOMS

Dr. Yaryura-Tobias talks about some of the peculiar characteristics of obsessive-compulsive behavior: "It usually takes about seven years or so for a patient to come in for a consultation, which tells us that the condition tends to occur gradually, becoming a part of the patient's behavioral system in a very, very slow manner. It occurs with equal frequency in males and females. Fifty percent of obsessive-compulsive patients manifest their sickness during childhood or adolescence. Later on—primarily after the age of 40—it fades away, and it becomes very rare after age 50.

CONVENTIONAL TREATMENT

According to Dr. Robert Atkins, there is some common ground between conventional Western medicine and more holistic approaches such as orthomolecular psychiatry, or what he refers to as "complementary" medicine. "Both orthodox medicine and complementary medicine, which is the nutrition-based alternative to orthodox medicine, recognize that if a certain neurotransmitter is in short supply, certain syndromes will result. A classic example is that a serotonin-deficient person will often be an obsessive-compulsive. These are the people who can't get out of the house because they've got to make sure the light switches are off or the gas jet isn't on, the people who have to wash their hands 20 times a day, and the people whose desks have to be perfectly neat. These people are serotonin-deficient."

The difference between the conventional and the alternative medical communities lies in how they address the problem. Dr. Atkins describes the conventional approach: "Now there are drugs that block the degradation of serotonin and allow the serotonin level to lift, but those drugs do a lot of other things: They poison a lot of enzyme systems, and that's why so many people got into trouble with Prozac and drugs like that."

BEHAVIORAL THERAPY

To treat obsessive-compulsive disorders, Dr. Yaryura-Tobias uses conventional behavioral therapy and an amino-acid approach, such as the use of L-tryptophan, along with some other nutrients.

"We basically treat with behavioral therapy. We try to use thought-stopping, exposure (flooding), and response prevention to prevent the brain from repeating the same thought. That is difficult, so we also use cognitive therapy to explain the reasons we think the things we do and try to modify the thoughts.

"Compulsions are the area where behavioral therapy is most effective. We expose the patient, either in reality or in her imagination, to what she is afraid of. If you have fears of AIDS or of blood, you are exposed to blood or taken to the hospital where there might be patients with AIDS. Or you will read articles on the condition.

"If it is contamination from dirt the patient is afraid of, we teach that person how to touch objects and not to be afraid of them. Then we prevent the patient from washing her hands; in other words, she must remain unclean for a while. I'm talking about patients who, when they are seriously ill, might completely use up one or two bars of soap per day. They might engage in rituals of washing for many hours. They may wash their hands sometimes a hundred or more times a day. Some of these patients will also clean their hands with alcohol or other substances. Sometimes their skin becomes extremely raw. I've seen cases where patients require plastic surgery.

"Overall, the treatment takes about six months. With medication there is improvement up to 60 or 70 percent of the time."

AMINO ACIDS AND OTHER NUTRIENTS

People with obsessive-compulsive and anxiety disorders often improve on the amino acid tryptophan. But, as Dr. Robert Atkins explains, "since the FDA [U. S. Food and Drug Administration] ban on tryptophan, pure tryptophan has not been available in the United States, even by prescription. However, some pharmacies will compound capsules of 5-hydroxytryptophan. This compound is an intermediary between tryptophan and 5-hydroxytryptamine, which is serotonin, the neurotransmitter you are trying to build up. The whole idea of supplying a precursor to build up a neurotransmitter that is in short supply is a fruitful approach to treating psychiatric disorders and should, in my opinion, be considered before the use of nonphysiological psychotropic drugs, which have more potential for toxicity."

Dr. Yaryura-Tobias adds, "My colleagues and I were the first to use tryptophan, and with it we were able to reduce and almost eliminate completely the use of drugs for this condition, and we obtained very good results. We were using between 3,000 and 9,000 mg per day.

"Then we used vitamin B$_6$, 100 mg, three times a day. Vitamin B$_6$, pyridoxine phosphate, is a vitamin that is very important for the breakdown of tryptophan into serotonin. The idea behind this was that these patients didn't have enough serotonin in their brains or were very dependent on serotonin or that the normal conversion of tryptophan into serotonin was not occurring.

"When we found by measuring that there was a lack of serotonin, this could be reversed by the administration of L-tryptophan with niacin and vitamin B$_6$. Some medications also accomplish this result, but with medications we face many types of side effects.

"About 30 percent of patients do not respond to any form of therapy. But it is not a closed chapter for these patients either. An investigation has to be conducted. Now that we have brain imaging, we are able to visualize the brain. We can measure, for instance, the metabolism of sugar in the brain. We find, for instance, that the frontal and temporal lobes and the basal ganglia, which are related to Parkinson's disease, are disrupted. We see the metabolism of the breakdown of sugar and also images of an abnormal brain. The same can be seen with some electrophysiological measurements of brain wave tests and so forth.

"Interestingly, work has been going on using pure behavioral therapy before and after measuring serotonin. With just behavioral therapy, we were able to modify the levels of serotonin in the body. In other words, we may not need medication to change or challenge the presence of a neurotransmitter such as serotonin. Behavioral techniques alone may have an effect."

Depression

Depression is a major health problem that can leave an otherwise healthy person unable to cope with the even the simplest everyday situations. It affects roughly 10 percent of the American population, perhaps 25 or 30 million people. This does not include the many individuals who function normally for the most part despite frequently finding themselves in low moods. Two-thirds of those who suffer from true depression are never treated and live their lives in misery without being recognized as sufferers of a mental illness. Often women bear the brunt of the depressive tendencies in families and other societal groups, since women still tend to be in the caregiving roles.

CAUSES

BIOCHEMICAL FACTORS

For the past 30 years psychiatry has been aware that certain biochemical changes which take place in the brain can both influence and reflect fluctuations in people's moods. A change in the delicate biochemistry of the brain is capable of governing how a person feels at any given moment. A physical deficiency in any of the chemicals responsible for maintaining "good moods" may lead to depression, just as a psychologically stressing factor in a person's life may manifest itself in the body by altering the sensitive chemical balance in the brain, also causing depression or low moods.

While psychiatry has recognized this mind-body connection in general terms for the past three decades, it is only in the last 10 to 15 years that it has actually isolated some of the specific brain chemicals involved. Especially important among these chemicals are substances called neurotransmitters, which are released at nerve endings in the brain and allow messages to be relayed throughout the rest of the brain and the body. Perhaps the most commonly known neurotransmitters are the endorphins. They are responsible for pain relief within the body and are thought to be responsible for the "high" that runners experience after exercise.

Mood swings can be traced to a similar mind-body relationship. Scientists have found that a large number of depressed people have significant deficiencies of the neurotransmitters norepinephrine and serotonin. These neurotransmitters belong to a chemical group called the amines which are responsible for the control of emotions, sleep, pain, and involuntary bodily functions such as digestion. Almost 90 percent of these amines are found deep in the brain; because of their importance, the normally functioning body has developed a recycling system, called reuptake, by which the nerve cell takes back 85 percent of a neurotransmitter for future use once the chemical reaction has been completed. Only the remaining 15 percent is destroyed by enzymes.

The metabolism of the neurotransmitters is intricate, and deficiencies can occur for many reasons. Dr. Priscilla Slagle, a board-certified orthomolecular psychiatrist who practices in southern California, states that age or genetics may cause one person to use up amines more rapidly than someone else might. She also points out that a defective receiving cell or reuptake mechanism, or a deficiency of the amino acids, vitamins, and minerals that make up amines, may be the culprit here. The nutrient deficiencies involved may result from excessive intake of caffeine, sugar, alcohol, or tobacco. Sugar and coffee can destroy the B vitamins and the minerals magnesium and iron, all of which figure significantly in neurotransmitter formation. Alcohol and tobacco also deplete almost all the B vitamins, vitamin C, zinc, magnesium, manganese, and tyrosine. These nutrients are essential to maintaining a good mood.

STRESS

Stress is another factor which can contribute to depression. Most people tend to associate depression with what are called major stressors, such as the loss of a loved one, being fired from a job, or another circumstance which upsets one's life in a significant way. However, even the stress associated with everyday living can directly deplete the vitamins, minerals, and amino acids that are so important in maintaining a good mood.

Dr. Slagle explains: "We have found very high levels of the hormone cortisol, which is secreted by the adrenal glands, in severely depressed patients. Indeed, scientists have devised a test which measures the levels of this hormone in the body to determine the degree of depression. When people are depressed and highly stressed, their adrenal glands may secrete higher levels of cortisol, triggering certain enzymes in the body that destroy tyrosine and tryptophan. One would think that under extreme stress the body would compensate for this breakdown by facilitating the survival of these important amino acids. Instead, for whatever reason, these amino acids are used up. I believe that high cortisol levels induce depression in certain people."

SIDE EFFECTS OF MEDICATIONS

Dr. Slagle also points out that depression as a side effect of many prescription medications is common. The list of medications that can cause depression is quite extensive; it includes antibiotics, antiarthritis pills, antihistamines, blood pressure medication, birth control pills, tranquilizers, and even aspirin. When people are given these medications, they often are not warned that they may experience depression as a side effect. Dr. Slagle, together with most other orthomolecular psychiatrists, believes that rather than ignoring the fact that such side effects exist or waiting for them to appear, whenever a prescription drug listed in the *Physician's Desk Reference* (PDR) is given that has side effect such as depression, a nutritional program should accompany the prescription in order to replenish the vitamins and amino acids which may be depleted by the medication.

ENVIRONMENTAL FACTORS

It is common for depressed people to have a family history of depression. In addition to the genetic factor, such family histories may also be due to common environmental factors, shared experiences in depressed families, and poor eating habits that are passed on from one generation to the next.

Environmental factors may play multiple roles as causes of depression. For example, being raised in a family in which one or more people are depressed may often be associated with poor nutrition. As Dr. William J. Goldwag reminds us, "Just being exposed to depressed people can be an influence, since children learn how to behave by imitation. Also, family members are eating the same food, and if, for instance, the mother is depressed and is cooking for and serving her family, that food is apt to be sparse in nutrients since she is interested in just getting the meal over with and has difficulty finding enough energy to prepare it."

Often the children of depressed parents are themselves abused physically or verbally. As a way of handling abuse, a child may withdraw and become depressed and inactive as a defense against very harsh treatment from the parent.

Dr. Doris Rapp, a board-certified pediatric allergist and specialist in environmental medicine, adds that mood disorders often lead to battering of family members and intimates: "Husbands batter wives, wives batter husbands, they both batter the children, and boyfriends batter their girlfriends. Mother battering, I might add, is very common. Many of the children I treat beat, kick, bruise, bite, and pinch their mothers. When some individuals have typical allergies and environmental illness, if they have a mood problem, they can become nasty and irritable and angry. All I ask is, 'What did you eat, touch, and smell?'

"To help find the cause I try to discover whether the change in behavior occurs inside or outside, after eating, or after smelling a chemical. It might be a food, dust, mold, pollens, or chemicals, which affect not only the brain as a whole but also discrete areas of the brain. As a result, the allergen or food or chemical exposure may make you tired or, if it affects the frontal lobes, make you behave in an inappropriate way. It could affect the speech center of the brain so that you speak too rapidly or unclearly, or stutter, or don't speak intelligently. It's just potluck as to what area of the brain or body will be affected when you are exposed to something to which you are allergic."

MAGNESIUM DEFICIENCY

According to Dr. Lendon Smith, a specialist in nutrition-based therapies and the author of many books on that topic, including *Feed Your Body Right: Understanding Your Individual Body Chemistry for Proper Nutrition Without Guesswork,* craving chocolate is also a sign of depression. It usually means that people need magnesium, because there's magnesium in chocolate. The day before their menstrual periods women often find themselves searching through the cupboards for chocolate. They find a big can of Hershey's and drink it down before feeling better from the magnesium.

"I often had the delightful experience of giving an intravenous mixture of vitamin C, calcium, magnesium, and B vitamins," Dr. Smith says. "Usually it has more magnesium than calcium. Afterward I asked patients whether they would like some chocolate and they told me they didn't need it. It really is connected.

"Women in the sixth month of pregnancy will often send their husbands out for ice cream because the baby is starting to grow fast. The woman has a conscious need for dairy products because she knows they will bring her the calcium she needs, but she also says, 'Don't forget the pickles.' She knows somehow that she needs to acidify that calcium source for the baby. She will not get much out of it and she will suffer from leg cramps.

"The chemist I work with in Spokane discovered something about GGT, a liver and gallbladder enzyme called gamma-glutamyl transpeptidase. The range that the lab has is anywhere from 0 to 40. They find these values all over the place. The mean would be about 20.

"What we've found is that if their level is below 20, they're more likely to have some of these magnesium deficiency symptoms: short attention span, trouble relaxing or sleeping, little muscle cramps in the feet and legs, and a craving for chocolate. Most of these people don't like to be touched. They may be a little crabby. Those symptoms go with low magnesium."

Dr. Smith explains that once food has been processed, magnesium is one of the first minerals to disappear. "Magnesium is also one of the first minerals to leave the body when there is stress, which accounts for how many women behave a day or so before their periods. They feel stressed because they're losing their magnesium.

"We need to supply magnesium to these people. We can determine who needs it by the blood test and by the sense of smell. If people smell a bottle of pure magnesium salt—magnesium chloride is a good one—and it smells good or if there's no smell, then the person needs it. The blood test we usually use is the 24-chem. screen, the standard blood test.

"Many symptoms of depression, hyperactivity, headaches, loss of weight, and other conditions are related to genetic tendencies. If there is a tendency to be depressed in the family, a magnesium deficiency will allow that tendency to show up. If there's alcoholism, diabetes, or obesity in the family, low magnesium may allow those things to show up in a person. There are reasons for all these things, and nutrition is basic. These patients don't have an antidepressant pill deficiency; they usually have a magnesium deficiency."

The first thing Dr. Smith does when he sees patients is ask what they're eating. "If I find that they're eating a lot of dairy products and that as children they had their tonsils taken out and that they had a lot of strep throat and ear infections, I know they're allergic to milk and they're looking for calcium. Sure enough, the blood tests will show this. That's the first thing they have to stop. Whatever they love is probably causing the trouble because food sensitivities can cause low blood sugar."

TOBACCO

Orthomolecular psychiatrist Dr. Abram Hoffer tells the story of a classic case of a misdiagnosis corrected, enabling one man to start anew after his life had seemingly been ruined. "A high school teacher and principal about 45 years old developed a severe depression. In fact, I believe he was misdiagnosed as a schizophrenic. He exhibited what we call a straightforward, deep-seated, endogenous depression. He was in a mental hospital for about a year or two and was then discharged. He was so depressed that no one could live with him. His wife divorced him and eventually he was living with his aunt, who looked after him as if he were a child. As a last resort, he was referred to me.

"When he came to see me, which was many years ago, I had just started looking into the question of allergies. At that time, I wasn't very familiar with food allergies, but I thought he was a very interesting case and I said to myself, 'He is a classic case of a depression, maybe schizophrenic. He'd be the last person in the world who would respond to this antiallergy approach.' At that time I was using—and I still do—a four-day water fast. This is a way of determining whether or not these allergies are present. He agreed that he would do the fast, which also involved refraining from any smoking or consuming of alcohol; he had to drink about eight glasses of water a day and nothing else. His aunt said she would help make sure he complied. When he came back to see me two weeks later, he and his aunt explained that at the end of the four-day fast, he was normal. All of the depression was gone.

"This man then began to get tested for food allergies, and he found that not a single food made him sick. But now he began to smoke again. Within a day after he resumed smoking, he was back in his deep depression. The ironic thing was that he had a brother who was a tobacco company executive, who kept sending him free cartons of cigarettes. When we made the connection to his cigarette smoking, he stopped smoking. Thirty days later, after he had been depressed for four years and hadn't been able to work, he was back in school teaching. I remember this clearly because the insurance company that was paying his monthly pension was so astounded at this dramatic response that it sent one of its agents to see me, to find out what the magic wand was that I had waved to get this patient off their rolls. This is a classic case of an allergy to tobacco that was causing this man's depression."

DIAGNOSING THE PROBLEM

Traditional psychiatrists diagnose depression according to the criteria set forth in the DSM-IV (*Diagnostic and Statistical Manual of Mental Disorders*, 4th edition), which essentially defines depression as a condition that includes at least five of the following symptoms during the same two-week period:
1. Depressed mood
2. Markedly diminished interest or pleasure in all or almost all activities
3. Significant weight loss or gain (when not dieting)
4. Insomnia (a constant inability to sleep) or hypersomnia
5. Psychomotor agitation (a hyperanxious state) or retardation
6. Fatigue or loss of energy
7. Feelings of worthlessness or excessive or inappropriate guilt
8. Diminished ability to think or concentrate or indecisiveness
9. Recurrent thoughts of death

While orthomolecular psychiatrists may use this definition as a starting point, they do not confine the diagnosis to these criteria. Orthomolecular psychiatry views depression or any other illness as a unique and individual condition. While there may be certain guidelines, such as those set forth in the DSM-IV, a diagnosis which rigidly adheres to these criteria can arrive at a wrong conclusion either by missing the diagnosis altogether because the person's symptoms are not those normally associated with depression or by falsely diagnosing a person as being depressed simply because he or she has the textbook symptoms.

Often a depressed patient is not aware of the condition, especially when it is complicated by associated physical symptoms. If you suffered from chronic back pain, indigestion, or neck stiffness, would you immediately think that you might be manifesting symptoms of depression? Probably not. You might go to several doctors in search of relief, and there would be a very good chance that none of them would ever consider depression as the root of your problem. Even if someone were to ask whether you were depressed, you might quickly protest if, as Dr. Priscilla Slagle puts it, you "have 'somatized,' that is, put [your] emotional feelings into the body, thereby inducing bodily symptoms."

Sometimes a patient may develop responses to medication that are misinterpreted as purely physical. "For example," Dr. Slagle says, "an acquaintance of mine who lost her daughter through death a year ago became so anxious that her doctor started her on tranquilizers. Although she was on tranquilizers for six months, she got worse and worse. When I visited her, it was readily apparent to me that she had severe depression. It was difficult to convince her of this because she could relate nly to the anxiety and the insomnia she was having. I started her on a nutrient program, and she improved dramatically in two to three weeks. Of course, I tapered her off the tranquilizers, because if they are stopped abruptly, one can have withdrawal symptoms which can aggravate the anxiety."

TRADITIONAL TREATMENTS

Orthodox treatments for depression range from counseling and psychotherapy to medication and electroshock therapy. However, when a traditional psychiatrist arrives at a diagnosis of depression, more likely than not the next step will be to put the patient on antidepressant medication. Some of the most common of these medications are Elavil (amitriptyline), Sinequan (doxepin), Tofranil (imipramine), and Nardil (phenelzine). They are all designed to increase the concentration of the neurotransmitters in one way or another, thereby prolonging their biochemical reaction. Although the manufacturers claim that there is no evidence of addiction to most of these drugs, they are not without serious side effects. The PDR entry for amitriptyline (Elavil), for instance, mentions many contraindications, warnings, precautions, and adverse reactions, including severe convulsions and possibly death if this drug is used improperly with other drugs, complications in patients with impaired liver function, hypertension, stroke, disorientation, delusions, hallucinations, excitement, tremors, seizures, blurred vision, dizziness, fatigue, baldness, and elevation and lowering of blood sugar levels.

Because suicidal tendencies are a common characteristic of depression, perhaps one of the most serious problems associated with antidepressants is the potential for drug overdose. The potential for suicide caused by the very medication prescribed to prevent it is further enhanced by the synergistic interaction of antidepressants with alcohol, barbiturates, and other central nervous system depressants. A glance through the PDR indicates that the quantity and magnitude of the dangers associated with Elavil are equally present with the other antidepressants.

ALTERNATIVE THERAPIES

DIET AND NUTRITION

It is surprising how often diet and nutrition are factors in depression and how effective enhanced or improved nutrition can be in helping someone suffering from depression to improve his or her mood. According to Dr. William J. Goldwag, "Often the quality of the diet suffers in depressed people. If the depression is profound, the individual doesn't even feel like eating. Depressed people who live alone or who are major providers or cooks in the home may not feel like preparing meals or even shopping. They're apt to restrict their nutrition to fast food or anything just to get eating over with." In many cases, weight loss is a symptom of severe depression. In others, there is substantial weight gain.

Dr. Goldwag notes that significant weight loss is likely to bring about "marked deprivation of the essential nutrients, including the amino acids needed to manufacture the proper proteins, as well as a deficiency in many vitamins and minerals. That in itself can aggravate the depression."

Dr. Goldwag suggests straightforward solutions to at least some of the challenges associated with depression: "There are some simple ways to prepare food in advance so that the food has to be prepared less often. I recommend preparing a raw salad once a week. Certain fresh vegetables keep well for quite a while in a refrigerator. There are a whole variety to choose from: carrots, celery, radishes, cauliflower, broccoli, peppers, red cabbage, green onions, snow peas, string beans. They can all be cut up and mixed together. They can be stored in a plastic bag or sealed container. When mealtime comes, a person can take a handful of these vegetables and then perhaps add some other ones that don't keep as well, such as tomatoes and sprouts. You then have a fresh salad that is already prepared with a lot of important nutrients. This is just one way of having food prepared in advance. It's good for people who are depressed and don't have the energy to make a whole meal."

Dr. Goldwag believes that the B-complex vitamins are especially important. "One of the major groups of vitamins to incorporate is the B-complex family. Years and years ago, when people suffered from severe vitamin deficiencies, some of the resultant diseases, such as pellagra, were characterized by accompanying psychotic reactions. That is, the thinking process was the most obvious one to be affected by the vitamin deficiency. Simply providing the proper vitamin, in this case vitamin B_3, or niacin, was the treatment. It cleared up the psychosis.

"There's no doubt that brain function is very dependent on nutrients such niacin and others, because when they're absent there is apt to be some very disturbed thinking. Depression is one of the symptoms that can occur with this.

"It is important to get all the B-complex vitamins, since they work together. Thiamine, B_1, is important, as is riboflavin to a lesser extent. Another important one is B_6, pyridoxine. B_{12} is still another one that can affect the mental processes.

"Niacin is often used in much higher doses than the others to accomplish some of these changes. Niacin is a ubiquitous vitamin. It is being used to improve cholesterol levels, to increase the good cholesterol and reduce the bad. The doses being used are much greater than those used to simply overcome a deficiency."

At the same time, there are plenty of foods that should be avoided. Fast foods can affect mental symptoms by causing blood sugar abnormalities. People who have tendencies toward hypoglycemia, or low blood sugar, should avoid eating too many simple carbohydrates, such as candy bars, which are converted very rapidly to sugar in the blood. As Dr. Goldwag says, "Simple carbohydrate foods temporarily raise the blood sugar, but then they drop it to a very low level several hours later, resulting in depression. This encourages the individual to repeat the cycle of taking sugar or some simple carbohydrate that's converted to sugar in order to feel that high again. This constant seesaw from a high to a low mood can account for many episodes of depression in individuals."

Both alcoholics and chronic dieters often have depressive tendencies. Alcoholics often suffer from symptoms of low mood, and although alcohol may appear at first as a stimulant and mood enhancer, it is in fact a depressant and substantially decreases the ability of the body to extract nutrients from the food we eat. Dieters tend to eat very few B-complex-containing foods, and they often suffer from depression as well.

AMINO ACIDS

A leading authority on the treatment of depression with amino acids and nutritional therapy, Dr. Priscilla Slagle, became interested in the treatment of mood disorders as a result of her own depression, which lasted for many years and did not respond to traditional psychoanalysis or psychotherapeutic treatment. Disinclined to use antidepressant medications because of the adverse reactions which so commonly accompany them, Dr. Slagle discovered that "there are natural food substances that will create the same end effects, that is, elevate mood in the same way without causing side effects or toxicity. I started myself on [a program using certain single amino acids to control mood] and achieved very dramatic results. Although I have had tremendous stress over the past 10 years, particularly the past year, I have not had one day of a low mood. This has been a marvelous reprieve, since I have had and therefore understand the pain that low moods can create for many people."

In her book *The Way Up from Down,* Dr. Slagle outlines a safe and easily implemented program of treatment for depression using amino acids and other precursors required for the production of norepinephrine and serotonin. She is careful to emphasize that people should follow the program under the supervision of a physician. For those already on antidepressant medication, it is not advisable to stop abruptly since they may experience withdrawal symptoms.

Dr. Slagle explains the basis of the program: "It consists of taking an amino acid called tyrosine, which in the presence of certain B-complex vitamins, minerals, and vitamin C will convert into norepinephrine in the brain. This neurotransmitter not only sustains positive moods but also helps our concentration, learning, memory, drive, ambition, motivation, and other equally important qualities. Additionally, it helps to regulate food and sexual appetite functions. Thus it is a very important chemical. The other amino acid used in the program is tryptophan, which forms serotonin in the brain if the requisite cofactors–the B vitamins, minerals, and vitamin C—are present. In addition to sustaining mood, tryptophan has other functions, such as controlling sleep and levels of aggression. People who are quite aggressive, irritable, or angry are often suffering from a marked deficiency in serotonin. Indeed, very low levels of serotonin have been found in the brain of suicide victims at autopsy.

"With these two amino acids, a good multivitamin-mineral preparation is taken to provide all the nutrients necessary to catalyze or promote the conversion of the amino acids into the neurotransmitters."

Dr. Slagle suggests the following dosages for the two amino acids: around 500 to 3,000 mg of tyrosine taken twice daily and about 500 to 2,000 mg of tryptophan. Public sale of tryptophan was banned by the FDA in March of 1990, but the supplement is now available by prescription through most compounding pharmacies. Dr. Slagle recommends that tyrosine be taken first thing in the morning on an empty stomach and then also sometime in the midmorning or midafternoon. Tryptophan, because of its sleep-inducing effects, is taken before bed. Any amino acids used therapeutically must be taken separately from other protein foods, because protein interferes with their utilization. Dr. Slagle also specifies that the amino acids be taken in capsules (tablets can pass through the body undigested) or in the "free form," a preparation in which the amino acids are ready for immediate absorption by the body.

OTHER SUPPLEMENTS

Nutrients that enhance brain function, such as the ones listed below, can improve mental and emotional states:

ACETYL-L-CARNITINE. This nutrient crosses the blood-brain barrier and provides the brain with more energy. The energy it provides is a gentle, not jittery, type energy, and it is especially important for older people, who tend to lose brain cells due to a lack of energy. Between 500 and 1,500 mg should be taken on an empty stomach.

LIQUID ZINC. Dr. Alexander Schauss, clinical psychologist, certified eating disorder specialist, and author of *Anorexia & Bulimia,* describes his studies with liquid zinc: "In our eating disorder studies, we used a multidimensional design and evaluated the affective or mood state of our patients for five years. One of the first things to improve in patients treated with liquid zinc was the degree of depression that they were experiencing based on psychometric instruments such as the Beck Depression Scale, the Profile of Mood Scales, and other indexes of depression. This suggests that we might consider using zinc as an antidepressant. There is a growing concern among many patients, and even therapists, that antidepressant drugs, such as Prozac, may not be safe, and we are looking at viable alternatives. We have discovered this antidepressive effect and have documented it in patients under blind conditions."

PHOSPHATIDYL SERINE. This nutrient is produced by the body but lessens with age. Taking 200 to 500 mg improves the ability of brain cell membranes to receive signals and improves their function. That, in turn, can elevate mood levels, help overcome winter depression, and enhance short-term memory.

HERBS

St. John's wort extract is an herbal remedy for depression that has made it into the mainstream media in recent years. Other plants containing chemicals with antidepressant properties include the following:

Pastinaca sativa (parsnip)
Myrciaria dubia (camu-camu)
Malpighia glabra (acerola)
Lactuca sativa (lettuce)
Amaranthus spp. (pigweed)
Portulaca oleracea (purslane)
Nasturtium officinale (berro)
Chenopodium album (lambsquarter)
Cichorium endivia (endive)
Spinacia oleracea (spinach)
Brassica chinensis (Chinese cabbage)
Brassica oleracea (broccoli)
Lycopersicon esculentum (tomato)
Avena sativa (oats)
Raphanus sativus (radish)
Anethum graveolens (dill)
Phaseolus vulgaris (black bean)
Cucurbita foetidissima (buffalo gourd)
Corchorus olitorius (Jew's mallow)

HOMEOPATHY

Homeopathic remedies can be quite effective in lifting depression. Dr. Gennaro Locurcioas, a homeopathic physician, says that while money does not create happiness, the king of remedies for treating depression is gold, also known as aurum metallicum. Here he describes this and other remedies for treating depression in women (men can benefit as well).

AURUM METALLICUM. Gold is for a perfectionist woman who has set high goals for herself but is unable to meet them. At first she will become irritable, a state that can last for several months. She feels as if she has lost the love of those around her and that it is her fault. This leads to feelings of frustration, accompanied by a strong sense of guilt, which may push her to suicide in extreme cases. Dr. Locurcioas observes, "At first sight, this woman appears perfect and polished. When we start talking to her, we get the idea that there is an abnormal focus on career and achievement. Being a workaholic just covers up the emptiness inside."

ARSENICUM. This remedy is for depression accompanied by anxiety. The woman is restless day and night. She fears being alone and is constantly calling her friends. She wakes up at night and walks around the room thinking about her fears and anxieties. She is afraid of a poverty-filled future and of death. "Arsenicum is from arsenic," says Dr. Locurcioas. "If we give that to a person, he person dies. But giving homeopathic arsenic to a person is completely safe and better than Xanax."

IGNATIA. This helps depression associated with grief. A woman has lost her child or her mother, or has been disappointed by a romantic relationship. The patient may exhibit physical characteristics such as a tic on the face, numbness, a lump in the throat, and sighing. "According to the homeopathic literature, if the patient says that she gets aggravated when she eats sweets and she improves by traveling, these are signs that ignatia is indicated," notes Dr. Locurcioas.

SEPIA. Sepia is a good example of how homeopathic healing uses substances that relate to a person's symptoms. According to Dr. Locurcioas, "This remedy is made from a black mollusk that emits a black ink. Black is the ink from which the remedy is prepared, and black is the color the depressed woman sees around herself. She sees black in her future. This little sea creature, at some point in its life, will deposit about 300 eggs, which are incredibly big for the size of this little animal, and then it will die. This is the housewife who has had a job and has also hdd to come home and prepare dinner for the husband and children. For years, she has given the best of her energy to her family and children. Now she is 40, 45, or 50. The children are gone, and she feels as if her mission in life is over. She sees no purpose in her life anymore. She does not hate her husband, but feels indifferent toward him. She does not want to be touched sexually, and cries many times during the day without knowing why. Inside she feels despair and isolation. Physically, she has a dull, inexpressive face, and the muscles of the body have lost their tone. The woman has varicose voinoj oho io oonotiputcd. Ocpiu io u rcmcdy for the exhausted housewife.

ACUPUNCTURE

Acupuncture frees blocked energy, and in so doing naturally lifts depression. Look at what one woman has to say about her experience: "When I was in my twenties, just after finishing college, I would go into a depression whenever I was about to get my period. It came on so suddenly that it was frightening. I went to see a doctor about it and was given a referral to an acupuncturist.

"After I was in treatment for six months, my practitioner and I sat down to talk about how I was feeling. I realized then that the depression was gone.

"That was 12 years ago. I've stayed in treatment, although not as regularly as when I first started. It's my primary form of health care. My eating habits and sleeping patterns have become totally regulated. I have been able to lose 40 pounds and maintain my weight without dieting. I also quit smoking without ever trying. I never get sick anymore. I never get colds or flus. In general, I'm much more balanced.

"The whole experience of being brought into harmony keeps me from going to extremes. I don't work too hard, I don't play too hard, I don't rest too hard. I manage to stay pretty much in the center of my life. It's a huge improvement. I often wonder how people live without going through a treatment process like I did."

EXERCISE

Physical exercise is another key to lifting depression, especially when accompanied by a nutritious diet, meditation, and vitamin and mineral supplementation. According to Dr. William J. Goldwag, exercise is one of the most profound aids in the treatment of depression: "One of the major errors in the thinking of patients and therapists is the notion that in order to be active, you have to feel better. This is exactly contrary to our approach.

"We recommend that you do first, and then the feeling comes later. In other words, you must do what you have to do regardless of how you feel. This aids in feeling better. You can't wait until you feel good to do something, because in depression that may take days, weeks, months, or even years. You want to accelerate the process.

"Those of us who exercise regularly have had days when we just didn't feel like it. That's the way depressed people feel about everything. They just don't feel like it. They don't have the energy, the motivation, the stimulation to do even the ordinary things. When it's severe, you may not even have the will or desire to get out of bed in the morning.

"The exercise may consist of very, very simple things, like just getting out and walking, getting up and doing some simple movements, some mild calisthenics, any kind of physical movement that gets the body in action. For some people just getting out of bed and getting dressed is a big accomplishment. That may be the first step.

"Another benefit of exercise is a feeling of accomplishment. Even doing a little bit of exercise will make you feel more energized later on. Finishing an exercise routine, even one that's fatiguing, after a brief period of rest will give you a feeling of revitalization and of energy and a psychological feeling of accomplishment. It gives a feeling of 'I've done it. It's completed.'"

YOGA AND MEDITATION

Dr. Michele Galante, a complementary physician in Suffern, New York, overcame depression in adolescence by learning how to center energy with yoga and meditation: "When I was in my late teens, I went through a period of depression where my energy was low. My whole being was unhappy. My parents and others I loved thought I should try seeing a psychiatrist for a while. I went a few times, but that wasn't satisfying to me. I thought nutrition might help, so I started drinking raw vegetable juices and became a vegetarian. I started eating to detoxify myself and to get myself back to feeling stronger again.

"Then I got into meditation and kundalini yoga. I learned about energy centers and started to learn how inner energy flows through the system. I began to sense blockages and to identify emotions and limiting thoughts that were holding me back. Through practice, I was able to center energy into the emotional center in the chest and into the abdomen where stabilizing rootedness can occur. That started to awaken inner energies and to strengthen me.

"The important thing is to not get too hung up in the head, where we have all these conflicts. Our center is the lower abdomen, where a baby grows in a woman. The Japanese call this the *hara*. In Zen we concentrate the mind and the whole being there. That's the hub of the wheel. The mind can be clearer when you do that, and you don't get hung up living in the realm of thought.

"Set aside 10 to 20 minutes daily to quiet the mind, let tensions drain, open up, and resonate with the environment. Everyone does it in a different way. You can do it with meditation or biofeedback. You can do it with music, yoga, a hobby, it doesn't matter what. Anything that takes you to a creative, quiet place and allows you to recharge. Learn to take the time to express your inner needs.

"I like to ask my patients the question, 'Why do we have a physical body?' My answer is always that we exist as a physical entity to carry around our minds and our hearts, in a sense our spirits, so that we can fulfill ourselves. We can then learn and grow and do what we need to do in life. We are nothing without our emotions. Yet we neglect and suppress our feelings. We don't consider nourishing ourselves in a spiritual way. We need some sort of daily practice.

"We have a lot of outward pressures. We have rules made by corporations which are fulfilling needs for profits and ruining resources. There is a huge lack of wisdom across the board. The only thing that can make you happy is looking inward. Bring your mind and energies inside. Sometimes, when you start out, all you see is unhappiness and tension. But if you keep at it, sitting down, breathing quietly, not moving, and slowly bringing the mind inside, you will start to feel a sense of peace, relaxation, and buoyancy. That is recharging your battery. That is the most profound thing you can do to bring your energy up."

Patient Story: Maria

Depression and anxiety are very difficult. You get up and do the things you feel you have to do. But you don't feel like you are in the flow of life. My conditions were probably not that apparent to the rest of the world, but I experienced them as very uncomfortable, and they took away from my quality of life. I felt stressed much of the time. I had difficulty concentrating. At times I would forget things. Someone would ask me to do something, and I would forget to do it. I knew there wasn't something wrong with my mind. I felt my lack of focus was due more to my being so hyped up and tense.

I felt overwhelmed by ordinary, everyday demands, and I felt exhausted by the end of the day. Many times, after lunch, I would feel really tired, almost like I needed to have a nap. Anxiety and depression seemed to gobble up my energy very quickly. By the end of the day, I was not in the mood for recreational activities. Work wore me out. I would just go home and bug out in front of the boob tube. And I wanted more than that.

Once in a while, I would have a drink and notice a difference; I would be able to focus much better. The reason was that the drink helped me relax. But I didn't want to relax that way. I wanted to find an alternative that would really work for me and help me to feel more joy in my everyday experience.

I went to several physicians, and they prescribed various medications for me. But I couldn't take medicines. They had all kinds of strange side effects, which were just as bad as the anxiety or the depression. The drugs masked my conditions, but underneath they were still there. All they did was make me feel very sleepy much of the time. I would be sitting at a meeting, dozing off, and I couldn't afford to do that. So I took only medications briefly.

I was looking for help when I happened to hear a Gary Null lecture at the Learning Annex. I was very impressed with some of the things I heard about limiting belief systems and how difficult it is to see beyond them. I liked the talk on vegetarianism as well. As a result, I went to see Dolores Perri and was very impressed.

Dolores went over my history and concerns. I really enjoyed talking to Dolores because, unlike most physicians I've encountered, she was very relaxed. I didn't get a sense that we were limited by time; we were done when we were done. Basically, I asked my questions and expressed my concerns. It was a very good experience. After we talked, she recommended certain foods, herbs, and supplements.

I have been following a nutritional routine for about two and a half months now, and I have definitely noticed a very dramatic shift. In particular, my hypoglycemia has disappeared. That's mostly from getting rid of refined sugars and processed foods. I used to feel very restless and nervous if I didn't eat. That's been stabilized, and I feel much calmer now.

My energy level is much, much better with a vegetarian regime, supplements, and herbs. The aloe I've been using is outstanding at perking me up at the beginning of the day.

I feel clearer as well. There are subtle differences in my ability to concentrate. And when I go through the day, I feel much calmer. A couple of days ago, I was late for a meeting through no fault of my own. I had to be late for something I thought was very important. Normally, I would be a complete wreck about it. But because of my new regime, I was calm and centered, and I didn't run up the stairs. I just walked in, explained what had happened, sat down, and joined in.

In the past, I would have been practically shaking from anxiety. This is a real departure, which I attribute largely to my change in diet as well as to my holistic orientation.

I think it's important to know that it's not only a shift in diet that has helped me. I became involved in meditation to clear my mind and help me reach that stillness. I do that in the morning before anything else. In addition, I take a greater interest in the holistic world and participate in seminars. All these different elements help enhance my well-being.

Chapter 22

Migraines

T wenty-three million Americans suffer from migraines. One in five women is affected, compared to only one in twenty men, making women four times more susceptible to this widespread health problem.

Causes

It is now believed that migraine headaches occur when a sudden dilation of the blood vessels creates pressure on the brain. There are numerous triggers for migraines. Dr. Mary Olsen, a chiropractor from Huntington, New York, who specializes in craniosacral adjustments and applied kinesiology, gives the eight most common reasons for their occurrence.

ALLERGIC REACTIONS

Dr. Olsen states, "Allergies can be dietary or environmental. Dietary triggers can be foods, food combinations, or additives in foods. Alcoholic beverages, particularly red wine and beer, are among the most common causes of migraines. Tyramine, a chemical found in cheese, smoked fish, yogurt, and yeast extracts, may be involved. Monosodium glutamate (MSG), which is found in Chinese cuisine and most processed foods, is often implicated, as is sodium nitrate, which found in cold cuts and hot dogs. Aspartame, a commonly used artificial sweetener, may lower serotonin levels in the body. Some researchers believe that this contributes to severe headaches. Chocolate and other foods containing caffeine can also be dietary triggers. In addition, people can have allergies to such common foods as wheat, dairy products, corn, and eggs. A person can have environmental allergies to toxic fumes emitted from modern products found in the home."

HORMONAL FLUCTUATIONS

Dr. Olsen explains, "Women suffer from migraines to a much greater extent than do men. Among women who suffer from migraines, approximately 60 percent correlate headaches to their menstrual cycle. The major contributing factor is the hormone estrogen. We know that women who take oral contraceptives are more susceptible to severe migraines and that women experience a lower frequency and severity of headaches after menopause, when there is a sharp reduction of estrogen. Unfortunately, the widespread use of estrogen replacement therapy has resulted in many women having a return of these headaches. Although the exact relationship between migraines and estrogen is unknown at this time, we do know that estrogen affects the central nervous system, including the systems involving serotonin, which can be involved in the development of migraines."

CRANIAL FAULTS

"Malposition in cranial bones or cranial faults is another factor contributing to migraines. Trauma to the head, such as striking the head on a car door or birth trauma, may be enough to lock a bone into a particular position. A whiplash injury may also result in cranial faults."

MERIDIAN IMBALANCE

"Applied kinesiologists and acupuncturists check for a meridian imbalance. Meridians are 12 bilateral electromagnetic channels of energy in the body identified within the Chinese science of acupuncture. Blocked energy, or *chi* (*qi*) within a meridian causes dysfunction, including migraine headaches."

UPPER CERVICAL SUBLUXATION

"Another common cause of migraine is cervical subluxation in the upper part of the neck. This is especially prevalent among people who use the telephone as a regular part of their work. The tendency to hold the phone between the neck and the shoulder forces the vertebrae in the opposite direction. You also see this with people who tend to read in bed. Propping the head up in one direction causes the vertebrae to shift, which puts stress on the nerves and contributes to the migraine."

LOW MAGNESIUM LEVELS

"A number of studies have noted that many people suffering from migraines have low levels of magnesium in their blood. This is also true of people who suffer from fibromyalgia, a myofascial condition that can cause severe pain to the head, mimicking a migraine."

DRUGS

"If you use aspirin, acetaminophen, mixed analgesics, or other acute care medications to get rid of your headaches, you actually may be causing them. The use of these painkillers is the single most common reason for migraines. They are called rebound headaches, and this is why they occur. When you take a painkiller often, the body gets used to having a certain amount of that drug in the bloodstream. When the level falls below that threshold, the body begins to experience withdrawal symptoms. One of these symptoms is headaches. If this situation exists, any preventive treatment for migraine will be undermined."

STRESS

Finally, Dr. Olsen cites stress as a factor in migraines: "Although stress is not a cause in itself, it can exacerbate the effects of a headache or cause an increase in the frequency of headaches."

Symptoms

Migraines differ from regular headaches in that they usually occur on one side of the head. They can be accompanied by nausea, vomiting, sensitivity to light and sound, fatigue, weakness, irritability, and vision problems. An aura sometimes precedes a migraine. Usually, this is a visual phenomenon that may appear as flashes of light or visual distortions. However, other sensory systems can be disturbed, causing the aura to manifest as numbness, tingling, odor hallucinations, language difficulties, confusion, or disorientation.

Clinical Experience

Although the exact treatment depends on a patient's individual needs, Dr. Olsen suggests general guidelines for treating migraines brought on by different factors. Of course, combination approaches are often indicated as well.

THE EIGHT MOST COMMON CAUSES OF MIGRAINE

FOOD ALLERGIES

As Dr. Olsen explains, "Since migraines don't necessarily follow immediately after ingesting a food, it may be difficult to make a connection between a particular food and the resultant headache. We often have patients keep a food diary to record what is eaten and their physical reactions. That makes it easier to correlate foods with delayed reactions. If we suspect that a particular food is troublesome, the patient is asked to place a sample of that food under the tongue. If there is a sensitivity, a muscle that tested strong previously will weaken.

Pulse is also evaluated for such changes as increases in intensity or frequency. Treatment can be as simple as removing the offending food from the diet."

ENVIRONMENTAL ALLERGIES

Dr. Olsen states, "If the migraines appear to be caused by environmental allergies, the British Migraine Association recommends keeping houseplants. Different plants have the ability to absorb different toxins. For example, spider plants absorb the formaldehyde released from particleboard, plywood, synthetic carpeting, and new upholstery, while chrysanthemum protects against the toxic effects of lacquers, varnishes, and glues. If you don't feel like keeping a lot of chrysanthemums around the house, the same effect comes from drinking an herbal tea made with this flower."

HORMONAL IMBALANCE

Dr. Olsen suggests that supplementing the diet with vitamin B_6 and evening primrose oil around the time of the menstrual period may help restore hormonal balance enough to forestall migraine attacks.

CRANIAL FAULTS

Dr. Olsen says, "Since migraines involve the cranial nerves, patients suffering from migraines should always be examined for cranial faults. These faults are extremely difficult to evaluate, due to the subtle movement of bones, but correcting them can be key to healing.

"One of my patients responded only partially to treatment after we corrected other findings that contributed to her headaches. Although the frequency decreased, she still reported migraines. At first, she had a general examination for cranial faults; there were no positive findings. Finally, after examining every single sutral point (or area of articulation) along the frontal bone in the forehead, we found the problem and corrected it. Her headaches stopped. In this case, the patient had an internally rotated frontal bone. Applied kinesiologists find this to be the most common cause of migraines from a cranial fault. This is particularly true if the patient reports eye pain with the migraine.

"The correction for this is done in three steps. First, pressure is applied to the posterior aspect of the palate on the side of internal rotation. Then light pressure is applied on the lateral pterygoid muscle, located behind the upper molar in the mouth. Next, pressure is applied to the medial pterygoid on the opposite side. That completes the treatment."

MERIDIAN IMBALANCE

Dr. Olsen states, "The task of the practitioner is to balance the energy by stimulating the meridians. There are various ways of accomplishing this.

Acupuncturists use needles, while applied kinesiologists prefer to stimulate the meridians with a finger.

"Three acupressure or acupuncture points are helpful in treating migraines. Lung 7 is located about two finger widths from the crease in the wrist, on the thumb side of the anterior part of the arm. Bladder 67 is found at the nail point of the little toe, and gallbladder 20 is located between the mastoid and the occipital protuberance in the skull. These points are stimulated in a circular or tapping motion until there is an effective change."

UPPER CERVICAL SUBLUXATION

Dr. Olsen suggests that migraines caused by upper cervical subluxation will cease with chiropractic adjustment to the proper area.

LOW MAGNESIUM

Dr. Olsen says that for migraines caused by low magnesium, "I have found a combination of magnesium and malic acid to be helpful. A health care practitioner should be consulted because the dose varies with each patient."

MEDICATIONS

Dr. Olsen says that people whose migraines are triggered by medications "must gradually wean themselves away from drugs, with the help of their doctor. When they are no longer dependent on these medications, treatment can begin."

STRESS

According to Dr. Olsen, "Studies in England suggest that the herbal remedy feverfew can reduce the frequency of migraines. Feverfew has sedative qualities and can be taken as a tea. One cup per day is usually effective. In addition, relaxation techniques such as meditation, progressive muscle relaxation, and yoga can help to reduce stress. Regular moderate exercise, such as swimming or walking, also lowers tension and creates a psychological sense of well-being."

Dr. Jennifer Brett, of Stratford, Connecticut, also comments on the benefits of feverfew: "An important study reported by the British Medical Journal back in 1983 found that one to two capsules of a freeze-dried extract of feverfew would prevent most migraines from occurring."

SUPPLEMENTS

In addition to feverfew, Dr. Brett makes the following recommendations: "When feverfew is taken with magnesium in doses of 250 to 500 mg daily and *Ginkgo biloba,* most people notice a significant reduction in the number of migraines, even to the point of disappearance. This includes people who suffer daily migraines. Many people come to me who have had no success with more conventional treatments. After I start them on feverfew and magnesium, they get a significant reduction in the number of headaches and the severity of pain. Even when they have headaches, they tend to be less frequent and less painful. In my experience, this combination will work for more than 70 percent of migraine sufferers.

"Some people find that they need to add the nutrient niacin. Niacin causes flushing in many people, and it is exactly this flushing that stops the migraine headache. When the blood moves out of the head and into the skin in the form of a flush, the migraine can be aborted before it even starts."

BIOFEEDBACK

The July 14, 1998, issue of the *Canadian Medical Association Journal* reported that people using thermal control, a biofeedback technique, were able to control migraines by learning to raise their finger temperatures with a digital-temperature device. They learned the technique in the practitioner's office and from manuals and audiotapes at home. Generally people need about two months to learn the technique. It appears to work by increasing blood flow, which is decreased by nervous tension.

Another biofeedback technique places sensors on the temples, over the temporal arteries. People learn to change their pulse rates in order to diminish their migraines.

OTHER THERAPIES

A variety of therapies can help relieve or prevent migraines, says Emily Kane, N.D., in an article on the website of the American Association of Naturopathic Physicians (www.naturopathic.org). She cautions, however, that people with severe or frequent migraines should first have a physician rule out serious conditions that may be causing their headaches, including diseases that cause seizures, brain tumor, aneurysm of a carotid artery, Meniere's disease (which affects the inner ear), and hemangioma (a tumor composed of new blood vessels).

PHYSICAL MEDICINE

Aerobic exercise, says Dr. Kane, can lessen the frequency of migraines if it is performed regularly, three times a week for a minimum of 20 minutes.

There are many inventive forms of hydrotherapy which involve applying cold to the head and heat to the feet. For example, cold wet packs on the forehead, back of the neck, and head will constrict the blood vessels so that less blood flows into the head. Soaking the feet in a hot footbath in which peppermint and apple cider vinegar are added to the water will bring the blood away from the head and into the feet, and also cool and cleanse the blood. A hot hip bath will also bring the blood away from the head. When the headache is severe, try alternating hot and cold, using towels that are soaked and then wrung out and applied to the face and head. The last application should be cold. You can also alternate hot and cold hip baths.

An enema with cool water may give relief, since migraines are frequently related to wastes remaining in the colon.

HERBS

Many of the herbs that have pain-relieving properties are toxic even in small doses, so Dr. Kane recommends that you consult a qualified professional, especially since different herbs are effective for migraines with different causes. Some nontoxic recommendations are as follows. For migraines associated with poor digestion or depression, lavender, which calms the nervous system, can be added to your bath water or rubbed into your temples. Feverfew works for the kind of migraine that is relieved by applications of heat. Eating three leaves a day has been known to prevent migraines. Willow relieves pain and reduces inflammation.

Dr. Kane suggests that this herbal tea, by cleansing the system, can prevent or decrease migraines:

1 part hops
1 part chamomile
1/2 part oatstraw
1/2 part catnip
1/2 part skullcap
1/4 part peppermint leaf

You can make this formula yourself or order it from Frontier Herbs (1-800-669-3275). Add a heaping tablespoon to a cup of water that has just boiled and steep for three to five minutes. You can add honey to sweeten. Drink this tea two to three times a day.

DIET

One strategy is to fast for a few days to detoxify the body. A glass of water to which lemon juice and a half teaspoon of baking soda have been added can help eliminate waste in the digestive tract.

Certain foods, says Dr. Kane, tend to promote migraines and should be avoided. These include spicy foods; stimulating foods such as chocolate, tea, and coffee; alcohol; and fried food. Obviously, any food to which you personally have a bad reaction should be avoided.

HOMEOPATHY

Many homeopathic remedies can help relieve migraines; the remedy must be matched to the particular symptoms. Some of those mentioned by Dr. Zane include the following:

ARNICA MONTANA. Arnica montana is for treating migraines that feel as though the head is burning but the rest of the body is cool. There is aching above the eyes that radiates to the temples. Sneezing and coughing cause shooting pains. Arnica is also used for migraines caused by head injuries such as concussion.

LACHESIS. Lachesis is for a severe congestive migraine, usually on the left side, that involves vomiting and loss of sight. There is throbbing and a sense of bursting. The headache is induced by sun (chronic). It is relieved by pressure on the top of the head and gets worse if discharges are suppressed (e.g., with antihistamines).

NATRUM MURIATICUM. Natrum muriaticum (table salt) is particularly effective for chronic headaches that involve intense pain accompanied by a feeling of bursting or of compression, as if in a vice.

NUX VOMICA. *Nux vomica* relieves migraines associated with stomach, liver, abdominal, and hemorrhoidal conditions.

The migraine comes on when the person awakes or gets up, after eating, in the open air, or when the eyes are moved.

PHOSPHORUS. Phosphorus is used to treat congestive migraines in which the head throbs. These headaches are made worse by motion, light, noise, lying down, hunger, and heat; they improve with rest. The person feels cold but likes cold applied to the head.

PULSATILLA. Pulsatilla is used for congestive migraines in which the head throbs and is hot. The headache improves with applications of cold or walking slowly outside. It may be associated with overeating and menstruation.

RHUS TOXICODENDRON. *Rhus toxicodendron* is used in cases where the person feels intoxicated or stupefied, as though the head were being weighted down. When the person wakes and opens her eyes a violent migraine comes on. Children may get this type of migraine when they get cold or damp or have wet the bed.

SEPIA. Sepia is used for migraines, especially in women, that are related to nervousness, indigestion, or heartburn, and may be violent or periodic and improve when the person lies quietly. This type is often cured by sleep, by strenuous activity such as dancing, or by long walks outdoors.

SILICA. Silica relieves chronic migraines involving nausea and vomiting that begin at the nape of the neck and move over the crown of the head to the eyes. The headache improves with pressure, lying down, heat, and urination.

THUJA OCCIDENTALIS. *Thuja occidentalis* is used for the person who feels as though a nail were being driven into the top of the head and who has severe stitches in the area of the left temple and pulsation in both temples. *Thuja* is effective for severe headaches that follow vaccination.

ACUPRESSURE

Dr. Kane describes acupressure points which can be used to relieve different types of migraines. A point known as Wind Gate is effective for migraines related to the change of seasons. It is actually two points located at the highest point of the neck just below the hairline on either side of the muscles that run up the spine. You can press these points or put two tennis balls in a sock and lie on your back so that the balls press into these two points.

Another point is in the fleshy area between the thumb and forefinger. Squeezing it can reduce migraine pain and also stimulate a bowel movement, which itself often relieves the headache. A point below the bottom of the big toe can relieve migraines that affect the upper part of the face and the eyes.

A PSYCHOLOGICAL APPROACH

Dr. Kane suggests pondering some themes that make connections between migraines and a person's emotional or mental condition. Insight into hidden stresses that manifest physically as migraines may help you release the tensions that lead to the migraine. For example, Dr. Zane explains, some experts believe that migraines represent an attempt to live out one's sexuality through the head. On a physiological level, the pattern of tension manifested as constricted blood vessels releasing into relaxation when the vessels finally dilate and the pain is relieved can be compared to an orgasm. This type of migraine can frequently be relieved by masturbation, although it may require more than one orgasm to bring relief. Dr. Kane notes further that constipation and problems with digestion are often associated with migraines. This indicates a "closed-up" condition in the lower body.

COLORS

Finally, Dr. Kane describes the use of color to relieve migraines as well as other ills. You can wear certain colors or use gels placed over lamps or other light sources. The colors most effective during a migraine, she says, are purple and scarlet. Purple increases the ability to tolerate pain and makes a person drowsy when a purple light is shined on the chest, throat, and face. Scarlet can be shined on the face to raise blood pressure, though only for migraines caused by decreased blood flow. For migraines that affect the right side of the head, shine blue on the face or the liver for five minutes.

In between migraine attacks, use lemon (said to dissolve bloot clots) and yellow (which works on the lymphatic system and motor nerves) for two weeks. Then use lemon and orange, which act as decongestants, for four weeks. Repeat this pattern for as long a period as required.

REFLEXOLOGY

Applying pressure to the feet can alleviate migraines because specific reflex points correspond to the head area. Reflexologist Gerri Brill says that the greatest benefit comes from a routine that encompasses all body systems. Here she gives a detailed description of her program: All the quotations are by Brill.

CREATING A COMFORTABLE ENVIRONMENT. "I start off by getting you to feel relaxed. Sometimes I use a foot basin to soften and warm up the feet. Then I have you lie down on my massage table while I explain the anatomy of the foot and the idea that each part corresponds to an area of the body. The big toe relates to the head, and the little toes relate to the head and sinuses. Under the toes is a ridge that corresponds to the neck and shoulders. The chest-lung area corresponds to the ball of the foot. The narrow part is the waist area, and at the heel you have the small and large intestines, the sciatic nerves, and the lower back."

RELAXING BREATHING. "There is a special place on the foot that corresponds to the solar plexus. This is a little notch just below the ball of the foot. The solar plexus is the seat of the emotions. By placing my thumb in this little notch as you inhale and releasing as you exhale, I help you to let go of a lot of stuck feelings held inside. It helps promote relaxation and is good to do at the end of the session as well."

WRINGING THE FOOT. "As you lie down, I wring out your foot three times or so, as if I were wringing out a washcloth. That helps the foot relax."

LUNG PRESS. "This is where I press the fist of my right hand into your chest-lung reflex while holding your foot with my left hand. This area is on the pad of your foot, directly beneath the ridge of the toes. As I press, I slowly bring the flat of my fist down to the heel. I repeat this action three times. It is another relaxation technique."

FOOT-AND-TOE BOOGIE. "Next I do what is called the foot boogie. That means rocking your foot back and forth to loosen it up. Then I do the same with your toes. I place my hands around each toe as I shake your toes back and forth. It sounds silly but it feels great."

ZONE WALKING. "Zone walking is performed with the outer aspect of the thumb. If you place your thumb on your lap, it is the area that rests on your lap. It's important to keep the fingernails short to avoid digging into anyone. Using the outer aspect of my thumb, I start way down at the heel. I mentally divide the foot into five zones, with each zone leading to a different toe. Starting at the outside portion of the foot, the fleshier part, I bend the working thumb at a 45-degree angle and apply pressure as I creep up the foot ever so slightly. Each move is no more than a sixteenth of an inch. There are a lot of nerve endings in the feet, and I want to hit all of them. Applying steady pressure, I work my thumb upward all the way to the tip of the toe. When I reach the top of the toes, I go back down to the heel again to repeat the process. These steps are repeated for all five zones. By covering the whole body in this way, I help to create an equilibrium."

SPINE REFLEX. "Now I am at the inside aspect of the foot. That's the spine reflex, and it is very important because the spine supports you and holds you erect. I start at the bottom by your heel with my thumb. Again, I work with the outside corner of my thumb held at a 45-degree angle and walk up your spine. I go all the way up to the big toe. Then I turn around and thumb-walk down, using little steps and steady pressure. I don't want to hurt you, but I do want to exert a good amount of pressure since this is pressure therapy."

SHOULDER AND NECK REFLEX. "Now I move to the ridge underneath the toes. This corresponds to the neck and shoulder line, and it is important for headache relief because when people have tension and headaches, their neck and shoulders are usually tense. Again, I use the thumb-walk. I start at the outside of the big toe and thumb-walk to the ridge. I bend the toes back slightly to get inside. This is repeated until I get to the little toe. Then I turn around and thumb-walk back."

HEAD AREA. "The big toe relates to the head, so of course I want to work this area. I place the fingers of my right hand over my left hand and thumb-walk down the fleshy part of ther big toe. I divide the big toe into five zones and work down each area using very, very tiny bites or steps. My aim is for 25 bites on that big toe. That covers the whole area. I do that five times. This is very important."

BRAIN REFLEX. "Rolling my index finger over the top of the big toe stimulates the brain and relieves aches caused by migraines. Often this area feels sensitive because of crystal deposits that accumulate. These deposits need to be broken up."

HEAD AND SINUSES. "After finishing the big toe, I move to the little toes. Again, using my thumb, I divide each toe into three zones and thumb-walk, using little bites. This is repeated three times on each toe. This is another place where I feel tiny grains of sand. Breaking them up is the main way to relieve migraines."

CLOSING THE SESSION. "Just to make the session complete, I go back to the top of the foot while supporting the heel with the fist. I finger-walk with the right hand between the little bones on the top of the feet. This area helps the lymphatics, chest, breast, and part of the back. Massaging here helps you to achieve a state of balance. Then I work around the ankle areas. The ankles relate to the reproductive organs and alleviate headaches caused by PMS. That's just one foot. Now I wrap up the foot that was worked on and start over on the other side. Afterward, I massage both feet at the same time, which is very soothing. At this point, you know that the session is coming to an end. Once again, I massage your solar plexus area and have you take a deep breath. Finally, I do a nerve stroke to soothe the feet. This is where I ask you to imagine taking in peace and balance with each breath. This promotes a profound sense of relaxation. At this point the session is over, but you should rest a few moments instead of getting up quickly. Just relax and acknowledge how great you feel. Be sure to drink some water after the session to flush out the deposits."

Herbal Pharmacy

Plants containing phytochemicals with antimigraine properties, in order of potency, are as follows:

Myciaria dubia (camu-camu)
Malpighia glabra (acerola)
Momordica charantia (bitter melon; foo gwa)
Portulaca oleracea (purslane)
Phyllanthus emblica (emblic)
Rosa canina (rose)
Capsicum annuum (bell pepper)
Capsicum frutescens (cayenne)
Carya glabra (pignut hickory)
Nasturtium officinale (berro)
Spinacia oleracea (spinach)
Phaseolus vulgaris (black bean)
Carya ovata (shagbark hickory)
Oenothera biennis (evening primrose)
Helianthus annuus (sunflower)
Allium schoenoprasum (chives)
Chondrus crispus (Irish moss)
Basella alba (vinespinach)
Brassica chinensis (Chinese cabbage)

Patient Story: From Dr. Olsen

A patient of mine complained of having headaches once a month, two days before her period. They occurred on the left side of her head and were debilitating, resulting in extreme fatigue and irritability. During this time, she felt that she was of no use to herself or her family, and she would go into a depression.

We made several recommendations. The first was a regular program of exercise, which for her meant walking daily. Exercise helps raise the level of endorphins in the body. Endorphins are the body's natural pain reliever and tend to elevate mood.

Our diet recommendations included the restriction of salt, caffeine, alcohol, and sugar. We added 200 mg of magnesium glyconate and a gram of fish oils each day. Many patients respond well to this.

It is also important to allot extra sleep at this time, particularly for women who have hormonally related migraines.

Her treatment was completed with a balancing of the cranial bones, which allowed the pituitary, the master gland that influences the menstrual cycle, to function properly.

Chapter 23

Multiple Sclerosis

P
eople sometimes ask me a rather disconcerting question: "Gary, don't you get depressed by always concentrating on disease and the human body's weaknesses? Aren't you dispirited by always hanging around sick people?"

The flip answer would be to say, "Well, if they are hanging around with me, they won't be sick long. I won't let them be." If I said that, it wouldn't mean I'm a miracle worker, but more that I demand discipline of people who are in one of my recovery groups. I expect anyone who stays in my program to do the juicing, the vegan diet, the exercise, the stress reduction, and all the other things that are necessary to a healthy lifestyle. Anyone who takes up such a life-affirming way of being will certainly see a change for the better in her health.

But there's a more philosophical answer I might give. The more I study the human body, the more I see its delightful complexity and astounding self-healing powers.

Take myelin. A problem with myelin, the casing of the nerves, is what is resposible for multiple sclerosis. But think of how complex myelin is as a substance.

You know that the body grows in stages, and not just in the womb. It is not till puberty, for instance, that most sexual characteristics appear, such as a deeper voice for boys or breasts for girls. The myelinization of the brain is even more staggered. As Nicholas Anastasiow reports in *Development and*

Disability, "Major transitional stages of development [of the human] are associated with areas of brain maturation, usually accompanied by increased myelinization and arterial blood flow." These transitional periods occur not only in infancy and childhood; further developments happen at ages 14 to 16 and at about 22 and 33 years of age.

This is just one of the myriad examples of how complexly the body's growth is programmed. Now, when myelinization is not working properly, there will be problems, as with multiple sclerosis.

What Is Multiple Sclerosis?

Dr. Michael Wald, supervisor of nutritional services at Advanced Medical of Mount Kisco, New York, holds degrees in nutrition and chiropractic and is a certified clinical nutritionist. He has authored five books about health. "Multiple sclerosis is a syndrome of progressive nerve disturbances," he explains. "What we have is a gradual loss in myelin, which is part of the outer covering of the nervous system. The nervous system breaks down." The disease seems to target females; 60 percent of cases of the disorder are found in women. Moreover, it strikes them when they are young.

Dr. Wald elaborates, "MS is a condition that can be quite shocking when it first presents itself. A woman could one day be quite healthy—it's usually a young person between the ages of 18 and 23—and then she will have sudden problems moving her limbs, muscle weakness, and problems with perception and feeling things. Her vision could be blurred. She could be quite dizzy.

"Generally the person will go to a neurologist and the neurologist will take an MRI. Maybe he will take some of the patient's cerebrospinal fluid and look for things. Then the doctor says, 'You've got the disease.' Then the person is put on one of several steroids and that is the end of that.

"That's really not enough. There is enough nutritional and medical literature to support the use of a whole host of dietary and nutritional changes in the lives of these people. What we want to do in natural medicine is slow down and reverse the degeneration of myelin. When myelin breaks down, it's called demyelinization. In about two-thirds of the cases of MS, the onset is between 20 and 40. We are talking about the most fit people in the prime of their lives, being struck with this condition."

Possible Causes

No one pretends to know the causes of MS. Some postulate that it is due to a virus. Often, a person will have a viral problem and will get MS shortly thereafter. So that may be a cause or a trigger. Yet, Wald cautions, "Human beings are complicated, as we well know, so even if we knew the cause, we would still want to approach it from a natural medicine perspective by giving the body whatever it needs to help whatever it wants to correct. Whether it's MS or a headache or some other problem, the natural healer strives to give the body what it needs."

The theory that MS is caused by a virus is based on animal studies. "Certain viruses can be given to certain animals, for example, which will cause every single symptom of MS. So it's not unreasonable. The common viruses they think might be involved in causing MS are the rabies virus, herpes simplex virus, and the parainfluenza virus. So natural approaches should be antiviral in nature. We want to think of echinacea, astragalus, goldenseal."

Multiple sclerosis is classified as an autoimmune disease. An *autoimmune disease* is one in which the immune system fails to recognize a component of the body's systems as "self" and mounts an attack on that component. For example, says Wald, "The body may be breaking down the myelin, causing symptoms of MS. So anything we do to slow that down or reverse it should theoretically help."

He adds, "in autoimmunity, the problem with immune breakdown occurs eventually to everyone as aging happens, so we are really talking about a situation that will affect everyone."

Treatment

DIET

In terms of diet the first thing, in Wald's opinion, is to indentify and eliminate food allergies. He remarks that allergies also indicate problems with the immune system. "An allergy means that the immune system becomes hyper-responsive. We already have that going on in MS, so we don't want to create any other hyperresponsiveness with foods."

A number of foods commonly cause allergies, including gluten-containing foods such as barley, rye, oats, and wheat. "These are common offenders. Also milk products fit this category. In fact, the intake of milk in adolescents is cor-related with a far higher MS incidence. That much has been proven."

How would a woman determine if she was allergic and what she was aller-gic to? Wald says, "You can do what is called an IgG4/IgG1 combination test for allergy, which is a blood test. Ninety foods can be checked, and you can deter-mine quite quickly how your immune system hyperresponds to some of them. Then you eliminate the foods and use substitutes. Another way to approach this would be to look at your diet for the top 10 or 15 foods that you eat most often or that are your favorite and eliminate them, because those best-loved foods tend to be the allergy foods. Even allergists recognize this."

Wald adds, "Most people find it strange that their favorite foods are what are getting them into trouble. A woman will say, "But I eat the food all the time." Yes, but you are also causing some disruption of the immune function by doing that, particularly if you have a weak immune system to begin with."

By eliminating these foods, "You will reduce overall stress on the immune system. That means healing has a chance to take place."

Aside from allergens, other foods to be avoided in relation to this disease are animal fats. "A high intake of saturated fats in the diet, animal fats, is definitely linked to MS."

Wald notes that some studies have supported vegetarianism as a positive path for MS sufferers. "Dr. Roy Swank, professor of neurology at the University of Oregon Medical School, did one of the longest studies of MS ever done, which was about 26 years in duration. People who had MS symptoms were put on essentially a vegan diet, cod liver oil, and several other similar things. Over time he noticed that those on this diet who initially had symptoms had fewer exacerbations and less worsening of their condition over the years or had no exacerbations and did very well or better in comparison to those who had an initial MS diagnosis and were given the standard drugs."

SUPPLEMENTATION

Another important avenue to explore is supplementation. Wald told me about an unusual new supplementation therapy developed at Harvard. "One practical suggestion is something called myelin basic protein. This is something that you or anyone can buy in the health food store. Harvard has investigated reactions with MS patients, using oral myelin from a cow, actually. Basically, if you eat myelin, the stuff in the nervous system will attack the myelin you are eating, leaving your nervous system alone and giving it a chance to repair. The technical term for that is molecular mimicry. You are mimicking your myelin, so it's a distraction technique. That's very important."

Less experimentally, there are certain supplements of proven effectiveness, particularly the omega-3 and omega-6 fatty acids. Wald notes, "Most of the readers probably know something about these. Evening primrose oil is an example of an omega-6. We get that from grains and seeds. The omega-3s can be obtained from such things as flaxseed oil and fish oil. There are dozens of other types of fats that are important. I do recommend that those with MS have what is called an essential fatty acid blood test done, so you can find out exactly what oils you need and then simply put them back."

These oils control inflammation in the body and immune function. They also are needed for vascular function—in other words, all the things we need for healing MS. Dr. Wald says that even if you don't have these special tests done, you certainly would want to at least purchase a supplement that contains a reasonable balance of omega-3 and omega-6 oils. Probably, you should look for one that is heavier on the omega-3 oils, the flax and fish oils.

"I myself find that MS patients have difficulty metabolically breaking flaxseed oil down into what they need. So, rather than flax, I tend to recommend what is called ephedra, a supplement. For dosage, you should follow the directions on the bottle unless you are seeing a health care practitioner who can individually tailor the dose."

Another very important nutrient for MS is glutathione. This amino acid is the major immune booster in the body. If you are going to help your health, regardless of what the concern is, you have to somehow raise glutathione levels. Wald recommends anywhere from 250 to 500 mg orally.

Selenium helps the body utilize the glutathione. The recommended dose would be in the 200-400 mcg range.

Vitamin B_{12} is also extremely important. Dr. Wald says, "Alcoholics, for example, can have the shakes, which are caused by degeneration of their myelin, due to a B_{12} deficiency. This seems very similar to the problems of MS. So, though a B_{12} deficiency is probably not the cause of MS, many MS sufferers have a B_{12} imbalance, one that doesn't necessarily show up on a blood test. So every MS patient we see gets a B_{12} shot. Oral supplements might do it, but it really depends on the level of disability."

Enzymes are also extremely important. As Wald puts it, "Any conversation about autoimmune disease would not be complete without speaking about them. Bromelain and papain are plant-derived enzymes. They are pancreatic enzyme supports."

Wald notes that these enzymes are key to defending the body against autoimmune chemicals in the blood which irritate and break down tissues. Enzymes that you eat like bromelain, papain, and others found in fresh fruits or vegetables, as well as pancreatic enzymes, get into the blood and literally digest some of these irritating chemicals. It's a must to include lots of those enzymes.

"Lastly," Dr. Wald says, "some other supplements should be mentioned. One is N-acetyl-cysteine (NAC). Cysteine and methionine are sulfur-containing amino acids that help liver detoxification and overall body detoxification. So any anti-autoimmune approach should contain generous amounts of NAC, between 250 to 1,000 mg orally. It works really well orally. The NAC increases glutathione levels. As we said earlier, glutathione is the single most important immune-boosting chemical in the body."

HERBS, OXYGEN, EXERCISE

Wald also uses extracts of herbs that are standardized, meaning they have been assayed for the active ingredient. "In other words," he says, "what the bottle says is in there, is in there." The herbs goldenseal, astragalus, and echinacea are the ones most often recommended for autoimmune disorders.

He mentions a common criticism of herb use. "I do want to recall a question I often field about herbs. A person will ask, 'If MS is a case of the ultrasensitization of the immune system, would you want to take herbs that would bolster the immune system?'

"Well, the wonderful thing about how nature has worked this out is that these supplements will not enhance immunity. They are what are called biologic response modifiers. They work to balance what is wrong. If your immunity is too high, they will work to bring it low. If your immunity is low, they will bring it up. Of course, you can abuse these things to a certain point. But almost no one, if she follows the general directions on the bottles, will be caused any harm. The most the person will experience is a little gastrointestinal upset, and once she experiences that she will naturally decrease the dose." In taking herbs, no matter which ones, Dr. Wald recommends a four-day-on, four-day-off cycle, so the body doesn't become insensitive to the herbs, which could result in the herbs losing some of their effectiveness.

He also notes that work has been done with oxygen in aiding sufferers from this illness. "Something not commonly talked about in MS is hyperbaric oxygen. It is possible—and there are many studies on this with MS—for a person to get into a chamber and be exposed to clean, purified oxygen under pressure for health reasons. The purpose of the pressure is to increase oxygen levels in the blood so that healing can take place. As we age—and you can think of MS as accelerated aging of the immune and nervous system—we do not use oxygen well and so tissues break down, producing lots of free radicals. Anything that helps prevent or reverse that has to be healthy just in general. So for those with less severe cases of MS, hyperbaric oxygen will be quite valuable."

In his experience, the effectiveness of exercise for those with MS depends very much on the individual. "Sometimes exercise worsens MS and sometimes it helps it. I think the reason is that if someone's nutritional status is lousy, and the person is exercising, she is only increasing her stress. So, you want to have a complete holistic program where supplements, diet, exercise, and stress reduction are all combined intelligently."

Chapter 24

Osteoporosis

O steoporosis (the word means "porous bones") is a serious problem in which the skeletal system weakens and fractures easily. More females than males become afflicted, with postmenopausal women being at greatest risk. Osteoporosis is attributed to the gradual loss of calcium, a process which begins in a woman's mid-thirties at a rate of 1 to 2 percent a year, and which can increase during menopause to a rate of 4 to 5 percent a year.

Causes

According to Dr. Jane Guiltinan, the most likely candidates for osteoporosis share a number of characteristics:
Northern European ethnic origin
Small frame
Family history of osteoporosis
Diet high in meat, caffeine, sugar, refined carbohydrates, and phosphates (found in sodas and processed foods)
Cigarette smoking
Alcohol use
Sedentary lifestyle

It may surprise some people to learn that dairy foods, while rich sources of calcium, can also contribute to the condition of osteoporosis. Registered nurse and acupuncturist Abigail Rist-Podrecca notes, "When I was in China, we noticed that no dairy was used. We expected to see a high incidence of osteoporosis, rickets, and other bone problems. In fact, we saw the lowest incidence. In the West, dairy is used a lot and osteoporosis is rampant. Something is not quite right here." The main factors responsible for the Chinese not getting osteoporosis, she learned, are diet, weight-bearing exercise, and acupuncture. (See below.)

Symptoms

According to herbalist Susun Weed, author of *Menopausal Years the Wise Woman Way*, early warning signs of osteoporosis include: persistent backache, especially of the lower back: sudden or severe gum problems; sudden insomnia or restlessness; cramps in legs or feet at night; and a gradual loss of height. Osteoporosis is accompanied by continued pain, frequent, spontaneous fractures due to decrease in bone mass, and body deformity.

Clinical Experience

CONVENTIONAL APPROACH

Synthetic estrogen is the traditional drug of choice for postmenopausal osteoporosis prevention, but controversy surrounds its safety and effectiveness. (See Chapter 6, "Breast Cancer," and Chapter 19, "Menopause.")

NATUROPATHIC APPROACH

The first step in osteoporosis prevention is noting whether or not you are at high risk for the condition, says Dr. Guiltinan. Obviously, certain risk factors cannot be changed, but many can be addressed, and will prevent the destructive effects of the disease.

DIET

A diet that is low in animal products and high in plant foods promotes bone growth and repair. Green leafy vegetables contain vitamin K, beta carotene, vitamin C, fiber, calcium, and magnesium, which enhance the bones. Other calcium-rich foods include broccoli, milk, nuts, and seeds. Sesame seeds have high calcium content. The Chinese, who as mentioned earlier have low rates of osteoporosis, use sesame often in their foods, and cook with sesame seed oil.

Foods to avoid include sugar, caffeine, carbonated sodas, and alcohol, as these contribute to bone loss. Too much protein from chicken, fish, eggs, and meat are also contraindicated. These are high in the amino acid methionine, which the body converts into homocysteine, a substance that causes both osteoporosis and atherosclerosis.

VITAMINS AND MINERALS

Women over 25 need adequate calcium, approximately 1,000 mg in supplement form, and an additional 500 to 1,000 mg from the diet. After 40 years of age, 1,500 to 2,000 mg is needed. Women on estrogen replacement therapy require between 1,200 and 1,500 mg.

In addition to calcium, the following nutrients are critical for keeping bones strong:

Magnesium (500–600 mg in citrate form)
Vitamin D (400 IU)
Vitamin C (1,000 mg)
Vitamin K (100 mcg)
Beta carotene
Selenium (75–150 mcg)
Boron (3 mg)
Manganese (5 mg)
Strontium
Folic acid (1 mg)
Silica
Copper
Zinc

A balanced vitamin/mineral supplement will provide most of these nutrients. It is best to take zinc separately, however; otherwise, it can have an adverse effect on vitamin and mineral absorption.

NATURAL HORMONES

NATURAL PROGESTERONE. Research indicates that natural progesterone from wild yams is safer and more effective than estrogen in that it builds strong bones and has no harmful side effects. Dr. Guiltinan notes that "Estrogen minimizes calcium loss from bones, but progesterone can actually put calcium back into bones." Natural progesterone can be taken in pill form. It also comes as a cream. Half a teaspoon should be rubbed into the skin over soft tissue and the spine, twice a day, for two weeks out of every month.

DHEA. This precursor to estrogen and testosterone is important in preventing numerous chronic conditions associated with aging. As we get older, there is often a drop in DHEA. If blood levels are low, 5 mg a day can safely be taken as a supplement.

HERBS

Susun Weed recommends horsetail, taken as a tea every day, to restore bone strength and density. She adds that dandelion root tincture will promote absorption of calcium. The micronutrients that are also important for bone flexibility and strength are found in the greatest abundance in seaweeds, dandelion, and nettles and in organic vegetables and grains.

EXERCISE

Dr. Howard Robins, director of the Healing Center in New York City and coauthor of *Ultimate Training* and *How to Keep Your Feet & Legs Healthy for a Lifetime,* stresses the importance of weight-bearing aerobic and weight-lifting exercises for the prevention of osteoporosis

AEROBICS. Aerobic exercises use major muscle groups in a rhythmic, continuous manner. Weight-bearing aerobic exercises such as brisk walking, jogging, stair climbing, and dancing produce mechanical stress on the skeletal system, which drives calcium into the long bones. Non-weight-bearing aerobic exercises such as biking, rowing, and swimming are not as helpful in osteoporosis prevention, but they do promote flexibility, which is useful for women prone to arthritis. "Women as well as men need to perform aerobic exercises anywhere from three to five or six times a week," says Dr. Robins. "You need a day off every third or fourth day so that the body can heal and reenergize."

WEIGHT TRAINING. "Most women stay away from weight training because they are afraid of developing, huge muscles like Arnold Schwarzenegger," says Dr. Robins. "The good news is, that won't happen. No matter how hard you train, you will never get huge muscles as a woman unless you take steroids to alter your body's metabolism."

Not only is weight training safe, it is important for preventing osteoporosis. As muscles are pulled directly against the bone, with gravity working against it, calcium is driven back into the bones. It also stimulates the manufacture of new bone. This adds up to a decrease in the effects of osteoporosis by 50 to 80 percent. Women need to do weight training two to three times per week for 15 to 30 minutes. All the different muscle groups should be worked on. Give your body 24 hours between sessions to rest muscles. For best results, an exercise program should be started long before the onset of menopause.

WARM-UPS. A complete routine is more than aerobic and weight-training exercises only. It incorporates warm-ups at the beginning and cooldowns at the end of a routine. Warm-ups are not to be confused with stretches. Rather, they are gentle exercises that produce heat by getting blood to flow into the muscles. To warm up leg muscles, for example, one could lie down on one's back and move the legs like a bicycle, or walk gently in place. Moving the arms and joints gently in all their ranges of motion will warm up the upper body. Warming up the body helps prevent injuries.

COOLDOWNS AND STRETCHES. After exercise, when the body is loosest, stretching is performed. Stretches are long, continuous pulls, not bounces. Bouncing only tightens the muscles and can lead to injury. Robins's book *Ultimate Training* describes a holistic workout in detail.

AROMATHERAPY. Aromatherapist Ann Berwick adds that essential oils enhance a warm-up and cooldown routine. "Before exercise, use warming and stimulating oils, such as black pepper, rosemary, ginger, and sage. Additionally, eucalyptus helps to deepen breathing. After exercise, you can apply a blend of lemon, rosemary, and juniper. These help to carry away waste products and to ease any stiffness."

YOGA

Yoga prevents osteoporosis in four ways: it builds and fortifies bone mass; it keeps muscles strong and flexible; it improves posture; and it helps balance and coordination. Physical therapist and yoga teacher Bonnie Millen explains why this is important: "With yoga, the old adage 'Use it or lose it' applies. Building and maintaining bone mass is most important for preventing osteoporosis. Remember, bone is alive. Yoga is unique in that it incorporates weight bearing on the upper extremities. Fractures of the wrist, forearm, and upper arm are common in women because as they fall they tend to reach forward with outstretched arms. Yoga has postures that involve weight bearing on the arms.

"Also important is building and maintaining muscle strength and flexibility. Let's keep the muscles strong so that they can receive the stress before the fracture happens. Also if the body is strong and flexible, it can cushion falls when they occur.

"Good posture improves overall functioning and prevents osteoporetic fractures of the spine. I teach yoga to a lot of older women who tell me they are afraid of getting a dowager's hump. This is where the body slouches forward and there is a hump on the back. Just take a moment to get into that posture where your chest caves in and your shoulders slump forward, with your head looking down toward the floor. Try to raise one arm up as if you wanted to touch the ceiling, and see how high the arm comes up. Now let the arm down and come into a nice seated posture, as if someone were going to take your picture. Sitting very tall, raise your arm up and see how high it goes. You can see from that little exercise that the slouched posture really decreases your range of motion. That makes it difficult to function. This is why you want to keep a good posture.

"By placing great pressure on the spinal vertebrae, the dowager's hump often leads to compression fractures of the spinal column. This is very painful, as you can well imagine, and you do not have to do anything special for it to happen. Just going up and down stairs or taking a step can cause breakage.

"The fourth way yoga helps is by improving balance and coordination. When you are balanced and coordinated, there is less chance of your falling in the first place. You are quicker to respond. And that can help prevent fractures."

Millen says that the best time to begin yoga is before osteoporosis sets in: "The time to begin a yoga practice, or any exercise, is not when you've gotten to menopause, and all of a sudden you realize, 'Oh my gosh! I'm at risk for osteoporosis.' You need to build bone mass throughout your whole life so that you have bone stored up. It's like preparing for retirement. You build up bone mass through exercise, you eat right, you maintain a healthy lifestyle. Then, when you reach your menopausal years, you've got a good store of bone mass to help protect you."

Millen points out that there are several styles of yoga but that all systems have foundation poses that address the above needs. Here she outlines a few basic postures:

DOWNWARD-FACING DOG. This posture strengthens bone mass in the wrists and arms. In this pose, you stand and bring your hands to the floor so that the space beneath you is triangular. One part of the triangle is from your hands to your hips, and the other part is from your hips to your heels. The space on the floor between your hands and your feet is the third part. As you hold the position, you will feel that you are bearing weight on your arms.

WARRIOR POSES. These poses increase muscle strength and flexibility, as well as balance. Here you are standing with your legs 3 to 4 feet apart, depending on your height. With your legs apart, you work at the hip to turn one leg out to the side. The other leg is turned slightly inward. That really works the hip muscles, which is important in helping to prevent the all-too-common osteoporetic hip fracture. The arms are either held out to the side or up over the head, depending upon which warrior posture it is.

COBRA. This is a back-bending pose that helps posture and gives flexibility and strength to the paraspinals, the muscles of the back of the spine. To begin, lie face down on the floor. Using the back muscles, sequentially lift the head and chest away from the floor.

SIMPLE STRETCH FOR CHEST MUSCLES. This is another exercise for improving posture that is especially helpful for women who tend to slouch forward. Take a blanket and fold it to resemble a box of long-stemmed roses. Lie on your back along the length of this bolster, making sure that your head and your entire spine are completely supported. Place your arms out to the side or up to form a V-shaped position with the palms facing up toward the ceiling. Just allow gravity to relax the shoulders down to the floor (shoulders should not be on the blanket). Breathe deeply. That will expand the intercostals, the muscles between the ribs. This is important because the intercostals become constricted with slouching. That, in turn, decreases lung capacity and causes all the organs to become compressed. This is a wonderful pose where you don't have to actually do anything. You just allow gravity to work for you and your breath to move through you.

BODY ROLLING

This technique, developed by Yamuna Zake, a bodyworker in New York City, uses a 6- to 10-inch ball in a series of routines designed to elongate muscles and increase blood flow in all parts of the body. As you relax your body weight onto the ball, the ball applies pressure onto bone, stimulating even bone that has begun to ossify to "wake up." "To me," says Zake, "bone is like dried fruit. Just as a raisin plumps up after you put it in water, when bone is stimulated and becomes alive it undergoes a subtle change, acquiring a supple quality.

"Studies have found that, by stimulating bone, weight-bearing exercise can prevent and possibly reverse osteoporosis. Weight bearing is nothing more than pressure exerted on bone. Body Rolling is actually a mild form of weight-bearing exercise in which the pressure is never more than the person's own body weight. My clinical experience has been that, when women diagnosed with osteoporosis directly stimulate bone by rolling on the ball, the bone becomes less brittle and more flexible." It is important, however, to use a soft enough ball that exerts only as much pressure as feels comfortable.

ACUPUNCTURE

As mentioned earlier, in China, osteoporosis is the exception rather than the norm. When it is present, women are treated with acupuncture. Rist-Podrecca explains how this works: "The Chinese use an electrical stimulus along the spine. The electrical impulse actually helps the bone stem cells, which are the reproductive cells of the bone, to reproduce, thereby strengthening the bone mass. It was very exciting to see this because we have some Western studies proving that peripheral stimulation by electricity, especially in the long bones in the leg, helps this process also." She adds that women whose calcium levels are low need to use this technique so that their bodies will have the proper foundation for increases in bone density. When weight-bearing exercises are added, the benefits are remarkable.

HOMEOPATHY

Homeopathy can be used as an adjunct to the nutritional and lifestyle factors discussed above. Some remedies to consider are listed below.

Regarding the appropriate potencies for these substances, homeopathic physician Dr. Ken Korins says, "For acute conditions, meaning they come on suddenly, and they are very intense, use a 200c potency. That is a very dilute potency, but energetically speaking, it is very powerful. For more chronic conditions, where you will be giving the remedy for a longer period of time, you might want to start with 12c or 30c. In general, the remedies should be taken as three to four pellets placed under the tongue. Take them on an empty stomach. Do not take them within 15 to 20 minutes of eating or 15 to 20 minutes after eating. Avoid coffee and aromatic substances, such as mints, perfumes, and camphors, which can interfere with their effectiveness. Also, it is a good idea not to touch remedies with your hands because any residues from perfumes or other substances can interfere with their energy properties."

CALCAREA PHOSPHORIC. This may help where the bones are weak, soft, curved, and brittle. It can be taken over a long period of time.

CORTICOID. Homeopathic corticoid is for painful posttraumatic osteoporosis, especially when it affects the hip. Consider this remedy for an elderly person who has fractured her hip because of osteoporosis.

PARATHYROID. Parathyroid is good for diffuse pain in the bones, especially the long bones. Walking is very painful. Often, there is pain in the ankles, hips, and knees.

Chapter 25

Pain Management

O dd as it may seem, pain can have a valued place in life. If you look at Chapter 27 in this book, "Pregnancy," you'll see that the pain of pregnancy has a number of positive effects, including helping the mother to focus and ultimately bonding her to the child, who is also suffering as she or he makes the trip into the outer world.

In James Baldwin's *The Fire Next Time*, written during the time of the civil rights struggles, the author describes the courageous black men who participated in nonviolent civil disobedience in the South to win the equal rights granted in the law but never in practice. (Of course, black women, as well as white women and men, also played a part in this struggle, but Baldwin singles out black men to illustrate a contrast.) He compares those men to the white men who were defenders of segregation, who often resorted to violence, even against children, to defend injustice. Baldwin's point is that throughout this struggle, blacks were fully human, where their opponents were not, because, he says, blacks had a deep and intimate experience with suffering. Having seen and suffered injustice had, perhaps paradoxically, made them compassionate, giving them insight not only into cruelty but also into endurance and dignity.

Hegel makes a similar point in the slave-master section of *The Phenomenology of the Spirit*. As the German philosopher sees it, there is a "turnabout" relationship between slave and master. The master uses force to make the slave do his will. However, the slave, in working with and mastering environment and materials, becomes capable and aware of the shaping and creative powers of humanity, even while suffering under the lash. The master, in his indolence, is ignorant of the real capacities of the human.

This does not mean, however, that we must endure and accept being in pain. Every day tens of millions of Americans wake up knowing they are going to contend with pain, whether from arthritis, musculoskeletal problems, or a variety of other conditions that cause pain. Many do not realize that there are varied ways of treating pain naturally. In this country we need a different approach to acute and chronic pain. We need to go from treating just the symptoms to treating pain holistically through a mind-body approach.

Getting proper nutrition through sensible eating and by ingesting natural supplements such as minerals and herbs are key ways of treating pain, though other methods, such as the Trager technique, shiatsu, and acupuncture, also have a role to play. This chapter surveys a broad range of healing strategies that can be used by anyone suffering from chronic or occasional pain.

Food

One of the most important ways to combat pain is by guiding your diet to avoid abrasive foods and concentrate on those that build up the body's biochemistry. You should eat in the same way you should drive—defensively.

It seems that people are really taking a new look at diet, especially people who used to think that for relief from aches and pains could come only from a jar or bottle or from even more drastic remedies, like surgery. Not in every case, but in many cases, we're finding that diet can be the most powerful medicine.

Let me give you an example of what not only raw organic foods, but also juicing can do to help pain. I had a man in my study group whose whole family were physicians: his daughter, his son-in-law, his wife, and others. He had a 90 percent occlusion of a carotid artery and blockages in many of the other arteries. With no chelation, since that had not worked, and with no other kind of intensive therapy—just with exercise, stress management, a vegetarian diet with plenty of juicing, and proper supplementation—the blockage was completely eliminated.

The blockage was eliminated so quickly that the doctors wanted to do a second examination because they couldn't believe that in just a year the entire blockage was gone. He was so much improved in health that he was able to participate in a race in the 75- to 80-year-old group—this man is 75.

This is just one example of what diet, in combination with other lifestyle changes, can do. Yet people will say to me, "It's impossible. It can't be that it is that simple. It can't be that foods will really help, because if they did, someone in medicine would have figured it out." But this is not the case. They just were not looking. Those who do look, however, will frequently find.

One physician who has been looking is Dr. Neal Barnard, author of *Food*

That Fights Pain and president of the Physicians' Committee for Responsible Medicine, a nationwide group that promotes preventive medicine and addresses controversies in modern medicine.

As he sees it, there are three ways in which food fights pain and four ways in which pain is manifested in the usual course of an illness. He uses arthritis as an example.

Pain from sore joints has four separate causes. First, there has to be an injury to the joint. Second, there is an inflammatory response with redness, swelling, and stiffness. Third, the nerves that transmit the pain signals up to the brain must be irritated. Fourth, the brain has to perceive this. Dr. Barnard says that there are strategies to deal with all four causes.

THREE STEPS TO MANAGE PAIN THROUGH DIET

Barnard sees three steps that must be taken in using diet to help with health problems.

The first thing to look at in confronting a health problem related to diet is trigger foods. These are foods that commonly set off pain: dairy products, wheat or citrus for some people, tomatoes, meat, and eggs. "We want to do a little detective work and see which one is a trigger for an individual, because the triggers may be different for each person," Barnard counsels.

The second step is to find out which foods are safe to eat. "We focus on the pain-safe foods, which is fairly simple to do."

The third step, which Barnard believes is especially necessary for women, is to use foods to balance hormones, especially if the pain is associated with menstrual or breast pain. Because low-fat, vegetarian diets reduce hormone swings and stop the overly aggressive thickening of the uterine lining that is often aggravated by a bad diet, they can dramatically reduce pain.

Barnard summarizes: "If we put these all together, what we are going to do is tailor the diet intervention to the individual's condition. Getting away from the animal products is certainly very important if you want to open up the arteries again, but if you have migraines or arthritis, we want to look at the specific food triggers. Sometimes that can be a food that would otherwise be quite healthy, such as a tomato or a grapefruit. If you are sensitive to them, you should learn that."

The most striking thing in Barnard's plan is that a patient doesn't have to be resigned to making a difficult diet change for a long period of time. Positive results often occur quite quickly. If a person has migraine or arthritis, for example, it may take as little as 10 days on a a new diet to see a difference. To begin, you have to take all of the triggers out of your diet; Dr. Barnard says there are about a dozen different triggers. After the pain has cooled down, you bring the triggers back into your diet, one every two days, and see which one is triggering the pain. Once you know what your triggers are, you will have more control over your migraine or arthritis pain.

TRIGGER FOODS

Foods that often trigger migraines include, in order of importance, dairy products, chocolate, eggs, and citrus fruits, followed by meat, wheat, nuts, tomatoes, onions, corn, apples, and bananas. The triggers for arthritis include dairy products, corn, meat, wheat products, eggs, citrus, potatoes, tomatoes, nuts, and coffee.

Of course, Barnard reminds us, "Many people will say, 'Wait a minute. What could be wrong with bananas or apples? These are healthy foods, aren't they?' Well, sure they are. They don't have fat in them, or almost none. They have no cholesterol. If they are not a pain trigger for you, go ahead and eat them. That said, we know people who are allergic to strawberries. They get a rash on the skin. What if the sensitivity is not on the skin but shows up, for example, in the blood vessels that go to the brain or in the linings of the joints or elsewhere? It's important to know that. So there is nothing necessarily wrong with tomatoes or bananas or strawberries, but if you are sensitive to them and you get symptoms, you need to know that."

FOODS THAT WEAKEN RESISTANCE TO PAIN

In contrast to normally innocuous foods such as strawberries, which may trigger a pain reaction in certain people, some foods may weaken the body's ability to resist pain. Coffee is one of those foods. People who drink coffee tend to have more headaches. On the other hand, coffee can have an analgesic effect and stop migraines. In fact, caffeine is one of the ingredients in Excedrin.

Dr. Barnard mentions sugar as another substance that lowers a person's pain tolerance. "Sugar never gets good press, and I'm sorry I have to add to the list of its problems. In a research study, people have taken volunteers and put a little metal clip on the web of skin between the fingers. Then this clip is hooked up to an electrical generator. The participants are given a little bit of electrical energy, which is gradually increased, and asked when they can feel it and when it becomes intolerable. Those numbers are written down. Then they are given sugar and the progression is repeated. These studies find that after ingesting the sugar, they feel the pain sooner and it becomes intolerable sooner.

"The same is true with people with diabetes. If you have adult-onset diabetes, when you have high blood sugar, you are more likely to feel pain more acutely. You are more likely to feel it sooner and find it intolerable at lower levels. Something about sugar changes brain chemistry so that pain is more intense."

He ends by saying, "I've been so struck by the fact that people would start their breakfast with a cup of coffee, which reduces pain, then add a little sugar, which will increase pain sensitivity. It goes on for the rest of the day, where we are mixing up foods that cause and reduce pain."

PAIN-SAFE FOODS

Pain-safe foods you should look for are rice—any kind of rice, but especially brown rice—and cooked green vegetables such as broccoli, Swiss chard, and spinach, which tend not to trigger migraines or other problems. If you get an upset stomach from broccoli, cook it a little longer; this knocks out some of the vitamins, but the proteins in the broccoli are what cause stomach irritation in some people. Also, cooked orange vegetables such as sweet potatoes and carrots are pain-safe. Cooked yellow vegetables such as squash are also good. For fruits, pick the noncitrus ones, especially dried or cooked.

PAIN-REDUCING FOODS

Barnard has also found that some overlooked foods are especially good for dealing with pain. "One of the things that we like to use is hot peppers, jalapeno peppers. The zing in the jalapeno is from a chemical called capsaicin. This doesn't just make your mouth hot, it actually changes what happens in the nerves. It stops the nerves from being able to conduct pain. Pharmaceutical manufacturers have taken this capsaicin straight out of the pepper and mixed it into a cream which is applied externally. Two brands of capsaicin cream in the United States are Capsin and Zostrix.

Capsaicin can be useful if you have superficial pain, such as the pain of shingles, which can be just miserable, or if you have mastectomy pain. At first when you put on the capsaicin, it tingles and may even burn a little just as a hot pepper would. Do it day after day, and gradually the pain will diminish. You will still feel touch and pressure, but you won't feel pain. Give it a couple of weeks to work."

PAIN RELIEF FOR VARIED CONDITIONS

Barnard uses diet to manage pain from various disorders where pain is a major factor.

MENSTRUAL PAIN

In June 1998, Barnard, working with Georgetown University, completed a study of menstrual pain reduction. Women with severe menstrual pain were put on a vegan diet with no animal products. This eliminated all animal fat and reduced total fat. Vegetable oils were also removed from the diet. When you do that, the amount of estrogen in the blood diminishes quite quickly. As a result, the pain lessens or goes away. Barnard reports that about two-thirds of the women in the study had a substantial reduction in pain.

DIABETES

For diabetes, Barnard uses a combination of diet and exercise. "Ideally, I suggest a vegan diet so that you can avoid all the animal fats. This is a Dean Ornish type of diet, the kind we use to reverse heart disease. But one special thing we found with people who have diabetes is that we are not going to be using white bread, white rice, or white pasta. To tell the truth, with most heart patients, they can eat these things and still reverse the cholesterol. But with diabetics, when a white bread or pasta is digested, it releases sugars a little too quickly. So we want to keep the fiber in there by eating whole-grain bread and brown rice (not white rice). White pasta is okay, but throw some beans and vegetables and other fiber-rich foods on top, because the fiber will slow the absorption of the sugars."

SICKLE CELL ANEMIA

Doctors are just starting to use diet to treat sickle cell anemia. Dietitians have known for a long time that they must make sure there are plenty of B vitamins in the diet of these patients, because the blood cells are getting destroyed and rebuilt, and that uses up the B vitamins, especially folic acid.

According to Barnard, researchers only recently found out that there is a natural compound called cyanate, which, if taken in pill form, will cut the frequency of sickle cell crises by about 40 percent. However, this compound also can cause nerve problems.

Barnard says, "What we have been interested in is that this natural compound occurs in some foods. A lot of times when you get a substance in the food you eat, it won't cause the side effects that occur when you concentrate it and isolate it in a pill. The foods that contain cyanate are yam, cassava, sorghum, and millet.

"If you look at countries where these foods are consumed as a normal part of the diet, such as Jamaica, these are places where a sickle cell sufferer can live a normal life. This is unlike the United States, where a person with sickle cell anemia is likely to have his or her life shortened by this condition, which can be a miserable experience. In contrast, there are people in Jamaica who have lived decade after decade, well into old age, physically fine. They do have the genes for the sickled cell, but we believe that something in their diet may be helping them. Before we jump on this bandwagon, of course, we need to have more research showing whether or not it will help and who it will help. To my mind, it means using the natural foods, putting them in a diet in a serious way, and seeing if we can get rid of some of these painful crises."

CIRCULATORY PROBLEMS

For circulatory disorders, Dr. Barnard focuses on getting to the root of the problem. "If a person has crushing chest pain," he says, "that means the person is headed for a heart attack. Our goal there is not to shut out the pain but to reopen those arteries so that we restore blood flow. Once you do that, the pain will go away and you will also correct the underlying damage."

Interestingly enough, he adds, back pain also may be partially accounted for by circulatory problems. Some back pain occurs when the little leathery discs between the vertebrae have started to degenerate. When they break, the interior herniates out and presses on the nerve, resulting in pain. According to Dr. Barnard, this may not start in the back, but rather in the arteries leading to the back. As the aorta courses down the spine toward the back of the leg, it branches off into the lumbar arteries, the first place in the body where artery blockage occurs before it forms in the heart. By age 20 or so, about 10 percent of Americans have one completely blocked lumbar artery. So," he reasons, "if you don't get blood supply to your back, it can't recover from the wear and tear of everyday life. It gets no oxygen and no nutrients, and you don't have a blood supply to carry away the waste."

He believes that there is now abundant evidence that back pain starts with the same artery blockages that come from the kind of diet that many people grow up on: bacon and eggs for breakfast, baloney sandwiches for lunch, and a chicken dinner. When we go to the Ornish type of proper diet (See Chapter 14, "Heart Disease"), "we believe that is going to be the answer for back pain."

CONCLUDING THOUGHT

Dr. Barnard adds a final note: "In preparing my book, I wanted to have recipes. I asked Jennifer Raymond, who did all the recipes for my earlier book, not only for the low-fat, vegan recipes that work with heart patients, but also for some trigger-free recipes that don't have—obviously—the dairy, but also no wheat, tomatoes, and other catalysts. She thought, 'Good heavens. How am I going to do this?' She eventually came up with marvelous soups, main dishes, desserts, and so on, with none of the trigger foods. She sent them back to me with a little note that said, 'You know, Neal, I have to thank you because in the process of testing these recipes, my own joint pain and digestive system problems went away.' And she had been following what we would all think of as a healthy diet before that. But by eliminating the triggers and really boosting the pain-safe foods, she made her own pain go away."

Herbal Remedies

Herbs eliminate pain by dealing with the underlying causes. There are different types of pain. Some are inflammatory, hot, and pounding. Some are due to toxins in the body that need to be cleansed. Proper herbal treatment can help the body do away with both the pain and the causes of the pain.

For women, herbalist Letha Hadady offers the following recommendations: "We must approach the pain of PMS (premenstrual syndrome) from both the emotional and physical sides. Emotionally, there are two types of PMS. One is the angry type. Aloe root is recommended for this. It cleans the system and cleanses the liver. It may taste a little bitter, but it is easy to take when added to a little apple juice. A stronger gall bladder and liver cleanser that lessens the impact of 'angry' menstrual pains is the Chinese preparation *lung tanxieganwan*. Twenty percent ginseng, it aids digestion and reduces anger. It also calms and quiets headaches and other pains.

"The second type of PMS is weepy. It comes from sadness and excess phlegm brought on by eating foods that are too rich, sweet, and oily or by drinking too much milk. Eating radishes, parsley, or barley soup will cut down on the phlegm. A remedy for this type of pain is homeopathic pulsatilla."

To treat both types of menstrual pain, warming herbs such as cinnamon and myrrh are invaluable. Capsules or drops taken in tea will increase blood circulation and clean the uterus, inducing a more complete period that does not start too early, stay too long, or finish early only to begin prematurely. A warming and cooling remedy for the pain is as follows:

1/2 cup of aloe vera gel

10 drops or one capsule of myrrh

Apple juice

This combines the cleaning action of myrrh with the cooling of aloe.

Vitamins, Minerals, and Other Supplements

Most people know that minerals are essential for building up the body, maintaining the body's fluid balance, and helping with many chemical reactions. Let us look specifically at how minerals and vitamins have proved effective in treating pain.

Dr. Luke Bucci, the author of *Pain Free: The Definitive Guide to Healing Arthritis,* states that for handling spinal column disorder, carpal tunnel syndrome, or arthritis, an antidepressant may prove helpful. Carpal tunnel syndrome occurs when, because of repetitive tasks, the tendons in the wrist become inflamed; this squeezes the nerves, which then tingle and go numb. About one-third of the cases of this syndrome can be cured by the administration of vitamin B_6 (100 mg/day) to which can be added vitamin B_2 (50 mg/day). To deal with the pain of the condition, one should take St. John's wort (*Hypericum perforatum*). This substance has a molecule that works like a pharmaceutical drug without any of the drawbacks or side effects.

Magnesium salts are also useful for those with pain from torso or joint aches. Many people are already deficient in magnesium. This calmative mineral is obtained from nuts and seeds that are raw and unroasted. Nuts are also beneficial in that they contain essential oils, including the omega-3 fatty acids, which also have mild anti-inflammatory properties that help reduce pain. For torso and joint problems, the dosage of magnesium citrate salts should be 400 mg per day, divided into doses of 100 to 200 mg.

Sound sleep is an essential part of good health. For people who have trouble sleeping due to headaches or other pains, there are a number of useful supplements. Valerian, hops (the same element found in beer), skullcap, or passion flower can be used. These supplements, which can be mixed, should be taken a half hour before going to sleep, in either capsule (one or two) or tincture form. One might also try taking 1 mg of melatonin before sleep.

For the pain arising from PMS, GLA (gamma-linolenic acid) is valuable. It can be obtained from evening primrose oil, black currant seed oil, or borage oil. The sufferer should take three to six pills per day. As an adjunct to GLA, vitamin E is helpful. Also to be taken is vitamin B_6 (100 mg/day) and magnesium, which smoothes muscle contractions.

Here as with all vitamin therapy, the patient must follow through, taking the supplements consistently for two or three months, to be assured of the effects.

The pain of sciatica, a pinched nerve running down the leg, can be reduced by reducing the inflammation at the nerve root. Here one should try a proteolytic enzyme such as bromelain, papain, trypsin, or chymotrypsin to support the body's natural healing properties.

Musculoskeletal pain, which may be due to too much lactic acid, can be relieved by a number of substances. L-carnitine allows the body to burn fats and soak up excess lactate. Also helpful with muscle aches are the methyl donors, such as DMG (dimethyl glycine) and TMG (trimethyl glycerin), taken in a dose of 100 mg per day.

To reduce the soreness after exercise, one should take vitamin E (400 to 800 IU/day), which prevents the leakage of enzymes from the muscles.

A final way to approach pain is to modify the way the brain perceives it. DL-phenylalanine (DLPA), which is a synthetic amino acid, slows down endorphins, making the ones you have work better. Taken in a dosage of 500 mg three times a day, it reduces chronic pain while getting the sufferer off analgesics.

Thus, there are many ways to nutritionally enhance the body without using pharmaceuticals that overwhelm the receptors.

Exercise

There is also a role for exercise in pain relief. As important as diet is, diet is not everything. When people with fibromyalgia become physically active, they do much better. That's true for just about any kind of pain. Dr. Barnard notes, "When you have a finely trained athlete—someone who can run a 5- or 10-kilometer race—running the race is the equivalent for deadening pain of having 10 grams of morphine in the blood. The effects are that powerful. You can actually test the athlete's pain tolerance. You put his or her hand into a bucket of ice water and see this dramatic reduction in pain sensitivity after a run."

Shiatsu

Shiatsu is based on the principle that a vital energy, called *qi* (*chi*), flows through the body. The primary cause of pain is an imbalance of this energy. The goal of the healer is to balance the client's energy so that pain and discomfort do not manifest or, if they do appear, will be relieved.

As Thomas Claire, a bodywork practitioner, explains, in performing shiatsu, he uses thumbs, fingers, palms, forearms, elbows, and even knees to apply pressure to specified points in the body to modulate the flow of energy. During a shiatsu treatment, the client lies on the floor on a comfortable padded surface, such as a futon, fully clothed or undressed to her or his level of comfort. What the client feels is pressure, which can be gentle or deeper at the places where the practitioner is working. As the pressure continues, the patient generally feels relaxed and energized at the same time.

Shiatsu is good for treating a variety of different pains. It is especially beneficial in combating chronic pain in the back, neck, or shoulders, but it has also proved effective in treating whiplash, herniated discs, and problems affecting the nervous system, such as Bell's palsy.

A shiatsu healer concentrates on certain pressure points that have metaphoric names that tell us something about what they do or how they are to be worked with.

The first point of interest is on the ankle and called Spleen 6. It is at the meeting of three *yin* meridians and is the most powerful point for tonifying the feminine energy in the body. It can be located by placing the little finger on the border of the inside ankle and counting up four fingers. At the very top of these fingers, and at the center, is Spleen 6. To modulate the energy, you can put pressure on this point with your thumb, pushing three times in succession for 7 to 10 seconds each time. This pressure will stimulate the feminine energy, helping a woman control PMS and irregular cycles. Moreover, since all people have feminine and masculine sides, use of this point can also be beneficial to men and can help with sexual problems such as impotence.

The corresponding point for male tonification is called Stomach 36. To locate this point, find the indentation just outside the kneecap. Put one finger at this indentation and go down four fingers. There you'll find Stomach 36, which is also known as Leg 3 Mile. This second name is given since, it is said, if you have a strong Stomach 36, you will have anough stamina to walk three miles with no trouble. Manipulation of this point can lead to a tonification of masculine energy as well as the whole body. For women, this point can be used to ease childbirth and labor pains.

A third important point, located at the middle of the web of the hand, is Large Intestine 4, also called Meeting Mountains. The latter name is derived from the "mountain of flesh" found jutting up between the thumb and index finger when you close your hand. To locate this point, find the highest point on that protruding flesh and then open your hand. This point should be pressed three times running for 7 to 10 seconds to tonify the upper body. Pressing this point can also help with nausea, vomiting, colds, and constipation.

Pericardium 6, or the Inner Gate, is found on the forearm. If you flex your hand, you'll find two tendons that pop up on the inside of your wrist. Go up these tendons and press. This point is particularly good for controlling nausea, such as that from morning sickness or motion sickness.

Another valuable point is found right in the middle of the palm. Pressing it can relieve tension such as that arising from a stressful work environment or relationship.

Runny nose, allergy, colds, and sinus infections can be treated by putting pressure on the point called Welcome Smell, so named since nearly any smell is welcome to a person whose nasal passages have been blocked. To approach this point, take the index finger and bring it in at a 45-degree angle to the crease under the nose. This pressure can be applied on either side of the nose, although it is not recommended that both sides be touched simultaneously because this might interfere with breathing.

In fact, all these pressures can be applied to either side of the body, since the meridians are bilateral and bring the same energies to each side of the body.

Acupuncture

Like shiatsu, acupuncture sees pain as being derived from blocked energy or *qi* (*chi*). In treating this blockage, the practitioner has to determine whether it stems from an overabundance of a deficiency in energy, so that treatment can be adjusted depending on whether it is necessary to strengthen or decrease *qi*.

The acupuncturist first records the patient's medical history in the manner of a conventional doctor. Then, with the patient lying down or seated, depending on the area to be treated, fine-gauge, stainless steel needles are inserted into significant points and meridians to exert different physiological effects on the body and induce both relaxation and energization. The patient will remain in this position for 20 to 30 minutes, though an appointment with an acupuncturist may last up to an hour, since part of the time will be spent consulting about the employment of other traditional and herbal treatments that might be recommended. Bodywork and massage may also be included in the session.

Dr. Christopher Trahan notes that the treatment will have analgesic and anesthetic effects, block pain, and accelerate recovery from motor nerve injury. Moreover, it enhances the immune system, which has a sedative effect; helps with muscular spasms or neurological problems; has a homeostatic effect in that it helps balance blood pressure; and has positive psychological effects, acting directly on brain chemistry.

If we look specifically at what acupuncture treats, we have to mention muscular, skeletal, and structural problems of the body; arthritis; TMJ (temporomandibular joint) pain; carpal tunnel syndrome; insomnia; asthma; headaches; digestive problems, such as ulcers and irritable bowels; menstrual cramps; and pleurisy.

Many patients with chronic low back pain find that acupuncture will not only help break the pain cycle, but also allow them to reduce pain medications and participate more vigorously in physical therapy. Dr. Emily Kane, a naturopath who practices in Juneau, Alaska, suggests trying acupuncture for low back pain. In an article on the website of the American Association of Naturopathic Physicians (www.naturopathic.org), she says that in experiments using animals such as rabbits, rodents, and cats, and in human experiments, it was shown that acupuncture stimulates the nervous system to release endorphins as well as other chemical pain relievers in the body. She adds that some people get immediate relief from low back pain after the first acupuncture session, but she recommends having six or eight sessions within a short period of time before assessing whether or not it is working for you.

Trager Technique

The Trager technique is a way of working with the mind and body simultaneously. According to the philosophy behind this technique, pain comes from the accumulated action of the patient frequently tightening his or her movements and posture. To correct it, the practitioner uses gentle motions to increase the patient's pleasure in the quality of the tissues and decrease the restriction and the sense of holding. The practice works by reaching into the functional subconscious with particular qualities of movement, posture, and sensation. Gentleness is emphasized so that no message will be sent to the body alerting it that pain is on the way or causing the patient to tighten up. The movement reaches into the central nervous system with a motion at once pleasurable, lengthening, softening, and opening, conveying this sensation to the tissues and joints. The movements can be very small and internal or can be done at the periphery of the body in the limbs. In the latter case, the limbs are used as handles to reach the core.

Roger Tolle, a Trager practitioner, says that some clients will feel results immediately as the touching allows them to release pain. In other cases, it takes a repetition of the information into the body and mind, which will gradually allow the client to relearn how to go about daily activity with a different quality of motion.

The Trager method works with the kind of pain we see in the neck and upper back, in migraines and sciatica, in holding patterns in the lower back, in the pelvic rotation muscles, in TMJ pain, and carpal tunnel syndrome. It also works with pains due to repetitive motion of a constrictive kind.

Rolfing

According to the practitioners of Rolfing, pain is due to chronic shortenings in the tissue. Correction of this pain can be accomplished through soft tissue manipulation. This manipulation acts to create order in the body so the client stands tall and free of restriction.

David Frome, a physical therapist, states that Rolfing is done in a 10-session series designed to address all the shortenings in the structure systematically. Each session works in a different area. In the first hour, for instance, concentration is on the trunk, shoulders, and hips. In the second hour, work is done on the back and lower leg. Going through the complete series allows the therapist to work through all the body's shortenings. During a session, a patient may experience a tingling sensation and a sense of release. The patient should strive to draw the deepest possible breath to aid in treatment.

The major goal of the treatment is not pain relief per se, but it has been found to help with TMJ pain, frozen shoulder, tennis elbow, carpal tunnel syndrome, chronic hip problems, sciatica, cervical neuropathies, and knee, foot, and ankle problems.

Craniosacral Therapy

The sacral region is at the bottom of the spine. Between it and the head there should be a balanced rhythmic motion maintained for the health of the organism. When pain arises, it may be due to a restriction that disturbs the harmony between these two regions or between them and the rest of the body.

In craniosacral therapy, the practitioner places his or her hands on the client's body in such a way as to try and bring the cranium (skull) and sacrum back into alignment, reestablishing a natural rhythm. Charles A. Kaplan, the founder and director of the Center for Pain Management, points out that this hands-on technique usually centers on touching the head or lower back but can be done anywhere, such as on the fingers or toes. Some patients will go through a first treatment and not feel anything, but most will leave the treatment table feeling very relaxed and stress-free.

Craniosacral therapy is recommended for dealing with muscular and skeletal pain, headaches, pains in the back and neck, sports injuries, sciatica, and nerve pain. It can also be beneficial to those recovering from pneumonia or bronchitis, helping by loosening the rib cage. This treatment is a tremendous stress reducer; it can eliminate back pain and improve the immune system.

Magnet Therapy

With an ancestry as old as that of acupuncture and shiatsu, magnet therapy also acts to influence the body's energy. Jim Joseph mentions that the healing power of magnets was known in China over 4,000 years ago. Such ancient fathers of medicine as Galen and Aristotle discussed magnets, as did Paracelsus, one of the founders of chemistry. The value of magnet therapy was a tenet of Mesmer and others in the 19th century and is still being developed and practiced today.

Down through history, magnets have been used to deal with the causes of various ailments. As Dr. Joseph remarks, "Pain is a messenger. We don't want to kill the messenger but find the cause."

Pain in the body can be caused by positive energy being drawn to the site of injury. To bring about this transfer, the brain sends out a negative signal. Using the negative side of a magnet can augment and assist that reaction. Furthermore, around an injury there will be an acidic buildup. The negative side of the magnet is an alkalizing force that can help alleviate the pain accompanying this acidity.

A second source of pain arises when a person is overworked or suffering from undue stress, causing that person's cells to be overly positively charged. Putting a negative magnet on a weakened area will repolarize the cells, restoring the balance between positive and negative charge.

The distortion of the cells' polarity and resultant pain may also be caused by our technological environment. We are swamped with positive electromagnetic pulses coming televisions, radios, electric clocks, and all the other electrical devices around us. The pulses of their fields are not congruent with the one found in our body and can throw us into disharmony and disease.

Magnets can be obtained in a plastiform case that can be molded and shaped for a particular area. They last indefinitely and are low priced. A medium-sized magnet may cost $20. Healing magnets are color-coded with the negative pole green and the positive red. The positive side of the magnet is active and sun-oriented; the negative side is relaxing and earth-oriented. All the treatments discussed here utilize the negative pole. One must be careful with the positive pole, since positive magnetism causes growth in any biological system, even cancer. Treatment should last from 20 minutes to overnight. The magnet's power should be from 1,000 to 6,000 gauss.

A magnet can be wrapped with Velcro on the area to be covered. Special wraps in which the magnets are inlaid in Velcro are available. These wraps can be placed on most parts of the body, though they should not be used on the eyes. Negative magnetism attracts fluids and gases, and a negative magnet placed near the eye would draw out its fluids. If work is to be done on the eyes, the magnet can be placed off to the side. From this position, magnetism can be exerted on cataracts to reduce oxidation and free radical development. The magnet's value in reducing oxidation is due to the fact that oxygen is paramagnetic. When you breathe, you are pulling negative energy from the earth into your body.

To deal with edema, a magnet is placed on the body, not at the site of the problem but near it and directed toward the heart so that it will pull the fluid causing the edema away from its place of occurrence. If you have edema in the calf, for instance, place the magnet above the knee to draw the fluid up from the site of the disturbance to the kidney. From the kidney, the fluid can be excreted.

For the pain of menstrual cramps, a magnet should be placed on the lower abdomen, two inches below the belly button. Do not, however, use this placement for one or one and a half hours after eating, since it will interfere with peristalsis. Also, a magnet should never be used by a person with a pacemaker or any kind of metal implant.

The negative side of the magnet is also good against parasites, which will stop eating when hit by the negative energy.

At night, it is useful to lie on a magnetic bed pad and put magnets behind the head, where they will bathe the pineal gland in energy. This will induce a restful night's sleep. By using a magnet, one can feel rested even after sleeping fewer hours than one normally does. The magnet has also been known to increase sexual abilities.

The magnet can help with shoulder pain, pain in the rotator cuff, and aches in the lumbar region of the back. Magnets can be attached to the head or neck to deal with hypothyroidism, depression, migraine headaches, and problems with the vestibular system. For depression, the magnet should be placed near the occipital lobe.

The Mind-Body Connection

Some therapists have recommended a more eclectic approach, one that looks for and relies on the often-overlooked synergies that flow between the mind and the body. Dr. Ron Dushkin brings up a number of points to consider in dealing with pain. He notes first the importance of relaxation, which will quiet and calm the nervous system. Remember that when we feel pain, we also are feeling a layer of stress on top of that pain. If the layer of stress is relieved, the pain will diminish significantly.

Human touch can also play a part in relieving pain. As babies we like to be touched and as adults we still find this important.

A third overlooked factor in healing is humor. The writer Norman Cousins tells the story of how he was hospitalized with a critical health problem. As he saw it, a lot of his physical deterioration was due to stress and negative thoughts from that stress. He reasoned that if we can create disease with stress, then by alleviating stress through means such as humor, we can cure disease. He had a movie projector brought into his hospital room and began showing Marx Brothers films and other comedies. Soon his room became a place of congregation for other patients who wanted to enjoy the shows. It got rather chaotic because so many people were coming into his room and laughing. You're not supposed to laugh in a hospital. Some people were scandalized.

Cousins said that the doctors would give him blood tests before and after he had been laughing at a humorous film and would find an improvement after the film. He also had less pain after laughing.

Guided imagery is also an element of the mind-body connection. With this technique, a sufferer places a hand over the injured area and invites the other cells in the body to go to the aid of the damaged area. After all, the body's cells always work together, and this is one way to encourage their interplay.

All the methods mentioned as part of the mind-body connection get the patient to take charge of personal recovery. Many people are strong in many areas of life—pursuing a career, forming good relationships, playing sports— but when it comes to their own health, they turn over all control to a doctor. To really escape pain, the patient must play a big role in the recovery process.

This can be said to inform all the strategies for dealing with pain that we have encountered in this chapter. Whether you are taking appropriate herbs or mineral supplements to reduce suffering or selecting a nontraditional, natural healer to help you redirect your energy or repolarize your cells, you have studied, meditated, and selected a natural way to diminish pain.

Chapter 26

Parasites

We all know what parasites are, and we also probably realize that some parasites, like the bird that picks the hippo's teeth, can be beneficial to the host. There may even be cases where a parasite that seems inimical to a body or society is actually making a contribution.

Quite a controversy erupted in 18th-century England with the publication of Bernard de Mandeville's *Fable of the Bees*, on just such a topic. He depicted a beehive in which discriminating study would show that everything that looked like parasitic vices, such as gambling, boozing, and whoring, although they usually ended in miserable consequences for the indulger, redounded to the benefit of society. For instance, gambling increased the circulation of money, drinking gave employment to taproom owners, and so on. This chapter, however, discusses parasites that take more than they give back.

If you are getting no relief from chronic fatigue, urinary tract infections, pelvic inflammatory disease, vaginitis, or candidiasis, consider the possibility of parasites as the root cause of the problem. "Statistics suggest that approximately 7 million Americans are infected with disease-producing parasites," states complementary physician Dr. Pavel Yutsis of New York, "which live at the expense of their hosts, human beings, and cause injury." He adds that these statistics probably underestimate the real incidence.

Parasites are represented by two main groups, worms and protozoa. Worms that invade the system include pinworms, hookworms, ringworms, roundworms, and tapeworms. They live off undigested food on the intestinal walls, especially sugar and refined carbohydrates. But the majority of people are affected by protozoa. Dr. Yutsis says these single-celled organisms multiply in the host and can survive and thrive in the face of the host's sophisticated defense forces: "Why are protozoa so resistant? It is because they live inside the cells, which makes them immunologically untouchable. Although immunity to protozoa exists, it is unstable, often getting fooled and missing the target. This is why attention to protozoa is so important."

Parasites and their Diets

Dr. Skye Weintraub is a naturopathic physician from Eugene, Oregon, who specializes in the diagnosis of food, chemical, and environmental allergies. She is the author of numerous articles and books on health, including *The Parasite Menace*.

She begins by noting that parasites are often overlooked as causes of disabilities. "Most people have never seen a parasite," she notes, "so they say, 'Why worry about them?'

"Since we have good sanitation in this country, you wouldn't think there would be such a problem with parasites. Most people think parasites only appear in distant, impoverished Third World countries. They really don't think we have a problem in this country. Because of this misconception, parasites are often missed as the cause of an illness and are not part of the medical evaluation. Many people have heard of pinworms or tapeworms, but they don't realize there are over 100 common parasites that could infect humans."

Why don't we hear more about them? She explains, "Most doctors are not trained in the detection or treatment of parasites, so they just don't go looking for them as the cause of an illness. Most parasites are not reported to the health department, so there aren't any records kept. Newspapers aren't shocking us with the details of parasitic infection. There aren't any fundraisers raising money for research on parasites. When you don't hear about a subject, it's easy to think that it just does not exist."

A parasite is an organism that lives in or on another organism, which is called the host. It lives at the expense of the host, and they often compete for nutrition. In any host-parasite relationship, the host will be injured in some way.

Says Dr. Weintraub, "Some parasites are microscopic, such as one-celled amebas. Others are very large, multicellular worms that can grow to several feet long. Many parasites have very long life spans. Some worms can live up to 20 or 30 years."

The diets of parasites vary, according to Dr. Weintraub. But, she says, "The ones that prey on humans usually like the same foods that you do. If you love sugar, you will have a parasite that also loves sugar or foods that break down into sugar easily, such as simple carbohydrates. Other parasites eat body cells such as skin or blood cells. They usually eat the nutrients in your body before you get to use them. They grow healthy and fat, and you get the leftovers. So your diet plays a big part in what parasites you might attract.

"Some of the most common parasites detected in stool samples are the one-celled protozoans, such as *Blastocystis hominis*. In fact, I probably see this particular amoeba more than any other parasite that we've tested. Others are *Endolimax nana, Entomoeba histolytica, Dientamoeba fragilis,* and *Giardia*. Some of these protozoa are not considered pathogens unless they are present in significant numbers. A relatively small number of them may not cause any symptoms. When there are enough of them, though, they can and will produce symptoms."

Causes

Parasites live everywhere. We can get them from food, water, insects, infected animals, fertilizers that haven't been sterilized, and other people, such as food handlers who don't wash their hands after they go to the bathroom.

Dr. Weintraub points out, "We are more at risk when we eat raw foods, believe it or not, even though they are healthier. Adequate cooking kills parasites, but if the food is not cooked or inadequately cooked, the parasites are right there. If you are in doubt as to where your food has come from or who has handled it, adequate cooking might be the best choice."

Parasites also get into the body when people put their hands in their mouths after coming into contact with something that has the parasite in or on it. So sharing drinks, kissing, sexual contact, and even inhaling dust that contains the oocysts of the organism are all ways that parasites that enter the body. We can also pick up parasites from our pets. It's important to have them checked for parasites, especially if they are going to be around small children.

Dr. Weintraub stresses the importance of diet. "Diets can also influence our bodies and how they deal with parasites, since most parasites love sugar, an acidic diet, and constipation." The amounts of processed sugars and refined foods are certainly increasing in our diets. Many parasites, such as roundworms, thrive in a body that consumes sugar, even from natural sources like juice. Parasites prefer a very acidic digestive system, so learn how to balance the pH of your foods.

According to Dr. Weintraub, "Diets high in processed foods, as well as pesticides, additives, and dyes, encourage an environment for parasites. This type of lifestyle is usually just part of other pollutants that weaken the body. No wonder the immune system can't fight back against parasites when it's so overloaded."

Contaminated water is another source of parasites. Dr. Weintraub says, "If you are in doubt about the safety of your drinking water, it may be time to invest in a good water filtering system for your home. Make sure the system can filter down to at least 3 microns to remove *Giardia* and *Cryptosporidium*. Always drink bottled water when traveling, and never use ice that doesn't come from bottled water. Distilled water may be even safer. If you are still in doubt about your water source, boiling the water is the best method to make sure that it is safe to drink. Bring the water to a vigorous boil and then allow it to cool."

Symptoms

The most common symptoms of parasites are diarrhea, abdominal pain, bloating, intense anal itching, foul-smelling stool or gas, loose stools, and constipation (which sometimes alternates with diarrhea). It's not unusual to see rashes on the body. There is also possibly joint pain or muscle pain. Parasites may drain energy, causing intense fatigue. Patients with chronic fatigue syndrome should look into the possibility of parasites. In women, cervicitis, vaginitis, pelvic inflammatory disease, and decreased libido may be present. Other general symptoms include hives, arthritis, colitis, food allergy, headaches, anemia, insomnia, loss of appetite, weight loss, night sweats, and fever. Dr. Weintraub is also "seeing a lot of symptoms of colitis or other inflammatory bowel diseases, such as Crohn's disease and ulcerative colitis caused by parasites. Other symptoms may be allergies that come on for no particular reason, and chronic digestive problems, such as irritable bowel syndrome."

She notes that when your doctor is stumped, that's the time to suspect parasites. "The doctors just can't find anything wrong with you. They do upper GIs, lower GIs. But they just don't find anything or they think it's stress. The next thing is that they want to put you on some kind of antidepressant."

Dr. Marjorie Ordene, a complementary physician from Brooklyn, New York, tells why parasites can cause such diverse symptoms: "They interfere with the vital processes of the host by the various things that they produce. For example, they can produce enzymes that erode the intestinal wall. This can cause what we call a leaky gut, in which toxins can go across the barrier of the intestinal tract and cause symptoms in all parts of the body. Parasites can also confuse the immune system and cause the body to react to and attack its own tissues, causing autoimmune diseases, such as rheumatoid arthritis."

Testing for Parasites

Many Western doctors have not been trained to diagnose or treat parasites, and you need to ask about your doctor's training and expertise with parasites and whether he or she uses laboratories that specialize in detecting parasites.

In Weintraub's opinion, "Most commercial labs just don't have the facilities to do a very good job. It's also important to send at least two to three stool samples, taken on different days. One sample only gives you about a 20 percent chance of detecting a parasite, where three stool samples can increase your chances to 65 percent.

"Sometimes, diagnosis requires multiple stool samples. We've had cases with *Giardia* in which we didn't get back a positive stool result until we took 9 to 12 stool samples. So just because a report comes back negative doesn't mean you don't have parasites. They just weren't found in that particular sample. You might want to call the lab yourself and ask about their testing.

"Ask the lab whether they use the rectal swab technique, since some parasites adhere to the sides of the rectum and are not found in the stool itself. You might also ask whether they do fluorescent staining. This makes the parasites highly visible under the microscope. Another test is the immunoassay test, which can detect the presence of antibodies to the parasites so that the technician doesn't actually have to see the parasite itself to know it's there. It should make sense that the more sophisticated the detection procedures, the higher the likelihood of finding the parasites."

With fluorescent staining, different types of stains detect different parasites. Various types of immunoassays look for monoclonal antibodies that attach even to small fragments of the parasite or its cysts. The attached antibodies are visualized under the microscope. These sensitive tests identify the biochemical markers of parasites, so that it is no longer necessary to literally find the parasites themselves. For example, this type of test can detect the marker of *Giardia* parasites, which primarily inhabit the duodenum and upper small intestine and are very difficult to diagnose using conventional visualization techniques. Also, sophisticated analysis of the stool with cultures for bacteria and other organisms yields important information regarding the ecology of the flora of the colon.

Detecting parasites that are not in the intestinal tract can be tricky, and may require biopsy, X-ray, MRI (magnetic resonance imaging), or sophisticated testing of the blood and/or urinary tract.

Treatment and Prevention

Once it has been established that a person has parasites, the next step is to knock them out. As mentioned, parasites thrive in an acidic, high-sugar environment, so as a long-term strategy it's important to so eat a diet balanced between acid and alkaline foods, while avoiding sugary products.

Weintraub gives some examples of acidic and alkaline foods. "All animal products are acidic. So are most grains, dairy products, and sugar. There are other acidic foods, but those are the majority of the really acidic foods which are part of all-American diet. It's important to balance the diet by also eating alkaline foods, such as green, leafy vegetables. In fact, most vegetables are alkaline. Beans, avocado, and soy are all alkaline. Even a lot of fruits are alkaline. Though they may taste acidic in your mouth, the way they break down in your body is very alkaline. The goal is to get at least a fifty-fifty balance on your plate. When in doubt, increase your alkaline foods."

That practice discourages parasites, but what about trying to expel them?

"This is what it usually takes to completely rid yourself of parasites," Dr. Weintraub explains. "You need to cleanse the intestinal tract, for example by having colonics. You have to modify your diet. Take the appropriate substances—drugs or herbs or other supplements—that will eliminate the specific parasites you have. Recolonize the intestinal tract with friendly bacteria."

There are some foods that parasites don't like. Dr. Weintraub says, "Eating three or four cloves of garlic a day for a week is one way to get rid of parasites. Of course, it may get rid of your friends as well. Garlic is one of the most effective body cleansers. Start with a garlic bud first thing in the morning on an empty stomach." You can also eat about 100 raw pumpkin seeds in the morning on an empty stomach. Then fast for about five hours and follow with a large glass of fresh carrot juice. Repeat this for several days. "In fact," says Dr. Weintraub, "eating raw carrot salads with large amounts of fresh garlic is very antiparasitic. You can also chew from a teaspoon to a tablespoon of fresh papaya seeds daily on an empty stomach. Do this for about a week, then stop for two days, then repeat again for another week. Finally, eat more horseradish, especially fresh horseradish. It tends to be very effective against some worms.

"Eliminate any risk factors to avoid reinfection. Remember always to wash your hands after going to the bathroom, since most people get parasites by the fecal-oral route. It's also important to have proper bowel movements before starting your treatments for parasites." According to Dr. Weintraub, you should have at least two bowel movements every day.

Dr. Weintraub warns that it is important to get professional help in the treatment of parasites. Many herbs that are used have to be taken in such high doses that they could become toxic. Be very careful when treating children, especially under the age of 4.

She says, "For a laxative you can use psyllium seed husks, a widely available remedy that is used primarily as a bulking agent, especially in cases of chronic constipation. Some people, I find, do better with flaxseed. It doesn't seem to cause as much bloating as psyllium does. Cascara sagrada also helps with waste elimination, particularly in cases of chronic constipation. Senna is also a safe and effective laxative, especially for the lower bowel."

Another measure is to eat fresh pineapple or papaya, which contain substances that break down the protein structures of parasites and help the body digest worms. It may be necessary to add other digestive enzymes, such as hydrochloric acid and pepsin, if you don't produce enough in your own body. These enzymes promote better digestion and absorption of nutrients, while breaking down the protein in the parasites. A good digestive aid may be very important as part of the treatment.

Parasites can also be fought with high doses of friendly bacteria, such as *Lactobacillus acidophilus* and *bifidus* bacteria; supplements of friendly bacteria are known as probiotics. However, Weintraub states, "It's important to know that many of the products available don't produce enough viable organisms to work. By doing before and after laboratory testing, we have found that many probiotics are simply not very good; the friendly bacteria don't tend to colonize in the digestive tract very well. So talk to the people at your favorite health food store and tell them that you really want to find the best product for your particular problem." She adds, "You always want to take a probiotic on an empty stomach at least 20 minutes before you eat. Take it with unchilled water, which tends to activate the organisms a little quicker."

You should also consider colonics. Some parasites, such as *Blastocystis hominis,* which is an amoeba, are very hard to get rid of because they hide out in the intestinal tract and can't be reached by medication. A colonic will get rid of encrusted fecal matter, allowing the medication to reach the parasite.

Asian Herbs to Consider

BAIBU. This Chinese herb helps get rid of pinworms. It is put on a piece of cloth containing alcohol and worn at night.

KU SHEN. When *ku shen* is used as a tea, it cleanses the lower intestinal and urogenital area.

LEI WAN. This powerful Chinese herb is for treatment of any parasitic infection.

LA JIAO (RED PEPPER) AND WU. These herbs may eradicate tapeworms from the intestines.

Herbal Formula

Dr. Weintraub suggests a prototypical herbal formula that has successfully treated many kinds of parasites. "The one I use," she noted, "has all the following ingredients in one capsule. You usually have to take at least four of these a day."

Black walnut (75 mg)
Oil of oregano (75 mg)
Quassia amara (75 mg)
Chinese wormwood (50 mg)
Pumpkin seeds (50 mg)

Berberine-containing herbs such as barberry, goldenseal, and the salt of this alkaloid, which is called berberine sulfate (about 25 mg)

Grapefruit seed extract (25 mg)
Male fern, 25 mg

Fennel, about 10 mg

Yellow gentian, 10 mg

Dr. Weintraub explains why each of the ingredients in her formula is important.

"Black walnut can kill many worms, including tapeworms. It's important to use the green hull of the walnut to be successful in treating parasites.

"Oregano is included in many formulas because of its ability to kill yeast as well as other pathogens. Many people who have parasites also have an overgrowth of yeast in their digestive tract.

"Quassia amara (75 mg) is used to kill protozoans such as amebas and *Giardia,* as well as pinworms and even some roundworms. It has an intense, bitter taste, so it is not something you want to take out of the capsule or crush if it's in tablet form. It seems that bitter herbs are the most effective against parasites.

"Chinese wormwood, also known as sweet wormwood, has been used in China for over 2,000 years against protozoans such as *Cryptosporidium* and yeast. It's also effective against liver and blood flukes. Since this herb can cross the blood-brain barrier, it's useful in amebic infections in the brain.

"Pumpkin seeds have traditionally been used for worms and are somewhat effective against tapeworms, roundworms, threadworms, and pinworms. The seeds paralyze and expel these intestinal worms." Dr. Weintraub adds, "Many herbs do not kill parasites. What they do is paralyze them, so it is important to then get them out of the digestive tract as soon as possible. Thus you may have to take a laxative or something that causes a purge in order to do this.

"Berberine-containing herbs, such as barberry, goldenseal, and the salt of this alkaloid, which is called berberine sulfate, have been used as natural antibiotics and natural antiparasitics for years. They've been effective against protozoans, including *Giardia, Entomoeba histolytica,* and even many viruses, fungi, and bacteria. They also inhibit the overgrowth of yeast that is a common side effect of antibiotic use."

She cautions, "In some of the testing I've seen, it seems that not only the parasites but the yeast and even an overgrowth of pathogen bacteria are becoming more and more resistant to the berberine-containing plants. So this might be something to consider in choosing which herbs to use. You may have to make other choices, such as bearberry, also called uva ursi.

"Grapefruit seed extract is absolutely fantastic. It seems to be effective against more pathogens than any other substance in this formula. It is antifungal, antiviral, antibacterial, and antiprotozoan, but it doesn't kill the healthy, good bowel flora. It's probably the most effective substance against amebas now available. This extract is also a good companion for the traveler. It's an exceptional alternative for killing parasites and other harmful organisms, especially the ones you are likely to come into contact with visiting foreign countries. Take one or two drops in a glass of water a couple of times a day, as a preventative for traveler's diarrhea. It's very bitter, so don't ever take it without diluting it. I read somewhere that a person put just a drop on his tongue to see what it tasted like. Don't ever do that. You can find grapefruit seed in capsules as well. An adult will need to take about 100 to 300 mg daily in capsule form to be effective. It is also a great food wash. You can add 7 to 8 drops of liquid to about 1 gallon of water.

"Male fern has been recognized for centuries as deadly to intestinal worms such as flatworms or roundworms. It's the herb of choice for the treatment of tapeworms because it so effectively paralyzes. Even though it doesn't kill the worms, they can be washed out by an active purge. It's probably wise, as mentioned, to use an herbal laxative when doing any treatment for parasites, especially if you tend to be constipated.

"Fennel, which is generally used as a flavoring agent in foods, is also a good digestive aid. It helps removes waste material from the body, including parasites.

"Yellow gentian improves digestion as well. It also is very effective against protozoans, especially *Entomoeba histolytica,* and it expels intestinal worms."

Dr. Weintraub says that the adult dosage of her formula is one capsule at each meal and at bedtime. She adds, "When you are out looking at different products, this formula description should give you some idea of what to look for. There are many different products on the market, and some of them cater to a particular type of parasite. What this formula tries to do is cover most of the ones we are seeing at this time."

One of the best times to treat worms is during the full moon, for most worms are at their most active then. Start taking the herbs about five days before the full moon and continue until you finish the treatment. Since new worms hatch every 22 days, it's important to continue through several cycles. Don't miss even one day of treatment. Many treatments can last anywhere from 30 days to three months. It can take even longer to rid the body of protozoans than it take to eliminate worms."

Dr. Weintraub concludes, "People may ask, 'Why use these natural treatments instead of drugs?' Many parasites have become so resistant that the drugs are no longer effective. Also, the treatment takes a lot longer than it used to, so the drug is more likely to cause adverse side effects. Many people just get too sick taking these drugs, so herbs or other natural treatments are a good alternative."

Chapter 27

Pregnancy

I rving Howe's authoritative *The World of Our Fathers*, relates the trials and travails of Russian and Eastern European Jews who began coming to New York City in the 1880s. Howe describes the way older resident Jews, who were often from Germany, looked down on "di grine," the greenhorns. Of course, these greenhorns were not as lacking in knowledge as their deriders believed.

I was reminded of Howe's tale when, sitting on a bench near a farmers' market in New York City recently, I met a young Russian Jewish woman, Olga Rakhminova, who had come to the United States four years ago and was now attending college. Eight months pregnant, she was having run-ins with her American doctor. She commented particularly on American doctors' practice of giving pregnant women drugs.

Her doctor kept urging her to accept epidural anesthetics during the birth. "I know at least five people who took epidural medication and they had back pain later," she said. "This pain now comes very bad at the time of their menstrual cramps. I think that to give that medication, they numb your nerves, which seems to damage them."

She wondered, "Why is it that 20 years ago people delivered babies without drugs? All drugs have side effects.

"When my sister gave birth," she went on, "she refused the epidural drugs. Even though she suffered during the birth, she felt wonderful afterward; but the lady in the bed next to her took the drugs and had pains after delivering.

My mother gave birth three times naturally in Tashkent [in the former Soviet Union]. She says three days after giving birth, she felt so fresh.

"When I refused to sign up for the drugs, my doctor told me, 'Nowadays, all people are taking it, so you don't feel the pain. You can watch TV while you deliver. If you don't take it, you'll be in pain.'

"But I told him, 'You need to feel when you give birth. Not watch TV.'

"As I got near my time, I had a pain when I eat. The doctor told me to drink Mylantin. 'Fine," I said, and he wrote me a prescription. When I got outside, I threw that prescription in the garbage. I didn't take any medicine when I was pregnant. Everything will affect the baby."

This recent immigrant's view of having a baby, drawn from her formative years in the Soviet Union, closely mirror the attitudes of the rest of the world in both developed and underdeveloped nations, which are quite different from U.S. attitudes. Most of the world (with our country a large exception) sees the natural way of giving birth—choosing midwives and eschewing drugs, for instance—as the sanest and healthiest way to bring a child into the world. After examining how American attitudes differ, and noting some of the underlying reasons for this, we will look at certain things you must avoid to have a safe pregnancy. Then we will turn to the many things you can do and foods and herbs you can take to make pregnancy as healthy and uncomplicated as possible.

Birthing Practices in the United States

What we in the United States accept as the safest, most acceptable way to give birth is a historical anomaly—something that has existed for only 75 to 100 years and is not practiced in the rest of the world.

Suzanne Arms is an independent researcher and activist who has published seven books on pregnancy and women's health and is producer of a video documentary called *Giving Birth: Challenges and Choices*. She is the author of the books *Immaculate Deception, Breast Feeding, and Seasons of Change*.

"In other parts of the world," she says, "childbirth is seen as a natural process. The only exceptions are areas where American obstetrics and neonatal approaches have been aggressively promoted and marketed. Many European countries and a growing number of Third World countries are gradually adopting these practices as they buy our wares, such as neonatal monitoring devices."

She compares the United States with Holland. "Holland is a highly modernized and industrialized country, not some primitive backwater, and yet it rejects the supposedly more modern ways of U.S. pregnancy care."

In the United States, the vast preponderance of women give birth in hospitals. They are led to believe, Arms explains, that the larger the hospital, the better the care. They are told that the more narrow the subspecialization training of their doctors, the safer the birth will be. So women don't want to go to a general practitioner (GP), but instead go to a perinatologist with a subspecialty in obstetrics. Says Arms, "Our home birth rate in 1998 was 2.5 percent, the lowest in our history. Although we do have midwives in hospitals and birthing centers outside hospitals, and we do legally permit home births, fewer than 5 percent of births are done with these resources, even if we count births done with midwives in hospitals."

In Holland, by contrast, there is a whole different system, which has historically understood the value of natural childbirth. Holland's national policy promotes natural childbirth because the Dutch have done the studies that show such birth is valuable, not only to the individual mother but to the culture. Over 30 percent of the births in Holland are done at home, despite concerted efforts by physicians in a number of cities there to bring in American obstetrics and turn midwives into obstetricians' assistants.

Arms notes one way the Dutch go about promoting natural childbirth. "They have free universal health care, either through insurance (through one's workplace, for example) or from the state. If you have a medical condition that calls for use of the hospital and its physicians for your birth, you can freely use them. However, if there is no such reason, you have to pay out of pocket for the privilege, because you are using something you don't need." She compares that situation to what goes on in this country, where you have to pay no matter what you do, whether directly or through insurance. Moreover, people here feel they have to go to the hospital because "society" considers that is the acceptable way to give birth.

The result of these differing sets of values is that in Holland, six times as many midwives as doctors do births. And the physicians who do handle births include GPs as well as obstreticians. In the U.S., by contrast, "we have 33,000 obstetricians and fewer than 6,000 midwives. So we have a 6 to 1 ratio in the other direction."

In Holland, when a woman becomes pregnant, the first person she sees is a GP or midwife, and, more and more commonly, she sees a midwife. The midwife will refer to the obstetrician if necessary. There is a whole list of protocols according to which she must consult or at least get information from an obstetrician. She has access to any hospital in the country. If the birth is taking place outside a hospital, she has direct access to a hospital in case of problems, without having to make an appointment with a doctor.

Note how different this is from the United States, where only a doctor can get you entry into a hospital. "Midwives," Arms informs us, "have fought for 30 years to get direct access, fighting on a one-to-one basis to obtain the privilege for each hospital. It may take a midwife 10 years to get access to one facility. In Holland, by law, all midwives have access to all the equipment in the hospital as needed."

Natural Childbirth: Is It as Safe as Hospital Birth?

One reason for the greater American preference for hospital births as compared to the rest of the world is that Americans have been led to believe you are risking the baby and the mother if you choose not to have a hospital birth. But, Arms points out, "If we look at the facts, we see this is not true." In the United States, there has been very little comparative study of the benefits of home delivery versus hospital births. She sees a a number of problems with making comparisons, such as the low number of home births, the fact that there are no national records kept of hospital births, and the inaccuracy of hospital records. For instance, a standard hospital delivery will be listed as "normal birth" in the records even if drugs may have been used to alter the labor and in some cases even if a forceps has been utilized. The notation will read "standard" whether the baby ends up in the nursery or the intensive care unit (ICU).

Therefore, to actually compare the safety of hospital and home births, she says, "We have to go to a place like England where they have very good national statistics on births and they have commissioned studies to see which are the safer methods."

Back in the 1970s, a controversial study appeared called the *Peel Report*. It was used to support a belief among politicians that home birth should be outlawed. At the time, Marjorie Tew, a statistician who was not involved in the controversy but happened to be analyzing statistics in a number of epidemiological areas, noted flaws in the report. She restudied the statistics on home births and found these births were as safe as hospital births. This was true not only for low-risk women—those who enter the process in a healthy state—but even for those with problems.

As a result of these findings, England has reversed its policy, which had been focused on eliminating home births and getting rid of midwifery. The country has gone back to supporting midwives, birthing centers and local home births. They are finding that hospitals are not the best place to give birth. "In fact," Arms concludes, "there is no study that shows a hospital is a safer place than alternative venues for giving birth."

THE AMERICAN BIAS AGAINST NATURAL CHILDBIRTH

This bias in the United States against natural childbirth can be traced back to our underlying world view, Arms believes. She explains, "We have to consider a number of things in relation to religion—and here I'm not talking about the spiritual aspects of religion but specifically about the orthodox doctrine of the West's institutionalized religions, Christianity and Judaism."

Historically, Judeo-Christian church doctrine has regarded pregnancy and childbirth as a curse. It is meant to cause suffering because women carry the seed of evil in their bodies. However, according to Arms, this view is not supported by anything in the Old Testament or by the teachings of Jesus. Rather, these ideas were developed by church authorities as part of a worldwide movement to spread the power of the church. Whatever their origin, eventually these ideas left women with a legacy of shame about their bodies and an extraordinary fear of childbirth. Organized religion had a lot to do with causing women to mistrust the birth process and the body's ability to come through pregnancy and childbirth in good health and without intervention.

PAINKILLERS AND THE BIRTH PROCESS

One aspect of women's fear of birth is that they think it will be unendurably painful. So, in many cases, they fill themselves with painkillers before the process even begins.

Arms recognizes this tendency. She says, "Those who advocate natural childbirth are often asked: 'Why should modern women experience painful childbirth rather than benefit from the painkillers modern medicine provides?'

The issue of pain is a complex one, in her view. "Our media tell us that we should be free of any pain and discomfort in our lives. If you look at TV advertising, billboards, and so on, you see there are a tremendous number of products geared to the elimination of the pain that occurs in pathological conditions. We are taught we shouldn't have to experience pain. Since we are used to taking drugs for everything else, why not for labor?

"But childbirth is not a pathology and the cause of pain during birth is not a disease." The size of the woman's pelvis and the baby's head are structured in such a way that the mother's tissues must expand to a much greater degree than occurs in most other animals. "A rabbit, for example, can spurt a baby out in one contraction, seemingly without much pain at all. This is not true throughout the animal kingdom, however. Cats, dogs, pigs, and horses experience labor as a tremendous effort with what looks like pain. We've come to believe that this pain is not pathological but the result of the body's stretching."

Remember that our Russian émigré informant seemed to sense that the pain was a necessary concomitant to the process of birth. Arms corroborates this: "Pain serves a function, which is to alert the woman to get herself out of harm's way to a private place where she can do the work of birthing the baby without any distraction." This is the most significant aspect of the pain. It's there so that, as Arms puts it humorously, "she doesn't continue shopping in the mall and drop her baby in the aisles."

The second reason for pain is to make the mother focus on her body and connect what is happening to her body with the baby who is about to be born. This baby is making the most important journey of his or her life up to that moment, moving through the mother's birth canal and out into the world. "The pain and effort cause the woman to focus on her baby and her body so she will move into a position that will help her baby come down."

Thus the pain of labor is the effort of connecting with the baby as it prepares to become a semiautonomous being and the woman prepares to welcome it. "Once she experiences relief after labor is over, the mother feels this surge of endorphins as she puts a baby to her breast and falls madly in love with it. Her love is virtually the only thing that is going to keep that baby out of harm's way as he or she grows up."

Beyond the fact that the pain of labor has value in the birthing process, the issue of the potential problems caused by drugs and anesthesia need to be addressed. Drugs and anesthesia always cause problems. They distort and warp the birth process and make it harder for the baby to do the work it's supposed to do. They complicate labor and make birth a pathological problem, something which we treat in the hospital.

THE IMPACT OF DRUGS ON PREGNANCY

Many drugs are given routinely by physicians during pregnancy and labor: sedatives, anesthetics, narcotics, and artificial hormones. The hormones are given to increase contractions, to strengthen the contractions, and to start labor. Hormones and the other drugs are dangerous. Almost no woman in the United States gets through a birth in a hospital without being given at least two of these, unless she specifically refuses them.

These drugs all enter the baby's nervous system and brain. This means the baby's liver and brain have to work hard at detoxification—from chemicals that shouldn't be there in the first place. This is especially difficult for the baby because, in the first weeks of life, its liver and brain are not fully functioning.

The baby is being drugged at 10 times the rate (on average) that the mother is drugged. And even though a local anesthetic such as an epidural may not get to the baby quite as quickly as a narcotic such as Demerol, all such drugs still reach the fetal circulation and the fetal brain.

Arms tells us, "Due to these drugs, you will find babies with sucking problems and with breathing problems. Each category of drugs carries different problems for the baby and tends to alter, lengthen, or cause complications in the labor. It's ironic that the very drugs we want to keep people from using as teenagers and that we want to get outlawed because we have such a drug problem in this country are given to babies at a sensitive time—before they've fully formed all the cells in the brain and before the cell migration in the brain has even occurred, we are drugging them."

What's the Best Birth Position?

Anthropological and comparative studies reveal that the United States is about the only place in the world where women lie on their backs for birthing. Everywhere else, women usually sit up in chairs, squat, or kneel to give birth. Lying on one's back is physiologically the worst position one can assume for giving birth because (1) it increases the pain, (2) it makes the contractions longer, (3) it is less effective (in this position, it is harder to open the cervix and push the baby down), and (4) it makes labor longer.

In a few hospitals, birth in an upright posture is being encouraged. Both manufacturers and midwives are also recommending the use of birthing beds and birthing stools as the best way to give birth. This is a growing but small trend, for 95 percent of births in the United States do not occur this way.

Being upright makes it easier for the baby to move through the inlet of the pelvis, move down, and negotiate its head and shoulders through the outlet of the pelvic bone opening. The baby goes through this long tunnel—it's only a few inches, but for the baby it seems long. The baby is very active in the process (unless the mother had drugs, in which case the baby also gets drugs, and this may cut down on its liveliness). Squatting or being upright makes it easier for the baby. As the baby's head emerges, squatting opens the mother's pelvic region to the widest possible dimension.

Arms comments: "We have so many women who are told by doctors that their pelvises are 'too small,' which is almost always untrue. Nature designs a baby's head to be soft and malleable to fit the mother's pelvis. The proof is that many women who have Cesareans because of 'too small pelvises' go on, if they have more children, to have vaginal births, and are able to give birth to a baby even a pound heavier without any trouble."

What Are the Differences Between Midwifery and Medicine?

The most important difference between midwifery and traditional medicine is that medicine treats disease, whereas midwifery is about preventing complications while going through a natural process. Obstetrics, a subspecialty of medicine, seems to consider birth "too unwieldy." Doctors need to get in and out of the hospital quickly, so they want to control the length of time a woman is in labor and how long it takes to give birth. However, the natural variability of giving birth does not conform to their standard. Each human body is unique, as is each human psyche. A 4-hour labor may be normal. A 36-hour labor may also be normal. But under a physician's management, a day and a half is too long.

Medicine focuses on giving drugs and doing surgery. Midwifery concentrates on following through the process normally, spotting problems as they arise and treating them as simply as possible before they become complications, while teaching people how to handle contingencies.

Are Cesareans Safe?

In 1990, the cesarean section rate in the United States was 25 percent, which is the third highest rate in the world. Upper-class women in Mexico have the world's highest rate, about 75 percent. The rate in the United States has now dropped to 22 percent; but many people in obstetrics say it is too low and should be around 50 percent.

But, Arms explains, contrary to popular mythology, a cesarean is major surgery. It involves three primary risks for the mother and one primary risk for the baby. For the mother, the risks are the same risks experienced for all major surgery, risks that doctors have never been able to eliminate: (1) bleeding that becomes unstoppable hemorrhaging; (2) infection; and (3) unexpected adverse reactions to medication. On this last point, note that we have over 160,000 deaths per year from drugs that have been given in the right dosage by the right people for the right diseases—that is, according to standard procedure—and yet the patient has died.

Depending on which study you read, a woman is five to seven times more likely to die as a result of a cesarean than she is from a normal birth. For the baby, a cesarean causes problems with breathing, because it denies the baby the experience of being squeezed through the birth canal, which prepares its nervous system and lungs to breathe. A baby born by cesarean is far more likely to end up in an intensive care unit than a baby who has not been born by cesarean. But there are other problems that have to do with the baby's need to go through the birthing process as part of its development, to complete the process that is natural for both mothers and babies. There is a bodily expectation that they will complete the process naturally. When that is denied, there are psychological effects, which is one reason women grieve after cesareans. It's a bodily grief.

Is Circumcision Necessary?

Sixty percent of babies born in hospitals in the United States are circumcised, which Arms sees as a wasteful and counterproductive practice. "The difficulty with circumcision," she believes, "is that it touches some of the most sensitive tissue on the human male body and takes a large amount of material from the penis. You are taking away all the natural protection of the penis, the tissue which keeps it from getting infected and getting diseases and which makes sexuality more exquisite."

She also says that in Europe, circumcision has never been routinely performed on infants, as it is in the United States. She believes that the U.S. practice of routine circumcism is one aspect of a cultural attitude that grew, in part, out of 17th-century Puritanism, which viewed sexual pleasure, including masturbation, as sinful, and advocated tying babies' hands to their cribs to keep them from touching their genitals, which might provide pleasure. (In the 1920s and 1930s, for the same purpose, clitoridectomies were performed on little girls in some parts of the country.) She regards circumcision as an outgrowth of such attitudes: it was done to prevent male babies from using their penises as organs of pleasure.

Arms says, "We can contrast this with the reason for circumcision under Judaic law. In that tradition, circumcision was done on the eighth day as part of a convenant with God. Many Jews now believe that circumcision can be done without cutting the boy."

She also argues that the medical reasons once given for this operation—for example that it prevents cancer—have turned out to be false. Circumcision has no medical value at all and has a lot of risks associated with it, including bleeding and other effects of surgery.

She continues, "It exposes newborn babies to what is for them excruciating pain. Some babies feel it less than others, but, by and large, it puts the baby into shock and trauma."

Many advocates of circumcision apparently feel it is a way to harden the boy. In the past, children to be circumcised were tied down on boards, six in a row. A baby would lie there unable to move, listening to the screams of the little boys next to him. This was considered a way to prepare boys to be ready as adults to give up their bodies in war.

Arms concludes, "I think it's very important that we begin to understand the shock and trauma from this process that we have called normal in the United States. And we don't even acknowledge this trauma, so how can we heal it? People are running around with the long-term effects in their nervous system of an unresolved trauma. Believe me, that is what we are seeing in this culture."

What are the Advantages of Breast-feeding?

For many of today's working mothers, breast-feeding is difficult because they can't be at home enough to be with their infants. However, women are further encouraged to neglect breast-feeding by the growth of fallacies about it, as well as a lack of full knowledge of its benefits.

The first major benefit of breast-feeding is the mother's milk itself: it gives the baby the appropriate nutrients. For the first nine months, Arms notes, the baby doesn't need any other food at all other than from breast milk, which helps establish and nourish the baby's immune system. Feeding the baby from the breast creates in the mother a feeling of calm, relaxation, and deepening love for her child. For the baby, just being there, skin to skin, with the mother, affords immune protection.

The components of breast milk actually change from feed to feed, and, for a mother who has more than one child, the milk changes from child to child. This is why formula can never mimic breast milk. Nor can the container that breast milk comes in ever be duplicated. There's a real difference between providing pumping stations at work and giving working mothers access on their job time to daycare where mother and baby can be together when the baby wakes up—not to mention allowing mothers to be home with their babies until the babies are old enough to be without milk for more than four hours at a time.

Breast-feeding does many things for the baby and the mother. It causes the mother's gut to secrete 23 hormones (that we know of), which bottle feeding does not do. These hormones cause a woman to lose weight as well as help her sleep better and feel calmer. If a mother is malnourished and underweight, breast-feeding helps her to get as much nutrient value out of her food as possible. More nutrient value is absorbed in her gut than would be if she were not breast-feeding.

Arms tells us, "All babies need to be breast-fed and almost all mothers, even those who have had breast surgery, can breast-feed, if we give them three months to get settled before we even think of having them go back to work. And then we need to create work situations where they can breast-feed during the day."

BREAST-FEEDING FALLACIES

The following corrections to common fallacies about lactation and breast-feeding are from K. G. Auerbach, "Breast-Feeding Fallacies: Their Relationship to Understanding Lactation," *Birth* 17, no. 1 (March 1990): 44–49.

Nipple soreness is not related to skin color.

The lactating breast is never empty.

All women do not experience pain during each breast-feeding.

Nipples do not get tougher with nursing.

Creams and oils on the breast are not encouraged for nipple soreness; vitamin E toxicity could be a concern because of liberal applications, and pesticide residues are a concern in sheep-fat-derived lanolin.

Engorgement may be experienced by newly breast-feeding mothers but is almost always indicative of inappropriate or infrequent suckling.

The let-down process is not a singular event, but occurs continually during suckling.

The human nipple is different from artificial nipples: it can stretch two to three times its nonsuckled length. It contains fifteen to twenty pores, which spurt a fine stream of milk. The milk ejection occurs in a rhythmic fashion. The nipple remains elongated only with active suckling. It does not drip continuously.

Noninfectious mastitis rarely requires antibiotic therapy; infectious mastitis includes temperature elevation and flulike systems as well.

Extra fluid intake is not needed for breast-feeding; drinking to quench one's thirst is sufficient.

The lactating mother's breasts become full usually between one and three days after the infant starts suckling.

Colostrum, which is a highly concentrated source of protein and antibodies, is produced as early as the third month of pregnancy.

Women with inverted nipples can breast-feed.

Healthy babies do not need supplemental feedings before the mother's milk comes in.

Breast milk helps reduce bilirubin concentrations by coating the small intestines, reducing bilirubin recirculation.

Additional water or glucose given to the infant reduces total caloric intake and diminishes the coating action of milk feedings.

Human milk is far superior in all aspects to artificial formula.

The Stages of Pregnancy

A woman's body undergoes numerous changes during each stage of pregnancy. These physiological changes are described by nurse practitioner and massage therapist Susan Lacina:

FIRST TRIMESTER

"The fetus grows rapidly, and the mother's body changes to support this swift development. Hormonal balance changes. Human chorionic gonadotropin hormone (HCG) is needed for development. As it is released, it causes many discomforts, such as breast tenderness, digestive problems, nausea, and vomiting. Progesterone levels increase and may cause mild hyperventilation, heartburn, indigestion, and constipation. Increased blood flow and its change in composition contribute to fatigue, overheating, and sinus congestion."

SECOND TRIMESTER

"The placenta takes over the hormone production, and the levels of HCG drop. Along with that, the discomforts of nausea and vomiting ease up. Physical growth of the fetus crowds the abdomen, and a woman's body expands to accommodate the growth. Fetal production of thyroid stimulating hormone (TSH) begins in the fourteenth week and causes the mother's thyroid level to increase. This can lead to irritability, mood swings, mild depression, increased pulse rate, and hot flashes. Adrenal hormones become elevated and remain that way until delivery. This may cause impaired glucose tolerance and swelling. Skeletal structure becomes softer and more flexible to allow for expansion. If a woman doesn't have enough muscle flexibility, she will have some pain, for tight muscles do not allow for these adjustments. She may experience sciatic nerve pain from the lower back down the back of her legs due to the extension of the pelvis, especially at the joint of the sacrum and the pelvic bone. The growing baby puts pressure on the inferior vena cava, which can cause light-headedness, nausea, drowsiness, and clamminess. Prolonged reduction of blood flow can cause backaches and hemorrhoids. Lying on the side decreases this problem.

"From the twentieth week on, the uterus expands by stretching muscle fibers. Abdominal muscles and ligaments stretch to support the uterus, and there may be abdominal pain. There is an increase in melanin production, causing darkening of the nipples and a line called the linea nigra down the abdomen. If the lymph drainage system is not functioning well, an excess of melanin in the skin can cause brown spots. A well-functioning lymph drainage system is believed to keep melanin levels down so that brown spots do not occur. Increased progesterone causes sinus congestion, postnasal drip, and bleeding gums. Increased capillary permeability may cause the hands and feet to swell."

THIRD TRIMESTER

"As the baby continues to grow, the expectant mother changes her posture to shift her center of gravity. Heavier breasts can cause shoulders to slump forward. The spine is pulled out of alignment, and this commonly causes backaches. The growing fetus also compresses the veins and the lymphatic system. That can cause ankle edema and varicose veins. There is increased pressure on the intestines and bladder, causing frequent urination and constipation. Pressure on the sciatic nerve can cause more lower back and leg pain. As the diaphragm starts to rise, breathing becomes more difficult. Insomnia is common."

What to Avoid During Pregnancy

Before describing the positive steps you can take to make your pregnancy, labor, and transformation after delivery as healthy as possible, I want to note some things, a few of which are normally benign, that you should avoid during pregnancy. Susun Weed is a herbalist and teacher with over 30 years of experience. She has taught at the Yale Nursing School as well as the National College of Naturopathic Medicine and at breast cancer institutes in Germany. She has written four books on herbal medicine, including *Wise Woman Herbal for the Childbearing Year*.

According to Weed, it is well known that the health of a baby's parents affects the health of the baby. If the mother has an overgrowth of *Candida*, so may the child. If the father is a heavy drinker, this may cause liver problems for the child. During the first two months after conception, women and their fetuses are the most sensitive to toxins, hair dyes, aspirin, and so on. Thus it is of paramount importance that a woman be aware of what things can have a detrimental effect on her growing fetus.

Drawing from her store of knowledge of American Indian lore, Weed tells us, "First of all, we need to be very aware of something that may come up before a woman is even aware that she is pregnant—because, of course, we are pregnant for two weeks before we miss that first period—something many women are not aware of, which is that high heat during these first few weeks can permanently damage the fetus." This heat may come from a hot bath, a sauna, or even a sweat lodge. This is one reason why, she elaborates, "in many native American traditions, women in their fertile years do not go into the sweat lodge due to the possible adverse effect to the fetus."

Women must also be careful about taking vitamin supplements. Women who take 10,000 units of vitamin A during the first six weeks of pregnancy are five times more likely to have a child with birth defects than women who don't take the vitamin. "I believe that during her fertile years a woman should be quite cautious in taking supplements," is Weed's opinion. "Of course, we want to get those good vitamins, but we want to try and get them from our fruits, our vegetables, our beans, and so on."

It is not only vitamin A that can lead to birth defects; vitamins D and E are also potentially dangerous. "Those three are oil-soluble vitamins," says Weed, "and they tend to be quite detrimental to fetal development when taken in pill form."

Smoking is not good for your fetus. Alcohol is not good for your fetus. Radiation is not good, so even a mammogram should be avoided during pregnancy or if you think you are going to get pregnant. Caffeine in any form should be avoided. Coffee and latte, tea (black, green, or twig tea), and many soft drinks contain generous amounts of caffeine and all can cause birth defects.

Avoid aspirin and certainly antihistamines. This last is a hard one, especially for women who are dealing with hay fever. Antihistamines have a fairly tarnished record when it comes to causing birth defects, Weed says. "I don't just mean drug antihistamines but herbal ones as well, such as *ma huang* or ephedra."

Laxatives are not the way to go. Unfortunately many people use them and, even worse, many misguided herbalists even suggest women use them to clean out. Of course, there's nothing to clean out. All laxatives, Weed believes, should be avoided by all people, but especially by women during their fertile years, or at least if they are having a baby or trying to get pregnant. This includes herbal laxatives like senna, aloe, castor oil, rhubarb root, buckthorn, and cascara sagrada. Even a bulk-producing laxative like flaxseed should be taken with some caution. To use it, buy the whole flaxseed, grind it up, and sprinkle a small amount into foods.

Generally, you should stay away from diuretics. A woman in her fertile years usually doesn't take them anyway, but anyone inclined to take diuretics should be aware that they can cause problems. Herbal diuretics such as juniper berries and buchu can also cause problems. Avoid hair dyes, all kinds of chemical stimulants and depressants, antinausea drugs, sulfa drugs, vaccines, and anesthetics, especially at the dentist's office.

Weed notes, "There is some question about what happens if we take steroidlike herbs. The more we look into steroids, the more widely we find them spread across the herbal kingdom. As a matter of fact, carrots, the regular carrots you find in the supermarket, contain so many phytohormones that generous use of carrots may prevent conception. We know that wild carrot seed, in fact all parts of the carrot plant, act to prevent contact between the egg and the sperm and prevent that egg from attaching to the uterine wall. So we often advise pregnant women to avoid drinking any carrot juice at all and to cut back on the amount of carrots they are eating."

There are a few other herbs which you need to avoid only if you have miscarried frequently. "Some women get very concerned about miscarriage," Weed states. "If you are concerned, there are some herbs normally used in cooking that you would do well to avoid during the first trimester of pregnancy. Don't go overboard in worrying about them; they will not harm the fetus, but they might, in a highly susceptible woman, cause uterine contractions." They include many herbs in the mint family, such as basil, thyme, sage, rosemary, marjoram, savory, and peppermint itself. The entire family of herbs in the carrot family, such as celery seed, parsley, cumin, coriander seeds, aniseeds, and fennel seeds may cause problems for the sensitive woman. Ginger, nutmeg, and saffron have been used to cause a fetus to leave the uterus. Of course, to achieve that effect, they must be taken in enormous quantities, but for a very sensitive woman, it is best to avoid even small amounts in foods for the first trimester.

One other herb that Weed thinks is especially important for pregnant women to avoid completely is goldenseal. She tells us, "I've been a herbalist for 35 years, and I've never once had the opportunity to use goldenseal. Where I live the native people used to give it to their enemies in order to torture them."

Nutritionist Gracia Perlstein adds two more items to avoid: "High on the list is chemical exposure to toxic household cleansers. Natural food stores are a good source for environmentally harmless cleansers of various kinds. You want to avoid fumes from paints, thinners, solvents, wood preservatives, varnishes, glues, spray adhesives, benzene, dry cleaning fluid, anything chemically based and questionable. Stay away from household pesticides. And *don't* go spraying for fleas, roaches, or ants with commercially available pesticides when you are pregnant or looking to become pregnant."

She also counsels women to avoid a toxic psychological environment. "As much as possible, avoid stress, negative people, and aggravating situations. Instead, try to spend quality time alone and with loved ones, people who are supportive. Spend time in nature. Read inspiring literature. Listen to beautiful music. This has a beneficial effect on your mental and emotional state. That, in turn, affects your baby's biochemistry."

Miscarriage

Surprisingly, two-thirds of all pregnancies end up as miscarriages. One reason is that many women miscarry before they even know they are pregnant. Most commonly, genetic abnormalities precipitate the problem. The embryo develops wrongly, and the woman's body naturally aborts the fetus. Endocrine system imbalances are also associated with miscarriages. Women in their late forties have an especially difficult time carrying to term, due to hormonal changes that accompany aging. Poor thyroid gland functioning can also interfere with pregnancy, as can intercourse during pregnancy. Another cause of miscarriages is low-grade infections, which are often the result of sexually transmitted diseases. The woman is not conscious that a problem exists, but the body knows, and rejects the fetus. Bladder infections are also common; as the uterus enlarges, it places great pressure on this organ. Miscarriages may also occur when women are too hard on their bodies. Women who push themselves to the limit by overexercising and undereating to the point of anorexia are risking miscarriage. They are not getting enough nutrition for their own bodies, much less for the fetus.

When a miscarriage occurs more than once, a woman needs to have a thorough medical workup. Once the problem is understood, it is often correctable. If a woman is having intercourse during pregnancy, for example, she may simply need to take precautions. Using a condom during intercourse can prevent a miscarriage because it keeps male prostaglandins out of the female system, which, in turn, prevents premature uterine contractions. Low-grade infections must be cleared up, and increasing the intake of liquids and vitamin C can sometimes do the trick. Mixing 4 oz of strawberry juice with 4 oz of water is an especially good source of vitamin C, which acidifies the urine and helps prevent bladder infections. More serious infections should be cultured and treated appropriately. Sometimes, this means taking antibiotics. Older women who are having a difficult time holding on to a pregnancy due to hormonal changes may need low doses of progesterone, about 25 mg, in suppository form.

Some herbs seem to prevent miscarriage. Midwife Jeanine Parvati Baker uses this formula. She mixes together 1 oz of wild yam root, 1 oz of *Mitchella repens* (also called partridgeberry, twinberry, squawvine or partridge root). Baker also adds 1/2 oz of false unicorn root and 1/2 oz cramp bark. She puts them together in a half-gallon jar, fills it to the top with boiling water, and lets it sit for about four hours. You can sip this brew slowly until you are over the symptoms of miscarriage or, if you are just worried about your pregnancy, drink a half cup each day. The half gallon will keep very well in the refrigerator.

Tonics and Herbal Preparations

Tonics are herbal preparations that keep your body in good trim, up and running for optimum performance and healthy living.

If you want to take such good care of yourself that you won't have any problems during pregnancy, there are certain herbs that will help you achieve your goals, Susun Weed explains. "One that all readers are surely familiar with is red raspberry, *Rubus idaeus*. It is probably the best known, the most widely used and the safest of all pregnancy tonics."

In Weed's opinion, "Tonics don't have too much effect unless they are brewed in water. My personal experience is that herbs in capsule form are basically placebos. They may release a person's fear because she thinks she is doing something rather than because of their ingredients. Now I have no quarrel with placebos; but I would rather use my herbs in a way that actually draws out their nourishing and tonifying qualities."

Taking red raspberry in capsules, then, is ineffective. So is taking a tincture of it, for in a tincture the alcohol fails to draw the minerals out of the plant. Minerals are crucially important to good health. What draws out those minerals is water.

To prepare red raspberry tonic buy dried red raspberry leaves in bulk. Weigh 1 oz of them in a quart jar, preferably a canning jar. If you don't have a scale, fill your jar about one-third full. Pour boiling water right to the top of the jar, set it aside, and let it steep for four hours or longer. Weed says: "Actually what I do is put up a nice infusion before I go to sleep at night. Then the next morning, it's ready for me. I strain the plant material, squeezing it to get the last of the good stuff out. Give that plant material back to the earth. The liquid is what I drink. I can heat it up, drink it at room temperature, or pour it over ice. Whatever I don't drink right then, I refrigerate and drink up within the next 36 to 48 hours." A quart a day of red raspberry tonic is usually not too much.

This tonic increases fertility in both men and women. It helps prevent miscarriage and hemorrhaging during the birth. It's one of the best herbs to ease morning sickness, and it helps provide a safe, fast birth, reducing pain during labor. It reduces afterbirth pains, helps bring down undelivered placenta, and increases the amount and quality of breast milk. The rich concentration of vitamin C, vitamin E, carotenes, vitamin A, calcium, iron, the B-vitamin complex, and the large amounts of phosphorus and potassium make taking red raspberry well worth it.

"One woman said to me," says Weed, "'You know, I took that red raspberry as strong tea in an infusion almost every day, and I had a very long birth. It took three days.'

"And I said, 'What happened after three days?'

"She said, 'I pushed the baby out.'

"I replied, 'That's because you had the strength of red raspberry in you. Most women, after three days of labor, wouldn't be able to push the baby out.'"

So red raspberry strengthens and tonifies the uterine muscle, promotes fertility, and benefits the whole body of the man and woman who are going to be the parents of this child.

Another tonic for early pregnancy is stinging nettle, which is one of the most nutrient-rich substances available. Ounce for ounce, it exceeds the amount of nutrients in any other plant from the ocean, land, or fresh water. It is loaded with carotenes, from which we make vitamin A; vitamins C, E, and D; the B vitamins; vitamin K; and calcium, potassium, phosphorous, and immune-strengthening sulfur.

Make a tonic the same way as for raspberry. Weigh out 1 oz of the dried herb, put it in a jar, fill the jar with boiling water, then tightly lid it and steep overnight. You can drink it warm, cold or in between, up to four cups a day. The chlorophyll in this brew is so high that the infusion will actually look black rather than green.

Nettle helps the kidneys, and the kidneys have to do a lot of work during pregnancy. Like red raspberry, nettle increases fertility in both men and women. It is an herbal vitamin and mineral supplement. Many women feel a little unprotected when they stop taking their daily supplement, but Weed advises them to drink their nettle infusion, which will give them as many minerals and vitamins as any supplemental pill.

Nettle is tremendously nourishing. It eases leg cramps and any other muscle spasms you have during pregnancy. Because of nettle's high calcium content, it diminishes labor pains and birth pains. It is such a superb source of vitamin C that it is one of the world's most highly favored herbs for preventing hemorrhaging after birth. It's also a wonderful way to reduce hemorrhoids. It can increase the amount and richness of your breast milk.

Herbs

Pregnant women who have fatigue, moodiness, and preeclampsia can benefit from herbs. Weed strongly advises women to take stinging nettle tonic, which is a power from the earth, for these problems.

"As an aside," notes Weed, "one thing I advise women to do is, at least sometimes, have a total freakout or tantrum. This will get your friends and family ready for what you are going to be like during labor, because in labor there are no holds barred. If a woman is planning to go through a natural labor, she may want to leave the door open to scream, cry, curse, whatever she needs to do. As midwives say, 'The holes all have to be open if we are going to get that baby out. The mouth has to be open too.'"

Mood changes in women are often mediated by hormone swings, as well as by blood sugar swings. And those hormones are going to be swinging around when you are pregnant. Other herbs, along with raspberry leaf and stinging nettle, can help avoid these swings. A very good one is dandelion. You can take it in any form. You'll probably find dandelion root tincture in any health food store. The usual dosage is 10 to 20 drops, taken before meals, in the morning, and just before you go to bed—a total of five times a day.

"I've also found," Weed informs us, "that the liver is very critical in maintaining a healthy pregnancy and in preventing preeclampsia." The kidneys have to do about 150 percent of their normal workload during the pregnancy. We also know that lack of nutrients, protein, salt, calcium, and potassium, as well as insufficient total calories, can push a woman into preeclampsia. Dandelion leaves, especially when eaten as a cooked green, provide tremendous amounts of potassium, calcium, and good-quality vegetable salt. They can even be used as a remedy for a woman who already has preeclampsia.

Here are a few more suggestions about herbs. Ginger is one of the best natural remedies for nausea. Ginger works best when the person taking it eats small, frequent meals and gets plenty of fresh air and rest. Ginger can be taken as a capsule or tea. A washcloth soaked in ginger or comfrey tea and applied to the area where an episiotomy has been performed promotes healing. Rosemary added to bath water relieves tension and back pain. Finally, adding jasmine and clary sage to a bath has an uplifting effect and prevents postpartum depression.

Other Aids to Healthy Pregnancy

Yogurt, like nettle and red raspberry, is high in calcium. A cup of nonfat yogurt has a staggering 450 mg of calcium. Generally, good organic yogurt has no lactose in it because the yogurt-forming bacteria have eaten the lactose. Those who have difficulty tolerating milk find that yogurt is a real mainstay in helping prevent preeclampsia and a great number of other problems. Weed reminds us, "I mentioned earlier that a woman who has an overgrowth of *Candida* is going to pass that on to the baby. But if she has a good amount of yogurt in her diet, it is virtually impossible for her to develop a *Candida* overgrowth. In fact, women who eat as little as half a cup of yogurt a day have a quarter of the vaginal infections and bladder infections of women who eat no yogurt. So this is one of the most critical foods for a healthy mother and a healthy baby."

Remember, too, that during pregnancy a woman's body is working very hard and she needs more rest. In Weed's view, "When you are pregnant, you have to set aside some time to work on the baby. So the first suggestion I make if a woman says she is tired during pregnancy is to take some more time off. Second, I suggest that she drink a nettle infusion. My third suggestion is that she not take any herb that would stimulate her, because she is going to wind up by being a lot more tired later."

Pregnancy Massage

Susan Lacina tells why a pregnant woman and her unborn child benefit greatly from massage. "We tend to think of a baby in utero as being cut off from the world," she says. "In reality, the child within is a conscious being that responds to sounds, emotions, and the inner environment that its mother creates, either through her sense of well-being or her lack of it." Here Lacina describes how maternity massage promotes a comfortable and healthy pregnancy:

HOW MASSAGE HELPS

RELAXATION AND STRESS REDUCTION

"This is the most important reason for a massage, and there are significant medical reasons why this is so. Research shows that prolonged stress builds up abnormal levels of toxins and chemicals in the bloodstream. These are passed through the placenta to the baby. Minimizing the buildup of toxins can be achieved by periodic deep relaxation. Relaxation increases the absorption of oxygen and nutrients by the cells of the muscles. When oxygen and nutrition increase, the woman has more energy. Some doctors also believe morning sickness and nausea are eliminated by lowering stress levels."

IMPROVED LYMPHATIC DRAINAGE

"Massage assists the lymphatic system in eliminating excessive toxins and hormones. Unlike the heart, the lymphatic system has no pump. It moves freely until muscles tighten up, but when muscles become too tense, either from the fetus or from stress, lymph movement decreases and the concentration of toxins rises. In the lower extremities, the growing uterus can inhibit lymph drainage, leading to swelling, varicose veins, hemorrhoids, and fluid retention. By relaxing the muscles, massage helps stimulate lymphatic drainage of toxins. It decreases the development of varicose veins by its draining effect and helps reduce swelling in the legs."

BETTER OVERALL MUSCLE TONE AND ELASTICITY

"A woman's body must expand to accommodate the growing fetus. Hips widen and abdominal, lower back, and shoulder muscles stretch. Legs must accommodate increased weight. Massage promotes flexible muscles, joints, ligaments, and tendons. It also helps decrease muscle spasms and leg cramps by getting rid of lactic acid buildup, and can alleviate the pain caused by sciatic nerve pressure. Added flexibility helps the muscles that are needed for labor."

HORMONAL BALANCE

"Massage balances the entire glandular system. An overactive thyroid gland becomes less active, thereby decreasing irritability, mood swings, and hot flashes. An underactive thymus gland is stimulated, which increases its ability to fight infection. The alternating relaxation and stimulation that massage provides helps a woman's body function in a more balanced manner."

MASSAGE DURING THE DIFFERENT STAGES OF PREGNANCY

Maternity massage lessens symptoms associated with each stage of pregnancy. Additionally, it eases and quickens labor, and helps afterward. Lacina points out, however, that there are instances when pregnancy massage should not be used. Contraindications include vaginal bleeding or bloody discharge, fever, abdominal pain, systemic edema (excessive swelling), sudden gush of water, severe headaches, blurry vision, excess protein in the urine, diabetes, high blood pressure, heart disease, and phlebitis.

FIRST TRIMESTER

"Massage must be gentle so as not to interfere with hormonal balance. Gentle pressure with the fingers on the bridge of the nose, under the eyebrows, under the cheekbones, and under the forehead can relieve sinus congestion."

SECOND TRIMESTER

"Concentration is on stimulating lymph circulation, decreasing edema in the hands and feet, and working on breathing problems by massaging the chest. Massage at this time also helps increase flexibility in the muscles, joints, ligaments and tendons. Additionally, it can reduce sciatic pain and muscle spasms. To alleviate hemorrhoids, pressure can be applied to the crown of the head for 15 seconds three times a day."

THIRD TRIMESTER

"Massaging the lower hips and the area near the sacrum helps reduce back pain. Stimulation of the lymph system and blood circulation continue, especially from the thigh to the abdomen. As delivery time approaches, the massage therapist can teach the mother and her partner shiatsu and acupressure points that stimulate and speed up delivery. At about 34 weeks, peroneal massage can be learned and applied."

PERONEAL MASSAGE

"This is a gentle stretch of tissues in the area between the vagina and rectum. Learning peroneal massage increases the mother's awareness of the muscles she needs to relax during the actual delivery and decreases her chances of having an episiotomy, an incision made to enlarge the vaginal opening at the time of birth. The actual procedure is as follows: Using warm vitamin E or vegetable oil, the mother places clean, oiled thumbs or index fingers an inch to an inch and a half inside the vagina and applies firm, gentle pressure downward and outward. Stretching continues until a burning sensation is felt. This is held for a few minutes. Performing this once or twice a day, up until the time of delivery, can result in an easier birth."

DURING LABOR

"Massage during labor helps to reduce pain and anxiety by offering relief from muscle contractions. The stimulation of certain acupressure points can speed up labor."

POSTPARTUM MASSAGE

"Postpartum is the name given to the six-week recovery period after birth. During this time, hormones readjust and the uterus involutes (returns to its prepregnancy size). Massaging the abdomen in a circular motion helps the uterus to contract and helps to expel blood. Massage also helps to stimulate milk flow. The following techniques can be applied for this purpose: (1) The pressure point at the base of the sacrum can be held for about 15 seconds, and then released. (2) Breast massage is another technique that can be used. Using some light oil, a woman circles her breasts with her fingertips. She places the hands flat on the breasts, starting at the nipple, and moves outward and up. That helps the glands to release milk. (3) Additionally, there is an acupressure point at the top and middle of the shoulder. Holding it for 15 seconds helps milk production. (4) Pressing the point between the sixth and seventh ribs (at the nipple level on the breast bone) helps to release milk."

ACUPRESSURE POINTS

Thumbs can be applied to the sacrum, at the bottom of the spine, and walked up the spine to the waist. Each point is held for about 5 seconds.

The point in the center of the buttocks is pressed in as the mother exhales and released as she inhales.

Thumbs can be pressed along the shoulder blades between the spine and the scapula.

On the legs, pressure can be applied to spleen 6, an acupressure point located approximately 3 inches above the ankle, on the inside of the leg right below the tibia bone. Holding this spot for 10 seconds and then releasing it helps to stimulate uterine contractions and speeds up labor.

The uterus point is on the inside of the foot, just under the ankle bone. The ovary point is on the outside of the foot, under the ankles, near the heel. Squeezing these points at the same time for about 10 seconds and then releasing them helps to speed up labor.

Breast and nipple stimulation helps create oxytocin, the hormone that helps the uterus to contract.

ALEXANDER TECHNIQUE

The Alexander technique differs from massage in that the pregnant woman is actively engaged. Kim Jessor, senior faculty member at the American Center for Alexander Technique in New York, makes an analogy to a piano lesson: "We talk about being Alexander teachers, the people who come to us are students, and the context is a lesson. So while the results are very therapeutic, I don't think of the work as a therapy but rather as a learning process. This is significant in that it empowers students to take charge in changing their movement habits."

The Alexander technique is based on the concept that all of us know how to move comfortably as children, but lose that natural flexibility over time. The method teaches people how to move freely again, which is especially valuable for women undergoing the stresses of pregnancy. Jessor explains this concept with a story: "I was watching my 15-month-old son in the playground as he squatted down to pick something up. There was something extraordinary in watching that particular movement. It was so easy, so organic, so direct. It's the kind of movement that most of us have lost contact with.

"That made me think of a film I saw of women in Brazil giving birth while squatting. They were working in harmony with gravity to push their baby out. While squatting is not a preferred method of delivering babies for Western doctors, it actually is one of the most efficient positions for a woman to be in to birth her baby and it is used in many cultures around the world.

"In an Alexander lesson with a woman who is pregnant, I actually work quite a bit on guiding her in and out of a squat. It's one of her movement options. Whether or not she, in fact, gives birth squatting, I think that it is a really useful way to begin to open up the pelvis.

"Young children have a certain freedom of movement that most of us lose contact with. One of the objectives of the Alexander technique is to restore that freedom of movement, which is important and wonderful for all of us, but particularly important for a pregnant woman dealing with the demands of pregnancy."

The Alexander technique is an experiential process. Real changes occur in the presence of a teacher who guides the student with hands-on training. "This is one of the special aspects of the Alexander technique," Jessor says. "You can learn a new way of moving because a teacher's hands give a new stimulus to your nervous system. After a lesson, people tell me, 'Wow, I feel so much lighter,' or 'I can't believe how easily I am moving.' This is because they are actively participating in the lesson. But it is also a function of the Alexander teacher's hands giving that experience."

Jessor describes some of the ways the Alexander technique helps women during and after pregnancy:

LOWER BACK PRESSURE IS RELIEVED

"In pregnancy, women are contending with additional weight in the front of the body, which creates more pressure on the lower back. I find that most people bend over from the waist, keeping the knees straight, and pulling the head back into the spine. This creates a lot of pressure in the back. If you do that over and over, day in and day out, it starts to wear on the body. Imagine trying to do that and being pregnant at the same time; there is even more stress. I might work with a pregnant woman on a movement like bending over. I actually put my hands on her, guiding her through the movement of bending, so that she gets an experience of moving in a new way. I have had two women come to me during their second pregnancy who had a lot of back pain the first time around. Both reported little or no back pain because they learned to move in new ways that no longer put pressure on the lower back. I really feel that back pain in pregnancy is not inevitable."

BREATHING IMPROVES

"Lots of pregnant women have breathing difficulties. There is a good reason for this; with the uterus growing and expanding, there is less space for the internal organs. The diaphragm has less room, so it is more difficult to breathe. The Alexander technique teaches students how to move with less downward pressure on the organs. This minimizes breathing constriction. A study on the Alexander technique and respiration performed by a Dr. Austin at Columbia Presbyterian Hospital in New York found significant improvement in breathing capacity after a course of lessons."

REST IS ENHANCED

"Fatigue and exhaustion are another issue in pregnancy, especially in the first and third trimesters. Women need to rest a lot, and there is an effective way to learn that in an Alexander lesson. This is not a movement component of the work, but involves lying down on the table. I have a woman lie down on her back in the beginning stages, and on her side as the pregnancy gets further along. I help her learn how to release unnecessary tension. It is easier to do this in the lying-down position because the student is not contending with gravity. The table lesson teaches the pregnant woman how to consciously release excess tension, which enables her to really rest and recuperate."

LABOR IS EASED

"Labor is an intense situation where a woman must learn to deal with pain and fear. The Alexander technique teaches the skill of releasing muscles between contractions. By fully letting go, the woman does not remain tense in response to the pain. Rather, she is able to conserve energy. When I gave birth, I worked with another Alexander teacher for labor support. She put her hands on me and gave me verbal direction. As a result, I was able to release more effectively between contractions. Husbands of pregnant students come to me for labor support lessons where they learn to be more available to women as they give birth."

STAMINA INCREASES AFTER DELIVERY

"There is a lot of very challenging physical labor in being a mother. Again, there is much bending. There is also a lot of lifting. It is very important to pay attention to how you are doing this. I work with a new mother on ways of bending efficiently to pick up her baby. Recently, I taught someone how to bend over and pick up a stroller while it had a 35-pound child in it. Also, the way that the baby is handled is very much affected by the way the mother is using her body. The better the use, the greater the sense of support and security for the child."

BREAST-FEEDING IS EASIER

"Breast-feeding also includes the component of bending. You tend to move toward the child as you are nursing, and there is the possibility of compressing your body. The Alexander technique teaches you how to maintain a sense of ease and balance while breast-feeding the baby throughout the day."

PSYCHOLOGICAL BENEFITS

Jessor concludes by saying that there are less tangible, but equally valuable, benefits from working with the Alexander technique during pregnancy. As a woman becomes aware of different options in movement, she simultaneously opens up to greater options in her thinking: "Women begin to realize that they can make different kinds of choices about the kind of birth they want to have, where they want to have it, and who they want to use for labor support. In the same way that they begin to find freedom in movement, they find greater options in terms of the choices they make about their pregnancy."

Diet and Supplements

The best insurance for a well baby is to follow a highly nutritious whole-foods diet. What you eat now will impact the health of your child later, according to nutritionist Gracia Perlstein: "When a woman is considering pregnancy, it is important that she address her diet to see how healthful it is, as many difficulties have their root in prenatal deficiencies. Scientific studies reveal that birth defects, and even problems that develop much later in life, can be prevented when the mother has excellent nutrition. I would like to include the father there too, because the quality of the sperm is also very important." Since the most crucial stage of embryonic development occurs in the first few weeks, before a woman realizes that she is pregnant, good-quality foods should be eaten all the time.

Eating properly means selecting unprocessed or minimally processed foods. A wide assortment of whole grains, legumes, vegetables, fruits, nuts, and seeds supplies multiple nutrients. "So many people eat the same 10 or 20 foods over and over again," Perlstein says. "In traditional cultures, people have much more variety. I would like to emphasize that supplements should only enhance an excellent diet. Make the effort to eat high-quality, nutrient-dense foods. That means whole foods, the way nature produced them."

The body intuitively knows what it needs to support new life, and paying attention to its messages can be a helpful guide. "A woman's body is very wise when she is pregnant. Many women can't stand the look or smell of coffee or cigarettes, even when they used to smoke or drink coffee several times a day," states Perlstein. She adds that worrying about eating the right foods all the time is stressful and can produce more harm than good. But nutrition education can benefit women with highly processed diets, who need to learn about better food choices. "Vegetarian women may crave animal foods or be drawn to dairy when they are pregnant. Usually it is good to pay attention to these cravings, but to respond in the most wholesome way possible."

Wholesome means organically grown. Pesticide-free fare is better for everyone, of course, but vitally important for young children and developing fetuses, according to recent research. Dairy and other animal products should be from creatures naturally raised. One reason for this is that pesticides and other contaminants tend to concentrate in an animal's tissues. The higher up the food chain, the higher the concentration of toxins. Fortunately, many health food stores, and more and more supermarkets, sell the healthful varieties.

Animal products, when a part of the diet, should be eaten in moderation. Although protein needs increase during pregnancy, they can be easily met from vegetarian sources, which are less toxic than their animal counterparts. Excellent vegetarian protein sources include fortified soy milk, tofu, tempeh, beans, nuts, and seeds, for example.

The increased need for calcium is similarly fulfilled in such a diet: "Many women do not realize that there are excellent sources of calcium other than milk and dairy. There are green leafy vegetables, fortified soy milk, tofu, almonds, and many other calcium-containing foods. If you eat a diet rich in fresh vegetables and fruits, you tend to get quite a bit of calcium. If you want a supplement, calcium citrate is easiest on the stomach. Other forms sometimes cause digestive upsets or constipation. Definitely avoid calcium-depleting foods: coffee, chocolate, and sodium."

Perlstein adds that eating several small meals throughout the day offsets common complications: "Hunger, not calorie counting, is the most reliable guide to eating during pregnancy. Five to six small, nutrient-dense meals per day is a sensible ideal. This is a good habit to develop in the last trimester of pregnancy, when the organs in your stomach are somewhat constricted, and good in the early stages to prevent nausea. It keeps the blood sugar from falling, and nausea has a lot to do with low blood sugar."

Water should be pure and taken in adequate amounts. Eight to twelve glasses are recommended to help flush out toxins from the liver and kidneys: "Many people do not drink enough fluids," notes Perlstein. "This is especially important during pregnancy because the woman is filtering the waste for two bodies."

Beyond an excellent diet, Perlstein recommends the following daily nutrients for pregnant women:

Multiple vitamin and mineral supplement

Vitamin C

B_{12}

Zinc

Vitamin E, 400 units

Folic acid

She notes that folic acid, which is also contained in green leafy vegetable and whole grains, is especially important in pregnancy because science has shown it to prevent neural tube defects. Even when included in the diet, extra folic acid should be taken in supplement form, since it is fragile and easily damaged by heat. Additionally, acidophilus helps prevent constipation and other types of colon problems.

Extra iron may be needed, but a woman should have her hemoglobin tested first, just to be sure it is really needed. Research shows that excess iron in the system can have damaging effects.

Exercise: General Guidelines

The American College of Gynecologists and Obstetricians (ACOG) endorses physical activity during pregnancy and has created specific guidelines for the dos and don'ts of exercise:

Pregnant women derive health benefits from a mild to moderate exercise routine. Exercising 60 minutes, three times per week, is preferable to intermittent activity, but some benefit can be derived from shorter durations as well. Sometimes little oxygen is available for aerobic exercise due to the body's increased oxygen demands. Therefore, a woman should begin an aerobic activity slowly, and gradually build to capacity. She should not push too hard, and certainly not to the point of breathlessness. Pregnant women should not exercise in the face-up position after the first trimester. This position limits blood supply to the baby.

Avoid standing for prolonged periods of time, doing heavy work in the standing position, and exercising at high intensities. These activities are associated with diminished birthweight in newborns. It's better for women to engage in non-weight-bearing activities such as cycling and swimming, rather than exercises like running. Non-weight-bearing exercise minimizes the risk of injury and allows activity levels to remain closer to prepregnancy levels, right up to delivery. A woman should be aware that her center of gravity is different, and that she might lose her balance when exercising. Anything that could involve falling over, or even mild abdominal trauma, should be avoided.

Pregnant women require an extra 300 calories per day in order to maintain their normal metabolic rate. Exercise increases the need for more calories.

A pregnant woman must be careful not to raise body temperature with vigorous workouts, especially in the first trimester. Excessive body heat in the mother can adversely affect the development of brain tissue in the baby. The threshold for this is a body temperature of about 39.2 degrees Celsius, which is 100 or 101 degrees Fahrenheit. To sume up: you should exercise, but never to the point of raising body temperature. Pool exercises help to dissipate heat. After delivery, gradually build up to prepregnancy exercise levels.

The overall benefits of appropriate exercise are enormous. According to chiropractor Richard Statler of Long Island, New York, "When a mother exercises, she gets more oxygen and is able to pass that to her baby. Better nutritional delivery, better oxygen, and better blood flow can only be helpful. There are also less complications during labor and birth, and that can mean a healthier baby."

Dr. Statler answers some commonly asked questions on the subject of pregnancy and exercise:

When should a pregnant women not exercise? "Basically, every pregnant woman can benefit from starting an exercise program at any point in pregnancy. However, there are certain exceptions to this rule. When any one of the following conditions is present, a pregnant woman should limit or avoid exercise: pregnancy-induced hypertension, premature rupture of membranes, incompetent cervix, persistent second- or third-trimester bleeding, premature labor during the prior or current pregnancy, and intrauterine growth retardation.

Other medical contraindications include thyroid, heart, vascular, or pulmonary conditions. Women with medical problems need a physician's evaluation to determine whether an exercise program is appropriate."

HOW MUCH EXERCISE SHOULD A PREGNANT WOMAN GET?

"How much exercise a woman is capable of largely depends on her fitness level before pregnancy. Someone who has never exercised should not begin a heavy program. Nor should someone who was an avid exerciser completely give it up. For a marathon runner to suddenly stop because she is pregnant can be as problematic as a nonrunner deciding to run marathons during her pregnancy."

WHAT ARE SOME SPECIFIC BENEFITS OF EXERCISING DURING PREGNANCY?

"Statistics show that women who exercise during pregnancy usually have an easier, shorter labor and safer delivery. There are fewer premature births. During pregnancy the woman feels more energetic and vital, and less stressed. Exercise alleviates a good portion of discomfort from back pain or sciatica. By stabilizing the blood sugar, exercise can even help women who are diabetic. Mothers who exercise see quicker recovery times after delivery.

"One benefit to exercising in a group program is the social aspect. An exercise group can provide informal support. First-timers speak to women who have been there, and get real-life input and suggestions. That's important in this day and age, when people no longer live with extended families who traditionally passed down such wisdom."

Specific Exercises

Dr. Statler says that exercises geared toward opening up the pelvis are particularly important in preparing women for delivery: "The pelvic area is where the baby sits. It must expand so that the baby can pass through. The pelvis has three contact points. In the front is the pubic bone area; in the back are two sacroiliac joints, one to the left and one to the right. Those joints can stretch and open up to allow the pelvis to expand. Although hormones secreted during this time allow the pelvis to open up tremendously, placing the woman in the typical birth position of lying on her back compresses the sacroiliac joints. We can potentially lock up two-thirds of her ability to stretch."

Stretching exercises are key for opening up this area. Here are three that Dr. Statler recommends:

HIP STRETCH

Stand with the feet shoulder-width apart. Rotate on the balls of the feet until the heels are turned out. In this position, do a half squat, keeping the back straight. It may help to do this while leaning against a wall. It can also be done on a supermarket line, while holding onto a shopping cart. An alternate way of doing the exercise is seated. Once again, feet are shoulder-width apart, and feet are flat on the floor. Shimmy forward slightly to keep from sitting back in the chair. Lean back a little bit to take the weight of the body off the hip joint. That allows for better movement. Place a child's volleyball or play ball between the knees and hold it there. Pivot on the balls of the feet to turn the heels out, keeping the heels flat on the floor. Now gently squeeze the ball while pushing the legs together and internally rotating the thighs toward the midline. Hold for 10 seconds and relax.

PUBIC STRETCH

This exercise, like the cat arch (see below) is great for opening up the hip and sacroiliac joints. Both prepare the mother for delivery by developing more stable joints throughout pregnancy. The pubic stretch helps the front of the pelvis by using motions that are opposite to those used in the hip stretch. Standing, with feet shoulder-width apart, turn toes and thighs out. Bend knees slightly. As before, this can be done in a supermarket while holding on to a shopping cart. In the seated position, sit on the floor with the soles of the feet together and knees apart. Use the back against the wall for support. Pull the feet as close to the body as is comfortable. Place the hands on the knees, and gently press the knees down and apart from each other toward the floor. Hold that for 30 seconds while breathing deeply. Repeat two or more times. Never do any bouncing or jerky motions. These are slow stretches.

CAT ARCH

The cat arch also opens up the hip and sacroilian joints. Kneel on all fours so that hands and knees are touching the floor. Arch the back like a cat, while slowly inhaling. Allow the back to return to the flat back position while exhaling. Do not curve the back in. Hold for a few seconds and relax. Repeat 10 to 15 times.

Aromatherapy

Ann Berwick reports that in Europe, where aromatherapy is scientifically studied and widely prescribed, hospital maternity wings utilize essential oils for their soothing and uplifting mind-body effects: "There is a report of one woman who had severe anxiety throughout her pregnancy. They gave her neroli oil, which helped to keep her blood pressure down and allowed her to go into delivery in a more relaxed state. During delivery, she was given lavender and clary sage to relax her uterus. Clary sage is also slightly euphoric, so it helped her to cope mentally with the birth." Here are some formulas to try before, during, and after birth:

As an antidote for nausea and vomiting, peppermint is effective when a very dilute amount is rubbed into the stomach or inhaled.

For relaxation, 8 oz vegetable oil, 13 drops lavender, 2 drops geranium, and 10 drops sandalwood can be massaged into the skin or used as a compress.

To clear nasal congestion, a teaspoon of eucalyptus oil can be added to a cold-air humidifier or pan of hot water. The steam inhaled lessens congestion.

To help heartburn, place two to three drops of diluted peppermint oil on the back of the tongue.

A good massage oil to use during labor consists of 5 drops rose oil, 12 drops clary sage, and 5 drops *ylang-ylang* in 2 to 3 oz of vegetable oil.

To prevent stretch marks, massage 2 oz wheat germ oil, 20 drops lavender, and 5 drops neroli oil into the thighs.

To soothe sore nipples, mix one pint cold water, one drop geranium oil, one drop lavender oil, and one drop rose oil.

After an episiotomy, a sitz (shallow) bath is helpful, especially when two drops of cyprus oil and four drops of lavender oil are added. Soak for 15 to 20 minutes.

To promote milk production, take two drops fennel oil with some honey water, every two hours.

Hemorrhoids will be helped by five drops of cyprus oil added to the bath.

The astringent action of cyprus and lemon oil constricts varicose veins. A few drops can be added to a body lotion and applied to the veins morning and evening.

Homeopathic Remedies

EARLY STAGES: MORNING SICKNESS

Homeopathic physician Stephanie Odinov Pukit lists a variety of remedies for all stages of pregnancy. She begins with treatments for morning sickness, noting, "Along with the dry biscuit in bed with a hot beverage, homeopathic remedies can be extremely important at this time."

SEPIA. Ambivalence is the key word here. There is a conflict between self-preservation and the urge to procreate, which makes wanting a child questionable. The woman becomes angry and irritable and feels as if a black cloud hovers over her. Although her appetite is insatiable, heavy pains worsen with smells or thoughts of food.

PULSATILLA. This is the opposite scenario. Pulsatilla is an excellent remedy for the woman who is cheerful, sweet, and somewhat helpless. The person is warm and may throw the covers off at night. She becomes worse with emotional excitement. Nausea comes and goes and is characteristically worse in early evening.

NUX VOMICA. This is a wonderful remedy for soothing the nerves after a woman has abused her body with alcohol, drugs, or coffee. She tends to be constipated. She tends to wake up at night to think about business because she is ambitious and driven.

ARSENICUM. The picture here is a person constantly anxious about her state of health. She always runs to the doctor fearing that something is wrong. The woman tends to have burning pains. She has great thirst and takes little sips. Symptoms are usually exacerbated at midnight.

COCCULUS INDICUS. This remedy specifically helps motion sickness. The woman tends to lose sleep and to be constantly exhausted. She may be nursing children or caring for someone. The woman feels dizzy standing and better when lying down. She feels worse in fresh air.

PETROLEUM. Petroleum may be indicated if there is a voracious appetite followed by persistent vomiting.

BRYONIA. The person has strong sensitivity to smells and may have connective tissue and arthritic problems. Nausea becomes worse with motion.

LATER STAGES

Dr. Odinov Pukit suggests these remedies for problems that occur in the latter stages of pregnancy.

SEPIA OR PULSATILLA. In the third to sixth month, the fetus presses high up in the abdomen, causing heartburn, shortness of breath, and indigestion. These remedies also help hemorrhoid problems. The one chosen depends on the other symptoms manifested. Sepia is for a gloomy disposition, while pulsatilla is for a sweet nature.

CARBO VEGETABILIS (CARBO VEG). The woman is slightly heavy and tends to have indigestion and shortness of breath due to poor oxygenation. Although she tends to be chilly, she prefers open windows with the air directly on her.

BELLIS PERENNIS. As the baby drops into the pelvis, pressure is felt on the organs in the lower part of the bladder. Pain and arthritis may occur as a result. *Bellis perennis* is specific for pain in the uterine area or groin. The woman might be walking when all of a sudden her legs weaken from a sharp nerve pain. After childbirth, when arnica has done its job (see below) and there are still some lumps remaining in the tissues, *Bellis perennis* is also excellent.

KALI CARBONICUM. Kali carbonicum is for women with back pain, especially those who tend to wake up between 2 and 4 o'clock in the morning. This individual's personality is somewhat crabby and closed. She is vague and evasive about answering questions. Pains are better with pressure and rubbing. The person tends to be anxious and chilly.

ACONITE. High-potency aconite is wonderful to use at any point in pregnancy when there has been shock or fright. Arnica and calendula may be useful for this purpose as well.

ABNORMAL PRESENTATION

In addition, Dr. Odinov Pukit works with abnormal presentation. She finds that homeopathic remedies can help turn the baby over when used between 32 and 36 weeks: "Pulsatilla works in 40 percent of the cases, and other remedies are used when they match the woman's constitution. A remedy that is wonderful for that woman in general may help in this specific area as well."

LABOR AND POSTPARTUM

Midwife Jeannette Breen finds homeopathy useful during labor and after birth. "I seem to be using more and more homeopathic remedies since I've been seeing the advantages." She also cautions that homeopathic remedies should not be used as a quick fix. "There is not always a pill to take care of every problem in labor and birth. Sometimes you have to be patient. That's what midwives are good at. They try to be as patient and supportive as possible during this time."

These are a few of the homeopathic remedies she recommends:

ARNICA. Starting a month before delivery, regular application of arnica directly to the nipples prevents later tearing and cracking with breast-feeding. After birth, arnica quickens recuperation. Calendula can be used in the same way.

CALIFILUM. Califilum may help a stalled labor. This is specific for a weak uterus or a uterus running out of steam. The woman often experiences weakness, exhaustion, trembling, and shivering. Sharp, brief, unstable, and painful lower uterine contractions fail to completely dilate the cervix and push the baby.

GELSEMIUM. Gelsemium may be indicated as a follow-up to califilum. It is also good for neuralgia, rheumatic discomfort, and pains in the bladder and vaginal area. The person tends to be thirsty and chilly.

CIMICIFUGA. Cimicifuga is good for stalled labor, especially when the woman is becoming fearful, hysterical, and exhausted, and the pains are becoming erratic. This tones the uterus, calms it down, and helps it to become more coordinated.

THE NEWBORN

Odinov Pukit adds that after-birth homeopathic remedies can help newborns as well: "If the baby is distressed, we might need arnica rescue remedy. Carbo veg is wonderful if there is cyanosis with some respiratory effect. And arsenicum if the baby is born lifeless."

Water Birth

Jeannette Breen is a great enthusiast for using water during labor: "It has a wonderful analgesic quality, which is much better than an epidural. Being immersed in water provides tremendous relaxation. It does not take the pain away, but women do report feeling less pain in the water. They feel less effect from the pull of gravity. Their movements are very easy, and there is much better tissue relaxation, which means there is almost no tearing in a water birth. It is also easier for the baby because the mother is more relaxed and moving freely. She is not stuck in one position. It is easier for the baby to negotiate the pelvis and to slip out in a warm, moist environment that is quite familiar."

Social Support

"Two keys to a normal healthy pregnancy and birth are a healthy diet and good social support," says Breen. "Those seem to be overlooked, especially in traditional maternity care in this country. The focus is on diagnostic testing, but not a lot of emphasis is placed on healthy diets, other than prescribing women prenatal vitamins and iron. There is no question that a high-quality diet rich in all the nutrients can make a woman's whole body work more efficiently and effectively.

"Social support creates an environment of love that is all-important but too often overlooked in hospital birthing environments that focus solely on technology. No one can have the baby for the pregnant woman, she has to do it herself. But if she is surrounded by love and support, rather than fear and technology, she is able to give birth in a very intuitive, instinctual way which is satisfying and safe."

Corrective Vaginal Surgery

In the United States, about 80 percent of women who give birth have an episiotomy performed. Of those operations, approximately 90 percent are improperly performed. "Doctors are just not instructed in how to do this surgery," says Dr. Vicki Hufnagel. "All you have to do is go to your local medical school, get out the textbook on obstetrics, and look at what an episiotomy is. It will have a drawing and a discussion that says to put one or two sutures here, and one or two there. They are teaching physicians to close an entire organ system in just one or two layers. If you were to close a laceration on your face in one or two layers, your muscles wouldn't work, your face wouldn't work. You'd be a real mess. We are teaching students how to close the vaginal vault area in a manner that is not allowable in other places. That is the standard of care that we have, and it is completely unacceptable."

Incorrectly performed episiotomies result in problems down the road. Without the support of the vaginal muscles, the cervix pushes through the vagina. It appears that the uterus is being forced out, when really it is not. Doctors mistakenly diagnose a prolapsed uterus and commonly recommend a hysterectomy. Tragically, 100,000 to 200,000 women with this misdiagnosis receive this operation each year.

Corrective surgery easily ameliorates the problem. Repairing the vagina is a simple procedure that can be performed in a doctor's office. It takes all of 45 minutes, and patients can go home the same day.

Postpartum Depression

Depression after childbirth affects thousands of women each year. Although the exact cause is unknown, hormonal shifts after birth, particularly drops in progesterone, may play a large role. Research also links the condition to low levels of the neurotransmitter serotonin. Emotionally, it is often connected to difficult labor and disappointments after birth.

Symptoms range in degree, but are generally worse than a temporary feeling of the blues immediately following childbirth, according to Dr. Marjorie Ordene, a complementary gynecologist from Brooklyn, New York: "Postpartum depression is defined as a gradually increasingly sullen mood and a loss of interest and enthusiasm starting around the third postpartum week. This is different from the 'baby blues,' which is a common occurrence in the normal population. The blues happens the first week postpartum, and basically goes away by itself. We are talking about something much more severe." In the worst-case scenario, women can become sick for years and lose touch with reality.

HOMEOPATHIC REMEDIES

Homeopathic physician Dr. Jane Cicchetti recommends that women try the 30c potency of the remedy that best addresses their symptoms. If this does not help, a visit to a homeopathic physician can provide more individual support.

SEPIA. Sepia may be needed after an exhausting delivery, after giving birth to two or more children at once, or after having several children. The woman feels completely worn out and depressed. Physically, she feels as if her uterus might fall out, and finds herself crossing her legs a lot. Often there is an actual prolapse of the uterus. Emotionally, a woman who loves her husband and children suddenly has an aversion to them. In fact, she has an aversion to everyone and wants to be alone. She becomes irritable and angry if anyone bothers her, and has an aversion to sex. The woman cries often but cannot understand what is wrong; in fact this problem is caused by a hormonal disturbance rather than an emotional one.

NATMUR. Natmur is for chronic grief. The woman is introverted and dwells on past, unpleasant memories but keeps them to herself. She tries to put on the appearance that everything is fine, and becomes aggravated if someone tries to comfort her.

IGNATIA. Ignatia is for postpartum depression brought on by emotions. It is needed when disappointment follows childbirth. A woman imagines an ideal pregnancy and birthing situation. When that does not work out, she feels extremely let down and depressed. These feelings may occur after a stillbirth or a miscarriage. There is uncontrollable sobbing and sighing, and a rapid change of emotions, which are often contradictory.

ARNICA. This commonly needed remedy is useful for depression, upset, and malaise brought on by bruising, soreness, and pain that lasts a long time. Arnica helps heal the physical trauma and improves the mother's energy and emotional state.

PULSATILLA. Pulsatilla is given when a woman cries a lot and wants to be taken care of. She needs to attend to her newborn baby, but feels as if someone should be attending to her. This individual will eat sweets and other goodies to alleviate overwhelming feelings of sadness and loneliness. The woman often is warm-blooded and enjoys the fresh air. She is happier walking around outside, and much happier if she can be with people.

CIMICIFUGA. This remedy is used less often, but is very important for those who need it. Cimicifuga is derived from black cohosh, a powerful herb for treating hysteria and female complaints. It is needed when a woman feels as if a dark cloud of gloom has settled over her. She fears losing her mind. Often this stems from a very difficult delivery. She may have had a mini-nervous break-down, feeling at one point as if she was going insane. This leaves her with a great fear of ever having a baby again. Often she alternates between different emotional states. When she is not under this dark cloud of gloom, she becomes excitable and talkative, jumping from one subject to another in an almost hysterical fashion. Cimicifuga heals the nervous system.

KALI CARBONICUM. This deep mineral remedy is indicated for women who become anxious and irritable after a delivery that leaves them feeling weak. Easily startled, they want to be left alone and have an aversion to being touched. They tend to be chilly and to have insomnia from 2 to 4 a.m. Further, they are regimented and have trouble going with the flow of caring for a new baby. Often these symptoms follow a delivery that primarily consists of back labor. Sciatica develops to some degree, which can lead to an emotional state like this.

PHOSPHORIC ACID. Phosphoric acid is helpful when a woman is extremely disappointed from physical or emotional shock. She may have lost the baby, or something might be wrong with the baby. A loved one may have died at the time of birth, or she may be affected from the loss of much bodily fluid during delivery. Indifferent to everything, the woman lies in bed with her face to the wall. It is as if her emotions have completely disappeared. She doesn't want to talk, think, or answer questions.

COCCULUS. This is a remedy for fatigue and emotional depression brought on by loss of sleep. The woman feels drunk and may go through the day feeling dizzy and staggering. These feelings are brought on by sleep deprivation.

AURUM METALLICUM. Arum metallicum is for profound depression characterized by total hopelessness, self-destructive behavior, and a longing for death.

These remedies can make a difference because they get to the root of the problem. Regarding conventional treatment methods that use antidepressants, Dr. Cicchetti says, "Women just suppress their symptoms, and their health does not really get any better."

NATURAL PROGESTERONE

"Studies show that postpartum depression can be prevented by treating women with progesterone," reports Dr. Ordene. "Companies that make natural progesterone cream recommend using a half teaspoon twice daily, starting a month after delivery. Since postpartum depression is supposed to start three weeks after giving birth, it makes sense to begin using natural progesterone at that time."

VITAMIN B$_6$

According to research, vitamin B$_6$ raises serotonin levels. Patients given B$_6$ for 28 days after delivery did not have a recurrence of postpartum depression.

Herbal Pharmacy

Plants containing phytochemicals with anti-morning-sickness properties, in order of potency. are as follows:

Persea americana (avocado)
Triticum aestivum (wheat)
Hordeum vulgare (barley)
Oryza sativa (rice)
Sesamum indicum (sesame)
Glycine max (soybean)
Lens culinaris (lentil)
Avena sativa (oats plant)
Zea mays (corn)
Avena sativa (oats seed)
Tamarindus indica (tamarind)
Pisum sativum (pea)
Theobroma cacao (cacao)
Gossypium spp. (cotton)

Patient Story: Laurie

I started massage about three years ago. I'm a nurse and I was working a twelve-hour shift in an intensive care unit, which really turned out to be thirteen- or fourteen-hour shifts. I was pregnant with my third child and having a great deal of back discomfort. A friend of mine, who had hurt her shoulder, recommended a massage therapist. I started to go and it helped tremendously. I felt wonderful.

After having the baby, I stopped going for a while because of finances. But then I started going again because I was having trouble with carpal tunnel where part of my fingers would get numb. And it helped tremendously with that.

To be honest, I had seen an orthopedic doctor about the carpal tunnel, and I didn't want surgery. I wanted to try to avoid that. I have to say, I feel perfect now just from going to the massage therapist for that problem.

Working in intensive care is very stressful, and I'm a wired type of person. The only time I sit down is to drive a car or go to the bathroom. This relaxes me and gets my whole mind clear for the week. It's really fantastic.

Patient Story: Darlene

I had severe back pain. When I became pregnant, I became quite worried about it. My chiropractor helped me to feel much better. He made the whole pregnancy easier.

My baby was colicky from birth, and my chiropractor suggested that I bring her in when she was seven days old for an adjustment. Every time she was a little gassy, I would bring her in, and he would adjust her. After that, she was a satisfied child who slept through the night. He really helped her.

As far as chiropractic treatment goes, I swear by it.

Abortion Aftercare

Although most women who have abortions do not have any serious medical complications from the procedure, the period after an abortion is a time for a woman to focus on herself; she may have a variety of physical and emotional needs that require attention.

READJUSTING HORMONE LEVELS

It's particularly important to remember that after an abortion your body's hormone levels have to readjust to the sudden change from a pregnant to a non-pregnant state. Dr. Susanna Reid, a naturopathic physician in Darien, Connecticut, who practices at the Center of Natural Medicine at the Center for Women's Health, describes the physical changes in a woman's body after an abortion.

"Hormone levels are elevated dramatically during pregnancy, and so the body has to readjust itself to its prepregnancy state," Dr. Reid explains. "One way to help the body to do that is by focusing on dietary factors that would be beneficial in regulating hormone levels. As well, you want to increase the circulation in the lower abdomen so that the body can heal itself. The more circulation in an area and the more nutrients that are in that area, the easier it is for the body to remove the toxic waste products. You'd also want to strengthen liver function, since the liver is essential to the balancing of hormones in the body; it functions to promote excretion of hormones. So if the liver isn't functioning correctly, you can have an imbalance of hormones."

To strengthen liver function she suggests eating foods that contain fiber, particularly fruits, vegetables, and whole grains. The gut needs fiber to prevent the reabsorption of hormones. "If there isn't enough fiber in the diet, the hormones are reabsorbed through the intrahepatic circulation. So fiber is very important. In the springtime, one can strengthen liver function by eating large amounts of fresh dandelions and other greens like cleaver. In other seasons, use yellow dock, nettle, dandelion, and cleaver with some red raspberry to make a tea. Red raspberry is a uterine tonic, so it helps to heal the uterus. You can put some peppermint in the tea to make it taste better and aid in digestion."

About two weeks after the abortion, she suggests using cold friction on the lower abdomen for 10 minutes at a time before going to bed or first thing in the morning.

PREVENTING INFECTION

One of the more common complications from an abortion is infection. It's important not to put anything into the vagina for several weeks after the abortion and to refrain from intercourse. Dr. Reid suggests several natural remedies to help prevent infections.

"If we enhance the immune function, we prevent infection. You can use an immune-enhancing diet that focuses a lot on fruits and vegetables. Fruits in particular are immune-enhancing." She also recommends echinacea, goldenseal, berberis, astragalus, and ligustrum to help immune function.

Dr. Allan Warshowsky, a board-certified obstetrician and gynecologist who practices holistic gynecology, recommends taking vitamins C, A, and E and other antioxidants to enhance immune function.

Dr. Reid also emphasizes fluid intake. She explains that an abortion creates many by-products, and one way the body can help eliminate them is through the exchange of fluids, so you should drink a lot of fluids.

EMOTIONAL ISSUES

Although each woman experiences abortion in her own way, it can sometimes create a strong emotional response, either positive or negative.

"If it is a desired pregnancy and it's a spontaneous abortion," Dr. Reid says, "then people are dealing with grief. Even if it is a therapeutic abortion, there can be many reasons for the abortion. It may be because the pregnancy isn't viable or wouldn't be viable or maybe it isn't the right time. So there are just a lot of grief issues for some women around abortion."

Dr. Warshowsky believes it is very important to deal with any negative feelings. He suggests that women who experience grief and other emotional and psychological consequences after an abortion may be helped by using meditation or visualization techniques.

Chapter 28

Premenstrual Syndrome (PMS)

P remenstrual Syndrome (PMS) refers to the symptoms that begin during or after ovulation and end with the conclusion of the menstrual flow. Because of diet and lifestyle, PMS is more widespread in Western societies than in Asian societies and in less developed countries. Jeese Hanley, M.D., in an article in Alternative Medicine magazine, says that PMS is an indication of imbalance in the body, either psychological, nutritional, or hormonal. Dr. Hanley sees PMS as "a wake-up call" signaling us to pay attention to these imbalances and fix them before they turn into a more serious condition.

Causes

Dr. Hanley points out that menstruation does not create pain and discomfort when a woman is healthy. However, we live in an environment full of synthetic chemicals, including herbicides and pesticides, that mimic estrogen once they get inside the body, enhancing the effects of natural estrogen and disturbing the hormonal balance. Further, an excess of estrogen in relation to progesterone causes problems of hormonal imbalance.

Symptoms

The effects of PMS range from mild to severe, and they vary from person to person. They may include bloating, cramps, headaches, swelling, fluid retention, low back pain, depression, abdominal pressure, insomnia, sugar cravings, anxiety, irritability, breast tenderness, mood swings, and acne.

Clinical Experience

DIET

Dr. Michael Janson, an orthomolecular physician from Cambridge, Massachusetts, and author of The Vitamin Revolution, says, "Sugar, caffeine, and alcohol precipitate or worsen symptoms and should be avoided. This is because a lot of patients with PMS have overt hypoglycemia. Their sugar levels fluctuate up and down. Eating sugar sends blood sugar levels way up, and the body responds by dropping sugar levels way down. Additionally, caffeine, even when taken in small amounts in the morning, can aggravate symptoms such as breast tenderness and sleep disturbances."

According to Dr. Janson, the best diet for lessening the symptoms of PMS is high in fiber and complex carbohydrates; meals should be small, with snacks in between. This helps to regulate blood sugar, and in many cases is enough to reduce or eliminate PMS symptoms. Herbalist Letha Hadady recommends eating a lot of cool green foods such as salads; avoiding hot, spicy, and acidic foods; and eliminating coffee from the diet. Some people, however, need more help and can benefit from vitamin therapy, exercise, and a stress management program.

Dr. Hanley recommends that a woman who suffers from PMS should completely avoid milk and milk products, for milk has a high concentration of pesticides and other estrogen-mimicking chemicals.

NUTRITIONAL SUPPLEMENTS

When symptoms are severe, diet alone may not be enough. The following nutrients may prove useful.

VITAMIN B$_6$ (PYRIDOXINE). Pyridoxine has a number of helpful properties for alleviating PMS. As a smooth muscle relaxant, it can decrease cramps. As a diuretic, it reduces fluid retention, swelling, and breast tenderness. Between 200 and 400 mg should be taken daily, and vitamin B$_6$ can be taken throughout the month, rather than just premenstrually. For the first two weeks of the cycle, take 100 mg a day in a B-complex vitamin; take an additional 250 mg the last two weeks of the cycle. Note that the more B$_6$ you take, the more magnesium you need.

MAGNESIUM. Magnesium calms the nervous system and relieves anxiety, depression, irritability, nervousness, and insomnia. As an antispasmodic, it alleviates cramps and back pain. Magnesium also helps reduce cravings for sweets. Between 500 and 1,000 mg may be needed.

GAMMA-LINOLENIC ACID (GLA). GLA is a precursor of prostaglandin-E1, a hormonelike substance that helps to regulate neurological and hormonal functions. Prostaglandin-E1 helps reduce muscle spasms, cramping, sugar cravings, mood swings, depression, anxiety, irritability, acne, and to some extent breast tenderness. It also reduces inflammation and decreases the stickiness of the platelets, which prevents blood clotting. GLA is found in evening primrose oil, borage oil, and black currant oil. Borage oil is the most concentrated source of GLA; it contains 24 percent GLA, the equivalent of six capsules of evening primrose oil. One 1,000 mg capsule of borage oil provides a daily dose of 240 mg of GLA.

EICOSAPENTAENOIC ACID (EPA). EPA, which is found in fish oil and flax seed oil, produces prostaglandin-E3, which helps to alleviate breast tenderness. Flax seed oil is fragile and should not be used for frying. It can be used in salad dressings or over cooked foods.

VITAMIN E. Vitamin E, 400 to 800 IU, can reduce cramps, breast tenderness, and fibrocystic breasts, which often swell up before a woman's menstrual period.

MULTIPLE VITAMIN AND MINERAL SUPPLEMENT

Dr. Hanley adds that women taking birth control pills need supplements high in the B-vitamin complex and in antioxidants (vitamins A, C, and E). That is because the pill can seriously lower the body's reserve of B and C vitamins, increasing the risk of cervical dysplasia and possibly cervical cancer.

EXERCISE

Exercise helps to improve mood, reduce cramps, eliminate excess fluid, and control sugar cravings. Aerobic exercises should be performed three to four times per week.

WESTERN HERBS

Naturopathic physician Janet Zand, in an article on the HealthWorld Online website (www.healthy.net), suggests two herbal programs for PMS, one a general program and one modified for women with PMS accompanied by flu and flulike symptoms. Zand says that with either program, if you have severe cramps during the fourth week, you can get symptomatic relief by taking homeopathic magnesia phosphorica in a 6c potency every 1 to 2 hours until cramps are relieved, then three times a day for three days.

GENERAL HERBAL PROGRAM

This program builds blood and balances hormones during the first two weeks, then decongests the liver during the second two weeks.

First and second weeks, or until ovulation occurs:

Combination of red raspberry leaf and *dong quai,* taken as tablets, capsules, tinctures, or tea, three times a day.

Third and fourth weeks (starting when ovulation occurs, until the menstrual flow begins):

Magnesium and vitamin B$_6$, two to three times a day. This combination helps decrease cramps and PMS symptoms.

Choline, methionine, and inositol, two to three times a day. These lipotrophic factors stabilize liver function by decreasing the amount of fat in the liver.

Bupleurum and dandelion, taken as tablets, capsules, tinctures, or tea, two or three times a day. These herbs comprise a liver-cleansing formula.

PROGRAM FOR PMS WITH COLD AND FLU SYMPTOMS.

Follow this program if you develop achiness and inflammation during the fourth week of your cycle. This indicates that your immune system has been weakened.

First and second weeks:

Same as previous program.

Third and fourth weeks:

Combination of goldenseal and echinacea, taken as tablet, capsule, tincture, or tea, three times a day. These herbs are antiviral, antibacterial, and anti-inflammatory.

Magnesium and vitamin B$_6$, two to three times a day, to decrease cramps and other PMS symptoms.

Inositol, choline, and methionine, two to three times a day. These lipotrophic factors help stabilize the liver.

Combination of bupleurum and dandelion, taken as tablet, capsule, tincture, or tea, two to three times a day, to cleanse the liver.

Zand adds that if you have severe cramps during the fourth week, you can get symptomatic relief with homeopathic magnesia phosphorica in a 6x potency. Take every 1 to 2 hours until cramps are relieved, then three times a day for three days.

CHINESE HERBS

Herbalist Letha Hadady finds the following Chinese herbs useful for alleviating symptoms of PMS:

LUNG TAN XIE GAN WAN. This Chinese remedy alleviates anger associated with PMS.

XIAO YAO WAN. This helps relieve PMS symptoms of depression, poor circulation, indigestion, and bloating.

WOMEN'S HARMONY. This herb increases circulation.

These remedies can be ordered from a mail order source in Oakland, California called Health Concerns (800-233-9355).

HOMEOPATHY

The homeopathic remedy chosen should correspond to the symptoms described; only one should be used for best results. Sometimes it's a matter of trial and error; if one does not work, try another.

DR. KEN KORINS'S RECOMMENDATIONS

Dr. Ken Korins, a classically trained homeopathic physician in New York City, recommends these remedies for PMS and lists the type of PMS symptom for which they are most useful..

LACHESIS. Lachesis helps most physical and emotional symptoms that accompany PMS, such as headaches, right ovarian pain, and breast tenderness. It may be indicated if PMS symptoms stop once menstrual flow stops. It is also indicated when symptoms get worse with heat and with constricted clothing around the abdomen. Emotional indications are restlessness, paranoia, and a tendency to be talkative.

LACCANINUM. Think of laccaninum when the only symptom is a painful, swollen breast, the pain leaves once the menstrual flow begins, and there is a tendency to be irritable.

BOVISTA. Bovista is indicated when gastrointestinal symptoms, such as diarrhea, occur before the period begins. There may also be traces of blood before the actual flow begins. Subjective and objective feelings of swelling occur throughout the body, even through the hands, resulting in a tendency for the women to feel clumsy.

PULSATILLA. Pulsatilla is good for emotional symptoms of PMS involving a weepy disposition and a need for consolation from others. It helps curb a strong craving for sweets.

NATMUR. Natmur is good when the woman's emotional state is melancholy and sad and worsens when others attempt to console her. Headaches occur before, during, or after the period, and there is a craving for salty foods and an aversion toward sex at the time of the period.

SEPIA. Sepia is indicated in the presence of symptoms such as sadness, depression, indifference, and feelings of discontent and discouragement about life. Often a colicky pain is felt before the menses. There may also be a sensation of the uterus dropping, as if it would fall through the vagina due to congestion in that area.

FOLLICULINUM. This is a new French remedy that can be given on the seventh day of the cycle in a 30 to 200c potency.

DANA ULLMAN'S REMEDIES

Homeopath Dana Ullman, in an article on the HealthWorld Online website (www.healthy.net), suggests some additional remedies. Take each one in the 6c, 12c, or 30c potency every two hours while symptoms are strong, then every four hours after symptoms diminish. When symptoms become mild, stop the remedy. If you experience no clear improvement within 12 hours, try another remedy.

BELLADONNA. Use belladonna when the major symptom is "bearing down" pains or cramps that appear and disappear suddenly. It is also useful when cramps are made worse by motion, a draft, or being jarred, and when they are associated with a headache.

MAGNESIA PHOS. Magnesia phos is recommended for cramps made better by warmth, by simply bending over, or by bending over and at the same time firmly massaging the abdomen, and made worse by cold and by being uncovered.

COLOCYNTHIS. Colocynthis is indicated for cramps like those just described when those cramps are accompanied by feelings of extreme restlessness and irritability.

IGNATIA. Ignatia is good for bloating accompanied by strong emotional downs, such as hysteria and grief, and when the woman experiences conflicting feelings.

CIMICIFUGA. Cimicifuga is used for bloating accompanied by sharp, laborlike pains shooting across the body, perhaps accompanied by sciatica or back pain, difficulty tolerating pain, hysteria, talkativeness, and a sense of everything being "just too much to bear."

NUX VOMICA. Nux vomica is used for Type A personalities who are often highly stressed, who experience bloating and nausea along with irritability, and who become quarrelsome and critical.

PROGESTERONE

To restore hormonal balance, Dr. Hanley advocates natural progesterone, preferably in the form of cream made from wild yam, which is rubbed into the skin. This is because only 10 percent of hormones taken by mouth actually reach the bloodstream; the liver filters out the rest, which stresses the liver and gallbladder and increases the risk of gallstones, gallbladder disease, and liver cancer. Progesterone cream is used between ovulation and the day before the menstrual flow starts.

Progesterone promotes youthfulness, and is beneficial against cancer and fibrocystic breast disease. Dr. Michael Janson says additional progesterone is especially important for women exposed to exogenous estrogens, found in pesticides, food additives, drugs, and other chemicals in the environment. These lead to an overload of estrogen and a deficiency of progesterone. Progesterone is extremely helpful for treating PMS symptoms when such an imbalance exists.

Dr. Hanley also cautions that women taking herbs to relieve PMS symptoms should be sure to include herbs that promote progesterone production. *Dong quai,* alfalfa, licorice root, ginseng, anise seed, garlic, fennel, papaya, red clover, and sage are all estrogenic herbs. They may relieve symptoms, but they may also lead to fibroids, tumors, and cancers. They should be balanced with progesterone-precursor herbs, including wild yam, sarsaparilla, and chaste berry (*Vitex agnus cassus*).

Dr. Hanley suggests a "hormone fast" in which you stop taking all hormone supplements for one week per month. Doing so simulates a woman's natural cycle, in which estrogen and progesterone are at low levels during menstruation.

LIVER DETOXIFICATION

According to Dr. Hanley, detoxifying the liver can relieve many female health problems. The first step is to reduce fat in the diet; and the second is to use a detoxifying formula that contains herbs and plant enzymes that work to remove toxins from the liver. The herbs and enzymes must be used together; neither should be used by themselves. Dr. Hanley recommends a liver detoxification program two or three months out of each year; women who suffer from severe PMS is severe can do the program for longer time periods and more frequently.

REFLEXOLOGY

Reflexology is a science and an art based on the principle that we have reflex areas in our feet that correspond to every part of the body. Massaging specific reflex areas in the feet helps to improve the functioning of specific organs and glands.

Laura Norman, a certified reflexologist from New York City, describes three reflexology techniques.

"Thumb walking can be used on the bottom, tops, and sides of the feet, although it is most often used on the bottom. The procedure entails bending the thumb at the first joint and inching along the bottom of the foot like a caterpillar, pressing from the heel up to the toe. The right hand is used on the right foot. Taking little tiny bites, press, press, press the whole bottom of the foot.

"Finger walking is similar to thumb walking, but is done by bending the finger at the first joint and using the tip of the finger on the outside edge.

"Finger rotation is where you rotate the finger into the foot."

Massaging the feet with thumb walking, finger walking, and finger rotation using a nongreasy, absorbent cream warms the feet and helps promote overall relaxation. For addressing specific problems, reflexology must be applied to specific areas.

Knowing where to massage is fairly simple because as reflex points on the foot correspond to the way the organs and glands are distributed within the body. Laura Norman explains, "If you were to imagine your body reduced, and superimposed onto your feet, the points would be laid out just as they are in your body, from top to bottom. The top of the body is the head, and the toes reflect everything in the head area—the eyes, nose, ears, mouth, teeth, gums, jaw, and brain. The ball of the foot represents the chest area—the heart, lungs, and bronchial tubes. The center of the foot represents the internal organs."

For PMS, of course, the points corresponding to the pelvic and reproductive organs are the points that need to be massaged. As Laura Norman explains, "The pelvic and reproductive organs are located in the heel and ankle area. The uterus point is midway between the ankle bone and the heel, on a diagonal. Thumb walking should be performed around the ankle on the big toe side of the foot. The thumbs should be pressed down, like a caterpillar, all over that inside ankle. After than, a circular rotation performed with the thumb can be done on that midpoint. Finger walking can also be used over that area.

"Next, work should be done on the reflex areas that correspond to the ovaries. Those are located on the outside of the ankle. With the right foot cradled on the left leg, find the high spot on the ankle bone. Square off the back of the heel and draw an imaginary diagonal line. Divide this line in half and that is where the ovary point is. This outside point of the foot will not be visible, and the correct point must be located by feel or by using the index or middle finger of the left hand as it wraps around the bottom of the heel. This reflex point is almost always more sensitive than the uterus point, so care should be taken not to use too much pressure. Done properly, this technique should help to get the blood circulating.

"Following this, the reflex point corresponding to the fallopian tubes should be addressed. That reflex point across the top of the ankle, from ankle bone to ankle bone, on the top of the foot. This connects the ovaries to the uterus. What you need to do is finger-walk from one ankle bone to the other across the top of the foot. Two fingers can be used here, one from each hand.

"Although the focus is on the reproductive organs and glands, all systems should be massaged, as the entire organism is interrelated. For whole-body relaxtion, therefore, it is important to massage and press on the entire foot. Sliding the thumbs across the bottom of the feet serves this purpose and feels wonderful."

Reflexology for PMS helps most when performed three or four days before, and during, menstruation. First the right foot is worked on, while resting on the left leg. Then the same actions are repeated on the left side.

Patient Story: Laura Norman

Twenty-five years ago, I had my first reflexology experience. My friend Judy came to visit me from California. At the time, I was suffering from terrible menstrual problems. I was premenstrual—bloated, headachy, achy, and feeling awful all over.

She said to me, "Laura, I've been studying something called reflexology that is such a powerful tool to help you feel better all over and especially with the menstrual condition." Judy had me take off my shoes and socks, lie down on my bed, and prop my feet up on some pillows. She pulled up a chair to the end of my bed, dimmed the lights, put on some music, and applied some hot, wet washcloths to my feet. She started to rub and press and squeeze my feet with the washcloths. It felt incredible to start with. Then she began massaging my feet with some cream, and this was heavenly. Next, she started to apply pressure to very specific parts of my feet, which she said corresponded to various parts of my body.

I felt fantastic. I was floating. I had never felt so deeply relaxed in my entire life. My symptoms completely disappeared. Afterward I was energized. I was so clear-thinking and productive. At that time I was in college studying for exams, and under a lot of pressure.

Judy continued to work on me, and I continued to find out more about reflexology on my own. The more I applied what I learned, the better the results that I achieved. It made a tremendous difference, and totally changed the course of my life. As a result of pursuing this technique for my own healing, I began to do reflexology professionally and began a whole new career.

Now I have been practicing reflexology for twenty-five years and have seen incredible results with all kinds of conditions in all walks of life—infants and children and seniors.

Chapter 29

Repetitive Strain Injuries

I n all the hoopla that has accompanied the manifestations of the computer revolution—from the original PCs to the World Wide Web—not much attention has been paid to how the installation of computers in offices has physically affected their users. What is talked about is how, at least in the industrialized countries, jobs that were grimy, dirty, and physically grueling, like those in steel mills and automobile plants, are being exported to nonindustrialized countries; while in their stead have come jobs in service industries—for the less educated, flipping burgers; for the more educated, sitting in offices at terminals processing and moving information.

Those who are infatuated with the world of computers see this exchange—back-breaking labor in the mills traded for work in sanitary, air-conditioned offices—as all to the good. However, although there are undeniably benefits to workers from this exchange, they do not necessarily fall in the area of occupational health and safety. It is undeniable that the owners and managers of plants that manufactured heavy industrial equipment were notorious for disregarding toxic chemicals and other dangers in the workplace, but it is also true that the managers of many light industries have exposed people to years of looking into computer screens and rattling out numbers on keyboards without ever taking a look at the possible health effects of this labor.

One of the better books to profile these effects on both physical and mental health is Barbara Garson's *The Electronic Sweatshop*. She moves up the job ladder, starting with lowly data-entry clerks and moving up to Wall Street traders and Pentagon officials, in order to show how their lives are impacted negatively by working with computers. In her interviews, she hears consistently about loss of autonomy and ill health. This chapter will look at a common type of health problem experienced by people whose jobs involve a lot of time at a computer terminal: repetitive strain injuries, and particularly carpal tunnel syndrome.

Repetitive Strain Injuries

Dr. Timothy Jameson, the author of *Repetitive Strain Injuries: Alternative Treatments and Prevention,* is a graduate of Los Angeles Chiropractic College and is certified as a chiropractic sports physician. He notes that many people today have repetitive strain injuries. "One unique thing about these," he points out, "is that they can affect every structure of the body, which is what sometimes makes them so hard to treat. Most people will start off with simple muscle fatigue, such as affects people who work on computers or on assembly lines. They fatigue the muscles because of the overexertion, that cumulative trauma."

To continue to put stress on already-fatigued muscle will eventually lead to problems with the connective tissue, or fascia, that forms a sheath around muscle. The fascia responds to repeated stress on the muscle by becoming harder and thicker. It can start getting "sticky" and begin to bind to the muscle and other neighboring tissues. The muscles and fascia become tight and restricted. Eventually, the nervous system gets involved.

A recent study in Great Britain showed that the sensory nerves, the nerves that pick up perceptions from the hands, the skin, and so on, are affected by repetitive strain. They are damaged by cumulative trauma. Cumulative trauma can also affect the tendons that connect muscles to bones. When this happens, the tendon and the sheath that holds the tendon may become inflamed. (When this occurs in the wrist, you have carpal tunnel syndrome.) This condition may lead to problems with the bursas, sacs which protect the joints.

These problems may even involve the spine, according to Jameson. "People with this type of injury tend to have a lot of pinched nerves that lead down to the arms. The process is very complex."

HOW SERIOUS ARE REPETITIVE STRAIN INJURIES?

As Jameson explains, repetitive strain injuries to various parts of the body can be extremely serious. "You become very limited in your ability to do any type of work, especially repetitive work. In severe cases, a person cannot work at all, cannot even get dressed in the morning. They cannot do the things they normally would do."

This type of injury is not like a broken bone. A fractured bone can be immobilized, and depending on the severity of the fracture, it will heal completely within a specific period of time. With repetitive strain injuries, multiple parts of the body are affected.

DIETARY FACTORS

If you are doing things that can lead to repetitive strain injury or are already suffering from this disability, there are foods you should cut from your diet. The number one items to avoid, which are major precursors of joint pain, are refined sugars, particularly high-fructose corn syrups. These increase sugar within the body, which sets off the whole process of the insulin reaction, with release of prostaglandins, which starts the inflammatory reaction.

Jameson recommends the book *Enter the Zone* by Barry Sears as a good source of information on proper nutrition. The book "goes into depth on how to prevent an inflammatory reaction. If you look through the aisles of the grocery store, you'll see that something like 50 percent of the products sold there use high-fructose corn syrup as an ingredient. The body has a lot of trouble digesting that. I know of cases where people cut it totally out of their diet, and their repetitive injury subsided within a few days."

Processed meats, such as corned beef, salami, and hot dogs, are very tough for the body to digest and can trigger an inflammatory reaction. Some of the more saturated oils, such as corn oil, palm oil, safflower oil, and butter, should also be avoided. Margarine, too, is bad. Many people think margarine is better than butter. However, margarine, because it has trans-fatty acids in it, is actually worse for the body than butter.

VITAMINS AND MINERALS

"When patients come in with this problem," says Dr. Jameson, "I put them on a number of vitamin supplements. I would recommend vitamin C, which is very important for tissue healing, starting out with about 1 g and going up to about 3 g a day.

"Also very important are the B-complex vitamins. These are used for nerve regeneration and nerve healing."

Minerals are another important supplement that can help in cases of repetitive strain injuries. As Jameson puts it, "You should never underestimate the power of minerals to rejuvenate cellular tissue." He puts his patients on a complete mineral regimen, with either colloidal or chelated minerals.

"A lot of people—especially people in jobs that involve heat, a lot of sweating, in the summer—are sweating out many of the minerals in their body. So if they are doing a lot of cumulative work and sweating they are depleting their body's mineral's resources." A list of the minerals and vitamins that Jameson finds useful for preventing and treating repetitive strain injuries follows. "I usually prescribe these substances in pill form," he notes, "but you can also get all these things in food."

CALCIUM. Calcium is very important for muscle activity and for bone growth; it is also a muscle relaxant. Take about 800 mg a day of calcium, a little more if you are pregnant or postmenopausal.

MAGNESIUM. Magnesium is also important for muscle relaxation and for coenzymes. It is required for the functioning of about 80 percent of the enzymes in the body. Good sources of magnesium are vegetables and whole grains. Jameson recommends starting out with about 200 to 300 mg of magnesium a day. He says. "That's a small amount, considering that magnesium is not well absorbed. However, I always like to start my patients out with small amounts to see how they react."

MANGANESE AND ZINC. Jameson says that zinc, in particular, is really important for enzyme function and for cellular healing. He recommends about 20 or 30 mg a day. Zinc is found in fish, meat, and poultry.

SELENIUM. Selenium, another valuable substance, is found in fish, wheat germ, and garlic. Take 50 to 200 mcg a day in the pill form.

VITAMIN E. Vitamin E is a very important antioxidant; Jameson recommends 200 to 400 IU per day.

BETA CAROTENE. "Beta carotene," Jameson remarks, "is a compound found in vegetables of a yellow-orange or dark green color. Carrot juice is a great source of beta carotene. I recommend that patients drink carrot juice to get a natural, fresh form of the compound."

COENZYME Q10. Dr. Jameson says coenzyme Q10 is particularly important for patients with underlying heart disease. It's also important to maintain cellular energy, which is vital in cases of repetitive strain injuries.

PROTEOLYTIC ENZYMES. "Proteolytic enzymes scavenge around the cells and rake up any cellular debris, aiding the healing process."

CARTILAGE GROWTH FACTORS. Jameson adds, "There is also some good research now on the cartilage growth factors glucosamine sulfate and chondroitin sulfate. A recent book called *The Arthritis Cure* describes them (see Chapter 4, "Arthritis"). I recommend them for patients who have a great deal of joint discomfort—joint pains, irritation of the elbow, the spine, or the hands and fingers."

HERBAL REMEDIES

Certain herbs help the body relax, which is important in overcoming some repetitive strain injuries. Although Jameson doesn't have specific dosage recommendations, he offers these ideas. "Valerian root can be used for reducing muscle spasms. It should be taken toward the end of the day, because it's a relaxant. You wouldn't want to take it throughout the day, because it might affect your ability to perform. Garlic is a natural antibiotic as well as antifungal. Some of these muscular problems can stem from an underlying fungal problem, something we also see in fibromyalgia. A third valuable herb is *Ginkgo biloba*, which increases circulatory function and brain function and enhances memory. It helps the blood flow get down to the extremities. Cayenne has also been found to help increase circulation. And ginseng is great for stress relief."

HOMEOPATHIC REMEDIES

In addition to vitamins, minerals, and herbs, homeopathic remedies can be of service. Try the ones you find in health food stores that are recommended for muscle and joint injuries and for rheumatoid arthritis.

Carpal Tunnel Syndrome

Carpal tunnel syndrome, a widely recognized type of repetitive strain injury, is a common disablity affecting office workers who sit at computer terminals. It is important that workers at risk for carpal tunnel syndrome not only follow the suggestions we make here but also to learn to sit and type with the correct posture and to use ergonomically designed chairs and keyboards.

CAUSES

The direct cause of carpal tunnel syndrome is the effect on the tendons of the lower arms of day-in, day-out use of the same muscles and nerves to perform a repetitive task. The result is numbness, tingling, and pain, which worsens at night. It's a miserable disorder.

In looking at the syndrome, Dr. Ray Wunderlich notes, "We also have to think about the various background factors which people bring to this syndrome." Dr. Wunderlich, who is board certified by the American Academy of Pediatrics and the College for the Advancement of Medicine, practices preventive medicine in St. Petersburg, Florida, and is the author of many books, including *The Natural Treatment for Carpal Tunnel Syndrome*.

When treating a case of carpal tunnel syndrome, he starts by looking for contributing factors. For women, he asks immediately, "Is she taking birth control pills?" The pill, in essence, "puts you in a simulated state of pregnancy, and we know that pregnancy is one of the risk factors for carpal tunnel syndrome. Birth control pills also diminish the nutrients in the body, some of the water-soluble vitamins. Morevover, many women who take them become bloated. They develop minor degrees of fluid retention." The carpal tunnel is a narrow space in the arm, which becomes too narrow if the tissues are swollen. Women who are taking birth control pills and who perform tasks likely to lead to carpal tunnel syndrome should consider some other form of birth control.

Two other contributing factors, says Dr. Wunderlich, are hormone replacement therapy (HRT) and thyroid deficiencies. With regard to HRT, Dr. Wunderlich says, "If the estrogen preparations are not in balance with the progesterones, this can cause problems."

Dr. Wunderlich finds that 75 to 80 percent of his patients have some kind of thyroid disorder. He says, "On top of the repetitive movement of their jobs, many people have thyroid disorders, which contribute to the syndrome and may be hard to diagnose. To pin this down, look for a pale, puffy person, edematous, which is to say retaining fluid. When there is swelling, especially in connective tissue and in the nine tendons that run through that carpal tunnel, that medial nerve in the tunnel is often screaming for more room."

Another background factor may be low adrenal states, which may occur for a variety of reasons. People who overwork themselves, who take caffeine and/or sugar, who have bombarded their body with these substances and are now faced with repetitive tasks and sedentary living, may wind up with low-functioning adrenals. In the workplace, they develop various allergies, sometimes combined with low blood pressure. These people often have swollen, edemenous tissues, which contributes to the problem.

Then, of course, there is diabetes. Type II diabetes in particular is often accompanied by edematous conditions. This may not be readily observed, Wunderlich cautions. "It may be microedema rather than pure edema. The ankles may not be swollen, for example, or the lungs congested, but the tissues may be slightly swollen.

"When the blood sugar is too high—which is almost a definition of diabetes—osmotic pressure rises. As we know from high school, osmosis is what controls the body's fluid pressure. The fluid should be in the blood vessels and in the lymph tissues. When it's outside in the body tissues, as happens in high blood sugar states or after we eat a lot of candy or, sometimes, fruits or juices in excessive quantities, the tissue may become water-logged. This too can cause problems in that narrow carpal tunnel. The medial nerve is screaming with numbness and irritability and pain every time we move our fingers."

Food allergies are another potential contributing factor to the development of carpal tunnel syndrome—and many other disorders. The repetitive, monotonous diets that so many people consume, especially with high-protein antigens—such as milk, cheese, and sometimes eggs—often produce food allergies. And a hallmark of the allergic response is swelling. Although the swelling is on the microlevel, the little cramped carpal tunnel reacts to the swelling, causing pain.

But even if you are not allergic to what you're eating, if you're on a typical American diet, you are headed for disaster. "The 140 pounds of sugar per person, per year, that the average American still eats is one problem," Wunderlich says. "We're not talking about a long time ago. It's still happening. And there are also the salt-laden diets, which could be improving as people are counseled by alternative nutritionists to take high-potassium foods over high-sodium foods. There are also animal foods, which are high on the inflammatory scale—they tend to accentuate the inflammatory cascade, or series of chemical reactions through which inflammation develops. Animals are on top of the food chain, and that is where all the refuse accumulates, all the toxic chemicals that get into the animals' fat. This is especially true if the animals are domesticated and not wild, which is the case with most of our animal food sources." Thus if you are not following a pristine, organic diet, which the majority of people are not, you may be contributing to the risk of carpal tunnel syndrome or worsening an already existing condition.

Finally, Wunderlich says, there are "the chemicals in the workplace. When you are sitting at your computer, you may be bombarded with pesticides they have sprayed around your place—every month they come in and do that, or every two weeks if they see a lot of roaches. All of this adds to the toxic load as background factors."

CONVENTIONAL TREATMENT

By the time a person with carpal tunnel syndrom consults a physician, the condition is often in a quite advanced stage. According to Dr. Wunderlich, "The person often has atrophy of the muscles and irreversible or nearly irreversible nerve damage. The doctors operate, often with excellent results. So it's very appealing." However, this is a drastic therapy and will result in a life with further impaired function.

For less severe cases, conventional medicine's procedure is less felicitous. "What ordinary medicine does is give pain relievers—aspirin, Tylenol, ibuprofen, and other nonsteroidal anti-inflammatory drugs, which in the long term are all counterproductive, damaging the gastrointestinal system, producing leaky gut, as well as actually destroying cartilage. But those are the standard therapies that are offered."

ALTERNATIVE TREATMENTS

Dr. Wunderlich's program is short, sweet, and sensible. "The number one approach in treating this problem," Wunderlich states, "is detoxification. We do a vitamin C bowel flush. That's the first step for bowel tolerance." The vitamin C flush gets all those accumulated toxins out of the body. Follow this up with the second step, taking your favorite bulking agent, rice powder or psyllium, for example. "Number three," he mentions, "is to support the liver. I like artichoke and thistle compounds. Maybe 100 mg of thistle, three times a day, and 500 mg of artichoke leaves three times a day. Those are basics, plus water.

"I also use infrared heat to have people sweat, carefully monitored, of course, so there is exchange of body fluids. Also, exercise is important. I do running."

In his program, then, he emphasizes detoxification of the body, shifting to a sensible vegetarian diet, exercising, and improving stress management.

It is a question of priorities, Dr. Wunderlich concludes. "Many people have kids, two jobs, and so forth, so they think they do not have time. But you have to sort out the priorities, which we are not doing. You have to have good air and an appropriate amount of sleep. You need to avoid toxic foods. It is also important to have regular bowel movements, and you have to use your body appropriately for you, hopefully in some sweating way."

The advice that Wunderlich gives about carpal tunnel syndrome also applies to people who have any type of repetitive stress syndrome. Ultimately, we need to make our workplaces more livable. This will involve the improvement of human interaction and of the machines we surround ourselves with. If we upgraded our environments as obsessively as we upgrade our computers, we might have very few occupational disorders with which to cope.

Chapter 30

Sexual Dysfunction

P sychologist Dr. Janice Stefanacci says that sexual dysfunction stems largely from a society that offers people no models of normal, healthy sexuality: "If we look to the media, we see things that are totally aberrant in terms of frequency and potency. We see relationships portrayed between males and females where there is power and domination, or submission and seduction. Role models of healthy sexual communication and actualization are virtually nonexistent. People need a sense of what is normal.

"They also need time to think about sexuality as an integrated part of their personality. Our culture is very fragmented in this regard. Many, many people, men and women, never spend time thinking about their sexuality. In fact, if you were to take an informal survey and ask people, 'What is sexuality?' a good proportion of them would say, 'It's sex. It's something you do, maybe in the bedroom, maybe at night.' Nobody is really sure how often you are supposed to have it or how long it is supposed to last. Most people don't realize that sexuality is a completely integrated part of their personality as much as actualizing in education or interpersonal relationships. Sexuality is very much a part of who we are, how we present ourselves in the world, what we do, and how we think of ourselves. Our adequacy and our self-esteem are tied up in our sexuality."

Causes

Our society defines sexuality entirely according to male standards: sex is a performance, and orgasm is the primary, and perhaps only, yardstick for gauging satisfaction and hence for assessing sexual "function." Some sex researchers are beginning to question the whole concept of sexual dysfunction, promoting broader and less rigid definitions of sexual response and pleasure. "The Masters and Johnson model of sexual response—excitement, plateau, orgasm, and resolution—is very performance-oriented," says Rebecca Chalker, a women's health activist whose book *Secrets of Women's Sexuality*(??) explores ways in which feminists are redefining male standards. "After desire and willingness, the only other compulsory element is pleasure," Chalker points out. "Pleasure and intimacy are the real goals of sexual activity, and if you look at it that way, the concept of sexual dysfunction simply collapses."

Nevertheless, women may worry when they have difficulty achieving orgasm, especially with a partner, and men become concerned if they have difficulty controlling ejaculations and getting or maintaining erections. Both women and men are also distressed when they don't feel sexual attraction. In fact, most people who seek out counseling do so for difficulties with sexual communication and the lack of sexual desire.

Early on, through regular masturbation, boys learn what feels good and how to reliably get orgasms. Girls often wait to begin sexual exploration until they engage in sexual activity with a partner; they miss out on the benefits of self-exploration. "Learning about sex from boys or men isn't the best thing for women," Chalker says. "Their efficient, orgasm-oriented model doesn't necessarily encompass women's needs and preferences. For example, the repetitive thrusting of intercourse is a pretty efficient way for men to get orgasms, but many women don't easily get orgasms this way. Many need very specific manual stimulation. Another problem is that men get their orgasms relatively quickly, and are then ready for a nap. On average, it takes women much longer to become fully aroused and able to have really strong orgasms." Chalker points out that the biggest difference between women's sexuality and men's is that women have an innate ability to have multiple orgasms. "But under the male standard, many women simply don't have the opportunity to discover this phenomenal facet of their sexuality."

Many sex therapists recommend that women explore their sexual response through masturbation, using a vibrator, sex toys, and sexy videos to stimulate sexual fantasies. You may also want to experiment with things like aromatherapy, oils, and herbs. After sufficient homework, you can try integrating these changes into sex with your partner. Another important change heterosexual couples can make is to try rewriting the "intercourse script." That is, plan to have sexual sessions where intercourse will not take place. Try giving each other maximum pleasure just with your hands. Men can also learn the time-honored technique of postponing intercourse, and hence delaying ejaculation. This ensures that women have time to become fully aroused and can get the maximum pleasure from a sexual session.

As a general rule, men under 40 don't have difficulties getting erections. In their forties, however, many men begin to find that erections are less reliable. This problem may in part be caused by lack of desire, but it is also caused by certain diseases, especially diabetes and multiple sclerosis; certain medications; excessive alcohol consumption; prostate surgery; hardening of the arteries, which is a normal part of aging but is greatly exacerbated by smoking; too much fat in the diet; and not enough aerobic exercise. Other than a healthier, more vigorous lifestyle, there aren't any quick fixes for erectile dysfunction. If, however, men begin to think about sex less as a performance than as an experience in which pleasure and intimacy are the ultimate goal, unreliable erections might become less of an issue. "For some men, taking the focus off erection and expanding it to include full-body stimulation may ultimately improve erectile ability," Chalker says.

Early ejaculation can also be a problem for some men, and is often the result of too much direct stimulation of the penis with both hands, or its insertion into the vagina. Men can retrain themselves to delay ejaculation by avoiding immediate penetration and/or direct stimulation of the penis for successively longer periods, or by varying the types of stimulation. Women can encourage their partners to avoid stimulation that brings them quickly to the feeling that orgasm is inevitable. Over time, maybe several months, the time between the beginning of the sexual encounter and ejaculation and orgasm should increase.

Chalker points out that there are two powerful aspects of our sexuality—the physiological and the psychological—and that "neither can live without the other." Unfortunately, it is the psychological problems which are the more difficult to deal with. Psychological problems manifest themselves in various ways. Single people suffer when they cannot find a suitable sexual partner, while people in long-term relationships may find that they are no longer attracted by their partner. In this regard, counseling, as well as exploring a variety of books that are available, can be very helpful. Many people search for aphrodisiacs to stimulate sexual desire, but many studies suggest that sexual images—in literature, photographs, or videos—are also quite helpful in stimulating the release of sexual hormones. The booming market in erotica would seem to support this research.

"Today, we have enormous resources available to help with sexual problems that we didn't have a few years ago," Chalker notes. "I've reviewed some of the herbal aids and remedies here, and I encourage the reader to explore the wide range of resources available in book stores or by mail order."

Of course, sexual dysfunction can also have physical causes. One, Dr. Vicki Hufnagel reminds us, is "improperly performed episiotomies" (see Chapter 27, "Pregnancy," the section on Corrective Vaginal Surgery).

In *Prevention* magazine, Dr. Tori Hudson lists a number of other factors that can affect the sex drive. She says that sexual problems can be related to menopause, non-menopause-related hormonal changes (often following pregnancy), medications (Prozac, Zoloft, Sertraline, and others), depression, relationship issues, a chronic health problem, fatigue," and others. "In order to diagnose the cause correctly, your health professional would have to ask you many specific questions." Hormonal factors may involve low levels of testosterone or DHEA, although it is not known precisely what effect these hormones have on the libido. If blood tests show that levels are low, supplementation may be in order.

In an article on the HealthWorld Online website (www.healthy.net), Dr. Michael Janson advises that a variety of health problems—sexually transmitted diseases, chronic conditions such as candidiasis, allergies, hypoglycemia, chronic fatigue syndrome—as well as various bad habits can affect sexual functioning. For example, smoking, obesity, stress, alcohol consumption, and fatty acid imbalance, which causes hormone imbalance, are factors.

Remedies

NUTRIENTS, HORMONES, AND SUPPLEMENTS

Studies show that a heightened libido and orgasmic intensity are related to blood levels of histamine. Women who have low histamine levels tend to experience low sexual excitement, while those with a high level are more able to sustain orgasms. Nutrients that increase histamine levels include vitamin B_5 and the bioflavonoid rutin. Broccoli, parsley, cherries, grapes, peppers, melons, and citrus fruits are good food sources of vitamin B_5 and rutin.

Dr. Tori Hudson says that oral testosterone (available only by prescription), and/or a testosterone cream applied two to three times a week or rubbed into the external genital area before sex have been used to stimulate sexual responsiveness. DHEA, the B-complex vitamins, adrenal extracts, and the herbs ginseng and damiana may also help improve sexual response. Dr. Hudson notes, however, that remedies that focus on sexual drive without addressing general health and emotional issues will not have a consistent effect.

Dr. Janson offers an example of a general supplement program that can be an initial step in treating sexual dysfunction:

Multivitamin, three capsules twice a day.

Vitamin C, two 1,000-mg capsules twice a day.

Vitamin E, 400 IU mixed natural, twice a day.

Ginkgo biloba tincture, 60 mg twice a day.

Gamma-lineolic acid, 240 mg in the form of borage oil, once a day.

Magnesium aspartate, 200 mg, twice a day.

Coenzyme Q10, 100 mg, once a day.

AROMATHERAPY

"Aromatherapy is fantastic for helping women regain their sense of sensuality," declares aromatherapist Ann Berwick. These are some of the oils she recommends:

Rose is wonderful for enhancing feminine qualities. It bring out the loving, tender side of us that wants to surrender. Men who have trouble showing their emotions or opening up to their partner can benefit from rose as well. *Clary sage* heightens sensation. It takes you out of your body and into a different realm, allowing you to relax and enjoy the romance. *Sandalwood* is a wonderful oil for people not in touch with their physical side. It is very earthy and very deep. *Jasmine* restores self-confidence in people who have been through traumatic sexual experiences. It can help women who have been abused or who are emotionally closed off from damaging relationships.

"By blending different oils, you can create a formula that enhances the sensual side of your nature," says Berwick. She suggests adding them to the bath or using them while massaging a partner or in self-massage. A personal perfume can be made and used daily. "Surrounding yourself with these glorious scents is a wonderful help."

NON-WESTERN REMEDIES

Registered nurse and acupuncturist Abigail Rist-Podrecca explains sexual dysfunction from an Eastern point of view: "Chinese medicine looks to the root of the cause, rather than just the symptoms, and the root seems to be the kidney. The kidneys are called the roots of life. Everything stems from the kidney, they say."

Weak kidney function can be diagnosed in Eastern medicine in multiple ways, including facial diagnosis: "Under the eye is the thinnest tissue in the entire body," explains Rist-Podrecca. "You can see through the skin there. If the blood is not being cleared by the kidneys and detoxified, you will see a darkness under the eyes. People will say, 'I haven't had enough sleep,' but it goes beyond that. In Chinese medicine, that darkness signals that the kidneys are not functioning optimally, so the blood isn't being cleansed."

She goes on describe various factors that can drain the kidneys. "Cold can deplete the kidneys. Many people can't tolerate cold. This is so because in the winter, the kidney's function becomes suppressed, much the same way as the sap in a tree runs to the core and into the roots. When people have a compromised kidney situation, where it isn't functioning optimally, they can't stand the cold weather.

"Overwork and tension can also weaken kidney function because the kidneys and the adrenal glands (the adrenal sits on top of the kidney) are considered one and the same in Chinese medicine. So too much stress, and too many chemical toxins, deplete kidney functioning." Hundreds of Chinese herbs nourish kidney function. Here Rist-Podrecca names a few:

HAR SHAR WOO. This is an essential herbal formula for nourishing kidney function. It is also said to darken the hair. Hair, bone, teeth, joints, and sexual functions are tied up with the kidney energies. When you energize the kidneys, you affect all these different areas. When combined with dong quai, har shar woo helps the type of kidney dysfunction that causes low back pain.

ROMANIA. Romania is a dark black herb that is high in iron and helps to nourish the blood and improve kidney function.

DONG QUA. *Dong quai* resembles a cross section of the uterus, and has an affinity for this area of the body.

Resources for Sexual Problems

BOOKS

Lonnie Barbach. *For Each Other.* New York: Penguin Signet, 1982.

Rebecca Chalker. *Secrets of Women's Sexuality.*(??) New York: Seven Stories Press, in press.

Mantak Chia. *The Multiorgasmic Man.* New York: HarperCollins, 1996.

Mantak and Maneewan Chia. *Cultivating Female Sexual Energy.* Huntington, N.Y.: Healing Tao Books, 1986.

Mantak and Maneewan Chia. *Cultivating Male Sexual Energy.* Huntington, N.Y.: Healing Tao Books.

Federation of Feminist Women's Health Centers. *A New View of a Woman's Body.* Los Angeles: Feminist Health Press, 1995.

Gina Ogden. *Women Who Love Sex.* New York: Simon & Schuster Pocket Books, 1994.

Cathy Winks and Anne Semans. *The Good Vibrations Guide to Sex.* Pittsburgh: Cleis Press, 1994.

VIDEO

Betty Dodson. *Sex for One and Selfloving: Video Portrait of a Women's Sexuality Seminar.* To order: Box 1933, Murray Hill Station, New York, N.Y. 10156; $45.00.

MAIL ORDER SUPPLIERS

Eve's Garden, 119 West 57th Street, #420, New York, NY 10019-2382.

The Sexuality Library, 938 Howard Street, #101, San Francisco, CA 94103: (800) 289-8423.

Chapter 31

Sexually Transmitted Diseases

S exually transmitted diseases (STDs) were once a scourge that could bring death or madness. As recently as the 1940s, they were deeply feared. The unpublished memoir of a well-known member of the film industry describes how, in 1940, still in high school, he ran off with his sweetheart. They rode the boxcars in hobo fashion from Chicago to California. Once in California, the couple lived happily and without guilt, until they came down with a venereal disease. The youth called and begged forgiveness of his father. They returned home because they were so frightened and because they didn't know how to get treatment for their illness.

These diseases are much better understood and more treatable than they were 50 years ago. However, although many people realize that there has been progress in the conventional medical treatment of STDs, what they may not know is that there has also been progress in using alternative, particularly herbal, treatments for STDs.

Gonorrhea

Gonorrhea is caused by the bacterium *Neisseria gonorrhoeae;* women are far more likely to become infected than men.

Carol Dalton warns that health practioners must be especially vigilant when it comes to gonorrhea, both in detecting the disease and treating it. Dalton has been a nurse practitioner, an RN, in women's health care for more than 25 years. In 1994, she helped found Wellspring for Women, a clinic that blends traditional and alternative medical approaches.

Because gonorrhea can cause pelvic inflammatory disease (PID) and other illnesses, as well as infertility, she believes in treating it by conventional means. "We don't want women who have the infection to pass it on. Gonorrhea can occur without any symptoms for a long time, so that you might be passing it on without being aware of it. We treat this very aggressively."

TREATMENT

The first recourse is antibiotics. However, Dr. Allan Warshowsky cautions that antibiotics must be carefully monitored. Dr. Warshowsky is a board-certified obstetrician-gynecologist whose specialty is holistic gynecology.

He says, "Most of my treatment of this disease is fairly conventional. I use antibiotics unless patients specifically ask me not to use them. But it is also important to maintain and restore gut bacteria while treating a patient with antibiotics. I use bifidum, acidophilus, and some of the Saccharomyces strains of beneficial yeast to maintain normal gut biosis. I think this is paramount."

He combines this with herbal treatment and psychological counseling. "It is also important, especially if a patient is having recurrent problems with STDs, to look at her relationships, because whatever is going on physically is a manifestation of a deeper energy problem in the individual. If the patient is amenable to examining these deeper problems, it can really help lead to a much more lasting cure than just taking antibiotics.

"There are certainly people I see who prefer not to have antibiotics and, then, as long as the patient is a willing partner in her own therapy and not just looking to me to cure the disease, I use some herbal products, such as echinacea and goldenseal, and other herbs and supplements that can be helpful in enhancing immunity and fighting off infection."

According to Dr. Linda Page, gonorrhea has recently been on the increase. Dr. Page, a doctor of naturopathy who received one of the first Ph.D.s in the field, is the author of *Healthy Healing*. At the Clayton College of Natural Healing, she is an adjunct professor supervising herbal Ph.D. work.

She has found a variety of herbs useful in treating STD's, including gonorrhea. She uses a combination that includes goldenseal, myrrh, pau d'arco, vegetable acidophilus, ginkgo, and dandelion. Another combination she uses is burdock, juniper, squawvine, bayberry, dandelion, gentian, and black walnut.

She adds, "You can see where we are going with these herbs. This is obviously a broad-spectrum approach—antifungal, antiviral and antibacterial. This is because these categories of STDs seem to exhibit symptoms of all these types of infections: fungal symptoms, such as discharge; bacterial symptoms, such as inflammation; and viral symptoms, in that these infections can migrate to other parts of the body."

Syphilis

Syphilis is caused by a bacterium called *Treponema pallidum,* which causes genital ulcers. Unlike gonorrhea, syphilis is not on the rise. Dalton remarks that she hasn't seen a case in her 25 years of practice. "To indicate how rare it is, in many places in order to get a marriage license, you used to have to get a blood test for syphilis. They haven't required that for 15 or 20 years, because we never pick up any cases of it."

TREATMENT

The treatment for syphilis is similar to that for gonorrhea. Dr. Page uses a blood-cleansing detoxification formula that includes gotu-kola, sarsaparilla, prickly ash, burdock, chaparral, licorice, and stillingia. "Stillingia has been very hard to get recently. Sometimes I use dandelion in place of stillingia." She notes that this formula has been used since ancient times.

She continues, "Chinese studies indicate that sarsaparilla alone has a 90 percent degree of effectiveness in treating syphilis. Even today, preparations with sarsaparilla as a major agent are regularly used in China to treat syphilis."

She also uses a calendula tincture on some of the sores.

Chlamydia

Amanda McQuade Crawford, an author and health expert whose new book is called *Herbal Remedies for Women,* describes chlamydia as one of the most widespread STDs in North America. The infecting organism, *Chlamydia trachomatis,* is a one-celled parasite with a rigid cell wall. Crawford notes that *Chlamydia* is harder to clear up with herbal agents than some other one-celled organisms, such as bacteria and yeast, which respond very well to herbal treatment. "It often goes undiagnosed and can cause an inflammation of the cervix in women. This is why it is one of the leading causes of more serious pelvic diseases, particularly PID."

SYMPTOMS

The symptoms of chlamydia can take a long time to appear, which is one reason it is such a commonly transmitted sexual disease. According to Crawford, "It's also quite hard to diagnose because the symptoms may not be the same for each woman. Sometimes there are almost no symptoms or there may be symptoms that look like any number of other conditions.

"Usually the first symptom is a painless bump that goes unnoticed, followed by swollen lymph glands and headaches. Some women get strange fleeting pains in their joints and muscles, as well as chills, and even weight loss, one to four weeks later.

"There will be a vaginal discharge that feels like mucus but has a bad odor. There may also be pain with sexual intercourse and some spotting after intercourse. If there is spotting between menstrual periods, a woman should see a licensed practitioner to look for signs of redness on the cervix.

"Other signs that women might experience are urinary frequency and painful urination, as well as some lower abdominal pain, although these symptoms may be caused by some other conditions as well."

Dalton emphasizes that chlamydia often leads to PID. "It can go up into the uterus, the fallopian tubes, and the ovarian area and cause very serious infections and scarring and, therefore, infertility."

As with so many diseases, early detection is essential. As Crawford notes, if left untreated chlamydia can lead to more serious medical problems, and as previously mentioned, it can cause infertility because of scarring. It can also cause problems in pregnancy, including premature or difficult delivery.

TREATMENT

In conventional drug treatment, antibiotics are used. Crawford explains, "Which antibiotic is chosen, if any, will depend on whether a woman is pregnant or not. There are often secondary infections with bacteria or viruses and that can complicate the picture. That's another reason why chlamydia is difficult to treat with simple remedies.

"In Dalton's practice, she uses antibiotics. "We use antibiotics because of the risk factor. I think in health care you always weigh the risks versus the benefits of treatment. In this case, you see that the risk is great. Even if someone isn't concerned about fertility, you still weigh the risk of damaging the woman's immune system because you have an active infection that could become very serious. So chlamydia is one of the things that we don't really fool around with. We treat it with antibiotics; and we recheck it to make sure it's gone."

Crawford has looked into herbal treatments for chlamydia. One is the anti-inflammatory herb calendula, or marigold—not the garden variety, but the medicinal single-flower kind. Demulcents such as plantain are also useful and often combined with herbs that help normalize the hormones. As she puts it, "Sometimes a hormonal imbalance will have led to a change in the reproductive tissues, so these rectifying herbs are needed to make it possible to clear up this infection."

Crawford explains how to make a tea of these herbs. "We use these herbs in combination. Start with the calendula, 4 oz—it's a very lightweight herb—and make a simple infusion by pouring a pint of boiling water over those 4 oz. It's going to make a strong brew, and be a deep, dark, golden color. Strain that and add 1 drop of essential oil of thyme. Take a teacup full of the mixture, followed by a glass of pure water. Drink this three times a day."

Herbal douches can also be of some help with reproductive infections, though, according to Crawford, they really can't get to the source of the problem. While the douche is rinsing out the infectious agent, it is also rinsing away the helpful bacteria, which is why you should be cautious about using herbal douches with any kind of infection. Still, the antimicrobial herbs used in the douches can help reduce the infectious organisms. "What we normally do," Crawford explains, "is follow each douche with a rest period, because these douches can dry out the tissue, making the irritated vaginal walls more susceptible to other infections. Even plain water douches will have that effect."

Crawford's douche formula uses 2 oz of organic grape root (also know as barberry bark root) and 1 oz of calendula flower. Steep 1 oz of this mixture in a pint of boiling water for about 45 minutes. Strain it and let the tea cool to a comfortable temperature for vaginal use. To this mixture, add about 7 drops of essential oil of tea tree. You can use a wire whisk to help mix them together. Make sure all the containers used are sterilized. Use this as a douche twice a week for up to three weeks. It's not necessary to rinse the herbs out of the vaginal canal afterward, but Crawford says that it feels very comforting to get rid of some of the bad-smelling discharge from chlamydia.

Dr. Page uses vaginal ointments to treat chlamydia. She suggests a combination of berberine-compound herbs: goldenseal, barberry, and Oregon grape. Mix this with vitamin A oil and apply directly to the cervix on a tampon.

Pelvic Inflammatory Disease (PID)

CAUSES

Pelvic inflammatory disease generally originates from an infection, like chlamydia, that spreads out of control. Dalton says that chlamydia is the primary cause of PID. Because PID can be a "silent" infection, someone can have it for years, without knowing she is infected. "So, it's easily transmitted. It can fester in the cervical canal, and then, when the immune system is low, can creep up into the other pelvic organs and cause a major infection."

She adds that it was a shift in birth control methods that played a big part in the rise of PID. "We really saw a lot of this disease when IUDs became popular, particularly when the Dalkon Shield was still being used. The Dalkon Shield had a multifiliment string; there were multiple threads within this string, and bacteria could climb up the threads more easily, and into the uterus. The problems with the Dalkon Shield brought about a greater understanding of PID: how to develop cultures for it, how to study it, and what treatment to use knowledge of the damage that PID could do."

SYMPTOMS

PID symptoms vary; some women have very severe symptoms, other women have symptoms so mild that they are unaware they are infected. The most common symptom is pain, which ranges from a dull ache to pain so debilitating that walking is impossible. Other symptoms are bleeding, a foul discharge, cramps, swelling in the abdominal area, fever, and chills.

In addition to damaging the internal organs, PID can also result in scarring, particularly of the fallopian tubes. As Dalton explains, "This is how PID causes infertility. Even after you have cleared the infection, even if it hasn't blocked the tubes completely with scarring, the wavelike, hairlike projections that sweep the sperm through the fallopian tube to the egg and which sweep the egg up into the fallopian tube to meet with the sperm are often damaged and flattened. So that even though you may have a good, clear tube, the system isn't working properly. When this happens, it's a very serious problem, particularly for young, fertile women. It's probably one of the major causes of infertility. That's why we have to be really aggressive in testing for chlamydia and in treating it. We can clear the infection. We can give women antibiotics, but if we don't catch it soon enough, it can do all of this damage may and result in infertility."

TREATMENT

Dalton explains that once a woman is at the point where PID has really taken hold, there is severe swelling and inflammation in the entire pelvic area. To heal properly, the woman has to rest her body completely, which means bed rest. "Because whenever we are standing or walking, just because of gravity and the weight of the body, the pelvic area is impinged upon and there is a lot of pressure. So we encourage a woman to go to bed and rest while she is being treated. We get a much better response, much better healing, quicker healing, and less reoccurrence when this is followed.

The other thing we advise patients to do is use diet and supplements to encourage healing. We use zinc and vitamins C and E to encourage good oxygenation and tissue repair. We have to remember that the antibiotic just kills the bacteria, it does not cause healing to take place. Those tissues have to heal on their own, and if you give them a little extra encouragement with extra nutrients they are going to do that in a quicker and better fashion."

Human Papilloma Virus (HPV)

Different strains of HPV (human papilloma virus) cause either genital warts, warts on other parts of the body, or cervical cancer. HPV is particularly hazardous, says Carol Dalton, because it often goes undetected. "People often have no idea that they have it because it's microscopic, so it's easily transmitted during sexual intercourse. One study showed that 75 percent of a group of women and men who were tested were positve for HPV, and most of them did not realize they were infected." HPV is diagnosed in women most frequently by a Pap smear. The pap smear results come back as "atypical, suspicious of HPV" or "dysplasia, suspicious of HPV," Dalton explains. She also underlines the possible consequences of getting HPV. "It's the primary cause of dysplasia. Probably over 90 percent of the time, dysplasia of the cervix or, eventually, cervical cancer, is caused by HPV. That's why it's so important to get a proper diagnosis."

The condition of the immune system is related to the health of a woman's vaginal and cervical cells. "Clearly, a woman can be infected with this, and we know it is in her system, but she is not having any problems. It's not invading the cells and growing and changing them into abnormal ones. Whether or not a woman will develop HPV depends on the response of the immune system.

"Once a woman develops abnormal cells, we diagnose it by doing a colposcopy and biopsy of any abnormal cells. A colposcope is an instrument we use to look at the cervix, vagina, and labia. It magnifies these areas so we can actually see the cells to identify the areas where abnormal cells are present. After we have identified the abnormal cells, we do small biopsies—pinhead size or smaller. The biopsies are sent to a pathology lab where they section them and examine them under a microscope to identify the cells and see what is going on there."

TREATMENT

There are several treatments for HPV. "The typical treatment can be to do nothing and watch for a while to see if the body can heal itself and reverse the process. Cryotherapy, freezing of the cells, may be used, as well as laser therapy or a procedure called LEEP (loop excisional electrosurgical procedure), which uses an electrical wire to cut out abnormal tissue. All of these destroy the abnormal cells."

The fortunate thing," Dalton continues, "is that the vagina and cervix produce a new surface of cells about every six to eight weeks. So if we can remove the cells that are abnormal, new, healthy cells will hopefully grow in. One reason it is important to remove the abnormal cells is that new cells tend to be like the cells next to them, so if abnormal cells remain in the body the new cells will grow into abnormal cells too."

The unfortunate thing is that just removing these abnormal cells often does not end the problem. As Dalton notes, "You can't kill off the virus completely, since it is in the surrounding tissue. You can't cauterize or remove the whole lining of the vagina. We only remove the cells that have become abnormal. There is a very high recurrence rate, with HPV causing the same abnormal cell growth all over again, unless you improve the woman's immune system and strengthen those normal cells."

Wellspring for Women uses oral supplements of zinc, vitamin C, beta carotene, folic acid, and general B complex, along with a multivitamin-mineral, to aid in this process. "We recommend larger than usual doses of these because we found that the new cell growth responds well to these nutrients. Moreover, many of these are antiviral nutrients. They help the woman's body fight the virus more readily and more systematically.

"We also use vitamin A suppositories. There's been a fair amount of work done on how cervical dysplasia can be treated with topical vitamin A. There are also suppositories we use called papillo suppositories that are made to fight the HPV virus topically. With these, we are treating the whole vaginal area and not just the cells that have become abnormal. We also use something called formula W, for wart virus, that contains herbs that help fight the HPV virus."

Her clinic uses both oral and topical treatments. They also examine patients' stress levels, their diet, and their lifestyle issues. This seems to be a successful approach, since, she maintains, "We have about a 1 to 2 percent recurrence rate with HPV, while the national average, when conventional methods are used exclusively, is 10 to 15 percent recurrence. So we feel that treating the whole person has made a huge difference in our ability to prevent recurrence, which is really the issue. HPV is not so hard to treat initially, but it's keeping it from coming back that is really the problem. I would encourage women who have this problem to look at the whole person."

HIV and AIDS have created a further difficulty in treatment."We've had to be very careful about screening for HIV and AIDS and treating those patients," Dalton points out, "because the immune system with HIV is so compromised that if a woman with HIV does contract HPV, it seems to grow at a very rapid rate. The cells can turn into cancerous cells much more easily on the vulva, labia, cervix and vagina. Practitioners treating patients who have HIV and AIDS need to be extremely cautious in doing colposcopies and biopsies. Even more than with the average patient, be aggressive with treatment and in building the immune system. Because having these other problems will greatly increase the risk factor of the abnormal cells turning into cancerous cells."

Genital Warts

Genital warts are caused by HPV. Symptoms of genital warts can take as little as three weeks and as long as eight months to develop after exposure to the virus. Genital warts are contagious, even before they become symptomatic.

TREATMENT

Dr. Page treats genital warts successfully with vitamin C therapy. "Up to 10,000 mg daily is used to enhance white blood cell activity and boost immune interferon. We use a mix of carotenes up to 200,000 IU daily." She also uses aloe vera gel as a topical application for genital warts. She particularly recommends an aloe vera/garlic mixture. "You steep garlic cloves in the aloe vera gel, so you have a very high sulfur mix. We ask patients to drink two glasses of aloe vera juice daily. We also use a 'vag-pack' for genital warts, which includes goldenseal, burdock, chaparral, and sarsaparilla. Blend the herbs and put them on a tampon and insert into the vagina. This is an internal poultice to draw out the infection. It is very effective, especially when you add B complex with extra folic acid. Both these supplements help normalize those abnormal cells."

She adds, "This is a virus, so you would want to take antiviral herbs. The ones I use regularly are lomatium, St. John's wort, and bupleurum. Occasionally, I also use myrrh. Any combination of these works. It's best to use them in an extract if you want antiviral activity."

Dr. Warshowsky notes that genital warts should be treated creatively and holistically. "When a woman is willing to do an entire body-balancing protocol, where she is looking at what is going on in her life that is making her susceptible to infection, balancing out her gut bacteria, eating a nutrient-rich diet, and employing some of these beneficial herbs and supplements, I think there is good success in restoring order, restoring balance, and getting rid of infection."

A Note on Another Use of Conventional Drugs: Tuberculosis

This chapter is one of the few in which you will find some alternative practitioners recommending antibiotics for treatment of infectious disease.

Accordingly I would like to interject a comment here on another such disease which many practitioners treat with conventional means: tuberculosis. I have found, however, that the best way to approach TB is with an alternative combination therapy. It comprises a detoxification program, along with 50 to 150 hyperbaric oxygen treatments, plus intravenous vitamin C. The hyperbaric oxygen treatment is given five days a week for an hour at a time, for around four months. Then you give the intravenous solution, which in addition to vitamin C includes glutathione, a water-soluble form of vitamin A, selenium, B_{12}, and B complex. You start at 50,000 IU and build up to nearly 200,000 IU, giving the drip twice a week. I've also found it helpful to give 1000 mg of alpha lypoic acid once a day and between 2,000 and 10,000 mg of vitamin C a day, plus 2,000 to 5,000 mg of quercetin a day and 100 mg of *ginkgo biloba* three times a day. All these treatments together constitute an effective approach to TB.

Chapter 32

Stroke

S trokes are the third leading cause of death in the United States; every 60 seconds, someone dies of a stroke. Strokes are also the leading cause of adult disability. One treatment that can both prevent and treat strokes is enzyme therapy.

Dr. Anthony Cichoke is a leading medical researcher in the field of enzyme therapy. Dr. Cichoke has taught at the University of Minnesota and the University of Rochester Medical School and is the author of hundreds of articles and seven books, including *The Complete Book of Enzyme Therapy.*

He explains that there are two different types of strokes: hemorrhagic stroke, which is a rupture in a blood vessel, and ischemic stroke, which is caused by a blockage in the blood vessels. The result of both types of strokes is a lack of blood flow to the brain and consequently insufficient oxygen for brain function.

Symptoms

Dr. Cichoke describes a stroke as "like a circulatory problem, but in the brain." Symptoms of stroke include dizziness, blurred vision and loss of sensation, slurred speech, loss of bladder control, and partial loss of hearing. Often a stroke will be accompanied by paralysis of an arm or leg on one side of the body. Strokes can cause swelling of the brain, stupor, and coma.

Treatment

Dr. Chichoke uses enzyme therapy to boost the immune system and detoxify the body. "Enzymes are catalysts," he explains. "Anything that is alive has to have enzymatic activity—whether it is in the grass outside or whether it is in your body. Enzymes are critical for every cell of our body. Nothing can go on in the body without enzymatic activity. Without enzymes there would be no breathing, no digestion, no growth, no blood coagulation, no reproduction. "Enzymes, he says, fight strokes by acting "as sort of a 'roto rooter' that helps break up cholesterol and toxins in your body.

"Strokes can be treated systemically with enzymes. They are used as digestive aids; they improve the absorption of other nutrients, herbs, health foods, whatever, Enzymes aid absorption and metabolism at the cellular level."

Dr. Cichoke uses enzyme therapy systemically, by having his patients take enzyme supplements orally between meals. He recommends enzymes such as bromelain, papain, trypsin, chymotrypsin, pancreatin, and microbial proteases, all of which have primarily proteolytic enzyme activity. Dr. Cichoke describes how enzyme supplements pass through the gut into the small intestine, where they are absorbed into the circulatory system. "These are all enzymes that work in the bloodstream and the various organs as well as at the cellular level of the body."

Enzymes aid in detoxification at the cellular level in various organs and in the bloodstream and digestive tract. He explains why it is important to have a well-ordered circulatory system. "The blood must get to the cells in order to bring nutrients to the body, and blood needs to help take the waste products away from the cells. Further, enzymes help break up the cholesterol and fibrin in the blood vessels." Dr. Cichoke pictures a blood vessel as a stream or river, with little curves and eddies. These curves fill up with fibrin and cholesterol which clog blood vessels so the blood and oxygen can't get through.

"Proteolytic enzymes help to break up the fibrin and cholesterol and allow the body to eliminate these waste products. Enzymes also improve circulation, They help keep the bloodstream normalized." He explains that it is important to have a balance between blood coagulation and blood thinning. "Enzymes help to keep this critical equilibrium in order."

Enzymes also help break up free radicals. "As part of the aging process, and also as a result of stress and illness and injuries, the cells of our body tend to oxidize—they rust. Think of the body's tissue as if it was like a lovely leather jacket. When you first buy that leather jacket it's soft and pliable. But then, as it gets older the leather oxidizes and it becomes cracked and hard. As we go through life, our body tends to oxidize. When you take antioxidant enzymes, such as superoxide dismutase, catalase, glutathione, and peroxidase, they fight free radical formation and work as antioxidants."

Enzymes can also dissolve large blood clots, which can cause strokes. Dr. Cichoke says that enzymes are currently being used both in and out of hospitals to break up blood clots and also to break up fibrin formations. "In hospitals, some enzymes used for this purpose are brinase, which comes from *Aspergillus oryzae*, streptokinase, which is of bacterial origin, and urokinase or prourokinase, which is actually from human urine."

Dr. Cichoke tells a story about a stroke patient in Portland, Oregon, who was treated with these enzymes. "They had given up on him. But as a last-ditch effort, nine hours after the stroke, they began to give him urokinase. Not only did he regain consciousness, he also regained the ability to move his arms and his legs. After six weeks of rehabilitation therapy he went home."

Dr. Cichoke cites an article in the *New York Times* science section of February 9, 1999, which stated, "Enzymes offer hope for reducing devastation from strokes." Currently, Dr. Cichoke notes, the Cleveland Clinic in Cleveland, Ohio, is using prourokinase to fight strokes. He stresses the importance of proteolytic enzymes as well as antioxidant enzymes. "I suggest taking 200 micrograms of antioxidant enzymes three times a day between meals and 8 to 10 tablets of combination enzymes three times a day, also between meals. If you take bromelain, take four to six tablets of approximately 230 to 250 milligrams every day.

"I know this can be fairly expensive," he goes on, "but how much does health mean to you? In 1960 medical services were 5 percent of our gross national product; by 1990 this figure was over 12 percent. We eat too much fat and too many refined carbohydrates, we smoke too much, we get virtually no exercise, and we overeat. For this reason, exercising, having a positive mental attitude, and eating fresh fruits are all very important. And enzyme supplementation is critical. This is the roadmap to better health."

Chapter 33

Temporomandibular Joint (TMJ) Dysfunction

The temporomandibular joints (TMJs) are hinged joints that open and close the jaw. The jaw is part of a wider system, the craniosacral system, which extends from the skull to the sacrum, which is the lowest segment of the spine. Disruption at any level of the craniosacral system can result in TMJ dysfunction.

Causes

The two most common causes of TMJ problems are poor bite and stress. Poor bite may be the result of new dental work that affects tooth alignment. Sometimes braces shift the palate, which affects the jaw. In recent years, more adults have been undergoing this procedure, which has resulted in an increase in the number of cases of TMJ disorders. Dentists who specialize in TMJ can diagnose bite problems.

Although TMJ dysfunction is not exclusively a woman's problem, it does affect larger numbers of females than males due to stresses brought on by hormonal changes. Dr. Deborah Kleinman, a chiropractor who works with TMJ patients, explains: "There are various stress factors we can talk about that are specific to women. First, we have premenstrual tension. This further weakens an already weakened system. I know women who have a problem with their jaw only three days before their period. As soon as their period comes, the pain goes away. This tells me that there is a weakness in the system and that the hormones are pushing the body past the point of being able to compensate for the weakness.

"Hormonal changes also occur during pregnancy and menopause. Pregnancy, in addition to hormonal changes and added stress, creates structural changes caused by weight gain and the loosening of ligaments. Hormones loosen the pelvis so that the woman is more flexible during delivery. These changes can further aggravate TMJ dysfunction.

"With nursing, postural changes can play a big role. Nursing places stress on the upper back muscles, especially if the woman doesn't use the proper pillows or if she gets lazy and slumps over while feeding her baby. These upper back muscles insert into the occiput, the bone at the bottom of the skull, which is part of this craniosacral system. Tightening or pulling on the occiput can affect the head, neck, and TMJ."

Symptoms

Pain can be isolated in the joint itself or it can radiate to the face, neck, ear, and shoulder. Headaches may be a part of the picture. There may be pain resembling that of a nagging toothache, even though the tooth is healthy. A person with TMJ problems may have difficulty opening the mouth all the way. Inflammation of the muscles around the joint may cause a spasm in those muscles, locking them open. Clicking, grinding, or popping noises may accompany chewing or movement of the joint.

Clinical Experience

CRANIOSACRAL THERAPY

Cranio means "skull"; *sacral* refers to the sacrum, which consists of the lowest five vertebrae of the spine, which are fused; the sacrum is also part of the pelvis. Craniosacral therapy is founded on an understanding of the relationship between these structures and several points in between, including the TMJ. Dr. Deborah Kleinman, who uses a specific form of craniosacral therapy called sacro-occipital technique, explains: "A chiropractor like myself who uses this technique understands that there is a balance between the nervous system and the musculoskeletal system, and a relationship between the pelvis and the sacrum and then the head and the cranium. Between both structures rests the spine, the shoulders, the neck. All of these structures react to shifts in the pelvis and the cranium. The TMJ is part of that." She adds that a stable pelvis balances the body and works in harmony with the cranium. This allows information to flow to the brain smoothly.

Dr. Kleinman says that with TMJ the first step is to have a doctor perform a series of tests to determine whether structural stresses exist, and, if so, where. Once the structural stresses have been identified, treatment can begin. "We place wedges or blocks under the pelvis. The muscles will relax and contract around these levers in an unforced way, based upon what these levers tell the brain. Then we incorporate breathing techniques to assist the brain in making musculoskeletal changes. This reestablishes the proper craniosacral flow." Sometimes secondary manipulations are necessary to readjust parts of the spine lying between the pelvis and cranium that get knotted up as a result of compensating for the pelvis and the cranium. Cranial adjustments, made specifically to the temporomandibular joint, also help to reestablish proper balance.

OTHER PHYSICAL THERAPIES

Regularly done isotonic exercise can help some cases of TMJ dysfunction. In addition to jaw exercise, self-treatment for TMJ problems may include jaw awareness, in which the patient tries to notice and avoid clenching and grinding the teeth, as well as biting on gum, ice, or fingernails. Eating soft foods and avoiding resting or sleeping on the stomach can also help, as can learning to rest the jaw and to adopt proper jaw posture. Other potentially helpful techniques include self-massage; relaxed rhythmic opening and closing of the jaw; alternating moist heat (15 minutes) with ice (2 to 3 minutes) to increase circulation; cool sprays and cryotherapy; bite guards; and splints. Surgery should be a last resort when dealing with TMJ problems.

Another physical therapy that can help relieve TMJ is Body Rolling, a technique developed by bodyworker Yamuna Zake, author of *Body Rolling: An Experiential Approach to Complete Muscle Release.* "Many of the muscles that run up the back and insert in the skull, as well as the muscles in the front of the neck, have attachments between the head and the chest. Thus the amount of tension in the muscles of the back, front, and sides of the neck can affect the level of contraction of the sutures (joints) and muscles of the cranium, and specifically the TMJ," she explains. In Body Rolling, a 6-inch-diameter ball is used to apply traction that lengthens and releases muscles. "The degree of tension in the TMJ is controlled by the tension maintained in the neck. By working the neck muscles with the ball to keep them at maximum length and minimum tension level, you can help reduce the buildup of tension in the TMJ." Zake has designed specific routines that use the ball to release the front and back of the neck, as well as an around-the-neck routine that helps break the holding pattern of tension that distorts head and neck alignment.

NUTRITION

Nutritional supplements may help in treating TMJ problems. Some of the most useful are listed here.

CALCIUM AND MAGNESIUM. These minerals are essential for proper muscular function and have a sedative effect.

B-COMPLEX VITAMINS. Take 100 mg of B-complex vitamins three times a day. B-complex vitamins are essential for combatting stress.

PANTOTHENIC ACID. The appropriate amount of pantothenic acid to take is 100 mg, twice daily. B-complex vitamins, like pantothenic acid, are for combatting stress.

COENZYME Q10. Coenzyme Q10 is another stress fighter.

OTHER SUPPLEMENTS. L-tyrosine and vitamins B_6 and C will improve sleep quality and alleviate anxiety and depression. It is also important to take a multivitamin and mineral complex.

Chapter 34

Thyroid Disease

This country's most important contribution to philosophy has been pragmatism. The basic principle of pragmatism, first outlined by Charles Pierce and then worked out in less technical language by William James and John Dewey, is that all concepts should be measured by their direct contribution to society. On first glance, pragmatism might seem a vulgar, anti-intellectual doctrine that might lead to arguing, for example, that any idea in a best-selling book must be good because it is making money for the author. This is a flawed analysis. The ideas of Pierce, James, and Dewey go deeper. For them, a true measure of an idea's value involves whether it contributes to the enhancement of a democratic polity and informed citizenship. Although a best-selling book may reap rewards for the author, if it undermines the knowledge and freedom of its readers, then, ultimately, it is not justified under the principles of pragmatism. The best thinkers who called themselves pragmatists, although they would throw stuffy, fussy academic trivia in the trashcan, would respectfully listen to alternative thought if it fostered the democratic ideals they held so high.

Like so many ideas, pragmatism has its vulgarizers. It has often been used to justify the American tendency to damn the side effects and repercussions of a practice as long as it gets results. In this chapter, which will look at thyroid disorders, we will note this tendency in the conventional treatment of hypothyroidism, a condition marked by deficient activity of the thyroid gland.

Although little is definitely known about the cause of the disorder, doctors seem happy to ladle out the drugs that suppress the symptoms, without being concerned that an afflicted person will be on these drugs for life, at ever-increasing doses.

Thyroid disease is about 15 or 20 times more prevalent in women than in men. About 1.5 million women are being treated for it in the United States, compared to only about 100,000 men. Thyroid disease is at once a hot-button issue and one of the most misunderstood illnesses facing us today. To cite just one example of the importance of thyroid disease: 70 percent of women with infertility and miscarriage have hypothyroidism.

Importance of the Thyroid

The thyroid gland is an important component of the immune system. Dr. Stephen Langer, who practices preventive medicine in Berkeley, California, explains that the thyroid gland is a small, butterfly-shaped organ at the base of the neck that releases about a teaspoon of hormone a year which affects the metabolism and acts as a cellular carburetor for every cell in the body—from our hair follicles down to our toenails. The thyroid can be implicated in just about any condition.

Dr. Langer says, "If a person's metabolism is hypo-functioning, every-thing is going to be slow. In a book I wrote called *Solve the Riddle of Illness,* I explain why upward of 40 percent of the population may have subclinical hypothyroidism and not detect it by the traditional blood chemistry work that is done at their general practitioner's office. The symptoms of low thy-roid include weakness, dry, coarse skin, slow speech, coarse hair, hair loss, weight gain, difficulty breathing, problems with menstruation, nervousness, heart palpitations, brittle nails, and severe chronic fatigue and depression. "If you have a patient with a constellation of symptoms like that, they're going to be sick and tired of feeling sick and tired. Plus they're going to feel depressed all the time because they're going from one doctor to another, sometimes with two or three or four pages worth of complaints, and the doc-tors tell them it's all in their head, or that they should go home and learn to live with it."

Dr. Hyla Cass, a holistic psychiatrist, emphasizes the importance of thyroid inflammation, or thyroiditis, as a root cause of a variety of emotional and physical problems. She also describes the difficulty today of establishing the diagnosis of thyroid disorder in the face of continuing skepticism from con-ventional physicians. According to Dr. Cass, "When the thyroid isn't working properly, the immune system is impaired, and this sets up a vicious cycle. You have a person whose immune system is depleted and who is anxious; they're told by regular doctors that the problem is all in their head, that there's noth-ing physically wrong with them. So then they feel worse."

Hypothyroidism

SYMPTOMS

Dr. Mark Lader is the supervisor of nutritional services at the Natural Wellness Center in New York. He's been in practice for over 10 years and is coauthor of *The Encyclopedia of Women's Health: Herbal and Nutritional Health.* He describes some of the history of hypothyroidism, a disease whose prevalence and dangers were already noted in the 1970s, although, since that time, it has remained a puzzle to scientists.

Lader says, "A milestone in the study of the disease was the publication of Broda Barnes's *Hypothyroidism: The Unsuspected Illness.* Back in 1976 when she wrote the book, so many of the symptoms that so many people were experiencing—ones which appeared to have no obvious cause—were called hypothyroidism. Some of those symptoms were tiredness, sluggishness, lethargy, weakness, slow speech, dry, coarse skin, bumpy skin on the back of the arm, intolerance of cold, puffy face or hands, loss of the outer third of the eyebrow, cramping, infertility, absence of period, excessive menstrual bleeding, loss of appetite, thinning of hair on the scalp, face, or genitals, swelling of the neck, gaining weight easily, and abdominal swelling. There are so many symptoms of hypothyroidism that are related to dysfunctions in so many organ systems of the body."

Broda Barnes was convinced that as many as 40 percent of Americans were affected by some form of hypothyroidism. But the effects of hypothyroidism go even beyond the multiple symptoms recognized by Broda Barnes. According to an article in the online magazine *Alternative Medicine* (www.alternativemedicinc.com), hypothyroidism can also aggravate many female problems, including miscarriage, fibrocystic breast disease, ovarian fibroids, cystic ovaries, endometriosis, PMS, and menopausal symptoms. All of these, the article asserts, can be caused or aggravated by hypothyroidism.

Although the exact cause-and-effect connection is not worked out, it is known that hypothyroidism is linked to hormonal imbalances, particularly an excess of estrogen over the other female hormone, progesterone. Normally, a woman's ratio of progesterone to estrogen is 10 to 1. If she has too much estrogen, this is bad for the thyroid, since estrogen inhibits thyroid production while progesterone promotes it. The connection between thyroid production and female hormones indicates that a disruption in one sphere will affect the other.

TESTING

In conventional medicine, hypothyroidism is diagnosed by serum testing of the hormones thyroxine (T4), triiodothyronine (T3), and thyrotropin or thyroid-stimulating hormone (TSH). The textbook explanation is that low T4 and T3 levels along with high TSH indicate hypothyroidism. Lader comments, "On the face of it, hypothyroidism seems to be a real simple illness. The symptoms and blood values seem to correlate very well to a hypothyroid case, and then when we give levothyroxin, the symptoms seem to go away."

However, these tests are not as accurate as they might seem, according to an *Alternative Medicine* article which points out that "most of the standard thyroid tests (for T3, T4, and TSH levels) often fail to pinpoint an underfunctioning thyroid, leading physicians to make erroneous diagnoses." The article goes on to say that doctors diagnose by symptoms, even while they remain unaware of the medical cause. So a patient with depression gets Prozac; one with weight gain is prescribed a weight loss drug; and one who is continually tired is said to suffer from chronic fatigue syndrome and gets no treatment.

In Lader's opinion, the standard blood tests do little to pinpoint the actual cause of the thyroid problem. Instead, he looks at the patient's overall environment to locate key problem sectors. The first step is ascertaining the patient's body temperature.

"For my own diagnosis, I ask the women about their symptoms and also use something called a basal temperature test, which is a very simple way to learn if the body is running cold. [Basal body temperature is a person's resting temperature upon waking up in the morning.] We ask the woman to use an oral thermometer. She shakes it down before she goes to sleep at night. The first thing upon arising in the morning, she puts it under her armpit for about seven minutes.

"The temperature should be above 97.8. If it's below that level, many doctors will say that is diagnostic for hypothyroidism. However, we must remember that some people have a lower body temperature than others. They tend to run a little cool but don't have the hypothyroid symptoms. Some people's underarm temperature doesn't even rise after they have a significant improvement in their symptoms."

Dr. Lader looks at the whole body and a person's whole environment. In his experience, most of the symptoms that people with hypothyroidism come in with are lethargy, weakness, dryness, and cold intolerance. By studying both the temperature and the patient's whole history, he is able to assess the patient's condition.

Conventional Treatment

Conventional treatment relies on prescription drugs. According to Lader, on the surface, it would seem reasonable to treat the symptoms of hypothyroidism with synthroid or armorthyroid, (the natural form of thyroid), or levothyroxin. These drugs make the symptoms disappear in a high percentage of cases. "But," he asks, "are we really getting to the true causes of the problem?" He cautions that there are certain drawbacks to these medicines.

Lader explains: "We know that in conventional treatment the patient will be on the medication for her whole life. Natural doctors believe we don't need to medicate people that long. Moreover, the increasingly larger doses these people are getting over the course of a lifetime cause more and more adverse symptoms."

If we look at the big picture, according to Lader, we see it's important to treat the whole body. "One of the true hallmarks of an alternative, natural practitioner is that she or he believes that eliminating symptoms is not really enough to determine if a successful therapy has been carried out." He adds, "Probably most readers realize that we have a medical tradition in this country of relegating hypothyroidism to the idiopathic trash heap. 'Idiopathic' is a term used when traditional medicine does not know what the cause is. In my opinion, though, it means we are not asking the right questions. Saying that this problem has unknown causes or ones that cannot be addressed nutritionally is really a copout. At the same time, many doctors just whip out the hormone replacement therapy prescription pad in order to treat the symptoms while ignoring the cause. To me this is sad, a sad commentary on our whole health care system in this country."

Dr. Lader notes that there are many different agents in our environment that decrease thyroid function, ranging from stress to food. And, says Lader, treating environmentally induced hypothyroidism by using hormones or drugs is an excuse for those who are not willing to do the right work to get people well. He argues that to treat hypothyroidism, "We have to use a natural approach to make the body stronger and healthier. To really give optimal treatment for hypothyroidism, we have to treat the ultimate cause of the illness. So we will have to deal with diet, nutrition, and all the environmental factors that can affect our thyroid gland."

Causes

Lader believes that nutritional deficiencies and stress are the two major keys to hypothyroidism. He says, however, that although iodine deficiency or excess has been fully documented as a causal factor, in the United States, unlike other countries, iodine deficiency is not a significant factor because most of the salt consumed in the United States is iodized.

Micronutrient deficiencies are important. Some of the major nutrients involved in thyroid metabolism are selenium, glutathione, and zinc, which are known to be required for proper conversion of T4 into T3, the form of thyroid hormone that is active in the tissues. Dr. Lader says that we also should examine protein, fat, and carbohydrate consumption to really get an idea of what's happening with the thyroid gland. With hypothyroidism, as with so many other chronic illnesses, excess carbohydrate intake can be a major contributing factor. Too much carbohydrate can push blood sugar high and stimulate cortisol production, leading to hypoglycemia, and this increases thyroid production.

Lader also notes that suboptimal intake of calories, especially in women, may contribute to hypothyroidism. He finds that this is a particular problem in young and middle-aged women who use calorie restriction as a misguided way to improve their health and lose weight. "Fasting is still a popular way to lose weight. I see that a lot of people who fast really go to excess and create problems. So we see over and over again that people are not eating enough food, which is causing problems." Diets high in caffeine may also adversely affect thyroid function. In addition, Dr. Lader notes, "Food allergies affect our thyroid glands, and that is why we see so many people with allergies who commonly have other systemic endocrine problems in their bodies. You also have to stop and look at chemical and medical toxicity. People whose cholesterol rises year after year may have hypothyroidism."

Other possible causes are pollutants, such as secondhand smoke or phthalates, which are used as softeners in some plastics and food wraps. The many plastics in our society may be related to decreased thyroid function, Lader believes. Since he believes that hypothyroidism is caused by stress and environmental factors, he says that it is essential to make an assessment of the role those factors may play in a woman's life and not get caught up in the quixotic search for a wonder drug. "A lot of people are looking for the magic bullet to treat thyroid disease, but I think one of the most important things is to look at a diet history of those who have thyroid problems. Diagnosing hypothyroidism is just the beginning."

He points out that toxins can hinder the natural thyroid cycle in the body. "There are many different environmental and chemical stresses that interfere with the conversion of T4 into T3."

The gut is another place where problems can start. Our body detoxifies and eliminates thyroid hormones through the gut, where certain enzymes in a healthy intestine help to break apart the soluble thyroid hormones so that we can reabsorb them through our intestines. Many people have had a lot of antibiotic therapy, and poor diet or intestinal problems have led to imbalances in microflora. This imbalance decreases the body's ability to reuptake active thyroid hormone. It's very important to establish a healthy environment in the intestines in order to maintain normal levels of thyroid hormones.

"We also have to look at the liver," he continues, "which is probably the most abused, overworked, and stressed organ in the body. Our liver is exposed to a number of toxins, which we have to make soluble so that we can excrete them out of our bodies. The same enzymes that break down many environmental toxins also break down thyroid chemicals. If our livers are overworked due to exposure to toxins, and those enzymes speed up, we are also going to be moving lots of thyroid hormone out of the body. This is really the X factor in thyroid illness."

Dr. Lader says that many drugs that people take also interfere with thyroid function. These include antidepressants and interferon, which is taken to treat hepatitis C but can affect thyroid function.

In sum, there are a staggering number of environmental stressors—including numerous synthetic pollutants—that can have a profound influence on thyroid function. "That's why," says Dr. Lader, "we are seeing so many thyroid problems. I'd say that 50 percent of the patients that come to see me, when they fill out thyroid appraisal questionnaires, have thyroid stress. And most of it is related to environmental pollutants."

TREATMENT

"The first thing I like to have my patients do is take the underarm temperature test," continues Dr. Lader. "Women who are menstruating need to do it on day two, day three, and day four of their blood flow. Remember if the temperature's 97.8 or below, they might have hypothyroidism.

"The next step is to keep a seven-day diary, which records foods eaten, stress, symptoms, and physical conditions. This diary can sometimes convert what appears to be a very difficult case into one that's obvious by giving you an idea of what is really happening in the body."

Next he concentrates on developing a healthier lifestyle. This includes eating right. "One thing I urge my patients to try to avoid is the brassica family foods—cabbage, broccoli, cauliflower." He acknowledges that these foods have many health benefits, but says that some people are eating way too many of them, especially if they are exhibiting thyroid symptoms. Stress management is also important. One of the major problems of hypothyroidism, as noted, is inadequate conversion of inactive thyroid (thyroxine) into active thyroid (triiodothyronine). Stress elevates cortisol, which inhibits this conversion process. Heavy activity, exercise, and different stress-reduction methods are needed. One also has to take a good, high-quality multiple vitamin and eat a healthy, balanced diet.

Another aspect of treatment is nutritional supplementation. The creation of a supplement program has to be handled carefully, Lader explains. "It comes down to the fact that every hypothyroid patient is different and requires a different approach. Supplemental programs need to be customized so that they address all the factors that have been ascertained during the diagnosis and the workup. In general, we have to make sure people are taking in adequate amounts of selenium, glutathione, and zinc."

Lader concludes, "People who are suffering from hypothyroidism should view the disease as a chance to make some positive changes in their lifestyle. especially in terms of stress and toxicity."

PATIENT STORIES: FROM DR. STEPHEN LANGER

Dr. Stephen Langer treats hypothyroidism by giving small doses of thyroid (powdered thyroid gland):

I put them on as little as a quarter or a grain of thyroid, which is a newborn infant dose, and this produces a radical change in the way a person functions. Of course, for someone who has low thyroid function, I also use orthomolecular nutrition and a lot of clinical ecology techniques along with treating the thyroid gland.

Recently I treated a patient who was the wife of a doctor and the mother of two young children. She basically came in and told me that she didn't want to go on living. She was so tired all the time, and so depressed, that she couldn't keep her head off the pillow after two o'clock in the afternoon. If she didn't go to bed, she would just fall apart. I did a history and physical on her and we made some dietary changes, but basically this woman was profoundly hypothyroid. We put her on a quarter of a grain of thyroid, which is what I start my patients with before building them up very gradually. A quarter of a grain is the smallest dose available. It's such a small quantity that most pharmacies don't even carry it, because when doctors order thyroid they don't even think to order so small a dose. But a quarter of a grain of thyroid was enough. Within a three-week period, not only did this woman regain her mental health, she was out taking tennis lessons, which was shocking even to me because although the treatment usually works it usually takes a longer period of time. So, just that amount of metabolic support was enough to turn this person's life around.

Another person I treated was a 62-year-old woman who was a member of the Catholic clergy. She had been a nun for at least 30 years when I met her, and I will never forget this woman. She came in bloated, profoundly depressed, and fatigued. The only thing that kept her going was basically overworking her adrenal glands. She came in and told me that when she was 12 years old, she went under a dark cloud. When I saw her it was 50 years later, and by that time she had been through 30 or 40 different doctors, including internists, endocrinologists, psychiatrists, and psychologists of various sorts. One of the first things that showed up in her—which I thought was a very positive sign—was that she was freezing all the time. When we did basal body temperature measurements on her, they never went above 95 degrees. However, when I did a blood workup on her, all her thyroid hormone levels were within normal limits. I empirically placed her on a dose of thyroid that we gradually built up to about four grains a day, which is quite a high dosage. She's one of the few people I've treated who has needed that high an amount. Within three months, her depression of 50 years' duration was totally gone.

Now, obviously she was bitter and angry that she had been suffering for all that time. But the organic feeling that she had of overwhelming fatigue totally disappeared within a three-month period of time, and I've seen that response in thousands of patients over the years. A small dose of thyroid, combined with things like nutritional support and eliminating food allergies, can really turn a person's life around.

Thyroiditis

Over the past 15 years or so, it has become apparent that some people with thyroid conditions have normal thyroid hormone levels and are suffering from another condition, known as Hashimoto's disease, or autoimmune thyroiditis.

What triggers an autoimmune response? Dr. Langer explains: "Imagine autoimmune thyroiditis to be like rheumatoid arthritis of the thyroid gland. A person can have rheumatoid arthritis, which is an autoimmune condition where the body puts out antibodies to the joints. Frequently people with rheumatoid arthritis can experience long periods of remission. When they are under a great deal of stress, the body puts out antibodies to the joints and all their joints swell up. A similar things happens with thyroiditis; if a person gets stressed out for any reason whatsoever, the body can start pumping out antibodies to the thyroid gland. The thyroid becomes acutely inflamed, and thyroid hormone which under normal circumstances would not be released starts escaping. It's almost like pumping speed into your system.

Dr. Langer notes, "There is a very precise blood test that any doctor can order called the autoimmune thyroid antibody test, and most of the people who I suspect have thyroid conditions and have normal thyroid hormone levels will have an elevation in their antithyroid antibodies. If they have an elevated antithyroid antibody level, they have the symptoms that go along with low thyroid, which can be any one of 125 symptoms that we enumerate in *Solve the Riddle of Illness.*"

Like hypothyroidism, thyroiditis can cause a number of psychological symptoms. Dr. Langer explains: "With thyroiditis people get anxiety attacks and panic attacks for no apparent reason. They could be sitting and reading a book. All of a sudden they will develop a cascade of heart palpitations and fearfulness.

I've had a number of patients who have been rushed, almost on a monthly basis, to the emergency room to be worked up by cardiologists because their heart was pounding over 200 beats a minute. Cardiologists would do EKGs and echocardiograms and then tell them to go see a psychiatrist. The psychiatrist would work them up, not find anything, and then put them on an antidepressant or a tranquilizer, and actually make the condition worse. When you have an undiscovered organic basis for a psychological problem, being put on psychotropic medication is like sitting on a thumbtack and being put on pain pills for the rest of your life. It has about the same effect. It wears the system down, and as a result the patient's condition not only does not improve but will in fact deteriorate, because the underlying cause is not being treated.

"To treat patients with thyroiditis, I put them on a trial dose of thyroid and continue to monitor their thyroid hormone levels. Most of these people wind up taking between one and two grains of thyroid a day and their thyroid hormone levels still stay normal despite the fact that their levels were supposedly normal to begin with. More importantly, they get a complete remission of symptoms, many of which manifest themselves as psychological symptoms."

A large number of Dr. Cass's patients also have thyroiditis. I really can't emphasize the importance of this problem enough," she says, "because thyroiditis often accompanies the mixed infection syndrome, which can consist of any combination of the following: parasites, candidiasis, and the viral syndromes, including Epstein-Barr virus and cytomegalovirus. Psychological components include depression, anxiety, and even panic attacks.

"To treat thyroiditis, I've done nutritional consults on people that were under the care of other physicians. When I suggested that they had thyroiditis and that it was to be treated with low doses of thyroid hormones, I was met with skepticism from the other doctors.

"When people have these long-standing chronic conditions, they can become extremely depressed. They feel like they can't go on anymore, particularly when their body has been so racked by the continuing illness. Also, some of the mixed infection of thyroiditis and the parasites or other viruses can actually affect the brain directly. Thyroiditis and its accompanying infections affect the central nervous system along with every other organ of the body. So people come in extremely depressed, both as a reaction to their prolonged illness and as a primary symptom of the illness, and this is usually totally overlooked. That's why it's crucial to do a good medical workup on a patient whose disorder may at first appear purely psychological in origin."

"There is one more connection to be drawn between depression and thyroid dysfunction," Dr. Langer adds, "poor libido. One of the classic symptoms of depression is a loss of interest in sex. Those people who in the past were sexually active, but who all of a sudden or gradually started to lose interest in sex, will be diagnosed as being depressed right away. Men come into my office by the score—many of them young—who have potency problems, and they can't figure it out because they have no apparent organic illness. As a result, they get performance anxiety, and if that continues long enough, they wind up getting severely depressed. But I have found that if you go to the root cause of their depression, very often it's the thyroid that's malfunctioning.

"If a person develops an acute depression that leads to a sexual dysfunction—which it frequently does—a doctor would be remiss if he or she didn't look for an imbalance in the thyroid. Patients have got to start taking their health destinies into their own hands and demanding that doctors do thyroid testing and look for autoimmune thyroid disorders and nutritional imbalances, which are frequently the underlying causes of sexual dysfunction and depression."

WHO IS AFFECTED?

"The constellation of problems associated with thyroid disorders occurs not only in middle-aged people but also in young people, and not only in women, but also in men," Dr. Langer says. "While thyroid disease, particularly autoimmune thyroiditis, is classically considered to be primarily a disease of women, this is just not true. I have seen as many men as women who are suffering from autoimmune thyroiditis and, I might add, from hypothyroidism. Men are really given short shrift and aren't even given the requisite diagnostic tests in many instances to rule out thyroid disease because the medical profession thinks that this is strictly a woman's disorder.

"Moreover, I have seen teenagers and children who are acting out, who are written off as hyperactive, when they may be suffering from a thyroid disorder. Very young children or teenagers express their emotions differently from adults. Sometimes they get written off as being mentally retarded or having minimal brain dysfunction. Then they're given any one of a number of different drugs and placed in special classes. Many times, these young people have thyroid disorders that can be easily treated. But because thyroid dysfunction often leads to frequent infections, these kids are placed on antibiotics. Then they wind up with an overgrowth of yeast in their gut that in turn causes a low-grade inflammation in their gastrointestinal system. As a result, they don't adequately digest their food, so the body starts regarding the food as a foreign invader and puts out antibodies to the food. The child starts exhibiting the classic symptoms of food allergies, which are psychiatric complaints: anxiety attacks, depression, forgetfulness, inability to concentrate, even full-blown panic attacks.

"In a lot of these cases, you can actually isolate and eliminate the foods that cause an anxiety attack, but merely removing the food is not enough to get to the underlying cause of the disorder. Frequently patients have food allergies because of a preexisting condition in their digestive systems which has to be addressed. The presence of such a preexisting condition can cause immune system alterations which result in autoimmune dysfunction. So this is a vicious circle. One of the chief target organs of autoimmune dysfunction is the thyroid gland. You get autoimmune thyroiditis."

ALTERNATIVE THERAPIES

"The question for holistic clinicians to ask themselves, regarding each individual patient, is where they're going to intervene," Dr. Langer says. "Different physicians will intervene at different places, depending upon their background and interests. I try, to the best of my ability, to get to the root cause of what's going on. If I am having difficulty figuring out the cause, then I try to intervene at a point in a person's imbalance that will cause the least disruption to their lifestyle and give them the best results for the least amount of money in the quickest period of time. Frequently, that turns out to be treating with small doses of thyroid and altering eating habits. In my clinical experience, I have found that with the thyroid and nutritional support, very often a person will get better. The thyroid is not a lifetime treatment and can be removed after the person's condition has been stabilized. Thyroid treatment is inexpensive, works rapidly, and when done properly it is absolutely nontoxic."

Dr. Allan Spreen, a general practitioner who specializes in nutrition-based medicine, reminds us that while thyroid supplementation is an important modality, it is not fail-safe. "I'd love to say that correcting thyroid function is a panacea. While it doesn't work 100 percent of the time, if a patient comes in complaining of fatigue and depression that is linked with the physical findings of foods not digesting well, and cold extremities, then an underactive thyroid may be the root cause. People come and say, 'Oh, my husband says, "Don't touch me with your feet at night because they're just ice cold."' These are the same people who are comfortable in a room when everybody else is boiling and who are freezing in a room when everybody else is comfortable. Their thinking seems to have slowed down. They just don't seem to be able to concentrate like they used to, and they don't remember lists the way they used to.

"In this kind of a situation, once I find that their blood levels of thyroid are normal, I go back to the old school of Broda Barnes, who, 40 or 50 years ago, did axillary temperature testing. I ask my patients to keep a record of their early morning basal body temperature. If their basal metabolic rate based on early-morning body temperatures is really low, then I consider them to be candidates for thyroid supplementation. In axillary testing, Broda Barnes talked about temperature ranges between 97.8 and 98.2 degrees Fahrenheit, which is lower than the 98.6 people think of as normal. But the axillary temperature is taken in the armpit first thing in the morning, using a mercury thermometer that stays there for 10 minutes before they get up. If their temperature is, much of the time, down in the 96.8, 96.7, 96.5 range, I at least consider the possibility that the person needs low doses of natural thyroid, which is still available.

"Thyroid is a prescription drug. Some doctors who use this type of testing use synthetic thyroid. I prefer to prescribe natural thyroid in very low doses. If a person responds—either their temperature rises or their symptoms lift—then I retest them to see if their blood levels of thyroid have changed. Many times a person with this profile of symptoms who takes thyroid begins to feel better, but their blood tests remain unchanged, including levels of thyroid stimulating hormone (TSH) and actual thyroid hormone. This means that the blood testing has missed the diagnosis, and yet the person feels well with the increased, but undetectable, dose of thyroid hormone."

Patient Stories

JENNY

I came to be treated by Dr. Spreen only after first following the conventional route in medical treatment. In 1988, I was in my fifth year of infertility treatments, had taken multiple infertility drugs, and wound up severely depressed, which caused me to lose 35 pounds in two months. I couldn't sleep, I had panic attacks, the whole horrible group of symptoms associated with depression. The doctors put me on the conventional Xanax treatment for three years before I met Dr. Spreen, who was helping me with some other related medical problems. I had hair loss, skin problems, nail-biting problems. I had aches all over my body, especially in my legs. Dr. Spreen got me on a vitamin regimen, which made me feel somewhat better.

Then Dr. Spreen put me on very low doses of thyroid and immediately—within two to three weeks—all the problems I just mentioned were gone. Now I had had thyroid checks three times during the whole time when I was being treated for infertility, and the blood tests had always come up negative. But I knew that in my family there were thyroid problems. There are at least six members of my family that I can think of who have thyroid disorders, but mine just never showed up on my tests. After taking these very low doses of thyroid, my skin problem cleared up, I stopped biting my nails, and my legs stopped aching. The mild depression I was still suffering from all of a sudden in August vanished. I felt great. I slept like a normal person again. I had energy. People started commenting on how I seemed to be like my old self again. It was like getting a new lease on life!

I feel rather fed up with the original doctors I went to see. They treated me like I was a hysterical woman who needed to get a grip on things. I have never told them about my recovery using alternative methods because I don't think they'd be receptive to it.

HELEN

I had hives, some kind of an allergic response, about five years ago and it progressed to the point where I had hives on my vocal cords. It was a pretty serious allergic reaction, for which I was first treated with antihistamines. Later, I was treated with prednisone. When small doses of prednisone given every other day didn't help, my doctor began increasing the dosage until I was taking 70 milligrams every day. After about six weeks I started declining physically from taking this tremendous dose. I gained about 50 pounds. I had conjunctivitis in both of my eyes. I had open sores.

I was so weak I was almost bedridden. I did find another doctor who slowly weaned me off of the prednisone. But when it was all over, my immune system had been damaged. I had a lot of viral illnesses that are usually associated with chronic fatigue syndrome. I could scarcely get out of bed, and I couldn't lose all the weight I had gained. So I went from doctor to doctor. I was living in the Midwest at the time and many of these doctors said, "Your metabolic system has been altered by prednisone. Too bad, but you will never lose that weight. And prednisone can damage the immune system. Too bad, but your immune system has been damaged." No one could offer me any help at all.

I first went to Dr. Atkins in New York and he was a lot of help to me. It was through Dr. Atkins and his association with Dr. Huggins that I learned about dental amalgams, because when your immune system is depleted you are much more susceptible to any kind of toxins, including mercury leaching from mercury amalgam fillings. It was causing me a great deal of trouble and I did have those removed.

Then I moved to California and I had heard, previous to my moving, about Dr. Slagle and her work with depression. In fact, I referred friends to her, friends I had made in California, and they had these miraculous cures from depression after two weeks of taking B-complex vitamins and amino acids. But I didn't think of going to her myself for quite a while because I thought of her as someone who only treated depression. In fact, like many alternative physicians, she treats the whole person. She had worked with fatigue a lot, and she first tested me thoroughly and found that my thyroid and, in fact, my whole endocrine system, was not functioning properly, most likely as a result of prednisone. She picked up subtleties in the test that other doctors ignored. She has the philosophy that a body should be healthy and whole. She doesn't need gross parameters of unusual test results to say something is wrong here. So she was able to discover that I had a rather unusual problem in my thyroid and she was able to treat it.

When I began seeing her I still had very limited energy. Even though Dr. Atkins had helped me lose weight so I looked normal, I still didn't feel normal. In one day, I could either go to the grocery store or go to a doctor's appointment. That was all I could do. The remainder of the day I had to rest. I went to Dr. Slagle and after she began treating my thyroid I had a leap of improvement. I regained my energy. She also gave me amino acids, which heightened my mood. Even though I hadn't thought I was depressed—and I still don't think I was—generally the amino acids made me feel healthier. And while I don't have the energy of a lot of people around me, I can pretty much function normally, which is a miracle. It has been a five-year struggle and I'm finally living practically a normal life.

Here's what I have learned from my experience. You simply cannot go to a traditional physician and carelessly allow that doctor to treat your symptoms with drugs. Traditional physicians tend not to look at the whole person, but to give drugs to ameliorate the symptoms, or to treat individual problems without regard to what that treatment does to the rest of the body. I learned to use tremendous caution when entrusting my body to someone. If you're going to trust your body to someone, you should know a lot about the physician. You should know whether the physician treats the whole person and sees you as more than an allergy or a gallbladder.

DR. HYLA CASS DESCRIBES A PATIENT

I recently saw a young woman who came in depressed, tired, unable to get up in the morning, and feeling overwhelmed by her work responsibilities. Her history revealed that she was often cold, especially in her hands and feet (she even wore socks to bed), had thinning hair, dry skin, constipation, and was losing the outer part of her eyebrows. I suspected an imbalance in her thyroid.

When I asked about thyroid disease, she said that it had been suspected before, but her tests had been normal. I checked her thyroid hormones, including thyroid antibody levels.

Often despite "normal" blood tests, there is an underactive thyroid. Dr. Broda Barnes's technique of monitoring thyroid function through body temperature is used by many alternative practitioners. Although this patient's thyroid hormone blood levels were normal, she did, in fact, have antithyroid antibodies, confirming a diagnosis of Hashimoto's thyroiditis. This is an autoimmune disease, treatable with thyroid hormone, antioxidants, and adrenal support. Her signs were those of hypothyroidism, indicating that the circulating hormone was being rendered ineffective. With Hashimoto's thyroiditis, there are often also intermittent signs of hyperthyroidism, or overactive thyroid, such as irritability or heart palpitations.

I prescribed thyroid hormone from natural (animal) sources, and asked her to monitor her body temperature, so I could adjust the dosage. She asked whether this supplementation would suppress her own thyroid function, and whether she would be taking it for the rest of her life. The answer was no on both counts. The treatment actually supported her own gland, allowing it to heal. Within 10 days of starting the program she was feeling alive again.

Chapter 35

Urinary
Incontinence

Causes

Eighty-five percent of the 13 million people who are incontinent are women. This is because urinary incontinence is related to childbirth and menopause. Gynecologist Vicki Hufnagel explains: "In many cases, women are given episiotomies after delivery, without proper closure. Since muscles are not put back together correctly, the whole area is unable to provide support." Dr. Hufnagel adds that during menopause, urinary incontinence occurs when a woman is not making enough estrogen. Too little estrogen enters the vaginal tissue, causing the area to become thin, inelastic, and weak.

Urinary incontinence can also be the result of brain and spinal cord lesions, trauma, multiple sclerosis, and allergies.

There are many causes of transient incontinence. Some common ones are infection, strophic urethritis or vaginitis, certain medications (sedatives, hypnotics, diuretics, anticholinergics, alpha-adrenergic agonists or antagonists, and calcium-channel blockers), psychological disorders (especially depression), endocrine disorders, hyperglycemia, restricted mobility, and stool impaction.

Smoking has been found to be the cause of 28 percent of cases of urinary incontinence in women. Smoking increases the odds of both stress and motor urinary incontinence, and with increased daily and lifetime cigarette consumption, the odds for genuine stress incontinence rise. A study of 606 women reported in the November 1992 *American Journal of Obstetrics* showed that genuine stress incontinence was twice as common for both former and current smokers as for nonsmokers.

Symptoms

Urinary incontinence is a partial or total loss of control over one's bladder and urinary sphincter muscles. Sometimes, incontinence is accompanied by a feeling of urgency. This is usually the result of a person's inability to empty the bladder completely. Coughing and other stressors can set off urinary incontinence. Overflow can occur when bladder capacity is small.

Clinical Experience

Women with urinary incontinence are often advised to get bladder surgery, even hysterectomies. But this drastic approach may be completely unnecessary, according to Dr. Hufnagel, who says that women need to be educated about more conservative treatments for this common problem.

OUTPATIENT SURGERY AND HORMONE REPLACEMENT

Women need to repair their failed episiotomy, or to receive hormones, Dr. Hufnagel explains. Often, they simply need outpatient surgery to put the muscles and tissues back the way they should have been restored at the time of delivery.

Regarding menopause, Dr. Hufnagel adds, "We can treat this locally, without surgery, by simply putting hormones into the vagina. One or two months later, we see normal, healthy tissue."

ELECTRICAL STIMULATION

This treatment became popular in Europe after it was learned that high voltages of electricity to the vaginal area caused muscles to contract. However, the effects were short-lived, and the technique was not without problems. Voltages had to be applied constantly, which sometimes resulted in tissue burning and nerve damage.

In the United States, electrical stimulation is being performed with lower voltages and a pulsing sequence of 1 second on and 1 second off to prevent muscle fatigue. The objective is to strengthen the urethral muscles and the puborectalis muscle, which control the opening and closing of the bladder muscles. This form of electrical stimulation, combined with pelvic floor exercises, has produced favorable results in trial studies. It allows for a retraining, toning, and strengthening of muscles so that a patient can regain continence.

One electrical product that looks promising is called Cystotron, put out by a company called Biosonics. More information about this system can be obtained on the World Wide Web at www.biosonics.com, or the old-fashioned way, by calling (800) 547-4357.

HOMEOPATHIC REMEDIES

Dana Ullman, who has an M.P.H. from the University of California—Berkeley, suggests in an article posted on HealthWorld Online (www.healthy.net) that homeopathic medicines can help prevent involuntary urination. He advises consulting a homeopathic practitioner who can individualize the treatment and work on strengthening the overall immune system, rather than just treating the bladder symptoms.

But there are homeopathic medicines that you can use on your own. One new, inexpensive homeopathic medicine he recommends is EnurAid, which is nontoxic and nonaddictive. Other homeopathic remedies that he recommends are listed below. Ullman recommends that someone who has not used homeopathic remedies before should start all the remedies suggested at the sixth potency and take the medication three or four times a day. If there is no improvement after taking a medication for a week, a different homeopathic remedy should be tried.

ARNICA (LEOPARD'S BANE). Arnica is good for involuntary urination after surgery.

BELLADONNA (DEADLY NIGHTSHADE). Belladonna is helpful for people who dribble urine and who sometimes have a burning sensation when they urinate.

CAUSTICUM. Causticum may help if involuntary urination gets worse in the winter and better in the summer. Often people with these symptoms lose urine when they cough or sneeze.

EQUISETUM (SCOURING RUSH). Equisetum is a general remedy for anyone who loses urine or is a bedwetter, with no apparent cause.

FERRUM PHOS (IRON PHOSPHATE). Ferrum phos works best for people who tend to lose urine during the day. Often people with this symptom have the strongest urge to urinate when standing; lying down lessens the urge.

KREOSOTUM (BEECHWOOD). Kreosotum is recommended for people who cannot control sudden urges to urinate. Ullman says that these people tend to wet their bed during the first part of the night, and may dream that they are urinating.

Chapter 36

Urinary Tract Infections and Inflammations

U rinary tract infections and inflammations are quite common, accounting for approximately 6 million office visits per year in the United States. Dr. Jennifer Brett, a naturopathic physician from Stratford, Connecticut, says only 60 percent of people with symptoms of urinary tract infections have true infections; the other 40 percent have inflammations. Three types of infections and inflammations that Dr. Brett commonly sees are true urinary tract infections, urinary tract inflammations, and interstitial cystitis, a more distressing form of inflammation that can last for months or even years.

Causes

The cause of urinary tract inflammations is unknown, but some doctors believe they may be caused by viruses, food allergies, *Candida* in the colon, hormonal changes, new sexual partners, or vigorous sexual activity. Interstitial cystitis may result from infection by *Candida* or allergic reactions to foods and additives. "These irritants inflame the pelvis and bladder, and the body responds by increasing blood flow to the area," Dr. Brett explains. "Pelvic congestion causes further irritation and pressure on the bladder. Again, the body responds by sending more blood. This becomes a vicious cycle."

David L. Hoffman, M.N.I.M.H., in an article posted on the HealthWorld Online website (www.healthy.net), adds that microcrystals of calcium phosphate in the urine may cause mechanical irritation to the bladder walls, resulting in inflammation.

HIGH-RISK GROUPS

David Kauffman, M.D., a specialist in women's urological problems at St. Luke's Roosevelt Hospital in New York City, says that there are basically four types of women at high risk: "The most common patients are young, sexually active females. Another large group at risk are postmenopausal women. In fact, 8 to 10 percent of all women over 60 will get a bladder infection at some point. We also see a lot of patients who are hospitalized. The risk of bladder infection increases about 5 percent per day for every day that a catheter is in place. For this reason, medical doctors try to get catheters out as quickly as possible. The last high-risk group are patients with neurological problems. An example would be multiple sclerosis; patients with MS do not completely empty their bladders."

Dr. Kauffman says, "Many sexually active women get cystitis as a result of intercourse because the bacteria that normally live in the vaginal vault area get pushed up into the urethra. A woman's urethra is only about an inch and a half long, while in men it is much longer. In females, it doesn't take too much for bacteria to migrate from the outside of the urethra to the inside of the bladder. That's why we see so many more young women with bladder infections than young men with bladder infections.

"It is very important for women to know that their partners are not giving them infections. The bacteria are already in the vaginal area and simply get pushed into the bladder during intercourse."

Dr. Hoffman mentions several other risk factors. One is being diabetic or eating a lot of sugars. Another is use of products such as douches, feminine deodorants, antibacterial soaps, and certain contraceptive creams or jellies that irritate vaginal tissue, making it vulnerable to infection. Using a diaphragm can also irritate the urethra. Excess use of antibiotics will promote growth of bacteria resistant to those drugs, which can make cystitis more likely. Finally, he says, eating foods containing pesticides can cause some types of interstitial cystitis.

HORMONAL IMBALANCE

Dr. Kauffman says there are many reasons that not all sexually active women get bladder infections. "One of the more interesting ones has to do with the woman's hormonal balance. We know that there are estrogen and progesterone receptors on the lining cells of the urethra. In some women bacteria sticks to these receptors, a condition that is related to hormone levels. Imagine bacteria as little organisms with Velcro hooks. Picture the lining cells of the urethra with the opposite kind of hooks. Bacteria hook on to the Velcro on the receptor sites. In most women, the urinary stream washes away most bacteria. But in women who have specific hormonal environments, the bacteria are not expelled that easily. These are the women we see in our office with recurrent bladder infections."

Dr. Kauffman adds that postmenopausal women tend to get urinary tract infections for this reason as well. Their low estrogen levels cause their urethral linings to be "stickier" for bacteria. "One way to treat that is simply to insert low-dosage estrogen cream into the vaginal vault, about once a week," he advises. "Many women are on estrogen pills, but that does not have the same protective influence on the urinary tract as does estrogen cream."

WEAKENED IMMUNITY

Linda Wharton, a naturopathic physician and acupuncturist from New Zealand and author of *Natural Woman Health: A Guide to Healthy Living for Women of All Ages,* says recurrent bladder infections reflect a state of lowered immunity and weakened vitality: "Remember that cystitis is an infection. As with all infections, individuals with lowered nutritional status, poor cellular health, and lowered immunity are much more susceptible to infection. Women don't always develop acute cystitis each time a stray bacteria finds its way into the bladder. Often, women play host to these potentially problem-causing bacteria for weeks or months or even a lifetime without ever experiencing acute symptoms. It is only when the health of the whole body is reduced that an explosion of this bacterial population takes place. This may occur, for example, when a woman goes through a period of great stress, such as a divorce or the death of a loved one."

STRUCTURAL PROBLEMS

Wharton adds that other causes of cystitis are often overlooked: "Pelvic floor muscles can weaken as a result of pregnancy and childbirth. When these muscles are weakened, the bladder may prolapse and bulge forward into the wall of the vagina. If the back part of the bladder droops below the neck of the bladder, it becomes virtually impossible to empty the bladder properly. This leaves an almost permanent reservoir of urine in the bladder. In time, the stagnant urine becomes a haven for bacteria to multiply, should they be present." Wharton also says that a prolapsed transverse colon—due to childbirth, age, abdominal fat, poor posture, or spinal problems—can eventually cause bladder problems. Over time the prolapsed transverse colon—which lies across the abdomen, sags, compressing the organs beneath it, including the bladder. Blood flow is impeded, and the oxygen-starved bladder becomes ripe for infection. She adds, "This same downgrading of tissue health can occur as a direct result of a chronic back problem. All the pelvic organs receive nervous impulses from the spine, and a chronic lower back problem can interfere with those nervous impulses from the spinal cord." Wharton advises women with chronic back problems to see an osteopath or chiropractor.

CONSTIPATION

Dr. Wharton says, "Waste materials are excreted from our bodies through several different channels. The bowels excrete in the form of feces; the lungs gets rid of toxins in the form of carbon dioxide; the skin eliminates toxins as perspiration; and the kidney and bladder pass toxins out in the form of urine. If any one of these waste disposal systems is functioning inadequately, it places an excessive load on the others. If you only manage a half-hearted bowel movement every two or three days, you are placing undue stress on your kidneys and bladder, as accumulated toxins are passed out this way instead. In a sense, then, there is actually a direct link between chronic constipation and repeated urinary tract infections."

Symptoms

Typical symptoms of urinary tract infections and inflammations are frequent urination, a sensation that the bladder is never quite empty, and a burning sensation upon urination. Often women get up at night to urinate. There may be cramps, and the urine may be dark and foul-smelling. In severe cases, there may be blood in the urine as well.

Clinical Experience

DIAGNOSIS

A diagnosis of cystitis is usually made by collecting a midstream urine sample and testing for the presence of bacteria. If the problem stems from an inflammation, no pathogenic bacteria will be found in the urine, nor will bacteria be found on a vaginal culture.

CONVENTIONAL TREATMENT

The usual treatment for cystitis is a course of antibiotics, and standard therapy for chronic cystitis generally consists of repeated rounds of the same therapy.

In the long term, this practice may actually exacerbate the condition rather than cure it. It is well known that broad-spectrum antibiotics are indiscriminate killers that destroy colonies of friendly gut bacteria along with problem-causing organisms. Once the delicate balance of the normal gastrointestinal microflora has been disrupted, less desirable organisms proliferate, virtually unchecked. These include *Escherichia coli,* the prime cause of cystitis, and *Candida* overgrowth, a suspected cause of inflammations.

Dr. Kauffman says that antibiotics should be a last-ditch effort, used only when various holistic protocols fail to achieve results. Even then, mild medicines should be used: "What of women who do all the right things, and still come back with bladder infections? In these cases, we need to turn to more traditional medical approaches. The gold standard for treating patients who do everything right and still get infections is a very gentle, bacteriostatic antibiotic. A bacteriostatic antibiotic does not kill the bacteria, but limits bacterial growth. It is gentler on the system, and generally does not cause yeast infections or gastrointestinal problems. I am not big on taking antibiotics, but this is a better alternative than constant infections."

Dr. Brett reports that radical therapies are sometimes used for persistent cases: "Treatments I have read about in recent medical journals include surgery to cut nerves to reduce irritation to the bladder, hormonal therapy, and even antidepressive medications to help women sleep better, even though this doesn't get at the root cause of the problem."

NATUROPATHIC TREATMENTS

DIET

It is important to drink plenty of pure water, about one 8-oz glass each hour. "If you are in agony and you don't know what to do, start drinking water, and don't stop," advises Dr. Wharton. "Stay away from tea, coffee, soft drinks, and alcohol, but drink plenty of water."

Cranberry, either in the form of unsweetened juice or capsules, changes the pH of the urine, making it more acidic and less hospitable to bacteria. Cranberries also contain powerful antibacterial substances. In fact, studies reveal that as little as 15 oz of cranberry juice results in an 80 percent inhibition of bacterial growth. Bacteria lose the ability to cling to the bladder wall, and must exit the system along with urine. Other research indicates that cranberry juice combined with vitamin C acidifies the urine further. The effect is therefore much greater when both are taken together.

Other drinks useful for temporarily acidifying the urine include lemon juice and water, buttermilk, and 2 teaspoons of apple cider vinegar stirred into a glass of water. Drink any of these substances three or four times a day.

During an acute attack of cystitis, the diet can be temporarily changed to further acidify the urine. Dr. Wharton warns that this is recommended only for short periods of time, during an acute infection: "Eat plenty of acidic foods, such as grains, nuts, seeds, fish, dairy products, meat and bread, and cut back on fruit and vegetables."

VITAMIN C

Any time the body is fighting an infection, it tolerates large amounts of C, sometimes as much as 10,000 to 15,000 mg orally each day (and even more intravenously). For cystitis, or for any infection, take vitamin C to bowel tolerance. (Bowel tolerance is where the stool becomes quite loose, almost to the point of diarrhea.) Vitamin C should be taken every two to three hours since it is water-soluble, which means that it is rapidly excreted from the body. According to Hoffman, recent studies indicate that ascorbic acid irritates the bladder. For this reason it is best to take vitamin C in the buffered form of calcium ascorbate. Aspartate also irritates the bladder, so avoid vitamins that contain it.

Dr. Wharton says that vitamin C fights infections in several ways: "Vitamin C concentrates in very high levels in the urine and exerts a direct bactericidal effect. It also supports systemic immune system function by helping to activate neutrophils, the white blood cells most involved in the front line defense against infection. It also works to stimulate the production of lymphocytes, which are important for coordinating immune function at the cellular level."

VITAMIN A

In addition to vitamin C, think about vitamin A. An easy way of supplementing with this vitamin is to use halibut or cod liver oil capsules, up to 25,000 IU a day, during acute phases of infection. Vitamin A helps protect the mucous membrane lining of the bladder and urethra from irritation during infection. It also improves antibody response and white blood cell function. Just a word of warning here: if you are pregnant, do not use such high doses of vitamin A, as they have been associated with birth defects. Beta carotene, with which the body can make vitamin A as it is needed, is a safer alternative.

ZINC

Zinc is essential for increasing white blood cell activity in response to infection. For acute cystitis, approximately 50 mg elemental zinc is needed daily.

HERBS

The classes of herbs used to treat cystitis include antiseptic herbs, demulcents, and diuretics. Antiseptic herbs for bladder infections include *uva-ursi*, buchu, goldenseal, juniper berries, and garlic. "Think garlic whenever you have any type of infection, including cystitis," says Dr. Wharton. Demulcents soothe inflamed mucous membranes inside the bladder and urethra, and include marsh mallow root, juniper berry, and corn silk. Diuretic herbs stimulate the production and excretion of urine, which helps to wash out bacteria. Common diuretics are parsley and goldenrod.

Dr. Wharton recommends these old naturopathic herbal remedies for treating burning urine: "Mix together equal parts of fennel, burdock, and slippery elm. Steep a teaspoon of this mixture in a cup of boiled water for about 20 minutes. Have one cup before each meal, and one before bed."

She also recommends flaxseed tea or a combination of *uva-ursi* and buchu: "For either tea, use one teaspoon of the dried herb(s) to a cup of boiling water. Again, let it steep for 15 to 20 minutes. Then drink one cup, three or four times a day. The results more than compensate for the awful taste."

Hoffman recommends the following formula for cystitis: Combine two parts of corn silk, two parts of *uva ursi*, and one part of buchu. Take 5 ml of this tincture three times a day. At the same time, drink an infusion of yarrow, another antiseptic herb, throughout the day.

Dr. Tori Hudson, a naturopath in Portland, Oregon, in her column for Prevention magazine recommends the following combination of herbs, either as capsules or in tinctures: pipsissewa, *uva-ursi*, echinacea or goldenseal, and buchu. For two days, take two capsules or 20 to 30 drops every 2 hours. For the next seven days, take the capsules or tincture three times daily.

Dr. Joseph Pizzorno adds this bit of advice: "After sexual intercourse, women should wipe the opening to the urethra with a dilute solution of Betadine or a strong solution of goldenseal tea to wash away any bacteria that may have been forced up into the urethra."

OTHER THERAPIES

HOMEOPATHY

Judyth Reichenberg-Ullman and Robert Ullman, naturopathic and homeopathic doctors in Edmonds, Washington, in an article posted on the HealthWorld Online website (www.healthy.net), recommend cantharis (Spanish fly), a frequently used remedy in cases in which extreme pain in the bladder occurs very suddenly and there is blood in the urine. *Staphysagria* (stavesacre) is the remedy to use when a bladder infection has developed after having sex ("honeymoon cystitis"). When cystitis is associated with pain in the kidney area, especially on the right side, they suggest *Berberis aquifolium* (Oregon grape).

HYDROTHERAPY

Hydrotherapy is another traditional naturopathic method for helping people overcome the discomforts of cystitis. Sitz baths or hot compresses stimulate blood circulation and remove toxins from the pelvic area. Dr. Wharton explains how this is done: "You can use a hot compress by dipping a small hand towel into a basin of water, as hot as you can possibly tolerate it. Wring out the water and quickly apply the cloth to the area just above the pubic bone. As the cloth cools, repeat the process. In total, apply the compress eight or nine times. Repeat this process two to three times throughout the day. It actually feels wonderful and gives quite a bit of local relief to the symptoms.

"Alternatively, you can try making a sitz bath. Fill a small tub with water, once again, as hot as you can bear it. Add six drops of bergamot oil, and sit in the bath so that water actually covers your pelvis and lower abdomen. Stay there for around half an hour. As the water cools, keep replenishing with fresh, hot water to keep the water up to a hot, even temperature. Just a word of warning: If you have a problem with a weak heart or high blood pressure, hot sitz baths aren't really for you. You are better off just using a local compress."

ACUPUNCTURE

Dr. Wharton reports impressive results in the treatment of chronic cystitis with acupuncture when it is accompanied by lifestyle and dietary changes: "Usually an acute attack of cystitis responds to two to four acupuncture sessions, spaced two or three days apart. Chronic cystitis sufferers often benefit from an extended course of acupuncture treatment to prevent the recurrence of their problem."

AROMATHERAPY

Essential oils can enhance any treatment program, according to aromatherapist Ann Berwick. To help clear up a urinary tract infection, 18 to 20 drops of juniper and cedarwood can be added to 1 oz of lotion and massaged into the lower abdomen. Also, six to eight drops of juniper, bergamot, or sandlewood can be added to a sitz bath or full bath.

A PSYCHOLOGICAL PERSPECTIVE

Judyth Reichenberg-Ullman and Robert Ullman caution further that it's important not only to rest but to pay attention to whatever message your body is giving you with this bladder infection, to avoid recurrences. Therefore, consider what might be its underlying cause. They add that breathing into the pain and relaxing can be remarkably effective: "We had one patient who cured a bladder infection solely through visualization and meditation."

Inflammations

For urinary inflammation not caused by bacteria, Dr. Brett suggests the following:

DIET

It is important to avoid foods that encourage the growth of *Candida*, such as wheat, simple sugars, white flour, pastries, candies, alcohol, aged cheeses, vinegar, and even fruit. Avoid known food allergens. It is a good idea to get a test to determine if there are any other foods in the diet that are acting as irritants.

WATER

As with bacterial infections, you should drink one 8-ounce glass of water every hour. It is also a good idea to drink a glass of water and to urinate immediately after sexual intercourse. This tends to reduce the bladder irritation that sexual intercourse may cause.

CLOTHING

Avoid tight-fitting pants, nylon underwear, and pantyhose. They encourage the growth of *Candida* in the vaginal tract, which irritates the bladder and urethra.

OTHER REMEDIES

For *vitamins,* take 2,000 to 6,000 mg of buffered vitamin C and 100 to 200 mg of vitamin B_6. Also take four to six capsules of evening primrose oil. *Herbs* that soothe the bladder include althea or marsh mallow, corn silk, slippery elm, and goldenrod. Finally, as with bacterial infections, the homeopathic remedy *cantharis* (Spanish fly) is often effective in reducing bladder and urethra irritations.

Interstitial Cystitis

"The basic way to treat interstitial cystitis," says Dr. Brett, "is to remove congestion from the pelvis." The therapies she suggests in cases of intersitial cystitis are listed below. "If you follow these basic guidelines," says Dr. Brett, "within three to four weeks, you are likely to notice that your ability to sleep through the night is improved and that your cramping and pain during the day is significantly lessened."

TESTS

It is a good idea to be tested for food allergies to see if some food is causing an antibody-antigen reaction and irritating the bladder. It is also important to test for *Candida* in the colon because *Candida* can cause irritations and antibody reactions that irritate the bladder. Next, check to see that the hormones are in balance. If they are not, use vitamin B_6, evening primrose oil, and herbs to restore hormonal balance.

EXERCISE

The two types of exercise that help in cases of interstitial cystitis are aerobic exercise and inversion exercise. Doing aerobic exercise every day helps to remove blood congestion from the pelvis. "Aerobic" means anything that gets the blood moving, such as walking briskly, jogging, swimming, and bicycling.

Specific exercises for moving the blood involve turning upside down. In yoga, this is accomplished with the headstand or shoulderstand. It can also be achieved by lying on the back, raising the legs up, and performing cycling rotations with the legs.. If there is a back or neck problem, however, a simple solution is to use a slant board, which can be made simply with an old door or a couple of one-by-four boards. One end can be placed on the couch, and the other end on the floor. Once it is stable, the person lies upside down, that is, with the head near the floor and the feet near the couch. The blood is automatically pulled out of the pelvis by gravity, and moved into the chest and head. Remaining too long can cause dizziness; 5 or 10 minutes works for most people.

HERBS

The soothing herbs previously mentioned are useful here as well: marsh mallow, corn silk, slippery elm, and goldenrod.

DIET

A low-acid diet decreases irritations. High-acid foods to omit are red meat, dairy, shellfish, and citrus fruits. The diet should include whole grains, beans, and vegetables. Essential fatty acids, such as those found in flaxseed oil, evening primrose oil, and fish oils, can help reduce inflammation. In interstitial cystitis, they are key for reversing the cycle of irritation and blood congestion.

PREVENTION

Long-term preventive changes obviously make a lot more sense than simply dealing with each acute infection as it arises. Here are some simple personal hygiene measures to reduce the likelihood of reinfection:

After a bowel movement, wipe from front to back, away from the vagina.

Encourage your partner to wash thoroughly before any sexual contact.

Avoid the transfer of bacteria from the anus to the vagina during lovemaking.

During a period, change pads and tampons frequently.

Do not wear tight-fitting jeans or nylon pantyhose or pants. Cotton pants and stockings with garters allow more air flow and ventilation.

Make a habit of drinking lots of water. Aim for seven to eight glasses each day. This keeps the urine dilute so that bacterial proliferation is less likely. It also prompts frequent urination, which washes out problematic bacteria. Reduce the intake of coffee and tea.

Make a habit of emptying your bladder frequently. Research shows that women who ignore their urge to urinate for long periods of time are much more likely to develop cystitis. The motto here is when you need to go, go right away. Urinate after sexual intercourse. This will help to wash out any of the bacteria that may have been pushed up into the urethra.

Try not to urinate before sex so that more bacteria is pushed out after sex. A glass of water right before intercourse will further increase the volume of liquid in the bladder for the washout of bacteria later on.

If infections are an ongoing problem, try this. Take a detachable shower and direct a stream of water into the vaginal area before sex. This will dilute the bacteria and decrease their numbers so that less bacteria gets pushed up into the bladder during intercourse.

Avoid chemical irritation to the urethra by staying away from perfumed or colored personal hygiene products. Diaphragms and birth control pills, as a means of contraception, often promote urinary-tract infections and should not be used by women who tend to get the condition. Condoms or a properly fitted cervical cap are better.

See a registered osteopath or chiropractor if you think you may have a spinal problem that can be contributing to your recurring cystitis.

Dr. Hudson suggests drinking one glass of cranberry juice (or the equivalent in capsules) and taking vitamin C every day to reduce the frequency of recurrent attacks of cystitis by creating an acidic environment in which bacteria cannot easily grow.

"Remember that your bladder health reflects your overall health," says Dr. Wharton, "so take a good look at your lifestyle. Ask yourself, "Do I eat a nutritious, balanced diet? Do I get enough relaxation and sleep? Am I under stress?" Maybe you drink too much coffee or alcohol or smoke or use recreational drugs. If your lifestyle is unhealthy, your body will be too."

ASIAN PERSPECTIVE

Dr. Brett explains that traditional Chinese medicine views cystitis as the end result of an accumulation of damp and heat in the bladder: "Often there is a weak flow of *chi* (energy) in the kidney and the spleen meridians. Weakness of spleen energy leads to the formation of damp in the body, which, in turn causes a stagnation of energy. As in nature, whenever anything builds up, there is friction. A stagnation of *chi* eventually leads to the development of heat, what we in the West interpret as cystitis.

"Spleen *chi* is easily disrupted through dietary indiscretion. Spleen *chi* can be damaged by any of the following: overeating; drinking with meals; overconsumption of damp-forming foods, such as dairy products, chilled foods or drinks, and raw fruits and vegetables; and eating greasy foods, such as takeout foods.

"What you do with your mind actually affects spleen energy as well. An overuse of the mind, particularly through chronic anxiety and worry, or through many years of overstudying, also tends to deplete spleen energy.

"When the cooling *yin* energy of the kidneys is weakened, cystitis becomes much more likely as well. Kidney *yin* is consumed naturally as we age, but it can also be prematurely diminished as a result of lifestyle. The long-term overwork, stress, and exhaustion that form a part of many American lives these days, along with an overconsumption of alcohol and too much sex, all deplete the vital kidney energy." Acupuncture, combined with lifestyle changes, can help to balance energy and eliminate cystitis.

Herbal Pharmacy

Plants containing phytochemicals with antibacterial properties, in order of potency, are as follows:

Coptis chinensis (Chinese goldthread)
Coptis spp. (generic goldthread)
Mangifera indica (mango)
Coptis japonica (huang lia)
Hydrastis canadensis (goldenseal)
Hamamelis virginiana (witch hazel)
Phyllanthus emblica (emblic)
Punica granatum (pomegranate)
Quercus infectoria (aleppo oak)
Berberis vulgaris (barberry)
Phellodendron amurense (huang po)
Argemone mexicana (prickly poppy)
Fragaria spp. (strawberry)
Rheum rhaponticum (rhubarb)
Glycine max (soybean)

Chapter 37

Vaginal Inflamation and Infection

One difficulty that has plagued diseases connected to the genitals is that in most societies sex is carefully regulated. Even private use of the sex organs—female or male masturbation—was strongly condemned until quite recently. We can now read with amusement the passage in Meyer Levin's brilliant novel of Chicago Jewish life in the 1930s, *The Old Bunch*, describing what happens when a doctor, Rudy, visits a friend, Lou, who is sick. There seems to be no cause for Lou's sickness and fatigue. Then: "In that moment, Rudy got the idea that maybe Lou was abusing himself. That might show in his general lassitude, the nervous abrupt movement of his hands. Hardly clinical symptoms, yet they gave Rudy the impression of hidden unhealthiness."

Because of the tone of medical/ethical disapproval displayed by passages such as these—an attitude still prevalent, although to a somewhat lesser degree, in some cultures—women and men have often been reluctant to come forward with even innocent medical problems related to the sex organs. In this chapter, we not only will give helpful information about dealing with vaginal infections, but emphasize the importance of treating these subjects frankly and thoughtfully as a natural part of life.

Vaginitis in General

CAUSES

Amanda McQuade Crawford, a medical herbalist whose latest book is *Herbal Remedies for Women*, explains, "There are many causes of vaginitis, which simply means an inflamed vagina. There's not always an infection. Many women use the term to refer to any number of situations where there's an irritation of the vagina. When it is caused by bacteria, it's called bacterial vaginosis. So we are talking about a number of different conditions.

"Though vaginitis isn't always caused by an infection, there are various microbes that commonly cause it. One of the microbes most commonly involved in nonspecific vaginitis is *Gardnerella vaginalis,* a bacterium that doesn't like oxygen. When men have *Gardnerella,* they don't show many signs or symptoms, so it may unsuspectingly pass to a female partner."

Some other common causes of vaginitis are *candida* (a yeast), *Trichomonas vaginalis,* a parasite, and a number of sexually transmitted diseases, such as gonorrhea, genital warts, and herpesvirus. When an infecting agent is not the cause of vaginitis, this condition may simply be caused by a hormonal imbalance.

Vaginitis can occur at many stages of a woman's life; for example, it is common when a woman's body adjusts to a lower level of estrogen at menopause. Vaginitis can be aggravated by stress, nutritional imbalance, a foreign object such as a diaphragm or a tampon, and problems that originate in the vulva, which can lead to a vaginal irritation.

Crawford points out, "Vaginitis is not a punishment. It is the body's way of signaling an irritation of the most tender gateway to the interior that leads all the way up to our heart, and of our relationship to the person we love and let into our body."

SYMPTOMS

One common vaginal symptom is a discharge, which can be of different types and colors. These differences can help determine the necessary approach for healing.

If the discharge is clear and has a normal smell, it may well be due to ovulation and does not require treatment.

If the color is a milky white and it has a creamy texture, but smells normal, this can also be a sign of ovulation.

If the discharge is white but sticky, it might be simply postovulation or an effect of taking the birth control pill.

When the discharge is brown and watery or sticky but has a normal odor, it can be spotting from the end of the menstrual period or, occasionally, spotting in between periods. If that is the case, it might be a good idea to consult a licensed practitioner to see why this is occurring.

When the discharge is watery and white, with almost a buttermilk quality, and smells fishy or foul—and especially when there's itching or other symptoms, such as fever—then you may have a case of BV (bacterial vaginosis), possibly from *Gardnerella*, which requires treatment.

Sometimes the discharge is white and flecked, like curds, and smells a bit like beer or rising bread dough with a yeasty smell, and is accompanied by itching. This could be from a yeast infection, which also requires treatment with antifungal, antiyeast herbs or other remedies.

When the discharge is yellow and frothy, sometimes with dots of red, has a very foul odor and is itchy, it may be from *Trichomonas*. See a medical practitioner to ensure that the infection is adequately treated, because it is persistent.

Crawford notes, "Be careful if the discharge is yellow to green, and there's a heavy, thick mucus discharge, with or without a bad odor that may be accompanied by other symptoms like abdominal cramps or pains, painful urination, and a fever. It could be evidence of PID or possibly gonorrhea. Even if there's no discharge, it still might be gonorrhea if the other symptoms are present. So, go to a medical practitioner for a clear diagnosis."

TREATMENT

In treating vaginitis, some very simple herbs can be used, such as the soothing, antinflammatory calendula flowers. Crawford also likes licorice root, which can be used as a douche externally. Another herb that is quite good is plantain (sometimes called ribwort). These should be used with an astringent herb. They will help pull the inflamed vaginal tissues together so the natural forces of your body can fight off whatever the infection or inflammation might be.

Crawford details, "An astringent herb which I use internally is anemone pulsatilla, or pasque flower. Take 3 ounces of that and combine it with 1 ounce of licorice root and 2 ounces of plantain. Mix those together. Over 1 ounce of the mixture, pour a pint of boiling water. Let that stand, then take a teacup full of this tea strained, three times a day. Alternatively, a woman can take extracts or tinctures of these herbs. The relative amounts would be the same. Take a teaspoon, diluted in 1 cup of water, three times a day."

Treat vaginitis for one or two weeks, then stop treatment and see if the condition is gone. "If there is a more deep-seated infection that doesn't resolve in that time period," Crawford says, "then I usually add 2 ounces of echinacea root to the other ingredients. Steep an ounce and use it in the same way as you did the previous tea, three to four times a day for at least 10 days. If that doesn't clear things up, it is necessary to reassess."

"There's always nutritional advice that goes along with herbal treatments," Crawford adds. "Avoid sugar, including honey, maple syrup on your pancakes, or fruit-juice-sweetened cookies, even if they are from the health food store. Lots of sugar is not going to help a woman fight off an infection."

Vaginal Yeast (Candidiasis)

Carol Dalton is a nurse practitioner who helped found the clinic Wellspring for Women. She explains that yeast infections are actually a general gathering of bacteria, a multiplicity of them, not just one organism. "Many of these organisms live normally within the vagina. If they are in the right balance and there are small amounts of them, they really don't cause any problem. But if they get out of hand and if the partner has a lot of bacteria as well, then it can really start to cause a lot of inflammation, itching, redness, and a foul-smelling discharge. Then it obviously is a problem."

She adds that just as we can be around someone who has a cold but not catch the cold if our immune system is good, a woman can come in contact with yeast but will not necessarily begin to grow it herself if her cells and immune system are healthy. On the other hand, if her immune system is depressed, she will pick it up and it will turn into a raging infection very easily.

CAUSES

A vaginal yeast infection has multiple causes, according to Dalton. She notes that the type of birth control you use will influence whether you can be infected. You may get the yeast infection from a partner, "if you are sexually active and particularly sexually active without any barrier protection or any spermicide—spermicide helps to kill off all of these things. So it may be passed more easily to women who are using the pill or the IUD, for example, and not using female or male condoms or a diaphragm. They will be at higher risk, because everything that comes into contact with the genital area can pass way up into the vaginal canal. That's one of the reasons we are seeing more of this and have been for the last 15 or 20 years: women are using more different kinds of birth control than we used to have. Women are tired of using the older methods, so they have switched to hormone injections (Depo-Provera), IUDs, and oral contraceptives, and those methods don't really offer any protection against yeast infections."

Dr. William Crook, author of *The Yeast Connection and Women,* says that taking antibiotics can lead to yeast overgrowth and that women are especially susceptible: "The yeast we're talking about normally live in the body of every man, woman, and child. It's called *Candida albicans.* When you are healthy, there are no problems, but when you take a lot of antibiotic drugs you begin to get complications. Antibiotics knock out the normal, friendly bacteria. As a result the yeast overgrows, and a woman may get a vaginal yeast infection, a child may develop thrush or diaper rash, and a man or woman may get bloating, constipation, and digestive symptoms.

"But that's not the major problem. This yeast puts out toxins that weaken the immune system. It so disturbs the interior membrane of the intestinal tract that you absorb food allergens that would normally be excreted. People truly become sick all over."

"There are several reasons why a woman is more susceptible to yeast infections than a man," says Dr. Crook. "Since her genitalia are internal, yeast is able to grow on the warm interior membranes of the body. The little tube going from the urinary bladder to the outside is only an inch and a half long in a woman, whereas in a man it is many inches long. This allows the bacteria to get up into the woman's bladder much more easily. Women have 50 times more urinary tract infections than men, and they are given antibiotic drugs as treatment. Birth control pills further promote yeast growth. So does pregnancy. And teenage girls with a few pimples on their face are much more likely to run to the dermatologist and get tetracycline, an antibiotic that makes yeast grow."

Nutritionist Gracia Perlstein adds these causes to the list: "Some women are susceptible at the end of each month's menstrual flow. There are low estrogen levels present at menopause, and also pregnancy, when the rate of infection can be as high as 20 percent toward the end. Also women who have diabetes have an increased risk.

"Stress is another factor. Many people have two or three jobs. They are running around, eating on the run, not really paying attention to their diet. When people do that, they tend also to overdo sweets and processed foods that weaken their immunity and set up a perfect environment for the *Candida* overgrowth."

Complementary physician Dr. Robert Sorge says *Candida* is the result of drug pollution. In addition to antibiotic overuse, mentioned earlier, he adds: "The most likely candidate for *Candida* overgrowth is a person who has been on steroids, hormone medication, cortisone, the entire gamut of prescriptions and over-the-counter drugs, especially ulcer medications like Tagamet and Zantac, and oral contraceptives. As far as I'm concerned, the sugar and junk food diet that most people have is also a drug."

SYMPTOMS

Classical symptoms of a yeast infection are itching, redness, irritation, and a cottage-cheese-like curdly white discharge. Symptoms are not always obvious, but a gynecologist can often confirm whether or not a yeast infection exists by looking at a smear under the microscope or creating a culture to see if yeast colonies form.

Clearing up immediate symptoms is relatively simple. Many over-the-counter preparations, including homeopathic remedies, exist for that purpose. The trick, according to Dr. Marjorie Ordene, a holistic gynecologist from Brooklyn, New York, is to treat the overall yeast syndrome, not just the local infection.

"Often the vaginal itching will be the impetus for the person to come to the doctor, but it is not the only problem they have. Unless the whole person is treated, the yeast is bound to recur." Dr. Ordene breaks down symptoms of a yeast syndrome into five categories:

GENERAL SYMPTOMS: low energy and fatigue, brain fog, depression, headaches, muscle and joint paints, memory loss, extreme sensitivity to chemicals, recurrent urinary infections, light-headedness.

DIGESTIVE SYMPTOMS: gas, bloating, intermittent constipation and diarrhea, indigestion, intestinal cramps.

RESPIRATORY SYMPTOMS: chronic post-nasal drip, frequent coughs, sore throats, colds, asthma, allergies.

SKIN PROBLEMS: eczema, itching, rashes, fungal infections.

HORMONAL PROBLEMS: menstrual irregularities, menstrual cramps, pre-menstrual syndrome, mood swings, problems with the endocrine glands, hypothyroidism, hypoglycemia or diabetes.

As already noted, the infection is more likely to take hold if a woman has a less than healthy immune system. "If the person who gets a yeast infection has a weak immune system, then the yeast, which comes out in the stool, can creep up. It grows like little tree branches, into the perineum and vaginal area. If the pH is off, it can cause an infection in that area," Dalton says.

DIAGNOSIS

Since the intestines serve as a reservoir for much of the yeast, a stool study may reveal an overgrowth. Excess yeast here indicates that yeast is present in other parts of the body, including the vagina, and causing recurrent yeast infections.

A simple skin test may reveal a yeast allergy as well. Red or itchy skin indicates a problem. Often the results are seen quickly, within ten to fifteen minutes, although sometimes there is a delayed reaction or none at all.

These tests are not always reliable, according to Dr. Crook: "Although we physicians generally like to have a test that can say you do or do not have a particular condition, such as a chest X-ray to see whether your heart is enlarged, there is not presently a single, simple laboratory test that can say whether you do or do not have a yeast-related problem. If a woman has a vaginal infection, a lab study of the secretion may help identify the yeast. Sometimes a culture may. But they are not 100 percent accurate. They may not be more than 50 percent accurate. There are studies done on stools because yeast grows there, but those are not reliable either. The best we can do is to suspect it, and then to note the response of a person to a sugar-free special diet, and oral antiyeast medication, both prescription and nonprescription."

ALTERNATIVE THERAPIES

YEAST-FREE DIET

A yeast-free diet is both diagnostic and therapeutic. If a woman feels better when following the diet, this indicates a yeast sensitivity. The diet should be observed for several weeks at a minimum, and may be followed indefinitely. Some people feel much better and choose to eat this way permanently. Foods can be added back gradually, however, to see their effect. If symptoms recur, the reintroduced food should be avoided.

There are two basic principles to follow on a yeast-free diet:

AVOID SWEETS. The relationship between sugar and yeast was seen in a study performed at St. Jude Hospital in Memphis, Tennessee, where mice who were fed sugar had 200 times greater yeast concentration than mice who were not. Yeast feeds on sugar, causing many symptoms, especially digestive problems such as gas and bloating. Avoiding sugar entails more than just not adding granulated sugar to cereal or tea; it means checking labels and staying away from corn syrup, maltose, artificial sweeteners, fructose, corn starch, sodas, and lactose, a milk sugar found in dairy products.

AVOID FOODS CONTAINING YEASTS AND MOLDS. These include baked foods such as breads, muffins, cakes, cookies, and other refined carbohydrates, commercial fruit juices, tomato sauce (unless homemade with fresh tomatoes), foods containing vinegar, pickled foods, smoked foods, alcohol, fermented foods, smoked meats, dried fruits, mushrooms (except for shiitake), pistachio nuts, and peanuts. Leftovers may be moldy as well.

What you can eat are healthful foods that do not contain yeasts and molds. Included are whole grains, such as brown rice, millet, amaranth, quinoa, and barley, as well as fresh vegetables. Lots of steamed green vegetables are particularly beneficial because they are abundant in purifying chlorophyll. Also allowed are sea vegetables, whole wheat matzo, sourdough rye bread, popcorn, tortillas, tofu, miso, plain yogurt, lean meats, fresh fish, organically fed, free-range poultry and eggs from free-range chickens. Organic extra-virgin olive oil, when used sparingly, can inhibit yeast overgrowth, according to recent studies. Raw garlic or lightly cooked garlic helps get rid of *Candida* in the intestines.

SUPPLEMENTS

Sometimes diet alone is not enough. After all, yeast has been in the body for years. These supplements provide additional needed help:

FLORA. The flora found in *Lactobacillus acidophilus* and *bifida bacteria* can be taken in powder form or as sugar-free yogurt. The effectiveness of flora was noted in a New York Medical School study of women with recurrent vaginal yeast infections. Those eating sugar-free yogurt had fewer infections than those who did not. Flora repopulate the intestinal tract with good bacteria, which in turn crowd out the yeast. The effects of flora are temporary, so the powder or yogurt should be consumed on a daily basis.

ANTIFUNGAL, ANTIYEAST AGENTS. Over-the-counter preparations, such as citrus seed extract, kyolic garlic, caprylic acid, pau d'arco, and berberine, may be helpful. Sometimes prescription agents such as nystatin are needed. These remedies get rid of excess yeast only. Since they are not absorbed into the blood, they are safe to take, even during pregnancy and while nursing.

HOMEOPATHIC CANDIDA. Helps desensitize the body to yeast.

GARLIC SUPPOSITORIES. Simple insertion of a clove of garlic into the vagina has a powerful healing effect. *The New Our Bodies, Ourselves* suggests that the clove should be peeled but not nicked, and then wrapped in gauze before inserting.

A strong body is better able to rebalance its health. In addition to supplements that target yeast infections specifically, these nutrients provide overall nutritional support:

MULTIVITAMIN/MINERAL SUPPLEMENT. Formulas containing zinc, magnesium, yeast-free vitamins, trace minerals, and essential fatty acids boost immune function and help prevent recurrent yeast infections.

CHLOROPHYLL. Cleanses the intestines and purifies the blood.

ESSENTIAL FATTY ACIDS. 3,000 mg of evening primrose, borage, or blackcurrant seed oil daily in three divided doses, or one tablespoon of organic flaxseed oil. (Never cook flaxseed oil, and keep refrigerated.)

VITAMIN C. 3,000-5,000 mg daily in three divided doses helps fight infections.

B COMPLEX. 50–100 mg with each meal combats stress.

HERBS

The following Asian and Western herbs can help alleviate yeast problems:

DIGESTIVE HARMONY AND HERBASTATIN. Digestive Harmony is a combination of bitter herbs that work together to cleanse the digestive tract and other internal organs of yeast infections.

Herbastatin gets rid of yeast caused by phlegm.

YU DAI WAN. This Chinese remedy helps to eliminate creamy discharges.

KU SHEN. Used as a wash to clean the vagina.

GARLIC. Excellent for fighting infections. Can be eaten raw or lightly cooked, or taken in capsule form. Odorless brands are sold in health food stores.

BLACK WALNUT TINCTURE. Thirty drops three times daily, added to water before meals.

PAU D'ARCO. This herb has wonderful immune-enhancing and antifungal properties. As a tea, take three to four cups daily.

SUMMA. This is another good herbal tea for helping the immune system.

Also helpful are goldenseal, bearberry, Oregon grape, German chamomile, aloe vera, rosemary, ginger, alfalfa, red clover, and fennel.

COLON THERAPY

"My battle with candida lasted a long time," says colon therapist Tovah Finman-Nahman. "I tried everything, including a strict diet, antifungals, and vitamin C drips. But I never got it under control until I started doing colonics. Then I saw quick results. The gas and bloating went away, and my chronic fatigue amazingly disappeared. I have seen similar results with a lot of people who come to see me. I can't stress how good colonics are."

What makes colon therapy such an effective treatment? First, it creates a clean internal environment. "We want a good environment so that flora can grow and flourish. That is paramount when we have *Candida* overgrowth," says Finman-Nahman. Second, colonics calm an irritated colon: "Herbs can be added to the water, such as pau d'arco, which has antifungal properties. Yellow dock can also be added to soothe any inflammation. Fennel can be used to dissipate gas and eliminate the bloating that a lot of people with *Candida* tend to get. Aloe vera gel is absolutely wonderful. It is very soothing to an inflamed colon. And of course, it can be taken orally in the form of aloe vera juice.

"In conjunction with colonics, psyllium can be taken orally. This moisturizes impacted fecal material in the congested colon, which further aids cleaning.

"People ask, 'How many colonics should I get?' That depends on the individual. The more the merrier. For a healthy person I recommend at least 10 in a series, and then a maintenance program. Sometimes, it can take as long as six months to get candida under control because it is a very hearty bacteria. When yeast is at the point of being candidiasis, it can grow through the colon walls and run rampant. The more we cleanse, the better our chance of getting it under control and regaining health."

AROMATHERAPY

Tea tree oil is scientifically shown to be antifungal, antiyeast, and antiviral. One tablespoon of the oil added to a pint of water, and used in a douche, helps eliminate yeast infections. Follow this by placing acidophilus tablets or capsules into the vagina to reestablish proper vaginal bacteria.

LIFESTYLE FACTORS

Nutritionist Gracia Perlstein notes these important habits for minimizing the incidence of vaginal infections:

Wear underpants with a cotton crotch so that air can circulate.

Avoid pantyhose or any tight-fitting clothing for the same reason.

Develop good toilet habits of always wiping from front to back. This keeps anal bacteria from entering the vagina.

Avoid feminine hygiene sprays and powders, which can cause irritation. Douching is not necessary; a healthy vagina is naturally clean.

Keep stress under control. Take a few deep breaths. Go for a brisk walk in the open air. Do something to alleviate the stress that builds up.

HOMEOPATHY

Since homeopathy treatments are chosen according to symptoms, deciding on a remedy depends on the quality of the discharge and the sensations, according to Dr. Ken Korins. Here he offers some of the major remedies for vaginal yeast infections:

PULSATILLA. This remedy is often indicated in vaginitis. The woman has a thick, yellowish-to-green discharge. Sometimes the consistency is milky or creamy. Mentally, she is often moody, gentle, and weepy, and craves sympathy.

SILICA. The main symptom is an itching of the vulva and vagina. It is sensitive to touch. The discharge tends to be thin, and sometimes curdly.

KREOSOTUM. The person has violent symptoms. Discharges are excoriating, burning is profuse, and there is a foul odor, as well as violent itching and a burning and swelling of the labia. Discharge tends to be yellow and may actually have a watery, bloody consistency.

HEPHERA SULPH. Symptoms are similar to silica, but more chronic. There is itching of the vagina, particularly after sexual intercourse, and it often has an odor similar to that of old cheese. Both hephera sulph and silica can be used to treat sores or cysts, particularly Bartholin cysts.

KALI BICHROMIUM. Here discharges tend to be thick, green, and sometimes jellylike.

ALUMINA. Discharge is thick and transparent.

NITRIC ACID. Helps when there are sores or ulcers on the vaginal mucosa. The sensation tends to be a sharp, sticking pain. Discharges are brown. Often, there is a stain on underwear that leaves a yellow perimeter.

MERCURIUS. The discharges are excoriating but greenish and bloody. There is a sensation of rawness.

MEDORRHINUM. Discharge is thick and acrid, with a sensation way up in the uterus.

WELLSPRING FOR WOMEN TREATMENT

The holistic program at the Wellspring for Women clinic treats chronic cases of yeast infection. As Carol Dalton points out, the conventional treatment for yeast is to prescribe antifungal medications. "If a woman went to a more traditional medical care facility, that would be the first choice. It would be an antifungal of some sort in either a vaginal or oral preparation.

"The problem with this approach is that you are not really addressing why this problem develops in the first place; why there is an unhealthy environment that allows this organism to grow. By prescribing these drugs, you are actually adding to the imbalance in the environment. This makes it even more likely that the person is going to pick it up again or that she will develop a yeast infection because you have killed her normal bacteria off and allowed yeast to overgrow there. Often that starts a cycle of bacteria, then yeast, sometimes even developing into bladder infection because the whole area gets so inflamed."

Dalton notes that she often sees patients who have had chronic infections for a long time. "What we try to do is establish what their general immune system looks like. Then we try to help them systemically to try to get that into balance.

"We look at their diet, their lifestyle, their stress factors, their supplements, all those things, and try to help them create a healthier, better balance. For example, if the woman was low on protein in her diet and eating a lot of sugar and carbs, then we might recommend a lower-carb, lower-sugar diet so we are not feeding the yeast.

"If the woman is not doing any kind of supplementation, we would tend to recommend things to raise the immune system and to help balance the flora in the vagina. We might suggest B complex vitamins, zinc, beta carotene, vitamin C, all of those things which seem to help the immune system in general."

Dalton also uses natural suppositories to treat the yeast, as well as oral antifungal remedies including garlic. This is a traditional treatment. "I've even had patients who were told to tie some dental floss on garlic or thread it through a garlic clove and insert the clove in the vagina. It is very antifungal, so it probably does work."

"There are many ways to treat this, but the basic premise when you have developed a chronic problem should be to look at the whole body."

Describing the difference between acute versus chronic yeast infections, Dalton says, "If somebody gets a one-time infection, then perhaps she has a new partner and is having more sex than usual. In that case I would recommend she get some over-the-counter Monistat cream or use a little antifungal vaginal gel for a few days, to get rid of it. However, if it's an ongoing problem, we try to look more at the whole person and why she is having infections over and over."

For chronic yeast problems, Dalton looks at the digestive system, because there is likely a yeast imbalance in the digestive system. That means the woman is getting more vaginal contamination than average. "Often you'll see symptoms such as gas, bloating, constipation or diarrhea, and rectal itching."

In chronic cases, it is important to determine what strain of yeast is present. At Wellspring for Women, Dalton says, "We do tests through our local lab or, more often than not, through Great Smokies Lab in North Carolina. The patient gets a kit from the clinic and takes a stool sample, and it's sent to North Carolina to be analyzed. With chronic yeast, the problem is that over time the yeast will mutate into a form that becomes resistant to most if not all of the medications typically used to treat yeast. The lab does not only cultures but also tests the strain or strains that are found for sensitivities to medications and natural treatments. "We have sometimes found yeast that has become resistant to garlic, for example. Though garlic in general is considered a great antifungal, there are some yeast strains that have mutated into a form in which garlic doesn't bother them at all—in fact, they probably thrive on it. And the same is true for resistance to various types of medication.

"So for chronic problems, we not only look a little deeper into the person's situation—into her lifestyle and habits—but we try to identify the exact organism we are dealing with and find out what that organism is sensitive to, so that we can help the person get rid of it completely."

PATIENT STORY

Carol Dalton recounts, "I had a patient who had a chronic yeast infection for about 12 years. It developed out of chronic bladder infections. She was given so many antibiotics that they ended by killing off the normal bacteria in the gut, which allowed the yeast to overgrow. Eventually that developed into vaginal yeast infections. We worked on it systemically. We tested to find out what organism she had and what it was sensitive to. We looked at her diet and her stress levels, which were high. After medication as well as natural treatments, we thought we'd gotten rid of it.

"Recently she had to be on antibiotics for 12 weeks for an abscessed tooth, so we wanted to check her. We found that she was fine. She had gone three months on antibiotics and there was no sign of yeast at all. We felt that she was really clear of it, since, being on the antibiotics that long, any average woman would have gotten a yeast infection. She was able to avoid it. So that was a very good sign that she was clear."

Trichomonas

Another vaginal infection, which Amanda McQuade Crawford labels as "tricky," is trichomonas, which is caused by a one-celled protozoan called *Trichomonas vaginalis.* Trichomonas, she says, "is usually sexually transmitted. It's a parasite, not a virus or a bacterium, and is not to be confused with trichinosis, the infestation of worms that can result from eating uncooked pork."

SYMPTOMS

Trichomonas causes an inflammation of a woman's vaginal lining. The symptoms, says Crawford, are intense vaginal itching, irritation and discharge.

These symptoms are worse than similar symptoms that appear with bacterial vaginitis or yeast infections. The thin vaginal discharge trichomonas produces is yellow or green, and occasionally gray, and has a bubbly or frothy appearance. This discharge produces a burning sensation; a raw feeling; and a characteristic bad, fishy smell. Sexual intercourse is painful.

Trichomonas is a very serious condition, and it is important to know how it is distinct from other vaginal infections. Some general medical symptoms are also present; fever, chills, nausea and fatigue. It can mimic a bladder infection (cystitis). The organisms that cause trichomonas can sit in the tissues of the vagina or the urethra or hidden away deep in some of the glands inside the vagina, which makes it difficult to treat with natural remedies. When the infection goes on long enough you need to consult a licensed health care practitioner.

TREATMENT

In herbal treatment, Crawford indicates, "We try to eliminate the parasite by optimizing natural immune system defenses and work on preventing a recurrence at the same time. This means eliminating risk factors, particularly unsafe sex. The woman's sex partners may need to be tested to see if they require treatment. If they test positive, they need to be tested until they are shown to be negative. It's not enough to just have the symptoms go away. The herbal treatment requires consistency and should be done for at least two months before a retest to see if the parasite has disappeared."

One of the best herbal antiprotozoals is cassia bark. Others are myrrh and barberry root. These herbs together are often used to kill off the parasite causing the infection. Tonics promoting long-term immune system health also offer benefits. Two herbs used for this purpose are relki, a Chinese mushroom, and astragalus root. This last has often been used to boost immunity, especially with long-term infections.

Crawford cautions, "The herbs that are strong enough to kill the organism are ones that taste particularly bad. I say that so women will know, when they are treating themselves for this, that it is not something like a beverage herbal tea. To take it will require some rigor and some willingness to gulp the things down." You can also take these herbs in capsule form. The dose would be about two double-0 size capsules with water and food at least four times a day for four to six weeks. It can take as long as two months to eliminate the infection.

To make a capsule, combine 4 oz of cassia with 3 oz of barberry root. Add to that 3 oz of reiki mushrooms and 2 oz of astragalus. All these herbs can be mixed together and put into capsules at home very easily. It's also very affordable.

If you don't want to take them as powdered herbs in capsules, you can take them in extracts and tinctures. The proportions would be the same, and the dose would be 1 teaspoon in 1 cup of water with meals 4 times a day for six to eight months.

Alternatively, you can take the herbs separately, although if you do, after three weeks you might encounter a little stomach distress. In that case, dilute them with even more water and be sure to take them with meals so that there is some food in your stomach. This will slow down the speed with which the herbs get into your bloodstream but will not neutralize their effects.

Don't forget that what you eat can also help the body heal. For trichomonas there is no one specific food that will make the difference. Crawford's recommendations are to decrease excess sugar and refined carbohydrates. Eat low-protein, high-quality whole foods with at least four to five servings a day of fresh fruits and vegetables in season. She says you must keep in mind that "We are eating foods that will nourish our whole being, not just the fruits or plants that will kill off parasites, because that won't get to the root of the whole problem."

Dalton also recommends certain supplements. She cites "good research on using fairly high doses of zinc, C, and beta carotene, which seem to systemically help the body throw off trichomonas."

Crawford uses douches in her treatment. One douche formula is cassia bark combined with equal amounts of licorice root bark to soothe the irritated, raw vaginal lining. Simmer 1 oz of each on low heat for about 15 minutes, then strain and use the tea as a douche.

A douche Dalton recommends contains aloe, vinegar, and tea tree oil. This is a drawing solution that helps get rid of the infection.

Crawford warns, "The thing to remember about douching is that it has some short-term benefits but also some long-term drawbacks. It should not be done every day, but only to relieve symptoms. At the same time, you must undergo a long-term treatment, such as taking the capsules, to deal with the root of the problem."

After six or eight weeks on the herbal treatment, get tested to see if the parasite has been eliminated. If it is still present, use the herbal treatment for an additional two weeks.

Crawford also notes that there's a need to counter the effect of the stronger herbal remedies. "If you are going to continue taking fairly strong herbs to kill off a small living organism, it's necessary to take some other herbs to help you counteract the negative side effects of these strong herbs. One of these counteracting herbs would be milk thistle. Take it as a standard extract, or in one of the many proprietary forms that are now in the marketplace. The dose would be 300 or 400 mg a day." Milk thistle can help the body develop long-term immunity as well as cope with the other herbs being used to treat the infection.

PATIENT STORY

Carol Dalton describes how she treated a drug-resistant case of trichomonas. "Trichomonas is generally treated with a drug called Flagyl. In traditional medicine, it's thought that Flagyl or other antiparasitic drugs are the only way to treat this. About 20 years ago I had a patient who had a resistant case of trichomonas. She had been in the university hospital in Denver and they had given her intravenous Flagyl. Still they had not been able to get rid of the trichomonas. We used the douche solution and oral supplements to boost her immune system, and, lo and behold, in about three weeks, the trichomonas was gone and never reoccurred. So the natural treatments really can work if people are willing to put forward the effort. Obviously, it's easier in many cases to take a pill or two a day than to do all of this regime. However, it helps the body be healthier in general."

Bacterial Vaginosis

BV (bacterial vaginosis) is caused by *Gardnerella,* a gram-negative bacterium that hates oxygen. An alternative treatment that has been used at women's health clinics across America is to mix 1 cup of distilled or sterilized water and 1 tablespoon of a 3 percent solution of hydrogen peroxide. Douche with this mixture once a day for a week. Then repeat every three days, for an additional two weeks. The hydrogen peroxide and distilled water increase oxygen in the vaginal canal and tissues, which is antagonistic to the *Gardnerella.* This douche is a noninvasive, effective way to treat the problem. If it doesn't work within a week to ten days, consult a licensed health practitioner for other kinds of help that might be appropriate.

Herbal Pharmacy

Plants containing phytochemicals with antibacterial/antifungal activity, in order of potency:

Coptis chinensis (Chinese goldthread)
Coptis sp. (generic goldthread)
Mangifera indica (mango)
Coptis japonica (huang lia)
Hydrastis canadensis (goldenseal)
Hamamelis virginiana (witch hazel)
Phyllanthus emblica (emblic)
Punica granatum (pomegranate)
Quercus infectoria (aleppo oak)
Berberis vulgaris (barberry)
Phellodendron amurense (huang po)
Argemone mexicana (prickly poppy)
Fragaria sp. (strawberry)
Rheum rhaponticum (rhubarb)
Glycine max (soybean)

Chapter 38

Varicose Veins

Varicose veins, a common condition that usually affects the lower extremities, is the result of damaged valves in the veins. Normally, these tiny valves ensure that the blood flowing through the veins will fully return to the heart. But when these valves are injured, and do not open and close properly, some of the blood runs backward in the veins, pools, and finally engorges the vessels. Varicose veins are large, contorted, unsightly, and sometimes even painful.

Causes

Three mechanisms help return blood to the heart, says Dr. Leon Chaitow, a naturopath, osteopath, and acupuncturist from England, writing in an article on the HealthWorld Online website (www.healthy.net): the action of muscles through which veins run, the pulsation of arteries that run alongside veins, and the movement of the diaphragm during breathing. Thus, he says, poor breathing function and lack of exercise, as well as various mechanical stresses, such as those resulting from occupations that require long periods of standing, will make venous return less efficient. Other factors that can increase the chance of developing varicose veins are inadequate fiber, vitamins C and E, and bioflavonoids in the diet; increased pressure in the pelvis, as from chronic constipation; and use of birth control pills.

Another cause of varicose veins, says Dr. Chaitow, is thrombophlebitis, a condition in which the veins are obstructed due to clot formation or an aggregation of platelets and fibrin, which restricts blood blow, causing inflammation and damage to the veins.

Herbalist David L. Hoffman lists several other reasons why the walls of the veins receive inadequate support, resulting in varicose veins:

OBESITY. A buildup of fatty tissue in the legs results in inadequate support for veins.

GENETIC PREDISPOSITION. In about 40 percent of cases, there seems to be an inherited tendency to varicosity.

AGE. Over time the connective tissue that supports the veins degenerates, and a decrease in exercise worsens the problem.

TIGHT CLOTHING. Tight clothing constricts and weakens tissue.

PREGNANCY. Pregnancy creates intrapelvic pressure that interferes with venous return.

Symptoms

According to Dr. Chaitow, the earliest symptom is feeling leg fatigue more often than usual. Other standard symptoms are an ache and heavy feeling in the legs, itching in the skin over the veins, and swelling, sometimes of the entire leg. The skin is discolored, and sometimes an eczema develops, with a breakdown of the skin that may lead to ulcers.

Clinical Experience

Standard procedures for treating varicose veins range are elevating the legs, wearing elastic stockings, and, in severe cases, surgery.

Many types of support stockings are available, but it is best to buy them at a pharmacy or surgical supply store, where they will be better quality. If you have a severe problem with varicose veins, you might look into custom-made surgical support stockings. In this country, two companies, Jobst and Sigvaris, make them. If you can't afford support stockings, sometimes an Ace bandage will give you the support you need. Wrap a 3- or 4-inch bandage around the leg where the varicosity is a problem. This may require wrapping your legs from the toes to the groin if the problem is severe.

With early intervention, the following natural remedies have a high rate of effectiveness.

NUTRIENTS AND HERBS

Certain foods and supplements may strengthen the integrity of the vein wall. These include dark-skinned fruits and berries, such as blueberries, cherries, and purple grapes. Vitamin C with bioflavonoids, especially quercetin or bilberry, improves elasticity, so that blood can return more effectively to the heart.

Dr. Chaitow also recommends vitamin E, in a daily dose of 500 to 800 IU, which is thought to help develop other channels of circulation, thus relieving the pressure in the veins. Vitamin E can also be applied direcly to leg ulcers. Selenium, which works together with vitamin E, should also be taken daily in a dose of 50 mcg. Essential fatty acids in the form of 500 mg of evening primrose oil and four to six capsules of EPA (eicosapentaenoic acid) a day will help decrease the likelihood of inflammation and lower the viscosity of the blood. Finally, he says, it is essential to consume enough fiber to keep the bowels functioning well so that no straining occurs.

Astringent herbs, such as horse chestnut, witch hazel, *gotu kola*, and butcher's broom, are good to take, although the first two should not be used when pregnant or lactating. Naturopathic physicians often recommend 1,000 mg of butcher's broom, two to three times daily, for pregnant women in their third trimester who are troubled by varicose veins or hemorrhoids.

Another factor to consider is dietary support for the liver. This is because a congested liver backs up venous circulation and places additional pressure on the veins, which can then damage valves. Foods such as beets and artichokes and herbs such as milk thistle and dandelion can improve liver circulation. At the same time, it is important to refrain from substances known to cause liver damage, such as drugs, alcohol, and other harsh chemicals.

David Hoffman offers the following lotion, which can be used as necessary to relieve irritation:

> 8 parts of distilled witch hazel
> 1 part of horse chestnut tincture
> 1 part of comfrey tincture
> Rose water, if desired

Hoffman also lists the herbs that provide all the effects needed to increase circulation and tone the tissue: prickly ash and ginkgo (to stimulate circulation); hawthorne, yarrow, horse chestnut (to tone the veins); witch hazel and yarrow (astringents); comfrey (to soothe irritation); comfrey (wound healer); and horse chestnut (anti-inflammatory).

EXERCISE

The main way to help relieve varicose veins is to do what you can to keep your blood flow up, in spite of the fact that the veins are not doing their job properly.

Helping the blood flow counteracts some of the problems due to the damaged valves.

Daily exercise is one of the keys to keeping the blood flow up. It is also important for keeping weight down. Excess weight creates stress on the body. Maintaining one's optimal weight lessens stress on the body, which, in turn, decreases the chance of damaging the valves in the veins. In addition, exercise improves overall circulation in the arteries and veins. Dr. Chaitow suggests exercises that involve contracting the leg muscles, circling the ankles, and upside-down bicycling movements.

Of particular benefit are maneuvers that take pressure off the legs. It is helpful to sit with your feet and legs elevated, waist-level or higher, whenever you can. This allows gravity to help the blood flow back to your heart. Inverted postures in yoga or even just lying on a slant board with the legs elevated for a few minutes a day are beneficial. (See Chapter 36, "Urinary Tract Infections and Inflammations," the section on Exercise.) You can also raise the foot of your bed by 6 to 12 inches. Medical magnets can be placed over the feet for added healing power. Maneuvers that take weight off the feet are particularly important for people who work in occupations in which they are constantly on their feet.

Another form of exercise to consider is *qi gong*, which strengthens the veins' ability to pump blood back to the heart.

CHELATION THERAPY

Many people know that chelation therapy improves arterial integrity, but few realize that it can aid venous circulation as well, thereby helping varicose veins. Chelation therapy also helps to overcome liver congestion and thrombophlebitis, two conditions that put women at risk for varicose veins.

ADDITIONAL SUGGESTIONS

Dr. Tori Hudson, a naturopath in Portland, Oregon, offers the following tips in her column in *Prevention* magazine:
    Eat a high-fiber diet.
    Avoid standing for long periods and lifting heavy objects.
    Use supplements: Every day take 1,000 mg of vitamin C; 1,000 mg of bioflavonoids; 150 mg of pycnogenols; and 400 IU of vitamin E.

Dr. Chaitow adds a few more suggestions:
    Instead of standing still, shift from one leg to the other, or walk gently back and forth.
    Don't cross your legs when you sit.
    Take warm, not hot, baths, and end by splashing cold water on the legs.
    Take regular sitz baths, alternating between hot and cold, but finish with cold; this stimulates circulation.

Alexander technique and osteopathic manipulation both improve body mechanics and thereby aid circulation. (For more information on the Alexander technique, see Chapter 27, "Pregnancy.")

Garlic is excellent for thinning the blood; Dr. Chaitow recommends the use of two or three capsules or raw cloves a day.

Chapter 39

Violence: Sexual and Physical Abuse

A key and revelatory point made by Susan Brownmiller in *Against Our Will* is that rape and sexual abuse have nothing to do with sex. They are about men trying to show their power over the so-called weaker sex. Moreover, she argues, assaults on women are committed by men as much to increase the perpetrator's standing among other males as to make a strong impression on the victim. Rape is a perverse kind of male bonding.

Note the striking power of her insight to shoot down still-pervasive media stereotypes that a woman who was raped is partly responsible because, by wearing a provocative oufit, for example, she aroused the criminal's undeniable sex desire. This is nonsense, if, as Brownmiller argues, the whole point is to assert dominance, not to get off erotically. In any case, abuse against women is a problem of staggering magnitude, and it occurs in every socioeconomic and ethnic group. In the United States, it is estimated that 1.8 million women are beaten every year by current or former partners. About 15 percent of women using primary care clinics have been assaulted by partners.

Sexual abuse, even more than physical abuse and battering, is a profound-ly invasive violation. It takes what is most pleasurable to us, our sexuality, and turns it into a nightmare of powerlessness and revulsion. Sexual abuse hap-pens to girls and boys, women and men, of all ages. If you have been sexually abused, the most important thing you can do is seek out a counselor, program, or support group that can guide you to recovery and help you become aware of the many resources now available. In addition, there are soothing, empow-ering products and therapies that may also aid the healing process.

No one deserves to be abused. If you have been abused, you are not the one who has done something wrong. Seek out local support groups, shelter, and legal help. Your state may have a hotline for abused women. Check the Yellow Pages under the following headings: Social Services, Battered Spouses, and Abuse. If danger is imminent, dial 911.

The National Coalition Against Domestic Violence may have a local branch near you. For assistance, or to find the branch nearest you, call the National Domestic Violence Hotline at 1-800-799-7233. It is staffed around the clock. You can also visit the coalition's website at www.NCADV.org.

Self-Defense: Model Mugging

Amy Ippoliti teaches a class called Model Mugging, intended not only for women but also for teens and men. Its purpose is to enable people to defend themselves against an assailant.

She explains: "Sixty percent of the population will freeze when they are confronted by an assailant or a scary situation. There is also another group that will just sort of flail and not accomplish anything useful or proactive. A very slim percentage, about 10 percent, will do something constructive and act rather than react. We strive to put people into that small percentage who, when under the adrenal surge, do something about the situation."

The class takes place in an emotionally supportive environment; the approach is therapeutic and very sensitive. Ippoliti notes, "We do have sur-vivors of assault taking the class, who use the class to work through their past histories of abuse or assault, whether that abuse be emotional, physical, ver-bal, or sexual. So we have a range of people taking the class for different rea-sons, but we all come together with the goal of being able to stand up for our-selves and learning a little about assertiveness as well as being able to defend ourselves full force in every possible attack scenario, including rape-specific stuff."

One principle that is stressed is "full force." That is, a woman has to be feel free to lash out with her complete power. "The instructor wears a sort of suit of armor that weighs 60 pounds. This allows the students to fight full force against the vital parts of the body without injuring the instructor." The instruc-tor presents real-life scenarios of assault so that students can experience actually being in a state of adrenal arousal in which they're under attack so they can learn to cope with this type of situation.

Model Mugging is not just another class in martial arts, however. Martial arts, Ippoliti explains, are based on Asian art forms, and are more an art form than a practical tactic of self-defense. "Often, in martial arts, you won't be fighting in the adrenal state. When you are sparring with your partner, you are not hitting full force, so you never feel in your body what it's like to follow through and go all the way with a strike because you are stopping short of your target.

"That's one of the main differences, as well as the fact that there are emotional and therapeutic benefits to the course that you don't associate with the martial arts or your basic YMCA self-defense class. We do a lot of re-creating of past assaults to work through old stuff that people bring with them. We work on assertiveness and empowerment training. It goes hand in hand with the self-defense, but, in this case, it is processed emotionally in a group discussion. People get a chance to share in the moment about what they have accomplished, what they fear, and how they are.

"From an emotional standpoint, it's very, very different from other practices, and from a physical one, there is the fact that we train in the adrenal state. We train full force. And we train from the ground, which is another huge difference in the course compared to other types of classes. And we use rape-specific stuff, such as what to do if you get pinned. What if you're sleeping in your room and an intruder comes in and you wake up and find yourself pinned? We teach how to get out of that from a lying-down position—how to wait for an opening to get yourself out of that."

The basic Model Mugging course totals 25 hours, spread over five sessions of 5 hours each. It spans anywhere from a week and a half to a month. Once students have graduated from the basic class, they can move on to upper-level training.

The class drills students in physical techniques. "In the first class, everything is in slow motion," says Ippoliti. "Then, as the class proceeds, we build up to street speed. Everything is clearly outlined and worked out, so each woman is totally familiar with the moves. Then we set up a realistic scenario, such as a woman being waylaid on a street. While one participant goes through the scenario, the other women form a line of spectators, encouraging her and cheering as she repulses her attacker. After the reenactment, we have a circle where everyone shares how it felt."

Another skill taught by the class is verbal deescalation. Students are taught not to curse or threaten the attacker, or call him names. "Just state over and over again, 'Leave me alone.' 'Back off.' Command statements that you just continually repeat even though the person is trying to negotiate or trying to intimidate you. You keep on saying what you need. Not yelling necessarily, unless you really need to project your voice, but not with an attitude. Just simply, 'Back off. I mean it.' Really strong statements, until that person walks away. Then if the person attacks, you have the physical skills to back you up."

Potential students go through a screening process to get into the course, both to make it clear to them what they're getting into, and to provide information to the staff. Students fill out confidential forms, "disclosing information about their physical health and any past history of assault that they may be bringing with them to the class. Also, we look at a history of family dysfunction. We ask what are their biggest fears about taking the course, what their fears are about being attacked, and things like that. Students then have the choice whether to share what is on their form or not with the class."

Male instructors are chosen for their sensitivity to women's issues; most have high ranks as martial artists, usually as black belts. They as well as the female instructors are tested for psychological and mental health, as well as psychological training, including going through therapy.

"The women have the same psychological preparation as the men. Typically it helps if the women have had some martial arts training, but it is not as necessary for them as it is for men. Then they go through anywhere from a year to two years' training to become instructors."

RESULTS OF MODEL MUGGING

Women who enter the program are frequently full of fear. "They don't want to become a statistic, or they have already become a statistic, and they are carrying around tremendous amounts of pain, fear, guilt, shame, and all kinds of stuff from their history. They get a chance in the class to work through that and share it and open up about it. Then they can get rid of some of the things they are holding in on an emotional level.

Once women lose some of these fears they blossom. "When they come out of the class, they have a feeling of freedom, of elation, and that they have gotten rid of something they have been holding in the cells of their body for years; now they are able to liberate it. Subsequently, I have gotten phone calls saying, 'I got promoted,' or 'I dumped that guy I was seeing who was really mean to me,' or 'I've accomplished something I wanted to.'"

Some people who took the course became celebrities—famous singers and others—simply from developing such confidence in themselves that they became assertive enough to get noticed. "Basically, they said, 'I would never have been able to embrace fame and embrace the success of having an album cut and hit the charts without this course. I never could have done that.'" Ippoliti has noticed that younger adults in particular "seem to embrace the work much more readily."

But one of the greatest successes has been that women do become able to fend off assault if it ever occurs. Ippoliti recalls graduates who knocked out assailants in less than 5 seconds, eight years after they had taken the training, without any review course or further practice in front of a mirror. "From training in the adrenal state," she notes, "they were able to retain everything that they learned in their muscle memory. There is just no comparison to actually following through full force on an instructor in the adrenal state in an attack scenario. There's no substitute because that imprints your reaction in your muscle memory so that you don't have to remember anything. You don't have to remember what move comes next because your body just does it, like riding a bicycle. That's why the work is so effective. That's why it continues to work. That's why I get calls continually from graduates saying, 'I used the technique and I was okay. It was scary and I survived. I'm all right.'"

Out of 30,000 graduates in the United States, about 62 have actually been attacked, Ippoliti says. "Thousands have been able to verbally deescalate situations. But out of those thousands, 62 were actually assaulted and 60 out of 62 knocked out their assailants in a few seconds or disabled them so they could get away. This was using the techniques from the course, including the follow-through till the knockout. That's just an incredible statistic to me."

WHERE TO FIND IT

There are chapters teaching Model Mugging throughout America and Europe, but during the second half of the nineties the nonprofit organization experienced a decline. Ippoliti says regretfully, "It seems the demand is not as high. Also the life span of an instructor is not that long because the work is so emotionally and physically draining." It's hard to keep the work going."

Part of the difficulty is that "you can't just go into a battered woman's shelter or a public school and offer this work. It costs money. To make it more accessible to people who don't have the money should be a goal. It used to cost about $500 for a woman to take the course. We would try to offer scholarships, but to make it accessible it really needs to be funded."

A substitute for a class in Model Mugging would be a class on women's empowerment and on deescalating techniques, one that focuses on "good, clear, assertive deescalation and voice work as well as physical techniques." Still, Ippoliti says, "there is no comparison with what Model Mugging can do."

Some chapters remain in existence, particularly in California, Colorado, and New York. In that city Ippoliti runs one class a year.

Traditional Chinese Perspective

When dealing with the trauma of sexual abuse, prayer, meditation, various forms of psychotherapy, and forgiveness are all important. However, Phyllis Bloom, who practices Chinese medicine, has special insight into how to handle the aftermath of such trauma with acupuncture and herbs.

Bloom received her training at the Tristate Institute for Chinese Acupuncture in the People's Republic of China. She currently practices acupuncture at day treatment programs for people living with AIDS. She has a private practice at the Center for Acupuncture and the Healing Arts in lower Manhattan. She explains the perspective of Chinese medicine on sexual abuse: "As you know, acupuncture and herbal medicine are based around energy, so we are dealing here with energy. I see sexual abuse as an attack on one's energy, which includes the body, mind, emotions, and, ultimately, the spirit.

"The framework I have developed, based on teaching and observation, begins with the idea that there are three levels of energy in the body: the protective level, the nutritive level, and the constitutional level. With sexual abuse, any and all of these levels can be affected. That depends, of course, on whether it's an acute situation or a chronic one. A chronic situation is when the abuse has gone on for a long time. Another important factor is whether the perpetrator is very intimately involved with the person who has been violated. Also, a very severe attack can cut through all layers. It depends upon where and how the person was violated." The most commonly affected levels are the protective and nutritive levels.

The advice Bloom gives depends on which level has been violated. "The protective level is the surface. It's what we use to defend ourselves and connect to the outside world, which sets boundaries against such things as viruses and flus. For example, I treated a person who continually gets flus, sinus problems, and illnesses, who was sexually abused. In this case, her protective level was overworked and really fell down. When that level is affected, people develop an armoring, depending on what kind of defenses they have had to use."

This level is the easiest to handle, and acupuncture is particularly effective. If a woman has been primarily affected on the protective level, Bloom will work a lot on the tendon or muscular meridians.

However, if the damage to the protective level is chronic, and the defenses must work constantly, where will the energy come from to keep that up? "The body delves deeper," Blooms explains, and brings energy up from the nutritive level. At this level, blood is created and energy and blood are moved through all the organs. The nutritive level, then, is concerned with daily functioning. "People who have problems on this level commonly seek acupuncture for digestive or respiratory problems. They have difficulties in all systems."

In working to heal damage at the nutritive level, Bloom looks at two factors. "One is the blood itself. The blood in Chinese medicine is the medium through which our energy expresses itself in the world. In other words, it is the medium through which we express ourselves. Of course, a person who has been sexually abused and traumatized is going to have a lot of difficulty in that area.

"Naturally, one blood problem that would show up for that person is pain, especially around periods, as well as tremendous dysmenorrhea or stabbing pains in the pelvic area that are unclear in origin. We say that when a person has been traumatized the blood is affected, just as when you are hit there are black-and-blue marks or scars. These same scars are affecting us on an energetic or blood level as well."

To deal with this blood problem certain herbal formulas are used. One of the most common formulas, used for many kinds of trauma, including psychic trauma, is called *Yunnan baiyao* (meaning the white medicine from Yunnan province). Bloom indicates that "this formula tries to help the body redirect the blood flow from areas where there has been trauma and the blood has been blocked, static, or stuck. New channels are created. That can be the beginning of a treatment. Once this flow is established we can get to other levels, other symptoms, and deeper layers of trauma."

Other formulas have the same effect of moving stuck blood. "If blood is stuck, you get pain, you get scars. You could also get masses such as fibroids and cysts. Many women who have been sexually abused have these masses. There are formulas particularly directed to stuck blood in the chest where there could be chest pain. There are formulas for areas below the diaphragm, where there are masses, and for the lower abdomen."

The common herbs that help move the blood and remove pain are corydalis, persica, and a formula called peropisin (??) bulrush, which is a cattail pollen herb. Another common one is called cinnamon emporia (??), otherwise known as cinnamon en ho lin (??). This last is used for masses or pain in the abdomen and for fibroids.

The second factor affected on the nutritive level is heat. "Chinese medicine is based on a five-element system," Bloom explains. "The elements are fire, water, metal, earth, and wood. The fire element in that system is basically responsible for relationships and intimacy as well as for boundaries in relationships. This element in our nourishing selves is very affected by trauma. The organs associated with it are what Chinese treatment refers to as the heart, the heart protector or pericardium, and the small Intestine. Each of these can be affected. Primarily, the heart is the center of who we are. In Chinese medicine, it is considered the emperor. So the heart has to be protected if at all possible."

Sexual abuse is a shock to the system that is absorbed by the heart. It can be treated using *Yunnan baiyao* and with acupuncture. The heart is also connected with memory, Bloom says, so that often when the heart is blocked, memory will be affected. The heart and the pericardium, its protector, if affected or damaged, can show signs of palpitations and arrhythmias. Insomnia is a very common symptom in those who have been sexually abused."

The major acupuncture meridians chosen to treat such abuse run outward from the chest along the inner side of the arm. One particularly important meridian is called the Spirit Gate.

Another formula that is useful in healing at this level is called an mian pian, which can relieve insomnia. Also useful, Bloom says, are some essential oils, such as sandalwood. "Just one drop in the center of the chest, on the chest's center of energy, can help with palpitations, nervousness, and insomnia."

Herbal Pharmacy

Plants containing phytochemicals with aphrodisiac properties, in order of potency, are as follows:

Vicia faba (broad bean)
Catharanthus lanceus (lanceleaf periwinkle)
Euphorbia lathyris (caper spurge)
Passiflora incarnata (passionflower)
Panax ginseng (Chinese ginseng)
Punica granatum (pomegranate)
Malus domestica (apple)
Zea mays (corn)

Appendix

Alternative Therapies

B elow you will find brief descriptions of alternative healing modalities that are referred to throughout this book.

Acupressure

Acupressure, also known as shiatsu, is based on the principle that a vital energy, called *qi* (*chi*), flows through the body. The primary cause of pain is an imbalance in this energy. The goal of the healer is to balance the client's energy so pain and discomfort do not manifest or, if they do appear, will be relieved.

The practitioner concentrates on certain pressure points that have metaphoric names that tell us something of what they do or how they are to be worked with. He or she uses thumbs, fingers, palms, forearms, elbows, and even knees to apply pressure to specified points in the body to modulate the flow of energy. During a treatment, the client lies on the floor on a comfortable padded surface, such as a futon, fully clothed or undressed to his or her level of comfort. What the client feels is pressure, which can be gentle or deeper at the places where the practitioner is working. As the pressure continues, the patient will generally feel relaxed and energized at the same time.

Acupressure is good for treating a variety of different pains. It is especially beneficial in combating chronic pain in the back, neck, or shoulders, but it has also proved effective in treating whiplash, herniated disk, and nervous problems, such as Bell's palsy.

Acupuncture

Acupuncture sees pain as derived from blocked energy or *qi* (*chi*). In treating this blockage, the practitioner has to determine whether it stems from an overabundance or deficiency in energy, so the treatment can be adjusted depending on whether it is necessary to strengthen or decrease *qi*. To accomplish this the acupuncturist will work to open blocked energy pathways, so healing energy can go directly to the point in the body where it is needed, thereby stimulating the body's natural healing capacities.

The acupuncturist first records the patient's medical history in the manner of a conventional doctor. Then, with the patient lying down or seated, depending on the area to be treated, fine-gauge, stainless steel needles are inserted into significant points and meridians (channels through which *qi* flows) to exert different physiological effects on the body and induce both relaxation and energization. The patient will remain in this position from 20 to 30 minutes, though an appointment with an acupuncturist may last up to an hour, since part of the time will be spent consulting about the employment of other traditional and herbal treatments that might be recommended. Bodywork and massage might also be included in the session.

According to Abigail Rist-Podrecca, a registered nurse, acupuncture works by "dilating the blood vessels, so that the vessels can open. You get more circulation, more of the nutrients, more oxygen flowing through the meridians."

Alexander Technique

Alexander technique is based on the concept that all of us know how to move comfortably as children but lose that natural flexibility over time. The teacher acts to help the student recapture this freedom and lightness of movement. Practitioners see themselves as teachers, and their sessions not as therapy but as teaching.

Each session is an experiential process in which the teacher guides the student with hands-on training to help her learn a new way of moving, by means of the teacher's hands stimulating the student's nervous system.

This technique can help mothers, for example, learn how to bend over and lift children in a new way that avoids stress on the back.

Applied Kinesiology

This discipline is related to Chinese acupuncture. Practitioners use it to determine which foods and herbs are best assimilated by the individual, in order to develop a healing diet and supplementation program that is finely calibrated to the person's own biology.

The patient extends her arm at shoulder level while holding a food or supplement in the other hand, and the practitioner pushes down on the extended arm. If the substance is appropriate for her, the arm will be strong and harder to force down. If the substance is not good for her, the arm will be weak. This is because the body can feel the value of the substance. Using various techniques, kinesiologists can study these reactions more precisely to determine proper individual diet.

Aromatherapy

Aromatherapy depends on the therapeutic powers of essential oils. These oils are commonly used in skin and body care products in the United States, but their medicinal properties have long been accepted in other countries, particularly France, where, in many instances, their antimicrobial properties make them acceptable replacements for drug therapy. Pure essential oils can be used to cure cold and canker sores, calm the emotions, diminish joint swelling, clear the nasal passages and lungs, balance hormones, and for many other applications.

Ayurveda

Ayurveda means "the science of life." It is a system of medicine widely used in India for the past 4,000 years. Ayurveda believes that balance is the key to perfect health. It basically determines which of three body/mind types a person belongs to and, based on that type, helps people choose the type of foods they should eat and the type of exercise best for them. For more information, read *Perfect Health* and *Ageless Body, Timeless Mind* by Deepak Chopra.

Bach Flower remedies

The Bach flower remedies were developed by Dr. Edward Bach during the 1930s. They consist of 38 plant extracts that are used to treat physical and emotional problems. The extracts used in each case are selected according to the individual patient's personality. For instance, for a person who cannot say no, the suggested remedy derives from the beech tree. For some with an unhealthy fear of the unknown, a remedy derived from the aspen would be perscribed. Bach flower remedies are said to have positive effects on the psychological and emotional stress that underlie many illnesses.

Biofeedback

Biofeedback is a technique that teaches a person to consciously regulate normally involuntary bodily processes, such as heartbeats, brain waves, blood pressure, and muscle tension. The bodily process, such as heart rate, may be monitored by electronic equipment or by natural observation, such as holding a finger against an artery. With practice, the patient learns to slow down the heart rate, relax tension, and so on. Biofeedback is helpful for conditions such as migraines, tension headaches, digestive upsets, and any other disorders that are aggravated by stress.

Body Rolling

Body Rolling, a form of bodywork developed by Yamuna Zake, uses a 6- to 10-inch ball in a series of routines designed to elongate muscles and increase blood flow in all parts of the body. As the body weight presses into the ball, the ball applies pressure onto bone and creates traction that allows the entire length of a muscle to release. Body Rolling is useful to relieve pain and tension in many parts of the body.

Chelation therapy

Chelation therapy flushes toxins out of the blood. A synthetic amino acid, EDTA, is administered to the patient through an intravenous drip. The EDTA moves through the blood vessels and attaches itself to heavy metals in the blood such as mercury and lead, holding onto these substances until they are washed out of the body in the urine. Chelation therapy is being used increasingly to treat heart disease as well as other illnesses.

Chiropractic

Chiropractic treatment involves the manual manipulation of vertabrae that have become misaligned, exerting pressure on nerves and blocking the flow of energy to various organs. The manipulation is called an adjustment. It involves the chiropractor's gentle and painless application of direct pressure to the spine and joints. The chiropractor may squeeze or twist the torso, pull or twist the limbs, or wrench the head or back. In this manner she or he is readjusting the spinal column to restore the normal relationship of one vertebra to another. This eliminates the body's energy blocks.

Chiropractic is effective in dealing with pain and as a preventive measure because it relieves nerve pressure as the spine is properly adjusted.

Colon therapy

Colon cleansing refers to washing out the colon in order to remove toxic buildups. First the colon is irrigated with warm water, washing out encrustations and old fecal matter. Next, healing substances to reduce inflammation and strengthen the colon wall are infused.

Craniosacral therapy

The sacral region is that at the bottom of the spine. Between that region and the head there should be maintained a balanced relation for the health of the organism. If a restriction is experienced at that point, pain will be felt and other problems may arise.

In craniosacral therapy, the practitioner places her or his hands on the patient's body in such a way as to bring the cranium and sacrum back into alignment and to reestablish a natural rhythm between them. Treatment usually centers on the head or lower back, although it may be done on many different parts of the body.

Enzyme therapy

Enzyme therapy uses enzymes to cure illness and enhance life. South American Indians used papaya as a healing agent, and medieval Europeans used the milky juice of plants of the spurge family for medical reasons. Today, many practitioners advocate enzyme supplementation to enable vitamins and other supplements, as well as food, to be properly absorbed.

There are many different types of enzyme therapy. One example is that which relies on the Wolfe and Benitez formulas, which combine animal and vegetable enzymes. The preparations are said to be powerful weapons aganist bacteria and other invasive microorganisms.

Feldenkrais

Feldenkrais is a practice that helps eliminate poor movement habits and relieve chronic tensions. It uses very gentle movements that the student does herself, guided by the instructor, while lying on the floor. Alternatively the student lies on a massage table and the teacher uses a hands-on approach, taking the student through gentle movements to enable the student to let go of a chronic holding pattern.

The goal is to learn to differentiate between parts of the body that are relaxed and parts that are still tense. Thus the nervous system learns a new way of functioning.

Guided Imagery

Guided imagery can be practiced either by an individual with a therapist or in a group setting. In the individual setting, the practitioner helps the client elicit her own mental images, which she then interacts with, perhaps in dialogue. For example, if the client is ill, she may call up images of the distressed part of her body and encourage it to heal through an imagistic interaction.

In a group, a facilitator helps the participants concentrate on building certain images whose healing power they can tap into. In this setting, the participant has the added benefit of being able to discuss the process with another participant afterward so as to further affirm and enrich the healing process.

Hellerwork

Hellerwork is a bodywork techinique derived from Rolfing (see below). Both modalities work to improve body structure with deep tissue work, but Hellerwork, unlike Rolfing, is not painful. The practice has three components. In the first, hands-on part, the practitioner finds a misalignment in the body and works with the client to release it.

The second part is movement education. The practitioner analyzes the patient's posture and movements, then gives her more relaxed and stressless ways to move. The third component is mind/body dialogue, whose purpose is to identify emotional patterns that underlie dysfunctional movement patterns.

Homeopathy

Homeopathy is based on the law of similars, the principle that what causes illness can also cure it. If a person has a head cold, you would give the person a substance that would cause cold symptoms in a healthy person, but in a sick person it helps to cure them. Homeopathy is limited in scope at this time in the United States, although 100 years ago it was the prevailing form of medicine-—until allopathic medicine and the American Medical Association in particular launched an intensive drive against it, which culminated in its being virtually banned in this country.

Recently, there has been a renewed interest in homeopathy, and growing numbers of physicians are using its principles. Homeopathy is particularly effective in the treatment of fevers, bacterial infections, toxicity, and the cumulative effects of alcohol, drugs, tobacco, caffeine, or sugar. It is not recommended for cancer, AIDS, or heart disease.

Natural Hygiene

Natural hygiene is the practice of creating optimal conditions for the body and its constituent cells, tissues, and organs to pursue and sustain health. This means environmental purity of air, food, and water; a balanced primordial diet based on natural foods; and stress reduction and management. It precludes the use of most drugs, since they are antithetical to a modality that perceives illness to be due to inappropriate nutrition and toxic accumulations (drugs are usually toxic substances). Finally, it means a symbiotic relationship of all humankind and harmony with God and nature.

Naturopathy

Naturopathic physicians can treat most conditions. They are not, however, allowed to perform major surgery (although they can perform minor surgery). Their very extensive background is centered in the botanical sciences, including the use of herbs and tinctures with a wide variety of natural immune-stimulating properties.

The naturopath practices a natural form of health care whose traditions precede the advent of modern medicine. In this the naturopath resembles the traditional Tibetan physician, who must be able to identify nearly 1,000 different healing herbs, mineral sources, and animal sources. The naturopath has years of extensive study in the healing potential of such substances. He or she is also able to understand muscular and skeletal bodily adjustment. Naturopaths use a much broader basis for diagnosis than do conventional allopathic physicians.

Orthomolecular Medicine

Orthomolecular medicine is an alternative approach to mental and physical health whose goal is to identify and treat the root cause of disease. The objective is to balance and rebuild the whole body, not merely to mask or suppress symptoms. To do this, orthomolecular physicians try to establish an equilibrium among the essential nutrients that may be lacking, present in excess, or are being poorly absorbed. Orthomolecular physicians are conventionally trained medical doctors who feel that such an imbalance is often responsible for psychiatric as well as physical disorders.

The physician looks at diet, glandular function, glucose metabolism, and a host of other biochemical factors which may play a role in the patient's mental health. Imbalances in the body are corrected through judicious use of vitamins, minerals, amino acids, and other naturally occurring nutrients. Orthomolecular physicians frequently use a very high-dose vitamin regimen.

Polarity Therapy

Polarity therapy is based on the belief that any stagnation or stopping of the natural flow of energy in the human body is the underlying cause of disease. The naturally occurring positive and negative energy fields of the body are in a polarity relationship with each other. However, when the energy is blocked, it turns neutral, and the surrounding tissues stagnate and become painful.

Practitioners use light forms of touch, gentle manipulation, and techniques such as rocking to restore the flow of energy, relieving stress and pain and encouraging healing.

Polarity therapy is particularly useful for depression, anxiety, fatigue, headaches, fibromyalgia, and other conditions involving emotional blockages.

Qi gong

The Chinese phrase *Qi gong* means air (considered the vital essence) and work. This traditional Asian practice utilizes aerobic exercise, meditation, relaxation techniques, and isometrics to control the vital energy of the body in the most efficient way. Like many Chinese practices, it emphasizes the unity of mind, spirit, and world.

The central practice is a combination of breathing, movement, and shallow meditation, in which the person is aware of what is going on but in a tranquil state in which positive images flow quietly through a relaxing mind. Once the person is in this state, the flow of the *qi* through the body is stimulated. This unobstructed flow will heal sickness or increase an existing sense of wellness.

Reflexology

Reflexology is based on the principle that people have reflex areas in their feet that correspond to every part of the body. The locations of the reflex points on the foot correspond to the way the organs and glands are distributed within the body. Massaging these specific areas on the feet thus helps to improve the functioning of particular organs and glands.

For example, the toes reflect the head area, the ball of the foot represents the chest area, and so on. The practitioner presses his or her fingers into the foot, using a variety of techniques, to massage and relax ill or stressed parts of the body.

Reiki

Reiki is a type of massage therapy or bodywork in which pressure-point techniques are used to move energy through the body in order to create balance and harmony. The practice, Japanese in origin, teaches the student to attain an attunement with the universal energy.

Whereas many Asian techniques involve learning a discipline to guide the flow of energy, in Reiki the student attains attunement from a Reiki Master, who transmits it during a ritual process. This single attunement can never be lost, although with further attunements one can move to a higher spiritual level.

Rolfing

According to practitioners of Rolfing, pain is caused by chronic shortenings in the tissue. Correction of the pain can be accomplished by soft tissue manipulation. This manipulation creates order in the body so the client stands tall and free of restriction.

Rolfing is generally performed in a series of 10 sessions, designed to address all the shortenings in the structure systematically. Each session works in a different area. The basic goal of Rolfing is not pain relief per se; still it has been found useful for TMJ, frozen shoulder, carpal tunnel syndrome, tennis elbow, chronic hip problems, sciatica, cervical neuropathies, and knee, foot, and ankle problems.

Therapeutic Touch

Therapeutic touch represents a reinvigoration of the old process of the laying on of hands, whereby the subtle touch of a healer on the patient's body will infuse her with positive energy. This therapy was orginally developed by nurses and emphasizes the nurturing aspect of the practitioner.

A key ingredient of the practice is compassion for the patient being touched. Unlike most of the therapies reviewed here, this technique requires minimal training, which is why it is widely practiced by both professional medical practitioners and laypeople.

Traditional Chinese Medicine

Traditional Chinese medicine is based on ancient Taoist philosophy, which treats the whole person. The philosophy is that body and mind are one; there is no separation between the two. When *qi*, or universal energy, flows freely through the meridians, a person is healthy, but when *qi* is blocked or disrupted, the person develops pain or illness.

Practitioners begin by examining the patient to identify patterns of disharmony. They then prescribe herbal remedies based on these patterns.

Trager Technique

According to the theory behind Trager technique, pain is caused when someone frequently tightens her muscles in movement and posture. To correct this, the practioner uses gentle motions to increase the patient's pleasure in the quality of her tissues and decrease the restriction and sense of holding. Gentleness is important, so that no message is sent to the body telling it that pain is on the way or causing the patient to tighten up.

The movement reaches into the central nervous system to convey the sensations of pleasure, lengthening, softening, and opening to the tissues and joints. This practice is used to relieve lower back, neck, and upper back pain, sciatica, migraines, TMJ, and carpal tunnel syndrome and other repetitive stress disorders.

Resource Guide

Dr. Peter Agho
175 West 72nd Street
New York, NY 10023
ph: (212) 501-8143

Dr. Majid Ali
The Institute of Integrative Medicine
95 East Main Street
Denville, NJ 07834
ph: (973) 586-4111

Dr. Majid Ali
140 West End Avenue
New York, NY 10023
ph: (212) 973-2444
e-mail: majidalimd@aol.com
www.fatigue.net

Dr. Richard N. Ash
The Ash Center for Comprehensive
Medicine and the Ash Heart and
Wellness Center
800-A 5th Avenue
New York, NY 10021
ph: (212) 758-3200
fax: (212) 754-5800

Dr. Robert Atkins
The Atkins Center
152 East 55th Street
New York, NY 10022
ph: (212) 758 2110
fax: (212) 751 1863
www.atkinscenter.com

Neal Barnard, M.D.
Physicians Committee
for Responsible Medicine
5100 Wisconsin Ave.
Washington, DC 20016
e-mail nbarnard@pcrm.org

Dr. Neil Block
60 Dutch Hill Road
Orangeburg, NY 10962
ph: (914) 359-3300

Dr. Eric Braverman
PATH Medical
185 Madison Avenue
New York, NY 10016
(212) 213-6155 or
1(888) 231-PATH

Hyla Cass, M.D.
1608 Michael Lane
Pacific Palisades, CA 90272
ph: (310) 459-9866
fax (310) 459-9466
e-mail: HCassMD@worldnet.att.net
www.doctorcass.com

Dr. Anthony J. Cichoke
P.O. Box 92094
Portland, OR 97292
e-mail: enzyme@hevanet.com

Dr. William Crook
International Health Foundation
P.O. Box 3494
Jackson, TN 38303
www.candida-yeast.com

Dr. Peter D'Adamo
2009 Summer Street
3rd floor
Stamford, CT 06905
ph: (203) 348-4800

Jerry Dorsman. B.A.C.
New Dawn
Box 71
Elk Mills, MD 21920
ph: (410) 392-9605

Michael Ellner
Chelsea Healing Center
216 West 23rd Street
New York, NY 10011
ph: (212) 645 6447
fax: (212) 645-8933
e-mail: revdocnyc@aol.com

Dr. Paul Epstein
School of Public Health
Cancer Prevention Coalition
University of Illinois Medical Center
2121 West Taylor
Chicago, IL 60612
ph: (312) 996 1374
fax: (312) 664 6250
e-mail: epstein@uic.edu

Dr. Martin Feldman
132 East 76th Street
New York, NY 10021
(212) 744-4413

Dr. Joel Fuhrman
ph: 1(800) 474-9355
www.drfuhrman.com

Dr. William Goldwag
ph: (714) 827-5180

Letha Hadady
Author of the book,
Asian Health Secrets
To order, call 1(800) 538-5856
e-mail: lethah@earthlink.net

Colette Heimowitz, N.S.
ph: (718) 261-1874
fax: (718) 261-2253

Dr. Hal A. Huggins
5080 List Drive
Colorado Springs, CO 80919
ph: (719) 522-0566
or 1(888) 843-5832

Susan Kolb, M.D., FACS
Millennium Healthcare
4370 Georgetown Square
Dunwoody, GA 30338
ph: (770) 390 0012
fax: (770) 457 4428
www.millennium-healthcare.com

Dr. Ken Korins
200 West 57th Street
New York, NY 10019
ph: (212) 246 5122
e-mail: kskorinsmd@email.msn.com

Dr. Mark Leder
330 East 70th Street #4H
New York, NY 10021
ph: (212) 737-6548
e-mail: drmleder@aol.com

Dr. Michael Lesser
www.newmedicinenet.com

Dr. Warren Levin
Comprehensive Medical Services
18 East 53rd Street
New York, NY 10022
ph: (212) 838 4926

Dr. Warren Levin
America's Medical Center
13 Powder Horn Hill
Wilton, CT 06897
ph: (203) 894-8370

Dr. Marshall Mandell
6721 Oakmont Way
Bradenton, FL 34202
ph: (941) 727 8506

Dr. John McDougall
Saint Helena Center
P.O. Box 250
Deer Park, CA 94576
ph: 1(800) 358-9195

Dr. John McDougall
McDougall Health Clinic
P.O. Box 14039
Santa Rosa CA 95402
ph: 1(800) 570-1654

Dr. John McDougall
Dr. McDougall's Right Food
ph: 1(800) 367-3844
www.drmcdougall.com

Dr. Marjorie Ordene
2515 Avenue M
Brooklyn, NY 11210
e-mail: ordene@rcn.com

Dr. Linda Page
Healthy Healing Publications
P.O. Box 436
Carmel Valley, CA 93924
ph: 1(800) 736-6015
e-mail: Barbara@healthyhealing.com
www.healthyhealing.com

Dolores C. Perri
Alternative Health Center
315 West 70th Street
Suite 1B
New York, NY 10023
ph: (212) 787-2404
askperri@webstan.net

Dr. William Philpott
Philpott Medical Services
Enviro-Tech Products
17171 South East 29th Street
Choctaw, OK 73020
ph: (405) 390 3009
Enviro-Tech ph: (405) 390-3499

Dr. Richard Podell
The Podell Medical Center
571 Central Avenue
Suite 106
New Providence, NJ 07974
ph: (908) 464-3800

Dr. Mitchell Proffman
144-02 69th Avenue
Flushing, NY 11367
ph: (718) 268-9080
e-mail: chiroprac8@aol.com

Doris Rapp, M.D., FAAA, FAAP, FAEM
8179 East Del Cuarzo Drive
Scotsdell, AZ 85258
ph: (602) 905 9195
fax: (602) 905 8281
e-mail: drrappmd@aol.com
www.drrapp.com

Dr. Richard Ribner
25 Central Park West
New York, NY 10023
ph: (212) 246-7010

Abigail Rist-Podrecca, O.M.D.
130 West 57th Street
New York, NY
abyryst@aol.com
ph: (914) 246-1387
or (212) 957-5266

Dr. Howard Robins
200 West 57th Street
New York, NY 10019
ph: (212) 581-0101
fax: (212) 582-7350

Dr. Michael Schachter
Schachter Center for
Complementary Medicine
2 Executive Blvd.
Suite 202
Suffern, NY 10901
ph: (914) 368-4700
e-mail: office@mbschachter.com
www.mbschachter.com

Sherrill Sellman
13707 East 31 Place
Tulsa, OK 74134
ph: (973) 772-2527
e-mail: golight@earthlink.net
www.ssellman.com

Dr. David Steenblock
26381 Crown Valley Parkway
Suite 130
Mission Viejo, CA 92691
ph: (949) 367-8870
fax: (949) 367-9779
www.strokedoctor.com

Dr. Michael Wald
Advanced Medical
of Mount Kisco, P.C.
213 Main Street
Mount Kisco, NY 10549
(914) 241-7030

Dr. Michael Wald
Avitar Industries Treatment Center
1867 Independence Square Ste. 155
Atlanta, GA 30338
ph: (678) 320 9933
fax: (770) 457 4428
www.avitar-industries.com

Dr. Michael Wald
Plastikos Surgery Center
4370 Georgetown Square
Dunwoody, GA 30338
ph: (770) 457 4677
fax: (770) 457 4428
www.plastikos.com

Allan B. Warshowsky, M.D.
2001 Marcus Avenue, Suite West 75
Lake Success, NY 11042
ph: (516) 488-2757
fax: (516) 488-3940
e-mail: abw88pe@aol.com

Dr. Yuan Yang
The Healing Center
175 West 72nd Street
New York, NY 10023
ph: (212) 501-7521

Jose A. Yaryura-Tobias, M.D.
Institute for Bio-Behavioral Therapy
and Research
935 Northern Blvd.
Suite 102
Great Neck, NY 11021
ph: (516) 487-7116
fax: (516) 829-1731
e-mail: Yaryura1@aol.com

Yamuna Zake
Body Logic
295 West 11th Street, Suite 1F
New York, NY 10014
ph: 1(800) 877-8429
e-mail: yamunazake@aol.com
www.bodylogic.com

Part II

Health
Empowerment
for Women

Barbara Seaman

So many of my friends recall sitting in rooms where secrets were shared among women. Typically, any shameful feelings we may have had lifted as we learned that our private experiences often turned out to be universal.

I remember the voices: "Yes, I had an illegal abortion." "Yes, I was raped." "Yes, my neighbor (brother, father, uncle, priest, doctor, therapist, teacher) hassled me sexually." "Yes, I fake orgasms." "Yes, every birth control method I've ever used was a disaster." "Yes, my gynecologist makes me uncomfortable, but I can't admit it, he's so esteemed. His pelvic exams are so rough it hurts to pee for the next three days."

Women talked, listened, and spread the word. We went back to our communities started our own women's groups, consciousness-raising groups, rap groups, know-your-body courses. By 1975 there were nearly 2,000 official women's self-help projects scattered around the United States, and countless unofficial ones.

Do women talk less to each other about health now than they did then? The very possibility is troubling.

If I have a single hope for this book it is that the women who read it be inspired to talk among themselves about health, more now than ever, since *women who talk to each other about health will go on to talk to each other about anything and everything.*

Our first chapter, "In the Beginning," tells how men wrested health care away from the women who originally provided it. Here in its entirety is Barbara Ehrenreich's and Dierdre English's "Witches, Midwives and Nurses," essential reading for women young and young at heart. Here too is "Motherhood" by Elizabeth Cady Stanton, "Rape in Great Art" by Audrey Flack, including many lovely pictures and some not-so-lovely impressions they can leave, as well as Kristin Luker on "Medicine and Morality in the Nineteenth Century" and Sojourner Truth's "Ain't I a Woman," among many other electric writings.

The next section, "Taking Our Bodies Back," concentrates on the 1970s—a highwater mark for health activism—with spotlights on such influential writers and activists as Byllye Avery, Susan Brownmiller, Phyllis Chesler, Angela Davis, Carol Downer, Shulamith Firestone, Germaine Greer, Shere Hite, Mary Howell, Patsy Mink, Norma McCorvey (aka Jane Roe of Roe v. Wade*), Letty Cottin Pogrebin, Alix Kates Shulman, Gloria Steinem, and many others. Chapters range from "Activism/Revolution," to "Sex and Orgasm," to "Women in White Coats," which spotlights and many more.*

Next, the "Body Parts," section, is organized by body part: "Breasts," "Face," "Hair," "Muscle," "Torso," "Womb," etc., in each case the body part signifies a whole state of mind and a body of literature. With selections ranging from a poem about aging by Erica Jong, to "Dreading It... Or How I Learned to Stop Fighting My Hair and Love My Nappy Roots" by Veronica Chambers, "Fat is a Feminist Issue" by Susie Orbach, "Women's Hearts at Risk" by Charlotte Libov, and "Science + Corporate Bucks = Health Revolution?", plan on surprises.

Our final section, "Still Taking Our Bodies Back," confronts the backlash, and illuminates important new issues unfolding for women in the 21st century. In addition to a look back at the history of Our Bodies, Ourselves *with Judy Norsigian, you'll find a chapter entitled "More Motherhood," where we look at some of the newer issues facing mothers through articles like "What Do You Love about Being a Lesbian Mom?" by Catharine Gund. Another chapter, "Conflict of Interest," spotlights how pharmaceutical companies and the medical establishment subjugate the interests of women for profit. And in chapter 73, "Feminism for the 21st Century," our final chapter, here are two dozen marvelous and inspiring writings on the challenges facing us as we forge ahead, including some of the new young feminist voices like Naomi Wolf, Leora Tanenbaum, and Paula Kamen that will lead us into the new millennium. And finally, closing out the chapter are interviews with and articles by important feminist activists; some pioneers (Marilyn Webb, Sheryl Burt Ruzek, Alice Wolfson, Belita Cowan, Betty Rollin) and some members of the new wave (Dr. Susan Love, Cindy Pearson).*

I hope, dear reader, you find all these writings to be both inspiring and familiar in the sense they speak to feelings you have already had. I hope also that this book can increase your ability to make informed decisions that will help you protect your own and your loved one's good health and best interests.—B.S.

Chapter 40

In the Beginning

On Motherhood

ELIZABETH CADY STANTON

Excerpted from Alice S. Rossi, ed., *The Feminist Papers: From Adams to de Beauvoir*, New York, Bantam Books, 1973, pp. 399–401. Originally published in *Elizabeth Cady Stanton: As Revealed in Her Letters, Diary, and Reminiscences*, New York, Harper & Bros., 1922. Reprinted by permission.

Her public cause was "votes for women," but her private mission and personal creed was "self-reliance," particularly in matters of health. Elizabeth Cady Stanton —the boldest and most brilliant of nineteenth-century American feminists— was born on November 12, 1815, in upstate New York. The family was prosperous; her father was a judge, and her mother was of aristocratic lineage. Of the Cadys' 11 children, only 5 daughters survived. As a girl Elizabeth studied homeopathy with her brother-in-law, Dr. Edward Bayard. In 1840 she married Henry Stanton—abolitionist, cofounder of Oberlin College, and a follower of Sylvester Graham, a charismatic lecturer, father of the Graham cracker, and, the record suggests, the Gary Null of his era, known for his passionate advocacy of daily excercise combined with a balanced, largely vegetarian diet.

A neighbor, Amelia Bloomer, once wrote on the envelope of a letter she forwarded to Elizabeth, "People have nothing to talk about when you are gone!" That was because Elizabeth usually acted on her beliefs, however unpopular. When her hometown refused to open its tax-supported calisthenics classes to

girls, she converted her barn into a gym and subversively offered instruction.
Armed with her homeopathic manual and her herbs, she "doctored" her own
and her neighbors' children through malaria, whooping cough, mumps, and
broken limbs, and even helped deliver some of them.

For more than 50 years, there seemed to be no impediment to women's full
equality that Elizabeth did not notice and attempt to rout: besides suffrage, she
campaigned for birth control, property rights for wives, custody rights for moth-
ers, equal wages, cooperative nurseries, coeducation, and "deliverance from the
tyranny of self-styled medical, religious, and legal authorities." In a famous
speech delivered in Rochester, New York, on August 2, 1948, she declared:

> *Woman herself must do this work—for woman alone can understand*
> *the height, and the depth, the length, and the breadth of her own degra-*
> *dation and woe. Man cannot speak for us—because he has been educated*
> *to believe that we differ from him so materially that he cannot judge of*
> *our thoughts, feelings, and opinions on his own.*

Through it all Elizabeth was a doting, hands-on mother of five sons and two
daughters, born between 1842, when she was 26, and 1859, when she was 43. It
was said that if she wasn't already pregnant or nursing, Elizabeth conceived
each time that Henry (a traveling man) came home. She so enjoyed the company
of her children (permissively raised, energetic and uppity like their mom) that
she moved her writing desk into their nursery.

The acid test of her maternal "self-reliance" occurred when her eldest,
Daniel (called "Neil"), was born with a dislocated shoulder. The doctors she
consulted set it in restrictive bandages, which made the condition worse.
"With my usual conceit," she told Henry, "I removed the bandages and turned
surgeon myself."

Here is the story in Stanton's own words, compiled by two of her younger
children, Theodore Stanton and Harriot Stanton Blatch, in their old age and
published in 1922, 80 years after their mother first drew her line in the sand to
protect and preserve their brother Neil.—B. S.

B esides the obstinacy of the nurse, I had the ignorance of physicians to
contend with. When the child was four days old we discovered that the
collarbone was bent. The physician, wishing to get a pressure on the
shoulder, braced the bandage round the wrist. "Leave that," he said, "ten days,
and then it will be all right." Soon after he left I noticed that the child's hand
was blue, showing that the circulation was impeded. "That will never do," said
I. "Nurse, take it off." "No, indeed," she answered, "I shall never interfere with
the doctor." So I took it off myself, and sent for another doctor, who was said
to know more of surgery. He expressed great surprise that the first physician
called should have put on so severe a bandage. "That," said he, "would do for
a grown man, but ten days of it on a child would make him a cripple." However,

he did nearly the same thing, only fastening it round the hand instead of the wrist. I soon saw that the ends of the fingers were all purple, and that to leave that on ten days would be as dangerous as the first. So I took it off.

"What a woman!" exclaimed the nurse. "What do you propose to do?" "Think out something better myself; so brace me up with some pillows and give the baby to me." She looked at me aghast. "Now," I said, talking partly to myself and partly to her, "what we want is a little pressure on that bone; that is what both of those men aimed at. How can we get it without involving the arm, is the question?" "I am sure I don't know," said she, rubbing her hands and taking two or three brisk turns around the room. "Well, bring me three strips of linen, four double." I then folded one, wet in arnica and water, and laid it on the collarbone, put two other bands, like a pair of suspenders over the shoulder, crossing them both in front and behind, pinning the ends to the diaper, which gave the needed pressure without impeding the circulation anywhere. As I finished she gave me a look of budding confidence, and seemed satisfied that all was well. Several times, night and day, we wet the compress and readjusted the bands, until all appearance of inflammation had subsided.

At the end of ten days the two sons of Aesculapius appeared and made their examination, and said all was right, whereupon I told them how badly their bandages worked, and what I had done myself. They smiled at each other, and one said, "Well, after all, a mother's instinct is better than a man's reason." "Thank you, gentlemen, there was no instinct about it. I did some hard thinking before I saw how I could get pressure on the shoulder without impeding the circulation, as you did." Thus, in the supreme moment of a young mother's life, when I needed tender care and support, the whole responsibility of my child's supervision fell upon me; but though uncertain at every step of my own knowledge, I learned another lesson in self-reliance. I trusted neither men nor books absolutely after this, either in regard to the heavens or the earth beneath, but continued to use my "mother's instinct," if "reason" is too dignified a term to apply to a woman's thoughts. My advice to every mother is, above all other arts and sciences, study first what relates to babyhood, as there is no department of human action in which there is such lamentable ignorance.

Why Elizabeth Isn't on Your Silver Dollar

BARBARA SEAMAN

November 12, 1895, Elizabeth Cady Stanton's eightieth birthday, found her enthroned on the stage of the Metropolitan Opera House, where 6,000 people had gathered to celebrate. Behind her, on the stage, red carnations spelled out her name in a field of white chrysanthemums, while roses banked her red velvet chair. Following three hours of ovations, tributes ("America's Grand Old Woman," "Queen Mother of American Suffragists"), and gifts—including an onyx-and-silver ballot box presented by a delegation of Mormon women from the Utah Territory—Stanton rose and gently reminded her admirers: "I am well aware that all these public demonstrations are not so much tributes to me as an individual as to the great idea I represent—the enfranchisement of women."

Two weeks later, she was in big trouble. Her book, *The Woman's Bible*, was published, and quickly became a best-seller, but, according to her biographer Elisabeth Griffith, she was branded as a heretic by a stunned public. *The Woman's Bible* argued that "the chief obstacle in the way of woman's elevation today is the degrading position assigned her in the religion of all countries—an afterthought in creation, the origin of sin, cursed by God, marriage for her a condition of servitude, maternity a degradation, unfit to minister at the altar and in some churches even to sing in the choir." Elizabeth, whose mealtime grace was addressed to "Mother and Father God," proclaimed her belief in an androgynous creator and declared that the story of the expulsion from Eden was a myth. Far from being cursed, woman had been the originator and ruler of Amazonian societies before man seized control and subjugated her.

Humiliated by Elizabeth's "blasphemy," the younger, more "practical" leadership in the suffrage organizations shunned her, convinced that she, their founding mother, had recklessly jeopardized their cause. "They refused to read my letters and resolutions to the conventions; they have denounced *The Woman's Bible* unsparingly," Elizabeth wrote. Susan B. Anthony, Elizabeth's protégé and junior collaborator, was now put forward as the symbol and standard bearer of suffrage. Susan's name, alone, would attach to the 1920 Constitutional amendment; her face, alone, to the commemorative coin and stamp.

Elizabeth died in 1902, 18 years before women got the vote, 54 years after she first demanded it, 51 years after she met Susan and recruited her to the cause. In the spirit of androgyny, Elizabeth's funeral service in her New York City apartment was conducted by a man assisted by the Reverend Antoinette Brown Blackwell. Her graveside service was conducted by a woman alone, the Reverend Phebe Hanaford.

Elizabeth was quite content in her old age despite (or perhaps because of) the controversy that her *Woman's Bible* inspired. As her biographer Lois Banner has written: "Politics was not really congenial to her. Independent by nature... the political mode of moderation, compromise, and slow progress did not fit her. Rather she preferred to shock her colleagues, to stir them out of complacency, to arouse their passions through introducing issues they had not considered.... Since the founding of the women's movement, she had seen her role as that of its radical conscience.... She had introduced suffrage in 1848 when the proposal had been new and shocking, [but now it was] accepted by all feminists and actually in force in the territories."

The following selections were written to stir readers out of complacency, to introduce issues they had not considered, and overall, to heighten our consciousness of woman's role in history.

Out of Conflict Comes Strength and Healing: Women's Health Movements

HELEN I. MARIESKIND

Adapted from Helen I. Marieskind, *Women in the Health System: Patients, Providers, and Programs,* St. Louis, Mo., C. V. Mosby, 1980. Reprinted by permission.

Helen Marieskind, founding editor of the journal Women and Health, *chose her surname to honor her mother, Marie. (*Kind *is the German word for "child.") With similar devotion she honors the names and the work of some superstar women healers in history. (Hey, girlfriend, how about that Hildegard of Bingen?!)* —B. S.

Conflict and activism in women's health care have a long history; ancient issues remain with us. In 3500 B.C. Egyptian midwives, *jatromaiai,* proudly protected their rights to practice surgery and internal medicine, distinguishing themselves from the strictly obstetrical practice of the *maiai.* Greece had many skilled women physicians, but by the third century B.C., their service as abortionists, the influence of Hippocrates, and the growth of the Pythagorean school combined to prohibit them from practice. Women "picketed the courthouse," winning the right to practice and acquittal of their favorite, Agnodice, arrested for practicing gynecology as a man.

The growth of Christianity led to a deepening conviction by men of the church that women should keep out of public and religious affairs, and major conflicts over women's role in health care delivery and in the nature of health care began in earnest. Saint Augustine had written, "educated women should take care of the sick," but by the Council of Nantes in 660, women were termed "soulless brutes." Thus began centuries of denying education to women and male dominance in medicine.

Only a few women—usually the wealthy, nobility, or clerics—were educated. Many of these women turned to monastic life, becoming medical missionaries with their monasteries as centers of healing. For example, the English princess Walpurga (c. 710–777), always depicted with a flask of urine and bandages, treated the poor at the monastery she founded in Germany. Hildegard of Bingen (1098–1179), who is best known today for her enchanting music, entered monastic life at age eight. In 1147, at age 50, Hildegard built a new convent near Bingen, on the Rhine. Hildegard wielded great power, corresponding with popes, emperors, and kings. Fiery and prophetic, she published her theories on the chemistry and circulation of blood, the causes of contagion and autointoxication, and the brain as the origin of nerve action. Obstetrician Trotula di Ruggiero of Salerno, Italy, is credited in the mid-1100s with the first description of the physical signs of syphilis and, prior to an understanding of sepsis, for advocating the use of protective pads to prevent fecal contamination during childbirth. Anna Comnena (1083–1148) served as physician-in-chief of an 11,000-bed hospital in Constantinople (Istanbul).

Conflict increased over the next centuries between the learned role of medical men and the widespread denial of education to women. Conflict was reinforced by church decrees in the early 1100s, the development of universities in most of Europe as primarily male preserves, the growth of essentially all-male guilds, and efforts at licensure by the church and state. Women's roles in health care were confined to nurses, midwives, herb gatherers, ecclesiastical and lay village healers, and occasionally empirics, who were lay women apprenticed to university-educated practitioners. Women (along with barber-surgeons) became providers of simple, direct care—treating wounds and infections and setting bones. This dichotomy between learned men and primary care–giving women laid the groundwork for a further division of labor in which women healers were essentially limited to nursing tasks while male practitioners commanded an elite, specialist role.

Jacoba Félicie de Almania's case illustrates the point. Brought to trial in Paris in 1322 for failing to comply with a 1220 licensure law, Jacoba was confronted not with a charge of incompetence but with witnesses and a detailed reading of her medical practices, showing her to be both practical and knowledgeable. She argued that the licensure law of 1220 was made for "idiots and ignorant persons" who knew nothing of the art of medicine and from which groups she was excluded because of her skill and expertise. Her eloquent pleas for the need for women to be treated by other women are recorded in the Charter of Paris, II:

> It is better and more honest that a wise and expert woman in this art visit sick women and inquire into the secret nature of their infirmity, than a man to whom it is not permitted to see, inquire of, or touch the hands, breasts, stomach, etc. of a woman; nay rather ought a man shun the secrets of women and their company and flee as far as he can.

Some outstanding midwives and women physicians did survive this period. Important female physicians were still emerging from Italy at a time when England and France were persecuting them. Dorothea Bocchi was appointed professor of medicine and moral philosophy at Bologna in 1390 and taught there for 40 years. A contemporary, Costanza Calenda of Naples, won high honors for her lecturing in medicine.

By the sixteenth century, exclusion of women from most European learning centers was firmly entrenched (Italy was a notable exception). Intense conflicts over women's health raged during the witch-hunts of medieval Europe, when thousands of people were slaughtered. Most of the women were lay women healers or "old wives" who served as midwives. This is an important distinction, because while accusations of witchcraft were also at times leveled at more recognized midwives, some separate provisions were made for them to be licensed. In England in 1587, for example, Eleanor Preade was licensed to perform the functions of midwife, including baptism.

Witchcraft trials had a lasting effect on women's place as healers, as the direct, primary, and often intimate caregiving roles had become so fraught with danger, that few women risked practicing for fear of being accused. The poor lost their village healers, and the professional control by church and state became firmly entrenched. Increasing corruption in the monasteries was matched by decreased interest in the medical and charitable aspects of clerical life, while the exclusion of women from the universities continued to effectively bar the participation of even upper-class women from medical practice. Moreover, by licensing some midwives and not others, stratifications and divisions formed among women healers, preventing a unified protest.

Again, there were exceptions. Outstanding French midwives practiced from the sixteenth to the nineteenth centuries. Louyse Bourgeois (1563–1636) set rules for handling each of the varied fetal positions. Angèlique Marguerite le Boursier du Coudray (1712–1789) invented a model of the female torso and was ordered by Louis XVI to travel throughout the provinces, giving free instruction to all "unenlightened midwives." Yet even in France, England, and Germany, where the skills of all highly accomplished midwives were well-rewarded, their discoveries published, and their talents sought after by the noblest and humblest of citizens, conflict still surrounded their licensure and entry into universities. "The midwives of the Academy have no desire of me," mocked Madame Boivin (1773–1847), midwife, decorated by the French crown and awarded an honorary M.D. degree by Germany in 1827, upon being denied entry into the (male) French Academy of Medicine.

By the end of the eighteenth century, conflicts over female practitioners, particularly midwives, were highly institutionalized throughout Europe. In France and Germany, although the status of some was diminished, the training programs organized led to an overall increase in competence and respect, resulting in the incorporation of the midwife into modern health care systems.

Midwives in England, however, were not only excluded from using rapidly developing technologies such as forceps, but were hampered also by their lack of organization, intragroup competitiveness, their assignment to obstetrics only, and by a wealthy and well-organized onslaught from the male physicians backed by church, state, and licensure laws. The ceaseless struggles of midwives such as Mrs. Elizabeth Nihell, Mrs. Sarah Stone, and Mrs. Elizabeth Cellier are colorful reading. It was not until Rosalind Paget founded the Midwives Institute in 1881 that the midwife once more became an integral part of the English health care system.

In the American colonies several midwives served their communities with great skill. The first midwife of record, Brigett Fuller, as her name is spelled on the land ownership register, reached the Plymouth colony in 1623 on the *Anne* and joined her physician husband Samuel, a *Mayflower* passenger. There was also Anne Hutchinson, a midwife, an organizer of women, and a religious dissident who cofounded a settlement in Rhode Island. We know of a Mrs. Wiat from her epitaph of 1705: "She assisted at ye births of one thousand, one hundred and odd children." The diary of Martha Ballard, midwife, converted to a contemporary book and film, aptly captures the poignant hardships and the joys of the midwife's role in colonial America.

In the United States, too, the midwife gradually lost her status, as did practicing female physicians—generally for the same reasons as in England. Women physicians, such as Dr. Mary Lavinder (1776–1845), who set up a pediatric and midwifery practice in Savannah, Georgia, in 1814, and Dr. Sarah E. Adams (1779–1846), also a practitioner in Georgia, were highly popular and successful even if not given equal status. Similarly, Harriet K. Hunt (1805–1875) gained a large following in her Boston practice, even though she had no degree. Oliver Wendell Holmes supported her application to Harvard Medical School, and the faculty could find nothing in the statutes to deny her admission. Nevertheless, Hunt was forced to withdraw her application when the students resolved: "That we object to having the company of any female forced upon us, who is disposed to unsex herself, and to sacrifice her modesty by appearing with men in the lecture room."

The greatest conflicts around women's health care in the United States arose during the popular health movement of the 1830s and 1840s, continuing well into the twentieth century. A current of liberal, democratic thinking hostile to professionalism, fostered the growth of the popular health movement, aided by lax or nonexistent licensing laws, a broad recognition of home cures and synergy between body and mind, and by a generally held belief that anyone who demonstrated healing skills should be permitted to practice medicine. Feminists, women practitioners such as Harriet K. Hunt, and working-class radicals joined together in the popular health movement to reject the perceived arrogance and incompetence of most doctors of the day.

During and following the mid-nineteenth century, women were widely regarded as inherently sickly, as documented by Ben Barker-Benfield in *Horrors of the Half-Known Life*. To help protect themselves, women at Ladies' Physiological Reform Societies, an outgrowth of the popular health movement, lectured on sensible—yet radical—ideas such as personal hygiene and frequent bathing, preventive care, elementary anatomy, loose-fitting female clothing (whalebone corsets worn by women of fashion disastrously cramped their internal organs), temperance, the importance of a healthy diet including whole-grain cereals, sex, and birth control. Birth control, and woman's right to it, continued to be highly controversial even up to the repeal of the last of the

Comstock Laws in 1965 in Connecticut. Female sectarian medical colleges established by branches of the popular health movement offered courses to women to improve both their own health and that of their families, while women graduates frequently taught through the societies. Lydia Folger Fowler (1822–1879) was one such teacher; in 1851 she was appointed professor of midwifery at the Rochester Eclectic Medical College, becoming the first woman to hold a professorship in a legally authorized medical school in the United States.

These and other topics, including abortion rights, the doctor-patient relationship, and overuse of drugs and surgical intervention, together with many of the historical issues of women's health care such as licensure, sparked the women's health movement of the 1960s and remain central to women's health issues today. We are still struggling over questions of licensure, of whether technological intervention of specialists is superior to the more natural healing methods of general practitioners and midwives, and while there are now almost as many women as men in medical schools, certain specialties are still dominated by men. Given today's advanced technology, the complexities have changed, but the fundamental conflicts surrounding women's health care—who determines and controls the right to practice and in what manner—remain the same. This sameness does not invalidate today's issues in any way, but shows us there are lessons to be learned from past struggles.

Women Healers in Shamanic Culture

SUZANNE CLORES

Suzanne Clores published her first book, Native American Women, *as she was graduating from college in 1995, whereupon she became the youngest member of the Authors Guild. Since then she has been collecting material for her forthcoming study on young woman and spirituality.—B. S.*

Ancient societies all over the world entrusted the health of the ir people to shamans. Shamanism is a system of healing that coexists with religion and is used to heal people suffering from spiritual sickness.

Healing techniques differ, depending on the perceived nature of the illness. The shaman may extract an invasive pathogen from the patient's body or use other rituals to recall the patient's lost or stolen soul to his or her body. In order to perform these rituals, the shaman enters a state of altered consciousness, a trancelike state in which the soul leaves the body and travels to various landscapes in the shamanic cosmology. In these subterranean or celestial landscapes, the shaman's soul is able to contact helper spirits who guide her to the information she seeks, either the whereabouts of the soul or the location and nature of the pathogen.

A shaman may play a number of other healing roles in a community: priest, magician, medicine man or woman. But these other roles alone do not make someone a shaman. It is the unique ability to escort the souls of the living and the dead to the otherworld that confers this status on a healer. The shaman is able to communicate with the spirits without being possessed by them or becoming their instrument, and can therefore take charge of the mystical and ecstatic practices of the community's religion, serving as a direct link between the living, their gods, and their dead.

Sickness or a religious crisis may indicate a shamanic vocation. Sickness is often regarded as a symbolic death for the shaman initiate, equivalent to a calling, and recovery is the first sign of resurrection, an indication from the spirits that the person called is open to the task.

In some cultures, only women or men may be shamans; in others, both men and women may fill this role. In Mircea Eliade's cross-cultural study *Shamanism: Archaic Techniques of Ecstasy,* the cosmologies of some shamanic cultures in Southeast Asia, the Arctic, and Africa portray women as great overarching mothers in charge of either celestial or infernal realms of the shamanic universe. Eliade suggests that these archetypes are remnants of an ancient matriarchy, in which the mothers granted permission to hunt, promised fair weather, kept the dead, and enabled shamans to do their work. Over time these indigenous societies fell under the influence of new cultures and religions, and changes occurred in their cosmologies.

The cosmology and practice of the Araucanian Indians of south-central Chile demonstrate many of these features of shamanism. For example, according to anthropological records dating from the early twentieth century, the Araucanians corresponded with a celestial Father God, but the art of shamanizing was in the hands of the women, indicating a religion in transition. Sudden illness in a young woman often informed the community of her candidacy as shaman. The Araucanian girl's initiation includes instruction from the spirits and older women shamans, symbolized in public ritual.

One account tells of a young girl who fainted and then reported upon awakening that she had been summoned to become a *machi* (a shaman) by a clear voice of divinity. During her initiation, she undressed and lay down on a couch made of blankets and sheepskins. The old shamans of the community began a ritual massage, rubbing her body with *canelo* leaves while repeating magical words. Other women attending the ceremony rang bells and sang. The older women then bent over the initiate and sucked her breast, belly, and head as if to extract illness. The modern explanation of shamanic sucking and spitting identifies the act as necessary symbolism for the removal of pathogens.

The following day a crowd of guests arrived at the celebration. They formed a circle around the altar and the initiate's family provided lambs to be sacrificed. An old *machi* invoked the celestial Great Shaman, or Father God, asking him to be favorable to them. After the animals were sacrificed, music began and dancing continued all night. At dawn the following day, the old shamans danced to the drums again, and several dropped into trance. An elder *machi* blindfolded the initiate and cut her fingers and lips several times with a white quartz knife. She then cut her own fingers and lips and mixed her blood with that of the initiate. The ritual cutting with a white quartz knife and the comingling of blood at these sacred points signifies the spiritual exchange between the old *machi* and the initiate. In some shamanic traditions, white quartz is considered to confer magical abilities of sight and the mouth and the fingers are thought to be places where the soul can pass into the body.

Finally, the candidate, and then the elder *machis,* climbed a nine-foot ladder-like tree trunk that had been positioned outside the initiate's house. This physical journey symbolized the psychic journeys the young *machi* would take as a healer. It also demonstrated publicly that the elder *machis* had passed on their knowledge and connection to the spirits, establishing the initiate's new, exalted social position.

When the initiate came down and her feet touched the ground, the crowd rushed toward her, wanting to be close to her soon after her symbolic ascent to the celestial realm. The initiate asked the Father God for the tools necessary for the work. Among her requests were the gift of clairvoyance (so she could see illness in a patient's body), the art of drumming (used to facilitate trance), and a striped or colored healing stone with which to purify a patient's body. (If it is projected into the body and comes out covered in blood, the patient is near death.) The old *machi* then promised the community that the young initiate would not practice black magic.

Shamanism can be traced back 30,000 years to Paleolithic drawings. In the last half-century, anthropologists have brought back a tremendous amount of information about its practice to the United States, and South American shamanic traditions have been adapted for use by non-Native Americans wishing to heal both psychological and physical ailments. The Foundation for Shamanic Studies, which is devoted to teaching and preserving shamanic traditions all over the world, estimates that 65 percent of its students and 60 percent of its certified practitioners are women. The foundation reaches nearly 5,000 people each year.

Shamanism remains a special system of healing that fills a gap between our modern therapies for mental health and institutions of religion. Sandra Ingerman, a psychologist and shamanic practitioner, has written several books on the shamanic concepts of soul loss and retrieval using contemporary psychological ideas as a bridge to public understanding. She estimates that 90 percent of her clients are therapists interested in incorporating shamanic techniques into their traditional method of psychotherapeutic healing.

Rape in Great Art

AUDREY FLACK

Art editor, Judith Kletter. Based on a slide lecture prepared and given by the author. Reprinted by permission

Many men—as well as women—attest that Audrey Flack's slide lecture on misogyny and violence against women in great art has deeply shaken, disturbed, and ultimately enlightened them. A world-renowned photo-realist painter and sculptor of contemporary, neoclassical goddesses, for years Flack was a persistent feminist voice at the American College Art Association. —B. S.

Looking at art in a great museum such as the Metropolitan Museum of Art can be a wonderful and uplifting experience, but the average woman doesn't realize that she is seeing rape all around her. She takes it for granted, looks at the paintings, and walks right on. Our vision has been so coerced that we accept scenes of brutality and abduction as part of out historical memory. What I am hoping for is an enlightened vision.

THE *VENUS OF WILLENDORF*

When I lecture or write on the Goddess, I go way back to ancient times and reference statues like the *Venus of Willendorf* (Fig. 1). The Venus has become a favorite of many women, including myself, but she must be examined more thoroughly and viewed through a new lens in order to be understood. She is one of the oldest goddesses to be uncovered, a small figurine with breasts so voluminous it would be hard for her to walk. Her belly is enormous and protrudes in front of her. She has something on her head, I have never been quite sure what, either a cap of curled hair or a tight-fitting hat, but in either case, she has no face. You cannot see her eyes or her expression—she just is.

Her feet are are very small, not unlike the big-breasted women with tiny feet that the famed sculptor Gaston Lachaise creates. There is one always on display in the garden of the Museum of Modern Art. It would be difficult, if not impossible, to support such a body with such malformed feet.

I am reminded of Chinese girls who for centuries had to endure their feet being bound in order to keep them from growing to a normal size. Tiny feet were considered a symbol of beauty. These women became cripples who could barely walk, all for the sake of male adulation. But it is more like male *domination,* for such a woman could not run away or protect herself. She is completely defenseless.

And so is the lovable *Venus of Willendorf.* People like her because she is not a threat, she is not a sexual object. Her body has been used a great deal. She is probably a very strong woman who survived childbirth without the help of a male obstetrician. And not just one birth: you can imagine how many women

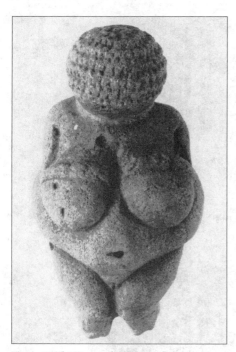

Figure 1: *The Venus of Willendorf*
[© Naturhistorisches Museum Wien.
Photo by Alice Schumacher]

died in childbirth in those days. Thin women, women with not enough fat or poor immune systems, probably perished immediately.

The *Venus of Willendorf* is a survivor, a giver of life. Her breasts nurtured many children, and she became an object of worship. I believe that the *Venus of Willendorf* was sculpted by a woman for other women, to be held and carried as a magic charm, transmitting much-needed healing energy during childbirth or other life-threatening situations. We love her because she is a survival object, delivering life forces to us even to this day.

But large, pendulous breasts ache and can cause back problems, and we all know the dangers of being overweight. Like tiny bound feet, big breasts burden us, tie us down; nevertheless, women put their own health at risk to enlarge their breasts with implants. I wonder if men would think about putting implants in their testicles. How would it feel having those testes hanging down to their knees? Would women find it attractive? I doubt it. Images of beauty must be reevaluated and reimaged. Double standards must be exposed and questioned.

THE EXPULSION OF ADAM AND EVE FROM THE GARDEN BY MASACCIO

In this wonderful painting by the fifteenth-century Italian master Masaccio, an angry angel is pointing a finger at the two sinners (Fig. 2). Adam is covering his eyes. Eve's face has a pained expression. She is covering her breasts and genitals in shame, but Adam remains exposed. What exactly is the terrible act she has committed? Let's think about it.

She took the apple from the tree of knowledge. She wanted information. She wanted to know what to do when she gave birth to her children. She needed to be informed about the process and what she was in for. It's the most basic question any woman can ask. A baby would grow inside of her and had to come out. She didn't even know what part of her body it would emerge from. Her desire for knowledge was considered a sin. Her only other alternative was to remain childlike and dependent, not in control of her body, her life, or her death. It is important to reassess early biblical and mythological stories and analyze how women are portrayed.

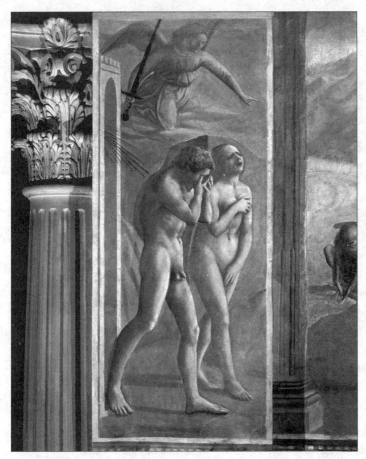

Figure 2: *The Expulsion of Adam and Eve from the Garden* by Masaccio
[Scala/Art Resource, NY]

LEDA AND THE SWAN BY MICHELANGELO

Myths about ancient goddesses are filled with tales of rape and violence. The male god is never held accountable. Why does Zeus, the most powerful of all the gods, have to deceive and rape women? Can't he get them any other way?

In this painting he transforms himself into an excessively long-necked swan and somehow manages to impregnate Leda (Fig. 3). While the image of a white-feathered giant swan twisting its body and elongated neck around a nude Leda may appear to be glamorous, imagine what a woman would *really* feel if she were penetrated against her will by an overgrown waterfowl.

THE RAPE OF EUROPA BY TITIAN

Here we see Europa lying flat on her back on top of a bull (Fig. 4). Her legs are spread wide apart facing the viewer in anticipation of receiving her abductor

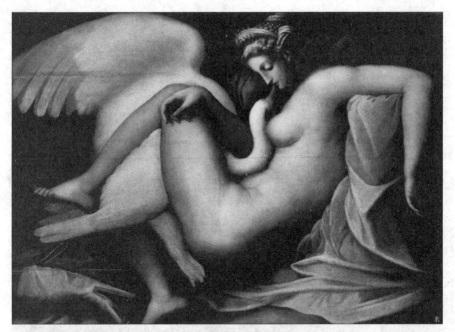

Figure 3: *Leda and the Swan* by Michelangelo [Alinari/Art Resource, NY]

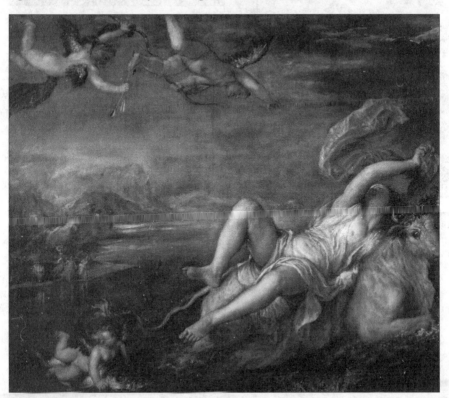

Figure 4: *The Rape of Europa* by Titian [Isabella Stewart Gardner Museum, Boston]

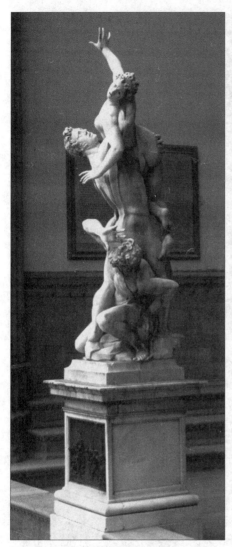

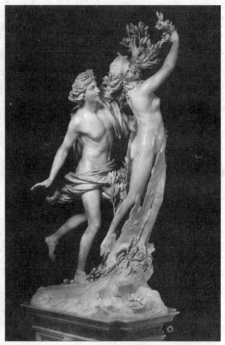

Figure 5: *Apollo and Daphne* by Bernini
[Alinari/Art Resource, NY]

Figure 6: *Rape of the Sabine Woman* by
Giovanni Bologna [photo by Manrico
Romano]

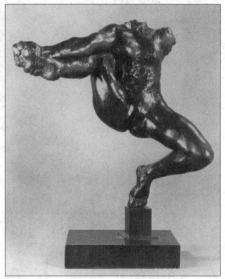

Figure 7: *Iris, Messenger of the Gods* by Rodin
[Los Angeles County Museum of Art, gift of
B. Gerald Cantor Art Foundation]

rapist. Europa's rapist is, once again, Zeus, who has transformed himself into a ridiculous, drooling white bull, decorated with garlands of flowers around his neck and horns, as if that would make him more appealing. The reality of being raped by a bull is grotesque, and yet this painting is considered delightful.

Museums all over the world are filled with images that glamorize and romanticize rape, and we have come to accept these images as part of the nature of things. Most often the woman looks like a helpless but willing victim. At other times she appears to be enjoying her situation.

In reality a woman confronted by a rapist will close her legs rather than open them, shield her body rather than expose it; she will fight her attacker using any means—scratching, clawing, kicking, gouging. She will not submit willingly. All rapists are ineffectual men who force sex in a misguided attempt to secure love. But even a rapist knows that no weapons or threat of power can force love from a woman against her will.

RAPE OF THE SABINE WOMAN BY GIOVANNI BOLOGNA

Rape is the subject of many great works of art—for example, Reubens' *Rape of the Daughters of Leucippus* or Bernini's *Apollo and Daphne* (Fig. 5)—though it may not be part of our conscious perception. The women's nude bodies are painted in pale tones, in sharp contrast to the ruddy, healthy-looking men who are either draped or fully clothed and armed with breastplates, shields, and swords.

I have looked at Giovanni da Bologna's *Rape of the Sabine Woman* (Fig. 6) for decades—I even saw the original in Florence—but only recently did I realize that this beautiful statue is a brutal rape scene. Throughout my entire art education I was taught to admire the lavish curves of the women's nude bodies, the graceful swing of their arms, and the expressiveness of the woman's hand in the air, but I was never once led to ask, "Why is her hand up in the air?" I will tell you why: she is imploring God, a patriarchal deity with a white beard, to descend from the heavens and come to her aid. He never does.

IRIS, MESSENGER OF THE GODS BY RODIN

This is another image that disturbs me (Fig. 7). Rodin exposes the model's genitals by spreading her legs apart as if she were on an examining table in a doctor's office. Rodin was a voyeur and a womanizer. This image is not surprising in our culture—we are used to women being displayed. Men would be embarrassed and upset to have their bodies portrayed in a similar manner. I'm not talking about nude statues. I'm talking about voyeurism and the double standard.

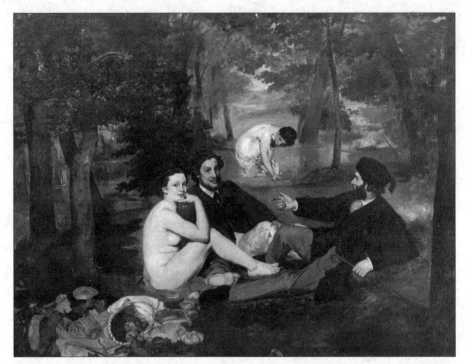

Figure 8: *Luncheon on the Grass* by Manet [Giraudon/Art Resource, NY]

LUNCHEON ON THE GRASS BY MANET

This is one painting that has always made me uncomfortable (Fig. 8). The men are sitting around fully clothed, having a picnic on the grass, and the woman with them is completely nude. The men are fully dressed, in suits and ties no less. Whenever I look at this painting, I think, isn't she cold? Her bare bottom is on the grass with all the bugs and dirt. Isn't the breeze affecting her? She is so vulnerable. Manet's purpose was to shock but also to titillate his male viewers.

PERSEUS WITH THE HEAD OF MEDUSA BY CELLINI

According to mythology, Medusa was a hideous gorgon with fangs, scales, and claws. Live snakes writhed in her hair. She was so ugly that any man who looked at her turned to stone. Freud even claimed that men were frozen with terror because Medusa's head looks like a huge bloody vagina, symbolizing castration.

In Cellini's sculpture, Perseus is stepping on Medusa's body as she writhes in pain, twisted and deformed (Fig. 9). He has just cut off her head by sneaking up behind her, not looking directly at her face, but instead looking at her reflection in his shield, which acts as a mirror. He holds her head up triumphantly as blood spurts from her neck. He is a hero. But look again—there is more to this story....

THE ANCIENT GORGON AND *COLOSSAL HEAD OF MEDUSA*

When I first began to research the story of Medusa and went back to Ovid, I found that a lot had been left out (Fig. 10). Medusa was one of triplets. Her sisters were hideous gorgons, but she was a beautiful sea creature with long, flowing hair. She looked like a goddess and sang like a siren.

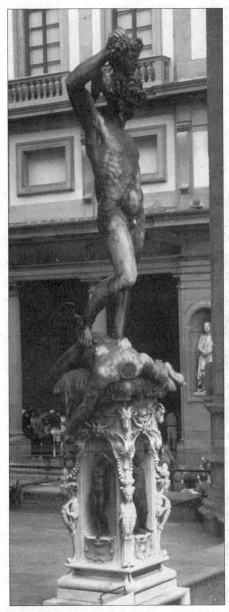

When Medusa was a young woman—I imagine her as a girl really, about 14 years old—Poseidon, god of the sea, fell in love with her. And he did what all gods do when they fall in love: he raped her. The violation took place in Athena's temple. According to myth, Athena was so angry that her temple had been defiled that she turned Medusa's hair into snakes. The innocent Medusa is thus twice victimized, once by rape and once by Athena's punishment.

I think that Athena was really trying to *empower* Medusa by guaranteeing that she would never be raped again: if any man harassed her, he turned to stone. But this empowerment is double-edged. Medusa never wanted to

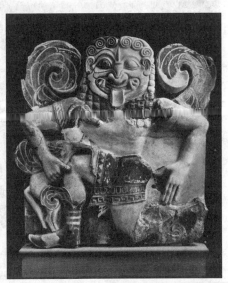

Figure 9: *Perseus with the Head of Medusa* by Cellini [Photo by Manrico Romano]

Figure 10: *The Ancient Gorgon* [Alinari/Art Resource, NY]

kill anyone, yet because men die at the sight of her, she can never again have sex. The same is true of victims of rape, who often cannot enjoy sex anymore, or at least not for a long while.

It took me 20 years to understand the story of Medusa from a woman's perspective, to see her as she truly was: a frightened young woman who had been brutally abused, so ashamed of the way she looked that she hid in her lair at the end of the world. But she isn't ugly; on the contrary, she is ravishingly beautiful. And this is how I portray her, waking up from her sleep just before the cowardly Perseus beheads her (Fig. 11).

There are wonderful men out there—considerate, kind, gentle men who know that the only way to save the planet is to share the power with women. But they need to base their masculinity on new role models, not on so-called heroes like Poseidon, Zeus, or Perseus. They need to be able to hear the women speak.

Very often I portray goddesses with their lips are slightly parted, as if they are about to speak. I want to give them a voice. It's time for them to speak out and show their true beauty. It's time to set these ancient myths straight.

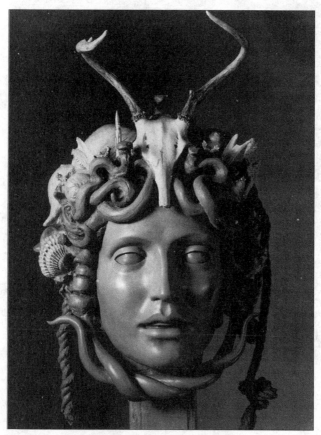

Figure 11: *Colossal Head of Medusa* by Audrey Flack
[Photo by Steve Lopez]

Forgotten Goddess History

SHERRILL SELLMAN

Excerpted from Sherrill Sellman, *Hormone Heresy: What Women Must Know about their Hormones,* Honolulu, GetWell International, 1998. Reprinted by permission.

In "Confronting the 'Goddess," a section in her already-classic 1979 book, Drawing Down the Moon, *Margot Adler comments that "the idea of 'Goddess' is fraught with problems and potentialities for feminists.... Western women have been excluded from the deity quest for thousands of years, since the end of Goddess worship in the West. The small exception is the veneration paid by Catholics to the Virgin Mary, a pale remnant of the Great Goddess. So, if one purpose of deity is to give us an image we can become, it is obvious that women have been left out of the quest, or at least have been forced to strive for an oppressive and unobtainable masculine image.... The obvious criticism is that the idea of a single Goddess, conceived of as transcendent and apart, creates as many problems as the male 'God.' Trading 'Daddy' for 'Mommy' is not a liberation."*

On the other hand, as Sherrill Sellman explains, a longing to know more about ancient cults of the moon Goddess, as well as a hope or even a conviction (!) that such understanding could be salutary for women's reproductive health, continues to pique the interest of many nature-minded women.—B. S.

Archaeological evidence suggests that thousands of years ago, human beings revered a female deity as the embodiment of the forces of life, death, and rebirth. These Goddess-oriented cultures were most likely matrilineal hunter-gatherer societies, in which there was relative harmony and equality between the sexes.

The art and artifacts that these early humans have left us scattered throughout the Old World suggest a religion that "embraced the constant and periodic renewal of life in which death was not separate from life," viewed the earth as a giver of life, and held the natural cycles of women in deep respect. In the societies where the Goddess was worshipped, "women held exalted roles as priestesses, leaders, healers, midwives, and diviners."

The moon held a special place in the worship of the Goddess. Noting the correspondence between women's menstrual cycle and the phases of the moon, early societies may have regarded the moon was feminine. Death was but "the precursor to rebirth," and the sex act was a source of "ecstasy, healing, regeneration, and spiritual illumination."

About 5,000 years ago warring tribes from northern Europe and central Asia invaded western Europe, the Near East, and India, conquering the indigenous cultures and supplanting the Goddess culture with their own patriarchal solar gods. "Women were stripped of their positions of political authority and their decision-making powers as leaders.... They were deprived of their spiritual authority as priestesses. Banned from functioning in their professional healing capacities, they were progressively disempowered from expressing their sexuality, intelligence, and self-sufficiency."

The major world religions that we know today "usurped the power of the feminine, declaring that which once was sacred to be taboo.... The patriarchy now ruled supreme. Inherent in this culture was blind obedience to the male principle, embodied by the father. It was based on the supremacy of the intellect, rigid rules, violence, control over others and the environment, efficiency, and suppression of spontaneity and emotions. Women were... considered the property of men. Women and all womanly functions... became synonymous with evil."

So great is the power of the patriarchal system that it is "encoded within the very psyches of women... passed down from generation to generation. It shapes [women's] behaviors, attitudes, and the very health of their bodies. It is the force that drives women to exhaustion, unable to stop long enough to attend to their own needs. It creates their obsession with a body that is never perfect enough. It is why women seek external authority to tell them how to live their own lives. It ensures that women remain economically, politically, and spiritually helpless and dependent."

And the patriarchal system affects our health, causing women to "feel shame, disgust, and guilt toward their bodies and normal female functions." Instead of being a revered and natural cycle, menstruation becomes "the curse" and causes millions of women to suffer each month with PMS and menstrual cramps, a symptom of women's rejection of the "feminine self." Because of the influence of the patriarchy, almost 50 percent of Western women have hysterectomies and 60 percent of women experience painful periods each month.

Sellman calls on women to "reclaim all that has been kept hidden from them. Reclaiming this wisdom begins with honoring the cyclic nature of women. Women are lunar in nature. Just as the moon continues to cycle through its changes each month, so, too, do women. The menstrual cycle is the most basic, earthy cycle women have. The flow of blood is a woman's connection to the archetypal feminine. In many cultures the menstrual cycle was viewed as sacred because it reconnected a woman with the creative principles of the universe."

Some believe that the menstrual cycle enhances creativity. Says Sellman: "The ebb and flow of dreams, intuition, and hormones associated with different parts of the cycle offer women a profound opportunity to deepen their connection to their inner knowing."

A Good Woman Is a Sacrificing One

STEPHANIE GOLDEN

Stephanie Golden, *Slaying the Mermaid: Women and the Culture of Sacrifice*, New York, Harmony Books. Reprinted by permission.

In her 1998 publication, Slaying the Mermaid: Women and the Culture of Sacrifice, *Stephanie Golden takes up some of the same themes as* The Woman's Bible, *and reveals how the theology of "female piety" encouraged (among other unpleasantries) eating disorders, self-mortification, and the withholding of pain relievers to women in labor.—B. S.*

D uring the later Middle Ages, an increase in religious institutions and movements provided new opportunities for women to express their piety, and the number of female saints grew. Although the culture told men and women equally that suffering—specifically "extreme self-mortification"—"was the way to salvation," the differences between women's and men's social circumstances dictated characteristic differences in their religious practices. Women's mysticism more often involved self-inflicted physical suffering, which was more likely to center on extreme fasting, sometimes to the point of self-starvation. The fourteenth-century saint Catherine of Siena, for example, began to fast as a child and by 16 was living on raw vegetables, bread, and water. She later became completely unable to eat, and died in her early thirties of self-starvation. Among her other penitential practices were self-flagellation and sleep deprivation. Other female saints inflicted equally flamboyant sufferings on themselves, often while struggling against male religious authorities suspicious of such extremism. Since women were considered morally weaker than men, it was feared that their austerities might lead to heresy or be inspired by the devil.

Psychological analyses of the female saints' behavior have focused on guilt, self-hatred, and family relations, but here it is more useful to relate their acts to the social context. A central theme of medieval religiosity was the imitation of Christ, whose purpose was a mystical fusion with his suffering on the cross and the offering of this suffering as a form of service for the salvation of the world. Because of the nature of their roles in medieval culture, women were particularly drawn to this form of piety, and to expressing it by rejecting food. Unable to control wealth and frequently forced into marriage, medieval women found their sphere of action limited. Their main activities were nurturing and serving; in medieval society, as in many other cultures, they were the preparers and servers of food—though not necessarily its eaters; they were generally expected to eat less than men and to eat lighter food. For them, suffering and fasting were symbolic acts that matched medieval notions ascribing to women a "suffering, giving self." Thus while male saints were seen as "models of action," female saints were "models of suffering and inner spirituality."

Women also chose self-mortification, especially through fasting, at least in part in reaction to a tradition that associated the female with nature and matter—that is, the evils of flesh—and the male with reason and spirit. Woman was "a very weak vessel" who had inherited the failings of Eve and was equally likely to harm man through her voracious sexuality. Fasting was a way to expiate the evils associated with the body and even to punish it. In later ages, women's relationship with food continued to be a significant component of their self-sacrifice. What is more, we can trace the exemplary suffering woman through vast cultural changes, right down to our own culture's fascination with a modern version of the female salvation-seeker: artists like Sylvia Plath and Frida Kahlo.

As the Middle Ages passed, the style of female piety changed: by the end of the sixteenth century, assertive, heroic asceticism like that of Catherine of Siena was frowned upon. The new Catholic model of female piety was a woman "visited by God with strange, painful maladies" that tortured her, deepening her spirituality until she died and could finally embrace the heavenly bridegroom. Unlike the earlier saints, whose self-mortification led them to a mystical wisdom that church authorities respected, holy women of this period achieved sainthood through suffering only. For example, Mary Magdalen de' Pazzi, daughter of a prominent Florentine family, refused to marry and entered a convent, where she ate very little and mortified her body. "Beginning in 1595 she prayed for… [an] atrocious death from painful illness" and eventually experienced "a three-year terminal illness marked by excruciating toothaches, head and chest pains, fever, and coughing." The "model of the suffering holy female, immobilized and racked by pain," appeared again in the nineteenth century, in a secular context. Despite its conformance to tradition, however, all this seemingly passive, pious suffering also had an active aspect: it conferred on a woman a kind of autonomy by eliminating the church and its priests as intermediaries between her and Jesus, while also enabling her to escape traditional roles, particularly that imposed by marriage.

In the seventeenth century, perhaps seeking a more active outlet for their piety, holy women turned to serving the poor and the sick. But meanwhile, suffering took on additional significance for ordinary women, as both Protestant and Catholic authorities became increasingly concerned by the "potentially destructive female nature" and the danger presented by female sexuality unless it was controlled within marriage, where the wife was supposed to be obedient to the husband, serve him, bear children—and suffer in the process. God's judgment on Eve in Genesis—"I will greatly multiply your pain in childbearing; in pain you shall bring forth children"—was taken literally. "Passive suffering and the archetypal female experience of childbirth have been seen as identical. Passive suffering has thus been seen as a universal, 'natural' female destiny, carried into every sphere of our experience," explains Adrienne Rich in her study of motherhood. The sixteenth-century Protestant theologian and reformer John Calvin asserted that woman was saved not by faith but by her suffering in childbirth, which erased the sin she inherited from Eve. So necessary was this suffering considered to be that in 1591 an English midwife was executed for giving pain relievers during labor. Even as late as the mid-nineteenth century, a French bishop, Félix Dupanloup, wrote: "It is quite evident that the mother is destined to an expiatory and holy suffering. She is great because she suffers." In the same period, the British clergy attacked the introduction by a Scottish physician of anesthesia during childbirth as "a decoy of Satan" that would "harden society." The clear implication is that women do the suffering for everyone else; if their pain is taken away, men lose the general redemption it provides. The theological context had changed since the fourteenth century, but the message was the same..

Witches, Midwives, and Nurses: A History of Women Healers

BARBARA EHRENREICH AND DEIRDRE ENGLISH

Barbara Ehrenreich and Deirdre English, *Witches, Midwives, and Nurses: A History of Women Healers,* New York: Feminist Press at the City University of New York, 1973. Reprinted by permission.

Barbara Ehrenreich and Deirdre English's Witches, Midwives, and Nurses: A History of Women Healers, *a 45-page pamphlet published in 1973, revealed some of the thuggish tactics powerful males often used to oust women (and alternative providers) from medical and midwifery practice, as well as the extreme—even lunatic—treatments offered by these more formally trained physicians. Defenders of orthodox medicine dismissed and tried to discredit Barbara and Deirdre's influential work, but a decade later, confirmation emerged in the form of a book that won the 1984 Pulitzer Prize for General Nonfiction,* The Social Transformation of American Medicine. The Rise of a Sovereign Profession and the Making of a Vast Industry *by Princeton University sociologist Paul Starr. Starr confirmed that in the U.S. colonies, "women were expected to deal with illness in the home and to keep a stock of remedies on hand; in the fall they put away medicinal herbs as they stored preserves. Care of the sick was part of the domestic economy for which the wife assumed responsibility... in worrisome cases perhaps bringing in an older woman who had a reputation for skill with the sick." Many guides to domestic medicine were available: "They argued that medicine was filled with unnecessary obscurity and complexity, and should be made intelligible and practicable."*

In contrast to home remedies, Starr recapitulates the teachings of Dr. Benjamin Rush, the revolutionary leader, who "greatly influenced future generations of physicians at the University of Pennsylvania." Rush maintained that there was but one disease, "morbid excitement induced by capillary tension," and its one remedy was "to deplete the body by letting blood with the lancet and emptying out the stomach and bowels with the use of powerful emetics and cathartics. Patients could be bled until unconscious and given heavy doses of the cathartic calomel (mercurous chloride) until they salivated."

"Heroic" therapy of this type "dominated American medical practice in the first decades of the 19th century," Starr reminds us, which helps explain why, by the 1830s, many states revoked the rights to licensure they had first granted to orthodox doctors around the time of the revolution.—B. S.

INTRODUCTION

Women have always been healers. They were the unlicensed doctors and anatomists of Western history. They were abortionists, nurses, and counselors. They were pharmacists, cultivating healing herbs and exchanging the secrets of their uses. They were midwives, traveling from home to home and village to village. For centuries women were doctors without degrees, barred from books and lectures, learning from each other, and passing on experience from neighbor to neighbor and mother to daughter. They were called "wise women" by the people, witches or charlatans by the authorities. Medicine is part of our heritage as women, our history, and our birthright.

Today, however, health care is the property of male professionals. Ninety-three percent of the doctors in the United States are men; and almost all the top directors and administrators of health institutions. Women are still in the overall majority—70 percent of health workers are women—but we have been incorporated as *workers* into an industry where the bosses are men. We are no longer independent practitioners, known by our own names, for our own work. We are, for the most part, institutional fixtures, filling faceless job slots: clerk, dietary aide, technician, and maid.

When we are allowed to participate in the healing process, we can do so only as nurses. And nurses of every rank from aide up are just "ancillary workers" in relation to the doctors (from the Latin *ancilla*, maid servant). From the nurse's aide, whose menial tasks are spelled out with industrial precision, to the "professional" nurse, who translates the doctors' orders into the aide's tasks, nurses share the status of a uniformed maid service to the dominant male professionals.

Our subservience is reinforced by our ignorance, and our ignorance is *enforced.* Nurses are taught not to question, not to challenge. "The doctor knows best." He is the shaman, in touch with the forbidden, mystically complex world of Science, which we have been taught is beyond our grasp. Women health workers are alienated from the scientific substance of their work, restricted to the "womanly" business of nurturing and housekeeping—a passive, silent majority.

We are told that our subservience is biologically ordained: women are inherently nurse-like and not doctor-like. Sometimes we even try to console ourselves with the theory that we were defeated by anatomy before we were defeated by men, that women have been so trapped by the cycles of menstruation and reproduction that they have never been free and creative agents outside their homes. Another myth, fostered by conventional medical histories, is that male professionals won out on the strength of their superior technology. According to these accounts, (male) science more or less automatically replaced (female) superstition—which from then on was called "old wives' tales."

But history belies these theories. Women have been autonomous healers, often the only healers for women and the poor. And we found, in the periods we have studied, that, if anything, it was the male professionals who clung to untested doctrines and ritualistic practices—and it was the woman healers who represented a more humane, empirical approach to healing.

Our position in the health system today is not "natural." It is a condition which has to be explained. In this pamphlet we have asked: How did we arrive at our present position of subservience from our former position of leadership?

We learned this much: that the suppression of women health workers and the rise to dominance of male professionals was not a "natural" process, resulting automatically from changes in medical science, nor was it the result women's failure to take on healing work. It was an active *takeover* by male professionals. And it was not science that enabled men to win out: The critical battles took place long before the development of modern scientific technology.

The stakes of the struggle were high: Political and economic monopolization of medicine meant control over its institutional organizations, its theory and practice, its profits and prestige. And the stakes are even higher today, when total control of medicine means potential power to determine who will live and will die, who is fertile and who is sterile, who is "mad" and who sane.

The suppression of female healers by the medical establishment was a political struggle, first, in that it is part of the history of sex struggle in general. The status of women healers has risen and fallen with the status of women. When women healers were attacked, they were attacked as *women;* when they fought back, they fought back in solidarity with all women.

It was a political struggle, second, in that it was part of a *class* struggle. Women healers were people's doctors, and their medicine was part of a poo ple's subculture. To this very day women's medical practice has thrived in the midst of rebellious lower-class movements which have struggled to be free from the established authorities. Male professionals, on the other hand, served the ruling class—both medically and politically. Their interests have been advanced by the universities, the philanthropic foundations, and the law. They owe their victory not so much to their own efforts, but to the intervention of the ruling class they served.

This pamphlet represents a beginning of the research which will have to be done to recapture our history as health workers. It is a fragmentary account, assembled from sources which were usually sketchy and often biased, by women who are in no sense "professional" historians. We confined ourselves to Western history, since the institutions we confront today are the products of Western civilization. We are far from being able to present a complete chronological history. Instead, we looked at two separate, important phases in the male takeover of health care: the suppression of witches in medieval Europe, and the rise of the male medical profession in nineteenth-century America.

To know our history is to begin to see how to take up the struggle again.

WITCHCRAFT AND MEDICINE IN THE MIDDLE AGES

Witches lived and were burned long before the development of modern medical technology. The great majority of them were healers serving the peasant population, and their suppression marks one of the opening struggles in the history of man's suppression of women as healers.

The other side of the suppression of witches as healers was the creation of a new male medical profession, under the protection and patronage of the ruling classes. This new European medical profession played an important role in the witch-hunts, supporting the witches' prosecutors with "medical" reasoning:

> Because the Medieval Church, with the support of kings, princes and secular authorities, controlled medical education and practice, the inquisition [witch-hunts] constitutes, among other things, an early instance of the "professional" repudiating the skills and interfering with the rights of the "nonprofessional" to minister to the poor. (Thomas Szasz, *The Manufacture of Madness*)

The witch-hunts left a lasting effect: An aspect of the female has ever since been associated with the witch, and an aura of contamination has remained—especially around the midwife and other women healers. This early and devastating exclusion of women from independent healing roles was a violent precedent and warning: It was to become a theme of our history. The women's health movement of today has ancient roots in the medieval covens, and its opponents have as their ancestors those who ruthlessly forced the elimination of witches.

THE WITCH CRAZE The age of witch-hunting spanned more than four centuries (from the fourteenth to the seventeenth century) in its sweep from Germany to England. It was born in feudalism and lasted—gaining in virulence—well into the "age of reason." The witch craze took different forms at different times and places, but never lost its essential character: that of ruling-class campaign of terror directed against the female peasant population. Witches represented a political, religious, and sexual threat to the Protestant and Catholic churches alike, as well as to the state.

The extent of the witch craze is startling: In the late fifteenth and early sixteenth centuries there were thousands upon thousands of executions—usually live burnings at the stake—in Germany, Italy, and other countries. In the mid-sixteenth century the terror spread to France, and finally to England. One writer has estimated the number of executions at an average of 600 a year for certain German cities—or two a day, "leaving out Sundays." Nine hundred witches were destroyed in a single year in the Wertzberg area, and 1,000 in and around Como. At Toulouse, 400 were put to death in a day. In the Bishopric of Trier, in 1585, two villages were left with only one female inhabitant each. Many writers have estimated the total number killed to have been in the millions. Women made up some 85 percent of those executed—old women, young women, and children.*

Their scope alone suggests that the witch-hunts represent a deep-seated social phenomenon which goes far beyond the history of medicine. In locale and timing, the most virulent witch-hunts were associated with periods of great social upheaval shaking feudalism at its roots—mass peasant uprisings and conspiracies, the beginnings of capitalism, the rise of Protestantism. There is fragmentary evidence—which feminists ought to follow up—suggesting that in some areas witchcraft represented a female-led peasant rebellion. Here we can't attempt to explore the historical context of the witch-hunts in any depth. But we do have to get beyond some common myths about the witch craze—myths which rob the "witch" of any dignity and put blame on her and the peasants she served.

Unfortunately, the witch herself—poor and illiterate—did not leave us her story. It was recorded, like all history, by the educated elite, so today we know the witch only through the eyes of her persecutors.

Two of the most common theories of the witch-hunts are basically *medical interpretations*, attributing the witch craze to unexplainable outbreaks of mass hysteria. One version has it that the peasantry went mad. According to this, the witch craze was an epidemic of mass hatred and panic cast in images of a blood-lusty peasant bearing flaming torches. Another psychiatric interpretation holds that the witches themselves were insane....

But, in fact, the witch craze was neither a lynching party nor a mass suicide by hysterical women. Rather, it followed well ordered, legalistic procedures. The witch-hunts were well-organized campaigns, initiated, financed, and executed by church and state. To Catholic and Protestant witch-hunters alike, the unquestioned authority on how to conduct a witch-hunt was the *Malleus Maleficarum* or *Hammer of Witches,* written in 1484 by the Reverends Kramer and Sprenger (the "beloved sons" of Pope Innocent VIII). For three centuries this sadistic book lay on the bench of every judge, every witch-hunter. In a long section on judicial proceedings, the instructions make it clear how the "hysteria" was set off:

---

*We are omitting from this discussion any mention of the New England witch trials in the 1600s. These trials occurred on a relatively small scale, very late in the history of witch-hunts, and in an entirely different social context than the earlier European witch craze.

The job of initiating a witch trial was to be performed by either the vicar (priest) or judge of the county.... Anyone failing to report a witch faced both excommunication and a long list of temporal punishments....

Kramer and Sprenger gave detailed instructions about the use of tortures to force confessions and further accusations. Commonly, the accused was stripped naked and shaved of all her body hair, then subjected to thumbscrews and the rack, spikes and bone-crushing "boots," starvation and beatings. The point is obvious: The witch craze did not arise spontaneously in the peasantry. It was a calculated ruling-class campaign of terrorization.

THE CRIMES OF THE WITCHES Who were the witches, then, and what were their "crimes" that could arouse such vicious upper-class suppression?... Three central accusations emerge repeatedly in the history of witchcraft throughout northern Europe: First, witches are accused of every conceivable sexual crime against men. Quite simply, they are "accused" of female sexuality. Second, they are accused of being organized. Third, they are accused of having magical powers affecting health—of harming, but also of healing. They were often charged specifically with possessing medical and obstetrical skills.

First, consider the charge of sexual crimes. The medieval Catholic church elevated sexism to a point of principle: The *Malleus* declares, "When a woman thinks alone, she thinks evil." The misogyny of the church, if not proved by the witch craze itself, is demonstrated by its teaching that in intercourse the male deposits in the female a homunculus, or "little person," complete with soul, which is simply housed in the womb for nine months, without acquiring any attributes of the mother. The homunculus is not really safe, however, until it reaches male hands again, when a priest baptizes it, ensuring the salvation of its immortal soul. Another depressing fantasy of some medieval religious thinkers was that upon resurrection all human beings would be reborn as men!

The church associated women with sex, and all pleasure in sex was condemned, because it could only come from the devil. Witches were supposed to have gotten pleasure from copulation with the devil (despite the icy-cold organ he was reputed to possess) and they in turn infected men. Lust in either man or wife, then, was blamed on the female. On the other hand, witches were accused of making men impotent and of causing their penises to disappear. As for female sexuality, witches were accused, in effect, of giving contraceptive aid and of performing abortions:

> Now there are, as it is said in the Papal Bull, seven methods by which they infect with witchcraft the venereal act and the conception of the womb: First, by inclining the minds of men to inordinate passion; second, by obstructing their generative force; third, by removing the members accommodated to that act; fourth, by changing men into beasts by their magic act; fifth, by destroying the generative in women; sixth, by

procuring abortion; seventh, by offering children to the devils, besides other animals and fruits of the earth with which they work much harm.…(*Malleus Maleficarum*)

In the eyes of the church, all the witch's power was ultimately derived from her sexuality. Her career began with sexual intercourse with the devil. Each witch was confirmed at a general meeting (the witches' sabbath) at which the devil presided, often in the form of a goat, and had intercourse with the neophytes. In return for her powers, the witch promised to serve him faithfully. (In the imagination of the church even evil could only be thought of as ultimately male-directed!) As the *Malleus* makes clear, the devil almost always acts through the female, just as he did in Eden:

> All witchcraft comes from carnal lust, which in women is insatiable.…
> Wherefore for the sake of fulfilling their lusts they consort with devils…
> it is sufficiently clear that it is no matter for wonder that there are more
> women than men found infected with the heresy or witchcraft.… And
> blessed be the Highest Who has so far preserved the male sex from so
> great a crime.…

Not only were the witches women, they were women who seemed to be organized into an enormous secret society. A witch who was a proved member of the "devil's party" was more dreadful than one who had acted alone, and the witch-hunting literature is obsessed with the question of what went on at the witches' "sabbaths." (Eating of unbaptised babies? Bestialism and mass orgies? So went their lurid speculations.…)

In fact, there is evidence that women accused of being witches did meet locally in small groups and that these groups came together in crowds of hundreds or thousands on festival days. Some writers speculate that the meetings were occasions for trading herbal lore and passing on the news. We have little evidence about the political significance of the witches' organizations, but it's hard to imagine that they weren't connected to the peasant rebellions of the time. Any peasant organization, just being an organization, would attract dissidents, increase communication between villages, and build a spirit of collectivity and autonomy among the peasants.

WITCHES AS HEALERS We come now to the most fantastic accusation of all. The witch is accused not only of murdering and poisoning, sex crimes and conspiracy, but of *helping and healing.*…

Witch-healers were often the only general medical practitioners for a people who had no doctors and no hospitals and who were bitterly afflicted with poverty and disease. In particular, the association of the witch and the midwife was strong: "No one does more harm to the Catholic church than midwives," wrote witch-hunters Kramer and Sprenger.…

When faced with the misery of the poor, the church turned to the dogma that experience in this world is fleeting and unimportant. But there was a double standard at work, for the church was not against medical care for the upper class. Kings and nobles had their court physicians, who were men, sometimes even priests. The real issue was control: Male upper-class healing under the auspices of the church was acceptable; female healing as part of a peasant subculture was not.

The church saw its attack on peasant healers as an attack on *magic,* not medicine. The devil was believed to have real power on earth, and the use of that power by peasant women—whether for good or evil—was frightening to the church and state. The greater their satanic powers to help themselves, the less they were dependent on God and the church and the more they were potentially able to use their powers against God's order. Magic charms were thought to be at least as effective as prayer in healing the sick, but prayer was church-sanctioned and controlled while incantations and charms were not. Thus magic cures, even when successful, were an accused interference with the will of God, achieved with the help of the devil, and the cure itself was evil. There was no problem in distinguishing God's cures from the devil's, for obviously the Lord would work through priests and doctors rather than through peasant women.

The wise woman, or witch, had a host of remedies which had been tested in years of use. Many of the herbal remedies developed by witches still have their place in modern pharmacology. They had painkillers, digestive aids, and anti-inflammatory agents. They used ergot for the pain of labor at a time when the church held that pain in labor was the Lord's just punishment for Eve's original sin. Ergot derivatives are the principal drugs used today to hasten labor and aid in the recovery from childbirth. Belladonna—still used today as an antispasmodic—was used by the witch-healers to inhibit uterine contractions when miscarriage threatened. Digitalis, still an important drug in treating heart ailments, is said to have been discovered by an English witch....

The witch-healer's methods were as great a threat (to the Catholic Church, if not Protestant) as her results, for the witch was an empiricist: She relied on her senses rather than on faith or doctrine, she believed in trial and error, cause and effect. Her attitude was not religiously passive, but actively inquiring. She trusted her ability to find ways to deal with disease, pregnancy, and childbirth—whether through medications or charms. In short, her magic was the science of her time.

The church, by contrast was deeply anti-empirical. It discredited the value of the material world and had a profound distrust of the senses. There was no point in looking for natural laws that govern physical phenomena, for the world is created anew by God in every instant. Kramer and Sprenger, in the *Malleus,* quote St. Augustine on the deceptiveness of the senses:

> Now the motive of the will is something perceived through the senses
> or the intellect, both of which are subject to the power of the devil....

The senses are the devil's playground, the arena into which he will try to lure men away from Faith and into the conceits of the intellect or the delusions of carnality.

In the persecution of the witch, the anti-empiricist and misogynist anti-sexual obsessions of the church coincide: Empiricism and sexuality both represent a surrender to the senses, a betrayal of faith. The witch was a triple threat to the church: She was a woman, and not ashamed of it. She appeared to be part of an organized underground of peasant women. And she was a healer whose practice was based in empirical study. In the face of the repressive fatalism of Christianity, she held out the hope of change in this world.

THE RISE OF THE EUROPEAN MEDICAL PROFESSION While witches practiced among the people, the ruling classes were cultivating their own breed of secular healers: the university-trained physicians. In the century that preceded the beginning of the "witch craze"—the thirteenth century—European medicine became firmly established as a secular science and a *profession*. The medical profession was actively engaged in the elimination of female healers—their exclusion from the universities, for example—long before the witch-hunts began.

For eight long centuries, from the fifth to the thirteenth, the otherworldly, antimedical stance of the church had stood in the way of the development of medicine as a respectable profession. Then, in the thirteenth century, there was a revival of learning, touched off by contact with the Arab world. Medical schools appeared in the universities, and more and more young men of means sought medical training. The church imposed strict controls on the new profession, and allowed it to develop only within the terms set by Catholic doctrine. University-trained physicians were not permitted to practice without calling in a priest to aid and advise them, or to treat a patient who refused confession. By the fourteenth century their practice was in demand among the wealthy, as long as they continued to take pains to show that their attentions to the body did not jeopardize the soul. In fact, accounts of their medical training make it seem more likely that they jeopardized the *body*.

There was nothing in late medieval medical training that conflicted with church doctrine, and little that we would recognize as "science." Medical students, like other scholarly gentlemen, spent years studying Plato, Aristotle, and Christian theology. Their medical theory was largely restricted to the works of Galen, the ancient Roman physician who stressed the theory of "complexions" or "temperaments" of men, "wherefore the choleric are wrathful, the sanguine are kindly, the melancholy are envious," and so on. While a student, a doctor rarely saw any patients at all, and no experimentation of any kind was taught. Medicine was sharply differentiated from surgery, which was almost everywhere considered a degrading, menial craft, and the dissection of bodies was almost unheard of.

Confronted with a sick person, the university-trained physician had little to go on but superstition. Bleeding was a common practice, especially in the case of wounds. Leeches were applied according to the time, the hour, the air, and other similar considerations. Medical theories were often grounded more in "logic" than in observation: "Some foods brought on good humors, and others, evil humors. For example, nasturtium, mustard, and garlic produced reddish bile; lentils, cabbage, and the meat of old goats and beeves begot black bile." Incantations, and quasi-religious rituals were thought to be effective: The physician to Edward II, who held a bachelor's degree in theology and a doctorate in medicine from Oxford, prescribed for toothache writing on the jaws of the patient, "In the name of the Father, the Son, and the Holy Ghost, Amen," or touching a needle to a caterpillar and then to the tooth....

Such was the state of medical "science" at the time when witch-healers were persecuted for being practitioners of "magic." It was witches who developed an extensive understanding of bones and muscles, herbs and drugs, while physicians were still deriving their prognoses from astrology and alchemists were trying to turn lead into gold. So great was the witches' knowledge that in 1527, Paracelsus, considered the "father of modern medicine," burned his text on pharmaceuticals, confessing that he "had learned from the Sorceress all he knew."

THE SUPPRESSION OF WOMEN HEALERS The establishment of medicine as a profession requiring university training made it easy to bar women legally from practice. With few exceptions, the universities were closed to women (even to upper-class women who could afford them), and licensing laws were established to prohibit all but university-trained doctors from practice. It was impossible to enforce the licensing laws consistently since there was only a handful of university-trained doctors compared to the great mass of lay healers. But the laws *could* be used selectively. Their first target was not the peasant healer, but the better-off, literate woman healer who competed for the same urban clientele as that of the university-trained doctors.

Take, for example, the case of Jacoba Félicie, brought to trial in 1322 by the Faculty of Medicine at the University of Paris, on charges of illegal practice. Jacoba was literate and had received some unspecified "special training" in medicine. That her patients were well off is evident from the fact that (as they testified in court) they had consulted well-known university-trained physicians before turning to her. The primary accusations brought against her were that

> ...she would cure her patient of internal illness and wounds or of external abscesses. She would visit the sick assiduously and continue to examine the urine in the manner on physicians, feel the pulse, and touch the body and limbs.

Six witnesses affirmed that Jacoba had cured them, even after numerous doctors had given up, and one patient declared that she was wiser in the art of surgery and medicine than any master physician or surgeon in Paris. But these testimonials were used against her, for the charge was not that she was incompetent, but that—as a woman—she dared to cure at all.

Along the same lines, English physicians sent a petition to Parliament bewailing the "worthless and presumptuous women who usurped the profession" and asking the imposition of fines and "long imprisonment" on any woman who attempted to "use the practyse of Fisyk." By the fourteenth century, the medical profession's campaign against urban, educated women healers was virtually complete throughout Europe. Male doctors had won a clear monopoly over the practice of medicine among the upper classes (except for obstetrics, which remained the province of female midwives even among the upper classes for another three centuries). They were ready to take a key role in the elimination of the great mass of female healers—the "witches."

The partnership between church, state, and medical profession reached full bloom in the witch trials. The doctor was held up as the medical "expert," giving an aura of science to the whole proceeding. He was asked to make judgments about whether certain women were witches and whether certain afflictions had been caused by witchcraft. The *Malleus* says: "And if it is asked how it is possible to distinguish whether an illness is caused by witchcraft or by some natural physical defect, we answer that the first [way] is by means of the *judgment of doctors*" [emphasis added]. In the witch-hunts, the church explicitly legitimized the doctors' professionalism, denouncing nonprofessional healing as equivalent to heresy: "If a woman dare to cure *without having studied,* she is a witch and must die."...

The distinction between "female" superstition and "male" medicine was made final by the very roles of the doctor and the witch at the trial. The trial in one stroke established the male physician on a moral and intellectual plane vastly above the female healer he was called to judge. It placed him on the side of God and law, a professional on par with lawyers and theologians, while it placed her on the side of darkness, evil, and magic. He owed his new status not to medical school or scientific achievements of his own, but to the church and state he served so well.

THE AFTERMATH Witch-hunts did not eliminate the lower-class woman healer, but they branded her forever as superstitious and possibly malevolent. So thoroughly was she discredited among the emerging middle classes that in the seventeenth and eighteenth centuries it was possible for male practitioners to make serious inroads into that last preserve of female healing—midwifery. Nonprofessional male practitioners—"barber-surgeons"—led the assault in England, claiming technical superiority on the basis of their use of the obstetrical forceps. (The forceps were legally classified as a surgical instrument, and women were legally barred from surgical practice.) In the hands of the barber-surgeons, obstetrical practice among the middle class was quickly transformed from a neighborly service into a lucrative business, which real physicians entered in force in the late eighteenth century. Female midwives in England organized and charged the male intruders with commercialism and dangerous misuse of the forceps. But it was too late—the women were easily put down as ignorant "old wives" clinging to the superstitions of the past.

WOMEN AND THE RISE OF THE AMERICAN MEDICAL PROFESSION

In the United States, the male takeover of healing roles started later than in England or France, but ultimately went much further.... By the turn of the century, medicine here was closed to all but a tiny minority of necessarily tough and well-heeled women. What was left was nursing, and this was in no way a substitute for the autonomous roles women had enjoyed as midwives and general healers.

The question is not so much how women got "left out" of medicine and left with nursing, but how did these categories arise at all? To put it another way: How did one particular set of healers, who happened to be male, white, and middle-class, manage to oust all the competing folk healers, midwives, and other practitioners who had dominated the American medical scene in the early 1800s?

The conventional answer given by medical historians is, of course, that there always was one *true* American medical profession—a small band of men whose scientific and moral authority flowed in a unbroken stream from Hippocrates, Galen, and the great European medical scholars. In frontier America these doctors had to combat not only the routine problems of sickness and death but the abuses of a host of lay practitioners—usually depicted as women, ex-slaves, Indians, and drunken patent medicine salesmen. Fortunately for the medical profession, in the late nineteenth century the American public suddenly developed a healthy respect for the doctors' scientific knowledge, outgrew its earlier faith in quacks, and granted the true medical profession a lasting monopoly of the healing arts.

But the real answer is not in this made-up drama of science versus ignorance and superstition. It's part of the nineteenth century's long story of class and sex struggles for power in all areas of life. When women had a place in medicine, it was in a *people's* medicine. When that people's medicine was destroyed, there was no place for women—except in the subservient role of nurses. The set of healers who became *the* medical profession was distinguished not so much by its associations with modern science as by its associations with the emerging American business establishment. With all due respect to Pasteur, Koch, and the other great European medical researchers of the nineteenth century, it was the Carnegies and the Rockefellers who intervened to secure the final victory of the American medical profession....

In western Europe, university-trained physicians already had a centuries-old monopoly over the right to heal. But in America, medical practice was traditionally open to anyone who could demonstrate healing skills—regardless of formal training, race, or sex. Ann Hutchinson, the dissenting religious leader of the 1600s, was a practitioner of "general physik," as were many other ministers and their wives. The medical historian Joseph Kett reports that "one of the most respected medical men in the late eighteenth century Windsor, Connecticut, for example, was a freed Negro called 'Dr. Primus.' In New Jersey, medical practice, except in extraordinary cases, was mainly in the hands women as late as 1818."

Women frequently went into joint practices with their husbands: the husband handling the surgery, the wife the midwifery and gynecology, and everything else shared. Or a woman might go into practice after developing skills through caring for family members or through an apprenticeship with a relative or other established healer....

ENTER THE DOCTOR In the early 1800s there was also a growing number of formally trained doctors who took great pains to distinguish themselves from the host of lay practitioners. The most important real distinction was that the formally trained, or "regular" doctors, as they called themselves, were male, usually middle-class, and almost always more expensive than the lay competition. The regulars' practices were largely confined to middle- and upper-class people who could afford the prestige of being treated by a "gentlemen" of their own class. By 1800, fashion even dictated that upper- and middle-class women employ male regular doctors for obstetrical care—a custom which plainer people regarded as grossly indecent.

In terms of medical skills and theory, the so-called regulars had nothing to recommend them over the lay practitioners. Their "formal training" meant little even by European standards of the time: Medical programs varied in length from a few months to two years; many medical schools had no clinical facilities; high school diplomas were not required for admission to medical schools. Not that serious academic training would have helped much anyway—there was no body of medical science to be trained in. Instead, the regulars were taught to treat most ills by "heroic" measures: massive bleeding, huge doses of laxatives, calomel (a laxative containing mercury) and, later opium. (The European medical profession had little better to offer at this time.) There is no doubt that these "cures" were often either fatal or more injurious than the original disease....

The lay practitioners were undoubtedly safer and more effective than the regulars. They preferred mild herbal medications, dietary changes, and handholding to heroic interventions. Maybe they didn't know any more than the regulars, but at least they were less likely to do the patient harm. Left alone, they might well have displaced the regular doctors with even middle-class consumers in time. But they didn't know the right people. The regulars, with their close ties to the upper class, had legislative clout. By 1830, 13 states had passed medical licensing laws outlawing "irregular" practice and establishing the regulars as the only legal healers.

It was a premature move. There was not popular support for the idea of medical professionalism, much less for the particular set of healers who claimed it. And there was no way to enforce the new laws. The trusted healers of the common people could not just be legislated out of practice. Worse still for the regulars, this early grab for medical monopoly inspired mass indignation in the form of a radical, popular health movement which came close to smashing medical elitism in America once and for all.

THE POPULAR HEALTH MOVEMENT The popular health movement of the 1830s and 1840s is usually dismissed in conventional medical histories as the high tide of quackery and medical cultism. In reality it was the medical front of a general social upheaval stirred up by feminist and working-class movements. Women were the backbone of the popular health movement. "Ladies' Physiological Societies," the equivalent of our know-your-body courses, sprang up everywhere, bringing rapt audiences simple instructions in anatomy and personal hygiene. The emphasis was on preventive care, as opposed to the murderous "cures" practiced by the regular doctors. The movement ran up the banner for frequent bathing (regarded as a vice by many regular doctors of the time), loose-fitting female clothing, whole-grain cereals, temperance, and a host of other issues women could relate to. And, at about the time Margaret Sanger's mother was a little girl, some elements of the movement were already pushing birth control.

The movement was a radical assault on medical elitism and an affirmation of the traditional people's medicine. "Every man his own doctor," was the slogan of one wing of the movement, and they made it very clear that they meant every woman too. The regular, licensed, doctors were attacked as members of "parasitic, non-producing classes," who survived only because of the upper class's "lurid taste" for calomel and bleeding. Universities (where the elite of the regular doctors were trained) were denounced as places where students "learn to look upon labor as servile and demeaning" and to identify with the upper class. Working-class radicals rallied to the cause, linking "King-craft, Priest-craft, Lawyer-craft, and Doctor-craft" as the four great evils of the time. In New York State, the movement was represented in the legislature by a member of the Workingmen's Party, who took every opportunity to assail the "privileged doctors."

The regular doctors quickly found themselves outnumbered and cornered. From the left wing of the popular health movement came a total rejection of "doctoring" as a paid occupation—much less as an overpaid "profession." From the moderate wing came a host of new medical philosophies, or sects to compete with the regulars on their own terms: eclecticism, Grahamism, homeopathy, plus many minor ones. The new sects set up their own medical schools (emphasizing preventive care and mild herbal cures), and started graduating their own doctors. In this context of medical ferment, the old regulars began to look like just another sect, a sect whose particular philosophy happened to lean toward calomel, bleeding, and the other standbys of "heroic" medicine. It was impossible to tell who were the "real" doctors, and by the 1840s, medical licensing laws had been repealed in almost all of the states.

The peak of the popular health movement coincided with the beginnings of an organized feminist movement, and the two were so closely linked that it's hard to tell where one began and the other left off. "This crusade for women's health [the popular health movement] was related both in cause and effect to the demand for women's rights in general, and at the health and feminist movements become indistinguishable at this point," according to Richard Shryock, the well-known medical historian. The health movement was concerned with women's rights in general, and the women's movement was particularly concerned with health and with women's access to medical training.

In fact, leaders of both groups used the prevailing sex stereotypes to argue that women were even better equipped to be doctors than men. "We cannot deny that women possess superior capacities for the science of medicine," wrote Samuel Thomson, a health movement leader, in 1834. (However, he felt surgery and the care of males should be reserved for male practitioners.) Feminists, like Sarah Hale, went further, exclaiming in 1852: "Talk about this [medicine] being the appropriate sphere for man and his alone! With tenfold more plausibility and reason we say it is the appropriate sphere for woman, and hers alone."

The new medical sects' schools did, in fact, open their doors to women at a time when regular medical training was all but closed to them. For example, Harriet Hunt was denied admission to Harvard Medical College, and instead went to a sectarian school for her formal training. (Actually, the Harvard faculty had voted to admit her—along with some Black male students—but the students threatened to riot if they came.) The regular physicians could take the credit for training Elizabeth Blackwell, America's first female "regular," but her alma mater (a small school in upstate New York) quickly passes a resolution barring further female students. The first generally co-ed medical schools was the "irregular" Eclectic Central Medical College of New York, in Syracuse. Finally, the first two all-female medical colleges, one in Boston and one in Philadelphia, were themselves "irregular."

Feminist researchers should really find out more about the popular health movement. From the perspective of our movement today, it's probably more relevant than the women's suffrage struggle. To us, the most tantalizing aspects of the movement are:

1. That it represented both class struggle and feminist struggle. Today it's stylish in some quarters to write off purely feminist issues as middle-class concerns. But in the popular health movement we see a coming together of feminist and working-class energies. Is this because the popular health movement naturally attracted dissidents of all kinds, or was there some deeper identity of purpose?

2. It was not just a movement for more and better medical care, but for a radically different kind of health care: It was a substantive challenge to the prevailing medical dogma, practice, and theory. Today we tend to confine our critiques to the organization of medical care and assume that the scientific substratum of medicine is unassailable. We too should be developing the capability for the critical study of medical "science"— at least as it relates to women.

DOCTORS ON THE OFFENSIVE At its height in the 1830s and 1840s, the popular health movement had the regular doctors—the professional ancestors of today's physicians—running scared. Later in the nineteenth century, as the grassroots energy ebbed and the movement degenerated into a set of competing sects, the regulars went back on the offensive. In 1848, they pulled together their first national organization, pretentiously named the *American* Medical Association (AMA). County and state medical societies, many of which had practically disbanded during the height of medical anarchy in the 1830s and 1840s, began to re-form.

Throughout the latter part of the nineteenth century, the regulars relentlessly attacked lay practitioners, sectarian doctors, and women practitioners in general. The attacks were linked: Women practitioners could be attacked because of their sectarian leanings; sects could be attacked because of their openness to women. The arguments against women doctors ranged from the paternalistic (how could a respectable woman travel at night to a medical emergency?) to the hard-core sexist....

The virulence of the American sexist opposition to women in medicine has no parallel in Europe. This is probably because, first, fewer European women were aspiring to medical careers at this time. Second, feminist movements were nowhere as strong as in the United States, and here the male doctors rightly associated the entrance of women into medicine with organized feminism. And, third, the European medical profession was already more firmly established and hence less afraid of competition.

The rare woman who did make it into a regular medical school faced one sexist hurdle after another. First, there was the continuous harassment—often lewd—by the male students. There were professors who wouldn't discuss anatomy with a lady present....

Having completed her academic work, the would-be woman doctor usually found the next steps blocked. Hospitals were usually closed to women doctors, and even if they weren't, the internships were not open to women. If she finally did make it into practice, she found her brother "regulars" unwilling to refer patients to her and absolutely opposed to her membership in their medical societies.

And so it is all the stranger to us, and all the sadder, that what we might call the "women's health movement" began, in the late nineteenth century, to dissociate itself from its popular health movement past and to strive for respectability. Members of irregular sects were purged from the faculties of the women's medical colleges. Female medical leaders such as Elizabeth Blackwell joined male "regulars" in demanding an end to lay midwifery and "a complete medical education" for all who practiced obstetrics. All this at a time when the regulars still had little or no "scientific" advantage over the sect doctors or lay healers.

The explanation, we suppose, was that the women who were likely to seek formal medical training at this time were middle-class. They must have found it easier to identify with the middle-class regular doctors than with lower-class women healers or with the sectarian medical groups (which had earlier been identified with radical movements). The shift in allegiance was probably made all the easier by the fact that, in the cities, female lay practitioners were increasingly likely to be immigrants. (At the same time, the possibilities for a cross-class women's movement on *any* issue were vanishing as working-class women went into the factories and middle-class women settled into Victorian ladyhood.) Whatever the exact explanation, the result was that middle-class women had given up the substantive attack on male medicine, and accepted the terms set by the emerging male medical profession.

PROFESSIONAL VICTORY The regulars were still in no condition to make another bid for medical monopoly. For one thing, they still couldn't claim to have any uniquely effective methods or special body of knowledge. Besides, an occupational group doesn't gain a professional monopoly on the basis of technical superiority alone. A recognized profession is not just a group of self-proclaimed experts; it is a group which has authority *in the law* to select its own members and regulate their practice, i.e., to monopolize a certain field without outside interference. How does a particular group gain full professional status? In the words of sociologist Elliot Freidson:

> A profession attains and maintains its position by virtue of the protection and patronage of some elite segment of society which has been persuaded that there is some special value in its work.

In other words, professions are the creation of a ruling class. To become *the* medical profession, the regular doctors needed above all, ruling-class patronage.

By a lucky coincidence for the regulars, both the science and the patronage became available around the same time, at the turn of the century. French and especially German scientists brought forth the germ theory of disease which provided, for the first time in human history, a rational basis for disease prevention and therapy. While the run-of-the-mill American doctor was still mumbling about "humors" and dosing people with calomel, a tiny medical elite was traveling to German universities to learn the new science. They returned to the United States filled with reformist zeal. In 1893 German-trained doctors (funded by local philanthropists) set up the first... German-style medical school, Johns Hopkins.

As far as curriculum was concerned, the big innovation at Hopkins was integrating lab work in basic science with expanded clinical training. Other reforms included hiring full-time faculty, emphasizing research, and closely associating the medical school with a full university. Johns Hopkins also introduced the modern pattern of medical education—four years of medical school following four years of college—which of course barred most working-class and poor people from the possibility of a medical education.

Meanwhile the United States was emerging as the industrial leader of the world. Fortunes built on oil, coal, and the ruthless exploitation of American workers were maturing into financial empires. For the first time in American history, there were sufficient concentrations of corporate wealth to allow for massive organized philanthropy, i.e., organized ruling-class intervention in the social, cultural, and political life of the nation. Foundations were created as the lasting instrument of this intervention—the Rockefeller and Carnegie foundations appeared in the first decade of the twentieth century. One of the earliest and highest items on their agenda was medical "reform," the creation of a respectable, scientific American medical profession.

The group of American medical practitioners that the foundations chose to put their money behind was, naturally enough, the scientific elite of the regular doctors. (Many of these men were themselves ruling-class, and all were urbane, university-trained gentlemen.) Starting in 1903, foundation money began to pour into medical schools by the millions. The conditions were clear: conform to the Johns Hopkins model or close. To get the message across, the Carnegie Corporation sent a staff man, Abraham Flexner, out on a national tour of medical schools—from Harvard right down to the last third-rate commercial schools.

Flexner almost singlehandedly decided which schools would get the money—and hence survive. For the bigger and better schools (i.e., those which already had enough money to begin to institute the prescribed reforms), there was the promise of fat foundation grants. Harvard was one of the lucky winners, and its president could say smugly in 1907, "Gentlemen, the way to get endowments for medicine is to improve medical education." As for the smaller, poorer schools, which included most of the sectarian schools and special schools for Blacks and women—Flexner did not consider them worth saving. Their options were to close, or to remain open and face public denunciation in the report Flexner was preparing.

The Flexner report, published in 1910, was the foundations' ultimatum to American medicine. In its wake, medical schools closed by the score, including six of America's eight Black medical schools and the majority of the "irregular" schools which had been a haven for female students. Medicine was established once and for all as a branch of "higher" learning, accessible only through lengthy and expensive university training. It's certainly true that as medical knowledge grew, lengthier training did become necessary. But Flexner and the foundations had no intention of making such training available to the great mass of lay healers and "irregular" doctors. Instead, doors were slammed shut to Blacks, to the majority of women, and to poor white men. (Flexner in his report bewailed the fact that any "crude boy or jaded clerk" had been able to seek medical training.) Medicine had become a white, male, middle-class occupation.

But it was more than an occupation. It had become, at last, a profession. To be more precise, one particular group of healers, the regular doctors, was now *the* medical profession. Their victory was not based on any skills of their own: the run-of-the-mill regular doctor did not suddenly acquire a knowledge of medical science with the publication of the Flexner report. But he did acquire the *mystique* of science. So what if his own alma mater had been condemned in the Flexner report, wasn't he a member of the AMA, and wasn't it in the forefront of scientific reform? The doctor had become—thanks to some foreign scientists and eastern foundations—the "man of science": beyond criticism, beyond regulation, very nearly beyond competition.

OUTLAWING THE MIDWIVES In state after state, new, tough, licensing laws sealed the doctor's monopoly on medical practice. All that was left was to drive out the last holdouts of the old people's medicine—the midwives. In 1910, about 50 percent of all babies were delivered by midwives—most were Blacks or working-class immigrants. It was an intolerable situation to the newly emerging obstetrical specialty. For one thing, every poor woman who went to a midwife was one more case lost to academic teaching and research. America's vast lower-class resource of obstetrical "teaching material" was being wasted on ignorant midwives. Besides which, poor women were spending an estimated $5 million a year on midwives—$5 million which could have been going to "professionals."

Publicly, however, the obstetricians launched their attacks on midwives in the name of science and reform. Midwives were ridiculed as "hopelessly dirty, ignorant and incompetent." Specifically, they were held responsible for the prevalence of puerperal sepsis (uterine infections) and neonatal ophthalmia (blindness due to parental infection with gonorrhea). Both conditions were easily preventable by techniques well within the grasp of the least literate midwife (hand-washing for puerperal sepsis, and eye drops for the ophthalmia). So the obvious solution for a truly public-spirited obstetrical profession would have been to make the appropriate preventive techniques known and available to the mass of midwives. This is in fact what happened in England, Germany, and most other European nations: Midwifery was upgraded through training to become an established, independent occupation.

But the American obstetricians had no real commitment to improved obstetrical care. In fact, a study by a Johns Hopkins professor in 1912 indicated that most American doctors were *less* competent than the midwives. Not only were the doctors themselves unreliable about preventing sepsis and ophthalmia but they also tended to be too ready to use surgical techniques that endangered mother or child. If anyone, then, deserved a legal monopoly on obstetrical care, it was the midwives, not the M.D.s. But the doctors had power, the midwives didn't. Under intense pressure from the medical profession, state after state passed laws outlawing midwifery and restricting the practice of obstetrics to doctors. For poor and working-class women, this actually meant worse—or no—obstetrical care. (For instance, a study of infant mortality rates in Washington showed an increase in infant mortality in the years immediately following the passage of the law forbidding midwifery.) For the new, male medical profession, the ban on midwives meant one less source of competition. Women had been routed from their last foothold as independent practitioners.

THE LADY WITH THE LAMP The only remaining occupation for women in health was nursing. Nursing had not always existed as a paid occupation—it had to be invented. In the early nineteenth century, a "nurse" was simply a woman who happened to be nursing someone—a sick child or an aging relative. There were hospitals, and they did employ nurses. But the hospitals of the time served largely as refuges for the dying poor, with only token care provided. Hospital nurses, history has it, were a disreputable lot, prone to drunkenness, prostitution, and thievery. And conditions in the hospitals were often scandalous. In the late 1870s a committee investigating New York's Bellevue Hospital could not find a bar of soap on the premises.

If nursing was not exactly an attractive field to women workers, it was a wide open arena for women *reformers*. To reform hospital care, you had to reform nursing, and to make nursing acceptable to doctors and to women "of good character," it had to be given a completely new image. Florence Nightingale got her chance in the battle-front hospitals of the Crimean War, where she replaced the old camp-follower "nurses" with a bevy of disciplined, sober, middle-aged ladies. Dorothea Dix, an American hospital reformer, introduced the new breed of nurses in the Union hospitals of the Civil War.

The new nurse—"the lady with the lamp," selflessly tending the wounded —caught the popular imagination. Real nursing schools began to appear in England right after the Crimean War, and in the United States right after the Civil War. At the same time, the number of hospitals began to increase to keep pace with the needs of medical education. Medical students needed hospitals to train in; good hospitals, as the doctors were learning, needed good nurses.

In fact, the first American nursing schools did their best to recruit actual upper-class women as students. Miss Euphemia Van Rensselear, of an old aristocratic New York family, graced Bellevue's first class. And at Johns Hopkins, where Isabel Hampton trained nurses in the University Hospital, a leading doctor could only complain that:

> Miss Hampton has been most successful in getting probationers [students] of the upper class; but unfortunately, she selects them altogether for their good looks and the House staff is by this time in a sad state.

Let us look a little more closely at the women who invented nursing, because, in a very real sense, nursing as we know it today is the product of their oppression as upper-class Victorian women. Dorothea Dix was an heiress of substantial means. Florence Nightingale and Louisa Schuyler (the moving force behind the creation of America's first Nightingale-style nursing school) were genuine aristocrats. They were refugees from the enforced leisure of Victorian ladyhood. Dix and Nightingale did not begin to carve out their reform careers until they were in their thirties, and faced with the prospect of a long, useless spinsterhood. They focused their energies on the care of the sick because this was a "natural" and acceptable interest for ladies of their class.

Nightingale and her immediate disciples left nursing with the indelible stamp of their own class biases. Training emphasized character, not skills. The finished products, the Nightingale nurse, was simply the ideal lady, transplanted from home to the hospital and absolved of reproductive responsibilities. To the doctor, she brought the wifely virtue of absolute obedience. To the patient, she brought the selfless devotion of a mother. To the lower level hospital employees, she brought the firm but kindly discipline of a household manager accustomed to dealing with servants.

But, despite the glamorous "lady with the lamp" image, most of nursing work was just low-paid, heavy-duty housework. Before long, most nursing schools were attracting only women from working-class and lower-middle-class homes, whose only other options were factory or clerical work. But the philosophy of nursing education did not change—after all, the educators were still middle- and upper-class women. If anything, they toughened their insistence on ladylike character development, and the socialization of nurses became what it has been for most of the twentieth century: the imposition of upper-class cultural values on working-class women. (For example, until recently, most nursing students were taught such upper-class graces as tea pouring, art appreciation, etc. Practical nurses are still taught to wear girdles, use makeup, and in general mimic the behavior of a "better" class of women.)

But the Nightingale nurse was not just the projection of upper-class ladyhood onto the working world. She embodied the very spirit of femininity as defined by sexist Victorian society—she was Woman. The inventors of nursing saw it as a natural vocation for women, second only to motherhood. When a group of English nurses proposed that nursing model itself after the medical profession, with exams and licensing, Nightingale responded that "nurses cannot be registered and examined *any more than mothers*" [emphasis added]. Or, as one historian of nursing put it, nearly a century later, "Woman is an instinctive nurse, taught by Mother Nurse" (Victor Robinson, *White Caps: The Story of Nursing*). If women were instinctive nurses, they were not, in the Nightingale view, instinctive doctors. She wrote of the few female physicians of her time: "They have only tried to be men, and they have succeeded only in being third-rate men." Indeed, as the number of nursing students rose in the late nineteenth century, the number of female medical students began to decline. Woman had found her place in the health system.

Just as the feminist movement had not opposed the rise of medical professionalism, it did not challenge nursing as an oppressive female role. In fact, feminists of the late nineteenth century were themselves beginning to celebrate the nurse-mother image of femininity. The American women's movement had given up the struggle for full sexual equality to focus exclusively on the vote, and to get it, they were ready to adopt the most sexist tenets of Victorian ideology: women need the vote, they argued, not because they are human, but because they are mothers. "Woman is the mother of the race," gushed Boston feminist Julia Ward Howe, "the guardian of its helpless infancy, its earliest teacher, its most zealous champion. Woman is also the homemaker, upon her devolve the details which bless and beautify family life." And so on, in paeans too painful to quote.

The women's movement dropped its earlier emphasis on opening up the professions to women: Why forsake motherhood for the petty pursuits of males? And of course the impetus to attack professionalism itself as inherently sexist and elitist was long since dead. Instead, they turned to professionalizing women's natural functions. Housework was glamorized in the new discipline of "domestic science." Motherhood was held out as a vocation requiring much the same preparation and skill as nursing or teaching.

So while some women were professionalizing women's domestic roles, others were "domesticizing" professional roles, like nursing, teaching, and, later, social work. For the woman who chose to express her feminine drives outside of the home, these occupations were presented as simple extensions of women's "natural" domestic role. Conversely the woman who remained at home was encouraged to see herself as a kind of nurse, teacher, and counselor practicing within the limits of the family. And so the middle-class feminists of the late 1800s dissolved away some of the harsher contradictions of sexism.

THE DOCTOR NEEDS A NURSE Of course, the women's movement was not in a position to decide on the future of nursing anyway. Only the medical profession was. At first, male doctors were a little skeptical about the new Nightingale nurses—perhaps suspecting that this was just one more feminine attempt to infiltrate medicine. But they were soon won over by the nurses' unflagging obedience. (Nightingale was a little obsessive on this point. When she arrived in the Crimea with her newly trained nurses, the doctors at first ignored them all. Nightingale refused to let her women lift a finger to help the thousands of sick and wounded soldiers until the doctors gave an order. Impressed, the doctors finally relented and set the nurses to cleaning up the hospital.) To the beleaguered doctors of the nineteenth century, nursing was a godsend. Here at last was a kind of health worker who did not want to compete with the "regulars," did not have a medical doctrine to push, and who seemed to have no other mission in life but to serve.

While the average regular doctor was making nurses welcome, the new scientific practitioners of the early twentieth century were making them *necessary.* The new, post-Flexner physician, was even less likely than his predecessors to stand around and watch the progress of his "cures." He diagnosed, he prescribed, he moved on. He could not waste his talents, or his expensive academic training in the tedious details of bedside care. For this he needed a patient, obedient helper, someone who was not above the most menial tasks—in short, a nurse.

Healing, in its fullest sense, consists of both curing and caring, doctoring *and* nursing. The old lay healers of an earlier time had combined both functions, and were valued for both. (For example, midwives not only presided at the delivery, but lived in until the new mother was ready to resume care of her children.) But with the development of scientific medicine, and the modern medical profession, the two functions were split irrevocably. Curing became the exclusive province of the doctor; caring was relegated to the nurse. All credit for the patient's recovery went to the doctor and his "quick fix," for only the doctor participated in the mystique of science. The nurse's activities, on the other hand, were barely distinguishable from those of a servant. She had no power, no magic, and no claim to the credit.

Doctoring and nursing arose as complementary functions, and the society which defined nursing as feminine could readily see doctoring as intrinsically "masculine." If the nurse was idealized woman, the doctor was idealized man—combining intellect and action, abstract theory and hard-headed pragmatism. The very qualities which fitted Woman for nursing barred her from doctoring, and vice versa. Her tenderness and innate spirituality were out of place in the harsh, linear world of science. His decisiveness and curiosity made him unfit for long hours of patient nurturing.

These stereotypes have proved to be almost unbreakable. Today's leaders of the American Nursing Association may insist that nursing is no longer a feminine vocation but a neuter "profession." They may call for more male nurses to change the "image," insist that nursing requires almost as much academic preparation as medicine, and so on. But the drive to "professionalize" nursing is, at best, a flight from the reality of sexism in the health system. At worst, it is sexist itself, deepening the division among women health workers and bolstering a hierarchy controlled by men.

CONCLUSION

We have our own moment of history to work out, our own struggles. What can we learn from the past that will help us—in a women's health movement—today? These are some of our conclusions:

➤ We have not been passive bystanders in the history of medicine. The present system was born in and shaped by the competition between male and female healers. The medical profession in particular is not just another institution which happens to discriminate against us: It is a fortress designed and erected to exclude us. This means to us that the sexism of the health system is not incidental, not just the reflection of the sexism of society in general or the sexism of individual doctors. It is historically older than medical science itself; it is deep-rooted, institutional sexism.

➤ Our enemy is not just "men" or their individual male chauvinism. It is the whole class system which enabled male, upper-class healers to win out and which forced us into subservience. Institutional sexism is sustained by a class system which supports male power.

➤ There is no historically consistent justification for the exclusion of women from healing roles. Witches were attacked for being pragmatic, empirical, and immoral. But in the nineteenth century the rhetoric reversed. Women became too unscientific, delicate, and sentimental. The *stereotypes* change to suit male convenience—*we* don't—and there is nothing in our "innate feminine nature" to justify our present subservience.

➤ Men maintain their power in the health system through their monopoly of scientific knowledge. We are mystified by science, taught to believe that it is hopelessly beyond our grasp. In our frustration, we are sometimes tempted to reject *science*, rather than to challenge the men who hoard it. But medical science could be a liberating force, giving us real control over own bodies and power in our lives as health workers. At this point in our history, every effort to take hold of and share medical knowledge is a critical part of our struggle—know-your-body courses and literature, self-help projects, counseling, women's free clinics.

➤ Professionalism in medicine is nothing more than the institutionalization of a male upper-class monopoly. We must never confuse professionalism with expertise. Expertise is something to work for and to share; professionalism is—by definition—elitist and exclusive, sexist, racist and classist. In the American past, women who sought formal medical training were too ready to accept the professionalism that went with it. They made *their* gains in status—but only on the backs of their less privileged sisters: midwives, nurses, and lay healers. Our goal today should never be to open up the exclusive medical profession to women, but to open up medicine to all women.

➤ This means that we must begin to break down the distinctions and barriers between women health workers and women consumers. We should build shared concerns: consumers aware of women's needs as workers, workers in touch with women's needs as consumers. Women workers can play a leadership role in collective self-help and self-teaching projects, and in attacks on health institutions. But they need support and solidarity from a strong women's consumer movement.

➤ Our oppression as women health workers today is inextricably linked to our oppression as women. Nursing, our predominate role in the health system, is simply a workplace extension of our roles as wife and mother. The nurse is socialized to believe that rebellion violates not only her "professionalism," but her very femininity. This means that the male medical elite has a very special stake in the maintenance of sexism in the society at large: doctors are the bosses in an industry where the workers are primarily women. Sexism in the society at large insures that the female majority of the health workforce are "good" workers—docile and passive. Take away sexism and you take away one of the mainstays of the health hierarchy.

What this means to us in practice is that in the health system there is no way to separate worker organizing from feminist organizing. To reach out to women health workers as *workers* is to reach out to them as *women*.

Childbirth in America

EDITED BY VICTORIA ENG AND SONIA LANDER

Excerpted from Richard W. Wertz and Dorothy C. Wertz, *Lying In: A History of Childbirth in America,* New York, Free Press, 1977; Margaret Charles Smith and Linda Janet Holmes, *Listen to Me Good: The Life Story of an Alabama Midwife,* Columbus: Ohio State University Press, 1996. Reprinted by permission.

Margaret Charles Smith, the subject of Listen to Me Good: The Story of an Alabama Midwife, *attended over 3,000 births; lost not one single mother and very few babies; and adapted to the mother's choice of birth position, however awkward it might be for Smith herself. In contrast, the experimental maternity techniques of nineteenth-century male physicians, as described here by Richard and Dorothy Wertz, seem needlessly bloody and barbaric. How these doctors lured some (by no means all) women to forgo midwives for the new "technology" remains a puzzle.—B. S.*

Richard and Dorothy Wertz's book *Lying In: A History of Childbirth in America* vividly illustrates the takeover of midwifery, and ultimately of women's bodies and health, by male physicians. Women in childbirth often suffered greatly because of the ignorant practices of male physicians.

These barber-surgeons often resorted to the use of horrific surgical tools. The following passage begins with an excerpt from Dr. Samuel Bard's *Compendium on the Theory and Practice of Midwifery* published in New York in 1815.

[The young doctor] will probably fail at first, for want of judgment, to discriminate accurately between one case and another, as well as for want of skill and dexterity in the application of his instruments; and finding himself foiled in the use of safer lever and forceps, he will become alarmed, confused, and apprehensive for his patient's safety, as well as for his own reputation. And now, deeming a speedy delivery essential to both, and that, having taken the case into his own hands, and began his work, he thinks he must not desist before he has accomplished it, he flies to the crotchet [an instrument for killing, cutting, and extracting a fetus lodged in the birth canal] as more easy in its application, and more certain in its effect—with this he probably succeeds; and although the poor infant is sacrificed, yet he persuades himself, perhaps honestly believes, this was necessary.

After 1750 American men began to return from medical education abroad to practice in colonial towns and cities. Perhaps the most notable medical attainment they brought, in terms of potentially widespread and concrete medical benefit, was new knowledge and skills to aid women in birth in ways that uneducated American midwives could not match. The doctors called their science and arts relative to birth by the traditional term "midwifery," but they realized that it constituted medical science's first major practical advance....

French doctors had come to regard the birth process as a natural process and defined midwifery as a science....

By defining birth as a natural process that followed its own laws, as a machine with shapes and movements of its own, the French reduced its potentially awesome aspects and removed its emotional and spiritual associations from their consideration. They could then look intently at what determined the success or failure of birth, and that would be their arena for further scientific and medical art.

They could have done this and have been wrong. It was common practice at that time to sever the sacred and the natural and to posit mechanical models for natural processes. But the mechanical model of birth was fortuitously accurate and adequate to describe many of the normal and abnormal events of birth.

The French achievement consisted primarily in finding a better understanding of birth rather than in discovering new techniques to aid it. Even their mechanistic view did not explain many of the pathologies of birth. It led some surgeons to make deep cuts to expand the birth canal or to open the abdomen, but, since the women usually died, they had to abandon such attempts to reshape or circumvent the birth medicine.... Often knowing that the canal was misshapen or inadequate only enabled them to announce that a woman would die....

The new midwifery had a different beginning in England. There it was not associated with medical institutions in which generations of birth attendants accumulated experience and formulated a new view of birth's processes. Rather, it began in the often desperate struggles of poorly educated medical empirics, the barber-surgeons, to save the life of the mother by extracting the child with whatever tools they could devise....

These empirical operators had a wide range of instruments—in fact, a real armamentarium—to extract the fetus, living or dead. They had blunt hooks to bring down the thighs in a breech delivery, sharp hooks (crotchets) and knives and perforators to puncture the fetus's head when it was completely impacted or dead, and the ancient device of the *speculum matricis* to dilate the vagina and make it easier to cut out obstructions or reach the fetus. Often they used the fillet, a strip of flexible but firm material, to slip into the uterus and loop around the child to pull it out. Most often the surgeons had to kill the impacted child in order to save the mother's life. Their efforts were not those of scientific observers but of desperate practical technicians, experimenting with various tools to aid delivery, rushing to save life often by killing life. (pp. 29–35)

In the mid-nineteenth century, after Queen Victoria elected to use chloroform during her own deliveries, it became acceptable to use anesthetics to relieve labor pain; from then on, the comfort of the patient was considered more important than the safe delivery of the baby. Class prejudice and Victorian notions of modesty played key roles in the development of clinical training in obstetrics. Male midwives, as they called themselves, went to great pains to protect the chastity and purity of their middle-class and upper-middle-class patients, often at the expense of good clinical practice.

The medical profession claimed that a doctor who could not practice "by the sense of touch alone" was incompetent in midwifery, and American textbooks on midwifery, drawing from French originals, obligingly illustrated that point by showing the doctor on one knee before his standing patient, feeling under her long skirts, with his eyes averted and staring abstractly into the distance.

The problem for modesty became not touch but sight, whether the male doctor could see the genitalia and whether the patient could see the doctor seeing her body. Exposure during physical examination and during delivery were the matters of most extreme delicacy in nineteenth-century America, for both doctors and patients. Exposure had been a problem in the previous century also, and British instructors in midwifery, such as [William] Smellie, had to resort to using a "mock-woman" to demonstrate the processes of birth to most students, although occasionally Smellie, [William] Shippen, and other instructors found poor women who were willing to allow male students to observe their deliveries....

A committee of the American Medical Association deprecated the exposure of a patient during delivery as unnecessary since a physician had to learn to conduct labor by touch alone or he was unfit to practice. Other national responses were more varied, some pointing out that clinical training in obstetrics had long been common in foreign countries and had contributed to new knowledge and better skills for complications of birth and other female conditions. Other doctors feared, however, that, if men could not perform obstetrical operations (including catheterization, forceps, and even embryotomy) "as well without the eye as with it," obstetrical practice would so offend women that they would choose female attendants and thus ruin many male doctors' practice.

The fit doctor was to be essentially a blind man....

Most doctors went forth to attend birth with no clinical experience; those from better medical schools associated with clinics or hospitals may have had experience of the touch alone. A desire to overcome the restriction on clinical training, which often created ignorance and mishap, prompted Dr. James White of Buffalo to demonstrate a delivery upon a living patient before a group of medical students in 1850. The woman was from the country poorhouse, was having her second illegitimate child, and was one of the recent Irish immigrants in Buffalo, a group of second-class citizens who had only shortly before won the right to enter the state legally. The presence of such a low-status female population may have been essential for clinical midwifery to proceed, for doctors could classify such women as not needing or deserving the same symptomatic treatment given to respectable women....

In the early decades of the nineteenth century in many cities doctors and philanthropic patrons did establish separate maternity hospitals as charitable asylums for poor or unmarried women who the doctors and patrons believed deserved a clean, comfortable, and moral environment in which to deliver and to rehabilitate themselves....

After the Civil War doctors realized that maternity hospitals provided occasions for clinical obstetrics; students might learn and professors teach and research. Doctors therefore struck a bargain with the charity patients in such hospitals; in exchange for medical treatment, the women would allow themselves to be exposed to the eye of medicine. Doctors could do this because respectable women patrons supported such institutions for the deserving poor, who were valuable to the patrons as object lessons about the redeemability of the poor and the value of charity.

The maternity hospital was an interesting example of the exchange of benefits between social classes, for what the doctors learned in treating the poor they could use in treating respectable women in their home. Doctors could study birth more intently… for they could disregard the scruples and feelings of poor charity patients more readily than those of respectable women. Since doctors acquired little status from treating the poor, the maternity hospital allowed obstetrics to transcend the barrier of modesty and to begin to transform itself into a science that looked primarily at the physical processes of birth rather than at patients. (pp. 84–100)

Despite these atrocities, professional, male-dominated, scientific procedures were considered safer and more socially acceptable than those of women's midwifery. Male doctors were largely ignorant of the midwives' methods, and perhaps because they felt competitive with these women, they set about to discredit and ultimately destroy the longstanding tradition of lay midwifery.

But the patients of barber-surgeons—the recognized pioneers in the practice of obstetric medicine—had much higher mortality rates than those of lay midwives. One such woman, Margaret Charles Smith, the subject of *Listen to Me Good: The Life Story of an Alabama Midwife* is notable for her sterling record: Smith attended over 3,000 births during her long career, and lost not a single mother and very few babies.

Lay midwives had no formal education and delivered babies for poor women (both white and Black); sometimes (probably because the care was considered so good) they delivered the babies of middle- and upper-middle-class white women as well. Over the course of time, laws were passed that strictly regulated the role of midwives. However, enforcement of these regulations did not extend into poor Black America—and that is why Smith was able to keep most of her methods intact.

The following passage, told in Margaret Charles Smith's own words, discusses many traditional birth techniques that midwives used.

When I first get to the mother's home, I'd see if I can find stuff to make a pad for them to deliver on. If they have some newspaper, I'd sit down and twirl that newspaper together and tack it so it won't slip and slide. If you put twenty sheets together, you won't have no trouble. See, you twirl them and fold them in a certain way, and then you tack it in each corner. I put that in the bed. That would catch the waste, so it won't get on the mattress, and it won't get on the sheet. I learned how to make the basket to catch the afterbirth out of newspaper. I learned that in Tuskegee.

Then sometimes, I'd tell the mother to go take a hot bath, and that hot water helps a lot. I sit their feet in hot water or let them sit in that tub, if they got it, a number three tub. I was willing to let them have their way until push comes to shove. Some of them would say, "I don't want to take a bath."

I'd say, "Just get in the tub, and I'll bathe you." I was right there to get them out, but some of them just wouldn't do it.

You are sitting there to do what you can for her, rub her or put something under her back, trying to rest her back some. That's what you are there for, talk to her. If you like tea, you can make them some hot tea, and that will pick them pains up. Then you can rub the stomach and make the pains start back. I'd put some grease in my hand or whatever the lady happened to have and rub it in. Sometimes I'd rub their back. That's where the misery was—in their back and stomach, but you know, if I go rub their stomach that would make some pains rise, and they'd want me to stop rubbing their stomach, so I'd rub their back, and some of them had all their pain in their back.

Sometime they want to get up, and I'd help them up. Walk around the room. Walk a pain off then get back in the bed. A lot of people get a kick out of walking. Go into different rooms and sit in different chairs, or get down on their knees—anywhere they think they can get ease. But there's no ease for birth till it's over with. It's good to walk, but you'll have to stop sometime. You can pretty much do what you want till you get down to the real nitty-gritty.

Now, some of the mothers be talking all this slack talk. But you're the midwife. So you, well, you got to take that. You could get up and tell them, "It doesn't make a difference. I don't care. It ain't no skin off my teeth."

I don't think that would be the words to speak. You are there. You just as well make the best of it you can, talking kind, giving kind words and rubbing her hands. That means a lot. That means all of it. Kindness whipped the devil. Kind words, that's right, and belief. If somebody is sick, and you start talking rash to them, that hurts their feelings, but if you talk kind to them, why, that makes a lot of difference.

I'd just tell them, "Well honey child, you're going to have to hurt before your baby's born. It ain't no way around that. You can expect that. Now the pains ain't hard now, but they're going to be hard. I want you to be aware of what's coming, and you'll have to learn to take it as it comes, and it will soon be over. If you are going to buck and ram and holler, you ain't going to help you none. You might as well settle yourself down and do the best you can."

See, a midwife just can't say, "You got to do so-and-so."

You know what you got to do, and you got to do it, but you can go around in a better way and make it more pleasant, the way I see it. You keep a-talking to them until they realize they got to bear to it. (pp. 88–90)

Women had more control over the process of their labor under the traditional practice of midwifery. This is in stark contrast to the procedures of clinical deliveries, which required women to be passive.

When it comes time to deliver, most of them want you to fold a quilt and put it down on the floor and turn down a straight-back chair like that one yonder with the cane-seat bottom. You put the pillows on back of it. Turn it down where they can be halfway kind of sitting up like, and their bottom part be scooted out. Somebody holds their bottom part, and somebody holds their knees. You take this chair and turn it down where she could feel the heat from the fireplace. The mother can't get cold, 'cause if she gets too cold, that's going to cut the pains down.

And then some of them get on their knees. If they're on their knees, they got some pillows on the back of the chair. They just open their knees out. Some people won't have a baby no other but that way. Mostly there be two or three women around. They use the back of the chair to support their back, and the people help them get down. (pp. 92–93)

Smith, however, was forced to submit to some of the regulations. Here, she recounts her decision to abandon the use of herbal remedies that were considered threatening by the medical establishment.

Now, the nurses didn't know what was good and what was bad. You can take too much of anything. You just need enough to warm you up inside and get those pains a-moving, if you done done everything you can do on the outside.

I had to stop fooling with teas and things in labor because my name was getting out.

"Miss Margaret, how come you are not using some of that stuff you used on Emma or Lucille. She was telling me about what good stuff you had. Why don't you give me some? Fix some for me so I can get through with this baby."

See, my name was getting where I could hear it. I stopped right then. I had been practicing a good while. I was going by what Miss Ella Anderson taught, but I stopped. I already knew about the teas 'cause I was going with this other midwife. They used to make teas for the mothers to pick the pains up.

The woman told us in the clinic, I think we had a meeting of all the midwives, the woman was from Selma.

She said, "No more pepper tea, no dirt dauber, no kind of root or nothing unless you give them some hot tea, regular. But not no roots and things like that."

They said, "They better not catch nobody giving nobody no tea of no kind. If they do, she was going to jail and from there to the pen."

You know, they're quick to think teas and things are going to kill somebody. One midwife told the nurse when we had the meeting, she just told her, "I think I'll bring my bag in and give it to you all because you all are not there when this labor is going on. You don't know how it goes. Rubbing helps and teas help. If I can't give them some hot teas which I know will help, I just well ought to give it up."...

So I quit. I quit trying to do anything but what they gave me to work with. I had been working a good while when I threw that root out my bag. (pp. 99–101)

Smith's account of her life and work paints a picture of the commitment and investment made by the midwife, qualities that were phased out of the medical profession with the invention of such tools of convenience as the early models discussed by Wertz and Wertz. There seem to be four main reasons why midwives had more success than medical doctors. Doctors, restricted by Victorian rules of modesty, practiced medicine blindly, whereas midwives were able to actually look at their patients as they treated them. Doctors practiced various types of medicine, but midwives were specialized in treating women. Doctors tended to rely on tools, while midwives relied on hands-on experience. Finally, and perhaps most importantly, doctors—ignorant of germ theory and basic aseptic techniques—were more likely to carry infection from one patient to the next.

Medicine and Morality in the Nineteenth Century

KRISTIN LUKER

Excerpted from Kristen Luker, *Abortion and the Politics of Motherhood*, Berkeley, University of California Press, 1984. Reprinted by permission.

Kristin Luker, sociologist at the University of California, San Diego, demonstrates how—beginning in 1859—the American Medical Association launched a successful campaign to ban induced abortions, not for the sake of their patients' health (to the contrary: more women's lives were lost) but to publicize themselves and call attention to their own "moral stature" and "technical expertise." —B. S.

Surprising as it may seem, the view that abortion is murder is a relatively recent belief in American history. To be sure, there has always been a school of thought, extending back at least to the Pythagoreans of ancient Greece, that holds that abortion is wrong because the embryo is the moral equivalent of the child it will become. Equally ancient, however, is the belief articulated by the Stoics: that although embryos have some of the rights of already-born children (and these rights may increase over the course of the pregnancy), embryos are of a different moral order, and thus to end their existence by an abortion is not tantamount to murder....

In the Roman Empire, abortion was so frequent and widespread that it was remarked upon by a number of authors. Ovid, Juvenal, and Seneca all noted the existence of abortion, and the natural historian Pliny listed prescriptions for drugs that would accomplish it. Legal regulation of abortion in the Roman Empire, however, was virtually nonexistent. Roman law explicitly held that the "child in the belly of its mother" was not a person, and hence abortion was not murder. After the beginning of the Christina era, such legal regulation of abortion as existed in the Roman Empire was designed primarily to protect the rights of fathers rather than the rights of embryos....

THE ORIGINS OF THE FIRST RIGHT-TO-LIFE MOVEMENT

At the opening of the nineteenth century, no statute laws governed abortion in America. What minimal legal regulation existed was inherited from English common law tradition that abortion undertaken before quickening was at worst a misdemeanor. *Quickening*, as that term was understood in the nineteenth century, was the period in pregnancy when a woman felt fetal movement; though it varies from woman to woman (and even from pregnancy to pregnancy in the same woman), it generally occurs between the fourth and the sixth month of pregnancy. Consequently in nineteenth-century America, as in medieval Europe, first-trimester abortions, and a goodly number of second-trimester abortions as well, faced little legal regulation. Practically speaking, the difficulty of determining when conception had occurred, combined with the fact that the only person who could reliably tell when the pregnancy had "quickened" was the pregnant woman herself, meant that even this minimal regulation was probably infrequent. In 1809, when the Massachusetts State Supreme Court dismissed an indictment for abortion because the prosecution had not reliably proved that the woman was "quick with child," it was simply reiterating traditional common law standards.

In contrast, by 1900 every state in the Union had passed a law forbidding the use of drugs or instruments to procure abortion at any stage of pregnancy, "unless the same be necessary to save the woman's life." Not only were those who performed an abortion liable for a felony (usually manslaughter or second-degree homicide), but in many states, the aborted woman herself faced the possibility of criminal prosecution, still another departure from the tolerant common law tradition in existence at the beginning of the century.

Many cultural themes and social struggles lie behind the transition from an abortion climate that was remarkably open and unrestricted to one that restricted abortions (at least in principle) to those necessary to save the life of the mother. The second half of the nineteenth century, when the bulk of American abortion laws were written, saw profound changes in the social order, and these provided the foundation for dramatic changes in the status of abortion. Between 1850 and 1900, for example, the population changed from one that was primarily rural and agricultural to one that was urban and industrial, and the birth rates fell accordingly, declining from an estimated average completed fertility for whites of 7.04 births per woman in 1800 to an average of 3.56 births in 1900. The "great wave" of American immigration occurred in this period, as did the first feminist movement.

The intricate relationships between social roles, moral values, and medical technologies that were associated with changing patterns of fertility simultaneously became both the cause and the product of demographic strains—strains between rural and urban dwellers; between native-born "Yankees" and immigrants; between the masses and the elites; and possibly between men and women.

But within this complex background against which the first American debate on abortion emerged, we can trace a more direct social struggle. The most visible interest group agitating for more restrictive abortion laws was composed of elite or "regular" physicians, who actively petitioned state legislatures to pass anti-abortion laws and undertook through popular writings a campaign to change public opinion on abortion. The efforts of these physicians were probably the single most important influence in bringing about nineteenth-century anti-abortion laws. (Ironically, a century later it would be physicians who would play a central role in overturning these same laws.) Even more important is the fact that nineteenth-century physicians opposed abortion as part of an effort to achieve other political and social goals, and this led them to frame their opposition to abortion in particular ways.

PHYSICIANS IN THE NINETEENTH CENTURY

Modern observers accustomed to thinking of the medical profession as prestigious, technically effective, and highly paid are sometimes shocked to learn that it was none of those things in the nineteenth century. On the contrary, much of its history during that century was an uphill struggle to attain just those attributes. Whereas European physicians entered the modern era with at least the legacy of well-defined guild structures—structures that took responsibility for teaching, maintained the right to determine who could practice, and exercised some control over the conduct and craft of the profession— American physicians did not. Because of its history as a colony, the United States attracted few guild-trained physicians, and consequently, a formal guild structure never developed. Healing in this country started out primarily as a domestic rather than a professional skill (women and slaves often developed considerable local reputations as healers), and therefore anyone who claimed medical talent could practice—and for the most part could practice outside of any institutional controls of the sort that existed in Europe.

From the earliest days of the medical profession in this country, therefore, physicians wanted effective licensing laws that would do for them what the guild structures had done for their European colleagues, namely, restrict the competition.

For the first third of the century, physicians had depended on a model of illness that called upon the use of drastic medical treatments such as bleeding or the administration of harsh laxatives and emetics. By the 1850s, a new group of physicians (including such luminaries as Oliver Wendell Holmes) rejected the use of this "heroic armamentarium" and earned for themselves the sobriquet of "therapeutic nihilists" inasmuch as they seemed to argue that anything a physician could do was probably ineffective and might be dangerous as well.

Two other developments in the course of the century kept the social and professional status of medicine low. First, as the effectiveness of "heroic" medicine was called into question by some physicians themselves, there was a proliferation of healers who advocated new models of treatment. Thomsonians, botanics, and homeopaths among others all developed "sects" of healing and claimed the title of doctor for themselves. These nineteenth-century sectarians flourished, perhaps in part because they intended to support relatively mild forms of treatment (baths, natural diets) instead of the "heroic" measures used by many doctors. Thus, regular physicians (those who had some semblance of formal training and who subscribed to the dominant medical model) found themselves in increasing competition with the sectarians, who they considered quacks....

ABORTIONS IN NINETEENTH-CENTURY AMERICA

With respect to abortion, as with respect to physicians, modern-day stereotypes about the nineteenth century can easily lead us astray. Contrary to our assumptions about "Victorian morality," the available evidence suggests that abortions were frequent. To be sure, some of these abortions may have been disguised (or rationalized) by those who sought them. Early in the century, a dominant therapeutic model saw the human body as an "intake-outflow" system and disease as the result of some disturbance in the regular production of secretions. Prominent among medical concerns, therefore, was "blocked" or "obstructed" menstruation, and the nineteenth-century pharmacopoeia contained numerous emmenagogues designed to "bring down the courses," that is, to reestablish menstruation. However, since the primary cause of "menstrual obstruction" in a healthy and sexually active woman was probably pregnancy, at least some of these emmenagogues must have been used with the intent to cause an abortion. Especially in the absence of accurate pregnancy tests, these drugs could be used in good faith by physicians and women alike, but the frequent warnings that these same drugs should not be used by "married ladies" because they would cause miscarriage made their alternative uses quite clear....

PHYSICIANS AND ABORTION

In the second half of the nineteenth century, abortion began to emerge as a social problem: newspapers began to run accounts of women who had died from "criminal abortions," although whether this fact reflects more abortions, more lethal abortions, or simply more awareness is not clear. Most prominently, physicians became involved, arguing that abortion was both morally wrong and medically dangerous.

The membership of the American Medical Association (AMA), founded in 1847 to upgrade and protect the interests of the profession, was deeply divided on many issues. But by 1859, it was able to pass a resolution condemning induced abortion and urging state legislatures to pass laws forbidding it; in 1860, Henry Miller, the president-elect of the association, devoted much of his presidential address to attacking abortion; and in 1864, the AMA established a prize to be awarded to the best anti-abortion book written for the lay public. Slowly, physicians responded to the AMA's call and began to lobby in state legislatures for laws forbidding abortion.

Why should nineteenth-century physicians have become so involved with the question of abortion? The physicians themselves gave two related explanations for their activities, and these explanations have been taken at face value ever since. First, they argued, they were compelled to address the abortion questions because American women were committing a moral crime based on ignorance about the proper value of embryonic life. According to these physicians, women sought abortions because the doctrine of quickening led them to believe that the embryo was not alive, and therefore aborting it was perfectly proper. Second, they argued, they were obliged to act in order to save women from their own ignorance because only physicians were in possession of new scientific evidence which demonstrated beyond a shadow of doubt that the embryo was a child from conception onward.

The physicians were probably right in their belief that American women did not consider abortion—particularly early abortion—to be morally wrong. But the core of the physicians' claim—the assertions that women practiced abortion because they were ignorant of the biological facts of pregnancy and that physicians were opposed to it because they were in possession of new scientific evidence—had no solid basis in fact....

MOTIVES FOR MOBILIZATION

Thus, the question remains: Why, in the middle of the nineteenth century, did some physicians become active anti-abortionists? James Mohr, in a pioneering work on this topic, argues that the proliferation of healers in the nineteenth century created a competition for status and clients. The "regular" physicians, who tended to be both wealthier and better educated than members of other medical sects, therefore sought to distinguish themselves both scientifically and socially from competing practitioners.

Mohr suggests that there were several more practical reasons why regular physicians should have opposed abortion. On the one hand, outlawing abortion would remove a lucrative source of income from competitors they called "quacks" and perhaps remove the temptation from the path of the "regulars" as well. In addition, the "regulars" were predominantly white, upper-income, and native-born; as such, they belonged to precisely the same group that was thought to harbor the primary users of abortion. As a result, they were likely to be concerned both about the depopulation of their group in the face of mounting immigration (and the higher fertility of immigrants) and about "betrayal" by their own women (because abortion required less male control and approval than the other available forms of birth control).

More broadly, Mohr argues that nineteenth-century physicians had a firm ideological belief that abortion was in fact murder. He asserts that they tended to place absolute value on human life and that having established to their own satisfaction that abortion represented the loss of human life, abortion became included in this more general value. The historian Carl Degler has made much the same argument: "Seen against the broad canvas of humanitarian thought and practice in Western society from the seventeenth to the twentieth century, the expansion of the definition of life to include the whole career of the fetus rather than only the months after quickening is quite consistent. It is in line with a number of movements to reduce cruelty and to expand the concept of sanctity of life."…

By the middle of the nineteenth century, American physicians had few if any of the formal attributes of a profession. The predominance of proprietary medical schools combined with the virtual absence of any form of licensing meant that the regulars could control neither entry into the profession nor the performance of those who claimed healing capacities. With the possible exceptions of the thermometer, the stethoscope, and the forceps, the technological tools of modern medicine were yet to come; and lacking the means of professional control, regular physicians were hard put to keep even those simple instruments out of the hands of the competition. Because they could offer no direct, easily observable, and dramatic proof of their superiority, regular physicians were forced to make an indirect, *symbolic* claim about their status. By becoming visible activists on an issue such as abortion, they could claim both *moral stature* (as a high-minded, self-regulating group of professionals) and *technical expertise* (derived from their superior training).

Therefore the physicians' choice of abortion as the focus of their moral crusade was carefully calculated. Abortion, and only abortion, could enable them to make symbolic claims about their status. Unlike the other medico-moral issues of the time —alcoholism, slavery, venereal disease, and prostitution

—only abortion gave physicians the opportunity to claim to be saving human lives. Given the primitive nature of medical practice, persuading the public that embryos were human lives and then persuading the state legislatures to protect these lives by outlawing abortion may have been one of the few life-saving projects actually available to physicians.

Physicians, therefore, have to exaggerate the differences between themselves and the lay public. Anti-abortion physicians had to claim that women place no value on embryonic life whereas they themselves ranked the embryo as a full human life, namely, as a baby. But these two positions, when combined, created an unresolvable paradox for physicians, a paradox that would haunt the abortion debate until the present day.

Water Therapy as a Women's Health Tool

DIAN DINCIN BUCHMAN

Adapted from Dian Dincin Buchman, *The Complete Book of Water Therapy: 500 Ways to Use Our Oldest Natural Medicine*, New Canaan, Conn., Keats, 1994. Reprinted by permission.

The American Medical Association, founded in 1847, excluded women and alternative practitioners. In her authoritative 1998 book Women's Health Care: Activist Traditions and Institutional Change, *Carol Weisman, professor of public health at the University of Michigan, explains that two alternative therapies particularly favored by women of that era were hydrotherapy and Thomsonian botanics:*

"Hydrotherapy was based on European methods that were introduced in the United States in the 1840s. Hydropaths used water treatments—ingesting water and various applications of water to the body—for the amelioration of many conditions, and stressed the importance of healthful habits such as exercise and proper diet. The water-cure establishments they administered were frequented by both women and men, but they offered specific benefits to women. These included respite from domestic responsibilities, female companionship in the residential treatment environment, care by female physicians, and relatively gentle treatments for a variety of women's health problems. Hydropathic training institutes actively recruited women for training, based on the belief that women had unique healing skills and that 'no Water-Cure establishment is complete without a qualified female physician.' Beginning in 1844, hydropaths also published the widely circulated Water-Cure Journal, *which included popular articles on a variety of topics related to women's health, such as diet and clothing reform.*

"Thomsonian botanics also emphasized gentle treatments and the role of women as caregivers. Samuel Thomson was a New England farmer who developed a patented system of botanics to be administered as home treatments and published a popular manual on his system in 1822. His followers were primar-

ily working class, and the sect appealed to women because of its reliance on herbal remedies, because it viewed women as the appropriate caretakers for their families' health, and because of its support for midwives, whom Thomsonians perceived as providing safer, less expensive care than physicians."

Because of renewed interest in alternative therapies, Dian Dincin Buchman's book The Complete Book of Water Therapy *is being reissued in 2000, under the title* The Complete Book of Water Healing.*—B. S.*

The water therapies used by women in the popular health movement of the 1830s and 1840s are rooted in ancient medicine. During a time when the medical profession was still developing, hydrotherapy's appeal to the masses represented the widespread desire to keep health care personal, safe, and effective.

One of the first written mentions of the use of water as medicine involves the temples of the Greek god of medicine, Asclepius. At the temples, bathing and massage were part of the treatment for the sick. Hippocrates, whom we consider the "father of medicine," is alleged to be a descendant of the legendary Asclepius. Hippocrates used water as a beverage in reducing fever and for treating many diseases. He also stressed the values of using various types of baths, each with a different temperature, as a therapeutic tool to combat illness.

Water's three forms—liquid, steam, ice—can be used in a wide variety of temperatures and, especially in the case of showers or whirlpool, can be used with different pressure. Water can be used internally by drinking it or by forcing streams of water into body orifices, as in an enema, a douche, or a nose or ear bath. Water can also be used externally in the form of full or partial baths; showers, even on minute spots of the body; single or double compresses; or in various simultaneous or alternating combinations.

AS A RESTORATIVE AND A TONIC Water not only restores the body's normal circulation and temperature, but intelligent water treatment, especially with cold water, can also act to restore and increase muscle strength and increase the body's resistance to disease. Cold water boosts vigor, adds energy and tone, and aids in digestion.

Techniques. Cold-water treading, whirlpool baths, cold sprays, alternate hot-and-cold contrast showers or compresses, salt rubs, apple cider vinegar baths, salt baths, partial baths.

TO REDUCE FEVER Water is nature's best cooling agent. Unlike drugs, which usually only diminish internal heat, water lowers the heat and removes it by conduction. In reducing fever, water is far more valuable than any medicine; it is the treatment of choice for fever, sunstroke, and heatstroke. The Brand cold-bath technique, a prolonged full cold bath, should be investigated as adjunct therapy for heat prostration.

Techniques: Short cold baths, prolonged tepid baths, dousings, sponging, cold-mitten massage, high enema irrigation, damp-sheet packs.

AS A STIMULANT Water applications can revitalize, awaken, or arouse parts of the entire body.

Techniques: Hot or cold baths, sponging, damp-sheet packs, enema or colon irrigation, whirlpool baths, salt rubs, salt baths, hot or cold showers, alternating hot-and-cold showers.

AS A SEDATIVE Water is a very efficient, nontoxic calming substance. It soothes the body and promotes sleep.

Techniques: Hot and warm baths to quiet and relax the entire body, salt baths, neutral showers to certain areas, damp-sheet packs.

FOR RELIEF OF PELVIC-AREA SPASMS Water therapy can relieve spasms of the bladder, rectum, or uterus in a variety of ways.

Techniques: Apply hot, moist compresses to the pelvic area for prolonged periods to relieve spasms of the bladder, rectum, and uterus and to increase menstrual flow. Sit in a cold, shallow bath to decrease the flow. Immerse feet in a hot footbath to relieve cramps. Showers on the shoulder area act by reflex on the pelvic area. For noninflammatory pelvic problems, sit in a hot, shallow bath or immerse feet in a hot footbath.

Women's Health and Government Regulation, 1820–1949

SUZANNE WHITE JUNOD

©1999 by Suzanne White Junod. Reprinted by permission.

Suzanne White Junod, a historian with the Food and Drug Administration, has compiled an original review of health issues over which women consumers organized to obtain government protection. In 1933, Eleanor Roosevelt was so impressed by an FDA "Chamber of Horrors" exhibit of dangerous drugs and cosmetics that she "moved it directly to the White House and showed it to anybody who would look," setting the stage for passage of the 1938 Food, Drugs, and Cosmetics Act.

On the other hand, "the first state statutes regulating abortion were, in fact, poison control laws. The sale of commercial abortifacients was banned but not abortion per se." In 1902, "the editors of the Journal of the American Medical Association *endorsed a policy of denying medical care to a woman who was suffering from abortion complications until she 'confessed.' This practice prevented women from seeking timely medical treatment. By the late 1920s an estimated 15,000 women a year were dying from abortions."—B. S.*

Women have always taken the lead in protecting themselves and their families from impure foods and dangerous drugs and medical devices. In the last two centuries, largely as a result of pressure from women, government agencies have taken an increasing interest in women's health issues: fertility, childbirth, menopause, geriatrics, and general nutrition and well-being. Following is a chronology of the regulation of products and devices affecting women's health.

THE NINETEENTH CENTURY

ABORTION During the nineteenth century, the abortion business, including the sale of widely advertised abortifacient drugs, was booming. Commercial preparations were so widely available that they inspired their own euphemism: "taking the trade." The first state statutes regulating abortion were in fact poison-control laws. The sale of commercial abortifacients was banned, but not abortion per se.

In June 1895, at the meeting of the Washington, D.C., Obstetrical and Gynecological Society, Dr. Joseph Taber Johnson encouraged his colleagues to begin a crusade against abortion. They had to convince both women and the medical profession that abortion was wrong. In 1902, the editors of the *Journal of the American Medical Association* endorsed a policy of denying medical care to a woman who was suffering from abortion complications until she "confessed." This practice prevented women from seeking timely treatment. By the late 1920s, an estimated 15,000 women were dying from abortions each year.

DRUGS AND UNSAFE ADDITIVES In 1880, Peter Collier, chief chemist at the U.S. Department of Agriculture, recommended a national food and drug law. Twelve years later, in 1892, the law (known as the Paddock bill) did pass the Senate, but it was not taken up by the House of Representatives.

By the turn of the century, women were actively agitating against the use of opium, morphine, and laudanum in so-called baby-soothing syrups, used to calm colicky babies. Women's groups (most notably the General Federation of Women's Clubs) and muckraking journalists also exposed the high alcohol content of most of the women's proprietary "tonics." Unlike men, who drank openly in saloons, women frequently became addicted to alcohol under the guise of self-medication and nursed their addictions surreptitiously at home.

The Women's National Labor League (later the National Women's Industrial League) decided to take matters into their own hands by putting direct pressure on the National Wholesale Druggists Association at their annual convention in Washington, D.C. They tried to present the association with a petition that, in effect, called for full disclosure and honesty in advertising.

Since the industrial classes could not always afford adequate medical care, said the league women, it was important that the proprietary remedies on which they depended should be reliable. Therefore, the products should be sold under fully informative labels that would show what was in them but not carry fraudulent claims about their therapeutic value. Furthermore, such products as Mrs. Winslow's Soothing Syrup, which contained morphine and was innocently given to babies, should be taken off the market entirely.

Haughtily the druggists told them that unless the reference to Mrs. Winslow's was struck out, they would not entertain the petition.

The women refused. They had drawn up the petition to express their own views, not to please the druggists; now they threatened to move on to Capitol Hill. Thoroughly alarmed, the druggists warned them that if they did anything of the kind and a clause directed against patent medicines found its way into the food and drug bill, the industry would spend half a million dollars to defeat the measure.

Despite the druggists' threat, the women went straight to Capitol Hill and informed members of Congress that it was not enough to prosecute the shippers who violated the law; their adulterated and misbranded merchandise had to be confiscated and destroyed as well. When the Food and Drug Act finally passed in 1906, it contained a provision for the seizure of illegal foods and drugs, largely as a result of the women's pressure. According to Ruth Lamb, who wrote *American Chamber of Horrors* in the 1930s advocating the need for a new federal food and drug statue:

> The full significance of this provision seems not to have been appreciated by anyone at the time, for it remained in succeeding food and drug bills and was finally enacted into law—to become the most hated and bitterly contested feature of the whole statute. To that perspicacious group of women in the 1890s, and their leader, Charlotte Smith, the public is forever indebted, for this single provision of the Food and Drugs Act has been, beyond all cavil, the government's most powerful weapon against dangerous or fraudulent products.

The drug-labeling provisions of the 1906 act required that the percentages of alcohol and other "dangerous" ingredients be clearly listed on the label. Although this early law did not make such products illegal, it did at least prevent them from being sold as "cures" for alcoholism. As a result, manufacturers generally reduced the amount of alcohol in their products and replaced the opium, laudanum, and morphine with less dangerous ingredients that did not have to be disclosed on the label itself.

THE EARLY TWENTIETH CENTURY

The Nineteenth Amendment granting women's suffrage was ratified on August 18, 1920. This was also a time of important medical discoveries.

> ➤ In 1922, Banting, Best, Macleod, and Collip at the University of Toronto announced the discovery of insulin as a treatment of diabetes mellitus. Their first patient was a 14-year-old girl, who, after initiating injections of insulin, lived to the ripe old age of 77.

➤ By 1922, radical mastectomy, introduced by William Halsted, had become the standard "cure" for breast cancer. Lung tissue, but not the soft tissue of the breasts, could be seen on x-rays.

➤ In 1927, Aurel Babes published an article in France discussing the possibility of cancer diagnosis from vaginal smears. His method was substantially different from the one developed later by George Papanicolaou, who published his "New Cancer Diagnosis" a year later in the *Proceedings of the Third Race Betterment Foundation.*

➤ In 1927, Congress enacted the Caustic Poison Act requiring warning labels to protect children from accidental death and injury caused by lye and 10 other caustic chemicals. The campaign for passage of the act was led by Dr. Chevalier Jackson and supported by the American Medical Association. The Food and Drug Administration (FDA) was given enforcement responsibilities.

➤ In 1928, Alexander Fleming discovered penicillin (which did not become available for widespread clinical use in civilian populations until 1945). Deaths from childbed or puerpheral fever dropped dramatically as a result of penicillin and other antibiotics.

WOMEN'S PRODUCTS CHAMBER OF HORRORS

During the 1920s, as women became more active outside the home, the cosmetics industry grew out of obscurity into a multimillion-dollar industry. Women's and consumer groups became concerned about the dangers of some of these new cosmetic products, notably hair dyes and rouges, as well as the safety of such devices as womb pessaries, bust enhancers, and nose straighteners; women's "tonics"; and the unrestricted use of amphetamines and other weight reduction drugs.

In the summer of 1933, the FDA set up an exhibit illustrating abuses in the sale of food, drugs, and cosmetics not covered by the Food and Drug Act of 1906. A number of the women's beauty and diet aids in the exhibit—hair dyes, depilatories, pessaries, skin whiteners—contained dangerous poisons such as lead, silver, pyrogallol, mercury, thyroid, thallium acetate, barium sulfide, and paraphenylene diamine. Other products made false or inflated claims.

After viewing the exhibit, Eleanor Roosevelt took up the cause. She had the exhibit moved from the offices of the FDA directly to the White House and showed it to anybody who would look. But, according to a Washington *Star* account, "the politicians paid absolutely no attention to her. They regarded her as a nuisance and didn't think that there were any votes involved in it, and she had no effect at all except as she worked through the women's organizations. And, of course, she did this a lot." She appealed to the nation's women to join the campaign for a new, more all-encompassing law. This set the stage for the passage of the 1938 Food, Drug, and Cosmetics Act.

The new law expanded the FDA's regulatory powers. Under the 1906 act, thyroid preparations were a drug, but because obesity was not considered a disease, the agency could not act against these preparations. But under the new law, the FDA could act against drugs designed *to change the structure of the body* (thyroid increased metabolism). The new law also allowed action against radium waters and radiopharmaceuticals (previously thought to be "natural") as well as nose straighteners and womb pessaries, all of which were now classified as drugs.

The new law also had a direct impact on the quality of prophylactics. The FDA announced that regardless of the nature of the products, or the methods in which they were used, all articles intended as "venereal disease preventives" were subject to the provisions of the act, and that articles depending for their prophylactic effect on preventing contact with infecting organisms should be free from defects. In an extensive survey of rubber and membrane prophylactics, 181 consignments seized from nine manufacturers were found to be defective. As a result, producers withdrew much of their outstanding stocks and made drastic changes in their manufacturing processes.

Another product that had a great impact on women's lives was the tampon. By 1921, there were at least 16 patents for tampons and one for a tampon applicator. Their use was limited to the treatment of disease. In 1933, Dr. Earle Hass patented the tampon that was introduced three years later in improved form as the Tampax tampon. Doctors and nurses actively promoted disposable sanitary pads and tampons in the increasingly "antiseptic" culture. Women viewed these products as practical and labor-saving. By 1947, 538 gross dozens, with a value of $11,099,000 were shipped to retailers. Tampons had been accepted.

THE 1940s: DIAGNOSING CANCER IN WOMEN

By the 1940s, 26,000 American women were dying of uterine cancer every year. George Papanicolaou and Herbert Traut published "The Diagnostic Value of Vaginal Smears in Carcinoma of the Uterus" in the *American Journal of Obstetrics and Gynecology*. This article presented their technique for obtaining a smear and their theory of exfoliative cytology, which allows the interpretation of the smears and the detection of malignancy. The National Cancer Institute estimates that between 1950 and 1970, deaths from cervical cancer dropped 70 percent. The decrease in cancer deaths was a direct result of the Pap smear.

Realizing the need for better breast imaging, Stafford Warren, a pioneer in radiation at the UCLA School of Medicine, developed a stereoscopic grid system for identifying malignant breast tumors. In 1949, John Wild applied ultrasound to distinguish malignant from healthy tissues. That same year, Paul Leborgne from Uruguay demonstrated the importance of high-contrast breast images in about 30 percent of the cases he examined, and established the value of breast compression in identifying benign and malignant breast tumors.

BRAVE NEW WORLD

In 1937, *The New England Journal of Medicine* carried an anonymous editorial discussing the possibility of conception in a watch glass as a future treatment of dysfunctional fallopian tubes. In 1940, Charles Huggins first reported the value of diethylstilbestrol (DES) in the treatment of prostate tumors. In 1944, after six years of intense experimentation, John Rock, a birth control pioneer, and a colleague claimed in vitro fertilization of a human ovum. The procedure and their results were accompanied with pictures and published in *Science*. In 1949, Barr and his colleagues noted that it was possible to distinguish male and female cells from the presence or absence of a small cellular body. Knowing the sex of the fetus had implications for families with histories of sex-linked diseases.

No one could have predicted where all this would lead in the second half of the twentieth century.

In their 1973 booklet, Complaints and Disorders: The Sexual Politics of Sickness, *a companion to* Witches, Midwives, and Nurses, *Barbara Ehrenreich and Deirdre English persuasively exposed the role of medicine in the social control of women:*

"Medicine stands between biology and social policy, between the 'mysterious' world of the laboratory and everyday life.... Biology discovers hormones; doctors make public judgments on whether 'hormonal imbalances' make women unfit for public office."

Before the nineteenth century, it was largely religion's task to portray the female as weak and incomplete, a 'misbegotten male,' but, with the blossoming of science, "nineteenth-century religious leaders happily supplemented religious justifications of sexism with newly developed infirmities won out over her moral defects as the rationale for male supremacy."

Women of the affluent classes were deemed too fragile, and too refined for strenuous activity, intellectual or physical, which might draw energy from the reproductive organs, where their destiny lay.... Popular medical authorities constructed the myth that working-class women were less vulnerable, almost a different species. In the words of Dr. Lucien Warner, in 1874, "the African negress, who toils beside her husband in the fields of the south, and Bridget, who washes and scrubs and toils in our homes at the north, enjoy for the most part good health, with comparative immunity from uterine disease." In the following selections, the voices of Sojourner Truth ("Nobody ever helps me into carriages or over mud puddles") and Charlotte Perkins Gilman ("Men have bred a race of women weak enough to be handed about like invalids, or mentally weak enough to pretend they are…") illustrate the double standard.—B. S.

Ain't I a Woman?

SOJOURNER TRUTH

Sojourner Truth (1795–1883) was born into slavery in New York State. She won her freedom in 1827, when that state emancipated its slaves. After working in New York City as a domestic for some years, she felt called by God to testify to the sins against her people. Dropping her slave name, Isabella, she took the symbolic name of Sojourner Truth. She spoke at camp meetings, private homes, wherever she could gather an audience. By midcentury she was well-known in antislavery circles and a frequent speaker at abolitionist gatherings.

Sojourner Truth consistently and actively identified herself with the cause of women's rights. She was the only Black woman present at the First National Woman's Rights Convention in Worcester, Massachusetts, in 1850.

The following year Sojourner Truth spoke at a women's convention at Akron, Ohio, presided over by Frances D. Gage. Since Truth could neither read nor write, all her words have come down through history interpreted by other people, usually white women, all of whom had their own agendas. As Nell Irvine Painter points out in her 1996 book, Sojourner Truth: A Life, a Symbol, *"Truth depended upon disparate amanuenses for the preservation of her identity. They represented her according to their own lights, often in dialect of their own invention."*

The Akron speech was written down by Gage 12 years after it was spoken as a response to an article in The Atlantic Monthly *by Harriet Beecher Stowe. Where Stowe's version of Sojourner Truth emphasizes her religion, Gage emphasizes or invents anger. Specifically, the phrase "ar'nt I a woman?," sometimes written in dialect as "ain't I a woman?," was Gage's invention.—B. S.*

Well, children, where there is so much racket there must be something out of kilter. I think that 'twixt the Negroes of the South and the women at the North, all talking about rights, the white men will be in a fix pretty soon. But what's all this here talking about?

That man over there says that women need to be helped into carriages, and lifted over ditches, and to have the best place everywhere. Nobody ever helps me into carriages, or over mud puddles, or gives me any best place! And ain't I a woman? Look at me! Look at my arm! I have ploughed and planted, and gathered into barns, and no man could head me! And ain't I a women? I could work as much and eat as much as a man—when I could get it—and bear the lash as well! And ain't I a woman? I have borne thirteen children, and seen them most all sold off to slavery, and when I cried out with my mother's grief, none but Jesus heard me! And ain't I a woman?

Then they talk about this thing in the head; what's this they call it? [Intellect, someone whispers.] That's it, honey. What's that got to do with women's rights or Negro's rights? If my cup won't hold but a pint, and yours holds a quart, wouldn't you be mean not to let me have my little half-measure full?

Then that little man in black there, he says women can't have as much rights as man, 'cause Christ wasn't a woman! Where did your Christ come from? Where did you Christ come from? From God and a woman! Man had nothing to do with Him.

If the first woman God ever made was strong enough to turn the world upside down all alone, these women together ought to be able to turn it back, and get it right side up again! And now they is asking to do it, the men better let them.

Obliged to you for hearing me, and now old Sojourner ain't got nothing more to say.

Excerpt from The Yellow Wallpaper

CHARLOTTE PERKINS GILMAN

Charlotte Perkins Gilman, *The Yellow Wallpaper*, Old Westbury, NY, The Feminist Press, 1973.

For Charlotte Perkins Gilman (1860–1935) the body of her work came almost directly out of her personal struggles. In her lifetime she was known around the world, although today she has been largely forgotten.

She was born Charlotte Anna Perkins on July 3, 1860, in Hartford, Connecticut. She was raised by her mother, Mary A. Fitch, because her father deserted the family soon after Charlotte's birth. From age 16 to 21 Charlotte lived primarily with her mother. During this time she initiated a new lifestyle that included health and dress reform and a commitment to reading, learning, and art.

In January 1882, Charlotte met Charles Walter Stetson. Within days he proposed marriage, and she refused. Ultimately, with grave reservations, she accepted his proposal.

Her fears and self-doubts, which had persisted during the courtship, led to despondency in marriage. She became so seriously depressed after the birth of her first child, Katherine Beecher, that she was persuaded by her husband to consult a specialist in women's nervous diseases. He prescribed extended bed rest, isolation, and near total inactivity. This treatment almost cost Charlotte her sanity.

Calling upon some inner sense of survival, she rejected both husband and physician and fled to the house of friends in California. Some time later she and Walter were divorced. Charlotte supported herself her daughter and mother (who stayed with her until her death by cancer in 1892) by running a boardinghouse.

In this difficult period Charlotte launched her career as a writer and lecturer. Her first major piece of work was the chilling short story "The Yellow Wallpaper," an intensely personal examination of her private nightmare. Her most famous book was Women and Economics, published in 1898. It was soon translated into seven languages and won her international recognition. Her other books include Concerning Children, The Home: Its Work and Influence, and Human Work. In 1935 Charlotte completed her autobiography, The Living of Charlotte Perkins Gilman. From 1909 to 1916 she edited and wrote The Forerunner, a monthly magazine.

In the spring of 1900, after a long and complicated courtship, she married George Houghton Gilman, and they remained together for more than three decades. When Houghton Gilman died suddenly in 1934, Charlotte moved back to Pasadena to live near her daughter. Charlotte died a year later.

"The Yellow Wallpaper" is based on Gilman's experience of 19th century medicine. Seriously depressed after the birth of her first child, Katherine Beecher, she was persuaded by her husband to consult Dr. Weir Mitchell, the leading specialist in women's nervous diseases. He prescribed extended bed rest, isolation, and near total inactivity. This treatment almost cost Charlotte her sanity and became the setting for her hallucinatory novella. To "cure" her "temporary nervous condition," the fictional narrator is confined to a bedroom in a country house, where the wallpaper begins to obsess her. She eventually decides that a woman is trapped behind the wallpaper, shaking it and trying to get out. In the end, the narrator strips the paper from the wall, freeing the trapped woman, who is clearly herself.—B. S.

As soon as it was moonlight and that poor thing began to crawl and shake the pattern, I got up and ran to help her.

I pulled and she shook, I shook and she pulled, and before morning we had peeled off yards of that paper.

A strip about as high as my head and half around the room.

And then when the sun came and that awful pattern began to laugh at me, I declared I would finish it to-day!

We go away to-morrow, and they are moving all my furniture down again to leave things as they were before.

[...]

I have locked the door and thrown the key down into the front path.

I suppose I shall have to get back behind the pattern when it comes night, and that is hard!

It is so pleasant to be out in this great room and creep around as I please!
[...]

(John) came in. He stopped short by the door.

"What is the matter?" he cried. "For God's sake, what are you doing!"

I kept on creeping just the same, but I looked at him over my shoulder.

"I've got out at last," said I, "in spite of you and Jane. And I've pulled off most of the paper, so you can't put me back!"

Now why should that man have fainted? But he did, and right across my path by the wall, so that I had to creep over him every time!

Women and Drug Addiction

STEPHEN R. KANDALL, M.D.

Excerpted from Stephen R. Kandall, M.D., *Substance and Shadow: Women and Addiction in the United States,* Cambridge, Mass., Harvard University Press, 1996. Reprinted by permission.

By 1782, it was common practice for the women of Nantucket Island to "take a dose of opium every morning." A century of so later, "although drug use was known to exist among women of all social classes, the stereotypical picture was that of a genteel white, middle- or upper-middle-class Southern lady much like the ennobled morphine-addicted Mrs. Henry Lafayette Dubose portrayed in Harper Lee's novel To Kill A Mockingbird.*" In every generation, physicians prescribe mind-numbing drugs to affluent female patients, but the roster of "respectable" products changes over time, depending, it seems, on who has the economic and political influence to determine what will be designated as "licit" or "illicit." In the nineteenth century, women relied on opiates, cocaine, chloral hydrate, and cannabis to numb their mental and physical pain; in the twentieth century, read Dexedrine, Nembutal, Valium, Prozac. In the twenty-first, self-medication with legal but "alternative" treatments such as herb-based pills tinctures and teas—including ginseng, St. John's wort, valerian, chamomile, ginkgo biloba, and kava—may overtake the prescription market.—B. S.*

The inability of contemporary society to deal with addiction in women in effective and comprehensive ways recapitulates the failures of the past. Historical information on women and drug use in the United States is far less accessible than comparable information on men. Precise statistical data on female addicts for the last half of the nineteenth century is lacking, and much of the available information is buried in physicians' anecdotes and pharmacy records. A few early surveys provide limited, if sometimes contradictory, information on this population Given the primitive epidemiology of the time, the easy accessibility of unregulated "patent" medicines, and the fact that women's opiate addiction was often unknown to their families, or if known, quietly tolerated, this scarcity is not surprising.

A number of major themes recur throughout the following chapters. The central one is that on a society where drugs have been available from early times, women have always made up a significant portion, and at times a majority, of America's drug users and addicts. Popular stereotypes notwithstanding, and socioecominic backgrounds, and these factors have affected individual patterns of drug use. If these women share any common bond, it is that their addiction has not yielded to treatment. Despite their intentions, guilt and shame, both self-imposed and societal, have pushed them to the margins of society.

A second theme is the inappropriated and often excessive medication of women by physicians and pharmacists, which, along with women's own self-medication, has been a significant component of the female addiction problem. Votaire once said that "doctors our drugs, of which they know little, for diseased, of which they know less, into patients—of whom they know nothing." Throughout recent history, women have been thought to need "special protection" and regarded as less able to bear pain and psychic discomfort, whether because of "women's diseases" and "neurasthenia," as in the Victorian era, or the modern-day stresses of running a busy household, competing in a male-dominated workforce, or attempting to conform to society's slender, youthful ideal. The fact that physicians, physicians' wives and nurses have been disproportionately afflicted by addiction, and are thus less likely to view it as a "problem, has resulted in the under-estimation of its gravity. In addition, the number of female physicians, who might be expected to be more sensitive to women's needs and life stresses, has increased only in recent years.

A third theme is the unique role of women as childbearers, child rearers, and child medicators. Throughout the nineteenth century, concerned voices called attention to the dangers of the opiate-laden homeopathic and allopathic (or "conventional") medications mothers and nurses gave to children at home. Until such drugs were regulated in the early years of this century, women were held increasingly responsible for their inappropriate administration. (This theme resurfaces with new virulence in the prosecution of women for drug use during pregnancy in the 1980s.)

A fourth theme is the link between female sexuality and drug use. The association is an ancient one. Within the context of the past century and a half, it has pervaded the issues of prostitution, the perceived or proclaimed sexual threats to women from minorities, the glamorization of drug-associated sex, the connection between psychedelic drug use and "free love," and the contemporary drug-using mother's "triple curse": minority status, HIV-positive diagnosis, and children who are "drug babies."

A fifth theme is that, although concern about women's drug use has been raised, and to some degree acknowledged, for over a century, the specific issue of helping drug-addicted women was not directly confronted until the early 1970s. Before the Second World War, much of the attention focused on women and drugs came from the less-than-objective press and from the movie industry, which, by sensationalizing the threat posed to women by socially marginalized groups such as Chinese immigrants, Southern black males, and Mexican migrant workers, both mirrored and shaped society's attempts to control these "socially deviant" groups. While it is true that some women were passive beneficiaries of such drug treatment efforts as sanitariums, drug clinics, and methadone maintenance programs, not until the 1970s, following the emergence of the Women's Movement and various self-help initiatives, did addicted women finally begin to receive attention in their own right. Even then, drug-using women, especially those belonging to racial and ethnic minorities, faced hostility, prejudicial reporting to legal and child protection authorities, and criminal prosecution for drug-related conduct during pregnancy. The story of women and drugs in the United States is an ongoing one and there is, unfortunately, no end in sight.

Parlor Massages

LEORA TANENBAUM

Adapted from "Parlor Massages," Leora Tanenbaum's review of *The Technology of Orgasm: "Hysteria," the Vibrator, and Women's Sexual Satisfaction,* by Rachel P. Maines, Baltimore, Johns Hopkins University Press, 1999, published in *The Women's Review of Books,* April 1999. Reprinted by permission.

A bizarre episode in the history of physician "manipulation" of female sexuality has been accidentally discovered by Rachel Maines in The Technology of Orgasm, *here reviewed by Leora Tanenbaum.—B. S.*

Many people equate sex with heterosexual intercourse. So widespread is the idea that oral sex, for instance, "doesn't count" as sex that teenagers who engage in it exclusively identify themselves as virgins. Indeed, in the "Sex in America" national survey of a few years ago, in which over 3,000 Americans were queried about their sexual practices, 95 percent said that they had had vaginal intercourse the last time they had had sex. Eighty percent said that they had had vaginal intercourse every single time they'd had sex within the past year. Despite the opportunity for variety, coitus is far and away the most popular heterosexual act.

Which is too bad. We females know all too well that intercourse is not necessarily—how shall I put this?—the most satisfying sexual act. As Shere Hite revealed in her *Hite Report* on female sexuality back in 1976, the majority of women simply do not experience orgasm through penetration alone. It is obvious that intercourse benefits men far more than women: for the heterosexual man, coitus nearly always leads to orgasm, regardless of whether he pays any extra-coital attention to his partner's pleasure.

So where is a sexually frustrated heterosexual woman to turn to relieve her frustration? The answer: the vibrator. Easy, quick, and practically guaranteed effective, the vibrator, as many of us know, is far more efficient than manual masturbation.

The vibrator has been around far longer than you might think. In *The Technology of Orgasm,* historian Rachel Maines traces the evolution of this sex aid back to the 1880s. She also finds that the precursor to the vibrator—midwife- or physician-assisted genital massage—dates all the way back to Hippocrates. For millennia, genital massage was a medically sanctioned procedure, designed to help supposedly ill or deviant women diagnosed with "hysteria." Maines uses the vibrator as a tool (so to speak) to expose Western medicine's long-standing preference for coitus and mistrust of women who are not sexually satisfied through penetration alone. In this original, witty, thoroughly researched, and eye-opening book (complete with photographs and drawings of old-fashioned vibrators), Maines skewers male-centered beliefs about female sexual satisfaction as well as the whole concept of "hysteria."

How Maines found her topic is almost as fascinating as vibrator history itself. She started out, she explains, doing graduate research on needlework history, which meant combing through turn-of-the-century women's magazines such as *Modern Priscilla* and *Woman's Home Companion.* But her attention kept wandering to the sides of the pages, which contained vibrator advertisements. At first Maines reacted to "their turgid prose" by assuming that "I simply had a dirty mind." Surely masturbation was not the purpose of these electrical appliances. (One, White Cross, was named after an 1880s British Episcopalian sexual purity organization to suggest virtue and chastity, she notes.) But her curiosity was piqued, and she investigated this sideline interest at the Bakken Library and Museum of Electricity in Life, in Minneapolis, which houses 11 turn-of-the-century vibrators (listed in their catalogue as "musculo-skeletal relaxation devices"). Encouraged by the museum staff, Maines dropped her textile history research to pursue the origins of this "capital-labor substitution innovation."

Beginning in the fifth century B.C.E., a woman was diagnosed with hysteria if she exhibited any or all of the following: anxiety, sleeplessness, irritability, nervousness, muscle spasms, sensations of heaviness in the abdomen, or "a tendency to cause trouble for others." Hysteria was believed to result from sexual deprivation. But "sex" meant "marital coitus"; any woman who did not reach orgasm through coitus, then, was potentially diseased. In the late nineteenth century, as many as three-quarters of the American female population were diagnosed with hysteria; it is one of the most frequently diagnosed diseases in history.

Maines observes that "hysteria"—a Greek word meaning "that which proceeds from the uterus"—essentially pathologizes all women, since "this purported disease... displayed a symptomatology consistent with the normal functioning of female sexuality." The American Psychiatric Association only officially eliminated hysteria from its canon of diseases in 1952.

The standard treatment for hysteria was genital massage to orgasm, conducted either by the physician himself or by a midwife. Masturbation was forbidden, since it was believed to cause disorders and diseases (in men as well as women). In the first century C.E., Galen noted that genital massage therapy resulted in the release of a fluid from the vagina, after which the patient was cured of her symptoms (at least temporarily). Soranus instructed physicians who practiced genital massage to "moisten these parts freely with sweet oil, keeping it up for some time." In the Middle Ages and Renaissance, physicians began to turn over the task of genital massage to midwives. Maines quotes from a 1653 medical compendium in which the author advises: "we think it necessary to ask a midwife to assist, so that she can massage the genitalia with one finger inside, using oil of lilies, musk root, crocus, or [something] similar. And in this way the afflicted woman can be aroused to the paroxysm."

The amazing thing is that no one seemed to notice that the paroxysm was in fact an orgasm. Since no penetration occurred, physicians did not recognize the treatment as being sexual in nature, nor did they realize that their patients derived sexual gratification from their "hysterical paroxysm." Maines does point out that occasionally, one or two physicians would publicly express concern about "whether to draw this harmful fluid out of the uterus by exciting and rubbing the private parts," but they seem to have been vastly outnumbered by their massage-happy colleagues.

In nineteenth-century Europe and the United States, it was widely believed that women were satisfied with intercourse regardless of whether they experienced what we now define as an orgasm, or even that "normal" women possessed no sexual desire at all. Either way, the sexual nature of genital massage was camouflaged, "since in the first case no penetration (and therefore nothing sexual) was occurring during the treatment and in the second case sexual pleasure on the part of the patient was theoretically impossible."

Lest you suppose that physicians performed genital massage for their own titillation, Maines is quick to point out that they did not enjoy the treatment. "On the contrary," she writes, "this male elite sought every opportunity to substitute other devices for their fingers, such as the attentions of a husband, the hands of a midwife, or the business end of some tireless and impersonal mechanism.... Like many husbands, doctors were reluctant to inconvenience themselves in performing what was, after all, a routine chore." Indeed, Maines titles her chapter detailing the history of medical genital massage "The Job Nobody Wanted."

The electromechanical vibrator was invented in the 1880s by a British physician: the first reliable treatment for hysteria. (Hydrotherapy, a precursor to the vibrator—the use of pumped water aimed at the pelvis—had been popular for "female disorders" during the previous hundred years, but the appliances were inordinately expensive.) The vibrator was eagerly embraced by doctors, who could now significantly increase the number of patients they could treat, and the income they could generate. (Women diagnosed with hysteria formed a particularly lucrative market: their "disease" was not deadly, and they required regular treatment.) By 1900 there were over a dozen vibrators available to physicians. The "Cadillac of vibrators," the 125-pound Chattanooga, cost $200 plus freight charges in 1904.

By 1905, many models were portable, allowing their use on house calls. Soon after, manufacturers began to bypass doctors altogether and targeted their wares directly to women's magazines such as *McClure's, Needlecraft,* and *Hearst's.* They were marketed as a health and relaxation aid, promising women that "all the pleasures of youth… will throb within you." In 1918 the Sears, Roebuck and Company Electrical Goods catalog offered six vibrator models, ranging in price from $5.95 to a deluxe model with numerous vibrators at $28.75.

In the 1920s, the vibrator fell out of use. The camouflage disappeared, revealing the sexual purpose of the device: Freud and others had correctly identified the clitoral orgasm as a sexual climax (though Freud mistakenly differentiated it from the so-called vaginal orgasm). Vibrators began to appear in erotic films. No longer was it possible to pretend that a vibrator-assisted masturbatory session at the local doctor's office was just another hum-drum treatment for a chronic disease. The vibrator only resurfaced in the 1960s as a sex aid. Today, you can purchase a vibrator quite easily: you can visit a women's sex store like Good Vibrations in San Francisco and Eve's Garden in New York City, or you can stop by your local electrical appliance store and pick one up, now sold (again) as a massage relaxation aid.

The Technology of Orgasm is a fun read. But it's frightening how many of the old attitudes about female sexuality continue to thrive. As recently as 1965, one medical authority said that he did not like to recommend clitoral stimulation to his patients because "most men… feel that the need to bring a woman to climax through clitoral stimulation is a burden." Maines observes that even today, heterosexual women are made to feel guilt if they cannot reach orgasm through penetration alone. Many men, eager to preserve their own hassle-free pleasure or worried that they may be sexually inadequate, or both, scoff when presented with the mechanical facts of female sexuality.

The male preference for penetration is so strong that Maines has been unable to carve an academic career in the area of female sexuality, despite her obvious research and analytic talents. In 1986, after she published her first article on vibrators, she lost her teaching job a Clarkson University, in part because the school feared that alumni would stop giving money if they discovered her line of research. She also tells us that after one early presentation of her findings, a male tenured professor told her that he was not convinced by her arguments, since "the sexual experience of women using vibrators and their predecessors was 'not the real thing.'"

Maines retails this reaction to illustrate that many men can't even fathom male-female sexual relations without penetration. But the comment is revealing in another way as well. Perhaps the professor intended to suggest that an act should not be classified as "sex" if those involved do not think of it as such. And he would have had a point. When a midwife genitally massaged a female patient as part of her workday routine, should that act be identified as a lesbian sexual experience? I would say no. Likewise, when a male physician masturbated a patient for medical reasons, the two could hardly be said to be engaging in sex, either.

As Maines so deftly shows, "sex" means different things to different people. Harm is done, however, when female sexual needs go unrecognized because of a narrow, male-oriented definition of "sex." So let's penetrate, if you will, the myth of penetrative sex and broaden women's sexual experiences.

Sylvia Bernstein Seaman (1900–1995)

KAREN BEKKER

Paula Hyman and Deborah Dash Moore, eds., *Jewish Women in America*, vol. 2, New York, Routledge, 1997. Reprinted by permission.

Sharon Batt, founder of Breast Cancer Action Montreal and author of Patient No More: The Politics of Breast Cancer, *remarked in 1999, "Many of the women who spoke out at the beginning... had been involved in activist politics before their diagnosis. But [other] women who wrote and spoke and lobbied had no such analysis. They just had breast cancer, and were more vulnerable to co-optation by vested interests."*

In that regard, I close this section in homage to my non so optable mother-in-law, Sylvia Seaman, who was born in 1900, played hooky from high school to participate in suffrage demonstrations, and helped introduce breast cancer activism in 1965 with the publication of her book, Always a Woman, *about the mastectomy she'd undergone a decade earlier. It was the first such book by a patient prying open the "closet door," as if in preparation for the transformative 1970s titles,* Why Me? *by Rose Kushner and* First You Cry *by Betty Rollin. Sylvia's book also publicized Reach to Recovery, the first and initially the most radical of breast cancer self-help organizations, which was acquired by the American Cancer Society in 1969 and then tamed down—if not co-opted. She died in 1995 when the breast cancer—diagnosed 40 years before—caught up with her as she was preparing her speech for the Diamond Jubilee of the Nineteenth Amendment.*

I like to remind my children that their paternal grandmother may well have been the last living link between the politics of Elizabeth Cady Stanton, and the activist health feminists of today.—B. S.

I'm still capable of marching. I marched sixty years ago. I just hope my granddaughter doesn't have to march into the next century." So said Sylvia Bernstein Seaman to a *New York Times* reporter on the occasion of the tenth anniversary of the 1970 Women's Strike for Equality and the coinciding sixtieth anniversary of woman suffrage (Fig. 1). During her long life, she was not only a witness to but a catalyst for the dramatic changes in women's roles and status over the course of this century.

Sylvia Bernstein was born on November 8, 1900, to Nathan Bernstein and Fanny (Bleat) Bernstein. She had one sibling, a younger brother, Steven. She was active in the women's movement from a very young age and first marched for suffrage in 1915. While a student at Cornell University, she marched in the celebratory parades of 1920 when the Nineteenth Amendment was passed and was arrested for publicly wearing riding britches. This was, however, only the beginning of her career as a feminist. After spending several years teaching high school English in New York City, and marrying chemist William Seaman, in 1925, she began writing professionally.

Her first books were novels written in collaboration with her college roommate Frances Schwartz and published under the pen name Francis Sylvin. In 1965, she published *Always a Woman: What Every Woman Should Know about Breast Cancer,* a book based on her own experience of a mastectomy. This was the first book written about breast cancer by someone outside the medical profession. The topic, about which Seaman also wrote magazine and newspaper articles, was rarely discussed publicly in the early 1960s. In a 1980 interview, Seaman recalled, "It was considered daring at the time, but it changed attitudes, I think.... As for me, I got so much fan mail on that book, you'd have thought I was a movie star."

How to Be a Jewish Grandmother (1979) is a humorous book of advice and anecdotes. Any topic was fair game for Seaman: vasectomies, daughters-in-law, even her own drinking habits. Besides the discussion of what it meant to be Jewish, a woman, and a grandmother, the book was an indication of the changes American culture had undergone in this century. *How to Be a Jewish Grandmother* is a record of the shifting social order of the 1970s, presented from the point of view of one who had herself rebelled against the norms of an earlier generation, but who may have been just a little bit bewildered by the transformations she was witnessing.

Seaman was not the only political activist in her family. Her son, Gideon Seaman, and daughter-in-law Barbara Seaman, coauthored *Women and the Crisis in Sex Hormones* in 1977; Barbara was also a cofounder of the National

Women's Health Network. It was she who had encouraged Sylvia to write *Always a Woman.*

It was breast cancer that many years later caused Sylvia Bernstein Seaman's death, on January 8, 1995.

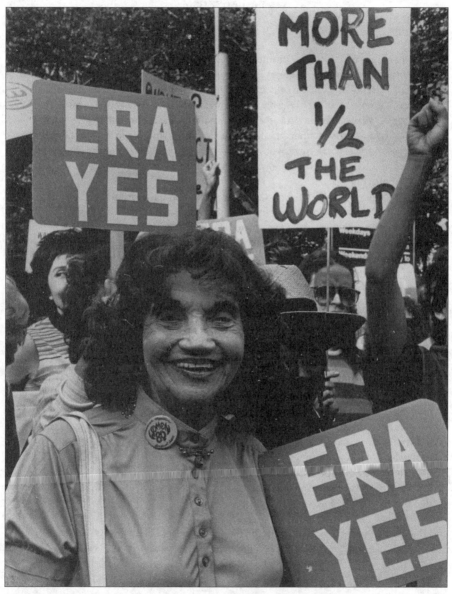

Figure 1: From marching for woman suffrage in 1915 to her groundbreaking book on breast cancer 50 years later to *How to Be a Jewish Grandmother,* Sylvia Seaman candidly and courageously explored a wide range of feminist issues. She is shown here in August 1980 leading a demonstration in celebration of 60 years of women's suffrage. [Carol Halebian]

A IS FOR ACTIVISM

by Byllye Avery

Just when does one decide to devote her life or some part of her life to activism? I can't recall ever hearing a child say, "I want to be an activist when I grow up." What transforms regular, hardworking citizens into dedicated, passionate activists? Perhaps it is anger fuming in the blood that makes us resist the injustices hurled at members of society. Perhaps it is the high standards of excellence that we hold for our society, to be better than the best, with integrity and respect for everyone. Whatever the cause, we never know when the moment will come that an issue emerges as a burning passion and we commit ourselves to making sure the world knows about "our" issue.

Activists help make the world a better place. Many important changes have been made because something clicked and made people see the picture more clearly, focusing on the vision of what could be, and how changes can lead to a better society. We must celebrate our activists. They are trailblazers who are not afraid to speak out, stand up, and challenge the status quo. They do their work today, and create a place for volunteers later. Activism leads and inspires change. The activist's passion provides a driving force for the rest of us.

I became and activist in the early '70s. The women's health movement was in full swing, making us all think about health in terms of personal involvement and control. My husband had a massive heart attack and died in 1970, and I realized that as an educated Black person I knew very little about health and taking care of myself.

I began to educate myself, and I dedicated more and more time to working on women's health issues. Before I knew it, health had become my issue and my full-time job.

We all have some parts of activism within us. Very few people don't have strong feelings about something. Some of us are quiet activists, keeping our feelings to ourselves and using our quiet strength and resources to advance our issues. We all need to seek ways to be activists and support activism.

As you add *activism* to your altar, think about and feel the passion of an issue that is important to you.

My actions are important and are
inherently powerful.
"Dissension is healthy, even when it gets loud."
—JENNIFER LAWSON

From *An Altar of Words. Wisdom, Comfort and Inspiration for African American Women*, New York, Broadway Books, 1998. Reprinted by permission.

Taking Our Bodies Back

"Each of us has the right and the responsibility to
assess the roads which lie ahead."—Maya Angelou,
WOULDN'T TAKE NOTHING FOR MY JOURNEY NOW

T aking Our Bodies Back, the title of this section, is borrowed from an extraordinary documentary produced in 1973 by Margaret Lazarus, then a
new graduate of Vassar. The film depicts a number of the topics that you'll
read about in these pages: home births, abortion, the insensivity of many male
physicians, racism, self-help gynecology, women of all ages meeting to rap and
to confide in each other on what they really feel about their bodies and their
healthcare. They are learning, "Don't agonize, organize," as Mother Jones
advised. The bad things that happen to women's bodies are often the system's
fault (due in large measure to this monster called sexism) than that of the individual—and the system can be changed.

The feminist movement galvanized in the '70s as women began talking to
one another and discovering that they had shared feelings and experiences.
They visited friends in other cities, went to meetings, and had their "pilots" lit.
They went back to their communities and started their own know-your-body

courses or consciousness raising self-help projects scattered around the United States. And every one of them was bent on improving women's lot.

These women had been the unpaid volunteers for everyone else's good causes —the civil rights movement, the peace movement, local charities or churches or reform politicians. It came to millions of us at once that our rights were also abridged, and the moment to stand up for them was—now.—B. S.

Chapter 41

Activism/ Revolution

A is for Avery, for Activism, and, as far as I'm concerned, for Awesome as well. The deserving recipient of a MacArthur Foundation "Genius" Award, Byllye Avery brought her unique spirit to the early years of the National Women's Health Network, spread her wings, founded the Black Women's Health Project, and set an example of dignity and leadership for all women of every conceivable background.

At least two of the women in this chapter are not only world-class revolutionaries but saints as well. In the approximately thirty years I have known each of them, Gloria Steinem and Judy Norsigian have unfailingly demonstrated the gentleness, goodness, and empathy we associate with the term. It goes to show— you don't have to chew up the carpet to shake up the world.

Shulamith Firestone and Gena Corea hold opposing ideas of women's reproductive goals. They represent the two feminist polarities. Shulie proposes "freeing women from their biology," while Gena is one of the world's most persuasive critics of reproductive technology.

There was then no feminist community, no slogans such as "the personal is political," or "Sisterhood is Powerful." Yet Terese Lasser—in 1952, following her mastectomy—and Sherri Finkbine—in 1962, seeking an abortion—each courageously drew their lonely lines in the sand with no community behind them, no peer group to assure them that society—not they—was in the wrong. But like later activists they were impelled, at any cost, to share what they knew with others in the same situation. I have called such women "transitional feminists," but Susan Brownmiller has a better term: These are our "heroic antecedents."   B. S.

Inside and Out: Two Stories of the Rumblings Beneath the Quiet

COMPILED BY SUZANNE CLORES

©1999. Original for this publication.

The Halsted radical mastectomy has been called "the greatest standard-ized surgical error of the twentieth century." Introduced in the 1880s by William Halsted, a surgeon at Johns Hopkins, it was debilitating, even crippling, and based on Halsted's unproven conviction that breast cancer was a local disease that could be fully—if brutally—excised. The Halsted radical was exacting. The woman was anesthetized and the doctor performed a "quick-section" biopsy. If the biopsy was positive, the doctor, without waking the patient, began his incision at the shoulder and removed the breast as well as the lymph glands, the muscles of the chest wall, and all the fat under the skin. The patient was left with a loss of feeling on that side of her body, a sunken chest, restricted movement, and probably some degree of "milk arm," the chronic and painful condition in which lymph fluid can no longer circulate properly and thus accumulates.

In 1954, Terese ("Ted") Lasser, founder of Reach to Recovery, became the first militant advocate for radical mastectomy patients. Recalling the Halsted radi-cal she had in 1952, she said, "You awake to find yourself wrapped in bandages from midriff to neck—bound like a mummy in surgical gauze, somewhere deep inside you a switch is thrown and your mind goes blank. You do not know what to think, you do not want to guess, you do not want to know." Lasser, the soignée, energetic (and imperious) matriarch in an affluent and well-connected family (J. K. Lasser, her husband, was author of the perennially popular *Your Income Tax*), was not accustomed to being patronized or hustled and had not been prepared for this drastic result. Nor did her surgeon (whom she described as a "brilliant but very busy man"), or anyone else at Memorial Hospital, give her the specific advice she craved on arm exercises, if, when, or how to resume sex relations with her husband, what to tell her children, or even how to shop for a prosthesis. Her epiphany occurred when she showed up at the department store where she normally bought brassieres, and the saleswoman screamed and fled, crying "People like us shouldn't have to wait on people like you."

As soon as Lasser discovered how to cope with these matters, a compulsion came over her to teach what she knew. She slipped into the hospital rooms of "mastectomees," bearing gift boxes with (1) a starter "falsie" for them to pin on the inside of their nightgowns; (2) a ball, a string, and instructions, which she demonstrated, for the painful but effective arm-restoring exercises that she herself had devised out of her desperation and genius; and (3) perhaps most daring, her famous "Letter to Husbands" about sex. Lasser maintained a pre-tense that she made these calls only at the request of the patient's doctor or family. However, she was often escorted out of the front door of Memorial Hospital when she was found visiting patients at random and without the consent of the responsible surgeon.

One consistent message from breast cancer activists has been that when cancer cells are "growing wild" inside, some sense of outer autonomy becomes imperative, even life-saving, for the woman. Dr. M. Vera Peters thought so, and is said to have treated her patients accordingly from the time she graduated medical school in Toronto in 1934. A world-class radiotherapist and oncologist before she reached the age of 40, she'd made a major contribution to the treatment of Hodgkin's disease. She argued for an aggressive approach; but regarding her second major interest, breast cancer, the evidence led her in the opposite direction.

Peters worked at a Toronto facility that admitted 7,261 patients for treatment of breast cancer between 1935 and 1960. On April 10, 1967, she published a paper in the *Journal of the American Medical Association* that reported the outcome for 825 of these women, including 200 who had only lumpectomies with radiation. All of the patients in the three other treatment groups had had some combination of mastectomy and radiation, but in only one group was the mastectomy performed immediately after a "quick-section" biopsy, eliminating patient choice.

Lumpectomy patients with stages 1 and 2 breast cancer survived fully as well, at five years, as those who had had mastectomies. With the chance to present evidence against the scourge of quick-section biopsies, she writes,

> It behooves us as cancer therapists to [find methods] which will not harm the self respect and good will of the patient. With quick section biopsy… the patients feel that they have been deprived of an opportunity to think positively about their treatment because the diagnosis had not been confirmed preoperatively.… If a preliminary local incision had been carried out routinely, the more radical treatment could then be discussed with the patient and the final decision in favor of either surgery or irradiation could safely be influenced by the patient's "special" fears.

Upon her retirement in 1976, Vera Peters was appointed to the Order of Canada, in recognition of her extraordinary contributions to the treatment of Hodgkin's disease and breast cancer, just as patents all over the world were beginning to seize their newfound opportunities to "think positively" for themselves.

In 1960, the judgment of Food and Drug Administration medical officer Dr. Frances Oldham Kelsey brought the widespread use of the drug thalidomide to a stop, but not before an epidemic of limbless babies were born to thousands of mothers who were sampling the pills purported to be mild sedatives. Kelsey refused to approve the drug, despite early news of the drug's success and pressure from the manufacturer, the Merrell Company, to distribute in the United

States. While thalidomide's effects on animals tested negative to malformation, Dr. Kelsey mistrusted the sleeping pill that did not cause sleepiness in animals.

In 1961, West Germany reported to the FDA that thalidomide had been associated with birth defects. The Merrell Company, who had furnished near-ly 1,100 doctors (almost 250 obstetricians and gynecologists) with samples of the drug, merely issued a letter of warning to just 10 percent of those physi-cians, hoping still for FDA approval and promising prescription sales. Thalidomide's danger to pregnant women was not made public in the United States until 1962. For her role in preventing distribution, Dr. Kelsey received the President's Award for Distinguished Federal Civilian Service in 1962.

The same year, Sherri Finkbine, a thalidomide-exposed pregnant woman, was denied the U.S. abortion she sought for medical reasons. Finkbine was not an abortion radical, believing an abortion should be undertaken only when absolutely necessary, but she thought herself the exception. She was disturbed that she had been given a drug that had destroyed her pregnancy, so the day before her scheduled abortion, she called a friend in the press and told her story. When the paper's headlines screamed of thalidomide's mutagenic effects, her scheduled abortion was canceled. She eventually did obtain one in Sweden, and her harrowing, well-publicized odyssey ultimately helped arouse sentiment for abortion law reform. Underneath her disclosure of the danger of the drug is the same vision for consumer well-being that prompted Dr. Kelsey's judgment. These two women acted in order to protect future female patients from medical industry politics—those of the FDA, pharmaceutical companies, or the medical community—which may not have the health and interest of the patient in mind.

Sisterhood

GLORIA STEINEM

Gloria Steinem, "Sisterhood," *Ms.,* Spring 1972. Reprinted by permission.

A very, very long time ago (about three or four years), I took a certain secure and righteous pleasure in saying the things that women are sup-posed to say.

I remember with pain—

"My work won't interfere with marriage. After all, I can always keep my typewriter at home." Or:

"I don't want to write about women's stuff. I want to write about foreign policy." Or:

"Black families were forced into matriarchy, so I see why Black women have to step back and let their men get ahead." Or:

"I know we're helping Chicano groups that are tough on women, but that's their culture." Or:

"Who would want to join a women's group? I've never been a joiner, have you?" Or (when bragging):

"He says I write about abstract ideas like a man."

I suppose it's obvious from the kinds of statements I chose that I was secretly nonconforming. (I wasn't married, I was earning a living at a profession I cared about, and I had basically—if quietly—opted out of the "feminine" role.) But that made it all the more necessary to repeat some Conventional Wisdom, even to look as conventional as I could manage, if I was to avoid the punishments reserved by society for women who don't do as society says. I therefore learned to Uncle Tom with subtlety, logic, and humor. Sometimes I even believed it myself. If it weren't for the women's movement, I might still be dissembling away. But the ideas of this great sea change in women's view of ourselves are contagious and irresistible. They hit women like a revelation, as if we had left a small dark room and walked into the sun.

At first my discoveries seemed complex and personal. In fact, they were the same ones so many millions of women have made and are making. Greatly simplified, they went like this: Women are human beings first, with minor differences from men that apply largely to the act of reproduction. We share the dreams, capabilities, and weaknesses of all human beings, but our occasional pregnancies and other visible differences have been used—even more pervasively, if less brutally, than racial differences have been used—to mark us for an elaborate division of labor that may once have been practical but has since become cruel and false. The division is continued for clear reason, consciously or not: the economic and social profit of men as a group.

Once this feminist realization dawned, I reacted in what turned out to be predictable ways. First, I was amazed at the simplicity and obviousness of a realization that made sense, at last, of my life experience: I couldn't figure out why I hadn't seen it before. Second, I realized, painfully, how far that new vision of life was from the system around us, and how tough it would be to explain the feminist realization at all, much less to get people (especially, though not only, men) to accept so drastic a change.

But I tried to explain. God knows (*she* knows) that women try. We make analogies with other groups that have been marked for subservient roles in order to assist blocked imaginations. We supply endless facts and statistics of injustice, reeling them off until we feel like human information retrieval machines. We lean heavily on the device of reversal. (If there is a male reader to whom all my prerealization statements seem perfectly logical, for instance, let him substitute "men" for "women" or himself for me in each sentence, and see how he feels. "My work won't interfere with marriage...." "Chicana groups that are tough on men...." You get the idea.)

We even use logic. If a woman spends a year bearing and nursing a child, for instance, she is supposed to have the primary responsibility for raising that child to adulthood. That's logic by the male definition, but it often makes women feel children are their only function or discourages them from being mothers at all. Wouldn't it be just as logical to say that the child has two parents, both equally responsible for child-rearing, and that therefore the father should compensate for that extra year by spending *more* than his half of the time with the child? Now *that's* logic.

Occasionally, these efforts at expelling succeed. More often, I get the feeling that we are speaking Urdu and the men are speaking Pali. As for logic, it's in the eye of the logician.

Painful or not, both stages of reaction to our discovery have a great reward. They give birth to sisterhood.

First, we share with each other the exhilaration of growth and self-discovery, the sensation of having the scales fall from our eyes. Whether we are giving other women this new knowledge or receiving it from them, the pleasure for all concerned is enormous. And very moving.

In the second stage, when we're exhausted from dredging up facts and arguments for the men whom we had previously thought advanced and intelligent, we make jokes, paint pictures, and describe humiliations that mean nothing to men, but *women understand.*

The odd thing about these deep and personal connections of women is that they often ignore barriers of age, economics, worldly experience, race, culture —all the barriers that, in male or mixed society, had seemed so difficult to cross.

I remember meeting with a group of women in Missouri who, because they had come in equal numbers from the small town and from its nearby campus, seemed to be split between wives with white gloves welded to their wrists and students with boots who talked about "imperialism" and "oppression." Planning for a child-care center had brought them together, but the meeting seemed hopeless until three of the booted young women began to argue among themselves about a young male professor, the leader of the radicals on campus, who accused all women unwilling to run mimeograph machines of not being sufficiently devoted to the cause. As for child-care centers, he felt their effect of allowing women to compete with men for jobs was part of the "feminization" of the American male and American culture.

"He sounds just like my husband," said one of the white-gloved women, "only he wants me to have bake sales and collect door-to-door for his Republican Party."

The young women had sense enough to take it from there. What did boots or white gloves matter if they were all getting treated like servants and children? Before they broke up, they were discussing the myth of the vaginal orgasm and planning to meet every week. "Men think we're whatever it is we do for men," explained one of the housewives. "It's only by getting together with other women that we'll ever find out who we are."

Even racial differences become a little less hopeless once we discover this mutuality of our life experience as women. At a meeting run by Black women domestics who had formed a job cooperative in Alabama, a white housewife asked me about the consciousness-raising sessions or "rap groups" that are the basic unit of the women's movement. I explained that while men, even minority men, usually had someplace where they could get together every day and be themselves, women were isolated in their houses; isolated from each other. We had no street corners, no bars, no offices, no territory that was recognized as ours. Rap groups were an effort to create that free place: an occasional chance for total honesty and support form our sisters.

As I talked about isolation, the feeling that there must be something wrong with us if we weren't content to be housekeepers and mothers, tears began to stream down the cheeks of this dignified woman—clearly as much of a surprise to her as to us. For the Black women, some barrier was broken down by seeing her cry.

"He does it to us both, honey," said the Black woman next to her, putting an arm around her shoulders. "If it's your own kitchen or somebody else's, you still don't get treated like people. Women's work just doesn't count."

The meeting ended with the housewife organizing a support group of white women who would extract from their husbands a living wage for domestic workers and help them fight the local hierarchy: a support group without which the domestic workers felt their small and brave cooperative could not survive.

As for the "matriarchal" argument that I swallowed in prefeminist days, I now understand why many Black women resent it and feel that it's the white sociologist's way of encouraging the Black community to imitate a white suburban lifestyle. ("If I end up cooking grits for revolutionaries," explained a Black woman poet from Chicago, "it isn't my revolution. Black men and women need to work together for partnership, not patriarchy. You can't have liberation for half a race.") In fact, some Black women wonder if criticism of the strength they were forced to develop isn't a way to keep half the Black community working at lowered capacity and lowered pay, as well as to attribute some of Black men's sufferings to Black women, instead of to their real source—white racism. I wonder with them.

Looking back at all those male-approved things I used to say, the basic hang-up seems to be clear: a lack of esteem for women—Black women, Chicana women, white women—and for myself.

This is the most tragic punishment that society inflicts on any second-class group. Ultimately, the brainwashing works, and we ourselves come to believe our group is inferior. Even if we achieve a little success in the world and think of ourselves as "different," we don't want to associate with our group. We want to identify up, not down (clearly my problem in not wanting to write about women, and not wanting to join women's groups). We want to be the only woman in the office, or the only Black family on the block, or the only Jew in the club.

The pain of looking back at wasted, imitative years is enormous. Trying to write like men. Valuing myself and other women according to the degree of our acceptance by men—socially, in politics, and in our professions. It's as painful as it is now to hear two grown-up female human beings competing with each other on the basis of their husbands' status, like servants whose identity rests on the wealth or accomplishments of their employers.

And this lack of esteem that makes us put each other down is still the major enemy of sisterhood. Women who are conforming to society's expectations view the nonconformists with justifiable alarm. "Those noisy, unfeminine women," they say to themselves. "They will only make trouble for us all." Women who are quietly nonconforming, hoping nobody will notice, are even more alarmed because they have more to lose. And that makes sense, too.

Because the status quo protects itself by punishing all challengers, especially women whose rebellion strikes at the most fundamental social organization: the sex roles that convince half the population its identity depends on being first in work or in war, and the other half that it must serve as docile ("feminine") unpaid or underpaid labor. There seems to be no punishment inside the white male club that quite equals the ridicule and personal viciousness reserved for women who rebel. Attractive or young women who act forcefully are assumed to be male-controlled. If they succeed, it could only have been sexually, through men. Old women or women considered unattractive by male standards are accused of acting only out of bitterness, because they could not get a man. Any woman who chooses to behave like a full human being should be warned that the armies of the status quo will treat her as something of a dirty joke; that's their natural and first weapon. She will *need* sisterhood.

All of that is meant to be a warning but not a discouragement. There are so many more rewards than punishments.

For myself, I can now admit anger, and use it constructively, where once I would have submerged it and let it fester into guilt or collect for some destructive explosion.

I have met brave women who are exploring the outer edge of human possibility, with no history to guide them, and with a courage to make themselves vulnerable that I find moving beyond the words to express it.

I no longer think that I do not exist, which was my version of that lack of self-esteem afflicting many women. (If male standards weren't natural to me, and they were the only standards, how could I exist?) This means that I am less likely to need male values to identify myself with and am less vulnerable to classic arguments. ("If you don't like me, you're not a Real Woman"—said by a man who is Coming On. "If you don't like me, you're not a Real Person, and you can't relate to other people"—said by anyone who understands blackmail as an art.)

I can sometimes deal with men as equals and therefore can afford to like them for the first time.

I have discovered politics that are not intellectual or superimposed. They are organic, because I finally understand why I for years inexplicably identified with "out" groups. I belong to one, too. It will take a coalition of such groups to achieve a society in which, at a minimum, no one is born into a second-class role because of visible difference, because of race or of sex.

I no longer feel strange by myself, or with a group of women in public. I feel just fine.

I am continually moved to discover I have sisters.

I am beginning, just beginning, to find out who I am.

Dear Injurious Physician

BARBARA SEAMAN

Barbara Seaman, "Dear Injurious Physician," *New York Times*, December 2, 1972. Reprinted by permission.

In 1957, pregnant with my first child, I told my doctor that I planned to breast-feed. "You wouldn't make a good cow," he said. To his mind that settled the matter, for he gave me a laxative that went straight to the milk and almost finished off my son.

In 1960, my oldest daughter was born "by appointment." All went well. In 1962, pregnant again, I chanced to fall into conversation with a public health pediatrician.

"When do you expect the baby?" she asked.

"My doctor is inducing her on October fifteenth."

"Why?"

"Why not?"

"Because it's dangerous," she explained. "Go back and ask him why he's doing it—and he better have a good reason."

I went back and asked him. He was hoping to go on a cruise in the late October.

If I had known then what I know now, having babies would have been a lot more enjoyable. Having miscarriages—and abortions—would have been a lot less terrifying. Some women want to let their doctors "do the worrying for them," but for those of us who don't, it has been extremely difficult to get honest health information.

Women are making a valiant effort to correct the situation. In recent months, several important health books by women have appeared, and there are more to come. I am thinking, for example, of *The Nature and Evolution of Female Sexuality*, by Dr. Mary Jane Sherfey; *Why Natural Childbirth*, by Dr. Deborah Tanzer and Jean Libman Block; *Vaginal Politics*, by Ellen Frankfort; *Our Bodies, Ourselves*, by the Boston Women's Health Book Collective; *Women and Madness,* by Dr. Phyllis Chesler. There will even be a book telling women that radical mastectomy is not necessarily the treatment of choice for breast cancer.

These books have been and will be misunderstood in many quarters. We do not expect men to be endlessly fascinated by the ins and outs of feminine plumbing, but it hurts when our sisters reject us. A reporter for *The New York Times* complained that she was tired of hearing feminists badmouth their gynecologists. Why don't they go to a woman doctor? she asked. She might as well have said, "Let them eat cake." According to the American College of Obstetrics and Gynecology, only 3 percent of its members are female. Furthermore, there are some male chauvinists among women doctors too.

Let those who doubt that women have cause to be angry at their doctors leaf through the ads in almost any medical journal. One of the worst offenders sells a widely and often irresponsibly used tranquilizer. A shrewish-looking woman is depicted, and the message seems to say: "Doctor, get her off your back.... Get her off her husband's back.... Shoot her up and shut her up with our product."

And let the skeptics, please, when the time comes, look up the January 1973 issue of the *American Journal of Sociology*. It will contain a study by Diana Scully and Pauline Bart on the images of women in gynecology textbooks. Even if the medical student starts out as a nice kid, he is bound to be a screwed-up sexist by the time he finishes memorizing these gems:

> ➤ "The traits that compose the core of the female personality are feminine narcissism, masochism and passivity." (Dr. James Robert Willson, 1971)
> ➤ "The frequency of intercourse depends entirely upon the male sex drive.... The bride should be advised to allow her husband's sex drive to set their pace and she should attempt to gear hers satisfactorily to his." (Dr. Edmund R. Novak et al., 1970)
> ➤ "If like all human beings, he [the gynecologist] is made in the image of the Almighty, and if he is kind, then his kindness and concern for his patient may provide her with a glimpse of God's image." (Dr. C. Russell Scott, 1968)

Amen.

Our Bodies, Ourselves: Remembering the Dignity

EDITED BY MEI HWEI ASTELLA SAW AND SARAH J. SHEY

Excerpts from *Our Bodies, Ourselves* (New England Free Press, 1971; Simon & Schuster, 1973, 1998); selections from Joanna Perlman's interview with Judy Norsigian, March 1999.

> Remember the dignity of your womanhood.
> Do not appeal, do not beg, do not grovel.

Take courage, join hands, stand beside us.
Fight with us…
   —Christabel Pankhurst, English suffragette, 1880–1958

In May 1969, Bread and Roses, a grassroots socialist-feminist collective in Boston, organized a one-day conference that included a workshop on "Women and Their Bodies." At the workshop, according to *Our Bodies, Ourselves* program director Judy Norsigian in a 1999 interview with Barnard College senior Joanna Perlman, the women were "struck by their level of ignorance about their own bodies." They decided to take action, and *Our Bodies, Ourselves* grew from there.

"The women decided to collect basic information about health care issues that concerned them—childbirth, pregnancy, contraception, abortion," Norsigian recalls. "They ended up drafting term papers and sharing them with one another. And they discovered that it was electrifying to share their own experiences. Women, in general, were not assertive and did not feel entitled to ask questions in the medical care setting. They realized that the key to getting good health care was to get as well-informed as possible."

Our Bodies, Ourselves was revolutionary on several counts. At the time, books on women's health issues were not easy to find. From the very first self-published issue of *OBOS*, in 1971, the Boston Women's Health Course Collective worked to make it accessible to all women who sought health information. Between 1971 and 1973, the collective paid for 11 printings altogether. When Simon & Schuster started publishing the book in 1973, the collective arranged for a special "clinic copy discount" of 70 percent off the cover price for nonprofit agencies. The collective also gave away free books to women in prison, and to others who couldn't afford to buy it, especially women in developing countries. This free book distribution continues to this day.

Existing texts tended to be "written in technical language that didn't really appeal or relate to women's lay experiences," says Norsigian. *Our Bodies, Ourselves* put information into language that was accessible. As Norma Swenson, a founding member of the Boston Women's Health Book Collective, pointed out in a *New York Times* article in 1997, "what was groundbreaking was the candor and honesty of women speaking about their experiences." The editors of the 1971 edition urged readers to "make suggestions, write up your own experience, or otherwise work on the course," reminding readers of a central fact of *OBOS*'s existence: "The course is what all of us make it."

In one of the early zine-like issues, the candor and honesty of *Our Bodies, Ourselves* is clear:

A few years ago an American woman with an unwanted pregnancy was doomed to a lonely and dangerous trip underground for an illegal abortion. Although things aren't perfect today, enough attitudes and state laws have changed so that *you can get a legal abortion*. If there is no chance of getting a legal abortion in your state, you can go else-where, probably to New York. *Do not risk your life by going to an illegal abortionist!* You don't have to do that anymore. Remember—early abortion (before 12 weeks since your last menstrual period) is safer and it is easier to obtain. So if you think you're pregnant and you don't want to be, don't delay in consulting one of the agencies mentioned below. And if you're pregnant and don't know how you feel about it, counselors at many of these agencies can help you think it out. (*OBOS*, 1971, p. 66)

Our Bodies, Ourselves dealt firmly and honestly with prickly issues like abortion, birth control, and sexuality, and also took it upon itself to bring to attention the troubling relationship between women and their doctors. "The feminist principles that were developing in the women's movement sort of collided with the dismay and distress women had with their medical and health encounters," Norsigian says.

"We looked at women's health and medical care, and saw how badly physicians were being trained," she says. "At that point, most of the physicians were men. Women were encouraged to think of their physicians as gods. In the period when *OBOS* was created, women were still reluctant to move out of the role of the passive obedient female in the presence of doctors. Women learned quickly that when they didn't ask questions and think 'What about me?' 'What are the side effects?' 'What are the risks?' they ended up having unnecessary surgery, and taking drugs they didn't know about, and wishing they hadn't done what they had done. That sense of entitlement I think OBOS has helped to facilitate in women—as well as the larger women's movement—was a great contribution."

Looking back today, one cannot help but notice the changes that *Our Bodies, Ourselves* has helped bring about in this area. Look at this account of the doctor-patient relationship in the 1971 edition...

Perhaps the most obvious indication of this ideology is the way that doctors treat us as women patients. We are considered stupid, mind-less creatures, unable to follow instructions (known as orders). While men patients may also be treated this way, we are worse because women are thought to be incapable of understanding or dealing with our own situation.

It is important for us to understand that mystification is the primary process here. It is *mystification* that makes us postpone going to the doctor for "that little pain," since he's such a "busy man." It is *mystification* that prevents us from demanding a precise explanation of what is the matter and how exactly he is going to treat it. It is *mystification* that causes us to become passive objects who submit to his control and supposed expertise. (*OBOS*, 1971, p. 134)

Now consider this woman's statement, from the 1998 edition.

> Friends now marvel at my close relationship with my current doctor and my ability to talk back, question, and disagree with him and his colleagues. He respects me and trusts me to tell him what is going on, and I in turn trust him to listen, make suggestions, and consult with me before any action is taken. When I don't want a procedure done or feel the psychological burden of making yet another trip to the lab or to his office is just too much for me on an occasion, I will tell him and he understands me most of the time. I have finally after many, many years found someone willing to take into account my whole medical history and apply it to my current situation. (*OBOS*, 1998, p. 686)

The 1973 edition included a chapter on sexually transmitted diseases, something that "had never been seen before," according to Norsigian. "We were among the first to talk about the fact that women were largely asymptomatic when we have STDs. We encouraged safer-sex practices before the term had even been coined. We saw the transition from when STDs couldn't be talked about to now when they're everywhere." In a manner that was now characteristic of *Our Bodies, Ourselves*, the writers conveyed medical advice and sound practical information, all the time urging women to take their health into their own hands.

PROTECT YOURSELF—PROTECT OTHERS

> If you notice any symptoms of VD in yourself, no matter how mild, you should go to a doctor or a clinic at once.
>
> ➤ Don't panic or feel guilty or embarrassed.
> ➤ Don't depend on one test only. If the first test for gonorrhea or syphilis doesn't show anything, make sure the doctor takes another one to be safe. Women should make sure the doctor takes smears from at least the cervix and the anus or urethra. Don't just accept what he says. Some doctors aren't careful enough—and it's your life, not his.
> ➤ Even if you are sure that you have had no contact with someone infected with VD, you may be saving other women's lives by demanding that your doctor routinely give you and every other woman tests for VD without attached moral judgment. (*OBOS*, 1973, pp. 104–105)

The 1979 edition proved that *Our Bodies, Ourselves* was not only a book that broke taboos but also a much needed medical reference and guide for women. The comprehensive chapter on venereal diseases revealed serious gaps in educating doctors about VDs and taught women how to recognize their own symptoms.

> VD education for doctors has been ignored by medical schools for the past 25 years and is only now being reinstated. Doctors who got their medical education during that period may not know enough about diagnosing and treating VD. Since doctors and health workers in clinics that regularly serve VD patients learn on the job, they probably have the best and most up-to-date VD information. Unfortunately, they are rarely informed about the preventive methods that women can use. (*OBOS*, 1979, p. 171–172)

This edition, and later ones as well, included a detailed drawing of a woman's body, illustrating sites where VD symptoms occur. A page-long table full of information about venereal diseases ("How you catch it"; "How to tell you have it"; "How to find out for sure"; and so on) enabled women to do a quick self-diagnosis before rushing to the doctor, thus putting vital medical information—and power—into their own hands.

As a tribute on its twenty-fifth anniversary, Vivian Pinn, director of the Office of Research on Women's Health at the National Institutes of Health, wrote to the Boston Women's Health Book Collective, "Your visionary call to action has inspired many women to take greater control of their lives, their bodies, and their health.... Women have come a long way from the time when they were afraid to ask their doctors questions concerning their health." Norsigian agrees, pointing out one of the main reasons for the early and continued success of *Our Bodies, Ourselves*: "The book meets many women where they are at. It doesn't preach. It doesn't say that something is wrong with you because you don't agree with what it says. The book tries to point out ways in which women are shortchanged and the ways in which women could be more fulfilled human beings."

In the 1970s, women certainly felt shortchanged, and found their way to *Our Bodies, Ourselves,* which took the role of wise and trusted friend for many a curious woman. It spoke honestly and openly about women's issues, many of which were strictly taboo. It was filled with first-person anecdotes. As the writers of the 1971 edition article on sexuality noted: "We felt that our own voices, our own histories, rang the clearest and truest and helped us reclaim the mysterious topic of sexuality." The effect was to normalize women's experiences. Here's one such example: a girl discovering masturbation.

> I was 14 or 15 years old, and a virgin. I was sitting cross-legged on my bed one day, and became aroused by memories of petting with my boyfriend, and having orgasms. I was also aroused by the sex smell I was exuding. I suddenly realized that I could do to my clitoris what he had done. I masturbated for the first time, had an orgasm, and wasn't so sure that what I had done was right. (*OBOS*, 1971, p. 13)

The writers followed with instructions on how to masturbate and achieve an orgasm—this at a time when doctors told many frustrated women that not all women had orgasms and that they would be better off forgetting about it.

One of the most famous pieces was published in the 1973 edition: an article entitled "In Amerika They Call Us Dykes" by the Boston Gay Collective. Their paper was made up of personal anecdotes that helped women begin to understand their own complicated sexuality. In this excerpt, a woman describes her gradual change in attitude about lesbianism.

> We had dancing classes in junior high. One night between dances a cold breeze started blowing through the open window. I reached over and touched Margaret's knee and asked her if she was getting cold too. She shrank back in mock horror and said, "What's the matter, Diana, are you a lesbian?" Everyone nearby started snickering. I didn't know what a lesbian was, but I knew I didn't want to be one. Later I found out; there was a lot of joking and taunting among girls in my class about lesbianism, which they viewed as sick and disgusting....
>
> I got into the women's movement, and felt an enormous relief that I would no longer have to play roles with men and act feminine and sweet, dress in skirts and heels, and do all the things I'd done on dates. Then I began to feel hatred for men for having forced me into these roles. During this time... I began to hang out with gay women, who turned out to be regular people, not the stereotypes I had imagined. On a gut level I was beginning to realize that gayness was not a sickness. One night I went out for a long walk, and when I got home I had decided that I was a lesbian. For me it was not a decision to become a lesbian. It was a question of accepting and becoming comfortable with feelings I had always had. (*OBOS*, 1973, pp. 58–59)

Twenty-five years later, *Our Bodies, Ourselves* includes articles on lesbians, transsexuals, bisexuals, and transgendered people. It still retains its personal approach, incorporating individual voices into the essays.

Since 1971, *Our Bodies, Ourselves* has grown from a quasi-underground, 138-page newsprint edition selling for 40 cents a copy to an 800-page tome the size of the Manhattan phone book. It is truly a historical, social, and cultural icon. According to a recent article in the *Journal of the American Medical Women's Association*, OBOS became a best-seller within five years of its first publication, in both the United States and internationally. More that 4 million copies have been sold to date; there are editions in Japanese, Russian, Chinese, Spanish, French, Italian, German, and a dozen other languages, including an edition in Braille. From a one-day conference in 1969, a movement was born. Just a group of women sharing their experiences forever changed the course of women's health care.

The Ultimate Revolution

SHULAMITH FIRESTONE

Shulamith Firestone, *The Dialectic of Sex: The Case for Feminist Revolution*, New York, Bantam Books, 1971. Reprinted by permission.

We have seen how women, biologically distinguished from men, are culturally distinguished from "human." Nature produced the fundamental inequality—half the human race must bear and rear the children of all of them—which was later consolidated, institutionalized, in the interests of men. Reproduction of the species cost women dearly, not only emotionally, psychologically, culturally but even in strictly material (physical) terms: before recent methods of contraception, continuous childbirth led to constant "female trouble," early aging, and death. Women were the slave class that maintained the species in order to free the other half for the business of the world—admittedly often its drudge aspects, but certainly all its creative aspects as well.

This natural division of labor was continued only at great cultural sacrifice: men and women developed only half of themselves, at the expense of the other half. The division of the psyche into male and female to better reinforce the reproductive division was tragic: the hypertrophy in men of rationalism, aggressive drive, the atrophy of their emotional sensitivity was a physical (war) as well as a cultural disaster. The emotionalism and passivity of women increased their suffering (we cannot speak of them in a symmetrical way, since they were victimized as a class by the division). Sexually, men and women were channeled into a highly ordered—time, place, procedure, even dialogue—heterosexuality restricted to the genitals, rather than diffused over the entire physical being.

I submit, then, that the first demand for any alternative system be:

1. THE FREEING OF WOMEN FROM THE TYRANNY OF THEIR REPRODUCTIVE BIOLOGY BY EVERY MEANS AVAILABLE, AND THE DIFFUSION OF THE CHILDBEARING AND CHILD-REARING ROLE TO THE SOCIETY AS A WHOLE, MEN AS WELL AS WOMEN. There are many degrees of this. Already we have a (hard-won) acceptance of "family planning," if not contraception for its own sake. Proposals are imminent for day-care centers, perhaps even 24-hour child-care centers staffed by men as well as women. But this, in my opinion, is timid if not entirely worthless as a transition. We're talking about *radical* change. And though indeed it cannot come all at once, radical goals must be kept in sight at all times. Day-care centers buy women off. They ease the immediate pressure without asking why that pressure is on *women.*

At the other extreme there are the more distant solutions based on the potentials of modern embryology, that is, artificial reproduction, possibilities still so frightening that they are seldom discussed seriously. We have seen that the fear is to some extent justified: in the hands of our current society and under the direction of current scientists (few of whom are female or even feminist), any attempted used of technology to "free" anybody is suspect. But we are speculating about postrevolutionary systems, and for the purposes of our discussion we shall assume flexibility and good intentions in those working out the change.

To thus free women from their biology would be to threaten the *social* unit that is organized around biological reproduction and the subjection of women to their biological destiny, the family. Our second demand will come also as a basic contradiction to the family, this time the family as an *economic* unit:

2. THE FULL SELF-DETERMINATION, INCLUDING ECONOMIC INDEPENDENCE, OF BOTH WOMEN AND CHILDREN. To achieve this goal would require fundamental changes in our social and economic structure. This is why we must talk about a feminist socialism: in the immediate future, under capitalism, there could be at best a token integration of women into the labor force. For women have been found exceedingly useful and cheap as a transient, often highly skilled labor supply,* not to mention the economic value of their traditional function, the reproduction and rearing of the next generation of children, a job for which they are now patronized (literally and thus figuratively) rather than paid. But whether or not officially recognized, these are essential economic functions. Women, in this present capacity, are the very foundation of the economic superstructure, vital to its existence.** The paeans to self-sacrificing motherhood have a basis in reality: Mom *is* vital to the American way of life, considerably more than apple pie. She is an institution without which the system really *would* fall apart. In official capitalist terms, the bill for her economic services*** might run as high as one fifth of the gross national product. But

---

*Most bosses would fail badly had they to take over their secretaries' job, or do without them. I know several secretaries who sign without a thought their bosses' names to their own (often brilliant) solutions. The skills of college women especially would cost a fortune reckoned in material terms of male labor.

Margaret Benston ("The Political Economy of Women's Liberation," *Monthly Review,* September 1969), in attempting to show that women's oppression is indeed economic—though previous economic analysis has been incorrect—distinguishes between the male superstructure economy based on *commodity* production (capitalist ownership of the means of production, and wage labor), and the preindustrial reduplicative economy of the family, production for immediate *use*. Because the latter is not part of the *official* contemporary economy, its function at the basis of that economy is often overlooked. Talk of drafting women into the superstructure commodity economy fails to deal with the tremendous amount of necessary production of the traditional kind now performed by women without pay: Who will do it?

***The Chase Manhattan Bank estimates a woman's overall domestic workweek at 99.6 hours. Margaret Benston gives her minimal estimate for a *childless* married woman at 16 hours, close to half of a regular workweek; a *mother* must spend at least six or seven days a week working close to 12 hours.

payment is not the answer. To pay her, as is often discussed seriously in Sweden, is a reform that does not challenge the basic division of labor and thus could never eradicate the disastrous psychological and cultural consequences of that division of labor.

As for the economic independence of children, that is really a pipe dream, realized as yet nowhere in the world. And, in the case of children too, we are talking about more than a fair integration into the labor force; we are talking about the abolition of the labor force itself under a cybernetic socialism, the radical restructuring of the economy to make "work," i.e., wage labor, no longer necessary. In our postrevolutionary society adults as well as children would be provided for—irrespective of their social contributions—in the first equal distribution of wealth in history.

We have now attacked the family on a double front, challenging that around which it is organized: reproduction of the species by females and its outgrowth, the physical dependence of women and children. To eliminate these would be enough to destroy the family, which breeds the power psychology. However, we will break it down still further.

3. THE TOTAL INTEGRATION OF WOMEN AND CHILDREN INTO ALL ASPECTS OF THE LARGER SOCIETY. ALL INSTITUTIONS THAT SEGREGATE THE SEXES, OR BAR CHILDREN FROM ADULT SOCIETY, E.G., THE ELEMENTARY SCHOOL, MUST BE DESTROYED. DOWN WITH SCHOOL! These three demands predicate a feminist revolution based on advanced technology. And if the male-female and the adult-child cultural distinctions are destroyed, we will no longer need the sexual repression that maintains these unequal classes, allowing for the first time a "natural" sexual freedom. Thus we arrive at:

4. THE FREEDOM OF ALL WOMEN AND CHILDREN TO DO WHATEVER THEY WISH TO DO SEXUALLY. There will no longer be any reason *not* to. (Past reasons: Full sexuality threatened the continuous reproduction necessary for human survival, and thus, through religion and other cultural institutions, sexuality had to be restricted to reproductive purposes, all nonreproductive sex pleasure considered deviation or worse. The sexual freedom of women would call into question the fatherhood of the child, thus threatening patrimony. Child sexuality had to be repressed because it was a threat to the precarious internal balance of the family. These sexual repressions increased proportionately to the degree of cultural exaggeration of the biological family.) In our new society, humanity could finally revert to its natural polymorphous sexuality—all forms of sexuality would be allowed and indulged. The fully sexuate mind, realized in the past in only a few individuals (survivors), would become universal. Artificial cultural achievement would no longer be the only avenue to sexuate self-realization: one could now realize oneself fully, simply in the process of being and acting.

Hidden Malpractice

GENA COREA

Gena Corea, *The Hidden Malpractice: How American Medicine Treats Women as Patients and Professionals,* New York, William Morrow, 1977. Reprinted by permission.

In 1975, 10 years after my stint as a nurse's aide, I sat in a Harvard Medical School building behind the Peter Bent Brigham. Medical writer Barbara Seaman was speaking during a conference on women and health. The portraits of twelve dignified white men, all former medical professors, looked down on Seaman as she proposed that, from then on, male medical students be barred from obstetrics and gynecology.

"It sounds a bit radical at first," she said, smiling, "but you get used to it."

Our Constitution, Seaman told us, guarantees us the right to privacy. Ever since the male incursion into midwifery in the eighteenth century, women haven't had it.

Listening to Seaman, I recalled the pelvic examination I had witnessed at the Brigham and I wondered:

Why were all the men right to be looking up vaginas?

Why were all the women wrong to be embarrassed?

Why didn't the men acknowledge that whether or not women "should" be embarrassed, the fact was that they were? Why didn't women insist that the medical system be changed to accommodate their feelings?*

Such questions had never occurred to me as a nurse's aide, but in the decade between my nursing and Seaman's speech, I had discovered much that disturbed me about woman's health care.

So I listened, shocked and intrigued, when Seaman declared, "On a gut level, I am now convinced that it is a most basic violation of our civil rights for the group that is not at any risk from reproduction (male) to control the group that is at risk (female)."

As a reporter for the Holyoke, Massachusetts, *Transcript* in 1971, I had learned myself how that violation of civil rights harmed women. For 18 months, I had investigated locally the charges feminists were making nationally. Medicine was one of the institutions I examined for sexism. When I began my investigations, I was not a feminist. By the time I had finished, the evidence I had gathered forced me to become one.

Seaman's proposal seemed radical to me at the time. It does not today. The truly radical proposals, I now see, were advanced in the seventeenth century, when

---

*A female physician who read this manuscript for me penciled in at this point: "Pelvic exam as a form of rape?" A second female physician, reading the same copy later, scribbled next to the question, "Yes!"

men took over midwifery, and in the nineteenth century, when "gynecology" was created as a specialty in which only men—with very few exceptions—engaged. Women did not like that situation then, as numerous physicians of the time testified, and many do not like it now. If enough of us feel this way, we must decide what we will do about it. It may not be enough to simply increase the number of female gynecologists, because, as Seaman points out, the few men remaining in the field will rise to the top, controlling hospital departments, research laboratories, and population agencies. This has already happened in socialist countries where many, if not most, gynecologists are women.

Pelvic Autonomy: Four Proposals

BARBARA SEAMAN

Barbara Seaman, "Pelvic Anatomy: Four Proposals," *Social Policy,* September/ October 1975. Reprinted by permission. Originally delivered as a speech, "Physician, Heal Thyself," at the Conference on Women and Health, held at Harvard Medical School, April 7, 1975.

M en have always said that because our bodies are different they are less, and they have used our biologic differences to legitimize other forms of discrimination. The very word *hysteria* is derived from the Greek for "wandering uterus." In this century, Freud said, "Anatomy is destiny," and Mussolini put it more starkly, "Genius is genitals."

During the past decade, many feminists have come to recognize that the reproductive or "body" issues may be central to the women's revolution. Various demands for piecemeal reforms have been issued, and expressive new slogans have been coined. Among these slogans are: "Abortion is no man's business," "Why isn't there a pill for men?" and "Happiness is knowing your (cervical) os from your elbow." Some feminists, including de Beauvoir, Firestone, and Atkinson, suggest that women will not achieve parity with men until infants can be produced by extrauterine methods. However, this writer, who has been a science reporter for 15 years, would not wish to surrender her ova to the male reproductive scientists she has observed. For example, in 1969, Dr. Frederick Robbins, a Nobel laureate, stated: "The dangers of overpopulation are so great that we may have to use certain techniques of conception control that may entail considerable risk to the individual *woman*." In 1971, Dr. Joseph Goldzieher, who gave dummy birth control pills to poor Chicana women who came to his clinic for a contraceptive, remarked: "If you think you can explain a double-blind study to Mrs. Gomez of the West Side of San Antonio, you haven't met Mrs. Gomez." Dr. Robbins is presently dean of the Case Western Reserve University School of Medicine. Dr. Goldzieher, after being graylisted by the Food and Drug Administration (FDA) for failure to observe ethical protocols, continues his pill research under grants from the Agency for International Development and the Department of Health, Education and Welfare.

While individual male researchers and clinicians may be free of sexual prejudice, these are rarely the ones who succeed to policy-making positions. Thus, while a woman may occasionally find a nonsexist doctor, the masculinist structure in which he operates remains unchanged. Dr. Louis Hellman, Assistant HEW Secretary for Population, has stated that *he* finds the diaphragm distasteful, and *he prefers* instructing women in other methods. When a reporter suggested to Dr. Hellman that *his* predilections might matter less than his patients', she was brushed aside. A comparable situation prevails in socialist countries where men make abortion available—or take it away—depending on their perceived population goals of the moment.

The individuals who determine health care policies are not responsive to the demands of feminists. One demand has been for an increase in female obstetricians, but instead, the number appears to be decreasing. Among the 16,500 Fellows of the American College of Obstetrics and Gynecology, 978 are women. Yet, in 1974, out of 3,750 obstetrics-gynecology residents, only 96 were women. While the ratio of women in the field is about 1 in 17, the ratio of women entering the field has declined to about 1 in 40. It is true that some female obstetricians are as contemptuous of their patients' rights as are their worst male counterparts. However, there is ample research to show that when women are permitted to enter a male preserve in token numbers only, they may deal with their cognitive and emotional dissonance by developing a "Queen Bee syndrome" or becoming "male-identified." The pressures to "think and act like a man" are particularly compelling in what are deemed "hard" (as opposed to "soft") areas of business and the professions. Within medicine, pediatrics is considered a soft preserve, suitable for women, while obstetrics-gynecology is deemed a surgical, or hard, specialty. It is often said that women are "too emotional" for the hard specialties or "lack the stamina" for them.

The tiny numbers of women permitted to enter obstetrics-gynecology have had to look to a male peer group, and to prove themselves as "one of the boys." It is not remarkable that some women in this specialty have become male-identified. However, when women enter in sufficient numbers to provide each other with a significant female peer group (15 percent to one-third appears adequate), most are able to rest comfortably with their female identity, and to question generalizations and clichés about women as a class, instead of deeming themselves exceptional.

Informed consent had become a central, critical issue in health care. Health feminists have long maintained that, whatever the arguments for concealing some drug or surgical side effects from some patients, there is no legitimate defense for concealing the side effects of modern contraceptives from the women who use them. In 1970, after a long struggle, the FDA agreed to place a warning to consumers in all pill packages. However, on June 23, 1970, a resolution opposing the warning was issued by the AMA House of Delegates, on the grounds that such a package insert would "confuse and alarm many patients." Instead, the warning was distributed to physicians to be given to pill users at the time a prescription is issued. However, for 100 million pill prescriptions, only 4 million warnings have been issued.

No new male contraceptive has been introduced since the condom and, feminist demands notwithstanding, little research effort is being channeled into male alternatives. Researchers concerned with the long-range safety of female methods are unable to obtain funds. Hospital delivery rooms are managed for the convenience of the staff, not the patients, and despite the protests of some conservative obstetricians, the use of potentially dangerous drugs to induce or speed up labor is increasing in the United States. The woman in labor is often unaware that such drugs are being given to her. Patients assume, on faith, that advances in modern obstetrics outweigh the drawbacks, but this assumption is difficult to prove. The infant mortality rate for the upper classes in the nineteenth-century Austro-Hungarian Empire was 19 per 1,000—precisely what it is in the United States today.

The author of this article is married to a male physician, and has a son, as well as two daughters. She does not deem herself a separatist, and like most feminists, wishes to abolish artificial sex-role stereotypes. She believes that such stereotypes have been crippling to men, as well as to women. Nonetheless, there is one difference between the sexes which is clearly not artificial: only women get pregnant. As Sandra S. Tangri, of the U.S. Civil Rights Commission, has written:

> Bearing children involves some or all of the following costs: invasion of the woman's body by the fetus; nine months of pregnancy; a period of restricted freedom while caring for the infant; risk of death, pain, disfigurement, major surgery (cesarean) and permanent or temporary disabilities such as job discrimination against pregnant women and mothers. None of these costs are borne by men, and none should be imposed unwillingly on anyone. It follows that the highest ethical priority for any intervention dealing with fertility is to secure to women the rights of personal security and freedom of action by giving them control over their bodies and reproduction.[1]

It may be a most basic violation of civil rights for the group that is not at any risk from reproduction (male) to control the group that is at risk (female). It is true that many groups or classes have arbitrary amounts of power over other groups and classes. Teachers and students are one example. However, every teacher was once a student, and any student may aspire to become a teacher. But no male has ever conceived or borne a child. There is an absolute difference between the risk bearer (a pregnant or potentially pregnant woman) and the males who wield control over her body, which is not paralleled in any other area of life. If male domination of obstetrics and related areas is a violation of our civil rights, we can legitimately demand that these fields be returned to women.

In their readiness to impose questionable contraceptive and obstetrics practices on women, the present controllers of reproduction may also be endangering the future of our species. Chemical birth control methods, for example, may have latent effects on the gametes and germ cells, but these crucial long-range questions are not being adequately studied. As Dr. Sheldon Segal has stated:

> The use of synthetic sex hormones has grown to an extent that makes this class of drugs a significant part of the chemical environment. The under-thirty generation has been raised on beef fattened with estrogen-laced feed, lambs born of estrus-synchronized ewes, chickens caponized with estrogen paste of pellets. They are the first generation to include a large percentage of post-pill babies born to mothers who used steroidal contraception prior to planned or unplanned pregnancies and are themselves prodigious consumers of steroidal estrogens and progestins on a steady basis... steroidal and nonsteroidal sex hormones... could reach and affect the gamete, embryo, or fetus... one serious hazard—the use of high doses of stilbestrol during pregnancy—has been disclosed.[2]

The following four demands were originally issued at a Women's Health Conference in Boston on April 7, 1975. Most of the women who attended are experienced health professionals who share the author's pessimism concerning reform.

FOUR DEMANDS

1. EFFECTIVE IMMEDIATELY, ONLY WOMEN SHALL BE ADMITTED TO OBSTETRICS AND GYNECOLOGY RESIDENCIES. MALES WHO ARE CURRENTLY IN TRAINING MAY REMAIN, AS MAY THOSE WHO ARE IN PRACTICE. We do not wish to be punative, or place undue hardships on any individuals. Gradually, however, these fields will be returned to women. If men wish to reciprocally exclude us from the practice of urology, they may do so. Our Constitution does guarantee the right to privacy. It has been suggested that some women might continue to prefer a male obstetrician. We do not wish to deprive such women of freedom of choice, and we shall kindly look the other way if a "civilly disobedient" group of male lay midwives, operating outside the official system at little financial profit to themselves, should emerge.

This writer would not wish to advocate any policies which are contrary to the equal rights amendment (ERA), which, according to the New York City Bar Association, "would permit sex-based discriminations only when they are grounded upon physical characteristics unique to one sex."[3] Feminist attorney Kris Glen argues that the demand for female obstetrician-gyneclogists can be construed as part of our right to privacy, like having women's bathrooms attended only by women, which *will* be continued under the ERA. Glen also suggests that femaleness can be claimed as a BFOQ (bona fide occupational qualification) for the practice of obstetrics and gynecology and the performance of reproductive research on women. Defending the BFOQ construction, Glen states that men are often socialized to think of women's bodies contemptuously, and that their record of past and present atrocities speaks for itself.

At the least, then, men who wish to enter this specialty should be required to demonstrate exceptional empathy toward women (see Demand 3), and the chiefs of obstetrics-gynecology departments should be required to show why women are not being accepted for training in their departments in the same proportions as they are presently graduating from medical school.

2. EFFECTIVE IMMEDIATELY, NO MORE FOUNDATION MONIES WILL BE AWARDED TO MEN FOR ANY KIND OF RESEARCH INTO THE FEMALE REPRODUCTIVE SYSTEM. FOR THE NEXT FIVE YEARS, ALL NEW GRANTS FOR REPRODUCTIVE RESEARCH WILL BE CHANNELED TOWARD TRAINING QUALIFIED WOMEN IN REPRODUCTIVE BIOLOGY. Men who have an interest in reproductive biology will be encourage to develop male contraceptives, perfect sperm banks, etc.

In justice, federal monies should also not be awarded to male researchers, certainly not those of the Goldzieher type who have publicly expressed their contempt for women. However, provisions limiting federal grants by sex might be in violation of the Fourteenth Amendment and various HEW regulations. Perhaps an empathy test (see Demand 3) for male researchers might be feasible. In any case, it is clear that compensatory aid for women scientists who have been the objects of discrimination which impeded their professional advancement and choices would be permitted under the ERA.

3. EFFECTIVE IMMEDIATELY, THE ESTABLISHMENT AND ADMINISTRATION OF LAWS CONCERNING FEMALE REPRODUCTION, ABORTION, AND STERILIZATION SHALL BE REMOVED FROM THE COURT AND LEGISLATIVE SYSTEMS. AN AGENCY MODELED AFTER THE NLRB, FCC, FTC, OR ATOMIC ENERGY COMMISSION SHALL HANDLE ALL SUCH MATTERS. Members of this agency would be required to demonstrate their empathy and capacity to understand the emotional and physical imperatives. It is likely that most or all of these commissioners would be women. A division of the agency will provide free advocates and legal aid for all women seeking help with any reproductive problem, or who have experienced malpractice in any form.

4. EFFECTIVE IMMEDIATELY, THE UNITED NATIONS AND THE UNITED STATES WILL NOT SPONSOR NOR PARTICIPATE IN ANY INTERNATIONAL POPULATION ACTIVITY

OR CONFERENCE UNLESS WOMEN ARE REPRESENTED IN PROPORTION TO THEIR NUMBERS IN THE POPULATION OF EVERY PARTICIPATING NATION. The United States will award no funds to other nations for research or other population activities unless women are represented on all projects in proportion to their numbers. Each project will be individually considered, and proof of compliance must be submitted.

In response to these demands, scores of women have now contributed comments and suggestions. Some urge that obstetrics be eliminated as a medical specialty altogether, in favor of female midwifery. Others believe that it may be feasible to immediately close obstetrics training to all males. Instead, a timetable might be established with a minimum of 10 percent women entering obstetrics next year, 20 percent the year after, and so on.

In any case there is now a small band of feminists, many of them quite influential, who agree with Dr. Pauline Bart that we must try to "seize the means of reproduction." If we succeed, let us hope historians will one day acknowledge, "Those women had *ovaries*!"

ENDNOTES

1. *Population Dynamics Quarterly* 11(4), 1974. Published by the Interdisciplinary Communications Program of the Smithsonian Institution, Washington, D.C.

2. From a paper delivered by Dr. Sheldon Segal to the FDA, January 23, 1975.

3. Personal communication from Kris Glen, Esq., March 10, 1975.

Chapter 42

Informed Consent

Y ou may know the lovely radio voice of NPR's Margot Adler, but she writes yet more beautifully. When I'm asked to give a presentation on informed consent to show what it isn't and why it's needed, I may read aloud from Margot's description of the deception surrounding her mother's death:

"B-e-n-i-g-n, she told all of her friends, is the most beautiful word in the English language. And then she could never understand why she wasn't getting better."

Could this happen today? Undoubtedly, but it would be the exception, not the rule. The laws have changed. Customs have changed. Doctors are expected to treat patients like adults.

Mental patients included. Ellen Frankfort, author of Vaginal Politics and columnist for the Village Voice, was a major popularizer of the movements for patient rights. Due in part to her sympathetic reporting, mental patients and their families became well organized, and now, at times, successfully impact on research and on treatment.

In part two (1950-1980) of her three-part report on Women's Health and Government Regulations, FDA historian Suzanne White Junod describes the AMA's resolution opposing a warning on the Pill because it would "confuse and alarm many patients." I had expected opposition to the warning from manufacturers, but had hoped that doctors would appreciate the potentially life-saving benefits. It wouldn't be until 1996 that I would grasp the unspoken reason behind the AMA's unrelenting stand against informed consent on prescription drugs. To be continued.—B. S.

It's Only Once Around the Merry-Go-Round

MARGOT ADLER

Margot Adler, "It's Only Once Aound the Merry-Go-Round," *Heretic's Heart: A Journey through Spirit and Revolution,* Boston, Beacon Press, 1997. Reprinted by permission.

M y mother, Freyda, has been dead for 25 years, but her exuberant energy was so intense that she still receives mail. A skeptic might say that it's the persistence of junk mail in our society that is remarkable, that explains why civil rights groups are still asking her for donations and banks are still offering her credit cards. But as I recently began to go through personal and family documents—journals and letters dating from the 1930s to the 1960s that I'd kept over the years—I came to realize that much of my life has been animated by my mother's persistent spirit, and that she, more than anyone, has a claim on setting and naming the parameters of my political and spiritual journey.

My mother died in January of 1970. She was 61. She had been a heavy smoker who quit too late in life (actually, one of her friends recently hinted to me that she never really quit). Her illness was diagnosed just months after the end of a bitter New York teachers' strike in which my mother, in deep turmoil, had crossed a picket line for the first time in her life—that of her own union— to support a group of Black parents. Her illness also happened at a time when she was truly happy and in love, perhaps for the first time. Just a year before her diagnosis, she confided to me that she had finally experienced "going over the rainbow." I always wondered if a small voice inside her said that she came from a suffering people and had no right to such happiness. She developed lung cancer which quickly metastasized to her brain and then her liver. The end was a lingering, unpleasant death that she only partly comprehended.

In the late 1960s, most patients with cancer were not told the truth of their situation. In my mother's case, many doctors, including a psychiatrist, decided that she did not really want to know. Their policy of disguising the truth was taken to such and extreme that when my mother asked to see her medical records, one of her doctors served up a phony piece of official-looking paper that said her tumor was benign. "B-e-n-i-g-n," she told all of her friends, "is the most beautiful word in the English language." And then she could never understand why she wasn't getting better.

Among those of my parents' generation, illness and death were rarely discussed. When I was a teenager my father waited a full week to inform me that my grandmother had died, not wanting to "ruin my vacation." And when my aunt went into the hospital some years later for cancer, I was told "it was a heart problem."

Most of my mother's friends also accepted the wisdom of the time, believing that she either did not want to know or in fact knew everything on some deeper level. At the time I felt intuitively that this policy was hellish, that my mother, a woman who planned so well for everything, would have despised such paternalism. She would have desired the truth in order to prepare for the end of her life with dignity. But I did not feel I could fight the combined judgment of seven male doctors single-handedly. I acquiesced. And I raged, silently, confused that I, a mere 23-year-old, *knew*, while the most powerful figure in my life was kept from the truth, infantilized. I knew I would never again take a doctor's statement at face value and all institutional documents would remain suspect. For several years after my mother died I would take a longer route to avoid the hospital that had deceived her. And when my mother told me, several months after she'd been told her tumor was benign, "I feel like I am in a dark tunnel, and I can't see the end," I did not find myself reassured that my own silence was right.

Informed Consent

ELIZABETH SIEGEL WATKINS

Excerpted from Elizabeth Siegel Watkins, "Oral Contraceptives and I.C.," *On the Pill: A Social History of Oral Contraceptives, 1950–1970*, Baltimore, Johns Hopkins University Press, 1998. Reprinted by permission.

In September 1969, the head of the information and education department of Planned Parenthood sent memos to the directors of the medical department and to the president of Planned Parenthood about the imminent publication of a book called *The Doctors' Case against the Pill* by Barbara Seaman. The memos warned that "the effect of the book… will be to destroy consumer faith in the efficacy of the pill" and advised the Planned Parenthood leadership to "put balance and background in the hands of reviewers to offset the impact of this book in all media before the bomb hits." The following month, days before the scheduled release of Seaman's book, Planned Parenthood sent a memo to all of its affiliates' executive directors and medical directors to alert them to "books attacking the pill." The memo contrasted portions of text from *The Doctors' Case against the Pill* with sections of the 1969 FDA Advisory Committee's *Second Report on the Oral Contraceptives* to illustrate the "distorted picture" presented by Seaman. It urged the affiliates to respond to queries from local media by "report[ing] your own clinic[']s experience to add the very impressive positive side of oral contraception." What did this book say to elicit such a strong reaction from the nation's largest family planning organization?

   The Doctors' Case against the Pill presented a wealth of evidence against the safety of oral contraceptives. Barbara Seaman had written dozens of articles during the 1960s about issues related to women's health for magazines such as *Bride's and Ladies' Home Journal*. Her book marshallled the testimony of physicians, medical researchers, and women who had used oral contraceptives to build her case against the pill and to indict the medical-pharmaceutical establishment that developed and marketed it.

Seaman's critique of hormonal birth control in particular and the medical-pharmaceutical complex in general lent support to the two renascent social movements of consumerism and feminism. The consumer movement, which originated in the United States with efforts to regulate the manufacture of food and drugs in the late nineteenth century, entered a new phase in the 1960's with the publication of books such as Rachel Carson's *Silent Spring* (1962), Jessica Mitford's *The American Way of Death* (1963), and Ralph Nader's *Unsafe at Any Speed* (1965).

Whereas Carson took on the chemical industry, Mitford the funeral industry, and Nader the automobile industry, Seaman challenged the pharmaceutical industry and the closely allied medical profession. She demanded that pill manufacturers and physicians share all available information about the health risks of oral contraception with patients, so that the women themselves could make informed decisions about birth control. This demand for full disclosure represented an extension of the relatively new concept of informed consent in medicine beyond the operating room to include all doctor-patient interactions.

Seaman's charge that women received inadequate care from their physicians, particularly obstetrician-gynecologists, mirrored a growing concern among feminists about women's health issues. *The Doctor's Case against the Pill* inspired feminists to vocalize the shared perception that the medical profession was "condescending, paternalistic, judgmental and noninformative." In part owing to the publication of this book, the controversy over the safety of the pill galvanized the women's health movement of the 1970s.

The book created little stir when it was released in 1969. Seaman recalls that "it didn't make a big splash when it came out, not in the first few weeks." When the *New York Times* finally got around to reviewing the book, two months after its release, the reviewer dismissed it as "disorganized" and "scatterbrained." However, the publisher, Peter Wyden, believed that the message deserved a wider audience. He hired a publicist in Washington who passed along a copy of *The Doctors' Case against the Pill* to U.S. Senator Gaylord Nelson.

HEARINGS ON "COMPETETIVE PROBLEMS IN THE DRUG INDUSTRY"

By the time Nelson received Seaman's book, he had already led his Subcommittee on Monopoly of the Select Committee on Small Business through sixty-four days of hearings over two and a half years on a broad range of topics, including drug pricing, testing, and advertising; brand name versus generic drugs; the relationship between the drug industry and the medical profession; and investigations into the use and misuse of specific kinds of drugs. One year earlier, the U.S. Congress had approved the Medicaid and Medicare amendments to the Social Security Act, which used federal tax dollars to provide health care for the poor and the elderly. Since the federal government spent more than half a billion dollars annually to purchase prescription drugs, Nelson, as a member of the legislative branch, felt it was his duty to expose the pharmaceutical industry to public scrutiny.

After the first year of hearings, Nelson concluded that since both the medical profession and the Food and Drug Administration depended on pharmaceutical companies for information about drugs, neither doctors nor government officials could rely on promotional literature to be completely objective. The industry, not the FDA, was responsible for conducting and/or arranging for tests and clinical trials of new drugs. Since pharmaceutical firms wanted to earn FDA approval quickly for their products, to reach the market as soon as possible, they often compromised the quality of new drug evaluations. Nelson also questioned the professional and ethical implications of close relations between medicine and the drug industry as in, for example, industry-sponsored medical publications and physician-stockholders in drug companies. Since doctors relied in part on drug detailmen, promotional literature, and free samples provided by drug companies for their continuing education in pharmacology, Nelson worried that physicians could not make intelligent decisions about prescription drugs because of the commercially biased information they received.

Thus when a book describing the hazards of a drug taken by millions of women each day landed on his desk, the senator took notice. He and the staff economist for the Senate Committee on Small Business, Ben Gordon, interviewed Barbara Seaman several times during the fall of 1969. She passed the test, and on December 22, 1969, Nelson released a statement to the press announcing his intention to hold public hearings on the oral contraceptives, to " present for the general public's benefit the best and most objective information available about these drugs. First, whether they are dangerous for the human body, and, second, whether patients taking them have sufficient information about possible dangers in order to make an intelligent judgment whether they wish to assume the risks."

THE PILL HEARINGS, PART I

The two issues of oral contraceptive safety and informed consent corresponded closely to Senator Nelson's larger concerns about medicine and the pharmaceutical industry. The adverse health effects of oral contraceptives cast doubts on the merit of the drug tests and clinical trials conducted prior to FDA approval, and thus deepened his suspicions about the integrity of the drug manufacturers. The question of whether women could make informed decisions about using the birth control pill reflected Senator Nelson's misgivings about the ability of physicians to obtain objective information from the pill manufacturers and in turn to pass that information on to their patients.

To evaluate the alleged health risks of oral contraceptives, Nelson and Gordon assembled a group of expert witnesses to testify about the biochemical, physiological, and psychological effects of the pill. Many of the scientists and physicians who appeared before the committee had also appeared on the pages of Seaman's book, and their testimony provided little, if any, new information about the biological effects of oral contraceptives. However, as a result of the intense media coverage of the hearings, the medical controversy over the safety of the pill reached a much wider audience.

Although Gordon relied heavily on Barbara Seaman for advice in choosing witnesses, he did not invite her to appear before the committee, "because she wasn't a primary source." Nor were any women who had experienced pill-related adverse health effects asked to testify. Seaman, by contrast, recognized the importance of women's voices and experiences in the pill debate, and included in her book heart-rending stories of women who had died or suffered serious consequences as a result of taking oral contraceptives.

In a way, Seaman and Nelson represented the ambivalence toward science and medicine in American society at the end of the 1960s. On the one hand, they questioned the merit and safety of the pill, a product of medical science and technology, and criticized scientists and physicians for their incursion into family planning. On the other had, they relied on scientists and physicians for evidence on which to base their critique. Nelson never acknowledged this inconsistency, at least not in public. Seaman, however, underwent a significant transformation after the publication of *The Doctors' Case against the Pill.* She had written the book as a "reformist" feminist, hoping to influence changes within the existing system of medical care. Later, after coming in contact with more radical feminists, she became critical of the medical establishment and its (mis)treatment of women's health care needs.

Seaman's enlightenment began on the first day of the Nelson hearings. Although not invited to testify, she attended the hearings as a press correspondent. In the middle of testimony from the second witness, some women in the audience interrupted the hearings. Seaman vividly recalled the disturbance:

> All of a sudden, these women started standing up and yelling... I heard my name, "Why isn't Barbara Seaman testifying?" And then somebody else was saying, "Why isn't there a pill for men?" And someone else was saying, "Why aren't there any patients testifying?"... Then they were cleared out of the room... So, I went outside. I followed them out. This was my story. What these guys were saying that I'd been writing about for years wasn't my story... So I went out and introduce myself to them... When I said that I was Barbara Seaman, they fell all over themselves... It turned out that it was my book that had inspired them to demonstrate.

The demonstrators belonged to a group called D.C. Women's Liberation, which had come together in 1969 to protest illegal abortion; their work soon led to a broader interest in women's health care. Alice Wolfson, a member of D.C. Women's Liberation and later one of the founders of the National Women's Health Network , explained how the demonstration got started:

> We were sitting at a meeting—which we did all the time in those days, nobody worked, I don't know what we did for money!—in the middle of the afternoon, and we had heard that there were going to be these hearings on the birth control pill on the Hill, so about seven of us went... When we got there, we were both frightened, really frightened, by the content and appalled by the fact that all of the senators were men [and] all of the people testifying were men. They did not have a single woman who had taken the pill and no women scientists. We were hearing the most cut-and-dried scientific evidence about the dangers of the pill... Remember all of us had taken the pill, so we were there as activists but also as concerned women... So while we were hearing this, we suddenly said, "My God," and we—because in those days you did things like that—raised our hands and asked questions.

The women quickly organized themselves and held militant demonstrations at every subsequent hearing . A group of twenty women arrived early each day

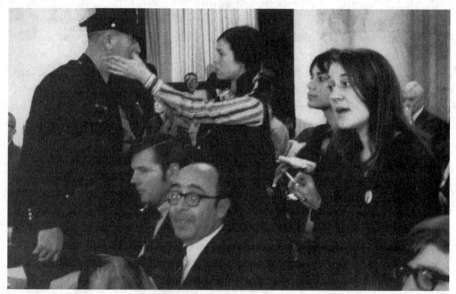

A pregnant Marilyn Webb (slapping the police officer) is one of a group of women who disrupted the 1970 Senate monopoly subcommittee hearings on the birth control pill, protesting the fact that no women had been called as witnesses. [AP/Wide World Photos]

and strategically placed themselves at the end and in the middle of every other row of seats. They came prepared with questions to interrupt the hearings and with bail money tucked inside their boots.

Ironically, both the feminists and Senator Nelson agreed on most issues. They believed that the FDA had allowed the drug companies to market the pill without adequate tests of its long-term safety. Neither the feminists nor Nelson advocated a ban on the oral contraceptives; both argued that women needed access to all available information so that they could make intelligent decisions about birth control. They agreed that the lack of informed consent stemmed from the problem of poor communication between doctors and patients.

At this point, the opinions of the senator and the feminists diverged. For Nelson, the issue of informed consent could be solved by improving the channels of communication among the manufacturers, the FDA, physicians, and patients. The more radical feminists saw the pill as the tip of the iceberg of much larger problems in women's health care; they doubted that these problems could be solved within the context of the contemporary system of male-dominated medicine.

The members of D.C. Women's Liberation took umbrage at the absence of female witnesses. Nelson's attempt to placate the demonstrators after the first interruption—in which he referred to them as "girls" and counseled them against disruptive behavior—only exacerbated the women's anger and increased their resolve to protest. Although they supported increasing public awareness of the health risks of oral contraceptives, they could not tolerate the established format of the Senate hearings.

Nelson also faced criticism from within his Senate subcommittee, mainly from a freshman senator from Kansas named Bob Dole. Dole professed concern that women would be unduly alarmed by public hearings of medical testimony regarding the safety of the pill. In his opening statement (read in his absence by the minority counsel), Dole warned: "We must not frighten millions of women into disregarding the considered judgments of their physicians about the use of oral contraceptives... Let us show some sympathy for the beleaguered physician who must weigh not only the efficacy and safety of alterative methods for a particular woman, but the emotional reactions of that woman which have been generated by sensational publicity and rumored medical advi[c]e." As a conservative Republican, Dole's ulterior interests probably agreed with those of the pharmaceutical industry, as well as the "beleaguered physician." When he joined the hearings on the third day, he remarked: "I think we probably have terrified a number of women around the country... I would guess they may be taking two pills now—first a tranquilizer and then the regular pill—because of our erudite investigation."

The controversial nature of the pill hearings did not go unnoticed by the media. All three national television networks covered them on evening news broadcasts in January 1970. Of the eight witnesses who testified during the first two days, seven voiced serious concerns about the safety of oral contraceptives, and excerpts from their testimony were televised to the American public. On ABC, Sam Donaldson reported, "Doctors do not agree on the relative safety of the pill. But on this first day of Senator Gaylord Nelson's hearings, the emphasis was on the dangers." On CBS, Walter Cronkite reported, "Almost nine million women in America, and ten million elsewhere, are taking the pill each day, in the words of one expert, 'as automatically as chickens eating corn.'" NBC's Chet Huntley led that network's evening news: "The pills have been on the market for ten years, but today was the first time Congress has seen fit to investigate them." The television cameras also captured the disturbance created by D.C. Women's Liberation as well as the impromptu news conference held by the women after the hearings.

Despite repeated invitations from Nelson, no industry representative ever appeared before the committee. G.D. Searle & Company chose to defend the pill by allowing one of its spokesmen, Dr. Irwin Winter, to be interviewed on television in his office at Searle's headquarters in Skokie, Illinois. Dr. Winter complained, "I thought when we brought out the pill several years ago that we were doing mankind [sic] a great favor and that this is a thing that women had been wanting from time immemorial. Now, from the headlines and the way this is being reported, or being presented… one would think we had unleashed a monster on the world." Nelson's invitations to the drug companies contrasted dramatically with his disregard of the feminists who had asked to testify. On January 23, D.C. Women's Liberation again interrupted the hearings, demanding to be allowed to appear.. All three networks featured the protest on the evening news, in which different women in the audience shouted:

> Why have you assured the drug companies that they could testify? Why have you told them they will get top priority? They're not taking the pills, we are!

> Why is it that scientists and drug companies are perfectly willing to use women as guinea pigs in experiments to test the high estrogen/low estrogen content of the pill, but as soon as a woman gets pregnant in one of these experiments she's treated like a common criminal! She can't get an abortion!

> Women are not going to stay quiet any longer! You are murdering us for your profit and convenience!

ABC reported that after Senator Nelson ordered the room to be cleared, he readmitted the press, but "the public and its virago element were not welcomed back." The other networks were more generous in their characterizations of the demonstrators and their intentions.

By the end of the first round of hearings, the television-viewing public knew a great deal more about the controversy surrounding the safety of the pill, but no more about whether the pill was safe to take. The *Washington Daily News* captured this uncertainty in a cartoon of a woman in a Hamlet pose holding in one hand a birth control pill and in the other a newspaper head-lined, "Scientists say pill is unsafe but safe enough." The cartoon's caption read: "To take or not to take…" On February 9, *Newsweek* reported the results of a Gallup poll of women between the ages of twenty-one and forty-five. News of the hearings reached an extremely wide audience; 87 percent of American women had heard or read about them. The survey found that 18 percent of the eight and a half million women with pill prescriptions had stopped taking the pills in recent months, and another 23 percent were considering stopping. One-third of those who had quit or thought about quitting directly attributed their recent or imminent abandonment of oral contraceptives to the Nelson hearings; another one-fourth cited side effects—experienced personally or by friends—as the reason for their doubts about the pill.

Perhaps the most disturbing finding of the survey addressed one of Senator Nelson's initial questions in the pill hearing: Were women being adequately informed by their doctors about the adverse health effects of the pill? The answer was a resounding "no." The poll revealed that two-thirds of women on the pill were never told by their physicians about the potential health risks of oral contraception. Millions of women chose to take birth control pills without knowing the whole story; the lack of communication between doctor and patient precluded informed consent in decision-making about birth control. This discrepancy between their doctors' actions and the expectations of the Senate committee heightened women's concerns about the wisdom of taking birth control pills in particular and about the quality of their medical care in general.

Data from Planned Parenthood clinics mirrored the trend away from the pill identified by the *Newsweek*-Gallup poll. In Detroit, during the month from January 14 to February 13, the clinic reported a tenfold increase in diaphragm requests, a doubling of requests for IUDs, and an "astounding increase" in requests for tubal ligations and vasectomies, all resulting from patients dis-continuing the pill. At the New York City clinic, almost one-fifth of oral contra-ceptive users switched to either the IUD or the diaphragm. *Business Week* reported an "almost hysterical cry for diaphragms" in January and February, resulting in a five-fold increase in sales of the device. A urologist in Rhode Island reported that vasectomy requests had tripled since the hearings began. Women all over the country telephoned their physicians demanding informa-tion on whether they should continue to take the pill.

Some doctors regretted the public forum of the hearings because of the alarm generated. An article in the *New York Times*, written by a physician, described the results of the hearings as "an epidemic of anxiety that has spread like wildfire." The author likened the scientific debate in the Senate Caucus Room to medical rounds in a hospital: "Unless the physician explains to the patient in words of one syllable and with understanding and sensitivity the facts in simple lay language, the consequences are anxiety and often real fear.".

By 1970, fewer patients were willing to accept that kind of paternalistic treatment. As consumer advocates turned their attention to professional services, such as medicine, they criticized the unequal balance of power in the doctor-patient relationship. Friction between doctors and female patients was further compounded by emerging feminist critiques of the male-dominated medical profession and of male-dominated society in general.

THE PILL HEARINGS, PART II

The second round of hearings presented testimony from witnesses both in favor of and opposed to the birth control pill. Many witnesses devoted their testimony to bemoaning the results of the first round of hearings held a month earlier. These experts generally approved of the pill as a valuable means of fertility control, and they lamented the anxiety and alarm produced by the hearings and concomitant media coverage. Not coincidentally, several of the pill advocates were affiliated with large-scale family planning agencies, such as the Margaret Sanger Research Bureau, or population control organizations, such as the Population Crisis Committee and Planned Parenthood/World Population. One witness, Phyllis Piotrow, formerly of the Population Crisis Committee, anticipated that one hundred thousand unwanted "Nelson babies" would be born in the coming year as a result of women discontinuing the pill because of fear generated by the hearings. In an article for the *Progressive*, journalist Morton Mintz ridiculed this eponymy and its supporters (notably Senator Dole) by suggesting pill-related diseases be called "Piotrow strokes" or "Dole thromboembolisms." The media immediately reported the concern about more unplanned pregnancies. In one of its articles on the Nelson hearings, *Time* printed a cartoon that showed one pregnant woman greeting another in an obstetrician's waiting room with the caption, "Corinne... You didn't tell me you gave up the pill, too?"

Once again, Senator Nelson found himself in unexpected opposition to his usual allies. Nelson prided himself on being an environmentalist; he helped to originate the idea of Earth Day (which took place just two months after the pill hearings). He worried about the effects of overpopulation and supported most fertility control programs. However, his doubts about the safety of oral contraceptives and his leadership of the public hearings on the pill alienated him from the population control community.

By the last days of the hearings, the central issue had boiled down to informed consent. Most physicians and scientists agreed that no new biomedical evidence had been presented ; the debate over whether the pill caused cancer, for example, would have to wait for more data in order to be resolved. They disagreed, however, on how much of this information should be presented to patients. Some concurred with Nelson, who insisted that women should be given all available information so that they could make up their own minds. Others sided with the witness who testified: "A patient cannot reasonably be expected to make a profound professional judgment—she is not a doctor."

The issue of informed consent crystallized on the final day of the hearings, when FDA Commissioner Edwards announced that his agency planned to require pill manufacturers to include information for patients in every package of birth control pills. This pamphlet, written in lay language and directed to the patient, would outline the health risks associated with taking the medication. Dr. Edwards explained that the insert was "designed to reinforce the information provided the patient by her physician." In the absence of good doctor-patient communication (which, according to the *Newsweek*-Gallup poll, characterized two out of every three women's experiences), the leaflet would supply the patient with the facts necessary to make an informed choice.

The hearings in February brought the first female witnesses to appear before the subcommittee. In total, four women testified: three physicians and the immediate past executive director of the Population Crises Committee (Ms. Piotrow). All of the women strongly advocated the use of the pill under a physician's supervision; none of them acknowledged the concerns expressed by the D.C. Women's Liberation protesters.

Dr. Elizabeth Connell, unlike many others, could afford the simultaneous luxury of a large family and a professional career. Given Connell's generously sized family, her interest in overpopulation and pollution could be interpreted as classist. However, she also felt concern and sympathy for women with unwanted pregnancies, and annoyance with a system that did not allow women to make their own reproductive choices. Connell argued for legalized abortion and relaxed sterilization laws, as well as for the availability of a wide variety of contraceptive options, so that every individual could be free to decide how many babies to have and when to have them. Connell offered powerful rhetoric, in a style reminiscent of that of Margaret Sanger, to make her case for oral contraceptives:

> As a physician who began practice before the advent of the pill, I am
> constantly aware of the immense difference it has made to the lives of
> women, their families, and to society as a whole. The look of horror on
> the face of a 12-year-old girl when you confirm her fears of pregnancy,
> the sound of a woman's voice cursing her newborn and unwanted child
> as she lies on the delivery table, the helpless feeling that comes over you
> as you watch women die following criminal abortion, the hideous
> responsibility of informing a husband and children that their wife and

mother has just died in childbirth—all these situations are deeply engraved in our memories, never to be forgotten. With the advent of more effective means of contraception, the recurrence of these nightmares was becoming blessedly less frequent.

It would be inaccurate to dismiss Connell as insensitive to women. Her distance from the younger generation of activists pointed instead to their differing agendas, which precluded consensus on the best way to fight for women's reproductive rights.

In February 1970, D.C. Women's Liberation held a press conference to announce their intention to hold their own hearings. They specifically invited women who had suffered ill effects on the pill to testify. The women's hearings took place in March, three days after the Senate hearings ended, in a church in Washington, with child care provided. Flyers advertising the hearings read, "The Pill: Is It a Menace, A No-No, or a Girl's Best Friend?" About a hundred people turned out to hear testimony from Barbara Seaman; Sarah Lewit Tietze, a research associate at the Population Council (and wife of Dr. Christopher Tietze, also affiliated with the Population Council); Elaine Archer, a women's health care advocate; Etta Horn, a welfare rights leader; and others.

In their opening statement, the women of D.C. Liberation made their position clear:

> We are not opposed to oral contraceptives for men or for women. We are opposed to unsafe contraceptives foisted on uninformed women for the profit of the drug and medical industries and for the convenience of men. It is not our mission to have all women of the pill discard it and change to another form of contraception. Our mission, if such it can be called, is to rise up, as women, and demand our human rights. We will no longer let doctors treat us as objects to be manipulated at will. Together we will ask for and demand explanations and humane treatment by our doctors and if they are too busy to give this to us we will insist that the medical profession must meet our needs. We will no longer tolerate intimidation by white coated gods, antiseptically directing our lives.

Doctors did not have to be male to fit the model of "white coated gods." Women doctors, such as Elizabeth Connell, who did not disclose all information to patients about the side effects of the pill, were subjected to the same sort of criticism from the new health feminists. Connell set her sights on the more reformist goal of helping women to achieve reproductive control as a means to greater economic stability and personal fulfillment; she viewed the pill as a beneficial—but not perfect—technological solution to family planning. The members of D.C. Women's Liberation, by contrast, rejected reformist feminism because it did not address what they perceived as the underling ills of a patriarchal system. Their objective was nothing less than the redistribution of power in society. In the realm of medicine, these feminists wanted women to participate as equal partners in their health care, which included the necessary prerogative of informed consent.

Thus, when FDA Commissioner Edwards announced the requirement for package inserts, many feminists regarded this as an important victory. After all, such an insert was a novel idea; oral contraceptives would be the first orally administered drug to carry a detailed warning directed at patients. However, as feminists and other advocates of the package insert soon found out, the road from promise to reality was not easily navigated.

FDA AND THE PATIENT PACKAGE INSERT

The 1938 the federal Food, Drug, and Cosmetic Act obliged pharmaceutical manufacturers to make information about the safety of drugs available to physicians. In 1961, an amended version of the law required this information to be listed on the label of the package in the interest of "full disclosure," and within a few years most prescription drugs included a detailed package insert directed to physicians. These pamphlets contained instructions for using the medications, as well as information on indications, contraindications, efficacy, and side effects. An editorial in the *Journal of the American Medical Association* pointed out that the drug companies composed and paid for the package inserts, thus making them little more than "promotional items." Indeed, the FDA did not participate in the preparation of these pamphlets; the agency left decisions about their specific content to the manufacturers, so long as they met the basic requirements for drug labeling as outlined by the legislation.

The extended FDA regulations created a new category of drugs available by prescription only. While government regulation was designed to protect consumers from unscrupulous drug manufacturers, it also removed a significant amount of decision-making about medical treatment from the patient's, or consumer's, domain. After 1938, patients relied on physicians to instruct them on which drugs to purchase and to use. The doctor controlled not only the patient's treatment, but also the degree to which the patient understood the complexities of that treatment.

The day after the FDA Commisssioner announced his intention to require the insert, the *New York Times* published the proposed text. Entitled "What You Should Know About The Birth Control Pill," the 600-word document described in lay language the health risks, side effects and contraindications of oral contraceptives. Although Edwards indicated that the insert was necessary because doctors did not adequately inform patients, the leaflet assured women of the competence of their doctors: "Your doctor has taken your medical history and has given you a careful physical examination. He has discussed with you the

risks of oral contraceptives and has decided that you can take this drug safely."
Ten of the fifteen paragraphs in the proposed text referred to the doctor as the
proper authority on oral contraceptives; the leaflet encouraged the woman to
consult her physician in no fewer than six different situations.

In spite of this deference to the doctor, the medical profession strongly
opposed the insert, claiming that the pamphlet would intrude upon the doctor-patient relationship. The pharmaceutical industry contended that the proposed leaflet overstated the potential risks and overlooked the benefits of oral
contraception. Even the Department of Health, Education, and Welfare
(HEW), which housed the Food and Drug Administration, argued that the
leaflet needed to be revised to satisfy somewhat murky legal issues. (The *New
York Times* reported that HEW was irked at having been left out of the loop on
the development of the insert.)

In response, the FDA backed away from its initial proposal and substituted
a much shorter, less detailed version. The revised text, 100 words in length,
mentioned only one complication of oral contraception, blood-clotting disorders. Whereas the first draft had included statistics on increased risk and mortality rates from thromboembolism, the edited version omitted this information. It encouraged women to see their doctors if they experienced side effects,
listing just five symptoms and conditions whereas the earlier draft had listed
more than twenty-five.

Outraged, women from D.C. Women's Liberation staged a sit-in at the
office of HEW Secretary Robert Finch to protest the watered-down version.
They came with their children and they sang, making up pill songs to the tunes
of nursery rhymes, like "The doctors give the pill, the doctors give the pill,
heigh ho the derey-o, the women take the pill, the women they get ill, the doctors send their bill." Alice Wolfson, organizer of the demonstration, said,
"Those of us who had babies... we brought them everywhere, and when anyone would say, 'take the kids out of the hearing room' or this or that, we would
say, 'well, that's fine, where's the day care center?' All of these issues were
always linked."

Secretary Finch did not see the feminists that day, but agreed to meet with
them a few days later. On March 30, 1970, Secretary Finch, FDA Commissioner
Edwards, and Surgeon-General Jesse Steinfeld met with six representatives of
the feminist group, including Barbara Seaman and Alice Wolfson. Wolfson
reported in the feminist newspaper *off our backs* that after an hour of discussion, "Finch stormed out of the room, tailed by Edwards and Steinfeld, claiming we were just wasting his time."

The feminist petition to reinstate the stronger version of the package insert
did not sway the officials of HEW and FDA. On April 10, 1970, the FDA published the abridged draft in The *Federal Register* and invited all interested parties to respond with comments. Letters from more than eight hundred individuals and groups flooded in. About a third requested more information

about the insert and about the oral contraceptives in general. Many had not read the actual notice in the *Federal Register,* but had heard or read about it in the news. More than half wrote to object to the abridgement of the text. Most of these were copies of form letters distributed by women's and consumers' groups which complained that the insert did not provide full disclosure on the adverse effects of the pill and called for public hearings on the matter. Over a hundred women and men wrote their own letters to protest the reduction in the length and scope of the insert. Some of them objected to the unequal distribution of power in the doctor-patient relationship:

> I have inadvertently received the physician's copy of facts and cautions now included in each 3-pack of Ortho-Novum pills; the first time I told the people who had given it to me they said, "You're not supposed to see that. That's only for doctors." I was outraged and insulted at this; the only reason I can see for doctors or other parties withhold medical information from patients is the desire to maintain their psychological and monetary power over us.

Others added their concern about the integrity of the pharmaceutical industry and its control over government agencies:

> In the *Chicago Daily News,* March 24, 1970, I read that the FDA has called for toning-down the wording of the precautionary literature on oral contraceptives which HEW has in the planning stage. It was clear from the article the HEW is bowing to pressure from the drug industry, the AMA, and many private physicians, all of whom feel that a precise report will harm the Pill's market and their own pocketbooks.

Still others expressed the opinion that women had the right to full disclosure on medical matter: "I DEMAND, that as a woman, having the option to take the pill or not, I have *all* the facts in front of me!"

Much of the public interest in the oral contraceptives can be attributed to the publicity generated by the Nelson hearings and the consistent coverage by the news media. It is less easy to explain why people moved beyond mere interest to direct action—in this case, writing letters of protest. Most likely the climate of the times spurred many individuals to act. In a society attuned to the issue of rights and conducive to political activism, people felt empowered to speak out against what they perceived as a denial of the right to informed consent. During this time, many Americans felt angered by the secret policies of the government in the Vietnam War: by 1970, the demand for public information extended to a broad range of government activities. In addition, Congress had recently passed the Freedom of Information Act (in 1967), which both entitled and emboldened citizens to seek information previously withheld from them.

Doctors also wrote to the FDA. The majority opinion of the medical profession was represented in letters from the American Medical Association and other national and state organizations. With very few exceptions, doctors strongly opposed the patient package insert, which they claimed would interfere with the doctor-patient relationship. Excerpts from physicians' letters reveal their indignation at regulation from outside the medical profession:

> I deeply resent the Government of the United States coming between me and my patients in the matter of a single class of prescription items...

> This practice can serve no useful purpose accept [sic] to frighten patients. Furthermore, it represents an undesirable entry of government into the practice of medicine.

> I would sincerely hope that before such a proposal becomes an accomplished fact, strong consideration be given to the far-reaching [e]ffects such legislation [regulation] will have on the medical community of this country, which has been so frequently maligned... The determination of appropriate use of medications must continue to rest in the hands of the physician... To remove this clinical relationship would be just another method of eroding the foundation of American medicine.

A few physicians expressed approval, agreeing with consumer advocates that the patient should be fully informed before making the decision to use birth control pills. One doctor argued that the insert would "serve as a protection for the doctor rather than as a cause for initiating lawsuits." One would think that this reasoning would appeal to the pharmaceutical industry as well; by 1970 more than a hundred lawsuits had been filed against birth control pill manufacturers.

However, drug companies vehemently opposed the inclusion of an FDA-mandated warning. The president of the Pharmaceutical Manufacturers Association (PMA), which represented 125 drug companies, articulated the industry's objections; four companies also wrote letters supporting the PMA position and offering additional comments on the proposed wording. The drug industry sided with the medical profession in preserving the sanctity of the doctor-patient relationship.

The content of the insert that became a requirement in June 1970 was significantly modified from the version proposed in April. The *New York Times* reported that the change resulted from pressure from physicians; clearly, the FDA bowed also to the interests of the powerful pharmaceutical industry. Although it did describe abnormal blood clotting as "the most serious known side effect," the insert did not list any symptoms; instead, it told the reader to "notify your doctor if you notice any physical discomfort." Four of the seven sentences in the insert described the availability of an information booklet, which the patient could request from the physician.

This 800-word booklet was written by the American Medical Association in conjunction with the FDA and the American College of Obstetricians and Gynecologists; it resembled in scope and content the original insert. The package insert merely informed the patient that further information was available; the onus fell on the patient to ask her doctor to give her the booklet.

In late June, a woman announced that she planned to sue the FDA and HEW under the 1967 Freedom of Information Act for disclosure of all clinical and toxicological records on eight different brands of oral contraceptives. According to HEW, release of the data from laboratory and clinical tests "would only confuse the average citizen." The plaintiff sought to challenge that assumption. In another lawsuit, an associate of the consumer advocate Ralph Nader lost a battle to have the booklet included directly in packages of birth control pills in lieu of the shorter insert. Barbara Seaman was "very shocked when we learned that it was going to be distributed to doctors' offices, not by pharmacists, and that the prescribing physician would give out the booklet... I spent a lot of time buttonholing women and asking them if they had received this, and I invariably found that if they'd been to a clinic, the chances were very good they had gotten it. Private physician, forget it! I don't know if I ever found one person whose private physician gave it to her."

The battle over the patient package insert demonstrated the influence and power of the medical profession and the pharmaceutical industry over the FDA. Yet, in spite of its watered-down wording, the insert still represented an important turning point in the doctor-patient relationship. Patients had demanded the right to know about the medications prescribed for them, and the package insert legitimized this claim.

Eight years later the FDA ordered the minimal package insert replaced by a lengthy information leaflet. In 1977, the FDA issued patient information requirements for estrogens used in hormone replacement therapy. In the wake of this mandate, the FDA revised the oral contraceptive requirements to be consistent with those of other estrogen products. This 1978 version of the patient package insert represented what consumer and feminist groups had wanted all along

THE WOMEN'S HEALTH MOVEMENT

Oral contraception was not the first reproductive health issue to engage women activists in the decades after World War II. The La Leche League began to promote breastfeeding as a better alterative to infant formula in 1956, challenging the authority of "scientific motherhood" and advocating the return of mothering to the mother. At the same time, women dissatisfied with the anesthetized experience of hospital childbirth turned to the "natural childbirth" techniques of Grantly Dick-Read. Another early feminist health issue centered on the promotion of physical therapy for radical mastectomy patients to prevent the loss of mobility in their arms. All of these initiatives sought to redress problems created by the medicalization of women's health in the twentieth century.

By the late 1960s, women around the country gathered in informal "consciousness raising" groups to share their experiences as women in a sexist society. Many of these groups focused their discussions on medicine, health, and the body. In Boston, women frustrated with the existing system of medical care decided to do research on health-related topics; the resulting papers written by members of this Boston Women's Health Book Collective formed the basis for the bestselling *Our Bodies, Ourselves.*

A rallying point for the early health feminists was the legalization of abortion. Members of D.C. Women's Liberation became more interested in women's health issues as they fought for legalized abortion. Alice Wolfson recalled: "We found that one of the leading causes of maternal death in D.C. General Hospital, which is the only public hospital in D.C., was botched abortions. So when we began to scratch that surface, we began to find out lots of other things about health care for women, and also began to develop a kind of analysis of the health care system and the relationship of women to power and the health care system as being kind of a microcosm of women's place in society in general at the time." It was only a short step from activism on abortion and sterilization abuse to activism on a broader range of health-related issues. In 1970, many abortion rights advocates were still working at the state level. The pill hearings, however, took place on Capitol Hill and attracted national attention.

At the Nelson hearings, Barbara Seaman met Alice Wolfson, thus bringing together the "uptown" and the "downtown" feminists on the issue of the safety of the pill. Seaman used the term "downtown" to describe the more radical feminists who belonged to militant groups such as the Redstockings, Bread and Roses, and D.C. Women's Liberation. "Uptown" referred to those feminists who belonged to more mainstream organizations such as Betty Friedan's National Organization for Women. Seaman described herself as an uptown feminist... until she met Wolfson: "I instantly struck up a friendship with Alice. I just thought everything she said was right, putting her political analysis on all of this. I thought, yes, yes, why didn't I see it this way, why didn't I understand it this way all along? But of course, if I had seen it that way, I wouldn't have been suitable to write for the *Ladies' Home Journal* or to write the kind of book I wrote. So in the scheme of things, it's just as well that I saw it from my particular lens up until that moment in January, 1970, when I met Alice."

The two women remained in close contact after the hearing; Wolfson lived in Washington and could keep track of the developments at the FDA. Soon thereafter, she invited Seaman to testify at the women's hearings on the pill, to meet with HEW Secretary Finch, and to "sit in" at a closed meeting of the FDA's Advisory Committee on Obstetrics and Gynecology: "Alice and I went down there [to the FDA] and we walked in [to the room where the Advisory Committee met] and we sat down and everybody said to us, "What are you doing here?" And Alice said, "Well, why shouldn't we stay? It's our bodies you're discussing." They told us we had to go out, and they would discuss whether we would be allowed to stay. We sat on the floor in the hallway right outside for about a half an hour, and then somebody came out and said okay, we could stay. I think that was the first time that the advisory committees were made open to the public." For both women, full disclosure and informed consent remained at the heart of all of their battles.

Wolfson and Seaman were in the vanguard of what became the women's health movement. In 1975, they joined with other health activists to form the National Women's Health Network. The network acted as an information clearinghouse for women's collectives around the country. It represented women's health interests in hearings held by Congress and the FDA and published a newsletter on health policy and legislation. Twenty years later, the organization remains actively engaged in women's health issues.

The goals of health feminists in the 1970s differed dramatically from those of their predecessors. A generation earlier, Margaret Sanger and Katherine McCormick lobbied for women's right to reproductive control. To achieve their goal, they enlisted the help of scientists and physicians and encouraged these experts to develop a solution to the problem of birth control. Sanger and McCormick hailed the oral contraceptive as a scientific triumph for women and gladly entrusted contraception to the hands of physicians. In contrast, the women's health movement rejected the hegemony of the medical-pharmaceutical complex and instead advocated lay control over the delivery of health services. Health feminists objected to the birth control pill on several grounds: insufficient clinical trials, potentially fatal side effects, and a lack of informed consent among its millions of users worldwide. In 1970, feminists interpreted the pill as representative of patriarchal control over women's lives; it was this issue that catalyzed the rise of the women's health movement.

Although not as well organized nor as powerful as the established medical profession and the pharmaceuticl industry, health feminists were determined to take on these male-dominate institutions and their traditional assumptions and practices. In the decades to follow, the interests of feminists, female patients, physicians, drug manufacturers, and government officials would clash many times over issues such as diethylstilbestrol (DES), intrauterine devices, Depo-Provera, Norplant, and abortion. All of these debates had their own unique set of concerns; however, in each one the matter of informed consent, as articulated in the controversy over the safety of oral contraceptives, remained central.

Julie Is Not a Statistic

BARBARA SEAMAN

Barbara Seaman, "Julie Is Not a Statistic," *The Doctors' Case against the Pill*, New York, Peter H. Wyden, 1969. Reprinted by permission.

To five blue-eyed little girls, she was "mommy." To her husband, she was "the heart of our home." To her older sister, she was a "born mother. That was the thing God meant her for."

Whatever she was meant to be in life, Julie Macauley was not a statistic. She became a statistic only when she died at the age of 29 from a pulmonary embolism and left her beloved husband, Tom, a widower and her children motherless.

Julie had been on the pill for less than a year. Her husband is convinced that it killed her and he is bitter against the doctors and drug manufacturers who he feels let death come so unnecessarily to his Julie.

"They say, 'Oh, it's only one in a thousand that's going to have trouble,'" he scoffed. "But this one in a thousand is my wife. She was the mother of five children. She was a real person. She was not a statistic."

Dr. Wood, a gynecologist in the large Midwestern city where Julie lived, placed her on the pill to regulate a long-standing menstrual irregularity. He testified in court that he had read drug company pamphlets and medical literature reporting more than 400 cases of clotting and 37 deaths among pill users through 1964. Nevertheless, he had placed Mrs. Macauley on the pill in 1965 without warning her of its possibly dangerous side effects.

The doctor said that he considered the statistical evidence of clotting to be "quite small.... I think the physician is supposed to exercise judgment. That's what I did. I felt I would be doing the lady a disservice to report it to her. You can scare a patient to death."

The fact is that Julie would not have been "scared to death" if the doctor had come straight out and told her the risks she was facing. She was not the type to be stampeded. Her sister Peggy described her to us as a "solid, steady sort of person—very quiet, very determined. She just went her own way."

She had been independent even when she was a baby, Peggy said. "She was tall for her age, but when she was 3 and 4, she always walked around with a little chair so she could get things she couldn't reach without having to ask for help. She was very tall and gangly by the time she reached her teens. She was really awkward then. And those long, gangly legs! They were always bent over chairs and things like that."

When Julie outgrew the gangly stage, she turned out to be a real beauty. She was tall, slender, blond. Her friends told her she should be a model. "She was a good student," her sister said, "but she didn't really like school. She didn't date much at first, but when she started to blossom, she dated quite a bit. And then she met Tom the summer right after she graduated from high school."

RHYTHM DIDN'T WORK

Anybody who knew Julie at all knew what was going to happen to her. She was going to get married and have a big family and live as happily ever after as real people ever do in real life.

"I met Julie when I was a sophomore," Tom Macauley told us. "We went together for two years before we got married, but I knew from the first that we were going to get married. When we were courting, we used to talk about the children we were going to have. We decided we wanted a large family, perhaps seven or eight children."

Julie and Tom got married while Tom was still in college. Their first daughter, Anne Marie, arrived within the year. The Macauleys decided that they should wait until Tom was through college before having another child. They turned to the only form of birth control acceptable to them as Roman Catholics.

"We practiced rhythm," Tom explained, "but it was very difficult." Julie had had very irregular cycles all the way from the time when she started having her periods. "It would vary between, say, 28 days up to 55 or 60 days," Tom recalled. "Well, we kept track of it. We took her temperature every morning and recorded it versus the day of the cycle. We tried to avoid relations during the period when she would have ovulated and been fertile."

Despite their meticulous recordkeeping and their careful study of the charts, the result had been four more blond, blue-eyed girls in seven years. With such a history, Julie should have acquired the right in her obstetrician's office to be regarded as a human being with a very human problem. Instead, she was just an anonymous white record card. Her doctors were a team of three specialists who shared a suite of offices and practice. Tom described it as "a big assembly line."

When Julie made an appointment to see one of the doctors, she pointed out to him that the rhythm method of birth control obviously wasn't working for them because her periods were so extremely irregular. The doctor suggested that she take the pill. "Julie told him right away that she was a Catholic," Tom said. "And he said, 'Well, I'm giving it to you for medical reasons. I won't prescribe if for you until you go first and tell your priest.' He said that the pill had a tendency to adjust the hormone system of the body in some way so that the cycle became more regular.

So Julie "went to Monsignor O'Hara," Tom said, "who was our pastor. He said that it was a strictly medical matter. Julie called the doctor back and he phoned the prescription to the drugstore so we could pick it up."

"OH, WE HAD PLANS"

Tom paused and recalled softly: "I remember, I think the most joyful look I ever saw on her face was when our first child, Anne Marie, was born. The nurse brought the baby into the room. It was the first time she saw the baby, you know, and fed it. I never saw such a look of joy on a person's face as I saw that time. I got a little of an understanding of what this means to a woman from the expression on her face."

Tom recalled: "Julie was always happiest when we were working together or doing something as a family. "One particular incident I remember. We went out and bought one of those outdoor swing sets that were so popular for the backyard. All the kids had to stand around, of course, and watch Daddy put the swing set together. Lots of giggles and laughs. Of course Mommy and Daddy had to do a little clowning around. I think kids get the greatest kick out of their parents clowning around.

"I got the camera out and took a few pictures. And Julie took one of me sliding down the sliding board. I was obviously too big for the sliding board. It's things like this that I remember as our happiest moments, that I keep remembering.

"She was always busy. She liked to knit. And she did all the mending. We were thinking about buying a sewing machine and had started looking at the different models... "

He paused and shook his head.

"In 1963, we moved into this house. It was September that we moved in and she died just two years later.

"We had so many plans. We used to sit back and plan and say, 'Well, some day we'll have a couch here and a new rug. We'll get a new dining room set.' Oh, we had plans."

Peggy knew the pride her sister took in the new house and spent many hours talking with her about how it should be furnished as soon as there was enough money. "The sad part of it," Peggy said, "she was just beginning to reap the benefits of all their struggles and sacrifices so that Tom could get his degree. Life was just beginning to be a little more easy. They had a nice home now, but she never lived to see it the way she wanted it."

For a time, it seemed that Julie and Tom were indeed destined to live happily ever after, but when Julie started taking the pill to control her menstrual irregularities, their life began to change. Tom tried to recall exactly what had happened. "Julie would become very upset and cry. It seemed like it didn't take anything at all to set her off. She would kind of go into a mood and it would last for a day of two.

"And then her attitude toward things changed. She became pessimistic. For example, she would feel that we were in real bad financial shape and things were not going to improve. She used to talk about our financial condition before, but she wouldn't get depressed and pessimistic. Our finances were typical for someone in our position. Naturally we weren't putting a lot of money in the bank or anything like that. But we were paying our bills. There were a lot of time payments, but I think any young married couple with five children has a lot of time payments."

"ALL OF A SUDDEN... "

Julie was depressed, on and off, for several months. But neither of them connected this change in her normally cheerful disposition with the pill. Tom was accustomed to doing a fair amount of traveling in connection with his job. Sometimes he would be away just overnight; other times, it would be for as long as a week. On the Tuesday before Julie died, he had to go on a trip.

"I returned Friday afternoon and found my wife sick," he told us. "She had been trying to get hold of the doctor. She had called the three rotating physicians, but they couldn't come out to see her.

"She told me she had had several incidents where she would be going about her business and all of a sudden, she would get very dizzy and break out in this cold sweat, become pale and feel very sick. This occurred once when she went shopping, and I think it happened another time when she went to get her hair fixed. When she went shopping, she had a whole cart full of groceries and she felt so bad, she couldn't even bother with the groceries. She just told the girl to put them back and she got in the car and came home.

"She had been taking bed rest and trying to get hold of a doctor all day. I finally succeeded in getting one to come out Friday night." The doctor checked her over and recommended that she go down to the hospital in the morning so that he could run some tests. He mentioned a chest x-ray, blood tests, and a urinalysis.

"The next morning," Tom recalled, "Julie wasn't feeling real well. There were no episodes of this dizziness, though, during the night. When we got ready to go down to the hospital, she wanted me to help her walk. She felt a little unsteady. I was surprised at how weak she was. We got to the hospital about 8:30."

The doctor came out to talk to Tom after the tests on Julie had been completed. He seemed cheerful and unconcerned. "He said that he didn't see any reason to admit her to the hospital," Tom said. "The x-ray didn't show anything particular. He said something about a broken blood vessel showing up on the x-ray, but later on he said, 'I was mistaken about that.'

"He told me there was some pus in the urine and there was some indication of infection. But it wasn't anything that couldn't be cured with bed rest and a little bit of medication."

"I thought there was something more serious," Tom said. "And so did my wife. The doctor saw that we were uneasy about it. I said something to the effect that I thought she ought to be admitted to the hospital anyway or something like that. He came back and said there is nothing in these tests that indicates any reason for having your wife admitted. And I felt a little bit relieved when he said, 'Just bed rest and take this medication. It's just a mild infection.'"

So Tom and Julie went home. He fixed up the sofa in the living room for her with pillows and a blanket and they watched a football game on television together.

"I fixed her a steak, a broiled steak," Tom said. "She ate well."

But she stayed close to the sofa all afternoon. They started watching Jackie Gleason and Julie suddenly became very sick.

Tom remembered every moment of it. "She became pale and she broke out in a sweat. She started to breathe real hard. She told me, 'Quick! Call an ambulance!' They arrived 15 minutes later.

"She asked me to fan her," Tom went on. "She was having trouble getting her breath. And she was white as a sheet, kind of a bluish white, I guess you'd say. And then all of a sudden her chest heaved up and her eyes rolled back in her head and she passed out."

Julie's mother had come over that day to care for the children, and she pitched in trying to help. She joined Tom at the sofa, fanning Julie. Her daughter looked up at her, just before she passed out and said, "Oh, Mommy, I don't think I'm going to make it."

"The ambulance came," Tom said, "and I held the oxygen on her mouth and we got her to the hospital. She was put in the emergency room. I was in the waiting room. The doctor came out later. I don't know exactly how much later it was, about 45 minutes or so. And he said it didn't look too good. And then the nurse came up to him and I could see from the look on her face that she was dead...

"The doctor said, 'I don't understand it. I don't understand it.'"

Tom was not the sort of man who was ready to leave without understanding. He signed the release for an autopsy. And then he made an appointment with a well-recommended internist.

HAD JULIE DIED IN VAIN?

The first thing the doctor asked was, "Was she taking birth control pills?"

Tom was surprised. "Yes, does that have anything to do with it?"

"I'll bet," said the doctor, "that the autopsy will show a pulmonary embolism, a thrombus in the ovarian vein."

And he was right. The attending doctor told Tom later that Julie had died from "a thrombus in the right ovarian vein, which caused an embolus which eventually caused the pulmonary embolism."

Tom was not only stunned by the suddenness of Julie's death. He was determined to find out what had really happened. He made a point of researching the effects of the pill. He read everything relevant that he could get his hands on. He pored over the medical journals and talked to whatever experts were available. He became increasingly convinced that his wife's death had been unnecessary, that just a little time and a little interest would have made the crucial difference as to whether or not the doctor would have prescribed the pill for medical reasons.

He particularly resented that his wife had not been warned of the dangerous side effects. Slowly, quietly, he became angry. And the more he learned, the angrier he became. Tom sued the drug company that had manufactured the particular pill. He lost the case.

The jury of four women and eight men sat for two weeks while pathologists, blood coagulation specialists, gynecologists, and other authorities testified whether or not, in their opinion, the blood clot that killed Julie was unquestionably caused by the pill. Some of the experts maintained that the clot was indeed pill-induced; others, testifying for the drug company, dismissed the idea and voiced their opinion that an upper respiratory infection was more likely to have caused Julie's death.

The jury decided in May 1969 that the manufacturer was not guilty. But this group of responsible men and women had obviously been moved to worry deeply about the medical testimony they had been hearing. Indeed, they had become so concerned that they accompanied their verdict with an unusual and urgent comment. They said that they felt that the manufacturers of this oral contraceptive should make it a regular practice to warn doctors and patients that these pills may be dangerous.

Tom had sought $750,000 in damages from the drug company, but to him the money was not principally at stake (although it can be very expensive to bring five children up without a mother). Tom's crusade had been a valiant attempt to ensure that Julie had not died in vain, that her death would become widely known and turn into a warning to other women.

And perhaps it will. The trial was covered by the major news services and many newspapers sent their own reporters. Reports of the testimony and proceedings appeared in newspapers from coast to coast.

Today Tom tries not to look back. His life and that of his daughters is in the future. But it is hard. He keeps remembering—how they all ate together at the big dining table, the baby in the high chair beside Julie, how they all piled in the car for a week's visit to his folks to show the girls off to the relatives.

He keeps telling people, "She was a real person, the mother of five, not a statistic. And she was an important part—she and a thousand other mothers—of what we call the human race."

Excerpts from Women and the Crisis in Sex Hormones

BARBARA SEAMAN AND GIDEON SEAMAN

Excerpted from Barbara Seaman and Gideon Seaman, *Women and the Crisis in Sex Hormones,* New York, Bantam Books, 1978. Originally published by Rawson in 1977. Reprinted by permission.

THE AMAZING STORY OF DES

One day, a Virginia woman named Grace M. was reading the newspaper when she noticed an article concerning a drug called DES—diethylstilbestrol, often called simply stilbestrol. The article pointed out a newly discovered danger associated with this drug: The daughters of some of the women who had taken it during their pregnancies had developed vaginal cancer as a result, said the author of the report, Dr. Arthur Herbst.

"I became alarmed and called my doctor immediately," recalls Mrs. M. "I had first taken DES in 1949 when I was pregnant with one daughter, and again in 1955 before the birth of another. So I took both my daughters to the doctor, and from the examinations, Marilyn, the 14-year-old, was found to have cancer of the vagina.

"Three weeks later, she had vaginal surgery in New York City. She was four weeks in the hospital. The doctors told me they had gotten all of it, there was no problem, everything was taken care of, this type of cancer rarely ever spreads beyond the female organs.

"And so, reassured, we went back to Virginia. A year later, Marilyn developed cancer of the lung and also three tumors on her trachea and her bronchial tubes. The doctors operated and removed the lung and tumors.

"About four months later, Marilyn started having severe head pains. The cancer had spread into her head. She had whole-head radiation, and from hip radiation she went on to the arms and legs, and eventually she went blind and died, two and a half years after we had discovered the cancer. It is a horrible, terrible thing to watch your child suffer, and eventually, when she dies, you think it is a blessing—the death is far easier to accept than the actual suffering."

Today, Mrs. M.'s other daughter, Patty, who is in her twenties, is under constant care. She is checked every three months because she has adenosis, an abnormal condition in her vaginal tract associated with prenatal exposure to DES and thought to be a precursor of cancer of the vagina.

On December 16, 1975, a 21-year-old woman named Sherry L. spoke on the steps of the Food and Drug Administration in Rockville, Maryland, at a National Women's Health Network memorial service that was held for all the women who have died from unnecessary estrogen products. Sherry herself is a "DES daughter"—like Marilyn M., and *an estimated 1.5 million other young U.S. women.* She has cervical abnormalities that were discovered in a routine checkup at a women's health center and in tests at Massachusetts General Hospital's DES screening program. She has to undergo continual monitoring. Sherry is anxious about the outcome of her life.

"I relieve a lot of my anxiety by working on DES projects, but it's still hard to live with," she says.

Mothers suffer equally. On Long Island, New York, many are active in an organization called DES-Action. This is a group of mothers and daughters who were exposed to the drug and who have banded together for mutual support, advice, and possible action. Similar activist groups are organizing in other areas. DES women in California have prodded the state health department to publish material alerting women and doctors to the dangers of DES, and to offer doctors one-day courses in the use of the colposcope, an instrument that aids in the discovery of vaginal abnormalities. Other women exposed to DES have themselves filed suits against the drug companies who make it—or have joined in filing class action suits.

Why are these tragedies, connected to a relatively small group of people, receiving so much attention? In terms of the population as a whole, the cause of a group of mothers and daughters who, over a 30-year span, were given a drug that proved dangerous to many does not seem of imminent concern to the rest of us.

But these women are not the only ones at risk. Abnormalities are now beginning to show up in some of the sons of women who were given DES during pregnancy. And in spite of the alarming track record of this synthetic hormone in after-the-fact testing, *DES is still being given today in the form of the morning-after pill, a favorite contraceptive handed out at many university health services. It is also being given as a milk suppressant to new mothers* who do not wish to nurse their babies.*

And on top of all that, this known carcinogen *is in the meat we eat.* The fact is that today—man, woman, or child— *we are all chemically medicated to some degree with DES, without our permission and usually without our knowledge.*

MORE NORMAL THAN NORMAL

DES is the grandmother product of all synthetic estrogens, as well as being the loss leader. (Leader to the pharmaceutical industry, loss to the women who have taken it.)

Synthesized by Sir Charles Dodd in England in 1938, it was the first hormone product that was both cheap to manufacture and effective to take by mouth. DES has been defined as a "synthetic compound capable of producing feminizing effects similar to those of the naturally occurring feminizing hormone estrogen." Similar to, but not identical with, as Dodds himself pointed out.

Nearly thirty years later, in 1965, Sir Charles made this comment about his brainchild: "It is interesting. . . to speculate on the difference in attitude toward new drugs 30 years ago and today. Within a few months of the first publication of the synthesis of stilbestrol, the substance was being marketed throughout the world. No long-term toxicity tests on animals such as dogs were ever done with stilbestrol. . . . It is really surprising that we escaped major pharmacological disasters until a few years ago."

THE BOSTON DISEASE: ITS ORIGINS

Paul Rheingold is an attorney specializing in malpractice and drug liability cases. He is planning a class action suit against the drug companies to pay for the health care of the daughters of women who were given DES while they were pregnant. He also handles individual DES lawsuits. "You know," he

---

*This was true as of 1977, seven years after the Herbst findings. It was only after the Surgeon General convened a task force on DES in 1978 that steps were taken to sharply restrict its use.

mused when we interviewed him in 1976, "it's almost like a Boston disease. The closer you get to Boston, the more DES daughters you find, and the farther away you get, the fewer."

He could have said Harvard because, in point of fact, the tragic story of DES begins at Harvard University. The first promoters of DES as a therapy for pregnant women were Dr. George Van Siclen Smith, head of Harvard's gynecology department from 1942 to 1967 and now professor emeritus, and his wife, biochemist Dr. Olive Watkins Smith.

George and Olive Smith married in 1930 when he was a fellow in gynecology at Harvard Medical School, and she was a young Ph.D. out of Radcliffe. Today they are a handsome enough couple to star in a leisure village advertisement, except that leisure is the one thing they don't have. He is still in private practice, and she performs research—70 hours per week—at the Fearing Research Laboratory of the Free Hospital for Women in Brookline.

They are tall, the two of them, and blue-eyed. They chuckle a lot together, and they are proud of their grown daughter and son. They also adopt a parental attitude toward the doctors they trained—"our boys"—such as DES investigators Arthur Herbst, Philip Corfman, and John Lewis.

Philip Corfman, of the National Institute of Health's Division of Child Health and Human Development, has given grants for several studies on the aftermath of DES. Dr. George said of Corfman, "He's too young to be an administrator. He was a good resident. We wanted to keep him here."

George and Olive Smith "started right in on the ovary" in 1928, and have been working on it ever since. As Dr. George puts it, "We have just lived ovarian hormones—pituitary and placental—for years and years." The Smiths were among the first to demonstrate how pituitary and ovarian hormones function over the course of the normal menstrual cycle, and, with the help of a tip from their friend Dr. Gregory Pincus, inventor of the birth control pill, were the first to demonstrate estradiol as one of the naturally occurring forms of estrogen.

THE FIRST DES STUDY

From the mid-1930s on, Dr. George and Dr. Olive, together and separately, published many important papers on estrogen excretion in normal pregnancy. It was in 1941, based on their observation of low hormone levels in mothers spontaneously aborting, that they conceived the idea of using the newly developed DES to help pregnancies that seemed threatened by miscarriage. Dr. Olive stated in her landmark report, published in the *American Journal of Obstetrics and Gynecology* in November 1948, "It was found... that diethylstilbestrol... might theoretically... provide an ideal agent for progesterone deficiency in pregnancy."

The report described a study of 632 DES-treated pregnancies, which dated back to 1943. The earliest DES mothers were not all Bostonians, for 117 obstetricians from 48 cities and towns in New York, New Jersey, Pennsylvania, the

District of Columbia, Illinois, North Carolina, Virginia, Texas, New Mexico, California, and all of the New England states cooperated in the study. Presumably the cooperating doctors gave the pills to pregnant patients who seemed in danger of miscarrying, although possibly some gave them to women who merely had problems with previous pregnancies.

By 1948 the Smiths were convinced that DES could be effective against many complications of pregnancy, including threatened miscarriage and diabetes. In addition, the babies of DES-treated mothers were said to be unusually rugged; the placentas were found to be "grossly more healthy-looking."

THE BIG BOSTON SUCCESS

The following year the Smiths completed their second major study at Boston Lying-In. This study, which had begun in 1947, included 387 women who received DES throughout pregnancy, compared to 550 who did not. All of these women... were observed to be having *normal first pregnancies.* Those who did not receive DES got no special treatment, or even a placebo. Women with known illnesses such as diabetes or hypertension were excluded from the study, in spite of the Smith's claims that DES had proved effective in pregnancies threatened by diabetes. Those in the study were all normal and healthy first-time mothers. What was the reason for giving them a powerful drug, except in the name of research? *Yet the women who were given DES were never informed that they were part of a highly controversial experiment.* Some DES mothers recall that they were told the pills were "vitamins."

The Smiths had a dream—a dream of helping women with problem pregnancies achieve motherhood, and then, as their experiment unfolded, a yet more daring dream of making normal pregnancies more normal!

Nowadays, a well-designed drug study must handle both treated and untreated patients in exactly the same way. The untreated patients are given placebos and the same kind of care as the treated. Codes are kept secret so that the doctors and staff (as well as the patients) never know who received the real medication until its all over.

The regional battle lines concerning DES were drawn on a day in 1949 in Hot Springs, Virginia, at the Seventy-second Annual Meeting of the American Gynecological Society. In general, the New Englanders supported the Smiths— and Harvard—while the Midwesterners did not. Dr. William J. Dieckmann of the University of Chicago and Chicago Lying-In Hospital pointed out that the untreated control group in the Smiths' study was not given a placebo, which he considered essential for scientific accuracy. He proposed a plan for testing DES at Chicago Lying-In, using a placebo as a control.

TROUBLESOME NEWS FROM NEW ORLEANS AND CHICAGO

A New Orleans obstetrician, Dr. John Henry Ferguson of Charity Hospital and Tulane University, also attempted to replicate the Harvard DES work. Like

Dieckmann, Ferguson believed that the Smiths had erred in not giving their control patients an inert pill. Alternate pregnant patients at Charity Hospital were given tablets called "white stilbestrol" and "yellow stilbestrol," but only the white ones contained the real stuff.

Ferguson's study was the first to show stilbestrol had no more effect than the placebo. In fact, more DES patients than placebo patients had miscarriages and premature births, while the control-group babies (and placentas) were slightly bigger and healthier. The only diabetic patient in the study, a DES mother, lost her baby! Dr. Ferguson had, in the words of one admiring contemporary, "driven a very large nail in the coffin that we will use someday to bury some of the extremely outsized claims for the beneficial effects of stilbestrol."

The Dieckmann Chicago study was begun on September 29, 1950... and completed on November 20, 1952. The DES babies in this study did not do better in any respect. To the contrary: Twice as many of the DES mothers had miscarriages; they had more hypertension... and smaller babies than the mothers on placebos. Dr. Dieckmann and his associates concluded that DES *actually favors premature labor.*

But even more serious in its implications was the testing of DES for carcinogenicity by animal researchers. At the National Cancer Institute, for example, Michael B. Shimkin and Hugh C. Grady dissolved the new DES in sesame oil and fed it to male mice. These mice were of a strain called C_3H, which is so highly susceptible to cancer that most of the virgin females develop breast cancer spontaneously, though the males do not.

The DES males *did.* When the Smiths were conceiving their human experiments, DES had already been proven carcinogenic in mice.

The Smiths were aware of this research, for as Dr. Olive said in 1976, "Before we even started any clinical work at all, we went through all the literature."

"However," said her husband, "you can do all kinds of things to rats and mice by giving them overdoses."

The New Orleans and Chicago reports must have convinced many obstetricians then that there was no value in using DES, though apparently not some of the sons of Harvard. In 1953, when the bad news from Chicago was brought to the Lake Placid meeting, one doctor was quick to quip: "As a former Bostonian, I would be entirely lacking in loyalty if I had not used stilbestrol in my private practice."

THE HERBST REPORT

Back in Boston, while the Lake Placid meeting was taking place, a young New Yorker named Arthur Herbst was graduating *cum laude* from Harvard College, class of '53. Herbst got his M.D. from Harvard Medical School in 1959, trained in obstetrics and gynecology, and became one of the Smith "boys." In 1966, a 15-year-old girl with clear-cell adenocarcinoma of the vagina came to his attention. It was the first time that this type of cancer had ever been seen at Massachusetts General Hospital in any woman under 25.

(Adenocarcinoma is cancer that occurs in *glandular tissue*. In normal women, the vaginal lining has no such tissue, but we now know that the vaginas of most daughters of women who took DES while pregnant, including those who are thus far free from cancer, have many tiny glands.)

Within the next three years, six similar cases of clear-cell adenocarcinoma in young women turned up at Massachusetts General Hospital. The youngest patient was 15, the oldest 22. The patients and their mothers were all questioned about possible causes, such as douches, tampons, birth control pills, and sexual activity. "Finally," says Herbst, "*one of the mothers made an intuitive guess that the cause might be the DES she was given in pregnancy.*" The researchers then added prenatal hormones to their list of questions.

And that was the connection. The mothers of the young women with adenocarcinoma had all taken DES while pregnant.

Today George Smith says, sadly: "We've been in on that from the beginning because we're close friends with Dr. Herbst. Of course he felt terrible about it, but a lot is being learned as the result of it, and who could predict 30 years ago that anything like this would develop? I mean, regardless of the rat and mouse work."

Herbst's relationship with the Smiths did not prevent him from publishing his findings in *The New England Journal of Medicine* on April 22, 1971, in an article he authored with Drs. Ulfelder and Poskanzer. At this point, Herbst had examined eight cases of adenocarcinoma in young women. All but one were DES daughters.

The frightening implications for these findings go far beyond DES because for the first time, Herbst showed that estrogen products can be cancer-producing in humans. It had been known since 1896, when surgeons started removing ovaries of breast cancer patients, that hormones—even the hormones produced by a woman's own body—could speed up the growth of an existing malignancy.

It had been known since 1932 that breast cancer could be produced in *male* mice by giving them estrogen injections, that sex hormones could *produce* cancer in laboratory animals, serving as "seed" as well as "fertilizer" in *susceptible* strains.

DES was the first hormone product to be named a human carcinogen. The work of Herbst and his colleagues was a crucial "missing link" concerning estrogens and the *initiation* of cancer in humans, for all estrogens have a similar way of behaving biologically.... In 1971, the millions of hormone-using women all over the world should have been warned of the significance of Herbst's DES findings. They should have been warned that estrogens *cause* cancer as well as *help it to grow.*

They were not. Only in 1975, when additional hormone products, such as

Premarin and the sequential pill, were also linked to cancer, did the U.S. Food and Drug Administration start to acknowledge that estrogen products must be viewed as a group.

Herbst himself understood the sweeping implications of his 1971 report concerning the DES link among the young women with cancer. In March 1971, the New England Journal of Medicine sent galleys of Herbst's article to the FDA. Herbst also shipped the FDA his raw data sheets. Then he waited . . . and waited.

THE GREENWALD REPORT

But while the FDA dallied, health officials of one state—New York—swung promptly into action. Dr. Peter Greenwald, the 34-year-old director of New York's Cancer Control Bureau, was a 1967 graduate of the Harvard School of Public Health. His specialty was epidemiology. He quickly collected data on five young New York women (aged 15 to 19 at the time of diagnosis) who had adenocarcinoma of the vagina. Three had died of advanced disease, and two were doing well post-operatively. The mothers of four of the young women had taken DES, and the fifth a series of different estrogens and progesterones.

In Dr. Greenwald's opinion, the symptoms of abnormal pregnancy in some of these mothers had been minimal. One mother had no symptoms, only a history of a previous miscarriage. Greenwald and his colleagues, Drs. J. J. Barlow, P. C. Nasca, and W. S. Burnett, quickly submitted their findings to *The New England Journal of Medicine*, which published them on August 12.

Meanwhile, on June 22, 1971, Dr. Hollis S. Ingraham, New York's Commissioner of Health and Greenwald's boss, sent an individual letter to every physician in his state telling of the Herbst findings and the confirming evidence collected by Greenwald. New York physicians were urged to report all similar cases immediately (Greenwald's phone number was enclosed) and to stop prescribing DES to pregnant women at once. Dr. George Himler, president of the Medical Society of the State of New York, and Dr. Eli Stark, president of the New York State Osteopathic Society, both endorsed Ingraham's appeal.

Though New York saw the situation as urgent, Washington did not. Earlier in June, Ingraham had written a letter to Dr. Charles Edwards, commissioner of the FDA, which said in part: "On the basis of our findings, we are officially notifying all physicians in New York State of the danger of estrogen administration during pregnancy. We also recommend most urgently that the Food and Drug Administration initiate immediate measures to ban the use of synthetic estrogens during pregnancy."

THE FOUNTAIN COMMITTEE

It was *two months* before Commissioner Edwards so much as acknowledged Ingraham's letter. In November, when Congressman L. H. Fountain held a congressional committee hearing on DES, he asked Edwards *why* he had dallied. Edwards said, "Well, I have no response to the delay . . . obviously when I received it, I sent it on to the Bureau of Drugs. I must, however, say that I do not agree with Dr. Ingraham's action. I think he was premature . . . not that his actions are necessarily wrong, but I think he could well have studied it a little bit more than he did."

Herbst had to wait even longer than Ingraham. The FDA did not get back to him until late October, some seven months after receiving galleys of the "missing link" report. During that seven months, many thousands of pregnant women continued to get DES.

In 1967, the National Academy of Sciences–National Research Council (NAS–NRC) had rated DES *possibly effective* and had sent the FDA the following report:

> The panel feels that estrogens are not harmful in conditions such as threatened abortion, but that their effectiveness can't be documented by literature or its own experience.

This statement gave the FDA a clear mandate, and obligation, in 1968 to prohibit DES in pregnancy cases *unless* the manufacturers came up with new evidence.

Under the circumstances, with the proof of the drug's effectiveness three and a half years overdue, it is astonishing that the FDA did not take action the moment that the Herbst galleys were received.

Let us examine the results of the FDA's inaction: During the 1940s and especially the early 1950s (after the Boston studies had been published, but before they were challenged in Chicago and New Orleans), DES was enormously popular as a pregnancy treatment. It has been estimated that estrogens were prescribed for nearly 6 million pregnant women between 1943 and 1959, resulting in the birth of at least 3 million children who had been exposed *in utero* to estrogens. On the basis of research that has been done on pharmacy records from 1960 to 1970, let's assume that some 30,000 unborn females were exposed to DES in 1971, an average of 2,500 a month. Had the FDA acted decisively upon receiving the Herbst galleys in March, instead of waiting until November, 20,000 young women who are now in danger of developing adenocarcinoma could have been spared.

Don Harper Mills, a physician and lawyer who serves as a medico-legal expert on the editorial board of the *Journal of the American Medical Association* (*JAMA*), advises all physicians who have ever used DES in pregnancy to search their records and send a notice to all such patients at their last known address. Few physicians are complying.

Incredibly, not only have a great many doctors failed to notify their patients, but some still prescribe DES for pregnant women.

Neither the drug companies, nor the government, nor any professional medical societies such as the AMA or ACOG have offered to finance the search for and treatment of DES daughters. Who will?

AFTER THE MORNING AFTER

Despite the 1971 bulletin to physicians warning against the use of DES in pregnancy, which Congressman Fountain had wrested out of FDA in November 1971, DES sales rose by 4 percent in the next nine months! Now that DES had proved carcinogenic in humans, doctors were prescribing it more than ever. The DES market had been salvaged in the nick of time by a new application, the morning-after pill.

THE MICHIGAN HEALTH SERVICE

In the late 1960s, the morning-after pill was being prescribed tentatively by some physicians. But by 1972, an official at the National Institutes of Health announced: "Most university health services are giving the morning-after pill."

How did this happen and why?

Some of the credit must go to the health service at the University of Michigan. On October 25, 1970, just two weeks before the FDA took action *against* DES as a pregnancy booster, *JAMA* published a report on 1,000 women in and around the university who had used it as a morning-after contraceptive. "No pregnancies resulted," according to the author, "and there were no serious adverse reactions"—an amazing statistic considering the fact that no contraceptive, *not even sterilization,* has ever been 100 percent effective in a population of 1,000 people. The report was like a green light to thousands of health service doctors.

THE COWAN STUDY

But something embarrassing happened. Local women in Ann Arbor, who were patients at the student health service, chanced upon the *JAMA* report. They didn't believe it. It didn't fit the facts. A few women who had been given the morning-after pill were pregnant, although they acknowledged it could have been from exposure earlier in the cycle. Other pregnant women treated at the health service had not had any earlier exposure, but were unable to finish the five-day course because the DES pills made them vomit. Then there was a third group: Women who had not had earlier exposure, were not too nauseated to swallow their medication, but were nonetheless . . . pregnant.

But how could the student health service know of these pregnancies when in fact it had *never followed up most of the DES patients?* The Ann Arbor DES patients were pioneers because, as disbelievers, they performed their own surveys. They continued to monitor the effects of DES, and repeatedly found facts that contradicted those in the *JAMA* report.

On February 27, 1975, Belita Cowan, a health instructor, testified at Senator Kennedy's hearings (the senator broke precedent for congressional health hearings by seeking opinions from patients and consumer advocates, as well as physicians and scientists):

"Last summer, I conducted a survey of over 200 women, ages 18 to 31, who had taken DES as a morning-after pill in Ann Arbor, Michigan, between 1968 and August of 1974. Twenty-nine percent of my sample stated that they had taken the morning-after pill at least twice within a year's time.

"The study showed that DES is being prescribed with carelessness and casualness. Forty-five percent were not given pelvic or breast exams. Fifty-six percent stated that the doctor did not take a personal and family medical history. Eight women said that they got the morning-after pill not for themselves but for a friend or roommate. Only 26 percent were followed up to see if they were pregnant.

"The study also revealed that DES is being given to women for whom estrogens are contraindicated. Women who cannot take birth control pills are being given the morning-after pill. They are not aware, nor are they informed, that the morning-after pill is estrogen.

"Fifty-seven percent of the sample were unaware that the morning-after pill did not have FDA approval and that it had not been proven safe and effective.

"Further, the study revealed that many women are not being told of the possible cancerous effects to the fetus if the woman is [already] pregnant. I could not find a single case where a pregnancy test was given prior to and after the DES regimen.

"Six percent of those in the survey stated that they themselves were DES daughters; that is, their mothers took stilbestrol when they were pregnant in the early 1950s. Of all the doctors I interviewed, only one expressed hesitation about giving the morning-after pill to DES daughters. Dr. Ann Pfrender of the University of Michigan Health Services stated that, 'We don't know the effects of the morning-after pill to DES daughters, so I don't give it to them.'

"The most interesting finding of the study is that 24 percent of the women stated that they did not take all 10 pills in the series. As one woman put it, 'I got so sick from the first pill that I never took the rest. I couldn't stand to be that ill!' And not surprisingly, 65 percent stated that if they had been fully informed about DES, they would not have taken it [the morning-after pill] in the first place."

SECOND THOUGHTS ABOUT THE MORNING-AFTER PILL

The drug companies themselves are patently uneasy about morning-after DES. As FDA commissioner Alexander Schmidt admitted in 1975: "DES is a generic drug and is made by many manufacturers, none of whom came forward with data to support the use of DES as a postcoital contraceptive."

They didn't come forward—they backed off!

In the *Physicians' Desk Reference*, 1977 edition, the Eli Lilly Pharmaceutical Company's thousand-word description of its diethylstilbestrol tablets starts out with the warning in oversized capital letters: "THIS DRUG PRODUCT SHOULD NOT BE USED AS A POSTCOITAL CONTRACEPTIVE."

At this writing, the University of Michigan is still using the DES pill, and so are thousands of other health services and private doctors. Doctors, the guardians of health, are prescribing a product for a purpose which its major manufacturer, a frankly profit-making concern, is publicly warning against.

PROMISE HER ANYTHING, BUT GIVE HER... CANCER

THE SELLING OF ERT

By 1947, a dazzling array of estrogen products, some combined with thyroid, were competing for a place on the American doctor's prescription pad. DES and other female sex hormones were available, from dozens of companies, by mouth, by vagina, and by long-acting and short-acting injection.

In ads in the medical journals, the early Premarin woman was shown waltzing with Arthur Murray's double, while the patient who liked her nightly "nip" could have Lynoral Elixir, "The Most Potent Oral Estrogen in a Pleasant-tasting Cordial" (and in a 14 percent alcohol base).

GUSBERG'S WARNING

In the midst of all these cheery advertisements—six full pages of the December 1947 issue of the *American Journal of Obstetrics and Gynecology*—an alarm was sounded by S. B. (Saul) Gusberg, who was then a young gynecologist and cancer researcher at the Sloane Hospital and Columbia University in New York.

"Another human experiment has been set up in recent years by the widespread administration of estrogens to postmenopausal women," Gusberg said. He went on to point out that the relatively low cost of oral estrogen and the ease of administration had made its general use "promiscuous." Uterine bleeding provoked in patients by this medication had become so commonplace that at Gusberg's hospital the expression "stilbestrol bleeding" was employed to describe those cases admitted for diagnostic curettage.

What did all these curettages (uterine scrapings) in ERT patients reveal? The pathology reports showed that ERT overstimulates the endometrium, or lining of the uterus, producing among other effects, "crowding of the glands into a lawless pattern."

Gusberg speculated that it was not the dosage of ERT, not the specific product, but *long-term exposure* that causes harm. (Research completed in 1975 showed Gusberg to be correct on two points out of three: Duration of use and high-dose levels are both significant in producing cancer, while product differences appear to be inconsequential.) Early as it was in the ERT game, by 1947 Gusberg had collected 29 cases of women whose endometria were profoundly disturbed by estrogen therapy—20 with a possibly premalignant condition called hyperplasia, which often necessitates hysterectomy, and 9 with cancer itself.

The scholarly gynecologists, those who had read the articles as well as the ads in their monthly journals, responded swiftly to Gusberg's work. They also collected cancer cases, and the promiscuous use of ERT slowed or at least stabilized . . . that is, until January 1966, when the M. Evans Co. published a book called Feminine Forever, by a handsome, avuncular Brooklyn physician named Robert Wilson.

WILSON VERSUS LIVING DECAY

Feminine Forever, which was excerpted in Look and Vogue and sold 100,000 copies in the first several months, promised that menopause could be averted and aging allayed with ERT.

Wilson was wholly dismissed as a quack by his more sober colleagues, but rarely in public and always off the record. Even good friends of estrogen, or at least the pill, were growling among themselves. Sherwood Kaufman of Planned Parenthood fumed at a medical meeting: "The situation has gotten ridiculous. Women come in asking for the 'Youth Pill,' and they say 'Check my estrogen levels.' From what they've read, they think it's as simple as driving into a gasoline station and having their oil checked."

Wilson, in the short space of an article in Look magazine, listed 26 symptoms that the Youth Pill would avert. These included nervousness, irritability, anxiety, apprehension, hot flashes, night sweats, joint pains, melancholia, palpitations, crying spells, weakness, dizziness, severe headache, poor concentration, loss of memory, chronic indigestion, insomnia, frequent urination, itching of the skin, dryness of the eye, nose and mouth, backache, neuroses, a tendency to take alcohol and sleeping pills, or even to contemplate suicide.

"While not all women are affected by menopause to this extreme degree," Wilson conceded, "no woman can be sure of escaping the horror of this living decay."

Reporters at The New Republic and the Washington Post called attention to the money Wilson received from drug companies. In a 1969 book, The Pill, An Alarming Report, Morton Mintz of the Post summarized:

"The Wilson Research Foundation, headed by Dr. Wilson . . . received, in 1964, $17,000 from the Searle Foundation . . . $8,700 from Ayerst Laboratories and $5,900 from the Upjohn Company."

By November 1966, the FDA was on to Wilson. They formally notified the Searle Company that he was unacceptable as an investigator for Enovid in menopause because he was disseminating promotional material claiming that the drug had been shown to be effective for conditions for which it had never been proved to work. And to this day, neither the FDA nor any other scientific body has ever approved Premarin or other hormone products as a preventive to aging.

When we interviewed Robert Wilson in 1976, he commented truthfully enough: "There are some people who don't like me. They say I shouldn't do what I'm doing. They say that menopause is a natural process. We should grow old gracefully and enjoy it."

Then he warmed to his topic: "They say we should do nothing to retard menopause. Just think of that. Isn't that dreadful? The estrogen regimen should start at age 9—*9 to 90*. It's necessary to begin then, and to check your estrogen level all through life, so that it never leaves you. Don't allow it to."

We asked Wilson to comment on endometrial cancer. "That's the worst lie in the world," he said, "the worst fallacy. I have over 40 doctors working all over the world, Switzerland, Czechoslovakia, all over the world, and we haven't seen one case of cancer."

THE SERVICE FOR MEDIA

Other pro-ERT books followed Wilson's, including *After Forty* by Sondra Gorney and Claire Cox, published in 1973.

On the jacket of *After Forty,* Sondra Gorney is identified as "Executive Director of the Information Center on the Mature Woman." What the cover fails to mention is that the Information Center, formerly located in New York City, and finally closed in 1976, was a "service for media" thoughtfully provided by the Ayerst Laboratories, manufacturers of Premarin.

The Pharmaceutical Manufacturers Association, to which Ayerst belongs, has a code of ethics which maintains that prescription drugs will not be directly promoted to the public. Ayerst, in violation of the code, hired the talented and energetic Ms. Gorney to provide free filler items, lauding ERT, to magazines, newspapers, and other mass media—rarely, if ever, with any indication that the source was a drug company.

A typical "background paper" from Ayerst Information Center states: "It was once believed that the change of life meant every woman had to resign herself to years of anguish and suffering. . . . When ovarian production stops, a woman's endocrine system is thrown into disarrangement. . . . Emotional problems can affect entire families. If not overcome, they can cause lasting harm to a woman's personality."

CLOUDS ON THE HORIZON

Ayerst's slogan "Keep Her on Premarin" succeeded.

Millions of normal woman were staying on Premarin for an average of a decade or longer. Most stopped only when they had to stop, because of side effects, such as the uterine bleeding so long ago noted by Gusberg.

Others, many others, were taken off Premarin because of changes in the breast tissue, or allergic reactions, or edema, or metabolic disturbances, or gallbladder disease. A standoff developed between the physicians who prescribed long-term ERT, most often gynecologists, and those who mopped up after it.

Even so, in all the years since Gusberg's brilliant early report, no well-controlled studies comparing cancer frequency in human ERT users and refusers has been completed. Thus, defenders of ERT argued that a cause-and-effect association had not been proven, and that the extent of risk, if any, remained unquantified. Cancer specialists knew it was just a matter of time.

THE BUBBLE BURSTS

The time came. In the fall of 1975 rumors were flying in the drug industry and among knowledgeable physicians and science reporters. *The New England Journal of Medicine,* it was whispered, was to publish a series of articles comparing ERT users and non-users, and showing that the risks of endometrial cancer in the former increased five- to fourteen-fold!

However it came to them, Ayerst knew the specific content of *The New England Journal* articles before publication.

This gave Ayerst time to tool up its propaganda machine. Ayerst sent a "Dear Doctor" letter concerning Premarin to physicians across the United States.

The letter was reassuring, making it appear that *The New England Journal* articles were "weak studies," and that the link between ERT and cancer was not really established. Meantime the physicians who advocated the Youth Pill found it hard to retreat:

"I think of the menopause as a deficiency disease, like diabetes," a San Francisco gynecologist told *The New York Times.* "Most women develop some symptoms whether they are aware of them or not, so I prescribe estrogens for virtually all menopausal women for an indefinite period."

"Everything in life is a trade-off—there are risks and benefits, and you must weigh one against the other," said another gynecologist.

However, these male physicians, unlike their patients, were not personally at risk. We wonder: Would they take a drug—and for symptoms they were "not aware of"—that greatly increased their chances of cancer of the penis?

ERT AND CANCER

The 1971 findings concerning cancer and DES came from Arthur Herbst and his colleagues at Massachusetts General Hospital. By contrast, the 1975 ERT studies were the work of *many* investigators, which all coalesced, or came together, in December. So many scientists dot the cast of characters that a summary of the contributions of each seems the clearest way to tell the story.

1. PENTTI SIITERI, UNIVERSITY OF CALIFORNIA MEDICAL SCHOOL IN SAN FRANCISCO, AND PAUL MACDONALD, UNIVERSITY OF TEXAS SOUTHWESTERN MEDICAL SCHOOL: Since cancer is more prevalent in older than younger women, it was formerly argued that high levels of natural estrogen might *protect* against it. Siiteri and MacDonald, with various associates, were first to demonstrate that postmenopausal women continue to manifest high levels of estrone (a type of estrogen) which is synthesized in body fats from precursors formed in the ovaries and adrenal glands. They later demonstrated that women with cancer produce twice as much natural estrone as healthy women.

Premarin, which stands for PREgnant MARes' urINe, is composed principally of estrone, the very estrogen that postmenopausal women who get cancer have too much of naturally. The work of Siiteri and MacDonald, which dates back to 1966, gives the lie to comforting theories, espoused by ERT promoters, that high levels of estrogen protect against cancer in older women. Siiteri and MacDonald provided the framework that helped all the 1975 studies to fall into place.

2. HARRY ZIEL AND WILLIAM FINKLE OF KAISER-PERMANENTE MEDICAL CENTER IN LOS ANGELES: In a study that cost only $1,900, Ziel and Finkle gathered the hospital records of 94 Kaiser-Permanente patients who had endometrial cancer. These were matched with 188 carefully selected control women—two for each cancer patient—who were much like the cancer victims in age, area of residence, and general health.

The records were evaluated by "blind" analysts who did not know which patients had developed cancer. Women who had used conjugated estrogens for seven years of longer, it was demonstrated, developed endometrial cancer at a rate *14 times as high* as comparable women who had never used it at all. Women who had used such products for one to five years developed this cancer at a rate that was about *five and one-half times as high as non-users.*

The overall risk, including longer and shorter term ERT patients, was computed to be almost eight times as great as normal.

ERT, according to Ziel and Finkle's research, may be more dangerous than heavy smoking. If you smoke for 20 years of longer, your risk of lung cancer increases 17- or 18-fold. Your risk of endometrial cancer increases 14-fold *after only seven years of ERT use.*

Other key researchers whose work helped clarify the estrogen/endometrial cancer risks included:

3. DONALD SMITH AND ASSOCIATES AT THE MASON CLINIC, UNIVERSITY OF WASHINGTON, SEATTLE: Smith and his associates compared 317 endometrial cancer patients with an equal number of women who had other female cancers, concluding that ERT increases the odds of endometrial cancer most in healthy women who lack other risk factors. Thus it may be more dangerous to a slim woman than a heavier one, who has a greater risk to start with.

4. THOMAS MACK AND ASSOCIATES AT THE UNIVERSITY OF SOUTHERN CALIFORNIA: Thomas Mack and his colleagues studied the residents of a southern California retirement community. Here again the odds of developing endometrial cancer increased eightfold among ERT users, the same average figure arrived at by Ziel and Finkle. And, like the Smith group in Seattle, the Mack group also noted that the dangers of estrogen therapy appear most striking in healthy women with no other risk factors.

While Ziel and Finkle brought in evidence concerning *length* of ERT use, the Mack group was interested in *dosage*. They report that higher doses of estrogen also enhance the risk. Thus, dose and duration of ERT are implicated in different studies.

We know now that the length of ERT use increases the risk of cancer, and that size of dosage adds to this effect.

5. DONALD AUSTIN, CHIEF OF THE CALIFORNIA TUMOR REGISTRY: Austin informed the FDA on December 16, 1975, that among white women 50 and over living in California, there was an 80 percent increase in uterine cancer during the years 1969–1974. The increase was noted in 75 hospitals, and was most pronounced in areas of greatest affluence where ERT use is high. In Alameda County, Austin reported, the annual incidence of endometrial cancer has *tripled*.

This unfortunate trend is now confirmed in other states that keep good registries, including Washington and Connecticut. Since 1969, endometrial cancer has steadily and rapidly increased.

FDA spokesman Crout has commented: "The chronic users tend to be middle- and upper-income women, the kind of people who go to doctors and the kind of people who would most value the longed-for youthful appearance. It's an interesting example of the poor being spared, if you will, some of the adverse effects of estrogens that are now coming to the fore."

6. BRUCE STADEL OF THE NATIONAL INSTITUTES OF HEALTH, BETHESDA, AND NOEL WEISS OF THE SCHOOL OF PUBLIC HEALTH AND COMMUNITY MEDICINE, UNIVERSITY OF WASHINGTON, SEATTLE: In an elaborate study of Seattle area residents, Bruce Stadel and Noel Weiss estimated that 51 percent of all women over 50 had, by 1973 to 1974, used ERT for over three months' duration. Most amazingly, of those who first responded that they had *not* used it, more than a quarter were found to be ERT patients after all. This was established during personal interviews at which estrogens were identified by a pill display, and by further discussion with the women's doctors.

The women on ERT were more apt to have suffered troublesome hot flashes before taking it—about two out of five reported this complaint—while the frequency in nonusers was less than one in seven. Clearly then, the flashes drove some women to ERT, but not the majority who took it. Weiss and Stadel conclude that "the frequency of menopausal estrogen use . . . is much higher than the estimated frequency of severe menopausal symptoms. . . . It appears that physicians in King and Pierce counties do not follow a conservative approach to hormonal treatment of menopausal problems."

THE STORY OF E

The earliest report on vitamin E therapy for menopause symptoms authored by Dr. Evan Shute, appeared in the *Journal of the Canadian Medical*

Association in 1937. Shute and his brother Wilfred continued their studies and published their work in many influential journals, including *The Lancet* and the *American Journal of Obstetrics and Gynecology*. Their research was confirmed by other less controversial investigators.

But in the 1940s vitamin E was far more costly than most estrogen products. And estrogens do curb flashes in women who fail to respond to E, or even to the more potent E, B-complex, bioflavonoids, evening primrose oil, and herbs.

We fear that another reason E was ignored by most doctors may lie partially in the way prescription and nonprescription remedies are regarded. Many women probably thought estrogen "better" than E because the hormone was available by prescription only. They may have been disappointed in doctors who told them to go out and buy a vitamin or eat wheat germ. In the wake of the Youth Pill craze, physicians forgot the research on vitamin E. Younger doctors may never have been introduced to it.

On the doctor's side, prescription drugs are sometimes more appealing because they give him or her *control*. Furthermore, vitamins, and especially E, fall under the same mantle of suspicion as some herbal remedies because they are claimed to have such a wide range of benefits. In his book, *The Heart and Vitamin E*, Evan Shute remarks: "No substance known to medicine has such a variety of healing properties." This, he concedes, is a major drawback to acceptance.

Finally, we must again refer to the second- or third-class citizenship status of the older woman. Her complaints do not attract the attention of many qualified researchers or the interest of many journalists. Thus, E's proven effectiveness in curbing hot flashes had been obscured by other dramatic claims for the vitamin, such as its possible benefits to the heart.

Vitamin E as a relief for menopause symptoms resurfaced almost by accident. In August 1974, *Prevention* magazine included a questionnaire on this controversial vitamin. Later, reporting the results, biochemist Richard Passwater, author of *Super-Nutrition*, explained:

"Actually, there was no mention of menopause on the questionnaire. *Yet 2,000 women volunteered that they found vitamin E to largely or totally relieve the problems of menopause.* The most frequent comments written in were (1) more energy and a better sense of well-being, (2) relief of leg cramps, and (3) relief of hot flashes and other problems of menopause."

Passwater searched the medical literature and found a number of studies that confirmed what *Prevention* readers said. One, written in 1945 in the *American Journal of Obstetrics and Gynecology,* reported that 25 women, all with severe menopause symptoms, responded to the vitamin E treatment and showed either complete relief or very marked improvement. No untoward aftereffects were noted.

In 1949 another investigator, Dr. Rita Finkler, described vitamin E treatment of 66 menopausal patients in the *Journal of Clinical Endocrinology.*

Good-to-excellent relief was obtained in 31 cases, fair in 16, and the remaining 19 women evidenced no improvement. The dosages used by Dr. Finkler were relatively low—about 20 to 100 units daily, the average being 30. In 17 cases, when the real vitamin E as replaced with dummy pills, symptoms soon recurred.

A PILL FOR MEN

The human male is a prodigious maker of sperm. In a single ejaculation he releases, to whatever destiny, some 80 million of these tiny life-bearing sex cells. Sperm are manufactured from precursor cells, in a process that takes about 70 days. Spermatogenesis is stimulated by two hormones, FSH and LH, which issue from the pituitary.

Once the female was also a prodigious bearer of eggs. She, or rather her fish and amphibian foremothers, deposited a milky "egg clutch" into sea water and tidal marshes. The male dropped off his sperm in the same neighborhood, and they merged.

Out of the primordial slime, the mammal, the primate, and humankind evolved. Evolution *depended on dramatic advances in female reproduction.* She reduced her cyclical egg release from an enormous quotient to a selected few or one. *She* retained the conceptus—the product of conception—within her own body, developed a placenta, and nourished her babies from her own blood and bones. The advances that make us humans rest, as modern embryology explains it, on adaptations that the female of the evolving species made.

Male reproduction—and this is not to minimize its importance—is still much like reproduction in the amphibian and fish. Sperm production is extravagant, not conservative, and the male role is biologically ended when sperm go on their way. The reproductive role of woman is longer, harder, and much more dangerous to her.

Revolution—often it is sounded to drama, drums, and discussion, but sometimes it just settles over us like mist. While some fortunate women always had access to vaginal spermicides (Cleopatra, for example, used a mixture of honey and dried crocodile dung) it was *male contraceptive methods,* first withdrawal, and later the condom, that drastically reduced the birth rate in modern times.

Carefully used, these are far more effective than modern people imagine, but each has obvious drawbacks. Although it requires skill and discipline, withdrawal was the sole method of contraception used by two-thirds of the couples in France and Hungary *until 1960!* The birth rate in these countries was admirably low. It shouldn't be overlooked as a method for emergencies.

Margaret Sanger, among other feminists, believed it was essential for birth control to be in women's hands, but, of the new devices, many have proved injurious to health. Senator Gaylord Nelson's hearings on the pill were forced to recess on January 23, 1970, after a raucous demonstration by Alice Wolfson and a group of young, articulate Washington, D.C., health feminists.

"Why are there no patients testifying?" the Wolfson women demanded. "Why is the press whitewashing all the adverse comments against the pill? *Why is there no pill for men?*"

EARLY WORK ON A MALE PILL

The fear that a pill for men might alter male libido or the sex organs has been a major deterrent to research. *Hormones can have this effect on some users of either sex.* Masters and Johnson have stated that when a woman who was previously orgasmic loses her ability, the first question they must ask is, "Has she been taking the pill?"

Scientists view diminished *male* sex drive more ominously than the female equivalent. After all, they argue, libido is needed to *put sperm into action* but *not* to position the ova in place. Species continuation rests on the libidinous male. One government population official recently put it like this:

"Many women don't have those orgasms you read about, anyway. A lot of that Masters and Johnson and women's lib stuff is about the extremes, almost the abnormal. I never heard any hesitation based on whether the pill would affect whether a woman would have an orgasm."

Among the early human subjects to be tested for male fertility control were 8 psychotic mental patients in a Massachusetts state hospital. They received an early form of Enovid in the 1950s. Ten milligrams a day of Enovid had a definite sterilizing effect. However, one young man was found—at the end of the five and one-half months' trial—to have shrunken testicles; his scrotum had become "soft and babyish," according to his doctor's report.

The sex drive of these patients—they can hardly be called volunteers—was not, in general, altered by Enovid. Their psychiatrists kept an eye on them, and they masturbated as much or as little as before.

Therefore, although Enovid was early shown to work for men, the fellow with the shrunken testicles put a damper on follow-up experiments. His side effect was viewed more seriously, we are sorry to report, than the unexplained *deaths* of three Puerto Rican women, during some of the early experiments with the pill.

Sex hormones, whether taken by implant, injection, or mouth, turn off sperm production, just as they do ova production, because they "fool" the pituitary into diminishing its natural output of the pituitary hormones FSH and LH. Within about two months' time (70 days), sperm will be gone from the semen. Any sex steroid may have this effect, but the pills used for women are too feminizing to be suitable for men. (In fact, it's a little startling to realize that experiments on human males, proving beyond any doubt that *various hormones produce infertility,* date all the way back to 1939.)

Why not use more malish hormones, the androgens? (Both sexes produce male *and* female hormones, actually, but in different proportions.) Testosterone-only contraceptives for men do not cause feminization but may pose other problems, such as heart attacks and an increase of red cells in the blood. (Pills for women also cause heart attacks and blood disturbances, but men fear the former more acutely since they are *normally* at greater risk.)

A logical solution is to find a combination of male and female hormones so balanced that they avoid feminization on the one hand, or immediate over-stimulation of the heart, blood cells, and prostate on the other. Such products are being clinically tested by, among others, Dr. C. Alvin Paulsen of the University of Washington, and Dr. Julian Frick from Innsbruck, Austria. Paulsen and Frick are investigating different combinations of drugs, which, inconveniently, involve taking *both* oral pills and monthly injections.

Any contraceptive that works through pituitary suppression is bound to have some long-range effects on the total system. The pituitary mediates *many* body functions, and it is always chancy to tamper with it. Thus, at best, male contraceptives *based on hormones* are unlikely to be safer than the current female pills. They "pool" the risks, but do not eliminate them, and should provide a fine sincerity test for men who claim they would die for love.

A MALE PILL THAT'S ALREADY HERE

The Paulsen and Frick formulations will not reach the market for years—certainly not, it is estimated, until the 1980s. But there are already products on the shelves of every drugstore that promise to be just as suitable.

These are the previously mentioned androgen and estrogen combinations, currently marketed as a treatment for osteoporosis, or bone loss, in aging individuals of both sexes and for the syndrome some people call male menopause. Their effectiveness as a bone treatment is disputed, but *hundreds of thousands of men have taken them, usually for long periods.* Some of the preparations include vitamins and mood brighteners, in addition to their dual sex hormones. *One also contains speed,* and is understandably hard to give up. More than a dozen brands are available, including Ayerst's Mediatric and Formatrix, Leferle's Gevrine, Reid-Provident's Estratest, Schering's Gynetone, Upjohn's Halodrin, and many more.

Far from being feminizing, such products usually contain substantially more androgen than estrogen (up to 500 times as much!) and so—while they are promoted as suitable for men or women—their manufacturers usually issue warnings such as the following:

"Watch female patients closely for signs of virilization. Some effects, such as voice changes, may not be reversible even when the drug is stopped."

Recently, Drs. Michael and Maxine Briggs of the Alfred Hospital, Melbourne, Australia, discovered that elderly men who use these products develop evidence of severely reduced sperm production without any such side effects as developing breasts, shrunken testicles, or grossly abnormal libido changes. They called for younger volunteers and selected five, who were instructed to take the osteoporosis pills twice daily with their meals.

At the end of the projected 70 days, or sooner, four of the five had stopped manufacturing sperm. The fifth patient took twice as long, but finally he stopped also.

The Briggs volunteers stayed on the hormones for 34 weeks, during 16 of which their wives gave up birth control. No pregnancies resulted. Sperm production returned to normal in all cases within 5 weeks after stopping the drug.

Three of the five men had occasional mild nausea, but there were no anatomical effects. Two complained of decreased libido in the first 8 weeks, which then returned to normal for the remainder of the trial. Another man had an increased sex drive, which leveled off when he stopped the medication. A fourth reported no changes while he took the hormones, but a decrease in sex drive when he stopped. This outcome might puzzle readers who are unacquainted with the aftereffects of the female pill. Any powerful drug suppresses some of our natural functions, which may in turn have some trouble reasserting themselves. As many of us have learned the hard way, we may all be too susceptible to a new infection right after taking an antibiotic.

What are the ethics of giving *an approved drug,* like these osteoporosis or male menopause remedies, *for an unapproved use,* such as contraception? Such questions are hotly debate among doctors, many of whom *do* prescribe hormones for purposes never dreamed of by the FDA or their own manufacturers. Two recent examples are the use of DES and Premarin as a morning-after female contraceptive, and a group of anabolic or "body-building" hormones, frequently prescribed to put flesh on athletes. Anabolic hormones could, in addition to building muscle, cause cancer of the prostate, breast cancer, and blood clots in athletes. They are rumored to have done just that to members of a professional football team.

Should any untoward effects occur, the doctor is in a weak legal position. However, he may get around it by asking the patient to sign a release.

This much can be said for the "new" male pill from Australia, limited as its contraceptive testing has been: A lot more is known about its side effects on men than was known about Enovid when *it* went on the market for women.

HIS SAFETY OF HERS?

In return for the wonders it may perform, any hormone is bound to have side effects. To pass off such potent pharmaceuticals as "natural" is nothing but fraud. The honorable way to prescribe drugs is to admit the risks, and let the patient decide whether he or she wants to take them. The Rx pad belongs to the doctor—but the body is the patient's alone. To prescribe a drug without informed consent is a violation of the Bill of Rights, we think—a kind of chemical assault.

The female pill was approved after little testing. The side effects of the pill are quite well known now, but 50 million women worldwide are willing to take it. The pill is still the preferred method of one in five fertile women in the

United States. Its male "twin," however chancy, will find a market a well, for, contrary to predictions of drug manufacturers and some researchers, men are not unwilling to share the risks. When Dr. Paulsen of Seattle ran a small ad in a college newspaper asking for volunteers, he was overrun with responses. He and others who supervise male programs get letters today by the handful.

Why has the research only just started? Why was male contraception ignored for 20 years (the 1950s and 1960s) while fortunes were being poured into finding new female products? Only in 1974 did funds for male studies start making any dent in the federal health budget. Nonprofit research groups, like the Population Council, are also supporting male projects, but not as generously as they might. Some $20 million is now being spent annually, *The Wall Street Journal* estimates, which is but one-fifth the amount needed to develop a contraceptive rapidly.

Unfortunately, drug companies have sharply reduced their efforts to deveop new contraceptives. Many projects have been abandoned. Executives say they are disenchanted with stringent federal test requirements (making it take longer than formerly to get a new drug on the market) and with costly lawsuits over the pill and the IUD.

A spur to research has been the arrival of a new medical specialty called andrology, concerned with male fertility. Another spur was the feminist charge of discrimination—denied, at first, by scientists who then rallied rather quickly to correct their course. The effort to find a male pill is hardly of crash proportions, but it exists. It is taken seriously. It may bear fruit.

Must a male pill rely on hormones? We hope not. There may be better ways of interrupting male fertility, *without involving the pituitary and higher brain centers*. Theoretically, a *safer* pill for men than for women might be devisable, but no one knows yet for sure. Discussion centers on the greater complexity of the female system. Sheldon Segal estimates that *there are 14 stages at which a woman's fertility might be interrupted, but only 7 in men*.

These male-female differences are looked at two ways. It can be argued, and is in some quarters, that woman's greater complexity affords more chances for interruption. It can be, and is, conversely argued that man's greater simplicity yields more opportunity to intervene *locally*, without widespread bodily effects. In women, reproduction is intertwined with many other functions, more so than in men.

Another debate centers on the natural history of ova and sperm. Unlike woman, whose lifetime supply of eggs is intact at birth, man produces new sperm as he goes along for most or all of his adult time span. It is feared that an imperfect fertility drug might allow a few damaged sperm to escape, producing defective fetuses. An opposing view is that permanent damage or latent drug effects on the sperm cells are less to be feared in the male. When he stops the pill he is set to manufacture brand-new sperm, whereas a woman's future-ripening ova might be residually influenced by a drug she once took.

OTHER SPERM INHIBITORS

The hypothalamus, a walnut-sized collection of brain cells, might be called the conductor of our endocrine symphony. In breakthrough research, Andrew Schally of New Orleans has recently isolated the hypothalamic chemicals that trigger the release of LH and FSH from the pituitary. Scientists in many laboratories are seeking hypothalamic suppressants based on his discoveries.

We mention Schally's work for its profound importance, as it much advances our knowledge of reproduction in both female and male. But we think it unlikely that a safe contraceptive will emerge from it. These hormones would affect both the hypothalamus and pituitary, and it is inadvisable to mess with them just for birth control. Local action in the genitals would be safer.

In England, Belgium, and Australia, scientists are working on a protein substance that might be able to block pituitary FSH secretion without altering LH. If the dream materializes, the protein may halt sperm production without at the same time inhibiting natural testosterone, or requiring supplements of the same.

Many drugs inhibit sperm formation in the testes or, if you prefer, testicles (the words are synonymous) without interfering with natural hormones. Thus far, all have exhibited unacceptable side effects, but the search goes on. One group, the nitrofurans, has had wide use as inhibitors of bacterial growth, but dosages high enough to sterilize are extremely toxic. Other sperm suppressants are found among cancer drugs (at least in mice) in a sugar analogue.

In 1960 a drug to treat intestinal amoebae was tested on prisoners and completely suppressed their sperm. When tried on men enjoying more normal circumstances, it was noted that the drug had the effect of Antabuse, causing dizziness and vomiting when alcohol was consumed. It might still have been marketed for teetotalers, except that during the two-month recovery period, abnormal and bizarre sperm and heart irregularities were reported.

Drugless intervention, such as heat, x-ray, diathermy, and laser beams, may also inhibit sperm and are being investigated.

Heat experiments were initiated, years ago, by Dr. I. Tokuyama of Japan, whose volunteer medical students submerged their scrota in hot water baths for half hour daily. Elevation of scrotal temperature by just a few degrees proved highly effective in sterilizing some men.

Next, Dr. John Rock, co-developer of the pill, got 75 of his students to either sit in hot water or wear insulated scrotal supporters—Rock's Hot Jock, they were nicknamed around Harvard. Now in retirement, Rock insists that the method *works*, but of course he was also the scientist who declared the pill to be safe.

In any case, Rock says that of his 75 volunteers only one complained of a side effect—sweating—and one other failed to show the usual reduction in sperm count. Subsequently, the wives of a number of these students conceived and bore normal children.

There is little question today that heat, including fever, reduces fertility some of the time. Hippocrates was aware of this, and today the first thing specialists tell their *infertile* patients is to stop wearing tight jockey shorts and trousers which, by generating heat in the scrotum, inadvertently sterilize some stylish men.

The great promoter of TMS (shorthand for "the thermatic method of temporary male sterilization") was Martha Voegeli, an indomitable Swiss physician using TMS in India since 1912.

Here is how she described her method: For three weeks, a man takes a daily 45-minute bath in water of 116°F. He then remains sterile for six months, after which normal fertility returns. If desired, the treatment can be repeated. (We suggest that men who try this get a sperm count done afterward to make sure it worked.)

At the University of Missouri, Dr. Mostafa Fahim, chief of Reproductive Biology, has been studying ultrasound for many years and has already designed a chair apparatus to administer ultrasound birth control in doctors' offices. He dreams that an ultrasound machine could become a standard home bathroom fixture. His trials on humans are mired down by requirements that, for the time being, he try ultrasound only on men with prostatic cancer, who (should the ultrasound prove dangerous) are already in line to have their testicles removed. At last report he'd located only one such patient—and he must find 10 before he can proceed with healthy humans. Fahim complained: "We inject hundreds of chemicals into the woman's uterus but we never touch the testes." Some of the most militant feminist supporters are men who are trying to do contraceptive research—on their own sex.

WHAT DES TAUGHT US ABOUT MALE FERTILITY

After leaving the testes, sperm move on to the epididymis, a compact 2-inch oblong tissue lying within the scrotum, against each testicle, and containing 6 or more yards of tubing. Here in the epididymis, where sperm remain for about two weeks, maturation and storage take place. The epididymis is highly sensitive to drugs, and in theory could be "selectively" treated without ill effects on other system. When epididymal function is altered, sperm may be produced in normal numbers, but won't be competent to fertilize eggs.

At Cornell University, Dr. C. Michael Bedford, a veterinarian-physiologist, is doing important research into these crucial but long-neglected components of male reproduction. We are still a long way from a safe epididymal suppressant, but if and when it arrives, it might be the ideal method we have all awaited.

Recently, the epididymis has been in the news for a most unfortunate reason. Sons of mothers who were given the hormone DES to strengthen their pregnancies have a 10 to 25 percent incidence of cysts of the epididymis, which impair fertility. The same effect has been observed in laboratory animals.

Most of these DES sons are perfectly normal in other respects, which reaffirms scientific belief that the epididymis is an especially susceptible target organ.

SPERM SWITCHES, SPERM BANKS

Sperm is found in the testes, matured in the epididymis, and transported in the vas deferens, the spaghetti-like site where male sterilization—vasectomy—is performed. *Reversible* vasectomies, or "sperm switches," involving clamps, plugs, and faucets, have been so discussed and prematurely publicized that many men ask for them, thinking they are available.

They are not. While research continues at ten universities and private laboratories, many observers are doubtful of success—ever. A narrow living channel like the vas is all too apt to scar over any temporary blockage, making the blockage permanent. No man should agree to be a test subject for one of these devices unless he is prepared to accept final sterility.

If "sperm switching" does not seem imminent, "sperm banking"—that is, preserving live sperm by freezing—prior to vasectomy may have a better chance. Animal sperm banks, especially for cattle, have been highly successful, but, in humans, the resurrection of frozen sperm still remains iffy. It is no more than 70 percent successful, tops. No one yet knows why some sperm can take freezing and others not.

Seminal fluid has an amazing composition, which includes trace materials such as iron, zinc, and magnesium, and carbohydrates that appear to be an important source of energy for sperm. An alcohol which may be oxidized into fructose, a sugar, is also present in the human variety.

Certain oral medication such as sulfonamides may be traced in seminal fluid. Thus it is possible that the right oral drug might so influence the fluid as to keep the sperm from "capacitating." Sperm are not fully competent (capacitated) until they traverse the cervical mucus and womb, on their way up the fallopian tubes to the ultimate egg. The apparent purpose of seminal fluid, the ejaculate, is to carry the sperm from male to female. Still, its chemical complexity, including so much nourishment, suggests that it also plays a part in the sperm's final development. Products that inhibit capacitation on the sperm's last journey might either be added to the seminal fluid, or given to the woman.

When a woman is fertile, the progress of sperm through her vagina, cervix, and womb has been likened to spinning along on a turnpike; other times in her cycle, the sperm's journey is more like slogging through a swamp. Altering of the chemical environment provided by *her vagina* as well as by *his seminal fluid* both offer possibilities for relatively safe birth control. Foundations and government bodies say that they want to develop new contraceptives for men. Until the 1970s they merely chortled at the notion, so it appears that genuine progress is afoot.

But, as Dr. Philip Corfman of the National Institutes of Health explains, a lot of research that *sounds* malish could just result in more new products for women to use. Sperm capacitation is an excellent example; contraceptives ensuing from these studies could well be vaginal suppositories or further female pills.

In the meantime, men who truly want to "participate" could experiment with TMS, according to Martha Voegeli's instructions. They could ask their doctors for one of the male menopause treatments, employed by Michael and Maxine Briggs; or they could buy quality condoms, thin ones, in Japan. They could go to France or Hungary for tutoring in withdrawal, and, of course, they can get a vasectomy, too.

Do Gynecologists Exploit Their Patients?

BARBARA SEAMAN

Excerpt from *Free and Female* by Barbara Seaman, "Do Gynecologists Exploit Their Patients?" as it appeared in *New York*, August 14, 1972, with changes. Reprinted by permission.

Just a few months ago, a friend of mine fled from a gynecologist's office in Brooklyn for excellent reason. In the waiting room, she fell into conversation with three sisters, all married, all in their forties. "We've just had our hysterectomies," boasted one. "It took some finagling, but the doctor got us all into the hospital at the same time, so we could keep each other company. He may be expensive, but for such a big doctor he's so understanding."

These sisters, like the majority of American women, were as worshipful of their gynecologist as Laraine Day was of Lew Ayres in the old *Dr. Kildare* movies. But that trust is often misplaced. Since women are told so little about the functions and malfunctions of their bodies, most have almost no way of judging whether their gynecologists are helping or hurting them.

Long ago, Plato made a sharp distinction between physicians treating slaves and free citizens. He urged that in treating a savle, a doctor should prescribe authoritatively, as if he were absolutely sure of himself and his potions. In treating a free citizen, the physician was expected to "enter into discourse with the patient" and was not entitled to proceed with any medications or surgery until the patient was "convinced." Unfortunately, many gynecologists today treat their patients more like slaves than like free human beings. The attitude too often is "don't worry your pretty little head—the doctor will take care of everything."

A gynecologist should be willing to listen to his patients and he should not pretend that he always has easy answers to their questions. The doctor and patients are partners in the patients' health. The doctor who acts like a master has psychiatric problems, in my opinion. He should realize that women are neither savles nor Barbie dolls and practice his medicine accordingly.

Many gynecologists are trying to carve out bizarre new areas of authority. One such area is family size. A prominent New York Hospital gynecologist, for example, told a married women in her late twenties that he would not refer her for an abortion because it was time she started a family. In contrast, a Mt. Sinai gynecologist boasted to me that he always tries to talk mothers of two or more into having abortions.

Once a decision is made to have a child, too many doctors want to tell their patients *how* to give birth. I would be equally wary of the gynecologist who practices natural childbirth exclusively and the gynecologist whose only philosophy is hit-'em-on-the-head-the-instant-labor-starts-and-don't-wake-'em-until-the-hairdresser-shows. Some labors will follow a course where natural childbirth is desirable and feasible—if that is what the mother wants. Others will follow a course where safe natural childbirth is not possible.

Some gynecologists even go so far as to decide *when* a woman will give birth, without consulting either the mother or nature. One study in Rochester, New York, revealed that a major cause of childbirth difficulty is the artificial stimulation of birth when there is no justification for it, except the gynecologist's own weekend schedule. Artificial means of labor induction such as oxytocin, the birth-stimulating hormone, have been established as something which should never be used frivolously. The Rochester study also indicated that impatient doctors sometimes use instruments when they should not, delivering children prematurely. Almost as a matter of course, some impatient doctors perform completely unnecessary cesarean deliveries. Most women who have cesarean sections are inclined to believe that their lives were saved by the procedure. However, when Dr. Alan Guttmacher, now director of Planned Parenthood, was asked to review the records of 13 typical cesarean sections performed on New York City women, he concluded that in 7 of the cases there was "serious question" about the necessity for surgery.

Needless authoritarianism is certainly a charge that can be aimed at many physicians in many different specialties, but it seems particularly pervasive in gynecology.

The "American" position for giving birth in many ways symbolizes the doctor's relation to his patient: the women is strapped on her back while the doctor towers above her. She is at her most helpless, he at his most "superior." There may be nothing intentionally condescending in this procedure, but at the same time it is suggestive of attitudes, and it may even be questionable medicine.

There are five basic positions women assume during delivery in various cultures: lying down, standing, sitting, squatting, and kneeling. The lying-down position is among the least popular in primitive societies. There are various natural advantages to some of the other positions, particularly squatting.

At the April 1970 meeting of the Society of Gynecologic Investigation, Gordon G. Power and Lawrence D. Longo reported the following: childbirth on one's back was introduced as a civilized innovation in sixteenth-century France, apparently for the convenience of obstetricians. This position has the tendency to raise the mother's blood pressure in the critical area of the placenta. As she lies on her back, the weight of the womb presses on the inferior vena cava, which is the venous trunk for legs and torso. As blood backs up, it can cut off umbilical circulation by creating distention in the placenta. This is called the sluice flow mechanism. In many cases the baby's heart rate slows down (a sign of fetal distress) when the mother is on her back. The treatment is simple, Drs. Power and Longo state: turn the mother on her side or let her use a birth stool.

Whatever the pros and cons of giving birth while strapped on one's back, it is indeed the rare doctor who suggests to a women that there is any other way. And other matters from birth control to nursing are often handled in the same single-minded way. What doctors should understand is that women use birth control more effectively if they understand how it works and if they have been allowed to select a method that pleases them, just as they have healthier and happier pregnancies and deliveries when they are allowed to be full decision-making participants.

Many gynecologists, for example, more or less force unnatural childbirth on their patients. Women should know, however, about such findings as those of Dr. Deborah Tanzer, who studied the pregnancy and birth experiences of 41 woman, 22 of whom had their babies by natural childbirth methods. The natural childbirth mothers had been taught what to expect when they started labor, and so they approached it more confidently. They experienced less pain and less fear. Their attitudes toward their husbands (who remained with them during labor) were more positive. Yet most doctors remain prisoners of the past, or of the way they have been taught, clamping women under sedation.

On the other hand, one hears occasional reports of physicians who are so devoted to the precepts of natural childbirth that they may fail to intervene as promptly as they should when circumstances warrant. A small, slim-hipped Manhattan woman was in heavy labor for 16 hours with her 11-pound, 5-ounce son, her first baby, before her doctor decided to perform a cesarean section. She is understandably bitter that her famous physician allowed her to suffer so long. It would be nice, of course, if more gynecologists were devoted to their patients, not their theories.

Another problem is the shy gynecologist. These kindly, paternalistic practitioners often wish to spare their young patients (and themselves) embarrassment. They are so delicate that they may fail to render the service they have contracted for.

A girl whom I shall call Joan had such a gynecologist. After college, she spent the summer in her hometown in Ohio. In September, she would be starting a new job in New York, and she decided to arrive prepared with a diaphragm. She visited her mother's gynecologist, the same doctor who had delivered her 21 years before.

"He seemed a little embarrassed," Joan recalls, "although he was very nice.

He didn't send me a bill. The trouble was, his instructions weren't too clear, and when I tried to practice using the diaphragm I never could be sure that I was finding the cervix. When I got to New York I went to the Margaret Sanger Research Bureau, where you practice putting it in, and then you have to come back and they give you a test. Not only was I using the diaphragm incorrectly, but the one that my mother's doctor had given me was two sizes too small! I guess he thought I was still a little girl."

Other doctors, who prescribed intrauterine devices for their patients, did not prepare them for cramps, occasionally severe, which may occur after insertion. "If I'd had any idea," recalls a Los Angeles woman, "I would have asked my husband to come with me, or my sister. But all the doctor said was, 'Don't worry, it only takes a few minutes, and then you won't even know you have it.' Driving home, I felt the cramps coming, as bad as labor pains, and I almost crashed the car."

Perhaps the most common and dangerous contraceptive negligence is the casualness with which many doctors hand out birth control pills. Despite the fact that there are hundreds of lawsuits pending against drug companies and doctors for deaths and permanent damage connected with the pill, and despite the fact that plaintiffs have won settlements of a half million dollars or more, some doctors continue to prescribe the pill as if it were sugar candy, without taking a careful patient and family history and without warning the patient of the serious danger signals to watch for.

A tragedy that could have been avoided occurred when Ann St. C., wife of a professor at an upstate university, mother of three and user of the pill, called her gynecologist and asked, "Is the pill safe? Should I be taking it?"

Dr. K. snapped, "Of course it's all right for you to be taking the pill. If it weren't, I'd never have prescribed it."

Ann never had a chance to clarify the reason she was calling. In the preceding two weeks she had experienced several attacks of dizziness and double vision. She had also suffered from stiffness in the neck. Ann had a stroke exactly eight days later. She spent two months in the hospital and then slowly recovered her speech and most of her physical functioning, except for weakness in the right arm and leg.

Most laymen are inclined to assume that medically, at least, if not psychologically, pregnant women in America receive the best care available anyplace. Sadly, this is very far from true. Our mortality figures, for mothers and babies alike, are substantially higher than in most fully industrialized countries. Sweden, Great Britain, Japan, Czechoslovakia, and Taiwan are among the dozen or more countries which outrank us, according to U.N. figures. In Sweden and the Netherlands, to name only two countries, infant morality rates are some 50 percent lower than they are here.

When questioned about our poor showing, a recent president of the AMA commented that if it weren't for our Black women (who, the theory goes, do not even know enough to seek adequate prenatal care), our comparative world standing would be very good indeed. However, in their October 1970 report on "Higher Education and the Nation's Health," investigators for the Carnegie Commission noted that our mortality rates for white mothers and babies are also very poor: "The rate of 19.7 infant deaths per 1,000 live births for white people in the United States in 1967 was above the overall rate for 10 other countries in that year."

It is generally (although quietly) assumed that about half the maternal deaths in this country are "preventable." We also lose some 20,000 babies each year and, among the survivors, an appallingly high number have cerebral palsy, mental retardation, and other nervous system impairments which can often be traced back to methods used at delivery.

While obstetricians and gynecologists may interfere with normal pregnancies more than they should, they are also failing to look to emergencies as sharply as they might. A study by Dr. D. C. Fraser of maternal deaths in the District of Columbia linked several mortalities to the "questionable use of oxytocic drugs" to bring on labor. Anesthesia was responsible for a number of deaths. Still others were the result of "delay in diagnosis and surgery."

But methods used at delivery are not the whole ugly story, for an astonishing new battle has arisen recently between gynecologists and nutrition experts. As any reader knows who has had a baby, American gynecologists tend to be quite determined on limiting weight gain during pregnancy. Many advise their patients that 15 pounds is "ideal" and anything more than 20 is "immoral." Not long ago, I had lunch with a friend who was in her eighth month of pregnancy. Her "meal" consisted of a diet pill and a few forkfuls of salad.

There is a growing body of evidence that excessive dieting during pregnancy may be extremely harmful to infants, for (as our grandmothers warned us) it leads to small babies, who have a far higher incidence of serious birth defects. A recent report of the National Academy of Science stated "low birthweight is the most important determinant of infant death, neurological abnormality, and intellectual development. Stillborns and newborn deaths are some 30 times more frequent in babies weighing under 5.5 pounds than in larger babies, and a firm relationship has even been established between low IQ at 4 years of age and low birthweight. An average maternal weight gain of up to 30 pounds is now estimated to be the most desirable for infant health and well-being. It is difficult to understand why gynecologists persist in torturing their patients about weight gain when there is so much evidence that they have been wrong on this score. Perhaps unnaturally slim mothers and small babies make the doctor's life easier at the time of delivery.

The three sisters who all had their hysterectomies at the same time so that they could keep each other company in the hospital are symptomatic of the freewheeling way in which uteruses are removed in this country. In the United States today, 516 hysterectomies are still performed annually for every 100,000 women. In England and Wales, the figure is only 213—well under half.

The Truslow Report, a study funded by the Teamsters Union Joint Council 16, which represents almost half a million New Yorkers, concluded that in the handling of gynecological disorders, "the grave suspicion of patient exploitation could be raised." The investigators noted that most of the unnecessary hysterectomies were performed by highly qualified specialists.

Dr. Alan Guttmacher reviewed the gynecology cases. He reported that "the surveyor felt that one-third had been operated on unnecessarily, and that question could be raised about the advisability of the operation in another 10 percent. The New York County Medical Society has attempted to answer Dr. Guttmacher's charges by conducting a study of its own. While citing many instances of sloppy gynecological practice and urging that hospital standards be "raised and enforced," the Medical Society concluded that "only" 10 percent of the hysterectomies performed in New York City are of dubious value.

I asked Dr. Arthur Greeley, who participated in the Medical Society's study, how he would explain the discrepancy between Dr. Guttmacher's findings and those of his own committee. He was disarmingly frank: "We tended to give the surgeons the benefit of the doubt sometimes," he admitted. "We've all been in error too, unwittingly. As clinicians we were all aware of that. The people involved with the Teamster audit were academic types who hold to more idealistic standards. I don't believe that gynecologists mean to exploit women, but as they are trained to do surgery, they want to operate—just like generals who are trained to fight and want to fight."

The perfect gynecologist, if he exists, is a very patient man. He plays a waiting game, reading and informing himself, keeping up in all the areas we have mentioned and more. But he uses his hard-gained knowledge and skills only occasionally because—and this is the crux of the problem—most of the patients who come to his office are *not ill.*

Nor are they children. Yet quite unintentionally, I am sure, gynecologists have been a significant force in keeping modern women infantile and immature, for their authoritarian attitudes deprive women of autonomy over their own natural functions. It is one thing to act like an authority figure with a sick patient who is frightened and lacks judgment, and quite another to frighten a healthy woman into believing that her destiny is not and cannot possibly be in her own hands.

Mental Patients' Political Action Committee

ELLEN FRANKFORT

Excerpted from Ellen Frankfort, *Vaginal Politics,* New York, Quadrangle Books, 1972. Reprinted by permission.

T he boutiquing of America. Somebody ought to write a book. No sooner does a major political event happen than Bloomingdale's sells it on the sixth floor.

In November 1971, the American Psychiatric Association did its boutiquing during its Seventh Biennial Divisional Meeting at the Hotel Biltmore in New York City. Throughout the weekend psychiatrists dropped by at Suite 1738 to "rap" with members of MP-PAC, the Mental Patients' Political Action Committee. Not only was there the thrill of crossing forbidden social barriers, but there also seemed to be a therapeutic component for the psychiatrists as one after another insisted that he, as an individual, was not guilty.

Outside the suite there was talk of a "newly formed coalition with America's *real* silent majority: mental patients." Strange talk for a group that excluded the former mental patients from panels, discussions, and cocktail parties, and even prevented them from obtaining official name cards. In fact, the boutique was there only because MP-PAC had gone to the trouble and expense of renting a suite; it had never been invited by the psychiatrists, who later were busy congratulating themselves on MP-PAC's presence.

MP-PAC is not a self-help group, a recovery group, or Schizophrenics Anonymous. MP-PAC is a group whose members have analyzed the mental patient's role from a political perspective and are dedicated to changing it. As they state in one of their papers, "In modern American society, two institutions of incarceration exist: the prison and the mental hospital. . . . In their essentials, they are quite similar; both are enclosed fortresses in which are incarcerated individuals who have come into conflict with society. In both, the restraints of walls, bars, and locks are used to keep their victims imprisoned. The patient, however, has an additional restraint not imposed on the prisoner, the restraint of *words... His* jailors are *doctors* and *nurses,* he is held in a *hospital,* all supposedly in order to *help* him... The prisoner who tells his guards that he hates the institution and longs to leave is seen by them as expressing a normal human desire for freedom; the patient who tells his doctor the same thing only adds on to the length of his indeterminate sentence The only way out of the mental hospital is to *appear* to cooperate with the semantic fiction while maintaining in the recesses of the mind the knowledge that it is fiction."

Propaganda from yet another activist group? Not quite. In December 1971, 31 staff members of the Ohio Hospital for the Criminally Insane were arraigned on charges brought by a grand jury. The charges included the beating of patients after they had been tied to doors or sedated, and sexual attacks on patients by attendants.

However much the psychiatrists wanted personal expiation, most weren't interested in real change. One, a psychiatrist from New York City's Fordham Hospital, wanted something—people with hospital experience willing to work without pay in an underfinanced, understaffed psychiatric ward... if they wouldn't upset the applecart, rock the boat, or cause any trouble.

"To the extent that injustice exists, I'm with you 100 percent," the psychiatrist said to MP-PAC.

"Then what are you doing about it?"

"I could ask you what you're doing about the war in Vietnam. When you tell me psychiatrists could be doing more, I'm with you 100 percent, as I said."

"Can we come speak to the patients in your hospital?"

"I told you that if you're a responsible, viable group with a constructive program."

"What does that mean?"

"That's for me to determine. When you live in an apartment and someone rings the bell, you have to decide whether he can be trusted to be let in."

"Look, the man is scared. He's fucking scared. He won't even let a small group of former mental patients into his hospital."

"Do you let anyone into your apartment?"

"If you're holding people hostage, it's not an apartment."

"You know, if you people were up on trends and directions in psychiatry, you'd know about patient meetings, governing boards.... "

"We *do* know about them. We've all been part of your meetings and your governing boards. Don't you understand?"

"Are you saying you want to work cooperatively or you want to bash my head in?"

Clearly the man was scared. MP-PAC was not exotica, a boutique, radical chic, or whatever you name it (and the naming is part of the boutiquing). MP-PAC members turned out to know more about what it's like to be a mental patient and what's wrong with mental hospitals than anyone else present. As the psychiatrist began to perceive that, he became concerned. You could almost see the visions of Attica racing through his head.

After three hours of polite dialogue with members of MP-PAC, the psychiatrist said he was not convinced that the group was "viable," that it wouldn't turn into another "fly-by-night affair," or that it wouldn't resort to "rantings and ravings once allowed inside." (All this from a man who decides in fifty minutes whether a stranger is to be committed to an asylum and stripped of all his rights, possibly for life.)

"But I want you to know, in principle I'm 100 percent sympathetic," the psychiatrist said as he got up to leave.

"How can you say that?"

"Why?"

"You don't even trust us to enter your hospital. Let's be honest at least."

"Look," he said, lifting the cuffs of his trousers. "See these? I'm a psychiatrist who wears boots." And then he, his wife, his colleague's wife all returned to the convention, officially entitled "Psychiatry: Explosion and Survival."

Women's Health and Government Regulation: 1950–1980

SUZANNE WHITE JUNOD

M any of the medical discoveries that were made in the first half of the twentieth century came to fruition in the second half. New techniques for detecting cancer and fetal abnormalities were developed. A number of new products were introduced into the market—not always with happy results. And women's struggle to make informed decisions about their own bodies often led to clashes with both the government and private industry. Some of these clashes took place in the courts; others, in the streets.

FETAL STUDIES

By 1955, four different research groups were credited with discovering that the sex of the fetus could be predicted through analysis of fetal cells in amniotic fluid. This information was important in cases of genetically transmitted sex-linked diseases.

In 1959, French cytogeneticist Jerome LeJeune discovered that one form of Down's syndrome was caused by trisomy of the 21st chromosome; this paved the way for a wider use of amniocentesis in diagnosing fetal genetic abnormalities. By 1966, the problems in culturing fetal cells obtained through amniocentesis were solved, and two years later, the first abortions after midtrimester amniocentesis and karyotyping were performed.

A cooperative registry was set up in 1971 to ascertain the safety of amniocentesis. By 1976, amniocentesis was shown to have favorable results in clinical trials. By the late 1970s, there were a number of successful lawsuits against obstetricians who had failed to refer a patient over the age of 35 for amniocentesis. As a result, amniocentesis came in to greatly expanded use.

Ultrasound, which Lars Leksell had used successfully in 1953 to diagnose a hematoma in an infant's brain, became a routine part of obstetrical practice after 1975, when improvements in gray-scale and real-time imaging made it commercially successful.

IN VITRO FERTILIZATION

The first successful use of follicle-stimulating hormone for ovulation induction was reported in 1958. The first pregnancy after treatment with human pituitary gonadotropin was reported in 1960; this led to studies of the hypothalamic-releasing factors that enable or block ovulation.

In 1969, Patrick Steptoe and Robert Edwards began collaboration on the human IVF project. Steptoe had improved the laparoscopy instrument in the 1950s and used it to operate on the fallopian tubes and to extract ova.

In 1973, Landrum Settles of Columbia University extracted an ovum from a patient with dysfunctional fallopian tubes, fertilized it with her husband's sperm, and incubated it in his lab in preparation for implantation in her womb. Horrified, the chairman of the Department of Obstetrics and Gynecology deliberately destroyed Settles' experiment, claiming that it was both unethical and a risk to the woman's health.

On July 25, 1978, Steptoe and Edwards reported the birth of the first "test-tube" (IVF) baby in England.

CANCER DETECTION AND TREATMENT

PAP SMEAR During the 1950s, cytology laboratories were established in the United States, signifying the medical community's growing acceptance of the Pap smear as a means of detecting cervical cancer, as well women's increasing demand for the test. The American Cancer Society was instrumental in educating physicians on its use. By the 1960s, the Pap smear was part of regular gynecology practice. Pap Check, a do-it-yourself test that had never received FDA approval was finally recalled in 1973.

MAMMOGRAPHY In 1960, Robert Egan at M. D. Anderson Hospital in Houston revolutionized breast imaging when he adapted a high-resolution industrial film to a mammographic technique. In 1962, Egan reported the discovery of unsuspected "occult carcinomas."

In 1963, Health Insurance Plan of New York tested Egan's breast-imaging technique and, in 1964, organized the first randomized controlled study to evaluate the effect of screening on mortality. Women who were screened were a third less likely to die from breast cancer than those who received physical examination only. This study served as a model for a national study sponsored by the American Cancer Society and the National Cancer Institute that included 250,000 women. In 1965, the American College of Radiology held its first conference on mammography.

Throughout the 1970s, however, there was concern about the side effects from mammography, especially in women who had undergone radiation treatment. Xerox Corporation replaced the film of the traditional x-ray with a selenium-coated aluminum plate prepared for exposure after being electrically charged. Xeroradiology reduced exposure and produced better quality images. Magnification mammography, which allowed better analysis of suspicious areas, was also introduced.

TAMOXIFEN Paclitaxel (Taxol) was first isolated from the Pacific yew in 1966. Dr. Craig Jordan, professor of cancer pharmacology and director of the breast cancer research program at the Lurie Comprehensive Cancer Center at Northwestern University Medical School in Chicago began studying tamoxifen as a graduate student in 1969. "It was the age of making love and not war, and everybody was looking for more contraceptives." Tamoxifen was a great post-coital contraceptive in rats, but it proved totally ineffective in women, so it went back on the shelf, at least temporarily.

But then Dr. Jordan found that tamoxifen could prevent breast cancer in animals, so in 1974 he began testing it in American women with breast cancer. In 1977, Tamoxifen was approved for patients with advanced breast cancer, and in June 1990, it was approved for node-negative patients.

NEW TREATMENTS, NEW PRODUCTS, NEW THREATS

DES In 1940, Charles Huggins first reported the value of a potent hormone, diethylstilbestrol (DES), in the treatment of prostate tumors. Over the next three decades, DES was prescribed to pregnant women, supposedly to improve the chances of a healthy delivery. A generation later physicians found that it caused adenosis (abnormal gland development) and vaginal adenocarcinoma (a form of cancer) in the daughters of women who took the drug. Genitourinary defects have also been found in sons, and more recent lawsuits allege harm to grandchildren as well. Since the 1970s, several thousand DES victims have sued pharmaceutical companies nationwide.

ENOVID In 1959, the FDA approved Enovid (produced by G. D. Searle) as an oral contraceptive. This profoundly altered the scope of the FDA's authority and established what evolved into a long-term interest in women's health issues. As FDA commissioner George Larrick pointed out, pregnancy was not a "disease." The agency had no experience in either approving or regulating a drug for such a purpose, and although the efficacy of the pill was not in doubt, its safety was soon rendered suspect when reports of associated thromboemolic problems began to surface. In 1967, British epidemiological studies confirmed the statistical link between thromboembolism and oral contraceptives. In 1968, the FDA instituted an Adverse Reaction Data Reporting Program on oral contraceptive drugs.

SILICONE IMPLANTS The first breast implant was in 1962.

In 1963, Dow Corning launched a national advertising campaign for Dow Corning Medical Fluid 360, a liquid silicone preparation that could be injected into the body "for removing facial wrinkles, recontouring women's breasts, and reshaping other parts of the body." FDA agents seized some of the product in the office of an osteopath and in the offices of two California cosmetic surgeons. The agents discovered that the California physicians had not only the Dow silicone "360" in their medical practice, but also a laboratory-grade silicone and an industrial-grade silicone, which the physicians had ordered through a furniture dealer.

In 1968, Dow defendants move to dismiss the government's criminal indictment against them, arguing that the product that they had shipped, silicone fluid, was not a "drug" or a "new drug" under the law. The court ruled that it could not make such a determination until the evidence was heard at trial. The defendants also charged that the statutory definitions of "drug," "device," "cosmetic," and "new drug" were unconstitutionally vague in regard to their product. The court also rejected this argument, saying "the choice of the proper classification is not as difficult as defendants make it out to be. With the guidance of the avowed Congressional policy of protecting the public health, when an item is capable of coming within two definitions, there is really only one answer, namely, that which affords the public the greater protection."

In 1971, Dow Corning and S. W. Rhode, former director of Dow's Medical Products Division, entered pleas of no contest to charges that they had sold a silicone product for rejuvenating middle-aged women in violation of the federal Food, Drug, and Cosmetic Act. The company acknowledged that it had failed to obtain premarket clearance for their product as a drug. Rhodes and Dow were subject to maximum fines of $8,000 and eight years in prison.

Four years later Dow Corning modified its original breast implant product. The FDA responded in a Talk Paper that it had "never approved injectable liquid silicone for breast augmentation or enlargement. Serious injury and at least four known deaths have been attributed to this procedure," and warned against medical use of nonsterile industrial-grade silicone. The FDA further noted that "there is another method of breast augmentation which is performed in the United States. It involves the use of silicone in a pliable plastic bag placed over the chest muscles. None of the problems connected with liquid silicone have been reported for this procedure."

On March 24, and July 6, 1978, the General and Plastic Surgery Devices Panel recommended that the silicone inflatable breast prosthesis be given a class II designation, but identified certain risks to health presented by the device.

DALKON SHIELD The Dalkon Shield, marketed by A. H. Robbins Pharmaceutical Company, was developed before passage of the 1976 Medical Devices Amendment and therefore did not go through a premarketing screening. Regulators had concerns about the device from the beginning, however, and it was targeted for investigation when reports of injury began to emerge.

Litigation began in 1974 and ultimately involved hundreds of thousands of claimants from among the 2.2 million women who had had the Shield implanted. By 1980, clear evidence of corporate wrongdoing and fraud had emerged, and juries routinely began awarding multimillion-dollar punitive damages. As a result, Robins entered bankruptcy court voluntarily in 1985, and in 1989 a plan was implemented to permit injured women to choose an administrative compensation scheme instead of litigation.

TOXIC SHOCK SYNDROME Toxic shock syndrome (TSS) was first identified in 1989. The earliest reported cases occurred among seven children; all were linked to the presence of *staphylococcus aureus*. Symptoms of the disease include vomiting, diarrhea, high fever, and a sunburn-like rash.

Before 1977 all tampon products were made of rayon or a rayon-cotton blend. Since 1977, 40 percent of tampon products have contained more absorbent synthetic material. In 1979, the FDA listed tampons as a class II device under the 1976 Medical Device Amendments and ruled that they must not contain drugs or antimicrobial agents. Today, 70 percent of menstruating women used vaginal tampons.

In 1978, TSS was identified as a distinct disease. A dramatic upsurge in cases reported to CDC occurred in 1980, when 890 cases were reported, 812 among women whose illness coincided with the start of their menstrual periods. The fatality rate among early TSS patients was around 8 percent. This striking association of TSS with menstruating women stimulated careful epidemiological analysis. When information collected by the Utah Department of Health suggested that a particular tampon brand, Rely, had been sued by many women with TSS, a detailed study was devised by the Centers for Disease Control in September 1980 to examine tampon brand use. This study found that 71 percent of a recent group of women with TSS had used Rely tampons.

On September 22, 1980, Procter and Gamble recalled all Rely tampons on the market, and all tampon manufacturers subsequently lowered the absorbency of their tampons. The FDA began requiring that all tampon packages carry information on TSS and advise women to use tampons with the minimum absorbency needed to control menstrual flow.

In 1980, the American Society for Testing and Materials organized a task force to develop uniform absorbency testing and labeling at the FDA's request.

Although cases of menstrually related TSS fell off dramatically after 1984, the overall number of cases is suspected to have risen as the staphylococcal bacteria that produces the deadly toxin has spread to more people. Today, only about half of the cases of staphylococcal toxic shock syndrome are connected with menstruating women. TSS has been reported in men, children, and older women, and in conjunction with surgery, a wound, influenza, sinusitis, childbirth, use of a contraceptive sponge, cervical cap, or diaphragm, intravenous drug abuse, an abscess, boil, cut, or even an insect bite.

THE WOMEN'S HEALTH MOVEMENT TAKES OFF

➤ 1969: Journalist Barbara Seaman publishes *The Doctors' Case against the Pill*, charging that women were not being adequately informed about dangerous side effects from the Pill, including stroke, heart disease, diabetes, depression, and other ailments.

➤ 1970: Senate hearings on the Pill; activist Alice Wolfson demanded to know why no women were being allowed to testify. TV cameras recorded the disruption as Seaman and other women joined the protest. The dissent helped to launch a political movement focusing on women's health.

➤ 1975: Seaman, Wolfson, and three other women activists went on to found the National Women's Health Network as an umbrella institution for nearly 2,000 women's self-help medical projects. The movement centered on the overuse of medical technology, insufficiently rigorous drug testing, and refusal to listen to patients (paternalism).

➤ 1970: Alice Wolfson took the first critical steps to open a dialogue between the FDA Obstetrics and Gynecology Advisory Committee and the FDA. The meetings were closed to the public, but Wolfson and several colleagues persisted in attending anyway. "What are you discussing that women shouldn't hear?" she asked. This was the occasion of the first sit-in at the FDA.

➤ 1970: The AMA House of Delegates passed a resolution opposing the PPI on the grounds that it would "confuse and alarm many patients." A compromise was reached wherein a modified version was mailed to physicians to hand out with every Pill prescription. Over the next five years, the AMA distributed only 4 million copies, although an estimated 10 million U.S. women per annum were taking the Pill. In time, the FDA went back to its original concept—distributing the PPI in the Pill packet through pharmacists. Again there was opposition from doctors and the drug industry. This time the consumer groups were more successful. It is likely that the PPI has contributed to the subsequent decline in Pill use.

➤ 1971: Self-help gynecology helped transform women's health and body issues into a separate social movement. The movement was born on April 7, 1971, at the Everywoman's Bookstore in Los Angeles. For some time feminists had met there to discuss health and abortion issues. After exhausting "book learning," Carol Downer, a member of the group, suggested empirical observation. After inserting a speculum in her own vagina, she invited other women present to observe her cervix.

➤ 1972: Police officers arrested Carol Downer and Coleen Wilson on charges of practicing medicine without a license. Margaret Mead observed that "men began taking over obstetrics and they invented a tool that allowed them to look inside women. You could call this progress—except that when women tried to look inside themselves, this was called 'practicing medicine without a license." (L.A. *Times,* February 5, 1974). Several months later, Downer was acquitted after two days of deliberation by the jury.

➤ 1972: Boston women organized Speakoutrage, a public hearing for women to testify about their experiences with abortion, forced sterilization, unnecessary surgery, and other forms of exploitation and mistreatment. Conditions at the Boston City Hospital ob-gyn clinic were especially decried. As evidence of medical abuse came to light in city after city and hospital after hospital generated a broader-based women's health movement.

Carol Downer, the "mother" of self-help gynecology, was arrested for using yogurt to treat yeast infections and for using a device called the Del-Em for menstrual extraction, also called "self-abortion." Her defense was eloquent and long-quoted as a cornerstone of the concerns of the women's health movement:

> In what has been described as "rape of the pelvis," our uteri and ovaries are removed, often needlessly. Our breasts and all supporting muscular tissue are carved out brutally in radical mastectomy. Abortion and preventive birth control methods are denied us unless we are a certain age, or married, or perhaps they are denied us completely. Hospital committees decide whether or not we can have our tubes tied. Unless our uterus has "done its duty," we're often denied. We give birth in hospitals run for the convenience of the staff. We're drugged, strapped, cut, ignored, enemaed, probed, shaved—all in the name of "superior care." How can we rescue ourselves from the dilemma that male supremacy has landed us in? The answer is simple. We women must taken women's medicine back into our own capable hands.

MEN, WOMEN, WHAT'S THE DIFFERENCE?

In 1961, news that the hypnotic drug thalidomide had been linked with an epidemic of malformed infants in Europe focused attention on women and pregnancy. Worldwide concern about thalidomide led to the passage of drug reform legislation in the United States which shut women out of the early phases of clinical drug testing and virtually orphaned clinical studies of pediatric drug efficacy and safety.

In the 1970s it was discovered that women taking the prescription drug Premarin to treat menopausal symptoms showed a lower risk of cardiovascular illness. As a result, in 1975 Rush-Cook County undertook a hormone therapy study—on *men* —to see what effects estrogen drugs had on heart disease. This study remains the only randomized, controlled scientific study about estrogen therapy and heart disease.

In 1977, the FDA published research guidelines that officially excluded women of reproductive age from early phases of clinical drug trials. As a result, drugs were routinely approved for general use that had not been tested on women. "Nobody was thinking much about how drugs might act differently in men and women," said Dr. Lainie Friedman Ross, assistant director of the MacLean Center for Clinical Medical Ethics at the University of Chicago. "Men are steady-state subjects. The problem is, about half of the people eventually taking the tested drugs were women with monthly hormonal changes."

The scratch-your-head logic of using men to test women's treatments helped garnish important support for the Women's Health Initiative in the 1980s.

Chapter 43

Toward a New Psychology of Women —the 1970s

I n a nine-year period from 1968, when Naomi Weisstein first presented her
paper "Kinder, Kuche, Kirche as Scientific Law," or, "Psychology Constructs
the Female," through the publication of Phyllis Chesler's Women and
Madness in 1972, which was followed by Jean Baker Miller's Toward a New
Psychology of Women in 1977, old conceptions of the female psyche and personality were swiftly and irrevocably overthrown. Changes in the actual treatment of women patients came slower, but also got off to a good start. Naomi and
Phyllis are both Ph.D. psychologists while Jean is an M.D. psychiatrist. Put them
together and it brings to mind a book titled Three Who Made a Revolution by
Bertram D. Wolfe.

Naomi Weisstein, an experimental psychologist and a founding mother of
the women's liberation movement, was teaching in Chicago at Loyola in the
1960s when she got involved politically with Shulie Firestone, among other
young radicals. After graduating Phi Beta Kappa from Wellesley, and ranking
first in her class when she received her Ph.D. from Harvard, Naomi was humiliated—and her consciousness raised through the roof—by her treatment at job

interviews. "How can a little girl like you teach a great big class of men?" was one question that she was asked. Sigmund Freud's belief that women are morally inferior to men also infuriated Naomi, specifically his claim that because she lacks a penis, a woman possesses an inadequate sense of justice, a predisposition to envy, weaker social interests, and a lesser capacity for sublimation. Beyond Freud, as we shall see, Naomi also rejected the popular theories of Erik Erikson and Bruno Bettelheim. Her audience at the University of California, Davis, where she first presented her findings in 1968, was electrified—and many were convinced—when she proclaimed, "Psychology has nothing to say about what women are really like, because psychology does not know."

Also represented in this chapter are Phyllis Chesler, Belita Cowan, Mary Howell, and Alice Wolfson, my cherished cofounders of the National Women's Health Network.—B. S.

Psychology Constructs the Female

NAOMI WEISSTEIN

Adapted from Naomi Weisstein, "Kinde, Kuche, Kirche as Scientific Law," *Women* 1(1): 15–20, 1970. Reprinted by permission.

It is an implicit assumption that the area of psychology that concerns itself with personality has the onerous but necessary task of describing the limits of human possibility. Thus, when we are about to consider the liberation of women, we naturally look to psychology to tell us what "true" liberation would mean: what would give women the freedom to fulfill their own intrinsic natures.

The central argument of my paper is this. Psychology has nothing to say about what women are really like, what they need and what they want, essentially, because psychology does not know. I want to stress that this failure is not limited to women; rather, the kind of psychology which has addressed itself to how people act and who they are has failed to understand, in the first place why people act the way they do, and certainly failed to understand what might make them act differently.

Psychologists have set about describing the true natures of women with an enthusiasm and absolute certainty that is rather disquieting. Bruno Bettelheim, of the University of Chicago, tells us that

> We must start with the realization that, as much as women want to be good scientists or engineers, they want first and foremost to be womenly companions of men and to be mothers.

Eric Erikson of Harvard University, upon noting that young women often ask whether they can "have an identity before they know whom they will marry, and for whom they will make a home," explains somewhat elegiacally that

Much of a young woman's identity is already defined in her kind of attractiveness and in the selectivity of her search for the man (or men) by whom she wishes to be sought....

Some psychiatrists even see the acceptance of woman's role by women as a solution to societal problems. "Woman is nurturance," writes Joseph Rheingold, a psychiatrist at Harvard Medical School." Anatomy decrees the life of a woman.... When women grow up without dread of their biological functions and without subversion by feminist doctrine, and therefore enter upon motherhood with a sense of fulfillment and altruistic sentiment, we shall attain the goal of a good life and a secure world in which to live it."

These views from men of high prestige reflect a fairly general consensus: liberation for women will consist first in their attractiveness, so that second, they may obtain the kinds of homes, and the kinds of men, which will allow joyful altruism and nurturance.

What we will show is that there isn't the tiniest shred of evidence that these fantasies of servitude and childish dependence have anything to do with women's true potential; that the idea of the nature of human possibility, which rests on the accidents of individual development of genitalia, on what is possible today because of what happened yesterday, on the fundamentalist myth of sex organ causality, has strangled and deflected psychology so that it is relatively useless in describing, explaining, or predicting humans and their behavior.

It then goes without saying that present psychology is less than worthless in contributing to a vision that could truly liberate—men as well as women.

The kind of psychology which has addressed itself to these questions is in large part clinical psychology and psychiatry, which in America means endless commentary on and refinement of Freudian theory. Here, the causes of failure are obvious and appalling: Freudians and neo-Freudians, and clinicians and psychiatrists in general, have simply refused to look at the evidence against their theory and practice and have used as evidence for their theory and their practice stuff so flimsy and transparently biased as to have absolutely no standing as empirical evidence.

If we inspect the literature of personality, it is immediately obvious that the bulk of it is written by clinicians and psychiatrists, and that the major support for their theories is "years of intensive clinical experience." This is a tradition started by Freud. His insights occurred during the course of his work with his patients.

In *The Sexual Enlightenment of Children* (1963), the classic document which is supposed to demonstrate empirically the existence of a castration complex and its connection to a phobia, Freud based his analysis on the reports of the father of the little boy, himself in therapy, and a devotee of Freudian theory. Now there is nothing wrong with such an approach to theory *formulation*; a person is free to make up theories with any inspiration that works: divine revelation, intensive clinical practice, a random numbers table.

But he is not free to claim any validity for his theory until it has been tested and confirmed. Consider Freud. What he thought constituted evidence violated the most minimal conditions of scientific rigor.

It is remarkable that only recently has Freud's classic theory on the sexuality of women—the notion of the double orgasm—been actually tested physiologically and found just plain wrong. Now those who claim that 50 years of psychoanalytic experience constitute evidence enough of the essential truths of Freud's theory should ponder the robust health of the double orgasm. Did women, until Masters and Johnson, believe they were having two different kinds of orgasm? Did their psychiatrists cow them into reporting something that was not true? If so, were there other things they reported that were also not true? Did psychiatrists ever learn anything different than their theories had led them to believe? If clinical experience means anything at all, surely we should have been done with the double orgasm myth long before the Masters and Johnson studies.

Years of intensive clinical experience are not the same thing as empirical evidence.

It has been a central assumption for most psychologists of human personality that human behavior rests primarily on an individual and inner dynamic, perhaps fixed in infancy, perhaps fixed by genitalia, perhaps simply arranged in a rather immovable cognitive network. But this assumption is rapidly losing ground as personality psychologists fail again and again to get consistency in the assumed personalities of their subjects and as evidence collects that what a person does and who he believes himself to be will in general be a function of what people around him expect him to be, and what the overall situation in which he is acting implies that he is. Compared to the influence of the social context within which a person lives, his or her history and "traits," as well as biological makeup, may simply be random variations, "noise" superimposed on the true signal which can predict behavior.

I want to turn now to the second major point in my paper, which is that, even when psychological theory is constructed so that it may be tested, and rigorous standards of evidence are used, it has become increasingly clear that in order to understand why people do what they do, and certainly in order to change what people do, psychologists must turn away from the theory of the causal nature of the inner dynamic and look to the social context within which individuals live.

Before examining the relevance of this approach for the question of women, let me first sketch the groundwork for this assertion.

There is a series of social psychological experiments which points to the inescapable overwhelming effect of social context in an extremely vivid way. These are the obedience experiments of Stanley Milgram, concerned with the extent to which subjects in psychological experiments will obey the orders of unknown experimenters, even when these orders carry with them the distinct possibility that the subject is killing somebody.

Briefly, a subject is made to administer electric shocks in ascending 15-volt increments to another person whom the subject believes to be another subject but who is in fact a stooge. The voltages range from 15 to 450 volts; for each four consecutive voltages, there are verbal descriptions such as "mild shock," "danger, severe shock," and finally, for the 435- and 450-volt switches, simply a red XXX marked over the switches. The stooge, as the voltage increases, begins to cry out against the pain; he then screams that he has a heart condition, begging the subject to stop, and finally, he goes limp and stops responding altogether at a certain voltage. Since even at this point, the subject is instructed to keep increasing the voltage, it is possible for the subjects to continue all the way up to the end switch—450 volts. The percentage of the subjects who do so is quite high; all in all, about 1,000 subjects were run, and about 65 percent go to the end switch in an average experiment. No tested individual differences between subjects predicted which of the subjects would continue to obey and which would break off the experiment. In addition, 40 psychiatrists were asked to predict out of 100 subjects, how many would go to the end and where subjects would break off the experiment. They were way below actual percentages, with an average prediction of 3 percent of the subjects obeying to the end switch. But even though psychiatrists have no idea how people are going to behave in this situation (despite one of the central facts of the twentieth century, which is that people have been made to kill enormous numbers of other people), and even though individual differences do not predict which subjects are going to obey and which are not, it is very easy to predict when subjects will be obedient and when they will be defiant. All the experimenter has to do is change the social situation. In a variant of the experiment, when two other stooges who were also administering electric shocks refused to continue, only 10 percent of the subjects continued to the end switch. This is critical for personality theory, for it says that the lawful behavior is the behavior that can be predicted from the social situation, not from the individual history.

To summarize: If subjects under quite innocuous and noncoercive social conditions can be made to kill other subjects and under other types of social conditions will positively refuse to do so; if subjects can react to a state of physiological fear by becoming euphoric because there is somebody else around who is euphoric or angry because there is somebody else around who is angry; if students become intelligent because teachers expect them to be intelligent and rats run mazes better because experimenters are told that the rats are bright, then it is obvious that a study of human behavior requires, first and foremost, a study of the social contexts within which people move, the expectations as to how they will behave, and the authority which tells them who they are and what they are supposed to do.

Two theories of the nature of women, which come not from psychiatric and clinical tradition, but from biology, can now be disposed of with little difficulty. The first argument notices social interaction in primate groups, and observes that females are submissive and passive. Putting aside for a moment the serious problem of experimenter bias (for instance, Harlow of the University of Wisconsin, after observing differences between male and female rhesus monkeys, quotes Lawrence Sterne to the effect that women are silly and trivial and concludes that "men and women have differed in the past and they will differ in the future"), the problem with the argument from primate groups is that the crucial experiment has not been performed. The crucial experiment would manipulate or change the social organization of these groups and watch the subsequent behavior. Until then, we must conclude that since primates are at present too stupid to change their social conditions by themselves, the "innateness" and fixedness of their behavior is simply not known. As applied to humans, the argument becomes patently irrelevant, since the most salient feature of human social organization is its variety; and there are a number of cultures where there is at least a rough equality between men and women. Thus, primate arguments tell us very little.

The second theory of sex differences argues that since females and males differ in their sex hormones, and sex hormones enter the brain, there must be innate differences in "nature." But the only thing this argument tells us is that there are differences in physiological state. The problem is whether these differences are at all relevant to behavior. Schacter and Singer have shown that a particular physiological state can itself lead to a multiplicity of felt emotional states and outward behavior, depending on the social situation.

In a review of the intellectual differences between little boys and little girls, Eleanor Maccoby has shown that there are no intellectual differences until about high school, or, if there are, girls are slightly ahead of boys. At high school, girls begin to do worse on a few intellectual tasks, such as arithmetic reasoning, and beyond high school, the achievement of women now measured in terms of productivity and accomplishment drops off even more rapidly. There are a number of other, nonintellectual tests which show sex differences; I choose the intellectual differences since it is seen clearly that women start becoming inferior. It is no use to talk about women being different but equal; all of the tests I can think of have a "good" outcome and a "bad" outcome. Women usually end up at the "bad" outcome. In light of social expectations about women, what is surprising is not that women end up where society expects they will; what is surprising is that little girls don't get the message that they are supposed to be stupid until high school; and what is even more remarkable is that some women resist this message even after high school, college, and graduate school.

In brief, the uselessness of present psychology with regard to women is simply a special case of the general conclusion: one must understand social expectations about women if one is going to characterize the behavior of women.

How are women characterized in our culture and in psychology? They are inconsistent, emotionally unstable, lacking in a strong conscience or super-ego, weaker, "nurturant" rather than productive, "intuitive" rather than intelligent, and, if they are at all "normal," suited to the home and the family.

In short, the list adds up to a typical minority group stereotype of inferiority: if they know their place, which is in the home, they are really quite lovable, happy, childlike, loving creatures.

My paper began with remarks on the task of discovering the limits of human potential. I don't know what immutable differences exist between men and women apart from differences in their genitals; perhaps there are some other unchangeable differences; probably there are a number of irrelevant differences. But it is clear that until social expectations for men and women are equal, until we provide equal respect for both men and women, our answers to this question will simply reflect our prejudices.

Demeter Revisited

PHYLLIS CHESLER

Excerpted from Phyllis Chesler, *Women and Madness,* Garden City, N.Y., Doubleday, 1972. Reprinted by permission.

ZELDA FITZGERALD (1900–1943)
ELLEN WEST (c. 1890–c. 1923)
SYLVIA PLATH HUGHES (1932–1963)—

All of these women were uncommonly stubborn, talented, and aggressive. All were hospitalized for various psychiatric "symptoms" which involved being socially withdrawn. They no longer cared how they "looked"; they refused to eat; they became sexually disinterested in their husbands. Ellen West and Sylvia Plath finally committed suicide when they were in their early thirties. Zelda Fitzgerald was burned to death in a mental-asylum fire.

These women share a rather fatal allegiance to their own uniqueness, which in each case was at odds with "being a woman." For years, they denied themselves—or were denied—the duties and privileges of talent and conscience. Like many women, they buried their own destinies in romantically extravagant marriages, in motherhood, and in approved female pleasure. Their repressed energies eventually struggled free, however, demanding long-overdue, and therefore heavier, prices: marital and maternal "disloyalty," social ostracism, imprisonment, madness, and death. They attempted to escape their enforced half-lives by "going crazy." In asylums, where they were treated as "helpless" and "self-destructive" children, they were superficially freed from their female roles. However, neither madness nor mental asylums offered them asylum or freedom.

Writing of her asylum experience, Plath found few differences between "us in Belsize and the girls playing bridge and gossiping in the college to which I would return. Those girls, too, sat under bell jars of a sort."

Perhaps she was right. She speaks of the bell jar as a glass cage of "femininity" and powerlessness in which many women sit, in and out of asylums, and from which many are trying to escape.

Ellen West was struggling to escape. She was a wealthy, sensitive young married woman. As a girl, she had preferred "trousers" and "lively, boyish games" until she was 16. Her childhood motto was "Either Caesar or Nothing," and, in a poem written when she was 17, she expressed the desire "to be a soldier, fear no foe, and die joyously, sword in hand." She became an ardent horsewoman, a diarist, and a poet. After feverishly and competently performing a variety of approved female activities (doing volunteer work with children, taking noncredit university courses, engaging in serious love affairs), she developed a fear of eating—psychiatrically interpreted as a fear of becoming pregnant—and finally stopped eating altogether:

> Something in me rebels against becoming fat. Rebels against becoming healthy, getting plump red checks, becoming a simple, robust woman, as corresponds to my true nature.... For what purpose did nature give me health and ambition?... It is really sad that I must translate all this force and urge to action into unheard words [in her diary], instead of powerful deeds.... I am 21 years old and am supposed to be silent and grin like a puppet.

Zelda Fitzgerald's "bell jar" was in many ways reinforced by her husband, writer Scott Fitzgerald, who was extremely jealous of and threatened by her considerable literary talent. He reacted with fury when Zelda completed an autobiographical novel before he had finished his own novel—a "story" of Zelda's life and psychiatric confinement. In a letter to one of her many male psychiatrists, Scott noted that:

> Possibly she [Zelda] would have been a genius if we had never met. In actuality she is now hurting me and through me hurting all of us.... [Zelda seems to think] that her work's success will give her some sort of divine irresponsibility backed by unlimited gold. It is still the idea of a high school girl who would like to be an author with an author's beautiful carefree life.

Nancy Milford, in her excellent biography, *Zelda*, reveals that Scott rather hysterically accused Zelda of being a "third-rate writer" and reminded her of his worldwide literary reputation. Milford notes that "Scott had some very fixed ideas of what a woman's place should be in a marriage," and quotes him in a conversation with Zelda:

> I would like you to think of my interests. That is your primary concern, because I am the one to steer the course, the pilot.... I want you to stop writing fiction.

Zelda says she does not want to be dependent on Scott, either financially or psychologically. Instead, she wants to be a "creative artist:" she wants to work. Only if she does good work can she defend herself against Scott's "bad lies." Her male psychiatrist asks her whether being an outstanding woman writer would "compensate you for a life without Scott"; if that accomplishment "would mean enough to you when you were sixty?"

But Zelda is, in Milford's words, "sick of being beaten down, of being bullied into accepting Scott's ideas of everything. She would not stand it any longer; she would rather be in an institution." (And yet, once she was hospitalized, Zelda's psychiatrists, according to Milford, all try to "re-educate her in terms of her role as wife to Scott.")

Sylvia Plath grew up in Massachusetts and began writing poems and stories when she was very young. Her poems and her autobiographical novel, *The Bell Jar*, describe her battle as an artist with the female condition—a battle she did not necessarily see in feminist terms. Plath attempted suicide, was psychiatrically hospitalized, finished college, published her work, got married, moved to England, and became the mother of two children—all before she was 30.

She was lonely and isolated. Her genius did not earn for her certain reprieves and comforts tendered the male artist. After separating from her husband, Plath continued to write and keep house for her children. On the night of February 10 or the morning of February 11, 1963, she killed herself.

Were these women really "crazy"? Are the women who continue to outnumber men in American psychiatric facilities at an increasing rate really "crazy"? And why are so many women seeking help, viewing themselves and being viewed as "neurotic" or "psychotic"?

There is a double standard of mental health—one for men, another for women—existing among most clinicians. According to a study by Dr. Inge K. Broverman, clinicians' concepts of healthy mature men do not differ significantly from their concepts of healthy mature adults. However, their concepts of healthy mature women do differ significantly from those for men and for adults. For a woman to be healthy, she must "adjust" to and accept the behavioral norms for her sex—passivity, acquiescence, self-sacrifice, and lack of ambition—even though these kinds of "loser" behaviors are generally regarded as socially undesirable (i.e., nonmasculine).

What we consider "madness," whether it appears in women or in men, is either the acting out of the devalued female role or the total or partial rejection of one's sex-role stereotype. When and if women who fully act out the female role (who are maternal, compassionate, self-sacrificing) are diagnosed or hospitalized, it is for "depression," "anxiety," and "paranoia." When women who reject the female role (who are angry, self-assertive, or sexually aggressive) are diagnosed or hospitalized, it is for "schizophrenia," "promiscuity," or "lesbianism." A woman who curses, or is competitive, violent, or successful, a woman who refuses to do housework is "crazy"—and "unnatural." A woman who cries all day, who talks to herself in low, frightened tones, or a woman who is insecure, timid, filled with self-contempt is a more "natural" woman—but she too is "crazy."

It is important to note that men, in general, are still able to reject more of their sex role without viewing themselves, or being viewed, as sick. Women are so conditioned to need and/or serve a man that they are willing to take care of a man who is "passive," "dependent," or "unemployed" than men are willing to relate to—much less take care of—a "dominant," "independent," or "self-centered" woman.

Researchers Barbara and Bruce Dohrenrend recently stated in "Social Status and Psychological Disorders" that men are really as "psychologically disturbed" as women are: "There is no greater magnitude of social stress impinging on one or the other sex. Rather [each sex] tends to learn a different style with which it reacts to whatever fact has produced the psychological disorder."

I would not so much disagree with this statement as qualify it in several important ways. Certainly, many men are severely "disturbed," but the form taken by their disturbance either is not seen as neurotic or is not treated by psychiatric incarceration. Men—especially white, wealthy, and older men— are permitted to act out many "disturbed" and many nondisturbed drives more easily than women can. American men who are young, poor, and/or Black are frequently jailed as "criminals" rather than "psychotics" when they attempt to act out the male role fully.

Women are seeking help because they are really oppressed and unhappy— really confined to a very limited sphere—and because the female social role encourages help-seeking, self-blaming, and distress-reporting behavior. This does not mean that such behavior is either valued or treated with kindness by our culture. On the contrary, both husbands and clinicians experience and judge it as annoying, inconvenient, stubborn, childish, and tyrannical. Beyond a certain point of tolerance, such behavior is "managed." It is treated at first with disbelief and pity, then emotional distance, economic and sexual depri- vation, drugs, shock therapy, and, finally, long-term psychiatric confinements.

Recent social trends also account for the fact that today more women are seeking psychiatric help and being hospitalized than at any other time in his- tory. Traditionally, most women performed both the rites of madness and child- birth more invisibly—at home—where, despite their tears, depression, and hostility, they were still needed. This is less true today. While women live longer than ever before, and longer than men, there is less and less use for them in the only place they have been given—within the family. Many newly useless women are emerging more publicly and visibly into insanity and institutions.

The treatment of women in mental asylums—and private therapy—both reflects and perpetuates the sexism in our culture. At their best, mental asylums are special hotels or college-like dormitories for White and wealthy Americans, where temporary descent into "unreality" (or sobriety) is accorded the dignity of optimism, short internments, and a relatively earnest bedside manner.

At worst, mental asylums are bureaucratized families, with the same degradation and disenfranchisement of self that is experienced by the biologically owned female child. In the institution, howere, degradation takes place in the anonymous and therefore guiltless embrace of strange fathers and mothers. In general, therapy, privacy, and self-determination are either minimal or forbidden in psychiatric wards and state hospitals. Experimental or traditional medication, surgery, shock therapy and insulin treatment, isolation, physical and sexual violence, medical neglect, and slave labor are routinely practiced. Mental patients are somehow less human than either medical patients or criminals. They are, after all, "crazy"; they have been abandoned by (or have abandoned) dialogue with their own families. As such, they have no way—and no one—to tell about what is happening to them. They can, of course, tell their father-confessor figures: their doctors.

According to the 1960 and 1970 membership figures of the American Psychiatric Association, 90 percent of all psychiatrists in America are men. These male psychiatrists and clinicians often repeat in treatment the authoritarian role women are taught to respond to in the family situation.

The mental asylum—and private therapy—are mirrors of the female experience in the family. This is probably one of the reasons why Erving Goffman in *Asylums* considered psychiatric hospitalization to be more destructive of self than criminal incarceration. Like most people, he was primarily thinking of the debilitating effect—on a man—of being treated like a woman (as helpless, dependent, sexless, unreasonable—as "crazy"). But what about the effect of being treated like a woman when you *are* a woman? And perhaps a woman who is already ambivalent or angry about just such treatment?

Those women who are more ambivalent about or rejecting of the female role are often eager to be punished for such dangerous boldness in order to be saved from its ultimate consequences—the complete ostracism by society. Many mental asylum procedures do threaten, punish, or misunderstand such women, thereby coercing them into real or wily submission. Some of these women react to such punishment (or to a dependency-producing environment) with increased levels of anger and sex-role alienation. If such anger or aggressiveness persists, the women are isolated, straitjacketed, sedated, or given shock treatment.

One study by four male professionals published in 1969 in the *Journal of Nervous and Mental Diseases* described their attempt to reduce the aggressive behavior of a 31-year-old schizophrenic woman by shocking her with a cattle prod "whenever she made accusations of being persecuted and abused; made verbal threats; or committed aggressive acts." They labeled their treatment a "punishment program" and noted that the "procedure was administered against the expressed will of the patient."

In addition, asylum life resembles traditional family treatment of the female adolescent in its official imposition of celibacy and its institutional responses to sexuality and aggression—fear, scorn, and punishment. Traditionally, all mental hospital wards are sex-segregated. Homosexuality, lesbianism, and masturbation are discouraged or forcibly interrupted. The heterosexual dances initiated in the late 1950s and 1960s were like high school proms, replete with chaperones, curfews, and frustration.

The effect of sexual repression and the shameful return to childhood are probably different for female than for male patients. Women already may have been bitterly, totally repressed sexually. Many, by "going mad," may be reacting to or trying to escape from such repression and the powerlessness it signifies. Male patients, on the other hand, may be "going mad" to escape the opposite pressure, the demands of compulsive and aggressive heterosexuality. Thus, the absence of opportunity for sexual expression is perhaps not as psychologically or physiologically devastating for men confined in institutions as it is for women.

In asylums, female patients, like female children, are closely supervised by other women (nurses, attendants), who, like mothers, are relatively powerless in terms of the hospital hierarchy and who, like mothers, don't really "like" their (wayward) daughters. Such supervision, however, does not protect the female as patient-child from rape, prostitution, pregnancy, and the blame for all three, any more than similar motherly supervision protects the female as female-child in the real world, either within or outside the family. From 1968 to 1970, there were numerous newspaper accounts of the prostitution, rape, and impregnation of female mental patients by male inmates at various psychiatric institutions. And, generally, the women must "bear the consequences"—enforced maternity—even though their "madness" may be due to just such pressures. A study published in 1968 in the *American Journal of Orthopsychiatry* documented a 366 percent increase in the recorded pregnancy and delivery rate among psychiatrically hospitalized women in Michigan state hospitals from 1936 to 1964. Sixty percent of the mental asylums in this study did not and/or would not prescribe contraceptives or perform abortions.

Behind such statistics are the misunderstood women themselves, I interviewed 24 of them, ranging in age from 19 to 65, who had been psychiatrically hospitalized at some time between 1950 and 1970. Twelve clearly reported exhibiting opposite-sex traits such as anger, cursing, aggressiveness, sexual love of women, increased sexuality in general, and a refusal to perform domestic and emotional-compassionate services. Four of these 12 also experienced "visions." The other 12 women reported a predominance of female-like traits such as depressions, suicidal attempts, fearfulness, and helplessness.

Some of these women had committed themselves voluntarily: their lives seemed hopeless, there was no alternative, and their parents or husbands insisted it would be "better" for them if they "cooperated" from the start. But most were committed wholly against their will, through physical force, trickery, or in a state of coma following an unsuccessful suicide attempt:

Carmen: "I was so sad [after my daughter's birth] and so tired. I couldn't take care of the house right anymore. My husband told me a maid would be better than me, that I was crazy... he took me to the hospital for what they called observation... "

Barbara: "My mother had me put away when I was 13. She couldn't control me. My father had left us; my mother was drinking and crying all the time. I kept running away from bad foster homes, and so she finally committed me to an institution.... "

All of the women received massive dosages of such tranquilizers as Thorazine, Stelazine, Mellaril, and Librium, and many received shock therapy and/or insulin coma therapy as a matter of routine, and often before they were psychiatrically interviewed:

Laura: "The first thing they did was give everyone shock treatment. It didn't matter who you were. You walked in and they gave you shock three times a week.... I was scared to death. I thought I was going to die.... "

Many of the women were physically beaten. Their requests for contact with the outside world were denied. Their letters were censored or not mailed. Legitimate medical complaints generally went untreated or were brushed aside as forms of "attention getting" or "revenge."

Barbara: "I got beat up lots of times. Then I learned the ropes, and they put me in charge of beating up the younger children if they got out of line... they were beating up 5- and 6-year-olds. If I complained about it, they'd do the same to me.... "

Those women remanded to state asylums were involved in sex-typed forced labor. They worked as unpaid domestics, laundresses, ward aides, cooks, and commissary saleswomen. If they accepted these jobs, and performed them well, the hospital staff was often reluctant to let them go. If they refused these jobs, they were considered "crazy" and "uncooperative" and punished with drugs, shock treatments, beatings, mockery, and longer hospital stays.

Susan: "I refused to peel potatoes in the kitchen. So they threw me in solitary for a few days."

Priscilla: "When I refused to mop up the ward and put the chronics' shit in the little coffee cans for them, they [the attendants] ganged up on me. They put a sheet over me, threw me down to the floor, and began punching and kicking me."

Only a few of these women received any psychotherapeutic attention. Therapy groups (and therapists) either interpreted their requests for information or release psychodynamically or counseled them to become more feminine and "cooperative."

Only two of the women had any awareness of their legal rights, and of course, both were defeated in court battles and "punished" by further psychiatric incarceration. Only one of the women did not consider herself crazy. Most of the women were humiliated, confused, fatalistic or naïve about their hospitalization and about the reasons for it. Most dealt with the brutality by (verbally) mini-mizing it and blaming themselves. They were "sick"—weren't they?

Lucy: "Whenever I'd question something they'd done, criticize them, espe-cially about how they treated some of the other patients, they'd yell at me and lock me in solitude. I'd get emotional and excited, I'm sick like that... They're not explicit about what's expected, but you find yourself locked up if you say too many things too loud that they don't like... I was sick, no question about it."

Why do these women think they are "sick"? *Are* they "sick"? Or are they just sick and tired of being powerless, of feeling hopelessly trapped in a Cinderella's slipper, a doll's house, or under a "bell jar"?

Dominants

JEAN BAKER MILLER

Excerpted from Jean Baker Miller, *Toward A New Psychology of Women*, London, Penguin, 1986. Originally published in 1977 by Beacon Press. Reprinted by permission.

Once a group is defined as inferior, the superiors tend to label it as defec-tive or substandard in various ways. These labels accrete rapidly. Thus, Blacks are described as less intelligent than whites, women are supposed to be ruled by emotion, and so on. In addition, the actions and words of the dominant group tend to be destructive of the subordinates. All historical evi-dence confirms this tendency. And, although they are much less obvious, there are destructive effects on the dominants as well. The latter are of a different order and are much more difficult to recognize.

Dominant groups usually define one or more acceptable roles for the sub-ordinate. Acceptable roles typically involve providing services that no domi-nant group wants to perform for itself (for example, cleaning up the domi-nant's waste products). Functions that a dominant group prefers to perform, on the other hand, are carefully guarded and closed to subordinates. Out of the total range of human possibilities, the activities most highly valued in any par-ticular culture will tend to be enclosed within the domain of the dominant group; less valued functions are relegated to the subordinates.

Subordinates are usually said to be unable to perform the preferred roles. Their incapacities are ascribed to innate defects or deficiencies of mind or body, therefore immutable and impossible of change or development. It becomes difficult for dominants even to imagine that subordinates are capable of performing the preferred activities. More importantly, subordinates them-selves can come to find it difficult to believe in their own ability. The myth of their inability to fulfill wider or more valued roles is challenged only when a dras-tic event disrupts the usual arrangements. Such disruptions usually arise from outside the relationship itself. For instance, in the emergency situation of World War II, "incompetent" women suddenly "manned" the factories with great skill.

It follows that subordinates are described in terms of, and encouraged to develop, personal psychological characteristics that are pleasing to the dominant group. These characteristics form a certain familiar cluster: submissiveness, passivity, docility, dependency, lack of initiative, inability to act, to decide, to think, and the like. In general, this cluster includes qualities more characteristic of children than adults—immaturity, weakness, and helplessness. If subordinates adopt these characteristics, they are considered well adjusted.

However, when subordinates show the potential for, or even more dangerously have developed other characteristics—let us say intelligence, initiative, assertiveness—there is usually no room available within the dominant framework for acknowledgment of these characteristics. Such people will be defined as at least unusual, if not definitely abnormal. There will be no opportunities for the direct application of their abilities within the social arrangements. (How many women have pretended to be dumb!)

Dominant groups usually impede the development of subordinates and block their freedom of expression and action. They also tend to militate against stirrings of greater rationality or greater humanity in their own members. It was not too long ago that "nigger lover" was a common appellation, and even now men who "allow their women" more than the usual scope are subject to ridicule in many circles.

A dominant group, inevitably, has the greatest influence in determining a culture's overall outlook—its philosophy, morality, social theory, and even its science. The dominant group, thus, legitimizes the unequal relationship and incorporates it into society's guiding concepts. The social outlook, then, obscures the true nature of this relationship—that is, the very existence of inequality. The culture explains the events that take place in terms of other premises that are inevitably false, such as racial or sexual inferiority. While in recent years we have learned about many such falsities on the larger social level, a full analysis of the psychological implications still remains to be developed. In the case of women, for example, despite overwhelming evidence to the contrary, the notion persists that women are meant to be passive, submissive, docile, secondary. From this premise, the outcome of therapy and encounters with psychology and other "sciences" are often determined.

Inevitably, the dominant group is a model for "normal human relationships." It then becomes "normal" to treat others destructively and to derogate them, to obscure the truth of what you are doing, by creating false explanations, and to oppose actions toward equality. In short, if one's identification is with the dominant group, it is "normal" to continue in this pattern. Even though most of us do not like to think of ourselves as either believing in or engaging in such domination, it is, in fact, difficult for a member of a dominant group to do otherwise. But to keep on doing these things, one need only behave "normally."

It follows from this that dominant groups generally do not like to be told about or even quietly reminded of the existence of inequality. "Normally" they can avoid awareness because their explanation of the relationship becomes so well integrated *in other terms*; they can even believe that both they and the subordinate group share the same interests and, to some extent, a common experience. If pressed a bit, the familiar rationalizations are offered: the home is "women's natural place," and we know "what's best for them anyhow."

Dominants prefer to avoid conflict—open conflict that might call into question the whole situation. This is particularly and tragically so, when many members of the dominant group are not having an easy time of it themselves. Members of a dominant group, or at least some segments of it, such as white working-class men (who are themselves also subordinates), often feel unsure of their own narrow toehold on the material and psychological bounties they believe they desperately need. What dominant groups usually cannot act on, or even see, is that the situation of inequality in fact deprives them, particularly on the psychological level.

Clearly, inequality has created a state of conflict. Yet dominant groups will tend to suppress conflict. They will see any questioning of the "normal" situation as threatening; activities by subordinates in this direction will be perceived with alarm. Dominants are usually convinced that the way things are is right and good, not only for them but especially for the subordinates. All morality confirms this view, and all social structure sustains it.

It is perhaps unnecessary to add that the dominant group usually holds all of the open power and authority and determines the ways in which power may be acceptably used.

Chapter 44

Self-Help Gynecology

C arol Downer and Lorraine Rothman are directly in the Elizabeth Cady Stanton tradition of self reliance based on practical study and physical dexterity. When Carol considered adding new self-help procedures to her repertoire, she normally weighed their level of difficulty compared to a familiar kitchen job. In 1977 she considered offering cervical caps—a barrier contraceptive imported from England—at her health centers. "We can do it," she concluded. "Women can do it…. It's not harder than stuffing a turkey."

In 1992, A Woman's Book of Choices—from which "Menstrual Regulation in the Developing World" is excerpted—was the object of a censorship effort by Andrea Dworkin and John Stoltenberg. They asked the authors to delete that prior to Roe v. Wade, some states permitted clean abortions if pregnancies resulted from rape, fearing, Dworkin and Stoltenberg said, that rape victims would be charged with making it up in order to secure abortions.

Carole now practices law in Los Angeles. Lorraine, now widowed, is taking it easy and honing her skills at folk dancing. Rebecca Chalker continues to write on contraception and female sexuality, as well as fitting cervical caps, in New York City.—B. S.

Self-Help Gynecology

EDITED BY KOFI TAHA

Excerpts from Carol Downer with Rebecca Chalker, "Through the Speculum" in R. Arditti, R. D. Klein, and S. Minden, eds., *Test-Tube Women: What Future for Motherhood?* Boston, Pandora Press, 1984; Lorraine Rothman, "Menstrual Extraction: Procedures," *Quest* 4(3), 1978; Lolly Hirsch, "The Curse: A Cultural History of Menstruation," *The Monthly Extract: An Irregular Periodical* September/October 1976; Rebecca Chalker and Carol Downer, "Menstrual Regulation in the Developing World," *A Women's Book of Choices*, New York, Seven Stories Press, 1992; Ellen Frankfort, *Vaginal Politics*, New York, Bantam, 1973. Reprinted by permission.

At the heart of the women's health movement in the early 1970s was the principle of self-help, which emphasized the importance of reclaiming women's bodies from the medical profession, re-examining conventional knowledge produced by patriarchal institutions about women's bodies, and removing the shroud of mystery, shame, and fear that is socially constructed and instilled in women around menstruation, childbirth, and reproductive health. The Feminist Women's Health Center in Los Angeles was at the forefront of this call for self-help gynecology and was also instrumental in developing a technique called menstrual extraction. Although menstrual extraction was mislabeled "self-abortion" by the mainstream media, was legally challenged in conservative states, and never enjoyed widespread practice, it represents perhaps the most revolutionary aspect of the women's health movement because it was created by women, for women, through research conducted by women, on women, in a nurturing group setting.

The following pieces attempt to recount the history of the self-help movement, explain the procedure and purpose of menstrual extraction, and discuss its applications, both in terms of its practical use and its theoretical challenge to patriarchy.

➤ In "Through the Speculum," Carol Downer, one of the founders of the Feminist Women Health Center in Los Angeles, describes the evolution of the center, the women's health movement, and the importance of information sharing in challenging the social control of women's sexuality and reproduction.

➤ "Menstrual Extraction," by Lorraine Rothman, inventor of the Del-Em menstrual extractor, details the procedures, materials, and methods of menstrual extraction.

➤ Lolly Hirsch offers, by way of a poetic description of the experience of menstrual extraction, a critical book review of *The Curse: A Cultural History of Menstruation*, written by Delaney, Lupton and Toth.

➤ In "Menstrual Regulation in the Developing World," Rebecca Chalker and Carol Downer discuss the related practice of menstrual regulation in developing nations and its potential implications for women's health.

➤ The final piece, from *Vaginal Politics* by Ellen Frankfort, discusses the nature of the resistance mounted against menstrual extraction and the theoretical underpinnings of the women's health movement.

AN EXCERPT FROM "THROUGH THE SPECULUM" BY CAROL DOWNER WITH REBECCA CHALKER. FROM: TEST-TUBE WOMEN: WHAT FUTURE FOR MOTHERHOOD? (LONDON, BOSTON, MELBOURNE AND HENLEY: PANDORA PRESS, 1984).

On April 7, 1971, a group of women met in a small women's bookstore in Venice, California. I had acquired a plastic vaginal speculum and wanted to share what I had seen with the group. After I demonstrated its use, several other women also took off their pants, climbed up on the table, and inserted a speculum. In one amazing instant, each of us had liberated a part of our bodies that had formerly been the sole province of our gynecologists. Afterward, in a consciousness-raising discussion, we observed that in this supportive, non-sexist setting, feelings of shame fell away, and we acknowledged the beginnings of feelings of power from being able to look into our own vaginas and see where our menstrual blood, secretions, and babies came from.

This meeting was the genesis of activities that spread and connected countrywide with other women engaged in similar pursuits which became known as the women's health movement. Collectively we worked to reclaim a huge body of knowledge that had been coopted by the medical establishment; through research and observation, [we] regained the technology for safe abortion, birth, and self-insemination and redefined our sexual anatomy, which had been distorted, put down, or simply ignored by mainstream sex educators and therapists.

Soon, we began doing referrals to illegal abortion clinics. Then we worked as assistants to physicians who were willing to do safe abortion procedures. By assisting at many abortions, we learned that the uterus is not such a remote, mysterious, inaccessible place and that early termination abortions by the suction method were far less technical and complicated than we had been led to believe. We planned to learn to do abortions ourselves, but the 1973 Supreme Court decision on abortion made the procedure legal to 24 weeks of pregnancy. Fifty-three days after that decision, we borrowed $1,200, rented a small house, hired a physician, and opened up the first woman-owned, woman-controlled abortion clinic in the United States.

This clinic became the Los Angeles Feminist Women's Health Center (FWHC). Within three years, similar clinics had started in Santa Ana, San Diego, and Chico, California, and in Atlanta, Georgia. Later, clinics in Portland, Oregon and Yakima, Washington, joined us on an affiliate basis.

The underlying principle of all of the work of the FWHCs is the strategy of undermining the patriarchal structure of society and male dominance by challenging the social control of women's sexuality and reproduction. The institutions of marriage and the laws which regulate divorce, abortion, prostitution, birth control, and homosexuality isolate women from each other and brutally repress their sexuality and reproductive rights. The FWHCs have worked in national coalitions to support the women's movement's impressive campaigns against these laws.

As we progressed in our understanding of the patriarchy, we saw that in addition to laws that maintain the patriarchal family, all institutions of a sexist society function to reinforce women's inferior status, but the male-dominated medical institutions have the special role of enforcing women's sexual and reproductive compliance. Further, we realized that the external oppressive controls and exploitation of women's sexuality has a subjective expression— intense shame—which deprives us of the strength and vigor to assert our most basic rights. This universal shame, felt by all classes of women, causes us to feel extremely humiliated when we expose our genitals, except in situations which we define as medical or sexually intimate. Even in such situations, women frequently need special surroundings, props or rituals to allow another person (nearly always a male) to see or touch her genitals. In our clinics, we have directly confronted the medical practice, peculiar to the United States, of draping women for exams, by dispensing with the drape altogether. The drape reinforces our feelings of shame we are supposed to feel and inhibits the free flow of information between a woman and her practitioner.

In the past 12 years, we have held thousands and thousands of self-help clinics and have repeatedly observed the immediate release of energy and the joy we experienced that first night in Venice. At the same moment the self-help clinic breaks down the barriers between women and strips away repression and inhibition, it also provides us with a realistic alternative to total dependence on the medical profession. Women can take direct control of their own bodies from the simplest ability to check an IUD string directly by looking, instead of blindly by feeling, to identifying and treating common vaginal conditions with safe, inexpensive home remedies. No one would dream of running to the doctor for every sore throat, yet women are expected to regard each vaginal infection as a problem only a doctor can know anything about.

Through information gained in early self-help clinics in Los Angeles, we were liberated from the oppression of misconceptions and misinformation. We learned that the structure of the cervix is beautifully simple. And by observing ourselves and each other on a regular basis, we learned that the medical definition of "the range of normal" is impossible narrow and restrictive. Such notions as "tipped uteruses," "eroded cervixes," "irregular menstruation," and "vaginal discharge," all considered health problems by our doctors, became obviously absurd. We found that everyone's uterus is "tipped" some way or other and that this term has no medical significance whatsoever. We realized that "eroded cervix" means irritated, although the medical term connotes actual disintegration. We soon discovered that very few women have "ideal" 28-day menstrual cycles. Unless noticeable signs of ill health are present, a woman's cycle can range normally from less than 20 days to 6 months, 9 months, or even longer.

The first technology self-helpers gained was the ability to perform safe, early abortions in a procedure we called "menstrual extraction." We chose this term deliberately to blur the distinction between removing a menstrual period and terminating a pregnancy. In our society, abortion is used solely as a means to control women's reproduction, but to a woman faced with the possibility of terminating a pregnancy, the important thing is to have her period on time. Lorraine Rothman, a member of our group, invented a simple suction device which we call "Del-Em" to extract the contents of the uterus. Through our observations of abortion procedures, we learned that a sterile plastic tube, about the circumference of a pencil, could be inserted into the uterus and the uterine contents, menstrual blood or an early pregnancy, could be suctioned out. Because menstrual extraction has traditionally been practiced in the watchful caring environment of small groups of women, the experiences of women having extractions have been profoundly positive, and few serious problems have been reported.

Medical domination and control of pregnancy and childbirth has been more subtle than oppressive abortion laws, but is virtually complete in Western countries. The normal human experience of childbirth has been entirely removed from daily life, so that most of us have no direct knowledge of it, and it has been transformed into a dangerous, pathological event, so much so that normal birth is no longer even taught in medical schools.

Self-helpers, other feminists and home-birth advocates have fought a monumental battle against the medical and legal establishments in the United States to retain the right to choose birth attendants and settings.

Through using the technique of self-examination and information-sharing, we reclaimed important and long-ignored information in the realm of women's sexuality. When we began to write about sex, we discovered a vast disparity between the way medical books and popular sex literature treated the sexual anatomy of men and women. The clitoris has always been considered to be the glands alone, while the penis is described as having many parts which function together to produce orgasm. We studied anatomical illustrations in both European and U.S. medical texts and took off our pants and compared our genitals to these illustrations, some of which date back to the nineteenth century. Our group, comprised of both heterosexual and lesbian women, shared experiences and made photographs and movies of masturbation. Putting all this information together, we *rediscovered* the entire clitoris, which encompasses structures of erectile tissue, blood vessels, glands, nerves and muscles. We learned that both visible and hidden structures of the clitoris undergo remarkable changes during sexual response including erection. The goal of the redefinition of the clitoris is to give women a concrete understanding of what actually occurs during sexual response and to offer clear explanations for various sexual phenomena.

After running clinics for a few years, we decided we needed to spread our ideas in written form. This decision has resulted in four books, each focused on a different aspect of women's health.

A New View of a Woman's Body (Simon & Schuster, 1981) differs from all other women's health books in that it was researched and written by lay health workers involved in day-to-day health care, and draws on the cumulative experience of more than 100,000 women who have visited our clinics over the past ten years. *A New View* also includes clear and detailed illustrations of women's anatomy, especially the redefinition of the clitoris, and the first color photographs of women's vaginas and cervixes to appear outside of a medical text.

How to Stay Out of the Gynecologist's Office (Peace Press, 1981) discusses in-depth problems that every woman is likely to encounter at some time in her life. We evaluated home remedies, over-the-counter preparations and medical remedies for effectiveness and possible harmful effects and compiled a glossary of over 1000 terms used by gynecologists. We also included information women might use when seeking to equalize the very unequal power relationship encountered in a gynecologist's office.

Woman-Centered Pregnancy and Birth (Cleis Press, forthcoming) [is] designed to give women more power and control over their birth experience. We included very detailed information to help women evaluate both the multitude of technological interventions they can be faced with in a medical setting. We also discuss self-defense techniques in the hospital, donor insemination and resources on how to work for political change in childbirth.

In 1979, in response to a request from Chilean women who were being raped while they were imprisoned, Suzann Gage and other women compiled information on self-abortion techniques. In 1979, we published this manuscript as *When Birth Control Fails,,, (How to Abort Ourselves Safely)* (Speculum Press). This book became the object of a heated public debate, both within the women's community and in the mainstream press. Nevertheless, feminists from around the worlds, especially in countries where abortion is illegal or difficult to obtain, ordered copies and the entire collection was sold in a very short time.

In researching and writing our books, we have found that our early belief in the power of self-examination has been reinforced and validated. Vaginal self-examination with a plastic speculum, when performed in a group setting, is a direct assault on the shame that has been inculcated in us regarding our genitals and is a powerful, positive act of trust and mutual support between women. After this barrier is broken, the information flows rapidly and voluminously. Myth after myth falls away. Using the format of the self-help clinic, women could rediscover all of the old knowledge which has been ripped away from us. Combining this knowledge with a group study of medical texts, we could question existing medical information and put it in a more sound empirical basis.

"PROCEDURES" BY LORRAINE ROTHMAN FROM MENSTRUAL EXTRACTION BY SUZANNE GAGE

Menstrual extraction is a procedure developed by the Los Angeles Self-Help clinic women in 1971 which gently removes the contents of the uterus by suction on or about the first day of menstruation.

MATERIALS AND METHODS

It was evident that women did not have equipment to do menstrual extraction, nor any way to get and safely use what was available. Vacuum aspirators are expensive, large and cumbersome, and produce much more vacuum than is necessary. We had practiced with a portable device used by Harvey Karman, and were impressed with its simplicity (the plastic cannula attached directly to a plastic syringe). We found it difficult to manipulate, however ,and it had the potential to accidentally reverse the suction, thus allowing menstrual fluid and possibly air into the uterus. We were concerned about potential complications that might result from reversing the suction. As a member of the Los Angeles Self-Help Clinic, I saw that we needed a simple and inexpensively-made device, which had build-in-safety features. I invented the Del-Em to suit the group's needs. Vacuum is created in a small bottle which is attached to a small cannula that is inserted into the cervical os. An automatic valve attachment controls the direction of the air flow and locks in the pressure, eliminating any possibility of pushing menstrual fluid or air back into the uterus.

Menstrual extraction occurs either at the woman's home or at the group's meeting place. A woman will usually choose to have an extraction on or about the first day her period is expected. However, some women have extractions as much as two weeks beyond the expected date of menstruation.

Three women are the key people involved with extractions: the woman who is to have the extraction (she sometimes controls the vacuum pressure), a woman who observes the equipment for proper functioning, and a woman who inserts and moves the cannula. At times, other group members participate in order to learn the procedure.

After the woman who is to have the extraction places herself comfortably on the table or bed, other women in the group perform a pelvic examination to determine the size, location, and characteristics of the woman's pelvic organs. Certain signs are watched for, such as advanced pregnancy, infection, or other problems. Because the group has frequent opportunities at regular meetings to become familiar with one another, a basis for comparison has been established so that any contraindications are more easily recognized.

The woman inserts her own speculum, examines her own cervix and talks with the group; has others in the group look at her cervix; and then decides whether or not she wants to have the extraction. She talks about her past experiences and purposes for extracting her period, such as relief of menstrual pain. If she suspects she is pregnant, she will discuss her subjective signs and these signs will be evaluated in light of her previous experiences with pregnancies, amount and frequency of exposure to sperm, and her fertility at the time of exposure.

The Del-Em consists of a plastic 50-cc syringe that has a valve on the end. The valve prevents air from being injected into the uterus. The syringe is pumped until it becomes difficult to pull the plunger. Air is removed from the bottle in this way creating a vacuum. The cannula is carefully inserted through the undilated cervical os. Often, the inner cervical muscle can be felt against the cannula. If the slender flexible cannula bends, forceps can be attached to the middle of the cannula giving it more stability. Sometimes a stabilizer is attached to the cervix so that the uterus does not move with the movements of the cannula.

The woman who is having the extraction will tell the other women when she feels the cannula touching the back wall of her uterus. she will continue to relate what she is experiencing as the cannula is moved back and forth making sure, however, that it remains fully inserted. The menstrual material appears within the cannula after a short time.

The cannula is moved within the uterus until either no more menstrual material comes out or the woman having the extraction says she wants to stop. The tubing attached to the cannula is clamped off to avoid any unnecessary discomfort of suction as the cannula is removed through the cervical canal.

RESULTS

Most women who do menstrual extraction do not experience excessive discomfort. Women experience different degrees of cramping during the extraction. Sometimes, women can feel strong cramping when the cannula is inserted through the cervical canal. Most women feel strong cramping at the end of the extraction as the uterus contracts. Menstrual extraction discomfort or pain is seldom as severe or intense as the discomfort or pain from abortions that are done by electrically powered suction machines.

Daily phone contact is the common follow-up method until the group meets again.

"REVIEW: THE CURSE: A CULTURAL HISTORY OF MENSTRUATION,"
BY LOLLY HIRSCH FROM THE MONTHLY EXTRACT: AN IRREGULAR PERIODICAL
(SEPTEMBER/OCTOBER, 1976).

No one can possibly describe a menstrual extraction who has not been there; who hasn't stood shoulder-to-shoulder with her sisters, breathing with the woman on her back, rubbing her forehead, rubbing her legs when they quiver, keeping silent except for interaction concerning the feelings of the woman on her back.

Who could ever describe the shock that happens when the syringe accidentally pulls out with the sound of an explosive rifle crack with everyone laughing in relief at the simplicity of the happening and the lesson of better control over the syringe, unless she's been there?

Who can know the best technique—whether the vacuum is best established before the extraction with a clamped-off tube—or better to assemble the tube, syringe, cannula, and bottle before entering the cervical canal—or after—unless she's tried both?

Who can describe a group who in unison holds back breathing as the cannula is gently, gently pushed through the cervical canal; the search for a method of keeping the cervix from wobbling or pulling back into the vagina, unless she's been there?

Who could ever describe the sensing of the cannula bumping the back wall of the uterus unless she's felt it—as the manipulator of the cannula and as the woman on her back, unless she's been there?

It's a learning experience unlike all the men's books ever written. It's pure learning; pure, unadulterated, uterine, menstrual knowledge. I can't imagine a group of three women who are an automatic beginning of a self-help clinic writing a book on menstruation who've obviously never been in a self-help clinic or done menstrual extraction.

No woman can know the empathy that flows through a group of women doing menstrual extraction; the exhilaration of control and power—whether it's just learning the extraction of menses process or whether it's terminating an unwanted pregnancy without suffering financial liability or physical trauma. The transcendental emotion of love, exalted in a group of powerful women demonstrating their power defies description.

The only comparable experience is that moment during a home birth when the baby's head exquisitely turns in the perfectly choreographed rotation at presentation while the mother is conscious and among friends.

These moments are holy.

These moments are moments of being overwhelmed with the powerfulness of being a *woman.*

No one can describe them who has not been there.

"MENSTRUAL REGULATION IN THE DEVELOPING WORLD," BY REBECCA CHALKER AND CAROL DOWNER FROM A WOMAN'S BOOK OF CHOICES.

At the same time that menstrual extraction was developing in California, international family planning activists began using a nearly identical method of fertility control in developing countries. The technique has had a variety of names: "minisuction," "menstrual induction," and "menstrual aspiration." However, the term most widely used today is menstrual regulation (MR). Like menstrual extraction, the procedure is often done without a laboratory test to confirm pregnancy. MR can also be used for teaching women about their anatomy and fertility, diagnosing uterine cancer, menstrual disorders, and infertility, and for completing self-induced or incomplete abortions.

One distinctive difference between the practices of menstrual regulation and menstrual extraction is in the equipment used. The Del-Em used in menstrual extraction is individually assembled, while the kit used in menstrual regulation is commercially produced and marketed. With this kit, the uterine contents are suctioned directly through the cannula into a syringe while with the Del-Em, the contents are suctioned through the cannula and a plastic tube about two feet long into a collection jar.

Early on, it became clear to medical professionals and family planning experts that paramedics and lay people with even minimal education could learn to use hand-generated suction devices safely and effectively. Today, training in most countries typically lasts from one to three weeks, occasionally longer, and is done on both a formal basis, including classroom lectures, demonstrations, and supervised practice; and on an informal basis often consulting demonstrations only. Trainees may observe from 10 to 20 procedures before beginning hands-on training, and then do up to 20 procedures under supervision before doing them on their own. Because of the lack of qualified trainers, and the demand for MR services, trainees sometimes begin doing unsupervised procedures without much hands-on instruction, but this is not recommended.

In developing countries where health education and contraception are not widely available, women who fear they may be pregnant often seek to induce miscarriages with sticks, wires or other instruments, by drinking toxic substances, or by douching with harmful concoctions. In Nicaragua, for example, women commonly use wire from telephone cables to induce miscarriages. Others resort to poorly trained abortionists who often use stiff, unsterile instruments. As a result, at least 200,000 women die each year, and many more are left infertile or with lifelong health problems. In addition, hundreds of thousands of children are left motherless or with a mother who may be too ill or disabled to provide for them adequately.

Many doctors who do menstrual regulation may use anesthesia, but in some clinics, the only anesthesia that is used is the comforting hand and soothing voice of a counselor. Zarina, a counselor at a woman's clinic in Bangladesh, reports that most of the women who seek MR have already endured childbirth; most say the discomfort from the procedure is quite tolerable, even without anesthesia.

In practice, menstrual regulation is performed up to eight to ten weeks from the last period, but in many countries, the procedure is also done up to twelve weeks from the last menstrual period. There are no reliable statistics on the rate of incomplete procedures in Bangladesh or other countries where MR is in use, but the rate of incompletes appears to be low, according to Zarina because "most women in these countries usually don't come in until they are eight to ten weeks from their last period, when it is easier to determine, by examining the tissue, whether or not an implantation has been missed."

Menstrual regulation is practiced throughout Latin America, Asia, in many African countries, and on a limited basis in the Middle East. In every setting in which this technique has become accessible, the complication rate for self-induced and poorly done abortions has been dramatically reduced. In Indonesia, for example, one study found that the rate of septic abortion was 80 percent higher in areas in which menstrual regulation (in this case, suction curettage) was not available, but that where MR was available, wards formerly reserved for cases of septic abortion were no longer necessary. Clearly, if menstrual regulations were employed more widely, the health of many women—and the lives of many others—would be saved.

In an era that is hostile to reproductive freedom, menstrual extraction and other home health care techniques are profoundly relevant. Women may consciously choose to use menstrual extraction or to take herbs for fertility control for a variety of reasons. When used properly, these techniques are far safer than childbirth, and can put an end to the makeshift methods that desperate women have often used to prevent unwanted pregnancies.

EXCERPT FROM VAGINAL POLITICS BY ELLEN FRANKFORT (QUADRANGLE EDITION OCTOBER 1972, BANTAM EDITION NOVEMBER 1973, PART 7: VAGINAL POLITICS: SECOND AND THIRD THOUGHTS, CHAPTER 22.

There are few genuinely original ideas that come along in a lifetime. Period extraction is one. The fact that no one conceived of removing the menstrual flow all at once and assumed that it was a process that had to take place over a "period" of time, until a group of women started doing it, indicates the revolutionary potential behind the women's health movement.

My own initial reaction to period extraction was concern about the immediate danger or risks of a totally new device being tried out by many women. In fact, I reacted as the medical profession responds to anything new: conservatively. In worrying about the crudeness of the first model, so to speak, I did not see what was truly original—the concept. I still worry about the risks... but the kinds of feelings inspired by the demonstration and the talk of the women who are extracting their periods are so impressive that I [have had] some second and third thoughts about period extraction, the whole self-help movement out of which it has come and the medical profession's response to both. For it is this response which has enabled me to see more clearly my own shortsightedness.

After describing the period extraction in "Vaginal Politics," in *The Village Voice,* I received dozens of letters from doctors about the number of women who would die if this thing caught on and how terribly dangerous and irresponsible it was for me to quote nonprofessional women in something that would be read by many women. (It was the "nonprofessional" that bothered them even more than the "women.") [It appears that] the doctor letter-writers were more upset at the independence that period extraction in particular and self-help in general gave women rather than at the dangers of either. Few argued or even considered that the device could be made safer; none remembered that the first camera or radio or airplane was not perfect and that only in time could a new invention be judged. Had women called in a board of doctors to set up a clinic for period extraction in which the doctors would be the ones to do it, I am sure they would have responded differently. But they saw, quite correctly, that period extraction was developed precisely to give women autonomy over their own bodies and that it was inseparable from the concept of self-help.

Carol Downer's History-Bearing Brushes with the Law

GENA COREA

Excerpted from Gena Corea, *The Hidden Malpractice: How American Medicine Treats Women as Patients and Professionals*, New York, William Morrow, 1970. Reprinted by permission.

Women's efforts to gain control of their bodies have been unsuccessfully challenged in court. In September 1972, ten policemen and a detective in Los Angeles raided the Feminist Women's Health Center. It had been under surveillance for six months. The lawmen issued arrest warrants for Carol Downer, the originator of the self-help concept, and Colleen Wilson, a clinic worker. Wilson pleaded guilty to fitting a diaphragm. She was fined $250 and put on two years' probation. (Fitting a diaphragm, Downer believes, is like fitting a shoe, only one fits it to a different part of the body.)

Downer was charged with practicing medicine without a license. She had practiced medicine, the police alleged, by helping a woman insert a speculum, by observing a vaginal infection, and by helping to apply a home remedy yogurt—to relieve the discomfort. (During the raid, the police tried to confiscate some yogurt as evidence but released it when a woman protested that it was her lunch.)

Downer went on trial November 20, 1972, at the New Courthouse in Los Angeles. Money for the defense and telegrams of support poured in from women around the country. Feminist Robin Morgan, referring to the police, telegraphed, "If they think they can burn witches and midwives again, they will be taught a bitter lesson."

As the trial progressed, feminists publicly asked for a definition of medical practice. Was it giving an enema? Was it diagnosing measles? If you decided yogurt might cure a cold or a sore and you put it in your mouth, would that be a crime? Then why did it suddenly become a crime when the yogurt was applied to the vagina? Is it a crime to tell a woman she has a sore on her lip? Then why is it a crime to tell her she has a sore—cervicitis—on her cervix? Is it criminal for a woman to look at her own vagina?

On December 5, after two days' deliberation, the jury found Downer not guilty.

"Women in California now have the right to examine their own and each other's bodies," feminist Deborah Rose commented, "... amazing to me that we have to win that right."

Women also had to win the right to give birth without a physician. In Santa Cruz, doctors had warned midwives at the Birth Center not to "catch" babies because that was practicing medicine without a license. The midwives ignored the warning, asserting that a woman delivers her own baby and has a right to do so wherever she wants.

On March 6, 1974, officials from the State Department of Consumer Affairs, the district attorney's office, the state police and the sheriff's office raided and closed down the Birth Center. They arrested one midwife there and two others in a private home, charging them with the unlicensed practice of medicine.

At their arraignment, the midwives refused to plead either guilty or not guilty. They demurred, arguing that the charge made against them—attendance at a normal physiologic function—did not constitute a crime. In January 1976, the Federal Appeals Court in San Francisco agreed. It ruled that pregnancy and childbirth were not disease states and that the midwives, therefore, could not have been practicing medicine. The court recommended that the state dismiss the charges. The prosecution is appealing.

Today, the Santa Cruz midwives continue to "catch" babies.

In Florida, roles switched. The Tallahassee Feminist Women's Health Center sued physicians, charging them with harassing its staff.

The Center provides abortions for a thousand women each year at its Woman's Choice Clinic, charging from thirty to fifty dollars less than private physicians. The Center prospered until 1975 when it lost three doctors in four months as a result, it alleges, of intimidation by the medical community. The Center maintained local physicians harassed the clinic doctors by (among other tactics) questioning the "ethics" of any doctor who worked at a clinic that advertised. The feminists suspected that physicians simply disliked competition. On October 1, 1975, the Center filed suit against six local obstetrician-gynecologists and the executive director of the Florida Board of Medical Examiners, accusing them of violating the Sherman Antitrust Act by "conspiring to restrain trade and monopolize women's health care in Tallahassee."

As of this writing, the case has not been settled.

In April 1976, the Center learned that women's health groups around the country were being harassed by physicians. So it joined with seven other health groups to form WATCH (Women Acting To Combat Harassment). WATCH will help women's clinics finance and file antitrust suits.

Chapter 45

Sex and Orgasm

I t's not surprising that feminism's foes liked to take comfort in the faux belief that these were women who "couldn't get a man." On the contrary, a high percentage of the early movers and shakers in the women's movement were young and good looking, as well as sassy and very smart. Of course a lot of them weren't glamorous by standards of the time. They rejected frilly clothes, hair dye, makeup, and flirtatious ways. In short, these were women who could have been sent by central casting for the purpose of portraying the "dowdy" schoolteacher or librarian before she removes her glasses, shakes her hair free, and takes off the bulky jacket that has concealed her glorious breasts.

The movement also had its unmistakeable beauties, and you are about to meet two of them: Anselma Dell'Olio and Shere Hite. Anselma, a stunning, statuesque brunette, and Shere, a porcelain-skinned strawberry blonde, could have played the star. After all these years they are both still stunning, both married to younger European men, and both living abroad. Anselma is a filmmaker; Shere continues writing books that are venerated in Europe, but not always available here.

It might seem "unfeminist" to dwell on the beauty of these two important authors, but I submit that it's relevant to the reception of their work. It was harsh enough for them to reveal how much women were dissatisfied, but that these critiques should have issued from such "objects of desire" made it especially disturbing and confusing for many men, which, in turn, helped precipitate vicious hostility toward Shere, and ultimately, her flight from New York.—B. S.

The Sexual Revolution Wasn't Our War

ANSELMA DELL'OLIO

"The Sexual Revolution Wasn't Our War," *Ms.*, Spring 1972. Reprinted by permission.

The women's liberation movement caught men off guard. They thought women had *already* been liberated by the sexual revolution.

According to most men, a liberated woman was one who put out sexually at the drop of a suggestive comment, who didn't demand marriage, and who "took care of herself" in terms of contraceptives. As far as men were concerned, that's all the liberation any woman needed. The bonus of bralessness and economically independent women simply fueled the misconception that the women's liberation movement was in some way a continuation of the sexual revolution, also known as the more-free-sex-for-us revolution.

In truth, women had been liberated only from the right to say no to sexual intercourse with men. Kinsey in the fifties, and Masters and Johnson in the sixties, contributed scientific ammunition for the sexual revolution which freed women from Victorian morality. This gift relieved us of centuries of moral and social pressure which had dictated that no *nice* woman would ever "go all the way" with a man until marriage.

But it destroyed the sanctuary of maidenhood, pressuring us to give our bodies without respite from late adolescence to old age, or until our desirability as sex objects waned. For the first time, we were shorn of all protection (patronizing as it may have been, and selective in terms of class privilege) and openly exhorted to prostitute ourselves in the name of the new morality.

We have come to see that the so-called sexual revolution is merely a link in the chain of abuse laid on women throughout patriarchal history. While purporting to restructure the unequal basis for sexual relationships between men and women, our munificent male liberators were in fact continuing their control of female sexuality.

With the advent of the new feminism, women finally began to ask, "What's in it for us?" And the answer is simple. We've been sold out. The sexual revolution was a battle fought by men for the greater good of mankind. Womankind was left holding the double standard. We're supposed to give, but what do we get? Kinsey's *Sexual Behavior in the Human Female* offered a priceless handbook for the revolution in its finding that (1) women could and did enjoy sex after all, (2) there is no such thing as a frigid woman, only inept men, (3) virginity in women was no longer considered important or particularly desirable by most men, and (4) women and men were now equals in bed and equally free to screw their bottoms off for the sheer fun of it.

What the popularizers of Kinsey's findings neglected to emphasize would have provided the seeds for a *real* revolution in the bedroom. We still remained ignorant abut the difference between orgasm and ejaculation, about the speed-of-response differential between male and female orgasm, about the fallacy of the vaginal-clitoral orgasm dichotomy, about women's multiorgasmic nature, and so on. Because of this deliberate or unconscious *excising* of Kinsey, and later Masters and Johnson, we have managed to survive into the seventies with the double standard intact, alive and well in the minds of average American males. And many females as well.

The new freedom of the sexual revolution was at best a failure, at worst a hoax—because it never caused significant changes in the social attitudes and behavior of men to correspond with this new morality being forced upon women. There has been no real revolution in the bedroom. For this crucial reason, the sexual revolution and the women's movement are polar opposites in philosophy, principles, goals, and spirit.

The real point is that there are not many women—liberated, unliberated, feminist, or otherwise—who are sleeping around for the sheer pleasure of it. The Achilles' heel of the sexual revolution is persistent male ignorance of the female orgasm.

Now, if there was anything that a sexual revolution should gave been able to accomplish, especially with the data made available by Kinsey as early as 1953, it should have been more pleasure for women during intercourse. Yet 19 years later, the majority of women have to put up with relatively infrequent orgasms during sexual—at least heterosexual—encounters.

Of course, before Freud, the question of orgasm was moot, because women weren't supposed to enjoy sex at all. Decent women submitted to it with clenched teeth. With Freud, female orgasm was rediscovered, and the high incidence of female frigidity was declared to be an emotional and psychological problem of "sexually immature" women. Vexed by the fact that women could reach orgasm freely and quickly through masturbation, but less frequently during standard intercourse, Freud though there must be two kinds of female orgasm: clitoral and vaginal. The clitoral orgasm, which worked for most women, but was difficult in the standard male gratifying positions, was defined as "adolescent." The vaginal orgasm was declared to be the only true, mature, womanly orgasm. It could only be achieved during intercourse through vaginal penetration by the penis. Since overwhelming numbers of women weren't experiencing the "mature" orgasm, Freud concluded that women, recognizing their inferiority to men, were loath to accept their femininity. For this dreadful condition he prescribed psychiatric assistance.

Over the decades psychiatrists have treated scores of us with little success, trying to get us to surrender to our destinies by transferring our orgasms from clitoris to vagina. Generations of women, including the present one, grew up masturbating in secret (men talked about masturbating long before women did), and faking orgasm during intercourse.

Kinsey and Masters and Johnson should have changed all that. Neither study produced a shred of evidence in defense of the double-orgasm theory. As a result of their extensive experiments, Masters and Johnson advanced four important conclusions:

1. The dichotomy of vaginal and clitoral orgasm is entirely false. Anatomically, all orgasms are centered in the clitoris, whether they result from direct manual pressure applied to the clitoris, indirect pressure resulting from the thrusting of the penis during intercourse, or generalized sexual stimulation of other erogenous zones, such as the breasts.

2. Women are naturally multiorgasmic. That is, if a woman is immediately stimulated following orgasm, she is likely to experience several orgasms in rapid succession. This is not an exceptional occurrence, but one of which most women are capable. In all of their students, Masters and Johnson found no incidence of a totally or clinically frigid woman.

3. While women's orgasms do not vary in kind, they vary in intensity. The most intense orgasms experienced by the research subjects were by masturbatory manual stimulation by the partner. The least intense orgasms were experienced during intercourse.

These findings were surely cataclysmic and should have been liberating, at least to the degree that they served to destroy established myths. Yet five years after publication, they still have had little or no impact on men's minds or women's lives.

Many women are still not having orgasms and still, as noted earlier, not sleeping around for pleasure—an unchanging fact despite the sexual revolution. In the meantime, men *are* pursuing sex for just that reason.

If pleasure is rarely the reward, women's continued willingness to have intercourse doesn't make sense. Why, then, are we doing it?

The truth is we are often pressured into it, and not only by the litany of the sexual revolution. It may be the need for affection and attention. Or the desire to please; the need for approval. It's no news to any of us that men can have intercourse with women they are totally disinterested in as human beings. For many women sex fail to bring physical satisfaction, and depersonalized sex denies women even the side benefits of communication and approval.

What the sexual revolution should have taught us is that *need* shouldn't be confused with *love*; that men and women can neither give nor receive love until we stop confusing it with a need for security and approval. The women's movement is trying to teach that lesson. Love is not getting high on fantasies of romance, the perfect lover, absolute happiness, and sexual ecstasy. Love is based on two-way communication and respect, and that only exists between equals.

When feminists are critical of romance, there is often a panicked reaction: "But you can't possibly want to get rid of love?"

No, we don't want to negate the emotion. We want a better definition. We want to get rid of the sick and hoary old illusions which women have pursued relentlessly at the price of our humanity. What is called love now is so clearly exploitative and unsatisfactory that it should make us suspicious that men want to preserve it at all costs. What is called love now is vital to the oppression of women.

Men have poured their creative energies into work; we have poured ours into love, and an unequal social and sexual relationship was the inevitable result. And because this was the situation the sexual revolution failed to correct, feminists are moving into an area they have won by default.

The problems are enormous. Whenever we manage to combat our sense of insecurity long enough to go out and actually do something, our attitude is betrayed by our conditioned belief that women's work is dispensable, our contributions secondary. When the man in our life complains about our absorption in work, we are apologetic. We turn somersaults to accomplish it at odd hours rather than claim our time as our own and risk his disapproval, anger, or complete rejection. Often, we apologize for our work even before a man has time to object—so thorough is our conditioning. And men most often accept our sacrifice as their due. The *droit du seigneur* of the sexual revolution.

Therefore, a sexually liberated woman without a feminist consciousness is nothing more than a new variety of prostitute for the sexual revolution. If we don't sell ourselves for money in the street or security in the suburbs, we sell ourselves in exchange for some measure of approval and (we hope) lasting affection.

Feminism was reborn in part to protest and correct the fact that, although women are no longer burdened by an old-fashioned morality (which is good), we are now saddled with the entire range of emotional and physical consequences of sexual availability (which is bad).

That old form of censure—every woman a virgin or else—was simply one side of the coin. The ancient epithet of "promiscuous" was always the other, and the coin has now been turned over. Promiscuity has lost none of its old sting. It has only acquired a whole new negative connotation with the aid and comfort of psychology, psychoanalysis, and psychiatry. Practitioners in these fields have taken to accusing the sexually active woman of "emotional" frigidity, inability to relate, nymphomania, etc. So even the apparent gain for women is illusory. If we are no longer expected to be virgins physically, we are still expected to be "practicing" virgins—mentally pure, and only "in love" with one man.

There are many women who have decided to challenge the hypocrisy of the sexual revolution by refusing to tolerate this double-standard nonsense and becoming at least as sexually liberated as men are. They soon find out that, emotional problems aside (and they are not insignificant), the physical obstacles are close to insurmountable. The physical price a woman stands to pay for sexual nonchalance is staggering. A woman's chances of getting pregnant are still good (meaning bad), and those chances get better (meaning worse) as the frequency of, and number of partners for, intercourse increases.

The pill is hazardous, and other forms of contraception are a drag, a distraction, and a nuisance, not to mention being failure-prone. Tampering with women's vastly more complex reproductive system is all right with men, but vasectomy, still the most practical, inexpensive method of birth control which can be performed in minutes in the doctor's office, is not; at least, not with most men. The virility-fertility connection is sacrosanct. And there you have the clearest evidence of why feminists view the sexual revolution as one more male ego trip. What kind of sexual revolution is it when, in the year 1971, the possibility of a practical male contraceptive still goes largely unresearched and unpublicized?

It's now clear that the dice are loaded and the women's movement is the one force that can make the game honest. The rising chorus of laments about a growing incidence of male impotence probably means that our feeble attempts to correct the situation are going in the right direction. It can't hurt for men to begin to experience a small dose of the medicine women have had to swallow for a century.

The sexual politics imbedded in the culture shows itself clearly through the language bias. When men don't function sexually, they are called "impotent," *without power.* When women don't, they are called "frigid," *icy cold.* The active-passive dichotomy is apparent. Men know a good thing when they have it, and they go to whatever lengths are necessary to protect their potency. If a woman is a threat to that potency, then her ego must be crushed. Notice that we never hear about females being "castrated" when our egos are destroyed and our potency denied. Such melodramatic symbolism is reserved for men. In fact, a woman's loss—her frigidity, her inability to derive pleasure from sex—is frequently described by men as "castrating." Frigidity is our fault, and male impotency is our fault too!

Perhaps the best evidence of the phoniness of the sexual revolution is the prevailing eighteenth-century attitude toward masturbation. For men, it is a fact of life. Locker rooms and little boys' habits have made it so. But for women, autoeroticism is a newly discovered secret. In view of the fact that there are women who still fake orgasm, women who feel embarrassed to request their own satisfaction in intercourse, or women who flatly tell a partner, "I don't come, so don't wait for me," it's about time we perfected the art of masturbation. Not as a substitute for intercourse, but as one means to pleasure and to the understanding of our own bodies.

These subjects remain difficult to discuss in plain language, and so the women's movement has rushed in where the sexual revolution feared to tread. And none too soon. As Susan Lydon says in *Sisterhood Is Powerful,* "Appearances notwithstanding, the age-old taboos against conversation about personal sexual experience haven't yet been broken down." This reluctance on the part of most people to discuss the issues openly and honestly has allowed the creation of many myths about sexual supermen and superwomen. Men who are inadequate lovers squirm out of their plight by claiming that a previous girlfriend was a real sexpot who had 14 vaginal orgasm in five minutes, so what's wrong with *you* anyway? Men strangle us with our sisters' lies. The next time you're tempted to fake orgasm, just think of the harm you may be doing to the next woman, if not to yourself.

A man with some respect for himself and you will not be turned off by your honesty. You may be the first woman who ever talked to him straight, and he may welcome the opportunity to clear up doubts of his own. And if he is turned off, you are well rid of him. As long as you allow yourself to be victimized, rest assured you *will* be—again and again. If female sexuality has been such a mystery to women for so long, think how mysterious it must be to men.

Men are severely troubled by women picking lovers with an awareness of self-interest. We are still ridiculed for wanting, after all this time, to reclaim our true sexuality. We are accused of *demanding* orgasms like spoiled children demanding sweets before dinner. Men are never accused of the same. For them, orgasm are regarded as necessary to health.

As often as we repeat the following story, it never seems to be enough: According to Ovid, Tiresias, the blind prophet of Thebes who had been both a man and a woman, was asked to mediate in a dispute between Jove and Juno as to which sex got more pleasure from lovemaking. Tiresias unhesitatingly answered that women did. Two thousand years and several sexual revolutions later, we still believe the opposite to be true.

Ideally, of course, we shouldn't have to *demand*, but we are going to have to start becoming more vocal and insisting on a sexual bill of rights if the situation is ever to change. Otherwise we will end up abandoning the idea of men as sexual partners or accepting our own mutilated sexuality. It's a radical truism that power is never relinquished, it must be taken—and potency is a synonym of power

The Liberated Orgasm

BARBARA SEAMAN

Excerpted from Barbara Seaman, *Free and Female*, "The Liberated Orgasm," as it appeared in *Ms.*, August 1972. Reprinted by permission.

Years ago Margaret Mead suggested that "the human female's capacity for orgasm is to be viewed… as a potentiality that may or may not be developed by a given culture."

We don't need to be anthropologists to realize that our Western culture has not only failed to develop that potentiality, but it has stifled and repressed it.

As a result, we women have been afraid to think for ourselves about our own sexual tastes and pleasures. We have tried to model our own preferences after the prevailing views of normality. We have been shy about telling our lovers what we want. We have feared it would be unwomanly to do other than let the male take the lead, however ineptly.

The modern sex manuals are filled with misinformation—for instance, the standard advice to men that they should flail away at the sensitive clitoris. But even when their suggestions are applicable to some women in some moods, they are rarely applicable to all women in all moods, and they foster a certain technical rigidity that is antithetical to really good sex.

Female sexuality is so easily bruised and buried in the myths and medical models of the prevailing culture that the self-awareness needed for liberation will be difficult to achieve unless women explore their own true sexual feelings and needs.

We know that all orgasms are similar on a motor level, and that all orgasms are different on a sensory level.

We know also that there is no ideal or norm, except in our own imaginations. The truth is that the liberated orgasm is an orgasm *you* like, under any circumstances *you* find comfortable. (The only qualification is that liberated persons don't exploit each other—that's just for masters and slaves.)

In the spring of 1971, my research assistant Carol Milano and I completed an informal but we think rather enlightening sex survey of 103 women. They were career women or students: models of the new woman who enjoys more than average sexual awareness and freedom.

In our survey all but six regularly achieved some sort of orgasm with relative ease. This is substantially higher than the figure for women in general in our society, especially when you consider that perhaps one-third of the women in our survey were under 25. (From the Kinsey report and more recent investigations, we know that while the majority of women do achieve orgasms sooner or later, for many it is later. It often takes years or even decades for adult women to achieve sexual satisfaction.)

[Some in our survey] could not comment on the clitoral versus the vaginal orgasm at all; to them, the whole debate seemed meaningless. These women simply did not experience their orgasms in one place more than the other. But with this group left out, there were the two extremes of women who stated a preference for, or more frequent experience of, one type or the other. Regardless of the actual physiology of the event, they *felt* most of their orgasms in either the vagina or the clitoris.

Women are so varied in their sexuality that even those who seem alike are different. Let us contrast two, whom I shall call Marie and Antoinette.

Both women are sexually informed and active, and both have given considerable thought to their sexual needs. To achieve orgasms, both require direct clitoral stimulation.

They are not militant clitorists, for neither doubts that some women obtain orgasms via vaginal stimulation, but it doesn't work for them. Marie says, "I know that lots of girls do *not* need as much direct stimulation as I do—but I think this is because they have larger and better placed clitorises." Antoinette says, "I don't think anyone really knows what percentage of women have orgasms during intercourse. It would seem to depend on individual anatomy and placement of the clitoris."

Although clitorises are highly variable in size as well as placement, Masters and Johnson say that in 11 years of research they found no evidence to support the belief that differences in clitoral anatomy can influence sexual response. This, however, must be viewed as a highly tentative finding since they were unable to observe any clitorises during orgasms. Masters and Johnson think that in certain women the thrusting penis does not exercise the traction on the labia and clitoral hood, that it does for others. So perhaps idiosyncracies of the vagina, rather than the clitoris, better explain the anatomical need for direct stimulation. Direct clitoral stimulation can be obtained in sexual intercourse, provided the woman is on top or the couple is side by side, and the pubic bones of the man and woman are touching.

What, in the experience of Marie and Antoinette, is the most common love-making error that men make?

Marie: "Not enough direct manipulation of the clitoris."

Antoinette: "Many men don't realize that the clitoris is the source of orgasms."

Analysts are undoubtedly telling us the truth when they report that they have "converted" thousands of women to vaginally experienced orgasms. The point is merely that, for some women at least, the strong desire to notice vaginal sensations makes these more noticeable. If Masters and Johnson are correct, all orgasms are essentially the same and quite sensibly involve all the pertinent parts God gave us.

But if all orgasms are the same, why do women not recognize the fact? Are we hopelessly stupid or recalcitrant?

Or are we complex human organisms whose responses are as varied and individual as we are ourselves? Some women noted a difference in their response to vaginal stimulation after childbirth. Several other women noted that they first experienced "vaginal" orgasm—that is, orgasm without direct clitoral stimulation—during intercourse with men who could either sustain vaginal thrusting for an exceptionally long period of time (compared to other lovers) or who had organs that seemed exceptionally large and "filling." One woman also noted a difference in male "sex rhythms": "With some of my lovers I need my clitoris fondled to reach orgasm, and with others I don't."

Several of the women who need direct clitoral stimulation gave what appeared to be very sound anatomical explanations of their preference. Here is one example: "Before the birth of my son, who weighed over 9 pounds and had an inordinately large head, I used to reach orgasm without needing to have my clitoris massaged. I don't believe that my vagina was repaired properly after childbirth. I think it must have gotten stretched out of shape because my same husband, with the same penis (and to whom I feel closer than ever), cannot bring me to orgasm so easily by his thrusting alone. I enjoy sex more than ever. My desire, if anything, has increased. But something is different about me, and if my understanding of Masters and Johnson is correct, I believe that the difference is that my vagina was slightly damaged, so that my husband's thrusting no longer provides as much traction on my clitoris."

So, allowing for the probability that there are anatomical differences that may have a strong bearing, what were the other differences between "vaginal" and "clitoral" women?

From [our] evidence, there were more women in the vaginal group whose early experience with men had been favorable and who had not had to struggle to learn to enjoy sex. These women, perhaps because they were more "trusting" or perhaps, more simply, because their earliest lovers were better controlled and had stimulated them vaginally for long enough periods to bring them to orgasm by that route, had somehow learned to experience "feeling" in their vaginas and to let themselves come to orgasms through vaginal stimulation alone.

The "clitoral" types generally had been exposed to more selfish or fumbling lovers, particularly in their early experiences. Some, of course, had themselves insisted on the practice of merely "petting to climax" in order to preserve a token virginity during their premarital years.

Outside or in, clitoral or vaginal, we are in no way as standardized as Hugh Hefner's airbrushed and siliconed playmates. For example, while 14 women in our survey complained that their lovers did not engage in enough physical foreplay, and 8 others complained that their lovers did not engage in enough verbal foreplay, pillow talk, or conversation, two respondents took the opposite position. They like to get down to the main business of sex more swiftly than their lovers. One observed: "I find foreplay detrimental." The second woman asks wryly: "I have very little interest in foreplay. Is that an inhibition or a total lack of it?"

Or consider the question of the handsome stranger, an alleged apparition in the dreams of younger females. Most of the women in my survey did not like sex with strangers. Over and over they emphasized the importance (to them) of warmth, intimacy, trust, tenderness.

Some women even deem it best to withdraw entirely from men. A prominent feminist confided: "I think it's wonderful that women have discovered masturbation, because it will enable us to keep apart from men as long as necessary. When you have work to do, you can't allow yourself to be diverted by sexual relationships. Masturbation is what male revolutionaries have always used to relieve themselves. Some of the women I know are so pathetic. They run around looking for a man, any man at all."

But what precisely is the female orgasm (which may or may not be developed by a given culture) and where does it take place? A women knows when she's had one (if she doubts it, she hasn't), but since her orgasm is not punctuated by the sure sign of ejaculation, men have felt free to develop lunatic theories about it, and women have not learned to trust their own bodies.

A woman's external sex organs consist of labia majora, or outer lips; labia minora, or inner lips; and the highly eroticized clitoris, the only organ known to man or woman whose sole purpose is to receive and transmit sexual pleasure. The hood of the clitoris is attached to the labia minora, which are directly affected by penile thrusting. Thus, intercourse causes the labia to exert traction on the clitoral hood, producing rhythmic friction between it and the clitoris itself.

Masters and Johnson have proved—or believe they have proved; their work has not yet been replicated—that virtually all feminine orgasms, however vaginal some of them may seem, do include indirect clitoral stimulation, the labia minora being the agent of mediation. Some Freudian analysts have long maintained that vaginal orgasms are entirely distinct from clitoral orgasms and are, indeed, the hallmark of a sexually mature woman. If clitoral stimulation, whether direct or transmitted through the labia, occurs in all orgasms, then distinguishing them is invalid. So is the complicated mystique attached to the distinction. Vaginal women have been said to be mature, feminine, loving, and happy, while clitoral women have had all the opposite traits attributed to them.

However, if I read Masters and Johnson correctly, they are saying that clitoral stimulation may occur in orgasm, but orgasm does not chiefly occur in the clitoris.

To the contrary, orgasm, which is a total body response, is always marked by vaginal contractions. No specific physiologic response in the clitoris has yet been recorded.

Let us review the physiology of the female sex cycle:

STAGE 1: EXCITEMENT. Within 10 to 30 seconds after erotic stimulation starts, the vaginal lining is moistened with a lubricating fluid. Nipples erect, and the breasts begin to swell, increasing in size by one-fifth to one-quarter in women who have not nursed a baby. (Breasts that have been suckled do not enlarge as much.) Other changes start to occur in the clitoris, labia, and vagina as vasocongestion (the engorgement of vessels and organs with blood) and muscular tension start to build. Late in the excitement phase, some women may start to develop a measles-like rash, or sex flush, across their bodies. (Seventy-five percent of the women evaluated by Masters and Johnson showed this response of some occasions.)

STAGE 2: PLATEAU. The tissue surrounding the outer third of the vagina engorges and swells, creating an "orgasmic platform." The deeper portion of the vagina balloons out to form a cavity. The uterus enlarges. The swelling of the outer third of the vagina reduces its diameter, allowing it to grip the penis better. The clitoris retracts, and it becomes harder to locate.

Just prior to the orgasmic phase, the labia minora undergo a marked color change called the sex skin reaction. In the woman who has not had children, the labia minora turn pink or bright red. In the mother, they turn bright red or deep wine (presumably because she has a greater number of varicosities). This coloration remains throughout orgasm, but disappears 10 to 15 seconds afterward. When a woman develops sex skin, she is almost certain to go on to orgasm. Women who are aroused to plateau levels but not brought to orgasm experience a prolonged and sometimes uncomfortable ebbing away of vasocongestion and muscular tension.

STAGE 3: ORGASM. The typical orgasm lasts only 10 or 15 seconds, if that long. Changes occur throughout the body. Muscles of the abdomen, buttocks, neck, arms, and legs may contract; pulse and breathing are more rapid; and blood pressure climbs. The woman experiences a series of rhythmic contractions in the outer third of the vagina and the tissues surrounding it and in the uterus. These contractions, each taking about four-fifths of a second, serve to discharge the accumulated vasocongestion and tension that have been brought on by sexual stimulation. A mild orgasm usually involves 3 to 5 contractions; an intense one, as many as 15.

From time to time a woman may experience what some Samoan Islanders call the "knockout" orgasm, and what Masters and Johnson term the "status orgasmus." Masters and Johnson suspect, but are not certain, that the woman is probably having rapidly connected multiple orgasms, over a time period of 60 seconds or so.

In prolonged intercourse a woman may have three, four, or five separate orgasms, and in a few primitive cultures, where men have good control of themselves, multiple female orgasms are apparently the norm. Some masturbating women can have up to 50 successive orgasms according to clinical observation.

Multiple orgasms are most apt to occur when intercourse is prolonged. Thus, while the much vaunted "mutual orgasm" has some very nice features, it also has some drawbacks from the woman's point of view. Or to put it another way, there is no need for a woman to hold back deliberately, for if the male can maintain effective thrusting for a long enough period, the woman will have several preliminary orgasms and, quite possibly, another when he reaches his.

Women who don't have multiple orgasms may fear that they are missing something, but women who do have them often report that these are not their most pleasurable experiences. "If I've had a great orgasm, I can't bear to go on," one such woman explained.

This mysterious thing called orgasmic intensity is measured, principally, in the number of contractions. Masters and Johnson maintain that females have the most intense orgasms when they are free to please themselves only— "without the distraction of a partner." But they do qualify it. "A woman might tell me that she had a delightful experience with the machine," Dr. Masters commented at the New York Academy of Medicine in 1968, "but the next night with her husband might have been even better, in her opinion, although we registered fewer orgasmic contractions."

STAGE 4: RESOLUTION. Blood vessels emptied and muscular tensions relieved, the various parts and organs return to their normal condition, some rapidly and some slowly. One woman in three develops a film of perspiration across her body.

According to Masters and Johnson, the clitoris contributes crucially to the buildup of sexual tensions, but orgasm itself is more correctly described as centering in the vagina. Tensions established, it is vaginal contractions that bring relief by emptying engorged organs and vessels. Masters and Johnson call these vaginal contractions "the visible manifestations of female orgasmic experience."

Yet, even for those lucky women who can fantasy to orgasm, the clitoris serves as receptor and transformer of sexual stimuli, while vaginal contractions punctuate the orgasm itself.

However, it is important to note that some women who do not possess a clitoris seem to be capable of orgasm. Dr. Michael Daly, a Philadelphia gynecologist, reports that he has studied in depth two patients in whom the total clitoris was removed because of cancer. Both continued to have orgasms, and both said that their sexual responsiveness after surgery was as great as it was before.

There also are established cases of women in whom an artificial vagina had to be created, because they were born without one. These women also are capable of reaching orgasm.

Apparently, it is lucky for us that most of our sex tissue is internal and can be stimulated by an almost infinite variety of methods.

It is clearly false to say "vaginal orgasm is a myth." But does the vagina contribute to sexual arousal? Or (as some sex researchers, most notably Kinsey, and some women have thought) does it have no feeling?

Yes, it does. Vaginal sensations are believed to be proprioceptive, which means that they are sensations resulting from a stimulus within our own bodies, not imposed from outside.

Close your eyes; extend an arm and bend it. If you can describe the position of your arm, if you know whether it is bent or straight, you are receiving and using proprioceptive information. Ordinarily, we do not pay much conscious attention to our proprioceptive intelligence, but without it we would not even be able to walk.

The vagina is most apt to develop proprioceptive abilities during states of sexual arousal and distention. In unaroused states, as, for example, when a gynecologist inserts a speculum, it may be quite unresponsive.

Obviously, there is a crucial distinction between motor experience (what's happening) and sensory experience (what we're aware of). Masters and Johnson do not always draw this distinction as sharply as many psychologists (and women) might wish.

Some orgasms seem to be experienced vaginally or deep in the vagina, while others seem to be in the clitoris. Some orgasms occur while direct clitoral stimulation is taking place, while others occur only with vaginal stimulation. The experts who have been discussing this have never even defined the terms "vaginal" and "clitoral" orgasm, and women could hardly be sure whether a clitoral orgasm meant an orgasm that was induced by clitoral stimulation, an orgasm that seemed to be experienced in the clitoris, or both.

The same woman may, at different times, experience orgasms in different locations or from different types of stimulation. Women know this, but as a rule men appear to have difficulty comprehending it. In 1968, Drs. Jules Glenn and Eugene Kaplan accused psychoanalysts of assuming, incorrectly, that clitorally stimulated orgasms are necessarily experienced clitorally. They said that their patients have reported a great variation in the location of the experienced orgasm. Occasionally, sites other that the vagina and clitoris (the abdomen, the anus) seem to be the focus of feeling. The area in which the orgasm is experienced need not be the area of stimulation, and there is great variation in the area or areas where orgasm is felt. The terms "vaginal orgasm" and "clitoral orgasm," according to Glenn and Kaplan have been "widely used but ill-defined."

The charge of technical rigidity is frequently leveled against not only writers of certain types of sex manuals, but also sex researchers, such as Kinsey, and Masters and Johnson.

There is a great deal that can be said against Masters and Johnson, and some of it has been said very well and very publicly. Among the many eloquent critics, Yale psychologist Kenneth Keniston has observed that Masters and Johnson are, although unintentionally, "helping to perpetuate rather than to remedy some of the more prevalent ills of our time—the confusion of human sexuality with the physiology of sexual excitement, naiveté with regard to the psychological meaning of the sexual act, and an inability to confront the ethical implications of sex." He also points out how little has been told of actual laboratory procedures and adds, "Masters and Johnson repeatedly reduce human sexuality to physical responses."

Dr. Natalie Shainess considers the Masters and Johnson view one in which "sex seems little more than a stimulus-response reflex cycle, devoid of intrapsychic or interpersonal meaning.... What is the attitude toward sex in a researcher who says, 'Masturbating women concentrate on their own sexual demand without the distraction of a coital partner'? Distraction! Is that the meaning of a partner in sex?"

But with all this, the fact remains that Masters and Johnson have recorded some sexual response cycles in women, and have done it in a way that helps clarify many issues for us. It is probably too much to ask that they be humanitarians and love advisers, as well as intrepid researchers.

Some of the anatomical details are interesting and useful to know, certainly for gynecologists and perhaps for women. And yet the interest we express in their work is, above all, a testament to the abysmal limits put on us by our own timidity.

Certain marriage counselors have long maintained that a loving wife is content merely to satisfy her husband, for instance, and that it need be of no consequence if she fails to achieve satisfaction. We have Masters and Johnson to thank for convincing them that sexual frustration can even give a woman cramps and headache. But how sad it is that we had to wait for sex researchers to demonstrate it. Didn't we know it all the time?

If there is going to be a breakthrough in human sexuality—and I think that such a breakthrough may be in the wind—it is going to occur because women will start taking charge of their own sex lives. It is going to occur because women will stop believing that sex is for men and that men (their fathers, their doctors, their lovers and husbands, their popes and kings and scientists) are the authorities. We need only study a little anthropology or history to understand that sexuality is incredibly plastic and easily repressed.

Women must discover and express their own sexuality, without shame or inhibition. And instead of following sex manuals or trusting the locker-room sexpertise of their fellows, men must learn to seek and receive signals from the women they love.

Shere Hite Debunks Freud's Vaginal Orgasm

SARAH J. SHEY

Excerpts from Shere Hite, *Women as Revolutionary Agents of Change: The Hite Reports and Beyond [WRAC]*, Madison, University of Wisconsin Press, 1993. Reprinted by permission.

With the publication of *The Hite Report on Female Sexuality* in 1976, Shere Hite killed Freud's notion of the superiority of the vaginal orgasm. Drs. William Masters and Virginia Johnson, Dr. Mary Jane Sherfey, Ann Koedt, Barbara Seaman, and, to some extent, even Dr. Alfred Kinsey had all challenged the "mature" orgasm that Freud popularized, but Hite's documentation—going beyond the handful of subjects Freud used to construct theories of women and distributing an essay questionnaire to 3,500 women on their sexuality—proved to be the psychoanalyst's undoing.

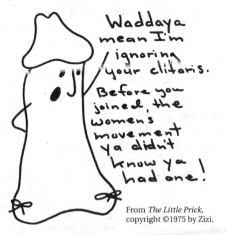

From *The Little Prick*, copyright ©1975 by Zizi.

Naomi Weisstein, scientist and author of *How Psychology Constructs the Female,* notes the astounding impact the Hite reports had when they were first published.

Hite... became involved with the feminist movement, and, taking seriously the idea that the personal is the political, undertook a major effort to find out what really happens in women's sexual lives.

From 1972 to 1976 she distributed a lengthy essay questionnaire to women all over the country; in 1976, on publication of the findings from the responses of 3,500 women, she explained her goals: "The purpose of this project is to let women define their own sexuality—instead of doctors or other (usually male) authorities. Women are the real experts on their own sexuality; they know how they feel and what they experience, without needing anyone to tell them.... In this study, for the first time, women themselves speak out about how they feel about sex, how they define their own sexuality, and what sexuality means to them. Hite's background in social and cultural history helped her to provide a cultural framework for this discussion, to see female sexuality for what it is, rather than how it fit into the prevalent patriarchal ideology.

Hite's basic finding was that 70 percent of women do not have orgasms from intercourse, but do have them from more direct clitoral stimulation. This testimony from thousands of women blew the lid off the question of female orgasm....

Hite's documentation with such a large sample of exactly how women do have orgasms easily—during self-stimulation—and that they do not usually have orgasms during simple intercourse without additional stimulation, as well as her declaration that there was nothing "wrong" with this, that if the majority of women said this, it must be "normal" for women—no matter what "professional sexologists" said— was, after an initial period of shock among some in the sex research community, accepted widely, and eventually Hite received the distinguished service award from the American Association of Sex Educators, Counselors and Therapists. (*WRAC,* 1993, pp. 1–3)

Hite herself enumerated the varied contributions of *The Hite Report on Female Sexuality* during a speech delivered to Harvard Forum in 1976, and again to the University of Pennsylvania in 1977.

The Hite Report on Female Sexuality is so long that very often it is understood on one level only. However, in reality there are three important levels on which to understand it. First, to hear women's voices on this subject is an historic breakthrough. Can you believe that, before this, we had almost no recorded descriptions of how orgasm feels to women, only how it feels to men? The second contribution of *The Hite*

Report on Female Sexuality is that it provides a new cultural and historical framework for the definition of physical relations as we know it, i.e., "sex." And finally, [it] provides many new findings for sex research, especially relating to how women achieve orgasm.

Perhaps one of the most widely publicized of those findings, and deservedly so, is that intercourse/coitus itself does not automatically lead to orgasm for most women. For centuries, women have been described as having "problems" with sex. However, it is now becoming clear that is not women who have a problem with sex, but the society that has a problem with its definition of sex, a definition that hurts both women and men, but a definition we can change. (*WRAC*, 1993, pp. 28–29)

It becomes useful, at this point, to look at some of the findings in *The Hite Report on Female Sexuality*, which would eventually become the first in a trilogy based on Hite's sex research.

1. MOST WOMEN DO NOT ORGASM AS A RESULT OF INTERCOURSE PER SE. The overwhelming majority of women require specific clitoral contact for orgasm. Women know how to orgasm whenever they want, easily and pleasurably, and women who masturbate can orgasm easily and regularly. Women are free to use this knowledge during sex with others. It is no more difficult for a woman to orgasm than for a man; women are not "dysfunctional" or slow to arouse—it is our definition of sex that makes women "dysfunctional."

In her latest book, *Women as Revolutionary Agents of Change*, Hite concludes that her earlier findings were essentially valid.

"If you don't have orgasms during intercourse, you're hung up." The influence of these psychiatric theories on women has been strong and pervasive. Whether or not a woman has been in analysis, she has heard these unfounded and anti-woman theories endlessly repeated—from women's magazines, popular psychologists, and men during sex. Everyone—of all classes, backgrounds, and ages—knows a woman should orgasm during intercourse. If she doesn't, she knows she has only herself and her own hang-ups to blame.

"I see my failure to have orgasms during intercourse as my failure largely, i.e., I've had plenty of men who were (1) adept, (2) lasted a long time, (3) were eager for my orgasm to occur, and (4) etc. but none of them were successful. I guess I have a fear of childbearing, a fear of responsibility—I don't know."

There was a lot of psychic jargon in the women's answers. The women may have been in therapy, but it's just as easy to pick up these terms from numerous articles by therapists and others in the women's magazines, and also from male "experts" with whom you may have "sex."

The idea that if we would "just relax and let go" during intercourse we would automatically have an orgasm is, of course, based on the fallacious idea that orgasm comes to us automatically by the thrusting penis, and all we have to do is to give ourselves over to what our bodies will naturally and automatically do—that is, orgasm. As one woman put it, "It's our fault that we can't be as natural as they are."…

Insisting that women should have orgasms during intercourse, from intercourse, is to force women to adapt their bodies to inadequate stimulation, and the difficulty of doing this and the frequent failure that is built into the attempt breeds recurring feelings of insecurity and anger. As Ann Koedt put it in *The Myth of the Vaginal Orgasm*: "Perhaps one of the most infuriating and damaging results of this whole charade has been that women who were perfectly healthy sexually were taught that they were not. So in addition to being sexually deprived, these women were told to blame themselves when they deserved no blame. Looking for a cure to a problem that has none can lead a woman on an endless path of self-hatred and insecurity. For she is told by her analyst that not even in her one role allowed in male society—the role of a woman—is she successful. She is put on the defensive, with phony data as evidence that she better try to be even more feminine, think more feminine, and reject her envy of men. That is: Shuffle even harder, baby."

Finally, there are two myths about female sexuality that should be specifically cleared up here.

First, supposedly women are less interested in sex and orgasms than men, and more interested in "feelings," less apt to initiate sex, and generally have to be "talked into it." But the reason for this, when it is true, is obvious: women often don't expect to, can't be sure to, have orgasms.

"I suspect that my tendency to lose interest in sex is related to my having suppressed the desire for orgasms, when it became clear it wasn't that easy and would 'ruin' the whole thing for him."

The other myth involves the mystique of female orgasm, and specifically the idea that women take longer to orgasm than men, mainly because we are more "psychologically delicate" than men, and our orgasm is more dependent on feelings. In fact, women do not take longer to orgasm than men. The majority of the women in Kinsey's study masturbated to orgasm within four minutes, similar to the women in this study. It is, obviously, only during inadequate or secondary, insufficient stimulation like intercourse that we take "longer" and need prolonged "foreplay." (WRAC, 1993, pp. 45–46)

2. DEFINING SEX AS "FOREPLAY" FOLLOWED BY INTERCOURSE TO MALE ORGASM IS A SEXIST DEFINITION OF SEX, WITH A CULTURAL, RATHER THAN A BIOLOGICAL, BASE. Historically, Hite wrote, this definition is only 3,000 years old. She reiterated this point in *Women as Revolutionary Agents of Change*:

There need not be a sharp distinction between sexual touching and friendship. Just as women described "arousal" as one of the best parts of sex, and just as they described closeness as the most pleasurable aspect of intercourse, so intense physical intimacy can be one of the most satisfying activities possible—in and of itself. (WRAC, 1993, p. 33)

3. **MEN MAKE THEIR OWN ORGASMS DURING SEX, AND WOMEN SHOULD BE ABLE TO ALSO.** Men should not be in charge of both their own and women's orgasms.

During "sex" as our society defines it both people know what to expect and how to make it possible for the man to orgasm. The whole thing is prearranged, preagreed.... But we can change this pattern, and redefine our sexual relations with others. On one level, we can take control over our own orgasms. We know how to have orgasms in masturbation. How strange it is, when you think about it, that we don't use this knowledge during so much of sex we have with men.... A man controls his own orgasm... [and] is not considered "selfish" or "infantile" because there is an ideology to back it up.

However, women, do not usually, are not supposed to, control their own stimulation:

"I have never tried to stimulate myself clitorally with a partner—I have always been afraid to."

"It seems too aggressive when I act to get the stimulation I want."...

There is no reason why making your own orgasms should not be as beautiful or as deeply shared as any other form of sex with another person—perhaps even more so. The taboo against touching yourself says essentially that you should not use your own body for your own pleasure, that your body is not your own to enjoy.... Controlling your own stimulation symbolizes owning your own body, and is a very important step toward freedom. (WRAC, 1993, pp. 61–62)

4. **AGE IS NOT A FACTOR IN FEMALE SEXUALITY.** "Older women are not less sexual than younger women, and they are often more sexual," she wrote. "Young women and girls are not less sexual than adults, but are often misinformed about the nature of their sexuality.... Girls are still being kept from finding out about, exploring, and discovering their won sexuality—and called 'bad girls' when they try. At puberty, girls are given information about their reproductive organs and menstruation, but rarely told about the clitoris!"

Ultimately, Hite wrote, the sexual revolution did not "free" women, but was, in many ways, a step backward for women:

The "sexual revolution" of the 1960s was a response to long-term social changes that affected the structure of the family and women's role in it. (Contrary to popular opinion, the birth control pill was more a technological response to these same social changes than their cause.) Up until the second half of this century, and throughout most periods of history, a high birth rate has been considered of primary importance by both individuals and society....

The change in the women's role was double-edged. In traditional terms, insofar as having many children had become less important, women's status declined. That is, since women had traditionally been seen almost completely in terms of their childbearing role, they themselves as a class became less important and less respected when that role was no longer so important. At the same time, it was said that, now that women were "free" from their old role, they could be "sexually free like men," etc.... However, as with the slaves after emancipation, becoming independent was easier said than done. In fact, women did not have equal opportunities for education or employment, and so they were stuck in their traditional role of being dependent on men. In spite of the so-called sexual revolution, women (feeling how peripheral, decorative, and expendable they had become to the over-all scheme of things) became more submissive to men than ever. This was even more true outside of marriage than inside, since marriage did offer some forms of protection in traditional terms. This increased submissiveness and insecurity was reflected in the child-like, baby-doll fashions of the 1960s—short little-girl dresses, long straight (blond) hair, big innocent (blue) eyes, and of course always looking as young and pretty as possible.... This situation eventually led to the women's movement of the late 1960s and 1970s, which was now trying to implement some of the positive potentials of the change in women's role, to make women truly independent and free. (WRAC, 1993, pp. 89–90)

Drawing from Hite's findings, Weisstein explored the traditional definition of sex and its lasting ramifications on women: "If women had been compelled to hide how they could easily reach orgasm during masturbation, then the definition of sex, it follows, is sexist and culturally linked.... *The Hite Report on Female Sexuality* linked the definition of sex as we know it to a particular society and historical cultural tradition, saying sex as we know it is created by our social system; it is a social institution." (*WRAC*, 1993, pp. 3–4)

Looking back, Hite says that she intended "not to create one new definition (i.e., redefinition) of sexuality but to allow for many—hence, 'undefining.'" *The Hite Report on Female Sexuality* allowed women to voice their opinions en masse on a subject that had been misconstrued for thousands of years. Women spoke—and women and men are listening. The revelatory undefining of sex is taking place.

The Sexuality Questionnaire

SHERE HITE

Shere Hite, ed., *Sexual Honesty: By Women for Women,* New York, Warner Books, 1974. Reprinted by permission.

INTRODUCTION

This book is a forum for our public discussion with each other of the nature of our sexuality, the first in a series intended for the reexamination and redefinition of our sexuality. We have never before attempted as a group to define or discover what the physical nature of our sexuality might be, and have in fact more or less just accepted the role which society handed to us. Never before have we tried to determine what feelings might lie buried beneath the layers and layers of myth we live by, or buried beneath the weight of the many "authoritative" books written by male "experts" who presume to tell us how we feel. It is time we made up our own minds, ended the ban on talking about sex, and came to terms with our own personal lives and how we intend to live them.

Most of the extant works on female sexuality contain distortions related to not knowing what female sexuality is about. The most damaging of this literature, often written by male doctors, is nothing more than the reiteration of "marriage manual" techniques for improving our "responsiveness," with some worn-out platitudes thrown in to "liberate" us from our "hang-ups." The most helpful of this literature has been the more scientific clinical studies, which, while in themselves valid and necessary, have also unfortunately been interpreted through the perspectives of unexamined preconceptions about our sexuality. There has rarely been any acknowledgment that female sexuality might have a nature of its own, which would involve more than merely being the logical counterpart of male sexuality. Actually, no one really knows much about the subject yet because women are just beginning to think about it. Therefore, even though some of these clinical efforts have been helpful, it is time women themselves spoke out and began to define their own sexuality.

What exactly is meant by "defining our own sexuality"? Perhaps we have become so submerged in our culture's idea of what we are supposed to be, that we have lost touch with what we really feel, and how to express it. So our first step, for which the questionnaires were designed, should be to try to get back in touch with our more instinctive feelings, and even perhaps to discover feelings never before articulated or consciously felt. Not only are we out of touch with ourselves, but we are also out of touch with each other, and with each other's feelings about sex, since no channels exist for communication on this subject. If we were lucky, our mothers or friends shared their experiences with us, but all too often this was not the case. Perhaps this lack of real information made us wonder if we were somehow "different" from other women. Furthermore, although the kind of material presented here is always part of the scientific investigation of sexuality, access to primary data is something the public is not ordinarily trusted with, and so even this possible channel of communication was closed off. With this book we have, perhaps for the first time, a means of sharing our feelings about sex and getting acquainted on a broad scale, a forum for discovering common experiences and needs, and for beginning the redefinition of who we are. Of course this book does not pretend to represent any kind of final definition of our sexuality, nor is it a statistical sample of all the replies received. It merely represents 45 out of the over 2,000 replies received to the questionnaires to date. Neither will this book be the end of our newly opened dialogue, but rather a beginning, as it will be followed by the publication of more of these answers, and eventually by the complete analysis of all the answers received. Therefore it is vitally important that you also participate in this discussion by sending in your own answers to the questions, and thus adding your own feelings to this redefinition.

The ultimate intention of this research is to formulate a critique of our current cultural definitions of sex, based on what we have all said. This book, to be published in 1975, perhaps together with some concluding original replies, will not be statistically oriented in that it will not attempt to correlate such things as age and background with attitude and "performance." Rather, it will attempt to answer the questions which formed the basis for this study, namely:

1. Insofar as we can possible know them, what are the "instinctive" (natural, not socially conditioned) physical expressions of our sexuality?

2. How do these compare with the basic physical activities we usually engage in?

3. What changes, based on the findings of (1) and (2), might we want to make in our sexual definitions and in our actual physical relations? What would be the implications of these changes for our present cultural definitions of sexuality, for the institutions related to them, and for men's perceptions of their own sexuality?

It does, even now, seem fairly clear that this reawakening of our sensitivity to what is instinctive and natural to us will be part of larger changes which involve not only such things as bedroom habits, but which will also have profound and far-reaching effects on all of our social relations.

SEXUALITY QUESTIONNAIRE II, JANUARY 1973

1. Is having sex important to you? What part does it play in your life?

2. Do you have orgasms? When do you usually have them? During masturbation? Intercourse? Clitoral stimulation? Other sexual activity? How often?

3. Is having orgasms important to you? Do you like them? Do they ever

bore you? Would you enjoy sex just as much without ever having them? Does having good sex have anything to do with having orgasms?

4. If you almost never or never have orgasms, are you interested in having them? Why or why not? If you are interested, what do you think would contribute to your having them? Did you ever have them?

5. Could you describe what an orgasm feels like to you? Where do you feel it, and how does your body feel during orgasm?

6. Is having orgasms somewhat of a concentrated effort? Do you feel one has to learn how to have orgasms?

7. Is one orgasm sexually satisfying to you? If not, how many? How many orgasms are you capable of? How many do you usually want? During masturbation? During clitoral stimulation with a partner? During intercourse?

8. Please give a graphic description or drawing of how your body could best be stimulated to orgasm.

9. Do you enjoy arousal? For its own sake—that is, as an extended state of heightened sensitivity not necessarily leading to orgasm? What does it feel like?

10. Do you like to remain in a state of arousal for indefinite or long periods of time? Or do you prefer to have arousal and orgasm in a relatively short period of time?

11. Do you ever go for long periods without sex? (Does this include masturbation or do you have no sex at all?) Does it bother you or do you like it?

12. How often do you desire sex? Do you actively seek it? Is the time of the month important? Do you experience an increase in sexual desire at certain times of the month?

13. Do you enjoy masturbation? Physically? Psychologically? How often? Does it lead to orgasm usually, sometimes, rarely, or never? Is it more intense with someone or alone? How many orgasms do you usually have?

14. What do you think is the importance of masturbation? Did you ever see anyone else masturbating? Can you imagine women you admire masturbating?

15. How do you masturbate? What is the sequence of physical events which occur? Please give a detailed description. For example, what do you use for stimulation—your fingers or hand or a vibrator, etc.? What kinds of motions do you make—circular, patting, up and down, etc.? Do you use two hands, or if not, what do you do with the other hand(s)? Where do you touch yourself? Does it matter if your legs are together or apart? Do you move very much? Etc.

16. What positions and movements are best for stimulating yourself clitorally with a partner? Do you have orgasms this way usually, sometimes, rarely, or never? Please explain ways your and your partner(s) practice clitoral stimulation. Can you think of other ways?

17. What other sexual play do you enjoy? Is it important for reaching orgasm? How important is kissing (mouth stimulation), breast stimulation, caressing of hips and thighs, general body touching, and etc.?

18. Do you like vaginal penetration/intercourse? Physically? Psychologically?

Why? Does it lead to orgasm usually, sometimes, rarely, or never? How long does it take? Do you ever have any physical discomfort? Do you usually have adequate lubrication? Do you ever have a decrease in vaginal-genital feeling the longer intercourse continues?

19. What kinds of movements do you find most stimulating during penetration—soft, hard, pressure to the back or front or neither, with complete oral partial penetration, etc.? Which positions do you find stimulating? Does the size and shape of penis or penetrating "object" matter to you?

20. Do you have intercourse during your period? Oral sex?

21. Is it easier for you to have an orgasm when intercourse is not in progress? In other words, do you have orgasms more easily by clitoral stimulation than intercourse? Are the orgasms different? How?

22. Do you enjoy cunnilingus? Do you have orgasms during cunnilingus usually, sometimes, never, or rarely? Do you have them during oral/clitoral or oral/vaginal contact or both? Explain what you like or dislike about it.

23. Do you use a vibrator to have orgasms? What kind of vibrator is it? At which body area(s) do you use it? Do you use it during masturbation or sexual play or intercourse or when? At other times?

24. Do you enjoy rectal contact? What kind? Rectal penetration?

25. What do you think about during sex? Do you fantasize? What about?

26. Does pornography stimulate you? What kinds? Which actions?

27. What do you think of sado-masochism? Of domination-submission? What do you think is their significance?

28. Do you prefer to do things to others or to have things done to you, or neither?

29. Which would cause you to become more excited—physical teasing, direct genital stimulation, or psychological "foreplay"?

30. Who sets the pace and style of sex—you or your partner? Who decides when it's over? What happens if your partner usually wants to have sex more often than you do? What happens if you want to have sex more often than your partner?

31. Do you usually have sex with the people you want to have sex with? Who usually initiates sex or a sexual advance—you or the other person?

32. Describe how most men and women have had sex with you (if there are any patterns, etc.).

33. Do most of your partners seem to be well informed about your sexual desires and your body? Are they sensitive to the stimulation you want? If not, do you ask for it or act yourself to get it? Is this embarrassing:

34. Do you feel guilty about taking time for yourself in sexual play which may not be specifically stimulating to your partner? Which activities are you including in your answer?

35. Are you shy about having orgasms with a partner? With only new partners or with everyone? Why?

36. Do you think your vagina and genital area are ugly or beautiful? Do you feel that they smell good?

37. Do you ever find it necessary to masturbate to achieve orgasm after "making love"?

38. How long does sex usually last?

39. Do you ever fake orgasms? During which sexual activities? How often? Under what conditions?

40. What would you like to try that you never have? What would you like to do more often? What changes would you like to make in the usual "bedroom" scene?

41. What were your best sex experiences?

42. How old were you when you had your first sexual experiences? With yourself? With another person? What were they? How old were you when you had your first orgasm? During what activity? At what age did you first look carefully at your vagina and genitals?

43. What is it about sex that gives you the greatest pleasure? Displeasure?

44. What can you imagine you would like to do to another person's body? How would you like to relate physically to other bodies?

45. Do you enjoy touching? Whom do you touch—men, women, friends, relatives, children, yourself, animals, pets, etc.? Does this have anything to do with sex?

46. How important are physical affection and touching for their own sakes (not leading to sex)? Do you do as much of them as you would like? Do you ever have sex with someone mainly to touch and be touched and be close to them? How often?

47. Do you ever touch someone for purposes of sensual arousal but not "real" sex? Please explain. (If desired, refer to question 9).

48. Is there is a difference between sex and touching? If so, what is that difference?

49. In the best of all possible worlds, what would sexuality be like?

50. Do you think your age and background make any difference as far as your sex life is concerned? What is your age and background education, upbringing, occupation, race, economic status, etc.?

51. Do you usually prefer sex with men, women, either, yourself, or not at all? Which have you had experience with and how much?

52. What do you think of the "sexual revolution"?

53. How does or did contraception affect your sexual life? Which methods have you used? Did you ever take birth control pills?

54. Do you feel that having sex is in any way political?

55. Have you read Masters' and Johnson's recent scientific studies or sexuality? Kinsey's? Others? What did you think of them?

56. Please add anything you would like to say that was not mentioned in this questionnaire.

57. How did you like the questionnaire?

Chapter 46

Motherhood

*S*ometimes a work of fiction may convey truths that are impossible to expli-
cate in a non-fiction form. Alix Kates Shulman's Memoirs of an Ex-Prom
Queen *remains one of the most beloved novels of women's liberation, and
expresses how obsessive and frightened a new mother may really feel. Her latest
book,* A Good Enough Daughter, *is about her parents. Letty Pogrebin, president
of the Author's Guild at this writing, has consistently given us lovely non-fiction
on many aspects of motherhood and childcare, and, by personal example, has
set the world on notice that feminists need by no means be anti-child or anti-
family. Barbara Katz Rothman, past president of Sociologists for Women in
Society, is another eloquent advocate for mothers.*

*Doris Haire is one more "heroic antecedent." In the early 1950s she delivered
her daughter by natural childbirth at a hospital in Pittsfield, Mass. She was able
to do this only because her husband worked for the Vanderbilt family, who were
hospital trustees. Part Cherokee, and born to a working class family in Oklahoma,
the special privilege she enjoyed made Doris feel "spoiled and guilty." "Why," she
asked herself, "must you be friendly with Ann Vanderbilt to get the right to natural childbirth?" Doris, an early president of the National Women's Health Network,
has devoted her life to safer childbirth and to childbirth choice.* The Cultural
Warping of Childbirth *is a tremendously influential document, the basis of FDA
actions, Congressional Hearings, and many popular books and articles.*

*Molly Haskell, the film critic, reminds us how much heat there used to be on
women to raise families. Another victory for the women's movement is that now
this matter is regarded as the woman's own business, not society's. "Yes, We Have*

No Bambinos," along with many other feminist pieces of significance appeared, oddly enough, in Viva, a sophisticated woman's magazine published in the 1970s by Bob Guccione. He hired feminists editors, most notably Patricia Bosworth, the biographer, and Betty Jean Raphael. The magazine also contained some extraordinary woman-oriented erotic art and photography.—B. S.

Motherhood

LETTY COTTIN POGREBIN

Letty Cottin Pogrebin, "Motherhood," *Ms.*, May 1973. Reprinted by permission.

I'd like to interview everybody," I announce at a recent meeting of our women's group. "I'm writing an article on motherhood."

"Oh God," my friends respond. "How boring! How old hat! How *could* you!"

One evening at the dinner table I question my children about their thoughts on motherhood.

"Is that like Robin Hood?" asks my 5-year-old son.

One 3-year-old daughter assumes an angelic expression and recites: "Motherhood is a great thing because a mother is a person's very best relative."

"A mother is someone who looks good in hoods," offers her twin sister, overjoyed at her own wit.

My husband shifts the conversation to a more pressing problem: "Now let's see if we can't all agree," he begins patiently, "that a family in midtown Manhattan has no business buying a hunting dog."

During the next several weeks I declare to every woman I meet that I need some input on motherhood. A couple of young unmarried friends admit that they're afraid to have children. It seems too difficult, too demanding.

A mother of teenagers confirms that kids are not easy but, for her, life would be incomplete without them.

"I don't think motherhood is for me," says a married woman who is childless at age 31. "At least not until I feel that fatherhood will really mean something to my husband."

"I want to have children whether I have a husband or not," declares a single woman who has given the subject much thought.

A mother who is also a lesbian states flatly: "I wouldn't have missed having and living with my child for anything in the world."

"I believe you can mother problems and projects if you're not the type who can mother kids," explains a busy activist. "But I admire someone who enjoys motherhood and does it well."

As I listen I think about how these statements would surprise the many people who seem to believe (with the aid of media distortion) that the women's movement is rabidly antimotherhood. In some minds, the all-purpose "women's libber" is either a self-serving single career girl who has an abortion every spring, or a Marxist lesbian who hates men, motherhood, and the flag.

Sure, there are a small number of radical women who argue that total biological equality between the sexes could be brought about by the development of test-tube pregnancies and the elimination of marriage, the nuclear family, and even "childhood" itself. However repellent this may seem to some, many people are intellectually engaged by the political ramifications of such visionary social changes. But the bottom line is that these few of our revolutionary sisters usually deliver themselves of opinions, not babies.

The rest of us, scores of feminists of every age, race, marital status, and sexual persuasion are talking seriously, thoughtfully, and candidly about motherhood.

We either have children already or wish to retain that option in our life spans. We care deeply about children whether we have our own or not. We work to improve educational curricula, child-care facilities, health services, and the childbirth experience. We are saying that men are parents, too; that fatherhood need be no less important or time-consuming than motherhood. We are examining the guilt feelings that force us into involuntary servitude in the home. Fears about the loss of our freedom; skepticism about our readiness for sharing that responsibility equally—all these serpentine doubts are writhing out in the open where we can get a grip on them.

We are trying, too, to make peace with the fecund wombs that have been used by sexist society to prove our weakness—sometimes a prideful peace and sometimes a peace of resignation. Most of us choose to see the female's "inner space" as a physiological reality, not an internal psychic or spiritual void. We refuse to believe that women are hollow shells unless and until we have brought forth issue.

Truly, feminists are talking about choice: about *making* the decision to become pregnant and *choosing* a motherly role that is right for ourselves and our children.

It sounds simple. And logical. Yet, in this area, the notion of choice is a new one for our generation. In the minds of so many women, motherhood is prescribed; nonmotherhood is deviate. Childless women are to be pitied. Motherhood is synonymous with womanhood (in a way that fatherhood has never been considered sufficient to fulfill a man or to prove manhood). Caring for a child is, in the old view, a shortcut to self-respect, maturity, and even martyrdom. For women who grew up believing in the inevitability of motherhood, the notion of choice is in itself disturbing and heretical. And so, when these women try to relate to the movement—no matter how much they may agree with its pragmatic goals—there is a point of alienation.

"Women's liberation makes me feel defensive about being a mother," my neighbor tells me. "I think feminists are looking at me and thinking: Is that all she can do?"

A woman at our local playground solemnly questions the loss of distinctions: "Once the nurturant role was woman's manifest destiny. Now psychologists are disproving the maternal instinct, and new fathers are demanding paternity leaves. Will there be anything special left for women?"

"I've come full circle right back to where my Victorian grandmother was," says a pregnant friend with a toddler on each hand. "Granny had to hide her condition out of modesty. My belly is embarrassing in 1973 because it labels me a population exploder or an exploited baby machine."

I am troubled by this new lament. It seems to proclaim that women are divided on the point that should most unite us. Right now, a discussion of motherhood can shake sisterhood to its roots. There is intransigence and enmity. The extremists' requiem for motherhood is premature; the traditionalists' Hallelujah Chorus is anachronistic. Yet no one seems able to orchestrate an ideology about motherhood that plays right for both audiences.

At this point in my investigations I become convinced that if anything can be said at this time about being a mother and a committed feminist, it must be no more ambitious and no less honest than a personal commentary—even if it comes out disconnected, vulnerable, and frankly sentimental.

I have found myself, now and then, in fierce arguments with people who can see no merit whatsoever in having children. These are not the proponents of zero population growth; they are arguing as if they believe in zero population. And no matter how I resolve never to proselytize parenthood, I find myself extolling the joys of a small child's smile in answer to their accusations that I produce offspring to guarantee my own immortality. (Since I have a profession, I am spared the aspersions about substituting procreative for creative energy. But those guns are at the ready for women not presently gainfully employed.)

The plot thickens. While the militant childless may have no ideological sympathy with the women's movement, they freely borrow and distort whatever feminist rhetoric is serviceable.

Under attack I begin to understand how, without its nuances explained, any monolithic party line can make women defensive and hostile. Because I am a mother of three, I make a clear target for the militant childless. And I realize that everything I say about the meaning of children in my life becomes a platitude echoing Sophie Portnoy or Rose Kennedy. It gives one pause.

Can we verbalize some of the components of motherhood or does analysis of the parts tend to trivialize the whole? If one has never known thunderous fear when a child is lost in a crowd, or shared the sweet intensity of a small boy's secret, or felt the blissful vertigo of a little girl's first bicycle solo, then explaining mother love—or father love, for that matter (though here I must speak only for myself)—will be rather like explaining the sea to a landlocked people. One puts sand in their palms and conchs to their ears and trusts the rest to human imagination.

I cry in natural childbirth movies. When the baby's head emerges, I want to cheer. The appearance of shoulders and arms makes me laugh, and finally the sight of the entire tiny creature bathed in primal slime moves me to awe, and more tears and whispered sobs about God and miracles. My emotional upheaval always peaks at that excruciatingly tender moment when the mother first sees her baby—still anchored to her by a twisted cord, but real, alive, and bawling triumphantly. It is a moment I profoundly missed in my first childbed.

Of necessity, cesarean sections are somewhat impersonal and antiseptic. So it was only after the total anesthesia wore off that my twins were brought to my hospital room in wheeled carts, and I saw my babies for the first time just as any visitor could have seen them: placid dolls sponged clean and swathed in neat bunting wraps. I remember nothing of their grand entrance into life; it could have been the stork that brought them after all.

Women who adopt their babies report that the life-cycle shock of motherhood can happen the instant your child is placed in your arms. In my case, missing the actual birth made the advent of motherhood seem remote and unreal. All I know is I badly needed a mother during 13 hours of labor. Next thing I was a mother myself. Perhaps the problem was that I was drugged during the drama of transition. Or maybe the fault lay with my preconceptions of what it would feel like to be a mother. Like many women, I had shaped a transcendent ideal out of my childhood image of my own mother. And I truly believed that ripeness, solidity, and wisdom would gestate within me along with the fetus, and that I would give birth to my own adult persona at the same time as I delivered my first child.

Well, it didn't happen that way. My first child was children, plural—which may have crowded out the gestating persona—and the fully mature mother I intended to be never quite materialized.

Next time around I refused to undergo childbirth *in absentia*. Although my third child also had to be delivered surgically, this cesarean was by appointment, and I insisted upon an anesthetic that would allow me to remain numb but conscious. My view was obscured by a tent of green sheets until the doctor yanked out the baby and hoisted him up in the air like a victory banner. True to form, I cried and laughed, clapped and whooped until the doctor warned that my display was making it impossible to suture the incision. He ordered a mask of gas to put me out of my ecstasy.

This time, because I had witnessed the birth I expected to wake up feeling transformed at last. But watching my son taken from my body like a vital organ did not change my perception of myself as unalterably unmotherly; motherhood as a state of mind was no more palpable than before.

Since then the years have passed cheerfully. I'm having a terrific time with my children and they claim I'm a good mother. I gladly answer when someone calls, "Mom." But I can't help feeling still that a mother is someone you *have*, not someone you *are*. Knowing myself since childhood, I simply cannot fit myself into my own abstraction of a Mother. I suppose the only one who ever could was my own mother. And perhaps that is as it should be after all.

If the truth were known, all parents have their favorite child-development state. Infancy was my least favorite period. I find that the more expressive and independent my kids become, the more I enjoy being with them.

Of course I know that nonverbal communication can be full of feeling and that caring and ministering to a baby is a kind of interchange. But personally, I have never been particularly gratified by dependency. I get no satisfaction out of being needed by someone who is totally powerless. (By contrast, one of my friends says she never thought of herself as independent until she had someone she knew was dependent on her. She views her babies as living proof that she is important and competent.) In my opinion, however, once a child can say "I think" or "I won't," the mother/child axis becomes more balanced, complex, and interesting.

Naturally, infancy is a period of justifiable dependency, and during my children's earliest months, I responded to their needs without resentment. But feeding, bathing, burping, or diapering aren't acts of love. They are functions one performs lovingly for a child (and I believe mothers, fathers, or surrogates can perform them); they are not the best that motherhood has to offer. To call them rewarding, or to romanticize them in Pampers, Gerber's, or Ivory Soap commercials is to mislead women (and men) and to risk starting parenthood with disillusionment.

The mother who glorifies and prolongs infancy may be clinging to her one opportunity to exercise control. In a world that disapproves of women in positions of authority, she is allowed and encouraged to be "in charge" of the children. Her helpless children are "her job." When they leave infancy, their growth toward self-sufficiency is a rebuke to the mother's indispensability and an erosion of her "job." Because the dependency mechanism can be habit-forming, it seems to me we must learn to love our children enough to let them grow away from us. And value ourselves enough so there is something left over when they leave.

Living with children has humanized me. Though I cannot claim an undifferentiated appreciation of all kids, the existence of my own children gives me a personalized empathy with the children of others.

The sterilized news of Vietnam couldn't disguise the fact that "defoliation" meant crops were being destroyed, and children were starving; "pacification" meant homes were leveled, families displaced; "accidental civilian casualties" meant babies had been maimed and slaughtered.

Everywhere—in the bizarre and the commonplace—I am sensitive to the discomforts of the children. In restaurants I see them hushed up and scowled upon. On public streets I see them slapped or dragged along disdainfully. In friends' homes I see them roughly scolded in the name of the parents' standards but without regard for the children's dignity. All too often, in the presence of the young, adults smile "Partridge Family" smiles and talk in condescending clichés. I don't remember noticing any of this eight years ago, before the children came.

Having children has also revitalized my sense of the future. I feel a greater responsibility for my own survival—not because "my children *need* me" but because I am deeply curious about the unseen scenario for all five of us. There is a difference, though, between my concept of future for the children and the one I attempt to contemplate for my husband and myself.

For example, since I am still in my early thirties, becoming 40 is an abstraction. I can only try to imagine how it will feel and what I will want to do and be. I have never been 40 before. But when my children turn 12 or 17 years old, I shall have a million points of reference. I have been there before. And no matter how the children choose to design those years for themselves, I will always have a sense of my own participation in an observed future that is more familiar than my own. I enjoy being a witness to the possibilities.

Which is not to say that I want to mold their lives in my image or to make my children, at 12 or 17, all the things I couldn't be. It seems to me one can share and enhance a child's life without dominating it. As one mother puts it: "I am not a sculptor who molds a child from clay. I'm the gardener who tends a seed that will grow to become itself." Another metaphor maker compares the process to apprenticeship: the protégée (child) lives with the sponsor (parent) in order to benefit from experience, minimize stress, and become professional at living in this world.

Childhood, I believe, is something one can experience twice. The first time directly, with growing pains and discovery, frustration and endless wonder. Living through childhood as a child is the universal purgatory, for our first real childhood is not ours to control. But our children's childhood is our second chance. And if we have kept our memories sharp and sensitive, we can help support a more endurable purgatory for our daughters and sons than the one we remember distilled in nightmares and dreams.

"Let's have a private talk, Mom."

It's an invitation I cherish. One child and I, without distractions; we banish other family members, close the door, lounge upon the big bed, and prop ourselves against the pillows. We are close. Trusting. A time for emotional refueling. Or for venting anger. Occasionally, one child simply wants to boast to me about something the others might call bragging or teasing. But most often we meet behind closed doors to discuss disappointment, confusion, and fear.

"When they said we had eight and a half players on our side, I knew I was the half, Mom, 'cause I was the only girl on the team."

I remember how it feels to be "just a girl" when boys are choosing up sides. (It still happens to me now, as a woman among men.) I remember once playing hide-and-seek. Secluded behind a wooden fence, I waited endless minutes for the boys to find me. Finally I understood that I had been tricked; they had run away to play without me.

After our talk I ask you to read aloud to me because it is your certain skill and I know no other child your age who can read with the exuberance that you give to a story you love. And a few days from now we will go to Central Park and we will throw baseballs and run and bat the ball into the trees until you feel strong and whole again.

"Mommy, I feel like sleeping with the lamp on tonight."

You were upset today when we saw war protestors lying in the street. And you were troubled when I explained that this was a symbolic reminder of real people dying in a faraway land. I know it is on your mind and you are frightened. Long ago, my father had an air-raid helmet, and my mother doused the lights, and we practiced being bombed in New York City. That was 1944, but I have not forgotten that a child doesn't always know how to tell what is real from what is make-believe.

"Did you get undressed in the bathroom when you and Daddy first had sexible intercourse?"

I tell you there are times when we display our bodies proudly, like poems that we have written to read aloud to someone we love. You confide your confusion: What about privacy? Why do women cover their breasts? Why do boys laugh when they see a girl's underwear? You ask why you sometimes feel ashamed. There's so much you want me to explain but, I suspect, in my way I'm as muddled as you. I teach you to feel food about your body, and yet I say you cannot lie naked in the sun. I explain that some people are perverted, and others are easily offended. Can I possibly make sense of it? In this second chance at childhood, I hack through a forest of sexual memories to clear a path for you that is not as tangled as my own was. I try not to fumble, although it's very difficult and I am not sure of myself. But for you, perhaps there should be less modesty so that there will be less shame.

I have often asked my mother-in-law for her secret.

"How did you raise him? What did you do that was different?"

I'm looking for a clue to explain why my husband is so easy to live with. It would be immensely helpful to me in raising my own son if I could know how my husband's mother produced a male with such a generous spirit, so innate a respect for women, such an absence of *macho* tensions, so much humor and love to give to me and the children. My mother-in-law shrugs. She claims the only secret she can pass along to me concerns the making of perfect stuffed cabbage.

When I ask my husband about his childhood, he tells me that he and his father always did the vacuuming.

I find both answers a trifle too glib. What I need is a signal that I'm on the right track with my son. While his father is a direct model, I also seek a special kind of relationship with our little boy. I'd like to avoid the classic conflicts and all the small-scale sex-role charades that I've seen mothers and sons act out over the years. So for the time being I have decided not to differentiate between my daughters and my son in the way I love and counsel them. With each of the three I have an organic mothering relationship that defines itself in new ways all the time.

Still, I wonder. How do you help a boy to be confident but not arrogant? How do you teach reason and compassion in a world where masculinity is equated with violence? As a woman, a feminist, and a mother, I have a certain mandate: what I transmit via example—and what my husband transmits via attitude—will affect my son's experience with women and men for the rest of his life. Together, his father and I will establish for him what we believe manhood is all about.

When my son bullies his two older sisters, I sometimes question whether aggression may be inborn after all. When he points a carrot at me and shouts, "Pow! You're dead!"—I feel I'm not getting through. And when he announces to our role-free household "Daddy's the boss," I'm totally baffled.

But there are times when he loses himself in painting or requests *The Nutcracker Suite* for his bedtime record or spends long periods playing gently with his infant cousin, that I decide he is a well-balanced short person indeed. The other day I even had a glimpse of a brave new world in which children will choose freely what they like to do and want to be; a world where competence and interest are not sex-typed quantities but are uncensored expressions of the self.

I had brought home several new things that the girls needed for school: paraffin, notepads, some colored yarn. My son looked up from his caravan of toy trucks, saw the haul of packages, and whined: "That's not fair! There's nothing for me." I told him we might get him something one day soon and asked what he'd like to have.

"A sewing kit," he said.

Time and again when I lecture, I am introduced as a "wife and mother of three." That credential precedes me to the podium like a disclaimer on the label of a dangerous drug—as though the audience could not tolerate a dose of feminist opinion without marriage and motherhood to make it palatable.

Isn't it obvious that by categorizing one another in opposing terms such as "career gal" or "working mother," we perpetuate the straitjacketing roles that limit women's lives? When was the last time we heard a serious male speaker introduced to an audience as "husband and father of three"? Who calls a businessman a "career guy" or "working father"? Sexist semantics is the verbal shorthand for sexist institutions. It's time we all kicked the habit.

I find it remarkable that traditional women's groups only ask to know that I am a mother—not whether I am a good mother or a happy mother. Once assured that I am one of them, however, an extraordinary thing happens: they then insist that I be *better* than they. If they can believe that I am superwoman and supermother, then they can exempt themselves from what I may say about self-actualization, expanded options, and women's participation in social change. They would like some proof that I am special—more educated, organized, energetic, younger, older, calmer—so that they can deny our commonality. It is a crafty device to protect themselves from identifying with what I have to say.

But I refuse to play that game. When they ask me how I "manage," instead of how I feel or think, I point out that their question betrays something like my own tendency to make motherhood fit an abstraction. I tell them that there is no right answer; I am not special; I don't have the formula for perfect motherhood. I am only trying to work it all out for myself and my children.

We all carry the secret fear that every other woman is doing a better job of it and only we are failures at "managing." It is one of our many common obsessions.

Pity. If only we could talk together about guilt and resentment, frenzy and frustration, devotion and love, then perhaps we could begin to arrive at the truth about our children and our lives. Unless we demythologize motherhood for all women, there will always be suffering for those who fear to be Gorgons, and despair for those who expect to be goddesses.

I came to terms with motherhood when one of my plainspoken daughters asked me the ultimate question. It was an average Saturday. Chaos was loose in the house. My husband was grumbling about a troublesome legal issue while trying to dress our son for a birthday party. I was alternately wrapping the birthday gift, working at the typewriter, and helping one daughter to make papier-maché.

Then the other daughter began complaining. She was bored. *No one* was paying attention to her. When would *somebody* have time to play with her. Totally frazzled, I explained that after her father took her brother to the party, he was going to the library to do some research. I had an article deadline to meet and would be at my desk all afternoon with the door closed. It was up to each girl to find activities for herself. No loud noise please. No interruptions. No fussing!

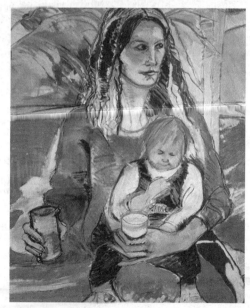

That was when she asked, "Did you ever wish you never had us in the first place?"

I think I became partially paralyzed. Guilt flooded my cheeks with blood. The glands in my neck seemed suddenly swollen. I've scarred her, I thought: I've made her feel like a burden—unwanted, unloved, rejected. Then I realized she was waiting for an answer. We both deserved to know the truth. I sorted my ragged thoughts and took her onto my lap. Gentleness

Lady Madonna by Jeri Drucker.

wrapped around us like a fog. When I finally spoke, I believe I was answering an unasked question in my soul.

"Sometimes my life is a little too full because I have you children," I said, "but, for me, it would be much too empty if I didn't."

The Cultural Warping of Childbirth

DORIS HAIRE

Excerpted from Doris Haire, *The Cultural Warping of Childbirth: A Special Report to the International Childbirth Education Association*. Originally published in *ICEA News*, Spring 1972. Reprinted by permission.

While Sweden, Finland, and the Netherlands compete for the honor of having the lowest incidence of infant deaths per 1,000 live births, the United States continues to find itself outranked by 14 other developed countries.

Several explanations for our poor national infant outcome have been advanced. Some try to explain our poor standing on the grounds that our statistics are more reliable, but according to the Statistical Office of the United Nations our statistics are no more accurate than those of other countries listed in all of which use the same U.N. standard for "live birth" without regard for gestational age or birthweight, and most of which collect their statistics on a uniform basis through their national health services. Analyses by Chase of the United States Public Health Service and more recently by Wegman, writing in *Pediatrics* acknowledge slight variations in the collection of this data but report that, when cross checked by other statistical data, the variations do not significantly alter the statistics.

In light of the fact that in most of the other listed countries there is no strong feeling of obligation to use extraordinary measures to preserve life when a live birth results in extreme prematurity, severe congenital malformation, or impairment, their incident of infant mortality should be greater than ours, not less.

No one will dispute the fact that socioeconomic factors play a significant role in any infant mortality statistics. However, research has demonstrated that among mothers of the lower socioeconomic groups infant outcome can be substantially improved by changing the pattern of obstetrical care offered these mothers during labor and birth.

There is no question that the welfare of their patients has always been the deep concern of American physicians, nurse-midwives, and nurses. The unphysiological practices which have become so much a part of American obstetric care—to the point where such practices have been generally accepted as normal accompaniments of birth—appear to have gradually built up as a result of social customs and cultural patterning. But cultural patterning can be changed if mothers can be helped to recognize the importance of their accepting some inconvenience and discomfort (and at times pain) in order to achieve the best possible birth and good health for their babies.

Educating mothers for the childbearing experience and improving the quality of emotional support given to mothers during labor and birth have been clearly demonstrated to lessen or eliminate the mother's need for obstetrical medication and obstetrical intervention during labor and birth. The benefit of individualized emotional support and care during this time of stress was made evident in a report by Levy, who notes that during a two-year medically directed, nurse-midwifery program carried out in California, in which nurse-midwives were employed to provide complete care for normal maternity patients, the incident of infant deaths decreased significantly. In order to avoid the inference that it was the additional access to prenatal care alone which made the difference in infant mortality Levy compared the incidence of infant deaths among women who had had *no prenatal care at all* before, during, and following the pilot program. He found that the incidence of infant deaths among mother who had had NO prenatal care at all, but who were attended during labor and birth by a nurse-midwife, dropped significantly during the nurse-midwifery program and then almost doubled when the nurse-midwifery program ended. Across the continent the success of the California nurse-midwifery program has been essentially duplicated by the Frontier Nursing Service in remote Leslie County, Kentucky, one of the poorest counties in Appalachia.

Obviously we cannot produce enough nurse-midwives overnight to fill the demand, but we can do much to improve our incidence of infant mortality and morbidity by maximizing the emotional support offered the childbearing woman in order that she may cope with the discomfort of labor and birth with a minimum of medication and its attendant hazards.

A spokesman for the National Foundation March of Dimes recently stated that according to the most recent data, the United States leads all developed countries in the rate of infant death due to birth injury and respiratory distress such as postnatal asphyxia and atelectasis.

According to the National Association for Retarded Children, there are now 6 million retarded children and adults in the United States, with a predicted annual increase of over 100,000 a year. The number of children and adults with behavioral difficulties or perceptual dysfunction resulting from minimal brain damage is an ever growing challenge to society and to the economy. While it may be easier on the conscience to blame such numbing facts solely on socioeconomic factors and birth defects, recent research makes it evident that obstetrical medication can play a role in our staggering incidence of neurological impairment. It may be convenient to blame our relatively poor infant outcome on a lack of facilities or inadequate government funding, but it is obvious from the research being carried out that we would effect an immediate improvement in infant outcome by changing the pattern of obstetrical care in the United States. It is time that we take a good look at the overall experience of childbirth in this country and begin to recognize how our culture has warped this experience for the majority of American mothers and their newborn infants.

As an officer of the International Childbirth Education Association (ICEA) I have visited hundred of maternity hospitals throughout the world—in Great Britain, western Europe, Russia, Asia, Australia, New Zealand, the South Pacific, the Americas, and Africa. During my visits I was privileged to observe obstetric techniques and procedures and to interview physicians, professional midwives, and parents in the various countries. My companion on many of my visits was Dorothea Lang, CNM (certified nurse-midwife), Director of Nurse-Midwifery for New York City. Miss Lang's experience as both a nurse-midwife and a former head nurse of the labor and delivery unit of the New York–Cornell Medical Center made her a particularly well-qualified observer and companion. As we traveled from country to country certain patterns of care soon became evident. For one, in those countries which enjoy an incidence of infant mortality and birth trauma significantly lower than that of the United States, highly trained professional midwives are an important source of obstetrical care and family planning services for normal women, whether the births take place in the hospital or in the home. In these countries the expertise of the physician is called upon only when the expectant mother is ill during pregnancy or when labor or birth is anticipated to be, or is found to be abnormal. Under this system the high-risk mother—the one who is most likely to bear an impaired or stillborn child—has a better opportunity to obtain in-depth medical attention than is possible under our existing American system of obstetrical care where the obstetrician is also called upon to play the role of midwife.

Deprivation, birth defects, prematurity, and low birthweight are not unique to the United States. While it is tempting to blame our comparatively high incidence of infant mortality solely on a lack of available prenatal care and on socioeconomic factors, our observations indicate that, comparatively, the prenatal care we offer most clinic patients in the United States is not grossly inferior to that available in other developed countries. Furthermore, the diet and standard of living in many countries which have a lower incidence of infant mortality than ours would be considered inadequate by American standards.

As an example, when one compares the availability of prenatal care, the incidence of premature births, the average diet of various economic groups, and the equipment available to aid in newborn infant survival in two such diverse countries as the United States and Japan, there are no major differences between the two countries. The differences lie in (1) our frequent use of prenatal and obstetrical medication, (2) our pathologically oriented management of pregnancy, labor, birth, and postpartum, and (3) the predominance of artificial feeding in the United States, as opposed to Japan.

If present statistics follow the trend of recent years, an infant born in the United States is more than four times more likely to die in the first day of life than an infant born in Japan. But survival of the birth process should not be our singular goal. For every American newborn infant who dies there are likely to be several who are neurologically damaged because the major differences in infant mortality between the United States and Japan are represented our by comparatively high incidence of infant deaths due to birth injury and respiratory distress, such as postnatal asphyxia and atelectasis, conditions which are more likely to occur if the mother has received obstetrical medication. The better records of infant outcome in Japan is even more dramatic when one considers that, according to a recent report by the Japanese Ministry of Health, the maternal death rate due to toxemia is 5 times greater in Japan than in the United States. Whether this is due to diet or lifestyle is not yet scientifically established.

Most American mothers do not, as yet, realize that the management of labor is even more important than the management of birth in determining how an infant will fare, not only during the first critical hours but perhaps throughout life. A poorly managed labor can result in an infant who shows no signs of respiratory distress and who scores well on the Apgar scale, while, in fact, a more scientific evaluation of the infant's condition may indicate lingering signs of oxygen deprivation in utero resulting from obstetrical medication administered to the mother.

Hellman and Pritchard state that the respiratory center of the infant is highly vulnerable to sedative and anesthetic drugs administered to the mother and that such medication may jeopardize the initiation of respiration of the infant at birth. They point out that sluggish respiration is observed to some extent in the majority of infants whose mothers received sedation during labor. The added burden on the newly born infant of having to detoxify indirectly acquired obstetrical medication as he adjusts to extrauterine life is the subject of abundant scientific literature in the past and present.

An outstanding monograph entitled "Effects of Obstetrical Medication on Fetus and Newborn," June 1970, published by the Society for Research in Child Development, makes it evident that we can no longer assume that the apparent recovery of an asphyxiated infant after successful resuscitation is a guarantee that the infant has come through unharmed. (This monograph should be required reading for all obstetrical personnel.) A baby with a heartbeat after cardiac massage may appear to be recovered but, in fact, may be irreversibly brain damaged. Virtually all obstetrical medications—nausea remedies, diuretics, sedatives, muscle relaxants, analgesics, regional anesthesia, and general anesthetics —tend to rapidly cross the placenta and alter the fetal environment as they enter the circulatory system of the unborn infant within seconds or minutes of administration to the mother. As Dr. Virginia Apgar bluntly puts it, the placenta is not a barrier but a "bloody sieve."

If prolapse of the umbilical cord or premature separation of the placenta occurs during labor, the fetus is compromised. If obstetrical medication is administered to the mother during labor and either of these conditions occurs, this compounds the danger to the unborn infant. No one can guarantee the mother that such conditions will not occur.

While respiratory distress is one of the more obvious hazards of obstetrical medication, the more subtle effects of such medications are now being noted. Sedatives containing barbiturates administered to the mother during labor have been shown to adversely affect the infant's suckling reflexes for four or five days after birth. The prolonged effects of some commonly used obstetrical medications, such as meperidine (Demerol), have been detected in the infant several weeks after birth.

Regional anesthesias appears to be an improvement over general anesthesia, but research indicates that even in the most dedicated hands regional anesthesias can compromise the mother and her infant. All regional anesthesias, including pudendal block, tend to alter the fetal environment and to inhibit the mother's ability to push her baby down the birth canal, which in turn, tends to increase the need for fundal pressure, uterine stimulants, and forceps extraction—conditions which should be avoided if possible in the best interests of the child. L. Stanley James, chairman of the Committee on Fetus and Newborn of the American Academy of Pediatrics, cautions, "Regional techniques are gaining popularity but they are not without problems." He points out that it is difficult to give spinal anesthesia—caudal, epidural, or saddle block—without any change in maternal blood pressure, and that even if pressure is restored by the use of vasopressors, there is no assurance that regional circulation through the uterus remains normal.

Because he must fill the role of both obstetrician and midwife, the overburdened American obstetrician frequently manages his maternity patient's labor by telephone and arrives at the hospital shortly before a birth is anticipated. This type of management must depend on reports from the mother's labor attendant, who may or may not have had specialized training in evaluating the effects of labor and obstetrical medication on both the mother and her unborn infant. But in countries which enjoy a lower incidence of infant mortality than ours it is the hospital-assigned, professional midwife who manages the prenatal care, labor, birth, and postpartum care of the normal mother and the care of the normal newborn infant. The professional midwife receives special training in maintaining the delicate physiologic balance between mother and child during labor and birth, and is trained to recognize conditions which require the medical expertise of the physician.

Because the professional midwife also is involved in the postpartum care of the infant, and not just labor and delivery, she is fully aware of the importance of providing individualized and skillful emotional support for the laboring mother as a means of reducing or eliminating the mother's need for obstetrical medication, with its possible narcotizing effect on the fetus and newborn infant.

The active encouragement of breast-feeding by the professional midwife also appears to affect the incidence of infant mortality in the various countries, for in those countries such as Sweden, the Netherlands, and Japan, where breast-feeding is still the predominant pattern of initial infant feeding, the incidence of infant mortality is significantly lower than in those countries where artificial feeding is the predominant initial form of infant feeding. It is interesting to note that in those older age categories, when the customary times for weaning occur, such countries as Sweden, the Netherlands, and Japan begin to lose their statistical advantages.

Unfortunately, the American tendency to warp the birth experience, distorting it into a pathological event, rather than a physiological one, for the normal childbearing woman is no longer peculiar to just the United States. In my visits to hospitals in various countries I was distressed to find that some physicians, anxious to impress their colleagues with their "Americanized" techniques, have unfortunately adopted many of our obstetrical practices without stopping to question their scientific or social merit.

Few American babies are born today as nature intended them to be. Among the 55,000 children included in the American Collaborative Prenatal Study carried out by the National Institute of Neurological Diseases and Stroke, there was no apparent effort made to include a control group of normal mothers who were educated to cope with the discomfort of childbirth without the use of medication. With rare exceptions, those mothers in the Collaborative Study who did not receive obstetrical medication were those who had a precipitous labor or those whose unborn child showed signs of fetal distress which precluded the use of obstetrical medication.

Although there is a tendency to think of paracervical and pudendal block anesthesia as relatively harmless, research indicates that they too can compromise the fetus and newborn infant. Rosefsky and Petersiel noted a drop in fetal heart rate in almost half of a group of 90 mothers who were observed after receiving paracervical block anesthesia. In another series the incidence of infant depression and Apgar scores (see Table 1) of 6 or less was almost 3 times greater among those infants whose mothers had received paracervical block than among the controls. The fetal hazards of depression with occasional death associated with paracervical block have been clearly demonstrated. Transient fetal bradycardia may appear to be relatively harmless, but an abnormal drop in fetal heart rate usually indicates a decrease in the oxygen saturation for the fetus. How much depletion of oxygen can be sustained by a given fetus or newborn infant before neurological damage occurs may not be recognized for several years, for the effect of even a relatively small decrease in oxygen saturation of the fetus and newborn has yet to be assessed. It is ironic that transient fetal bradycardia is taken so lightly, for no one would purposely inject medication or apply a device to a newborn infant which would possibly decrease his oxygen supply for even a few minutes without grave cause.

The relaxed attitude in the past toward the use of obstetrical medication was not due to a lack of concern for the fetus and newborn infant but to an unawareness of the problem. However, newer scientific methods of evaluating the immediate and prolonged effects on the fetus and newborn infant of

TABLE 1:
METHOD OF SCORING FOR APGAR SCORE

Sixty seconds and again at five minutes after the complete birth of the infant (disregarding the cord and placenta) the following five objective signs are evaluated and each given a score of 0, 1, or 2. A score of 10 indicates an infant is in the best possible condition. Infants with scores of 5 to 10 usually need no immediate treatment. A score of 4 or below indicates the need for prompt diagnosis and treatment.

SIGN	0	1	2
Heart rate	Absent	Slow (below 100)	Over 100
Respiratory effort	Absent	Slow, irregular	Good crying
Muscle tone	Limp	Some flexion of extremities	Active motion
Reflex irritability: response to catheter in nostril	No response	Grimace	Cough or sneeze
Color	Blue, pale	Body pink, extremities blue	Completely pink*

*American professionals are frequently amazed to see the consistency with which Scandinavian and Dutch newborn infants "pink up" to the very tips of their fingers and toes a few seconds after being born.

---

obstetrical medications and many of our common obstetrical practices now make it evident that they do, in fact, tend to alter the normal fetal and infant environment. The effect of minimal brain damage on the child's personality and his ability to learn and to cope with our complex society is only now beginning to be fully understood. Research by Lewis indicates that infants who were rated between 7 and 9 on the Apgar scale at birth were significantly less attentive than were those infants rated 10, and that the difference, in general, held true over the first year of life. It is not unlikely that unnecessary alterations in the normal fetal environment may play a role in the incidence of neurological impairment and infant mortality in the United States. Infant resuscitation, other than routine suctioning, is rarely needed in countries such as

Sweden, the Netherlands, and Japan, where the skillful psychological management of labor usually precludes the need for obstetrical medication. In contrast, in those European countries, such as Belgium, where the overall pattern of obstetrical care is similar to our own the incidence of infant mortality also approaches our own.

Obviously there will always be medical indications which dictate the use of various obstetrical procedures, but to apply the following American practices and procedures routinely to the vast majority of mothers who are capable of giving birth without complication is to create added stress which is not in the best interests of either the mother or her newborn infant.

Let us take a close look at our infant mortality statistics and then at some of our common obstetrical practices from early pregnancy to postpartum which have served to warp and distort the childbearing experience in the United States. While not all of the practices below affect infant mortality, it is equally apparent that they do not contribute to the reduction of infant morbidity or mortality and therefore should be re-evaluated.

After you have read each section below, check the appropriate box if the obstetrical care in your community includes the practice discussed. The total number of check marks that you record will provide some idea as to how far obstetric practices in your community have digressed from normal physiological childbirth.

WITHHOLDING INFORMATION ON THE DISADVANTAGES
OF OBSTETRICAL MEDICATION

Ignorance of the possible hazards of obstetrical medication appears to encourage the misuse and abuse of obstetrical medication, for in those countries where mothers are not told routinely of the possible disadvantages of obstetrical medication to themselves or to their babies the use of such medication is on the increase.

There is no research or evidence which indicates that mothers will be emotionally damaged if they are advised, prior to birth, that obstetrical medication may be to the disadvantage of their newborn infants. Offering the mother accurate, printed information (adapted from that which appears in the package insert of every obstetrical medication) on the relative safety and hazards of commonly used obstetrical medications and practices, prior to her confinement, may seem a nuisance, but such a precaution helps to protect the hospital, physician, or professional midwife from legal liability resulting from the mother's uninformed consent and allows the mother to share in the responsibility for her own well-being and that of her child in utero. To withhold information as to the possible complications of obstetrical medication is to delude the mother into assuming that there are no risks involved.

We must keep in mind that it is the mother who must ultimately bear the major emotional burden of a damaged or impaired child, even if that child is institutionalized. Under normal conditions no one should usurp the mother's prerogative by placing her unborn or newborn infant at a possible disadvantage without her informed consent. As the public becomes more aware of the possible effects of obstetrical practices on infant outcome, failure to disclose or inform the mother of the possible adverse consequences of some of the obstetrical practices discussed herein may become the basis of legal liability if or when those adverse consequences occur.

AMBIVALENT PRENATAL COUNSELING ON BREAST-FEEDING

In most of the countries of the world breast-feeding is actively encouraged during the prenatal counseling and during the mother's hospital confinement. Breast-feeding is particularly encouraged if birth is premature. If an infant is too premature or ill to suckle his mother's breasts, the mother is frequently asked to return to the hospital in order to express her milk in the presence of her baby, since the closeness tends to increase the mother's production of milk. In contrast, most American mothers are merely asked prenatally to state their preference for breast-feeding or bottle feeding, without being offered any information as to the relative benefits of breast-feeding to their babies. Once the mother has stated her preference to bottle-feed, little or no effort is made to suggest to her the advantages of breast-feeding. Yet the incidence of allergy among formula-fed infants is steadily on the rise in the United States.

While not all of the protective mechanisms of breast milk are understood, many scientists have demonstrated that there is significantly less incidence of illness among children who are breast-fed. A survey of over 3,000 children living in a housing project in England (postpenicillin) showed that the death rate was 9 times greater among children who were artificially fed from birth. All of the children in the project received their health care from the same doctors and nurses. Yet among those children who were breast-fed there was significantly less incidence of common colds, bronchitis, pneumonia, eczema, asthma, hay fever, colic, gastroenteritis, otitis media, mastoid, whooping cough, measles, German measles, and scarlet fever. Colostrum and breast milk contain antibodies against three strains of polio, Coxsackie B virus, two types of colon bacilli which can cause fetal infant diarrhea, pathogenic strains of *E. coli*, and gram-negative infections.

Diseases resulting from malabsorption, such as delicate syndrome, and sudden infant death syndrome (SIDS) rarely occur among completely breast-fed babies. Unfortunately, there are too few breast-fed infants in the high-incidence SIDS study areas to make up an adequate number of breast-fed controls.

Newborn infants who are breast-fed excrete more strontium than is ingested in breast milk whereas bottle-fed infants accumulate strontium.

There are now indications that the protective effects of breast milk may go far beyond the weaning period. Various researchers suggest that there is less incidence of dental caries, orthodontic disproportion and orofacial dental deformities, premature atherosclerosis, and ulcerative colitis among young people and adults who were initially breast-fed. One can only wonder about the future incidence of ulcerative colitis among adults whose initial food was foreign protein, fed at a temperature 25° below the temperature of breast milk, an infant's normal, species-specific food.

Research is strongly supportive of the use of breast milk for the premature infant. Mothers who breast-feed were noted by Paffenberger to show a decreased susceptibility to delayed postpartum hemorrhage. In light of the abundant research showing the medical value of breast-feeding it would seem that a statement such as "One is just as good as mother" can hardly be applied to the initial form of feeding of a newborn infant.

For additional information and references on this subject read, "The Nurse's Contribution to Successful Breast-Feeding," prepared by the author and available from ICEA's Education Committee or Supplies Center.

PERMITTING THE MOTHER TO FACE CHILDBIRTH UNINFORMED
OF WAYS IN WHICH SHE CAN HELP HERSELF TO COPE WITH THE
DISCOMFORT OF LABOR AND BIRTH

All mothers should be offered the opportunity to be physically and emotionally prepared to cope with the discomfort of childbirth because circumstances frequently preclude the use of obstetrical medication, even if the mother requests it. Dr. Charles Flowers, former Chairman of the Committee on Obstetric Analgesic and Anesthesia of the American College of Obstetricians and Gynecologists, states, "Gymnastics are not necessary in the preparation of the patient for childbirth but the ability of a person to know what to do and how to relax and how to breathe during labor is of fundamental importance."

A well-controlled research program by Enkin of Canada demonstrated that mothers who were prepared for the possibility of effectively participating in the birth process tended to experience significantly shorter labors, to require less medication and less obstetrical intervention, and to remember the experience of birth more favorably than did those mothers who were motivated to ask to be prepared to cope with childbirth but could not be accommodated in classes.

According to Dr. Pierre Vellay, a pioneer in childbirth education, the ability to relax is the key to pain relief during labor and birth and the breathing patterns act as a distraction from painful stimuli. Experience in several countries indicates that the type of controlled breathing patterns, either chest or abdominal, taught in class or in the labor room is relatively unimportant since it is the mother's intense concentration on the controlled breathing patterns, and not the breathing patterns in themselves, which makes her less aware of the discomfort or pain of her contractions.

The psychoprophylactic method of childbirth training, developed and still used successfully in Russia, involves no controlled breathing patterns. While controlled breathing patterns may be unnecessary in the future, such patterns serve a useful purpose at this point in our culture. The recent deemphasis on breathing patterns will help to avoid hyperventilation (according to McCance, hyperventilation rarely occurs in animals) and will help to bring childbirth educators into greater agreement.

REQUIRING ALL NORMAL WOMEN TO GIVE BIRTH IN THE HOSPITAL

While ICEA does not encourage home births, there is ample evidence in the Netherlands and in Chicago (Chicago Maternity Center) to demonstrate that normal women who have received adequate prenatal care can safely give birth at home if a proper system is developed for home deliveries. Over half of the mothers in the Netherlands give birth at home with the assistance of a professional midwife and a maternity aide. The comparatively low incidence of infant deaths and birth trauma in the Netherlands, a country of diverse ethnic composition and intermarriage, is evidence of the comparative safety of a properly developed home delivery service.

Dutch obstetricians point out that when the labor of a normal woman is unhurried and allowed to progress normally, unexpected emergencies rarely occur. They also point out that the small risk involved in a Dutch home delivery is more than offset by the increased hazards resulting from the use of obstetrical medication and obstetrical tampering which are more likely to occur in a hospital environment, especially in countries where professionals have had little or no exposure to normal labor and birth in a home environment during their training. We cannot justify deprecating a system of care which rarely produces a newborn infant with an Apgar score less than 9 when we in the US have a predicted yearly increase of more than 100,000 retarded infants. If the increasing American trend toward home deliveries is to be contained, it is imperative that an effort be made to make birth in the hospital as normal, as homelike, and as inexpensive as possible.

ELECTIVE INDUCTION OF LABOR

The elective induction of labor (where there is no clear medical indication) appears to be an American idiosyncrasy which is frowned upon in other developed countries. In discussing electric induction of labor in *Williams Obstetrics*, 14th ed., Hellman and Pritchard caution that the conveniences of elective induction are not without the attendant hazards of prematurity, prolonged latent period with intrapartum infection, and prolapse of the umbilical cord. They report that studies involving almost 10,000 elective inductions indicate that perinatal deaths due to premature elective inductions occur despite efforts to comply with specific criteria.

In reviewing the results of 3,324 elective inductions of labor at the University of Pennsylvania Hospital, Fields stresses the importance of caution in the selection of candidates for elective induction. He states, "Amniotomy carries with it the risk of injury to the mother or fetus and displacement of the presenting part, resulting in malposition, prolapsed cord, prolonged latent period and infection. The hazards of the use of oxytocin in labor are related directly to the dose for a given individual. Overdosage results in uterine spasm with possible separation of the placenta, tumultuous labor, amniotic fluid embolus, afibrinogenemia, lacerations of the cervix and birth canal, postpartum hemorrhage and uterine rupture. There may be water intoxication due to the antidiuretic effect of oxytocin. There may be fetal distress due to anoxia and intracranial hemorrhage, and trauma may result from tumultuous uterine contractions. Fetal and/or maternal mortality are, of course, ever present dangers."

The elective induction of labor has been found to almost double the incidence of fetomaternal transfusion and its attendant hazards. But perhaps the least appreciated problem of elective induction is the fact that the abrupt onset of artificially induced labor tends to make it extremely difficult for even the well-prepared mother to tolerate the discomfort of the intensified contractions without the aid of obstetrical medication. When the onset of labor occurs spontaneously, the normal, gradual increase in contraction length and intensity appears to provoke in the mother an accompanying tolerance for discomfort or pain.

Since the British Perinatal Hazards Study found no increase in perinatal mortality or impairment of learning ability at age 7 among full-term infants, unless gestation had extended beyond 41 weeks, there would be no medical justification for subjecting a mother or her baby to the possible hazards of elective induction in order to terminate the pregnancy prior to 41 weeks gestation. The elective induction of labor, when there is no specific medical indication, could be considered obstetrical interference in the normal physiology of childbirth and may leave the participating accoucheur legally vulnerable unless the mother is offered accurate information as to the possible hazards of elective induction of labor.

SEPARATING THE MOTHER FROM FAMILIAL SUPPORT DURING LABOR AND BIRTH

Research indicates that fear adversely affects uterine motility and blood flow, and yet many American mothers are routinely separated from a family member or close friend at this time of emotional crisis. Mice whose labors were environmentally disturbed experienced significantly longer labors, as much as 72 percent longer under some conditions, and gave birth to 54 percent more dead pups than did the mice in the control group. Newton cautions that the human mammal, which has a more highly developed nervous system than the mouse, may be equally sensitive to environmental disturbances in labor.

In most developed countries, other than the United States and the eastern European countries, mothers are encouraged to walk about or to sit and chat with a family member or supportive person in what is called an "early labor lounge." This lounge is usually located near but outside the labor-delivery area in order to provide a more relaxed atmosphere during much of labor. The mother is taken to the labor-delivery area to be checked periodically, then allowed to return to the labor lounge for as long as she likes or until her membranes have ruptured.

The rapid acceptance by professionals of permitting the mother to be emotionally supported by a family member during birth is perhaps the most dramatic change in obstetrical care throughout the developed countries. However, in some countries where multiple-bed delivery rooms are prevalent, such as in the eastern European countries and Asia, husbands are usually excluded.

CONFINING THE NORMAL LABORING WOMAN TO BED

In virtually all countries except the United States, a woman in labor is routinely encouraged to walk about during labor for a long as she wishes or until her membranes have ruptured. Such activity is considered to facilitate labor by distracting the mother's attention from the discomfort or pain of her contractions and to encourage a more rapid engagement of the fetal head. In America, where drugs are frequently administered either orally or prenatally to laboring mothers, such ambulation is discouraged—not only for the patient's safety but also to avoid possible legal complications in the event of an accident.

The disadvantages to the fetus resulting from the mother's lying in a recumbent position during labor have been recognized for several years. It is not unlikely that research will eventually find that the peasant woman who labored in the fields up until the moment of birth may have been well served by this physical activity.

SHAVING THE BIRTH AREA

Research involving 7,600 mothers has demonstrated that the practice of shaving the perineum and pubis does not reduce the incidence of infection. In fact, the incidence of infection was slightly higher among those mothers who were shaved. Yet this procedure, which tends to create apprehension in laboring women, is still carried out routinely in most American hospitals. Clipping the perineal or pudendal hair closely with surgical scissors is far less disturbing to the mother and is less likely to result in infection caused by razor abrasions.

WITHHOLDING FOOD AND DRINK FROM THE NORMAL UNMEDICATED WOMAN IN LABOR

The effect on the fetus of depriving a mother of food and drink for many hours, as is the custom in the United States, has not been sufficiently investigated. Intravenous feeding, as a substitute for light eating, only adds to the pathologic environment of an American hospital birth. In most developed countries one of the incentives for an expectant mother to take advantage of prenatal care is the fact that she will be allowed to eat and drink lightly during labor only if her prenatal examinations show her to be normal. Since anesthesia is not routinely administered during childbirth, light eating and drinking has not been found to increase the incidence of maternal morbidity or mortality in these countries.

The inhalation of gastric fluid by itself can be hazardous to the anesthetized mother. Therefore, to avoid this hazard obstetricians in most countries require that the mother's stomach be emptied or special precautions be taken if for any reason she must be anesthetized for delivery.

PROFESSIONAL DEPENDENCE ON TECHNOLOGY AND PHARMACOLOGICAL METHODS OF PAIN RELIEF

Most of the world's mothers receive little or no drugs during pregnancy, labor, or birth. The constant emotional support provided the laboring woman in other countries by the nurse-midwife, and often by her husband, appears to greatly improve the mother's tolerance for discomfort. In contrast, the American labor room nurse is frequently assigned to look after several women in labor, all or most of whom have had no preparation to cope with the discomfort or pain of childbearing. Under the circumstances drugs, rather than skillful emotional support, are employed to relieve the mother's apprehension and discomfort (and perhaps to assuage the harried labor attendant's feeling of inadequacy).

The fallacy of depending on the stethoscope to accurately monitor the effects of obstetrical medication on the well being of the fetus has been demonstrated by Hon. While electronic fetal monitoring is more accurate, the fact that some monitoring devices require that a mother's membranes be ruptured and that the electrode penetrate the skin of the fetal scalp creates possible hazards of its own. Therefore, obstetrical management which reduces the need for such monitoring is advisable.

Many professionals contend that a "good experience" for the mother is of paramount importance in childbearing. They tend to forget that, for the vast majority of mothers, a healthy undamaged baby is the far more important objective of childbirth. The two objectives are not always compatible. Human maternal response has not been demonstrated to be adversely altered by a stressful, unmedicated labor if the mother has been prepared for the experience of birth. To expose a mother to the possibility of a lifetime of heartache or anguish in order to insure her a few hours of comfort is misguided kindness, for while analgesia and anesthesia for the laboring woman may be the easier route for the nurse, midwife, or physician, the price of a narcotized mother may be a narcotized or damaged newborn infant whose ultimate potential for learning is forever diminished.

CHEMICAL STIMULATION OF LABOR

Oxytocic agents are frequently administered to intensify artificially the frequency and/or the strength of the mother's contractions, as a means of shortening the mother's labor. While chemical stimulation is sometimes medically indicated, often it is undertaken to satisfy the American propensity for efficiency and speed. Hon suggests that the overenthusiastic use of oxytocic stimulants sometimes results in alterations in the normal fetal heart rate. Fields points out that the possible hazards inherent in elective induction are also possible in artificially stimulated labor unless the mother and fetus are carefully monitored.

The British Perinatal Study appears to consider 24 hours as an outside limit for the first stage of labor, with a second stage of 2 or 3 hours or more. The average labor is about 13 hours for a primipara and about 7½ hours for a multipara. Shortening the phases of normal labor when there is no sign of fetal distress has not been shown to improve infant outcome. Little is known of the long-term effects of artificially stimulating labor contractions. During a contraction the unborn child normally receives less oxygen. The gradual buildup of intensity, which occurs when the onset of labor is allowed to occur spontaneously and to proceed without chemical stimulation, appears likely to be a protective mechanism that is best left unaltered unless there is a clear medical indication for the artificial stimulation of labor.

MOVING THE NORMAL MOTHER TO A DELIVERY ROOM FOR BIRTH

Most of the world's mothers, in both developed and developing countries, give birth in the same bed in the same hospital room in which they have labored. Since most European labor-delivery beds do not have adjustable backrests, mothers are supported into a semisitting position for birth by their husbands or a midwife. The midwife assists the mother, and if necessary, performs an episiotomy from the side of the bed, rather from the end of the bed. The suturing of an episiotomy is done by the side of the bed, or the bed may be "broken."

American nurse-midwives, especially those who have been trained abroad, are now beginning to permit American mothers the same privilege. This may seem innovative to many Americans until we realize that there is no research or evidence which indicates that a normal, essentially unmedicated mother should be required to give birth in a delivery room, rather than in a labor room which is equipped with portable or permanent sources of oxygen, suction, and high-intensity lighting. The pathological environment of the modern American delivery room is not conducive to a relaxed, normal childbirth experience.

The low temperature of the average delivery room has in the past been more suitable for the staff than for the infant. The American Academy of Pediatrics, acting as the infant's advocate, now recommends that the temperature of the delivery room should be maintained between 71.6 and 75.2°F.

DELAYING BIRTH UNTIL THE PHYSICIAN ARRIVES

Because of the increased likelihood of resultant brain damage to the infant the practice of delaying birth by anesthesia or physician restraint until the physician arrives to deliver the infant is frowned upon in most countries. Yet the practice still occurs occasionally in the United States and in countries where hospital-assigned midwives do not routinely manage the labor and delivery of normal mothers. One of the benefits of husband-attended deliveries noted by many chiefs of American obstetrical departments is the tendency for obstetrical coverage by attending physicians to immediately improve.

REQUIRING THE MOTHER TO ASSUME THE LITHOTOMY POSITION FOR BIRTH

Some contend that the low incidence of spontaneous birth among American mothers is due to the disparity in the size between the parents, resulting from the differences in their ethnic background. However, there is gathering scientific evidence that the unphysiological lithotomy position (back flat, with knees drawn up and spread wide apart by "stirrups") which is preferred by most American physicians because it is more convenient for the accoucheur, tends to alter the normal fetal environment and obstruct the normal process of childbearing, making spontaneous birth more difficult or impossible.

The lithotomy and dorsal positions tend to:

1. Adversely affect the mother's blood pressure, cardiac return, and pulmonary ventilation.

2. Decrease the normal intensity of the contractions.

3. Inhibit the mother's voluntary efforts to push her baby out spontaneously, which, in turn, increases the need for fundal pressure or forceps and increases the traction necessary for extraction.

4. Inhibit the spontaneous expulsion of the placenta, which in turn, increases the need for cord traction, forced expression, or manual removal of the placenta—procedures which significantly increase the incidence of feto-maternal hemorrhage

5. Increase the need for episiotomy because of the increased tension on the pelvic floor and the stretching of perineal tissue. The normal separation of the feet for natural expulsion is about 15 to 16 inches, or 38 to 41 centimeters, which is far less separation than is allowed by the average American delivery table stirrups.

Australian, Russian, and American research bears out the clinical experience of European physicians and midwives—that when mothers are supported to be a semisitting position for birth, with their feet supported by the lower section of the labor-delivery bed, mothers tend to purchase more effectively, appear to need less pain relief, are more likely to want to be conscious for birth, and are less likely to need an episiotomy.

The fact that the extended delivery table or bed spares the mother the common but often unspoken fear of involuntarily expelling her baby onto the floor before the doctor or midwife is ready to receive the infant, or the fear that the accoucheur might accidentally drop her baby may inhibit the mother's ability to relax her perineum during the second stage of labor.

The increased efficiency of the semisitting position, combined with a minimum use of medication for birth, is evidenced by the fact that the combined use of both forceps and the vacuum extractor rarely exceeds 4 to 5 percent of all births in the Netherlands, as compared to an incidence of 65 percent in many American hospitals. (Cesarean section occurs in approximately 1.5 percent of all Dutch births.) These differences are even more striking when one considers that in modern Holland, which has a population almost as heterogeneous as our own, the average pelvic measurements of the Dutch mother and the average circumference of her baby's head are the same as those of their American counterparts.

Manual removal for the placenta occurs in approximately 0.6 percent of all Dutch births despite the fact that oxytocin is not administered to mothers routinely.

Although the author knows of no specific research which verifies the incidence, clinical experience in the United States suggests that mothers who give birth in the semisitting position, with their legs resting on the bed, are less likely to sustain postpartum backache and fracture of the coccyx. A scientific investigation is long overdue.

THE ROUTINE USE OF REGIONAL OR GENERAL ANESTHESIA
FOR DELIVERY

In light of the current shortage of qualified anesthetists and anesthesiologists and the frequent scientific papers now being published on the possible hazards resulting from the use of regional and general anesthesia, it would seem prudent to make every effort to prepare the mother physically and mentally to cope with the sensations and discomfort of birth in order to avoid the use of such medicaments. Regional and general anesthesia not only tend to adversely affect fetal environment pharmacologically, which has been discussed previously herein, but their use also increases the need for obstetrical intervention in the normal process of birth since both types of anesthesia tend to prolong labor. Johnson points out that peridural and spinal anesthesia significantly increase the incidence of midforceps delivery and its attendant hazards. Pudendal block anesthesia not only tends to interfere with the mother's ability to effectively push her baby down the birth canal due to the blocking of the afferent path of the pushing reflex but also appears to interfere with the mother's normal protective reflexes, thus making "an explosive" birth and perineal damage more likely to occur.

While there are exceptions, the use of regional and general anesthesia usually dictates that:

1. The mother must be restricted from eating or drinking from the onset of labor.

2. The mother's uterine contractions must frequently be pharmacologically stimulated.

3. The mother must be moved to a delivery room which is equipped for obstetrical emergencies (obstetrical medication tends to increase the need for resuscitative measures for the infant).

4. The mother must be placed in the lithotomy position for delivery since she will not be in control of her legs.

5. Fundal pressure and/or the use of forceps and an episiotomy will be needed to facilitate the delivery of the infant.

6. The infant's umbilical cord will be clamped early to facilitate immediate resuscitative measures for the infant and to shorten the infant's accumulation of obstetrical medication.

7. Fundal pressure or manipulation, cord traction, pharmacological stimulation of contractions, or manual removal of the placenta be employed in order to facilitate the prompt delivery of the placenta to prevent maternal hemorrhage.

FUNDAL PRESSURE TO FACILITATE DELIVERY

Cooperman cites the past work of Pennoyer as he points out that the application of pressure on the fundus during delivery has been shown to depress oxygen saturation in the newborn infant. The use of obstetrical medications which tend to precipitate the use of fundal pressure should be avoided in the best interests of the mother and her infant.

THE ROUTINE USE OF FORCEPS FOR DELIVERY

There is no scientific justification for the routine application of forceps for delivery. The incidence of delivery by forceps and vacuum extractor, combined, rarely rises about 5 percent in countries where mothers actively participate in the births of their babies. In contrast, as mentioned previously, the incidence of forceps extraction frequently rises to as high as 65 percent in some American hospitals. Research in Europe, where there are more natural births to serve as controls, has demonstrated that, when forceps are used for delivery in order to relieve maternal distress, those infants so delivered are more likely to sustain intracranial hemorrhage and damage to the facial nerve or the brachial plexus. There are obviously times when indications of fetal distress dictate the use of forceps to facilitate the safe delivery of an infant, but there is no scientific support for the routine application of forceps during birth.

ROUTINE EPISIOTOMY

There is no research or evidence to indicate that routine episiotomy (a surgical incision to enlarge the vaginal orifice) reduces the incidence of pelvic relaxation (structural damage to the pelvic floor musculature) in the mother. Nor is there any research or evidence that routine episiotomy reduces neurological impairment in the child who has shown no signs of fetal distress or that the procedure helps to maintain subsequent male or female sexual response.

Pelvic Relaxation: The incidence of pelvic floor relaxation appears to be on the decline throughout the world, even in those countries where episiotomy is still comparatively rare. The contention that the modern washing machine has been more effective in reducing pelvic relaxation among American mothers than has routine episiotomy is given some credence by the fact that in areas of the United States where life is still hard for the woman pelvic relaxation appears in white women who have never borne children. Interviews with gynecologists in many countries suggest that the incidence of pelvic relaxation is strongly influenced by genetics. The condition, although comparatively rare in both Fiji and Kenya, occurs more frequently among Indian women in those countries than among black women, although the living habits and fertility rate of both groups of women are much the same. Whether a resistance to pelvic relaxation is due to diet, physical activity, practices or position used during birth, or any other factor is not clear. The fact remains, however, that susceptibility to pelvic relaxation appears to be a genetic weakness which has not been shown to be eliminated or reduced by routine episiotomy.

Neurological Impairment: Shortening the second stage of labor by performing an episiotomy when there is no sign of fetal distress has not been shown to be beneficial to the infant. The scientific evaluation of 17,000 children, born in one week's time and followed for seven years in Great Britain, indicates that a second stage of labor lasting as long as two and one-half hours does not increase the incidence of neurological impairment of the full-term, average-for-gestational-age infant who shows no signs of fetal distress.

Sexual Response: In developed countries where episiotomy is comparatively rare the physiotherapist is considered an important member of the obstetrical team—before, as well as after birth. The physiotherapist is responsible for seeing that each mother begins exercises the day following birth which will help to restore the normal elasticity and tone of the mother's perineal and abdominal muscles. In countries where every effort is made to avoid the need for an episiotomy, interviews with both parents and professionals indicate that an intact perineum which is strengthened by postpartum exercises is more apt to result in both male and female sexual satisfaction than is a perineum that has been incised and reconstructed.

Why, then, is there such an emotional attachment among professionals to routine episiotomy? A prominent European professor of obstetrics and gynecology recently made the following comment on the American penchant for routine episiotomy, "Since all the physician can really do to affect the course of childbirth for the 95 percent of mothers who are capable of giving birth without complication is to offer the mother pharmacological relief from discomfort or pain and to perform an episiotomy, there is probably an unconscious tendency for many professionals to see these practices as indispensable."

Interviews with obstetrician-gynecologists in many countries indicate that they tend to agree that a superficial, first-degree tear is less traumatic to the perineal tissue than an incision which requires several sutures for reconstruction. There is no research which would indicate otherwise. It would appear callous indeed for a physician or nurse-midwife to perform an episiotomy without first making an effort to avoid the need for an episiotomy by removing the mother's legs from the stirrups and bringing her up into a semi-sitting position in order to relieve tension on her perineum and enable her to push more effectively.

EARLY CLAMPING OR "MILKING" OF THE UMBILICAL CORD

Several years ago De Marsh stated that the placental blood normally belongs to the infant and his failure to get this blood is equivalent to submitting him to a rather severe hemorrhage. Despite the fact that placental transfusion normally occurs in every corner of the world without adverse consequences there is still a great effort in the United States and Canada to deprecate the practice. One must read the literature carefully to find that placental transfusion has not been demonstrated to increase the incidence of morbidity or mortality in the placentally transfused infant.

Routine early clamping or milking of the umbilical cord may appear to save the professional a few minutes time in the delivery room, but neither practice has been demonstrated to be in the best interest of either the essentially unmedicated mother or her infant. Placental transfusion resulting from late clamping, whereby the infant receives approximately an additional 25 percent of his total blood supply, is part of the physiological sequence of childbirth for most of the world's newborn infants in both developed and developing countries where the dorsal, squatting, or semisitting position is preferred for birth. The lithotomy position for birth, preferred by the American obstetrician because it is more convenient for him, makes placental transfusion inconvenient since there is no end of the bed on which the obstetrician can place the wriggling infant. The practice of "milking" the cord in order to save three minutes time does not appear to be in the best interests of the newborn infant.

Early clamping has been demonstrated by research to lengthen the third stage of labor and increase the likelihood of maternal hemorrhage, retained placenta, or the retention of placental fragments. The latter condition frequently necessitates the mother's return to the hospital in order to stop inordinate bleeding and to prevent infection. Because early clamping tends to interfere with the spontaneous separation of the placenta, making the need for obstetrical intervention more likely... , such a practice also tends to increase the incidence of fetomaternal hemorrhage or transfusion. Fetomaternal transfusion, which occurs when fetal blood cells pass into the maternal circulatory system, increases the likelihood of an Rh-negative mother of an Rh-positive baby developing antibodies. If a mother has already developed such antibodies, fetomaternal transfusion should be avoided in order to lessen any complications for any future Rh-positive fetus the mother might carry.

Whether early clamping increases the incidence of anemia in the rapidly growing child has not been sufficiently investigated, but research has demonstrated that the red cell volume of late clamped full-term infants increases by 47 percent.

ROUTINE SUCTIONING WITH A NASOGASTRIC TUBE

Although the use of a nasogastric tube attached to a deLee trap is now a widely used method for removing mucus from the newborn infant's nasopharynx, Cordero and Hon suggest that blind suctioning with a nasogastric tube is a hazardous procedure. They point out that the procedure can cause severe cardiac arrhythmias and apnea—conditions which do not tend to develop when the suctioning is accomplished by the use of a bulk syringe.

APGAR SCORING BY THE ACCOUCHEUR

No one can be completely impartial in judging his own skills, no matter how objective he or she may try to be. As one pediatrician put it, "Asking the person who delivers the infant to determine that infant's score on the Apgar scale is like asking a student to fill out his own report card." In countries where obstetrical medication is the exception rather than the rule the Apgar score of the majority of newborn infants seldom falls below 9. Therefore, it would appear that an infant's Apgar score is possibly more influenced by the management of labor and delivery than the physical condition of the mother.

Although there is a "maximum dosage" level and time interval recommended by the manufacturer of most obstetrical medications, there are no recommendations, guidelines, or restrictions on the use of several medications administered to the mother at the same time. Nor is there any recommendation or guideline for determining safe time intervals between administration of multiple medication. A review by the hospital joint obstetric-pediatric committee of any Apgar score of 7 or below would very likely tend to improve infant outcome.

Treatment of a slow learner or retarded child may be facilitated by knowing the Apgar score of the child under observation. Since the Apgar score of an individual is now always accessible several years after birth (many hospitals discard birth records after 7 to 10 years) parents should be given a copy of their baby's Apgar score for retention, even if the score is coded.

OBSTETRICAL INTERVENTION IN PLACENTAL EXPULSION

The most common mismanagement of the third stage of labor involves an attempt to hasten it. Cord traction, the use of uterine stimulants such as oxytocin, ergonovene, etc., manipulation of the fundus, and manual removal as a means of accelerating the expulsion of a reluctant placenta are pathological procedures which tend to increase the incidence of fetomaternal transfusion, maternal blood loss, and the incidence of retained afterbirth or placental fragments. Such obstetrical intervention is rarely found necessary when (1) the mother has received little or no medication, (2) she has been supported to a semisitting position for birth, and (3) placental transfusion has reduced the volume of the placenta.

SEPARATING THE MOTHER FROM HER NEWBORN INFANT

There is no evidence that the full-term infant of a relatively unmedicated mother will suffer an abnormal drop in temperature if he is dried off quickly, wrapped in a prewarmed blanket, and placed in his mother's arms during the recovery period. Experience at Yale–New Haven Hospital in Connecticut indicates that when the above procedure is followed and the mother is allowed to hold her baby for two hours or so, the infant's body temperature remains stable. In light of the present concern over the possible hazard of infant warming devices in the delivery room, perhaps we should recommend one of the most logical of warming devices—the mother's arms.

A mother-baby recovery room, staffed with skilled nursing personnel, makes it possible for even the high-risk or postoperative mother to be with her baby during the first hours of life.

Recent research by Klaus and Salk has demonstrated that the conventional hospital postpartum routine tends to inhibit rather than engender maternal response and nurturing. The first 24 hours following birth appear to be a critical period for the establishment of the normal mother-infant bonds. Separating the mother from her infant during this time tends to interfere with the mother's normal responses to her baby. Salk suggests that the mother's increased sensitivity to her newborn infant during the first 24 hours following birth may be a biochemical mechanism which is not yet understood. Both Salk and Klaus have demonstrated that maternal responses and nurturing are adversely affected a full one month after birth when the mother and her baby have been restricted to the usual hospital postpartum schedule (a glimpse of the baby shortly after birth, brief contact and identification at 6 to 12 hours, and then 20 to 30 minutes every 4 hours for feeding). How long this initial restrictive pattern of contact adversely affects maternal behavior is yet to be assessed.

As I visit hospitals throughout the world I am always impressed by the effort made in most countries to keep mothers and their babies together from the very moment of birth. Even when there are abnormal conditions which require adjustments to be made, there is still great emphasis placed on the importance of mother-baby contact during the immediate postpartum period.

DELAYING THE FIRST BREAST-FEEDING

The common American practice of routinely delaying the time of the first breast-feeding has not been shown to be in the best interest of either the conscious mother or her newborn infant. Clinical experience with the early feeding of newborn infants has shown this practice to be safe. If the mother feels well enough and the infant is capable of suckling while they are still in the delivery room, then it would seem more cautious, in the event of tracheoesophageal abnormality, to permit the infant to suckle for the first time under the watchful eye of the physician or nurse-midwife rather than delay the feeding for several hours when the expertise of the professional may not be immediately available.

In light of the many protective antibodies contained in colostrum it would seem likely that the earlier the infant's intake of species-specific colostrum, the sooner the antibodies can be accrued by the infant.

Research on several species of animals suggests that the earlier the newborn's intake of colostrum and maternal milk the earlier gut closure will occur. Gut closure, whereby the colostrum acts as a sealant to the intestinal lining, appears to prevent or lessen the passage of harmful bacteria or foreign protein through the intestinal lining. Although similar research has not been carried out on the human infant, it is not unlikely that such a similar protective mechanism exists.

OFFERING WATER AND FORMULA TO THE BREAST-FED NEWBORN INFANT

The common American practice of giving water or formula to a newborn infant prior to the first breast-feeding or as a supplement during the first days of life has not been shown to be in the best interests of the infant. There are now indications that these practices may, in fact, be harmful. Glucose water, once the standby in every American hospital, has now been designated a potential hazard if aspirated by the newborn infant, yet it is still used in many American hospitals.

It is a comment on the American penchant for the artificial that there has never been any research carried out in the United States which attempts to evaluate the safety of colostrum as the infant's first intake of fluid, yet nature obviously intended the initial fluid intake of the newborn infant to be of the same consistency as the relatively thick, viscous colostrum.

Whether the human infant experiences such as a gut closure, as is seen in animals, and whether the administering of water or formula initially to the infant who is to be breast-fed will interfere with normal gut closure has not been scientifically investigated. Experts in the raising of cows make great effort to see that species-specific bovine colostrum, not milk or water, is the first fluid received by the newborn calf. It is ironic that we do not give the same consideration to human newborns.

Unless the physician or the nurse can be absolutely sure that an infant has no familial history of allergy, it would be cautious to obtain the mother's permission before offering her infant formula in the nursery. Offering the infant formula in the nursery interferes with the normal progress of lactation in so many ways that the subject cannot be adequately discussed herein.

RESTRICTING NEWBORN INFANTS TO A FOUR-HOUR FEEDING SCHEDULE AND WITHHOLDING NIGHTTIME FEEDINGS

Although widely spaced infant feedings may be more convenient for hospital personnel, the practice of feeding a newborn infant only every four hours and not permitting the infant to breast-feed at all during the night cannot be justified on any scientific grounds. Such a regimen restricts the suckling stimulation necessary to bring about the normally rapid onset and adequate production of the mother's milk. In countries where custom permits the infant to suckle immediately after birth and on demand from that time, first-time mothers frequently begin to produce breast milk for their babies within 24 hours after birth. In contrast, in countries where hospital routines prevent normal, demand feeding from birth, mothers frequently do not produce breast milk for their babies until the third day following birth.

Widely spaced feedings, which limit the normal suckling stimulation of the breast:

1. Restrict the infant's normal intake of colostrum at a time when he is most in need of the protective antibodies in colostrum.

2. Increase the likelihood of dehydration in the infant by suppressing both the onset and production of breast milk.

3. Interfere with the maintaining of the normal, relatively constant level of glucose in the infant's blood which occurs when an infant is fed on demand

4. Increase the likelihood over overdistention of the breast by interfering with the normal clearing of colostrum from the lactiferous ducts before the onset of milk.

5. Increase the likelihood of poor "let down" of breast milk due to the mother's discomfort or pain resulting when the overly hungry infant tugs anxiously at his mother's engorged, unyielding breast which is overdistended with accumulated milk.

Physiological jaundice, which, if it does occur, usually appears about the third day of life, appears to be quite common among infants in those cultures where breast-feeding predominates. The switching of an infant from his mother's milk to foreign protein because he shows evidence of physiological jaundice is a practice which has not been justified by scientific research.

A scientific evaluation of the relationship of prenatal diuretics and other pharmacologic agents to the incidence of postnatal jaundice should be carried out.

PREVENTING EARLY FATHER-CHILD CONTACT

Permitting fathers to hold their newborn infants immediately following birth and during the postpartum hospital stay has not been shown by research or clinical experience to increase the incidence of infection among newborns, even when those infants are returned to a regular or central nursery. Yet, only in the eastern European countries is the father permitted less involvement in the immediate postpartum period than in the United States (eastern European fathers are usually not permitted to enter beyond the foyer of the maternity hospital and are not allowed to see their wives or babies for the entire seven- to nine-day stay). Research has consistently confirmed the fact that the greatest sources of infection to the newborn infant are the nursery and nursery personnel. One has only to observe a mother holding her newborn infant against her bathrobe, which has probably been exposed to abundant hospital-borne bacteria, to realize the fallacy of preventing a father from holding his baby during the hospital stay.

ASSIGNING NURSING PERSONNEL TO MOTHERS OR TO BABIES
(RATHER THAN TO MOTHER-BABY COUPLES)

The traditional American system of assigning postpartum nurses to mothers and nursery nurses to babies has done much to distort the normal pattern of initial mother-baby interaction. The European concept of assigning nursing personnel to care for mother-baby couples, then letting them care for their assigned babies in the mothers' rooms or in the nursery, has not been shown to increase the incidence of infection. The latter pattern of assignment has been approved by the Committee on Fetus and Newborn of the American Academy of Pediatrics.

RESTRICTING INTERMITTENT ROOMING-IN TO SPECIFIC ROOM
REQUIREMENTS

Throughout the world great effort is made to keep mothers and babies together in the hospital, no matter how inconvenient the accommodations. There is no research or evidence which indicates that intermittent rooming-in should be restricted to private rooms or to rooms which have a sink, or which provide at least 80 square feet for mother and baby. Such requirements are based on conjecture and not controlled evaluation. Nor is there any scientific support for requiring that each room used for intermittent rooming-in be supplied with a covered diaper receptacle. A simple system, whereby soiled diapers and baby linen are placed in plastic bags which are tied to the crib (for the mother's convenience) and then changed at the end of each shift, has been found to be safe. This system would appear less likely to be a source of infection than using communal diaper receptacles and is far less expensive for the hospital.

RESTRICTING SIBLING VISITATION

The common American practice of prohibiting toddlers and children from visiting their mothers during the hospital stay is an emotional hardship on both the mothers and their children and is unsupported by scientific research or evidence. Experience in other countries and in several hospitals here in the United States suggests that where sibling visitation is permitted a short explanation as to the importance of not bringing suspect illnesses into the hospital seems to be effective in controlling infection.

SUMMARY

As mentioned previously, most of the practices discussed above have developed not from a lack of concern for the well-being of the mother and baby but from a lack of awareness as to the problems which can arise from each progressive digression from the normal childbearing experience. Like a snowball rolling downhill, as one unphysiological practice is employed, for one reason or another, another frequently becomes necessary to counteract some of the disadvantages, large or small, inherent in the previous procedure.

The higher incidence of fetal, neonatal, and maternal deaths occurring in our large urban hospitals, as opposed to our smaller community hospitals, is undoubtedly due, in part, to the greater proportion of high-risk mothers in the urban areas. But we in the United States must stop looking for scapegoats and face up to the fact that by individualizing the care offered to maternity patients much can be done immediately to improve infant outcome without the slightest outlay of capital.

There is currently an increasing emphasis on consolidating maternity facilities. However, we in ICEA do not see the consolidation of community obstetrical facilities as being always in the best interest of the vast majority of mothers who are capable of giving birth without complications. There should, of course, be centers where those mothers who have had no prenatal care or who are anticipated to be obstetrical risks can be properly cared for. But to insist that every healthy mother must go to a major maternity facility which is unnecessary for her needs and inconvenient for her family, and where she is very apt to be "lost in the crowd," will only spur the growing trend in the United States toward professionally unattended home births.

Throughout the United States the current inclination of many expectant parents is to seek out, to "shop around" for the type of physician and hospital they feel they need in order to have the type of childbearing experience they want. They not only want a doctor who will support them in their efforts to have a prepared, natural birth, with a minimum of or no medication, they also want a hospital which offers education for childbearing and a supportive family-centered atmosphere. These expectant mothers appreciate the availability of such facilities as an early labor lounge, a dual-purpose labor-delivery room, a mother-baby recovery room, and a children's visiting room if they have older children. But most of all they want a supportive atmosphere in which they can share the childbearing experience to the extent that they desire and one which makes an effort to meet the individual needs of the mother, the father, and their newborn baby as they form their family bonds during the hospital stay.

By working together in an interdisciplinary effort the professional and lay members of the International Childbirth Education Association of the USA and Canada, the National Childbirth Trust of Great Britain, and the Parents' Centers of both New Zealand and Australia have served as catalysts to the improvement of maternity care throughout much of the world. We stand united in the belief that parents should be educated and prepared for childbearing and then be given the freedom to participate effectively in the birth of their children in order to insure the quality of life's beginning.

In which a Sensible Woman Persuades Her Doctor, Her Family, and Her Friends to Help Her Give Birth at Home

BARBARA KATZ ROTHMAN

Excerpted from Barbara Katz Rothman, "In Which a Sensible Woman,…" *Ms.,* December 1976. Reprinted by permission.

December 17

Dear Linda,

I need you to be fairly impartial, to act as a "sounding board." Hesch is as supportive and helpful as a husband can be, but he's just too involved. And I think everyone else thinks I'm crazy. So as sister (and aunt), you're elected.

I do not want to have the baby in the hospital. I've started to do some reading, and it does seem to me that the hospitals create as many problems as they solve—with too many drugs, and delivery tables that force you to give birth against gravity, and just too much interference.

I really don't feel ready to be thinking about all this so soon—I won't even look pregnant for another four months—but I know that if I don't start now, I'll surely end up in a hospital.

So—I made about 60 phone calls to obstetricians today, and I just may have found a doctor. She's never done it, but at least she'll talk to me about it.

My breasts are hurting. That's certainly planning ahead, isn't it?

Love, Barbara

December 29

Dear Linda,

It's been quite a day. We got into a strange kind of bargaining situation. She promised a "relaxed hospital environment," no prep (enema and shave), and I can go home as soon after the delivery as I want to—measured in hours, not days. All I have to do is go to the hospital. It took the wind out of my sails.

I don't know what to do. Maybe I ought to just be a good girl and go to the hospital like everybody else.

Love, Barbara

January 17

Dear Linda,

You're right. I don't know what a "relaxed hospital environment" is supposed to mean either. It's like that George Carlin routine on inherent contradictions: jumbo shrimp, military intelligence, etc.

I don't want my consciousness raised on the delivery table. I'm a feminist and I'm pregnant. That shouldn't be contradictory. There has to be a way of having a baby with dignity and joy—as a feminist, not in spite of being a feminist.

I've been reading about "natural childbirth." First off, they prefer to call it "prepared" rather than natural, there being nothing particularly natural about breathing and relaxation exercises you have to learn. I gather that if you're a very good girl and you show how cooperative you're being, then probably the nurses won't strap your hands down. If you're very polite and rational with your doctor, then maybe you won't be anesthetized when you don't want it. Terrific. It seems to me you should be able to make these decisions when you're at your best and be able to expect that nobody will double-cross you when you're defenseless.

Does that sound paranoid? We've been raised with the idea that hospitals are not just the best, they are the *only* place to give birth—and we lose sight of the fact that hospitals are a fairly recent invention, and like all institutions, they are run more for the comfort of the staff than for those they ostensibly service. And so when I remind people of that, they tell me: "We all have our hang-ups." It's an interesting, and frightening, way to dismiss my ideas.

Love, Barbara

March 12

Dear Linda,

I am now recognizably pregnant, and people are starting to respond to me differently. My belly is public property.

I'm getting basically two kinds of response to the idea of having the baby at home, now that people are beginning to believe I mean it. First, an astonishing number of women say they were talked out of it. I had no idea that so many women wanted it. It makes it all the harder for me to understand why nobody's doing anything about it.

The second response is for people to tell me that it's not safe. Some people tell me how they, or their mother or aunt or friend, would have died if they hadn't been in a hospital. And when I ask why, it so far has always turned out to be not as it first sounds. Some were in labor for frighteningly long times and needed medical assistance, even a cesarean. Long labors, by definition, are not sudden medical emergencies. Some were breech births, or RH problems—but those things you know about weeks ahead of time. When you have good reason to expect a problem, then you *do* go to a hospital.

But the best story was the friend who told me that her mother would have died without emergency care. Why? The hospital had given her the wrong drug and if she hadn't been in a hospital, they couldn't have corrected the error!

I started wearing maternity clothes. Did you ever look in a maternity department? One of my friends says that if a man from Mars arrived, he'd think that in pregnancy the breasts swell, the belly grows, and little puffs appear on your shoulders.

Maternally yours, Barbara

May 15

Dear Linda,

I'm getting bigger and bigger, and the time is getting closer. And I can't seem to get a real commitment from the doctor. I wrote her a letter, and I'm sending you a copy.

Barbara

Dear Marcia:

This has something very basic to do with questions of control, power, and authority. At home, I have it; in the hospital, it's handed over to the institution. I don't want this to come across in such a way that it is offensive to you, but the way I see it is that I am hiring you to do a service for me. In your office, I can hold on to that idea. Not so in other offices I have been to. The asymmetry of forms of address sets the tone for an entirely different relationship ("The Doctor will see you now, Barbara." "Hello, Dr. Stevens." "Hello, Barbara.")

I have read arguments for home rather than hospital delivery that spoke about privacy. I think it's less a question of privacy and more a question of authority. At home, nobody's coming in the door that I did not choose to have come in. I chose you and I am therefore delegating my control over my body to you, or pretty much anyway. I'll do what you tell me to do, and see you as the "expert." But that's because I expect you to be making decisions on the basis of your medical expertise, and not on the basis of "them's the rules" or what's most convenient in an institution that is simultaneously processing umpty-seven baby-making women.

Besides the authority/control issue, there are other reasons. As Hesch pointed out the other day, I am having a baby after all and not an appendectomy. It is a condition of health, not of illness. You do not put someone in hospital gowns on hospital tables under hospital lights with little bracelets on, and not create the image of patient.

At home I will go into labor and I'll call you and the nurse and eventually someone will show up and eventually the baby will be born and eventually you'll all leave. There is a continuum. The hospital alternative means, first I go into labor and then we have to decide when it's serious enough for me to be driven to the hospital. From there on I am processed through, in clearly demarcated states—labor room, delivery room, wherever one goes after, and then back home. It is partly a question of how the situation is defined and again partly a question of control over self and situation.

I think I first got the idea seriously about six or seven years ago. I saw two childbirth films. One was the Lamaze film with everybody running around and carrying on in French at this woman all draped in white on a table. The other was a film of a down-South Black midwife at work. The Black woman giving birth did not know from beans about panting in rhythm or any other fun and games. And she was definitely feeling pain sometimes. But she was in her bedroom with this one nice woman she knew, and sometimes they chatted and sometimes not, and the midwife dealt with her as an entire person; helping her get out of her nightgown when she was hot, and wiping her face and delivering her baby. Her husband came in sometimes, but it was definitely woman's territory only. And you could see the sun going down through the windows, and hear kids playing outside, and it was all of a piece.

Now, about safety. You asked how I am going to feel if something goes wrong. And that points up something very interesting I have to deal with. Anything that goes wrong is going to be my fault if we do it at home—is going to be perceived as my fault. I have to take on that responsibility personally—can't even really share it with Hesch. It's my problem. If this kid is born without arms or something, somehow it's going to be seen as my fault for having it at home.

It's a tricky question, maybe best dealt with through the sociology of knowledge, as to what we define as risk-taking behavior and what as normal, acceptable behavior. There are some risks I could take that are totally socially acceptable. I am not held accountable, for example, for how I choose a doctor. If I just chose the local doctor because I hate subways, that would be considered legitimate. And if he/she screws up, that's not my fault. Or, for another example, I could be asked to be drugged out of it completely, and I would not be held socially accountable for whatever risks that entailed. A friend's mother took diet pills all through her pregnancy because the doctor prescribed them. The pills have since been taken off the market for everybody, let alone pregnant people. A friend of my mother's was given that drug, diethylstilbestrol (DES), to prevent miscarriages, and they're still waiting around to see if the daughter by that pregnancy gets cancer. But none of these women are responsible, because they followed the doctor's orders. The moral is that the more control I give up, the more responsibility I give up for the consequences, and the more socially acceptable my behavior is.

That pretty much covers my ideological, philosophical, sociological arguments. And now, last of all: I don't want to act sentimental, but I am having a baby, and I do want it to be as positive and beautiful an experience for Hesch and me as we can make it.

See you on Thursday.

Barbara

June 1

Dear Linda,

She's going to do it. She read the letter, she understands, and she's going to do it. Hesch and I sat in her office and talked it all over. Even the baby picked up the vibes and jumped around!

We're going to do it without any drugs, without trying to deal with emergencies in the home that should be dealt with in the hospital. If anything is even questionable, we'll head for the hospital.

So, Linda, it looks like you get to do the whole staying-downstairs-and-boiling-water number. Try and come in soon—you won't want to miss this!

Love, Barbara

Around 3:30 on a Tuesday morning, the week before my due date, I woke to find myself in labor. It must be awkward and make a person feel silly to go rushing off to the hospital on a "false alarm," but to bring the doctor to me if I wasn't really in labor was unthinkable.

By 8:30 I decided it was time to get mobilized. I woke up Hesch, handed him the watch and the lists (things like make sure we had ice cubes, and clean the bathroom, make the bed, sweep—baby or no baby, we had company coming!). I left a message with Marcia's answering service that I was almost certainly in labor, and called my mother and asked her to drop off the cushions she was re-covering for my big platform rocker.

I sat in my rocking chair while Hesch cleaned up. He found pretty music on the radio, and chatted and timed contractions. On Hesch's list (we are crackerjack list makers) he noted that at 11:00 I was looking happy and self-satisfied, beginning to feel an outward, downward thrust to the contractions. But by 11:30 he noted that I was looking decidedly uncomfortable.

Marcia had returned our call and told Hesch to remind me that it really was going to hurt. It helps us understand what is going on when we speak of "contractions" rather than "pains," but the contractions of labor are painful, and I guess it's easier to deal with if your expectations are realistic. If I had been going to the hospital, that is probably the point at which we'd have gone. Contractions were strong and every three minutes. I was still sitting in my rocking chair, with Hesch sitting opposite me and very gently rubbing my belly, when Marcia arrived, at around two o'clock. By then we had given up timing, no longer able to sort the pain out into separate contractions. Marcia timed the contractions at two and a half minutes, with 10-second rests, and told me I could expect a "horrendous but short" labor.

All afternoon our family had been arriving, one by one. My mother sat tensed at the bottom of the stairs while Hesch's mother compulsively cooked chickens. Fathers and siblings sat around. When I cried out during a particularly painful examination, Marcia went out afterward to explain to them that I was okay—and came back with the message that they were all bearing up well.

Sometime after 4:00, I entered the phase of labor called transition, in which the last few centimeters of dilation takes place, the cervix opening up completely to let the baby come through. The contractions may have been more painful, I really don't know, but they started sorting themselves out into separate entities—maybe 90 seconds and 60 off. Again, I'm not sure. But they did have peaks and, blessed be, valleys. Hesch (who never moved from his seat opposite me) suggested I deal with the contractions by using two pants and a blow. That was the smartest thing I'd ever heard in my life. I was impressed by how clever and insightful he was—it sounds silly, but that's just the way I felt; how clever an idea. That, I gather, is what they mean when they say you need strong direction during labor.

I'd read that women get a "second wind" once they're fully dilated and ready to begin pushing the baby out, and it was certainly true for me. Pushing was the strangest, and in some ways the nicest, sensation I've ever had. I could actually feel the shape of the baby, feel myself sitting on the head as it moved down. Marcia said I looked comfortable enough on the chair, and I didn't have to get to the bed if I didn't want to. So there I was, on my rocking chair, with my feet up on two little kitchen chairs, with Hesch on one side and Marcia on the other, and pushing like crazy. I was like moving a grand piano across a room: so hard, but so satisfying to feel it move along.

Eventually, Marcia said I could have the baby in 2 pushes with an episiotomy (the small incision to widen the birth outlet), or maybe 10 pushes without. I said no thanks. I thought, Hell, I still wasn't sure it was happening, maybe I could accept the reality of it given the few extra minutes. I really needed the time to prepare myself, like the last-second cramming before the exam booklets are passed out.

So there I was, on my rocking chair with my feet up, pushing like crazy.

Hesch said my mother wanted to come in. My mother-in-law came in shortly after. It didn't take me 10 pushes, just 5. I heard noises coming out of my throat that I couldn't believe—like the soundtrack of a horror movie, but I had no time to laugh. And then I felt myself sitting on the head, felt myself opening, felt the head push through. A beautiful, total sense of opening and roundness. The shoulders seemed big and the shape was less comfortable than the symmetry of the head. And then slurp, wriggling, warmth, wetness, and there was a baby. He was up in the air, upside down, Marcia holding him over me. The longest few seconds in the world passed and then this gray-blue thing became alive and pink and breathing. Marcia handed him to my mother. I kept reaching out for him, but my mother was too dazed to move. I watched the cord being clamped and cut, and my baby, my son, Danny, was suckling by the time the placenta was out.

After maybe five minutes I stood, spilled blood all over the floor, and my mother walked me to the shower. As much as I had needed Hesch's support before, I felt the need for mothering then. I got the shakes—part physical, part emotional reaction, I guess. She bundled me up so I was warm and helped me put on a sanitary napkin—it was like the first time I got my period and was initiated into all the mysteries. Once I was changed and back into the rocker and Hesch and his mother had cleaned up the blood that had spurted from the cord, the whole world was in my room. Brothers and sisters and parents, suddenly aunts and uncles and grandparents. They brought with them champagne and flowers and a teddy bear and a silver spoon, and looks of wonderment and love. It was the best birthday party I had ever been to.

As much as I had wanted it, I don't think even I understood how good it can be to have a baby at home. I gave birth, freely and consciously—I was not *delivered*. And my baby and I were surrounded by love, not efficiency. Images pass through my mind—my mother-in-law helping me get my breast out of the nightgown and to Danny; my brother carrying a big plastic garbage bag down from the bedroom singing "afterbirth" to the tune of "Over There"; my mother and Hesch trying to clean up the meconium (the baby's first bowel movement) in the middle of the night without waking me. I am sure there are more efficient ways to do these things—but who needs them?

The pediatrician came the next day to examine the baby. She kept telling us we were crazy. The baby looked so big and healthy (he was 8 pounds, 5 ounces, and had been a 9+ on the Apgar newborn scale of 10) and I looked so good, dressed and walking around, up and down stairs, but still we were crazy.

Dr. Spock's Advice to New Mothers

ALIX KATES SHULMAN

Excerpted from Alix Kates Shulman, *Memoirs of an Ex-Prom Queen,* New York, Knopf, 1972. Reprinted by permission.

We made Andrea in the new year and I bore her in the fall, entering the park world in the winter, bundled up. The books I had taken from the library in preparation proved to be mere parodies of life; but there was nothing else to go on. Child care was neither discussed in society nor taught in school. However contemptuous I'd been of the prospect of Spock, I was grateful for him now. He had the latest word and a good index.

It would be good news for every baby weighing 10 pounds or more to be outdoors, when it isn't raining, for 2 or 3 hours a day, as long as the temperature is above freezing and the wind isn't bitterly cold. (Dr. Spock, *Baby and Child Care*, Section 244.)

The old lady who fed pigeons peered into the carriage, but otherwise I was alone on a deserted bench, paralyzed by the fragility of my overwhelming charge, afraid to move for fear of waking her, afraid to take my eyes off her lest she sleep and die. During her brief sleeps I studied her like a difficult text, trying to fathom each mysterious tremor and start, praying she would not wake too soon. When she did wake—always grievously ahead of schedule—I leaped to juggle the carriage as I had seen the neighbors do, trying to shake the sobs from her throat and the knots from my gut.

If you live in the city and have no yard to park the baby in, you can push him in a carriage. Long woolen underwear, slacks, woolen stockings, and galoshes make your life a lot more pleasant during this period.

In summer it would be different. She would be older then and I would not fear her death so much as her life. In my breast lay the power to soothe or torment her, but also dangers. If ten minutes of jiggling the carriage didn't get her back to sleep, that would be ten wasted minutes, six hundred useless sobs tearing at my raw conscience. It would take ten more minutes to get home from the park, and another ten to get the carriage up the stairs and our wraps and clothing off.

What do you do if he wakes as soon as you put him to bed or a little later? I think it's better to assume first that if he has nursed for 5 minutes he's had enough to keep him satisfied for a couple of hours, and try not to feed him again right away. Let him fuss for a while if you can stand it. (Section 127.)

The baby carriage turned out to be an unexpected aid in stopping traffic. But it was still a good half hour between whimper and feeding—a half hour that took months off my life and left yellow milkstains of my nursing bras.

It may start leaking from the breasts when you hear the baby beginning to cry in the next room. This shows how much feelings have to do with the formation and release of the milk. (Section 102.)

If I had stayed home with her instead of going to the park I could have put her to suck the instant she woke, forgot the clock and the dangers.

The treatment of fretfulness seems clear to me.... The baby should be allowed to nurse as often as every 2 hours, for 20 to 40 minutes. (Section 122.)

But I so wanted everything to be right for her, and the park was the preferred milieu. Constant feeding was contraindicated. If my breasts were never more than partially emptied, which could result from putting her to suck too often, then they would not be properly stimulated to fill up again and I would dry up with no comfort for my helpless daughter

> If the breast-milk supply is insufficient at all feedings, you will need a bottle at all feedings, whether you give the breast first or not. (Section 126.)

I knew I shouldn't be offering her bottles yet, but how could I risk starving her? Her life was in my hands. I nursed her around the clock every two hours for half an hour at least, watching her tiny fists clutch spasmodically at my long hair and her toes curl in the joy of sucking, until she fell asleep at my breast; then gingerly I tried to roll her onto her stomach without waking her.

> There are two disadvantages to a baby's sleeping on his back. If he vomits, he's more likely to choke on the vomitus. Also, he tends to keep his head turned toward the same side.... This may flatten that side of his head. It won't hurt his brain, and the head will gradually straighten out, but it may take a couple of years. (Section 248.)

During the mornings and late afternoons, when I had the diapers and laundry, the bottles and bedding to do, I let her sleep on our bed between feedings. I carefully slipped rubber padding between her diaper and our sheet, sometimes leaving her bottom bare to help her diaper rash. ("Jesus, Sasha, isn't there anything else you can use on her diaper rash besides Desitin Ointment? It smells worse than shit; our bed stinks of it," said Willy.) But at night, when I longed to share with her my brief interludes of sleep, I couldn't risk keeping her in bed with me. Even if Willy hadn't protested her little body coming between ours, it was a dangerous place for her. A carelessly flung arm could snuff out her fire like a breath a birthday candle; not to mention the

> chance that he may become dependent on this arrangement and be afraid and unwilling to sleep anywhere else. (Section 250.)

> No; better to follow (Section 251) the doctor's better sensible rule not to take a child into the parent's bed for any reason (even as a treat when the father is away on a business trip);

> better to suffer now than later.

The conspiracy of silence about motherhood was even wider than the one about sex. Philosophers ignored it and poets revered it, but no one dared describe it. The experts who wrote articles for magazines ("Ten Steps to Restore Muscle Tone"; "Before You Call Your Pediatrician"; "Take the Time to Stay Interesting: Six Shortcuts to Keeping Informed") spoke in euphemisms; as to the real dangers, their best advice was to consult still other doctors. Why didn't the women speak? Evidently they were too busy....

She purred and giggled as I suckled her. She had her preferences, did my daughter, and when something made her cry she broke my heart with her great stores of tears that flooded her enormous green eyes and overflowed their thick banks of black lash like swollen rivers. How, I wondered, could Willy bear to be away from us? Why did he leave us promptly every morning and return late every night?

"Sasha," called Willy, "she's started crying again. I was just sitting here with her and she started screaming for no reason."

I dropped the spatula and ran to the living room, oblivious of Spock's warning to parents who

> always anxiously pick him up when he fusses:... the more they submit
> to his orders the more demanding he becomes. (Section 282.)

"Give her to me, Willy, for God's sake, don't let her cry like that!"

> If your baby is sensitive about new people, new places, in the middle of
> his first year, I'd protect him from too much fright by making strangers
> keep at a little distance until he gets used to them, especially in new
> places. He'll remember his father in a while. (Section 348.)

I took my baby in my arms and walked her, patting her perfect back the way I had when she was a newborn. The sound of her crying was always absolutely unbearable to me.

> Many mothers get worn out and frantic listening to a baby cry, especial-
> ly when it's the first. You should make a great effort to get away from
> home and baby for a few hours at least twice a week—oftener if you can
> arrange it.... If you can't get anyone to come in, let your husband stay
> home one or two evening a week while you go out to visit or see a movie.
> (Section 278.)

The trouble was, Willy didn't get home most evenings till eight or so and couldn't have helped me then if he'd wanted to.

How could he relieve me if he left us in the morning and returned late at night, or if he were away, as the omniscient Spock had divined, on a business trip?...

Once every two weeks I hired a daytime sitter and tore myself from Andy as Spock advised. I planned to slip off to the library and read a book or arrange to meet a friend at the Museum of Modern Art. But somehow the hours were too precious to use up on personal frivolities, and instead I took to dropping in on Will for lunch (as in the old days), doing everything I could to live up to my photographs. Flat-stomached supermother uptown between feedings.

I took more care dressing for those office calls than when Will wrenched me away form Andy at bedtime to accompany him to the movies or a party at Hector's, where I watched the world go spinning on as though babies were a recent invention. Couples stood in line at movie theaters holding hands, oblivious of the consequences; old friends gathered at Hector's with new girlfriends to exchange news of charter flights and recent books, as though Dr. Spock's *Baby and Child Care* had not been written for them....

That first summer I took Andy to the crowded playground every day, carrying her up the slide and sliding her down on my lap.

From a park bench I watcherd her at my feet intently tearing up a leaf, her mouth open and brows knit in concentration, her pudgy fingers moving with careful grace. Though I always took a book to the park I didn't dare read for the dangers; couldn't read for the distractions. Anyway, most books were now irrelevant. Instead, I searched around to see which of the other mothers, multiparous and knowing, could tell me things about my daughter I ought to know. Some of them were limber and accomplished, some foul-mouthed and acne-scarred, no doubt with mean lives and husbands to match. I hung on every casual comparison they made of Andy with their own like revelations. My daughter's life was on my hands....

I began each day solemnly with resolutions:

Today I will make myself lunch; I'll brew myself a cup of tea between breakfast feeding and diaper delivery.

I will *not* pick her up whenever she cries today.

I will be *calm* when she spits out her food.

The horror of my predicament was: everything counts. Each tiny mistake I made was destined to reverberate through all eternity.

The first time I yelled at Andy she looked at me unbelieving; betrayed. Her chin puckered, her lip trembled, then tears gushed from those green eyes all over her hands. I sank into a week-long depression.

> It's possible that you will find yourself feeling discouraged for a while when you first begin taking care of your baby. It's a fairly common feeling, especially with the first. You may not be able to put your fingers on anything that is definitely wrong. You just weep easily. Or you may feel very bad about certain things. One woman whose baby cries quite a bit feels sure that he has a real disease, another that her husband has become strange and distant, another that she has lost all her looks. (Section 16.)

Exactly as I had once imagined but forgotten, when my child was born my fate slipped through my fingers into the bay. I was hers now.

> If you begin to feel at all depressed,... go to a movie, or to the beauty
> parlor, or to get yourself a new hat or dress.... (Section 16.)

A new locale, a new hair style, could solve nothing any more. We swam around
sifting plankton, hoping for some huge uplifting wave to come along and carry
us high and wide; but there were only the usual ripples and currents and erratic seismographic disturbances to be recorded on the precision instruments of
oceanographers....

Thinking her still asleep in her crib at naptime I had gone next door to borrow some diapers from a neighbor. When I returned, I heard her screaming in
her room. (Was it my fault? "Look, honey," Willy had warned, "this is the third
time you've run out of diapers. What happened to the emergency supply I got
you? You need better planning. If you won't increase the regular order, you'll
just have to use the ones you have more sparingly.")

An accident? Had I forgotten to raise the side of the crib?

> A baby, by the age he first tries to roll over, shouldn't be left unguarded on
> a table for as long as it takes the mother to turn her back (Section 349.)

I rushed to her room to find her standing in her crib clutching the bars terror-
stricken, her fat knees buckling.

"Standing! Look at you!" I cried. She sobbed with exhaustion and victory. A
star!

I unhooked her fingers one by one from the bars and scooped her up into
my arms, my bumblebee, pressing kisses all over her shining face. "You can
stand. You can do anything." I rejoiced. When she kicked to be put back again,
I sat her down in the crib; then up she climbed on her little legs once more,
crowing with pride.

She had learned to stand not for a moment or a day, but for all time. I knelt
before her crib. She looked so much tinier upright than sprawled across her
mattress. She was one of us now, though she didn't come up to my knees. As I
knelt adoringly before her, trying to kiss her nose through the bars, she began
to shake her little body furiously, rattling the bars, laughing until her chin
puckered, her lower lip protruded toward me, and once again, the deluge.

Down again with my help to sitting, then up on her own. For an hour and
more we did our joyful dance while the tide waited.

"William Burke, please."
"Just a minute, please." A new voice at the switchboard.
"Willy? She can stand up."
"Alone?"
"Yes. She holds on, of course, but she can get up by herself."
"Hey! That's great, Sash! Great! It's about time, isn't it?"
"No, Willy. She's only nine and a half months old. Spock says it happens any
time in the last quarter of the first year. I thought you'd want to know about it."

"Sure do, honey. Thanks a lot for calling me."

When I hung up I chastised myself for having phoned him with the news. And when he finally did come home, I overdid it, searching his face for a joy that could not possibly appear. And filled up like a Hoover bag with resentments.

The experts would have agreed I expected too much of Will: infants' progress is fit news only for ladies' magazines. Andy's triumphs were everything to me—elating, exonerating—and only bonuses to him, which somehow diminished them....

Willy tried. He brought home quince blossoms in the spring and roses often. But even with the living room a garden, he sat at the window and looked out. I could see he felt trapped inside with us, whereas I, trapped too, could barely be induced to leave.

On Sundays he was gallant, taking us to Central Park, first to the zoo cafeteria for pancakes, then to the carousel, where he waved to us from a bench each time Andy and I rode by. But in between, though I never actually caught him, I knew he looked at the carefree New York girls.

When I felt the flutter of life in me anew, I kept the thrill of it to myself. Something told me to be careful. I did my quota of nesting, washing Andy's outgrown layette and making extensive lists of details to attend to, but I was careful not to burden Will with them.

I did my best to avoid sensitive topics. I hid my child-care pamphlets among my recipes as I had once hidden my beauty charts and *Seventeen*s. I knew they were considered vacuous, like the talk of formulas and play groups that blighted cocktail party repartee—unless it issued from some doctor. But they dealt with matters too important to leave to chance. I knew I risked the worst contempt for reading them, but I had more than my own ego to consider: there were the children's. How else was I to learn the pitfalls of sibling rivalry or the symptoms and cure of croup? I had no models, no advisers for child care. Like housework, it was something charming people didn't discuss and rich people didn't do.

Once I had tried to read Will an urgent paragraph from the "Parent and Child" feature in the Sunday *Times Magazine* supplement. Tearing it away from me he had cried, "Why do you read that trash and let it upset you? It's just bullshit!" as, during my earlier pregnancy, he'd forbidden me to read about the limbless thalidomide babies, saying, "You'd be a nervous wreck if you didn't have me to protect you."

I too was protective. But however carefully I spared him our disorder, he still used every excuse to come home late. No matter how endearingly Andy greeted him at the door, once home, it seemed, Will couldn't wait to get out of the house again.

Men react to their wife's pregnancy with various feelings: protectiveness of the wife, increased pride in the marriage, pride about their virility....

But there can also be, way underneath, a feeling of being left out... which can be expressed as grumpiness toward his wife, wanting to spend more evenings with his men friends, or flirtatiousness with other women. (Section 18.)

Of all the experts I'd ever consulted, none—no Watson, Webber, or Spock—was unequivocally on my side. They made us do it, then blamed us for it, another case of damned if you do and damned if you don't. They found nothing more hateful than a clinging wife—except a dominating mom.

> Some fathers have been brought up to think that the care of babies and children is the mother's job entirely. But a man can be a warm father and a real man at the same time.... Of course, I don't mean that the father has to give just as many bottles or change just as many diapers as the mother. But it's fine for him to do these things occasionally.... Of course, there are some fathers who get goose flesh at the very idea of helping to take care of a baby, and there's no good to be gained trying to force them. Most of them come around to enjoying their children later "when they're more like real people." (Section 20.)

From the confines of my cell I tried to thwart Willy's wanderings. It was my duty. And when I ran out of coffee or snapped at him in my regular early morning panic, I kicked myself for driving him off to Riker's Restaurant for breakfast, the *Times* tucked under his arm as he walked out the door. And when I finally went to the hospital to give birth to Jenny, I could no longer hide my obsessive conviction that once Will was free of us, with me away and Andy gone to stay with his mother and nothing in the world to keep him at home, he would simply pack up his things and leave.

Yes, We Have No Bambinos

MOLLY HASKELL

Molly Haskell, "Yes, We Have No Bambinos," *Viva*, March 1975. Reprinted by permission.

I recently moved with my husband from a small apartment in midtown Manhattan to a larger apartment on the Upper East Side, in what is fondly referred to by everyone except me as a "family neighborhood." Eleven floors below, back to back with our building, is a boys' school called St. David's which seems to have staggered recess periods. There is at least one class of little boys shrieking and yelling in the courtyard at all times. I never would have thought prepubescent voices could be so loud or carry so far. When I tell my friends about it, or they hear it for themselves, they smile benignly and say that these are "life sounds," or "the music of human voices." The best I'm able to say, I'm afraid, is that I've grown accustomed to the voices (they often make the day begin, all too literally, well before the alarm clock rings). The very constancy of the noise turns it from an off-and-on intrusion into a background din, but I don't suppose I'll ever exactly relish it, or think affectionately of the little dears as they release their youthful high spirits.

What's wrong with me? Am I a female W. C. Fields? An infantophobe? A Lady Macbeth? No, I'm just a nonmother with what I like to think is a healthy balance of hormones and perhaps an above-normal quotient of husband-love and professional drive. I write, of course, and my powers of concentration, as you may have guessed, are not those of Jane Austen, who wrote at her little desk in the middle of the living room, surrounded by a huge family (and even she didn't have a child to contend with). But aside from the demands of a career, there are other features of my life that I would have to surrender were I to become a mother. I like to stay up and watch the late show or go with my husband to the movies or to a restaurant on the spur of the moment. I like to read the paper through in the morning and eat the kind of food children would gag at and take walks and choose my friends because of a natural affinity rather than because they have kids the same age as mine. I like to spend money—not extravagantly, but without having to think about each penny. I like not having money arguments with my husband, and I like not being forced into a conservative philosophy because of concern for the "future well-being" of my children. I like the idea that if my husband and I ever did divorce, the height of acrimony would be over the division of books rather than human beings.

Of all the rumblings and murmurings, tremors and upheavals that have taken place in the last few years, both within the wake of the women's movement and as a distant echo, the most radical is that women, in something that could be described as *numbers*, are deciding not to have children. Not to have children! This, more than any technological breakthrough or political movement, is a revolutionary idea. It reverses, or at least questions, the whole process, thought to be both instinctual and immutable, by which the human race reproduces and multiplies and woman fulfills her destiny as a woman. It goes against the supposedly automatic, heaven-decreed assignment of woman to marry and give birth and consign herself to 20 years of being more or less at the disposal of her offspring. And yet this radical option is being discussed and adopted by women who are not freaks or witches or "selfish bitches" or even necessarily obsessive careerists, but who are well-adjusted, sane, happily married women, some of whom do and some of whom do not have professions. The reasons, as I discovered from talking to women around the country, range from genetic weaknesses inherent in one member of the couple to concern with overpopulation to lifestyle choices. And it has happened— that is, the idea has become socially acceptable if not widely applauded— within an amazingly short time.

In January 1963, Gael Green wrote an article in the *Saturday Evening Post* entitled "A Vote against Motherhood," describing in quite reasonable terms the ways in which children had frustrated or crippled the lives of some of her friends and the reasons she and her husband had decided not to have any of their own. The resistance, the censure, and the horror that those around her felt at her decision was confirmed by the 3,000 pieces of hate mail provoked by the article.

Just four and a half years ago Betty Rollin wrote a piece entitled "Motherhood—Who Needs It?" that ran in *Look* magazine and drew a scandalized response. It was a lively, dispassionate, well-researched examination of all the myths surrounding and pushing women into motherhood. *Look* was inundated with what Betty says was one of the greatest floods of mail ever received, "most of which was hate mail."

Reaching the point where not having children has become an acceptable cultural choice couldn't have happened without the pressure of important social forces like inflation and overpopulation creating an atmosphere in which large families are discouraged. Sterilization has had an astonishing success with both younger and older couples as a way of limiting a family or preventing children altogether.

There is even a new organization dedicated to furthering nonparenthood. NON, the National Organization for Nonparents, brings together people who share an interest in curbing population either on a world scale or in their own homes, and in simply making the notion of nonparenthood acceptable.

But it is on married women in their early thirties that the burden of decision falls most heavily, for they (and we who have made the choice) must live with its consequences. There are feminists who feel, with some justice, that women shouldn't have to make such a choice. The *Ms.* ideal woman, for example, as analyzed by Hunter professor of communications Dr. Helen Franzwa, is a working mother *with* children. There is even a semantical feud with NON over whether women without children should be characterized as "childless (considered too negative by NON) or "childfree" (considered arrogant by *Ms.*)—hence my own positive-negative title for this article.

In a recent *Ms.* article, Ellen Willis expresses the opinion of certain feminists that an expansion of day-care programs and an increased delegation of responsibility to the fathers would and should permit women to combine work and children. Nonmothers are characterized as "militant," elitist snobs (little difference here from the white-collar view of them as "selfish bitches"), or dupes of a sexist society, which forces a choice upon women that no man ever incurs. It is this last charge that rings true and is almost unanswerable unless we shift our thinking entirely towards a more communal, socially shared form of child-rearing. When you suggest, as Willis does, that many of the drawbacks of motherhood are the result of a patriarchal, capitalist society, then you must pursue the political corollary: that motherhood itself, as practiced in our society, a proprietary, bourgeois-individualist institution. The dream of giving birth—of having *one's own* child, of nurturing him/her with "every advantage," of hoping he/she will surpass his peers—all of this not only sits quite well with the patriarchal capitalist system but is its very foundation, its means of perpetuating itself.

Couldn't Ms. Willis and others like her participate in the rearing of others' children? Why must she, particularly in a world endangered by overpopulation, have her *own* child? This would take a certain reordering of habits and institutions. But even without any kind of socialized child care many of the women I talked to are finding ways to involve themselves in caring for other women's children, becoming, in effect, unofficial godparents. The point is, it's a very complex issue, and no one can prescribe for anyone else.

As Betty Rollin says, "Not to have children doesn't mean a life without children. I have a part-time child [her husband's by a former marriage]. Often the people who contribute the most to children have none of their own, and they can do this because they are free. Just think—if Anna Freud had had her own family, she might never have done her remarkable work in child psychology!"

The popularity of sterilization—both laparoscopy and vasectomy—enabling women to enjoy sex without fear of pregnancy, is an acknowledgment of something that ten years ago was inadmissible—that adult women, whether mothers or nonmothers, continue to enjoy sex. One of the most crippling aspects of Momism (the cult of motherhood as it was defined in the fifties) was that the mother figure was purged of the "taint" of sexuality at precisely the time in her life when she might be expected to enjoy it most. In a culture obsessed with youth, a lusty, sexy woman in her thirties was an embarrassment, a figure of ridicule, and a woman's only claim to status was through her children. But women are fighting back, refusing to be prematurely put out to pasture by the next generation.

It is, perhaps, the image of motherhood as it has evolved in our society and been purveyed, rather unappealingly, in Hollywood films, that we are reacting against. We who identified with James Dean in *Rebel without a Cause* must suddenly cast ourselves in the roles of the villains—parents—or reject the part.

Several years ago, when there still seemed some hope that I might have children, my mother was trying to persuade me with the solace-for-your-old-age argument, emphasizing how much I'd meant to her.

"But, Mother," I protested, "how could I? We live 300 miles apart."

"It's just your being there, and my being interested in what happens to you," she said. But I kept thinking about her loneliness, made greater by the infrequency of our visits together. I happen to think I have one of the world's greatest mothers—so there's no reacting against a bad childhood on my part—and yet I have no desire to follow in her footsteps and bring up a selfish brat like me, who'll want to sprout wings and fly away at the first opportunity. If anything, it's not the model of motherhood that discouraged me from having children—it's the model of childhood… my own! And I think I'm not unlike many women in feeling, somewhere below the surface, this loss of connection between parent and child, a lack of concern for one's "elders," that might, one day, be turned against us as parents.

At this moment in history, both young and middle-aged middle-class couples seem to live in the worst of all possible worlds: close enough to parents to still feel the pressure of obligation and guilt, but not close enough to benefit from a sense of warmth and protection, or even the services they might offer.

We feel a pressure to "keep house" in the style of our parents, but without domestic assistance. And we feel social and psychological pressure to love and guide our children, to give them more attention than was given us, while we have less time to give. Our lives are completely different from our parents', but we continue to judge ourselves, or allow ourselves to be judged, by their standards and expectations.

In a scene from the Bergman film *Scenes from a Marriage* that burns a hole in the memory, Liv Ullmann, as a divorce lawyer, interviews an elderly woman who has made up her mind to divorce. Very slowly and methodically, the woman reveals that her relationship with her husband has been a sham for 15 years, that she feels she is losing her ability to respond to life, and, finally, that she doesn't love her children.

"I have never loved my children," she says, "I know that for sure. But I've been a good mother all the same.

This woman has uttered the most shocking words a woman can say, the unsayable, the unthinkable. It is one thing for a child not to love his mother and father; it is even permissible for a father to acknowledge reservations about his children. But for a mother to make such an admission! Is mother love not an absolute? The answer, of course, is No, it is not. And the sooner we admit it the less hypocrisy there will be.

The beatific aura in which motherhood has been sold to us has intimidated women from expressing even minor reservations, for fear they will be thought monsters. Only once in a while will you find a woman who admits that life with children is a flawed affair, who even admits that if she had it to do over she might do without.

Yet even after all the rational arguments have been made, the name-calling level of debate remains. Part of the charge is the oft-touted "selfishness" of not having children—which seems to me a childish issue. A case could be made for family life as the most *self*-centered institution ever conceived. But it's like the religious debates my friends and I used to have in the sixth grade, when we argued that believing in God and doing nice things for other people were selfish because the only reason you did them was to make *you* feel good.

Well, I don't have children, and I feel good. Possibly, if I had them I would feel just as good, for different reasons. Still, I find that even the most emancipated woman is reluctant to say, definitively, that she is not going to have children. "Not for the moment," she will say, as I used to say, knowing in the back of my mind I probably wouldn't but wanting to keep an escape hatch open. At least that was the reason I gave to myself. Now I think it's because I was still afraid of What People Would Think. That I was a monster. And ever perhaps, that what they were thinking about me, I was thinking about myself. Even now I haven't decided if I'm "right" or "wrong," "selfish" or "un-selfish"—only that whatever it is I can live with it.

And speaking of monsters, just listen to those voices—shouting, brimful of life, eleven floors below. I'm glad they're not in the next room.

How Late Can You Wait to Have a Baby?

BARBARA SEAMAN

Excerpted from Barbara Seaman, "How Late Can You Wait to Have a Baby?" *Ms.*, January, 1976. Reprinted by permission.

Men like to think they can all go on reproducing as long as Chaplin, and apparently some do. But where fertility is concerned, women fear that we must use it or lose it, that it's risky to delay having children. We worry about time running out on our bodies. We lose the luxury of postponing "the baby decision."

The reproductive capacity of women—and men—deteriorates with advancing age. But physically, there is no ideal time to have a baby, for mother and baby do not operate on the same trajectory of risk. Maternal risk is lowest in the late teens and twenties, rises slowly but steadily through the thirties, and after 40 may be as much as 10 times higher than for women in their twenties.

Infant mortality, on the other hand, is lowest when mothers are in their late twenties and only rises again very slowly thereafter. The infant mortality rates for mothers aged 35 to 39 are the same as the rates for mothers aged 20 to 24, while the rates for mothers over 40 are comparable to those aged 15 to 19.

A most dangerous time to have a baby, in terms of risk to *both mother and child*, is in the early teens, the years just after menarche. It's as if the female reproductive system were warming up, but is not yet ready to go the distance. Impoverished countries where very early marriage prevails have strikingly higher infant and maternal mortality figures than comparable countries where marriage occurs later.

Thus, for your child's sake there is much to be said for delaying mother-hood until your mid-twenties at least. The children of young mothers also have more health problems and accidents, and a higher mortality rate at ages 1 to 4. Mothers under 20, or even under 25, produce more babies of precari-ously low birthweight. Might the junk foods and crash diets in which adoles-cent girls indulge leave a deficit that takes some years to correct? If the female sexual response does not reach peak efficiency until the late twenties, or beyond, are our reproductive organs still, in some hidden aspects, short of their optimum maturity in the early twenties?

We have been oversold on the health advantages of starting our families early. This may sound coutrary to everything you've heard about Down's syndrome and malformed infants being born to older women, but here are the surprising facts.

The statistics on birth defects are exceedingly difficult to sort out, because they are recorded in so many diverse ways. Consider, for example, a handicap such as deafness, which is not usually diagnosed until the second year of life, or dyslexia (reading disability), which is not diagnosed until school age. These disorders, among many others, are not and cannot be reported on ordinary birth records. The figures, then, on the frequency of birth defects in *any population* range from about 1.5 to about 8 percent, depending on who's counting what—and how.

Birth defects are associated with a variety of causes, some of which are better understood than others. Of particular concern to older women is one group of defects called "chromosomal abnormalities," of which the best known is Down's syndrome. *It is only this special group of birth defects—the chromosomal abnormalities—which have been proved to occur with greater frequency to older mothers.* Malformations and birth defects that are *not chromosomal in origin* are rarely, if ever, associated with maternal age. A number of defects do appear to be associated with low birthweight (under 5 pounds), which in turn occurs most commonly in very young mothers, poorly nourished mothers, mothers whose pregnancies were spaced at less than 2 year intervals, and White, but not Black, mothers who have a history of mental illness. In recent years we have also become aware that some birth defects are *iatrogenic* (doctor-caused) are associated with the injudicious administration of drugs to pregnant women, excessive limitations on weight gain during pregnancy, misuse of anesthesia, the confined birth position, and other kinds of mismanagement of labor and delivery.

In 1959 it was discovered that children with Down's syndrome have 47 chromosomes in most cells of their body, instead of the normal 46. It is thought that the egg cells which give rise to babies with Down's syndrome have become overaged, so that their cell division does not function properly. The risks of Down's syndrome may be especially high in women who have already started menopause.

Another birth defect which is chromosomal in origin is Klinefelter's syndrome, afflicting 1 in 400 males. It is marked by small testes, which will not produce sperm, and is sometimes associated with mental retardation. Klinefelter's syndrome is associated with parental age, and some rarer chromosomal defects may be also, although the evidence is not conclusive.

All told, it is estimated that serious chromosomal defects, including Down's and Klinefelter's syndrome, occur once in every 200 births, regardless of maternal age. The number of *conceptions* involving such defects is considerably larger, but since many are incompatible with life, an estimated 88 percent abort spontaneously.

Chromosomal defects can now be detected during pregnancy, by means of a procedure called amniocentesis. The older mother who has "passed" her amniocentesis test may have no more reason to fear birth defects than a comparable woman many years her junior. At the centers which specialize in it, amniocentesis is better than 99 percent accurate.

At Columbia University, sociologist Amitai Etzioni and his former research associate, Nancy Castleman, have also been puzzled by the failure of many physicians to notify "high-risk" patients that amniocentesis is available. In their random sampling of 500 board-certified gynecologists, only two-thirds of the 40 percent who responded stated that they inform their older patients about the procedure. In 1973, a 42-year-old Brooklyn woman appealed to Dr. Etzioni for support in her malpractice cast against her obstetrician. Having already had a defective child, she inquired about amniocentesis, but her doctor dismissed her as "a worrier," and her child was born with Down's syndrome. The woman received a settlement.

At 36, Marlene Sanders, the television producer, became pregnant a second time. Sanders now explains, "I put off having children because I was getting established in my work. Then Jeff, my first son [born when she was 29], turned out to be a great kid."

In the third month of her second pregnancy, Sanders started bleeding. She was treated with hormones. "It didn't occur to me that it would be better to abort."

Her second son had Down's syndrome.

"Anyone who's had a baby with Down's syndrome in the family, who's seen these children, knows how essential it is for women to be informed. My son doesn't even know that I'm his mother. They say there are compensations in having a child with Down's syndrome, but I can't think of any—not one—except that I learned that life is unpredictable, and random bad luck can strike at any time."

Several years later, Sanders's 38-year-old sister-in-law took the test and was reassured that her unborn *daughter* had no chromosomal defects.

Amniocentesis does reveal the sex of the child, and this troubles some physicians who fear that parents may use the knowledge casually to preselect daughters or sons. Others are reluctant to suggest any procedure that could result in a midpregnancy abortion. Still others hesitate to send their patients to a colleague for amniocentesis, for fear that doctor switching may result.

Some geneticists have cautioned against amniocentesis on the grounds that it will "weaken our biological heritage," by encouraging parents who have already had one defective child to keep trying for a normal child. These normal siblings of Down's syndrome children, it is feared, may turn out to be carriers of the defect.

While the politicians and futurists slug it out (should the procedure be imposed on all women... or completely withdrawn?) only Etzioni and Castleman have thought to propose that medical specialists might simply be required to *inform* women and allow us to each make a personal choice.

Of equal importance is the question of what risks are faced by *mothers* over 40. In the United States there were 24 maternal deaths per 100,000 live births in 1972—good compared to the early 1950s figures of 83.3 deaths, but bad compared to the 1972 figures from countries such as Denmark and Sweden, whose rates were under 15 maternal deaths per 100,000 live births. Preliminary reports from the National Center for Health Statistics indicate that 1973 may have brought marked improvement in the United States, our figure finally declining to 15.2, which puts us in the same ballpark with other technologically advanced nations. Only 477 maternal deaths were recorded in the United States in 1973.

In one sense time is on a woman's side, for as she grows older and wiser, obstetrics does too. In 1940, the U.S. maternal death rate for women of *all* ages was 376 per 100,000 live births. By 1950, it had dropped to 83.3.

Physicians who feel comfortable delivering older women—and many do not—claim that the after-40 mortality figures are somewhat misleading. They point out that many more deaths from all causes occur in the forties than in the twenties, regardless of pregnancy, and that most maternal fatalities occur in women whose general health is poor.

Says Dr. Arthur Davids of Manhattan: "A lot of nonsense is published on this subject. The american woman is not old at 40. Physically she can pass for 30 if she's well-nourished and has good medical care... Kidney disease, hypertension, diabetes, cardiac disease, these have to be ruled out, but younger women can get them too. I can't remember ever telling a patient never to get pregnant *unless she had a chronic disease.* We're getting more women in their thirties having a first child, and more unmarried women deliberately getting pregnant."

Is the delivery process itself more complicated for an older woman? Statistically, the answer is yes. Her cervix may not dilate well, labor may be prolonged, and her chances of requiring a cesarean section are greater. A 1967 story by Dr. Sidney H. Kane entitled "Advancing Age and the Primagravida" indicated that abnormal fetal presentation (any position other than headfirst) was 18 percent among women aged 25 to 29, but 31 percent among women aged 40 to 44. Postpartum hemorrhage due to uterine inertia (weak contractions) rose from 2.7 to 6.2 percent for the same two age groups. Still, at an advanced medical center with conscientious attendants standing by, the absolute risks arising from such complications are not very high. I, who have long been a critic of (some) obstetricians for intervening when things are going normally, am happy that we have the good physicians—and, yes, even their fetal monitors and Brave-New-Worldish intensive care delivery rooms—when complications arise. I do not think that a woman in her forties should try a home delivery.

To mother *and* child, the order of risks is somewhat higher for a first pregnancy (whatever the mother's age) than for a second and third. However, after the fourth, the risks rise again.

First labors tend to be somewhat longer than subsequent labors, presumably because the uterus (up to a point) gets more efficient with practice. However, these statistics don't tell the stories of the women who, having had a grueling first experience, decline to repeat it.

Regardless of the mother's age, spacing children closely, at less than two- to three-year intervals, somewhat increases the risks. But spacing them far apart, at more than five-year intervals, somewhat diminishes the benefits derived from an "experienced" uterus. Generally, a woman's best labor is apt to be her second or third—if it follows more than two but less than five years after the one before. A woman who has deferred childbearing until 35 or after, may not have done so by choice. Many such women have had fertility problems, repeated miscarriages, or gynecological conditions such as fibroids, endometriosis, or cystic ovaries. Still others have systemic diseases which they were waiting to get under control. The risks to women who *had* to postpone a first birth for medical reasons are obviously higher than the risks to women who *chose* to wait. Actually, some of the complications associated with older pregnancy occur *more* frequently with later than with first births. Women past 35 are, for example, about three and a half times more likely to have placenta previa (a condition producing hemorrhage during labor) than those under 25. But, the chances of placenta previa in older mothers are lower if it's a first birth than if it's a later one.

No woman can be positively assured that she will remain as fertile at 40 as she was at 20. Besides aging, which does lower fertility in an absolute sense, infections such as venereal disease may intervene. So may drug effects, systemic diseases, and possibly radiation and other environmental influences. Age also lowers fertility in men, and while there are many exceptions, most women continue to select sexual partners who are their own age or older. (A biological imperative may be at work. Several studies reveal that, mysteriously, birth defects occur much more frequently when the age between mother and father is substantial.)

The woman who appears to have marginal fertility in her youth—as suggested, for example, in scanty and irregular menstruation—may find it especially hard to conceive in her thirties and forties. Frequent, repeated abortions may reduce fertility, as may use of the pill and perhaps the IUD. But one advantage of waiting to have a child is that some women discover they were not so keen on becoming mothers after all.

Finally, let's stop being so susceptible to what psychiatrist Ann Seiden calls "Old Doc's Tales," whether they be alarming, or falsely reassuring. Having a baby is never, strictly speaking, safe.

In a social sense, we who are at risk should determine the laws and practices surrounding birth control, abortion, and emerging reproductive issues such as amniocentesis. In a personal sense, we must inform and preserve ourselves.

For a healthy, affluent woman in 1976, the comparative risks of childbirth after 35 have been exaggerated—especially if she lives near a fine medical center. You can't expect objectivity from the sort of people whose textbooks, in this day and age, refer to women having their first child after 30 as *elderly primaparas.*

But the insults and patronizing suffered by affluent women are as nothing compared to the neglect suffered by the poor. The risks faced by poor mothers and their babies at the two extremes of the reproductive life span are inexcusable.

Given our current technology, and social trends, we would serve women and children better if we worried less about advancing age per se, and worried more about delivering medical and social services to mothers who are too poor or too young.

The optimum time for starting a family can be anywhere from 25 to 35. However, as Dorothy Nortman points out in her authoritative 1974 study entitled *Parental Age as a Factor in Pregnancy Outcome and Child Development,* "It cannot be stressed too often that, if other factors are favorable, age alone should not deter a woman who wants a child from bearing one."

Chapter 47

Abortion

I n 1994 Norma McCorvey (aka Jane Roe of Roe v. Wade) powerfully told her own story in collaboration with Andy Meisler. Later, she reconsidered and changed her mind about choice. An excerpt from her second book appears in Chapter 73. The pro-choice movement has too many martyred heroes who never received the recognition they deserved. Another example is Lucinda Cisler, a key New York figure; a full-time brilliant volunteer for choice; an architect who gave up her practice in service of her cause, scraping to get by, and, in the end, having some of her best writing and other work appropriated by others, without credit or compensation.

The sociologist Pauline Bart writes about the underground Jane Collective in Chicago where she lived and taught. The psychoanalyst Magda Denes reveals how sadistically some abortion clinics treat their clients, and instead of being thanked she is excoriated in the New York Times by a male reviewer who incorrectly perceives her to be anti-choice. Finally, a warning about Alix Kates Shulman's section on abortion in Memoirs of an Ex-Prom Queen: You will never forget it, and it will surely impact on you.—B. S.

I Am Roe

NORMA MCCORVEY

Excerpted from Norma McCorvey with Andy Meisler, *I Am Roe: My Life,* Roe v. Wade, *and Freedom of Choice,* New York, HarperCollins, 1994 Reprinted by permission.

I n February 1970 I was Norma McCorvey, a pregnant street person. A 21-year-old woman in big trouble. I became Jane Roe at a corner table at Columbo's, an Italian restaurant at Mockingbird Lane and Greenville Avenue, in Dallas. I'd suggested to Linda Coffee that we meet there.

Columbo's is gone now, which is a shame. It was an inexpensive place, clean, and made very good pizza. The tables had red-and-white checked table-cloths—just like the one I'd bought for Woody back in California. Columbo's wasn't very big. When I walked into the place that evening, I didn't have any trouble figuring out who was waiting for me.

Linda Coffee and Sarah Weddington, sitting together, stood out in Columbo's. Both were older than me, and both were wearing two-piece business suits. Nice clothing, expensive looking. One of them was tall and dark and thin. Delicate. The other was short and blond and a little plump, her hair in a stiff-looking permanent. Her hairdo was old-fashioned, even for then.

I was wearing jeans, a button-down shirt tied at the waist, and sandals. I wore my bandanna tied around my left leg, above the knee. That meant I didn't have a girlfriend.

I walked over to their table. It was obvious to me even from across the room that these women hadn't talked to a person like me for a long time, if ever. For a second, I felt like turning around and running out the door, writing the whole meeting off, and starting over again. But I didn't. Instead, I thought, Norma, they're just as scared of you as you are of them. Looking at the nervousness and doubt in their eyes, I almost believed it.

"Hi, I'm Norma McCorvey," I said.

The shorter blond woman came to life.

"I'm Sarah Weddington," she said.

Sarah Weddington reached out and shook my hand. Linda introduced herself, too, but it was apparent right away that Sarah was the one who would speak for both of them. For most of that meeting—in fact, for most of all our meetings—it was Sarah who talked, and it was Sarah who listened to me with the most concentration.

"Thanks for showing up," I said.

I don't remember much else about the first few minutes. Small talk was awkward for us, considering how little we had in common. I talked about Henry and how much I liked him. Sarah agreed. She told me that she and Linda were lawyers, which I already knew. The conversation died down.

I went to order our pizza and beer at the counter. While I stood there, waiting, I worked up the courage to ask these women the only question I was interested in getting an answer to.

I brought the beer back to the table.

"Do you know where I can get an abortion?" I said.

"No," said Sarah, "I don't."

Son of a bitch! I thought. I sat up in my chair and got ready to leave. I didn't want to hear the adoption spiel again.

But surprisingly, Sarah didn't begin to give it to me. Instead—and this is what kept me from leaving—she went off in another direction entirely.

"Norma, do you really want an abortion?" she asked.

"Yes," I said.

"Why?"

"Because I don't want this baby. I don't even figure it's a baby. And I figure it's making my life pretty miserable right now."

"Yes," said Sarah. "Go on."

I looked closely at her to see if what I'd said disgusted her. Or made her dislike me. But no, all I could see was that she was interested in my story. And maybe, just maybe, interested in helping me somehow.

"See, Sarah," I said, "my being pregnant, I don't think I'll be able to find work. And if I can't get work, I can't take care of myself. I don't want to be pregnant. I don't want this thing growing inside my body!"

By the end of my answer I was almost shouting. But Sarah didn't seem to mind.

"Norma," she said, "do you know what the abortion process is? Do you know what women have to go through when they get one?"

"Not really," I admitted. "But I kind of have a general idea."

Sarah told me, roughly, what a doctor did during a regular abortion. It sounded awful. But the truth was, it wasn't much different from what I had imagined all along.

Sarah leaned forward. "Norma. Don't you think women should have access to abortions? Safe, legal abortions?"

For the first time I realized that Sarah and Linda weren't just ordinary lawyers. For the first time *I* realized how interested she was in what I was interested in. Abortions. And in my getting one, too? Despite everything, my hopes rose a little.

"Sure," I said, "of course they should. But there aren't any legal ones around. So I guess I've got to find an illegal one, don't I?"

"No!" said Sarah and Linda, together.

"Why the hell not?" I said.

I felt a little flare of anger. First they were for abortions. Then they didn't want me to have one. What kind of mind games were these women playing with me?

"Because they're dangerous, Norma," said Sarah. "Illegal abortions are dangerous."

"Yeah, so?" I said.

Sarah shook her head. Then this woman in her nice suit, a woman I couldn't have imagined even going to a horror movie, began to tell me stories.

Terrible stories. Stories of women who'd had illegal abortions and lived to regret them. Or hadn't lived. Women who'd gone to gangsters, or shady doctors, and had their insides torn out. And who'd gone home and bled to death.

"These women were murdered," said Sarah. Then she told me about pregnant, unmarried women who had been so desperate to get rid of their babies that they'd tried to give themselves abortions with coat hangers. And killed themselves.

Then the worst story—one that made me shiver with fear. Sarah told me about a woman who didn't want anyone to know she had gotten the abortion—who was found, in a pool of blood, in a hotel room in New York City.

"They didn't find her for a couple of days," said Sarah. "And even when they did, she had no identification. So they didn't know who she was. They couldn't notify her family. All they could do was call her Jane Doe. And wait for someone to come forward and claim her body."

Jane Doe! That could be me.

An awful picture passed through my mind. Of me, alone—no friends, no lovers, not even a name—lying dead in that hotel room. Who would claim my body?

I began to cry, in front of strangers. Smart, rich strangers, who made me feel poor and ignorant. It was awful that they were seeing me cry. Embarrassing. Sarah handed me a Kleenex from her purse.

"Yes," she said, "it's really unfair and inhuman. And it shouldn't have to happen to any woman. Rich or poor. Anywhere." That's why, she said, she and Linda and some other people who thought just like them were working hard to overturn the Texas law against abortions. Their weapon was a legal project, a lawsuit, to challenge the law in the courts.

She wasn't sure if they would be successful, but if they could do it—and it would take a lot of hard work, plus a pregnant woman like me, who wanted but wasn't able to get an abortion, to put her name on their lawsuit—then abortions would be legal in the state of Texas.

"Would that mean that somebody like me would be able to get an abortion?" I said.

"Yes," said Sarah, "it would."

It would? New hope began to flood through me, even though I'd been crying my eyes out a few seconds ago.

"That would be great," I said, excited despite myself.

"Yes!" said Sarah, just as excitedly.

In her excitement, Sarah began describing the road the lawsuit would take—through district courts and appeals courts, state courts and federal courts. Early on, I lost the thread of what she was saying. But I kept nodding anyway. Sarah sounded so revved up, so intense, so passionate about her plans, that it was as if she were telling me her innermost personal secrets—instead of describing all sorts of complicated legal business, using words that I was certain only lawyers understood.

I thought, I don't really want to hear about courts. I've been in too many courts in my life. But I didn't want to interrupt her. This woman might be able to help me.

Finally, she stopped.

"That's great," I said, a little bit too late.

But I must not have fooled anybody, because there was an awkward silence. Then somebody, either Sarah or Linda, asked me to tell them all about myself.

Another silence. A longer one. All about myself? What would these women think about me if I told them all about myself? I didn't know much—anything at all, really—about their lives, but I was pretty sure they hadn't gone to reform school or dealt drugs or been beaten by their husbands or spent their days and nights in gay bars.

They might be shocked—or worse, maybe disgusted—by my story. On the other hand, they seemed to like me, wanted to connect with me, in their own way.

Would they still want to help me if I told them that my private life was none of their damn business? I took a deep breath and made my decision.

Over that red checkered tablecloth, I told them everything. Or almost everything. Louisiana and Dallas and Woody McCorvey. The whole miserable story. Over pizza and a pitcher of beer. While the people at the next table laughed and whooped it up.

Sarah and Linda hung in and listened sympathetically for a while. Then I got to the part of telling them I was a lesbian. That I liked girls. That I lived with women, get it?

Sarah and Linda looked at each other. They frowned. I felt the flashes of fear and doubt and confusion passing between them. I realized what they were thinking: how could this woman who says she's a lesbian have gotten herself pregnant all these times? It doesn't make sense. Maybe nothing she'd told us makes sense. But here's what does make sense: maybe she's lying to us. Or maybe there's something we don't understand about her. Something weird. Something dangerous. Something that will hurt our lawsuit. Hurt us.

No! Inside my head, I shouted back to them: You don't have to worry about my hurting you! I'm only dangerous to myself!

They didn't hear me. But how could I explain it all in words? I could sense them thinking about brushing me off and finding another pregnant woman. They were slipping away from me. And with them, my only chance for an abortion.

I panicked.

"You know," I said, "I was raped. That's how I became pregnant with this baby."

The horrible lie—this was the second time I'd used it—pulled at the insides of my stomach. But it got their attention. The two lawyers turned away from each other and quickly said they were sorry to hear this. That rape is a terrible thing. A crime.

"Was the rapist arrested?" asked Sarah.

"No," I said.

"Did the police look very hard for him?"

"No," I said, sinking deeper and deeper.

"Did you report the rape to the police?"

"No," I said, burning inside with shame.

Sarah stopped quizzing me. I tried to figure out whether she thought I was lying. This time, I couldn't read her.

She looked at Linda again. They seemed to come to some sort of conclusion.

"Well, Norma," she said, "it's awful that you were raped. But actually, the Texas abortion law doesn't make any exception for rape. So it doesn't matter in terms of our lawsuit."

"Oh, that's too bad," I said.

"Yes, it is," said Sarah.

A long pause.

"Well, anyway, we would like to have you as a plaintiff in our lawsuit. Would you like to help us?"

"Sure," I said, trying to be as cool as I could. A plaintiff. What was that? Well, I'd look it up in the dictionary later. At least I hadn't lost this chance.

We drank a beer toast to our lawsuit. Before she left, Sarah explained to me that they'd need me to sign some legal papers. With my own name, if I wanted to, but under a false name if I wanted to stay anonymous.

"Great," I said.

Sarah asked me if I had any questions. I said yes, I did.

"How much will I have to pay you two for being my lawyers?" I said.

Sarah smiled. "Nothing, Norma. We're doing this case *pro bono*." That meant, she said, that they were doing it for free.

"Then when can I get my abortion?" I asked.

"When the case is over, if we've won," said Sarah.

I was two and a half months pregnant. I didn't know how late you could get an abortion, but I did know that it was better to do it as soon as possible. How long could a lawsuit take? I remembered some of the trials I'd seen on television. The times I'd been in court myself. None of those occasions seemed to have taken much time at all.

"When will that be?" I said.

Sarah looked at me closely. I can see her sitting across from me, right now.

"It's really impossible to tell you that, Norma," she said. "We'll just have to let due process take its course."

It was a couple of weeks until I heard from Sarah and Linda again. In the meantime, I stayed at my dad's. I didn't tell him, or anyone else, about what had happened at Columbo's. Why risk being held up to public ridicule if the whole thing failed and we lost, and I still had to have a baby? Or worse, what if it was all some kind of harebrained scheme—or even a scam?

That's what made me decide to stay anonymous. To not put my own name on the lawsuit.

By the time Linda called me to come down to her office I was cleaning my father's apartment immaculately, several times a day, as if I was possessed by cleaning demons. I went downtown, and in front of Sarah and Linda signed a piece of paper. Not as Jane Doe—that reminded me of the woman who had been killed giving herself an illegal abortion—but as Jane Roe. The whole thing took only a few minutes. Sarah and Linda seemed very excited about it all. And so was I, despite myself, despite the feeling that I shouldn't be getting my hopes up too high.

And that was the start of *Roe v. Wade.* The lawsuit that would allow me, and millions of other women, to be in control of our own destinies.

To me, it didn't feel historic. Just a little confusing… and intimidating.

I didn't even know who Wade—Henry Wade, the Dallas district attorney who would be fighting the lawsuit against us—was. But that was all right. Sarah and Linda looked as if they knew what they were doing.

They both thanked me and said I could go home and let them do the legal work.

And then I waited.…

It was a strange pregnancy. It was a strange time, watching and feeling this baby—no, this *thing* I didn't want happening to me—growing bigger and bigger inside me. Some days, I looked very pregnant. Others, for some reason, I didn't look pregnant at all. I was out of work. Alone most of the day in a little apartment. I had all the time in the world to think about things.

My moods swung up and down, usually by the day, sometimes by the hour. When I was up, I was way up—I was the smartest thing on two legs. I wasn't just sitting around feeling sorry for myself, after all—I had taken action. I'd gotten a pair of wonderful smart young lawyers, and I was going to win my case and be the first girl in Texas to get a legal abortion.…

I was six months pregnant by the time the trial was over. When I called in, Linda told me to come right over. She sounded excited. After I finally arrived, hot and tired, she said that she had both good news and bad news to tell me. The good news was that we had won the case.

"That's wonderful," I said, holding my breath for the second part.

The bad news was that I had lost.

Even though the judges had ruled that abortion was now legal in Texas, Henry Wade had announced he would appeal the case—and until that appeal was decided, he would prosecute any doctor who performed an abortion on a woman.

"Well, then, Linda, how long will the appeal take?" I asked.

"A while," she said. "But, Norma, what does it matter? An abortion has to be performed in the first 24 weeks of pregnancy, and it's clearly too late for you now."

The world stopped.

The Jane Collective

PAULINE BART

Excerpted from Pauline B. Bart, "Seizing the Means of Reproduction: An Illegal Feminist Abortion Collective—How and Why It Worked," *Qualitative Sociology*, 10(4), 1987 Reprinted by permission.

The unique female capacity for reproduction has always been regulated. In no society and in no era have all women had control of their reproductive capacity. Yet, everywhere and in all times, women have attempted, with varying degrees of success, to obtain such control. Jane, or, the Service, began in 1969 as an abortion counseling and referral service, a work group of the Chicago Women's Liberation Union. Some of these women went on to do more than counsel and refer—they assisted the illegal abortionists. By the winter of 1971 they took over the entire process themselves. They decided to provide abortions for any woman, at any stage of her pregnancy, with or without funds.

Let us follow a woman through the steps she took to obtain an abortion from Jane.

1. A woman needing an abortion could get Jane's phone number from the Chicago Women's Liberation Union or personal networks or even Chicago police officers. She could call and leave her name and number on a message machine.

2. The messages would be collected every two hours and the call would be returned by a woman assigned to that task, called Calling back Jane. She would take a medical history and advise the woman that a counselor would call her.

3. The woman would be assigned to a counselor by the administrator, "Big Jane." The counselor saw the woman either individually or in a group. The woman would then receive the appointment time, date, and address where she was to go.

4. The woman would go to an apartment called "the Front" with her significant other(s). The Front was set up so that nonmembers would not know where the procedures were taking place.

5. The women, but not those accompanying them, were taken by a Jane driver to an apartment where the procedure, including a pap smear actually occurred.

6. They were returned by car to the Front.

In order to prevent complications and to treat any which occurred, the woman would phone her counselor during the following week. If she did not call, the counselor would call her, since it was important for an illegal organization like Jane to avert problems. Protection for "mistakes" available to physicians was not available to them.

The process for second trimester abortions varied. Leumbach Paste was inserted when available. Otherwise, the amniotic sac was ruptured or the umbilical cord was cut to induce labor. The woman was told to go to a hospital when labor started. She was given careful instructions on how to be admitted without the hospital calling the police. She was told her rights and what she did not have to reveal. Since women were "hassled" in spite of that information, a midwifery apartment was established with Jane women who specialized in delivering "long terms." The women aborted in that apartment.

A major logistic problem was disposal of the embryos and fetuses. At night "runs" were made to supermarket disposal bins. Sometimes this task was assumed by men who were friends, lovers or husbands of the Jane women.

Women in the collective also served as assistants, giving shots, inserting speculums and dilating cervixes. All these jobs, except abortionist, developed from the beginning of Jane's history.

WHY DID IT WORK?

The most important reason for Jane's effectiveness was the strong, radical and feminist sentiment pervasive in 1969 when the Service was initiated. Police brutality vis-à-vis antiwar protesters at the Democratic Convention the year before had radicalized the liberal and radical communities, leaving them angry and disenchanted with exciting institutions. It was in this climate that the Women's Movement began to attain momentum in Chicago.

The first national Women's Liberation meeting was held in Chicago in November, 1967. While many of the Jane women were not initially feminists and some were not "political," they wanted to do something for and with women. Since this was their first feminist activity, it was fueled by an enormous amount of energy, faith and hope, as well as anger towards men and patriarchal institutions.

The original members were primarily housewives supported by their husbands and with enough free time to organize the Service before there was enough surplus money to pay them. Babysitting was performed by some childless members and also was shared. When Jane women took over the Service from the professional abortionists and created paying jobs, it allowed the participation of more women who were young, single, and radical, and who could devote time to the Service only if they were paid.

Engaging in illegal activities made the group cohesive in the face of a common enemy. More important, the illegality of voluntarily terminating a pregnancy convinced Jane members that it was absolutely necessary to perform abortions. Jane members followed the tradition of civil disobedience to unjust laws with they had learned through participation in the civil rights and peace movements.

Because the group was illegal, it was cohesive and efficient, according to the women. No time was spent in what they termed hassling with the licensing agencies or maintaining bureaucratic forms. When some of the women subsequently organized a legal women's health center, they found bureaucratic restrictions to be constraining.

In contrast to other groups of people with equal good will, members of this group could actually solve problems—the women would walk in pregnant and leave no longer pregnant. In contrast, a worker on a woman's hotline stated that there was little she could do the battered women who called since at that time Chicago had no battered women's shelters

The collective supported itself and could pay salaries. Although no one was turned away for lack of funds, the average fee received was fifty dollars. The fact that women could be paid enabled a group of women to put much time into the Service who otherwise would have had to work at what they termed "shit jobs." By earning money in productive feminist work they were able to lead totally radical feminist lives. Financial self-sufficiency also ended the contradictions some women felt when supported by their husbands. Moreover, no energy was required for fund-raising or for grant-writing.

ORGANIZATIONAL THEORY

1. *The Goal of Providing Safe, Humane Abortions on Every Woman who Needed One Was Not Diluted by a Concern for Organizational Survival.* Some organizations have a vested interest in the continued existence or even exacerbation of their "problem" in order to justify and expand their funding.

2. *Authority Resides in the Collectivity as a Whole.* Jane's commitment to consensus meant that although they sometimes had to spend more time than they would have liked hammering out lines of their agreement, their eventual agreement allowed them to work smoothly under pressure.

3. *Minimal Stipulated Rules.* Although Jane members followed strict rules of medical procedure—e.g., if a woman was feverish, she was given an antibiotic—they had few formal rules of collective behavior. Their openness to the ad hoc decision-making of each member allowed flexibilityand a degree of autonomy for each member that helped them maintain their voluntary commitment of time and energy.

4. *Social Control through Homogeneity.* Jane's membership was homogeneous: over one-half of the women were between 20 and 30 years old, and all

but two were white. Most were born and raised in urban areas, particularly Chicago. When the Service was operating, about one-half of its members were single and one-half married, with two divorced or separated. The ratio of Protestants to Jews was approximately 1:2, and four women were Catholic. The typical Jane worker had postgraduate education.

Distressed by their own homogeneity, Jane workers, with only slight success, tried to recruit Black and Latino workers, the ethnic and racial characteristics of large segments of their clients. Although the women claimed ideological diversity, the diversity was within feminist and Left boundaries. Although they fought against it, the relative cultural homogeneity of the members of Jane was a blessing in disguise since it provided social cohesion.

5. *The Ideal of Community.* The search for community never replaced the goal of providing safe, humane abortions. Little time was spent "processing" relationships because of the urgency of the task of providing abortions.

6. *Recruitment.* The major pathway to Jane membership was through friendship networks. Some women became members after they or their friends had abortions with the Service. Recruitment procedures insured a relatively culturally and ideologically homogeneous group.

TRANSMITTING SKILLS

All skills were learned by observing other women and performing tasks under the supervision of women with greater skill. Skills necessary to perform abortions are not difficult to learn. One woman said:

> The thing itself [the curettage] was real easy. It's like making cantaloupe balls–the same motion with the curette.… The greater precision was in the handling of the dilator. You had to feel the woman's muscles through the instrument into your hand. So much of what you have to learn is sensitivity to the woman's body and that is what is unlearned in medical school.

Birth control information was offered and all the women received copies of *Our Bodies Our Selves, The Birth Control Handbook* and the *VD Handbook.* However, counseling was considered the heart of the procedure and everyone was supposed to counsel.

7. *Solidarity and Personal Growth Incentives Primary; Material Incentives Secondary.* Jane's appeal was to enacting symbolic values, such as a woman's right to control her own body. Moreover, all paying jobs paid the same, and many tasks, including counseling, were not remunerated at all. Because the Service was illegal, no one in Jane could use their experience in the organization to further their careers.

The individual autonomy and varied work that the organization provided had a major impact on the lives and self-images of the participants. In taking care of others, the Jane women fulfilled their own potential. Jane women also reported sharp increases in their feelings of identification with other women.

8. *Social Stratification: Egalitarian.* Jane had a strong commitment to equality. Consistent efforts were made to flatten the decision making and status hierarchies, especially after the paid professional abortionists were no longer present.

9. *Minimal Division of Labor.* The goal was to have every member perform every task. The Service exemplifies Marx's belief that "Only in a community with others had each individual the means of cultivating his [sic] gifts in all directions; only in the community therefore, is personal freedom possible."

CONCLUSION

Jane illustrates both the characteristics of a successful movement organization and the possibility of making abortion a less alienating experience for the women having them and for the medical personnel involved. To use Ehrenreich and English's phrase (1973), these women seized the "technology without buying the ideology"; that is, they used antibiotics and medical equipment but did not adopt the hierarchical system or the sense of entitlement that characterizes physicians. Since abortion has been legalized in this country, some physicians and nurses have expressed guilt over abortions they were performing. No women in Jane expressed such guilt, probably because they all had to counsel women who wanted the abortions and, therefore, knew the importance for the woman's life of not having a baby at that time.

When this research was begun, abortion was legal and poor women received third party payments. Now, however, third-party payments for abortions are almost nonexistent and a strong lobby supporting a "human life" amendment is trying to make abortions illegal again. Perhaps knowledge of the success of Jane will do more than expand the sociology of medicine, the sociology of social movements and organizational theory. Perhaps it will enable us to seize themes of reproduction.

The Abortion

ALIX KATES SHULMAN

Excerpted from Alix Kates Shulman, *Memoirs of an Ex-Prom Queen*, New York, Knopf, 1972. Reprinted by permission.

Roxanne told me about a way to abort myself with a speculum, a catheter and syringe, sterile water, and a friend. (Not till months later did I learn it could be lethal.) "There's nothing to it. I've done it twice myself. You just have someone squirt a little sterile water into the uterus, you wait, and in a few days you abort."

"What if you don't?"

"Then you do it again."

When I told Willy, he hit the roof. "Are you kidding? That's insane! We'll find a proper doctor to do it, thank you."

"But Roxanne's done it three times," I said exaggerating. "She says it's easy."

"Just thinking about it makes me sick."

"Come on, Willy. You'll help me, won't you?"

"Not that way. I'm going to find you a doctor."

Roxanne knew an intern whom she got to do it at his apartment in the Bronx. He pulled all the blinds and locked the doors while she boiled up the instruments.

"What a tight little twat you have," he said as Roxanne directed a flashlight between my legs. Each leg hung over a kitchen chair instead of being fitted into stirrups. I was ashamed. "It's a pleasure to work on you after the gaping smelly cunts that come into the hospital. If you could see them, you'd never want to have children."

"What do children have to do with it?"

"Believe me, having babies wrecks your plumbing. Now hold still a second. I don't want to hurt you if I can help it."

An instant of pain, and the catheter was in. "I wouldn't want to have children even if it was good for my plumbing," I said flatly.

"Don't you like kids?"

"I love kids. Other people's."

"Hey, will you relax? That's better. Don't you have any maternal instincts?'

"I have an instinct of self-preservation."

"You'll feel different when you fall in love. That's when they all want their babies. Now hold very still one more sec. Here comes the water."

"But I am in love."

"I doubt it," he said.

It was a familiar line, about love and babies. I'd been bucking it all my life. If it were true, as the scientists claimed, it would be smarter to live without love. The only power a woman had against a man was the possibility, never more than problematical, of leaving him; with babies even that defense vanished. No; plumbing aside, maternity was vulnerability itself, sentencing a woman at best to the plight of Mrs. Alport, and at worst to grubby isolation.

Sensation without pain, I felt the liquid enter me. "When I'm in love," I told him, "I rely on my convictions."

That very night, sometime after midnight, I awoke with unbearable cramps. I was exploding, coming apart at the seams. I rolled around and doubled up and moaned.

"What's the matter, Sash?" asked Willy in his sleep.

"Nothing. Go back to sleep."

I thought it was food poisoning or appendicitis. Then at last I felt I had to take an enormous crap.

"Where are you, Sash?" called Willy, feeling me absent from the bed.

I sat on the toilet and pushed and pushed. Then out it popped, my first baby.

I looked down. It was suspended over the water in the toilet bowl, swinging from my body, its head down.

"Oh my God! Oh my God! Oh Willy!" I cried. I covered my mouth and screamed.

A nightmare. I looked again. It hung there like a corpse.

"Willy, please! Come quickly! It's a baby!"

I couldn't understand what was happening. I had thought at two or three months it would be a fish with gills, or a tadpole. But it looked like a real baby, with a human head, only blue.

"Oh God! It's hanging here! Please help me."

"Now listen, Sasha," Willy was saying softly, "you've got to pull it out of you."

"Did you see it?"

"Yes."

"It's a baby, Willy!"

"I know honey, but you've still got to pull it out."

"Oh I can't." I was all atremble.

"You've got to."

"I can't."

It was too awful: the first baby I produced in this world I deposited like a piece of shit straight into the toilet.

"Try darling. Pull it out. Trust me."

At last, I pulled it out of me and dropped it into the water. It had always lived in a liquid medium. I couldn't look at it, my own child. I flushed the toilet. Then I dissolved on the bed in a shudder of tears and afterbirth.

"It was a baby. I can't believe it. It was a baby," I moaned. Will stroked my back as I wept and bled.

"Do you think you'll be all right for a few minutes while I get the car? I'm going to take you to a hospital."

"I'm all right," I sobbed. "I'll get blood all over the car."

"Fuck the car," said Willy.

"I'm all right," I repeated. "I don't need to go to a hospital."

"Do as I tell you!" he shouted.

When we got to the hospital, a doctor prescribed three kinds of pills and a bed in the maternity ward.

"Don't leave me here, Willy. I don't want to stay here."

"Don't worry, honey, I won't leave you."

"I'm sorry, sir, but you're not permitted on the ward," said the nurse. "You can visit her tomorrow."

"What are you going to do to her?" Will asked the doctor. "Can't you do something now so I can take her home?"

"Can't do anything till tomorrow," said the doctor.

"Why not?"

"I've ordered some pills to control the bleeding, and antibiotics and a tranquilizer. If she'll stop with the hysterics there may be a chance we can save your baby."

"But there is no baby, doctor," said Will. "She miscarried."

The doctor looked skeptical. "You sure?" he asked.

"Of course I'm sure. I saw the fetus myself."

"Did you bring it with you?"

"Bring it? No!"

The doctor shrugged and turned away.

"It's flushed down the toilet," said Willy frantically.

The doctor shook his head. "That's really too bad," he said, "If you'd brought it with you we might be able to clean her out tonight. But if she's not hemorrhaging and there's no fetus and I do a D-and-C at three A.M. with no one from the regular staff around, I could get into a lot of trouble. You understand. I wish I could help you out—"

"Take an x-ray," said Willy desperately. "You'll see there's no baby inside her."

"We can't take an x-ray."

"Why not?"

"An x-ray might damage the fetus."

Chapter 48

Rape

T here remain some evil voices in the world who still make light of rape, and mock the women who stand against it as shrill, obsessed, simplistic, and— humorless.

These two selections by Susan Brownmiller and Pauline Bart illustrate how subtle and how sensible the literature of rape can be. Here's an interesting story in connection with "Rape Doesn't End with a Kiss." Remember Viva? What delicious subversion. It was Bob Guccione who picked up the bills for this excellent rape exposé, conceived by Patricia Bosworth and B. J. Raphael, and executed by Pauline Bart.

In the summer of 1973, an unfortunate Supreme Court ruling called Miller v. California replaced obscenity guidelines with "Community standards." On the one hand a new wave of over-the-counter pornography was released in many communities. I remember trying to steer my daughters away from newsstands. Entering puberty, they didn't need to see women's breasts burned with cigarettes, a popular S&M magazine cover. But, simultaneously, news came to me from certain cities—Cleveland, for one example—that their banning boards were hatcheting the feminist books that dealt with body issues—medical and sexual. My Free and Female was newly out in paperback, as was Vaginal Politics. The Simon and Schuster edition of Our Bodies, Ourselves was climbing the bestseller lists. Our three books were pronounced a threat to community standards, as were Viva and a competing erotic magazine for women called Playgirl. But in these same communities, Penthouse and Playboy were allowed to stay.—D. S.

Against Our Will: Men, Women and Rape

SUSAN BROWNMILLER

VICTIMS: THE SETTING

The rape fantasy exists in women as a man-made iceberg. It can be destroyed—by feminism. But first we must seek to learn the extent of its measurements.

Male sexual fantasies are blatantly obvious in the popular culture. Female sexual fantasies are quite another matter. Rarely have we been allowed to explore, discover, and present what might be some workable sexual daydreams, if only we could give them free rein. Rather, our female sexual fantasies have been handed to us on a brass platter by those very same men who have labored so lovingly to promote their own fantasies. Because of this deliberate cultural imbalance, most women, I think, have an unsatisfactory fantasy life when it comes to sex. Having no real choice, women have either succumbed to the male notion of appropriate female sexual fantasy or we have found ourselves largely unable to fantasize at all. Women who have accepted male-defined fantasies are often quite uncomfortable with them, and for very good reason. Their contents, as Helene Deutsch would be the first to say, are indubitably masochistic.

What percentage of women fantasize about sex? Frankly, I do not know the answer, nor would I care to hazard a guess. I know of no objective studies that deal with the nature and prevalence of women's sexual fantasies. Kinsey did not delve into this area; nor, as yet, have Masters and Johnson. I am vehemently hostile to suggestions that some known, popular sex fantasies attributed to women are indeed the product of a woman's mind. I am thinking here of the scurrilous, anonymous pornographic classic *The Story of O* and its dreary catalogue of whips, thongs, bonds, and iron chastity belts that represents the pinnacle, or should I say the nadir, of painful masochism. I first became acquainted with *O* when it made the rounds of my college dormitory. It was during finals week, as I recall, and I was looking for some diversion. I nearly retched before I closed the book and handed it back to the giver. A few years ago, when I was working for one of the TV news networks, a fellow writer earnestly presented this same book to me as "the truest, deepest account of female sexuality" he had ever encountered. I am sorry I behaved with such civility at my second refusal of "O" and "her" story.

Because men control the definitions of sex, women are allotted a poor assortment of options. Either we attempt to find enjoyment and sexual stimulation in the kind of passive/masochistic fantasies that men have prepared us to have, or we reject these packaged fantasies as unhealthy and either remain fantasyless or cast about for a private, more original, less harmful daydream. Fantasies are important to the enjoyment of sex, I think, but it is a rare woman who can successfully fight the culture and come up with her own nonexploitative, nonsadomasochistic, non-power-driven imaginative thrust. For this reason, I believe, most women who reject the masochistic fantasy role reject the temptation of all sexual fantasies, to our sexual loss.

Given the pervasive male ideology of rape (the mass psychology of the conqueror), a mirror-image female victim psychology (the mass psychology of the conquered) could not help but arise. Near its extreme, this female psychosexuality indulges in the fantasy of rape. Stated another way, when women do fantasize about sex, the fantasies are usually the product of male conditioning and cannot be otherwise.

Two extreme examples of male fantasy that were commercially palmed off as female fantasy in recent years have been the pornographic movies *Deep Throat* and *The Devil in Miss Jones,* and I cannot deny I know a few women who claim they enjoyed seeing them. But I am not talking about such obvious junk, but of the normal run of books and movies with the theme of man as the conquering sexual hero, works that influence the daydreams of women, unfortunately, as well as men.

I do not mean to suggest that a woman's basic erotic fantasy, through cultural conditioning, is a fantasy of being raped. Rape is simply a noticeable marker near the end of a masochistic scale that ranges from passivity to death. And I do not intend to limit this discussion to specific erotic fantasies. At issue here is Everywoman's attitude toward her sexuality, her being, her attractiveness to men.

I owe it to Helene Deutsch to quote from her writings, since she was the first to define the female rape fantasy. Deutsch writes

> The conscious masochistic rape fantasies are indubitably erotic, since they are connected with masturbation. They are less genital in character than the symbolic dreams, and involve blows and humiliations; in fact, in rare cases the genitals themselves are the target of the act of violence. In other cases, they are less cruel, and the attack as well as the overpowering of the girl's will constitute the erotic element. Often the fantasy is divided into two acts: the first, the masochistic act, produces the sexual tension, and the second, the amorous act, supplies all the delights of being loved and desired. These fantasies vanish with the giving up of masturbation and yield to erotic infatuations detached from direct sexuality. The masochistic tendency now betrays itself only in the painful longing and wish to suffer for the lover (often unknown).... Many women retain these masochistic fantasies until an advanced age.[1]

The combination of perception and dogma contained in the above paragraph continues to amaze me no matter how many times I read it through. The conscious rape fantasy is offered as proof of inherent female masochism; masturbation is seen as an adolescent stage to be "given up." Yet despite these rigidities in her thought, Deutsch perceives that the female rape fantasy is no simple matter: For some, the rape of the will constitutes the erotic element; yet for others, the sufferance of a physical attack, or mental abuse, is a necessary prelude to the acceptance of love and affection. These two quite different sets of responses might have given Deutsch a clue that the most significant factor of all lies precisely in the lack of a uniform response. I would conclude that both sets of responses, or utilizations of the rape daydream, indicate a pitiful effort on the part of young girls, as well as older women, to find their sexuality within the context of the male power drive. This effort is the crux of woman's sexual dilemma.

ENDNOTE

1. Helene Deutsch, *The Psychology of Women*, vol. 1: "The Conscious Masochistic Rape Fantasies," New York: Grune Stratton, 1944–1945, p. 225.

Rape Doesn't End with a Kiss

PAULINE BART

Pauline Bart, "Rape Doesn't End with a Kiss," *Viva*, June 1975. Reprinted by permission.

In November 1974, *Viva* magazine published a questionnaire asking readers who had been victims of rape to help gather information about this widespread yet highly misunderstood crime. Dr. Pauline Bart analyzed the enormous response from over a thousand women—the most wide-ranging survey ever taken in this country.

Psychiatrists say a gun is a substitute phallus. After reading and analyzing the stories of 1,070 rape victims I find the reverse to be true. When it comes to rape, a phallus is a substitute gun. Rape is a power trip, not a passion trip. The rapist is more likely to rape in cold blood, with contempt and righteousness, than with passion. And women don't relax. They don't enjoy it. They don't much trust or like men afterward—a long time afterward. And they don't forget it. It haunts their lives.

As one woman wrote "The rape and attempted rape… have combined to foul up my relationships with men to the point where I react irrationally when angered. All men, my present husband and son included, lose their identity in my eyes and become walking penises."

Who gets raped? Every female is a potential victim, as are some men (the

1,070 cases include several men who recounted homosexual assaults). The ages ranged from 4 to 47 years, but the percentage increased dramatically between 12 and 16, with most rapes perpetrated on women between 16 and 20. Unmarried status was much more common in the group than in the U.S. female population at large. Twenty-two percent of the victims were under 15, with 7 percent under 12.

Ninety-seven women, or 9 percent, suffered gang rape. Although gang rapes were no more likely to result in physical injury than being raped by one man, the victims were more likely to feel hostility towards men afterward.

Eighty-four women (8 percent) were raped on more than one occasion, sometimes both as a child and as an adult. In some cases, two or even three rapes took place in adulthood. For seventy women, the rape was attempted but not completed. These women who were able to fend off the attempts were less seriously affected than those who were raped.

Who is the rapist? In the most frequent scenario, the rapist is a total stranger. When the attacker was known, he was most likely to be an acquaintance (23 percent) or a date (12 percent). But rapists could also be friends, men known by sight, relatives, ex-lovers, lovers or husbands. State laws are usually written in such a way that even the most brutal sexual attack by a husband is not considered rape. Nevertheless, four women named their husbands as their rapists.

Rapists averaged older than their victims. About 70 percent were white. Contrary to racist stereotypes, most rapes in the society at large are not perpetrated on white women by nonwhite men. Even in this selective sampling, 700 of the rapes were intrarace—71 percent of the white women being raped by white men and 68 percent of the nonwhite women being raped by nonwhite men.

Almost half the attackers were calm or matter-of-fact; about a quarter were contemptuous, angry, and righteous; on the other hand, 11 percent seemed frightened. While some victims mentioned that the attacker was drunk, very few noted that the attacker was sexually hungry or passionate.

Given the fact that the rapists averaged considerably taller and heavier than their victims, it is a tribute to women's courage that 99 percent of them resisted, 70 percent of them physically. Those who did not resist often gave reasons. "I allowed the man who raped me to do it without trying to fight him," explained one woman, "because he could have done me great physical damage." In many states, a woman must prove she resisted in order for the rapist to be prosecuted and convicted. Fortunately, feminist groups have succeeded in changing some such laws and are working to change others.

Where and when do most rapes occur? No time is safe. Rape takes place at all hours of the day and night. The fewest took place in the morning between 6 and 12 A.M.; fully half were in the 6 hours between 9 P.M. and 3 A.M. Over half of the women were attacked inside—one-fifth in their own homes and one fifth in the man's home. Only 161 of the women (15 percent) were actually raped outside—in the streets, alleys, and parks.

What happened to the victims as a result of the rape? Plenty. Almost half suffered a loss of trust in male-female relationships. About a third were affected sexually, had nightmares, and felt hostility toward men. About a quarter said they felt a loss of self-respect, and a similar number received psychiatric care. Sixteen percent had suicidal feelings, 16 percent felt a loss of independence, and 14 percent had physical injuries.

Not all the effects were bad. Over half of the women felt more strongly about standing up for themselves, 16 percent learned self-defense, and 6 percent joined women's groups.

More often, there is an aftermath of guilt and misery. "I was too ashamed to tell anyone in my family about it because of my puritanical upbringing," wrote one woman. "When I decided to tell my minister about my having been raped, I was told never to show my face in the house of God again."

Even when the woman is treated sympathetically after the rape, she still frequently suffers sexually. An 18-year-old was raped by her cousin when she was 15. As is frequently the case when the assailant is a family member, she didn't report the rape because it would cause a family scandal.

> The pain! For six months I didn't go out with guys at all. Later I could go out but sex was completely out of the question. After almost a year of that, I decided to block it completely out and make love with someone. It didn't work. Every time a guy and I would start to get it on, he would touch me in a certain way and flash! I froze. All I could see was my cousin on top of me, hitting me, hurting me—and it was all over for me and my guy. My boyfriends became frustrated, and eventually left me in search of girls not as "cold" as me.
>
> Now I can enjoy sex most of the time, but once in a while my partner touches me the wrong way and, baby, it's all over.

The more intimately the victim has known the attacker, the more likely she is to suffer sexual problems after the attack.

To be raped by a stranger is a violation of your body; to be raped by someone you know adds an even crueler violation of trust.

Young victims, those under 15, were much more likely to have their sexuality affected. This may be because they were more likely to be raped by someone they knew and thus more likely to have their trust violated.

Another factor affecting the woman sexually is whether or not the rapist is legally convicted. Forty-one percent of those women whose rapists were *not* convicted were affected sexually. One policy implication of this study is that in order to diminish the effect of rape on women's sexuality, more vigorous efforts should be made to apprehend and convict the rapists.

Women who reported the rape to the police were substantially less likely to lose trust in male-female relationships than women who did not. This result is probably dependent in part on whether or not the police were sympathetic.

Women who were raped by men who were righteous and contemptuous were substantially more likely to be hostile to men afterward than were women raped by men not holding those attitudes. The reason is probably that righteous and contemptuous rapists think they are *entitled* to sexual access regardless of the women's feelings.

The last factor significantly associated with hostility to men was the attitude of the police. A woman who was raped twice by the same man said: "I can only commend the Seattle police. I talked to 9 (at least 10 different people)... [They were] very sympathetic and willing to offer whatever aid or counseling I might find necessary." She reports that her feelings about the two incidents are "anger and rage against the man who raped me; *not against all men* [my italics]."

It is important not only that the police were sympathetic but that she was treated in a special rape relief center in the Seattle hospital. Such specialized centers at hospitals, most notably at Philadelphia General Hospital and Jackson Memorial in Miami, are performing a vital function, and the antirape movement is working hard to make such centers available in all cities.

About a quarter of the women lost self-respect as a result of the rape—a classic example of the way women are taught to blame themselves for whatever happens and to turn their anger inward rather than against the aggressor.

It is not surprising that almost a quarter of the women had psychiatric care of some type as a result of the rape. This does not necessarily mean that they were *helped* by the care; *35* percent of those who had such care said they were helped. The remaining 65 percent were not. Almost one-half were helped by other sources. For example, 132 women who reported they had had psychiatric care but were not helped by it received help from women's groups.

Quite possibly because of the greater number of antirape groups, hotlines for rape victims, and other women's support groups, more recent victims have alternatives to psychiatric care which were previously not available.

Women who resisted physically or by screaming were *more* likely to be physically injured than those who didn't—although it is unclear which caused which—and those who resisted by talking were *less* likely to be physically injured.

The following letter from a woman who was raped at knifepoint is an example not only of why women do not resist but also of the possible physical effects of rape—in this case, gonorrhea and severe pelvic infection. The letter also explains why she, like two-thirds of the women who answered the questionnaire, did not report the rape to the police:

> I tried to talk my way out of the situation, but he put his knife in his sleeve, put his arm around me, and ordered me to walk with him without a sound—I never once imagined that I was allowing this man to walk me right into my own rape!

I refused to go to the police out of fear. When I went to a gynecologist, I found I had become infected with gonorrhea. I was treated immediately with antibiotics.

The shame stayed. I talked to some friends—that seemed to help. Then one day I felt a terrible pain in my stomach. I realized I had a high fever and I rushed to the hospital, where I was found to have a severe pelvic infection resulting from the original gonorrhea. I was hospitalized for 10 days. It took me two years to get back on my feet physically —and I am afraid that I may never be able to have children.

Some women reacted constructively they felt more strongly about standing up for themselves, they joined antirape groups. Women belonging to antirape groups (which provide victims with the kinds of legal advice and emotional support necessary for them to endure the court ordeal and testify effectively) are more likely to report the rape to the police and the attackers are more likely to be arrested *and* convicted.

In order for the victim to be treated she has to see a physician, and in order for the rapist to be arrested she has to go to the police, and in order for him to be convicted she has to appear in court. Yet most victims don't do any of these things. Why? Perhaps this account, by a woman who was raped by her sister's ex-boyfriend, helps explain why so many women prefer silence to dealing with these institutions.

From the moment the police came it was just one question after another. After they got all the important information, I was taken to my family doctor. When he found out I had my period, he skipped most of the examination.

After five minutes at the doctor's office (most of it spent dressing and undressing), I was taken to the police station. I made a full statement, which took two and a half hours. I had to undress in front of four policemen to look for semen and bruises. They took pictures of me naked.

Now, the district attorney tells me that the man who raped me, thanks to a fancy lawyer who changed his plea three times, will more than likely get parole. I did my duty and reported the crime—and for my trouble they are going to set him free.

Everything I went through was for nothing. So help me God, if I ever get raped again I'll never lift a finger to help the police. It's just not worth what you go through. All this has taught me is that a lot of money and a good lawyer will get you out of any trouble.

Stories of official indifference are becoming less frequent. Our findings indicate not only that women *should* go to the police but that the police have become more sympathetic. Police are more sympathetic if the attacker is unknown and if the victim resisted by screaming. Perhaps surprisingly, we could not find any differences in police attitude associated with the race of either the attacker or the victim. Police, at least in this sampling, were just as likely to be sympathetic to nonwhite women, whatever the race of their attackers. The presence of policewomen is noted as helpful.

Hospitals, however, have lagged behind the police in sensitive treatment of rape victims.

> The hospital personnel. made it quite clear they were examining me only for presence of semen. The nurse rudely yanked my legs into the stirrups. The doctor who examined me stated, "You're lucky you take the pill." I was never told whether they found semen. I was never offered any tranquilizers, and the surface wounds were never examined or x-rayed. I was told to see my personal physician for a VD test.... The final coup came about two months later when I received a bill from the emergency room.

Why do I believe that rapes should be reported in spite of these horror stories? Because it makes a difference. Of those rapes reported to the police, 38 percent of the rapists were arrested. Of those arrested, 44 percent were convicted of rape. As word gets out that the police and courts are more sympathetic, more victims will choose to report their rapes, and as a consequence more rapists will be taken off the streets.

What can we learn from this study? It is amazing how insensitive our society has been to rape victims. The women's movement has been able to bring about changes in the victims and in the institutions with which they have to deal; but clearly, many men, often including the husbands of victims, are unaware of rape's impact. One respondent's husband crossed out his wife's responses to the question, "In what ways would you say your life has been affected?" and wrote: "I helped my wife fill out this form, and I don't believe she was honest about this." Women's feelings about their rapes must be seen as valid, and their reality supported. Men have to realize this for their own welfare as well as the welfare of the women they relate to. This kind of support is what the rape crisis lines, rape counselors, and feminist therapists provide.

Rape need not be always with us. It may simply be something that we are set up for because of the way our society is put together and the way boys and girls are brought up. The solution lies not in changing our biology but in changing our society so that, as one woman wrote, "God willing, maybe someday a woman can walk down a dark alley or sit in her home... without fear of rape."

Chapter 49

Women in White Coats

B orn in 1932, Mary Howell went to Radcliffe College and wanted to be a musician. Fortunately for women and the women's health movement, she decided to become a pediatrician after the birth of her first son, and ultimately wrote "Why Would a Girl Go into Medicine." Researching the slim booklet recalled for Mary her experiences in medical school: the slights, condescensions, jokes, and outright hostility she endured from school administrators, faculty members, and male students, in a time when even female patients thought female doctors inferior.

Written under the pseudonym Margaret Campbell (Mary acknowledged authorship only after resigning from Harvard in 1975), "Why Would a Girl..." was used by many groups pressing to gain a fairer role for women in the medical field. The prospects for women in medicine were altered drastically over a period of just a few years because Patsy Mink and Edith Green's Title IX (see Chapter 60) was passing Congress in the same year that Mary's research was being circulated. In 1969 the proportion of women in medical schools hovered around 8 or 9 percent. A decade later, women made up about 25 percent of medical school students.

In 1995 Harvard University hosted a week-long event to fête women in medicine; although Mary was mentioned on the timeline created for the event, she was not invited to attend. She died in 1998 of breast cancer.

Michelle Harrison still believes that the field of obstetrics/gynecology is not always scientific or ethical in its use of technology. What the Tuskegee studies of syphilis were to African Americans, the early birth control pill trials and child-

birth technological inventions were to women. An amosphere of mistrust was developed between women and their doctors. Controversy still exists within the medical community as to the usefulness of continuous fetal monitoring, developed in the mid-'70s, and now a mainstay of obstetrical care.—B. S.

Why Would a Girl Go into Medicine?

MARGARET A. CAMPBELL

Excerpted from Margaret A. Campbell (aka Mary Howell), *Why Would a Girl Go into Medicine?* New York, Ann E. O'Shea, publisher, 1973; Old Westbury, Feminist Press, 1973. New introduction by Ann E. O'Shea, 1999. Reprinted by permission.

I n 1973, ten years after the publication of Betty Friedan's *The Feminine Mystique,* nine years after passage of the 1964 Civil Rights Act, which prohibited discrimination in employment on the basis of sex, four years after Barbara Seaman's book, *The Doctors' Case against the Pill,* rocked the medical-pharmacutical industries,and one year after Congress enacted Title IX of the Educational Amendments Act, which banned discrimination against women in all federally supported educational institutions, a typewritten, 113-page book entitled *Why Would a Girl Go into Medicine?* by Margaret A. Campbell mysteriously appeared. The book, which the author described as "a survey of discrimination against women in U.S. medical schools, written to inform and encourage women medical students of the past, present, and future and to promote radical change in medical education and in the care of patients," began to circulate just as the women's movement and its outspoken feminist health advocates converged with the passage of dramatically far-reaching federal legislation making discrimination in employment and education against women and minorities illegal.

I was three years out of college and working with Barbara Seaman at *Family Circle* magazine. Barbara gave me a copy of the typewritten manuscript and asked if I would help her distribute it for the author, whose real name was Mary Howell, a dean at Harvard Medical School. This was an extraordinarily radical document, which detailed the insidious discrimination faced by women medical students at the most prestigious American schools, including Harvard. The need for a pseudonymous author was apparent, as was the need for an underground method of distribution. The feminist publications advertised the book and let readers know that copies could be obtained for $2 by writing to me at my New York City apartment. I remember making hundreds of photocopies of the book—many on *Family Circle*'s copying machines—and convincing Alan Handell (who would later become my husband) to run off hundreds more copies at his newly established printing company. I became the ersatz publisher of a radical underground book describing the discrimination suffered by women medical students and suggesting the larger issue of discrimination suffered by women consumers of health care. Mary Howell's book, together with Title IX, revolutionized medical education in the United States.

—ANNE E. O'SHEA, 1999

Why "girl"? The title of this booklet requires a word of explanation. It is a direct quotation from a woman medical student: "I have often been asked, "Why would a girl go into medicine?" It was chosen to symbolize the themes of this report. The wonder expressed in the question—that anyone of the female sex would want to, or could, become a competent physician—is half of the problem. The other half of the problem is found in the word "girl." Of course, one does not expect of "girls," nor of "boys," the maturity one hopes for in a physician. The denigration of the term "girl" used to describe a woman, an adult, tells us how we have all been socialized with regard to stereotypes of gender-role. This report is an attempt to inform all who are concerned about health care about the relationships between the prejudice that describes women as "girls," the effects of the prejudice on women being trained to become physicians, and the inappropriate attitudes and assumptions that color the behavior of many physicians toward their women patients.

We all know that discrimination against women exists, although we sometimes deny that knowledge because discrimination is painful to experience. Trying to change the sources of discrimination is a long, hard process, and in the meantime we must keep from being destroyed or poisoned as a consequence of what some people would have us think about ourselves. I believe the first three lines of defense are (1) information about the specific forms of discrimination in any situation, so we are never taken by surprise, (2) an understanding of ourselves and how we react to discriminatory attitudes and practices, and (3) strong support of each other, in formal or informal networks. That is what this document is about.

INTRODUCTION

This document has been assembled to assist women in selecting and surviving a medical school education.

Most of the information that students need to have before choosing a medical school is of course equally relevant and equally available to men and women. One set of questions has, however, been very difficult to answer: What is it like to be a woman student at X medical school? Are the various medical schools significantly different in their dealings with women? How do women who are now medical students feel about their experience?

The information collected for the report is "case study" data from women medical students. An exploratory questionnaire composed of open-ended questions was widely but nonsystematically sent to many (but probably not all) of the 107 degree-granting medical schools in the United States. Seventy-six questionnaires were returned from 146 women students at 41 medical schools. All data were collected between February and September of 1973.

What follows is an unremitting recital of Bad Things. Of course, there are also many positive aspects in the experience of being a woman medical student, as illustrated by the fact that 140 of the 146 student respondents urge other women to join them at their schools. This can in no way excuse the occurrence of the instances of discrimination cited here. These things should not happen.

INSTITUTIONAL DISCRIMINATION

The instances of discrimination described in this and following sections are only those that students are aware of and thought appropriate to describe. Evidence of institutional discrimination is difficult for students (or anyone else) to document, probably because it is blatantly illegal.

RECRUITING Because of the very large numbers of students now applying for a relatively few places in U.S. medical schools, little recruiting is done. Many schools do recruit (and compete for) students representing racial and ethnic minorities, and often some informal recruiting is done by faculty and alumni to attract especially attractive white male applicants. There is little or no school-supported recruitment of women, although women students some-times organize among themselves to encourage women applicants.

> Recruiting policies are not equal. Women are a minority in the school: 12 out of 125 in our class, equal or smaller percentages of previous classes. There is an active recruitment program for Blacks and Chicanos with the goal of equalizing population and enrollment percentages.*

ADMISSIONS Students have very little accurate information about admissions policies in action. In order to assess the possibility of discrimination in the admissions process we need to know, for each school, the qualifications of the applicant pools and of the accepted students, and the criteria used to judge students.

Until this information is made available, the AAMC data on admissions is limited but suggestive: we know only the proportion of women in the entering class of each school, and the proportion of women in the combined entering class of all schools taken together (the national mean). Schools that admit women in proportions less than this national mean may be presumed to be discriminatory until they supply data to disprove this presumption.

The admissions formula (compiled from weighted averages of grade point average, points for type and place of degree, MedCAT scores, extracurricular scientifically related activities) is equal on the surface. However, one's acceptance

---

*These statements are taken directly from student questionnaires.

also depends on how the applicant impresses two interviewers, who are of course male faculty members; this is probably the place where the discrimination takes place.

"MOTHERSTUDENTS" Only 16 schools—15 percent of the total number of schools offering M.D. programs—are known to have admitted 9 or more women students who were mothers in the years between 1956 and 1972. A discriminatory policy cannot be ascertained unless we know about the applicant pool and the number of "fatherstudents" admitted, but we should inquire whether those schools at which few or no motherstudents have been admitted have not made discriminatory prejudgments about applicants' capabilities based on traditional and stereotypic views of women and family life (i.e., that mothers care for children but fathers do not, that children cannot thrive unless their mothers care for them full-time, and that mothers cannot also be competent students and workers).

FINANCIAL AID Information about financial aid is also closely guarded, and students generally do not know how aid is distributed with regard to need; they could begin to find out, of course, by asking each other.

> One of the women could not get aid that would include her husband as dependent, although men with wives in the same position have no problem. Getting financial aid for children was almost impossible. They seemed to think I was asking for maid service, and that I was lazy.

LODGING The most frequent instances of discrimination against women have to do with on-call rooms at school-affiliated hospitals. Often the women students, with admirable flexibility, offer to make do by using the men's facilities—but the usual result is that the men students become angry and upset at the women.

> We asked for a lounge for women doctors and students because we can't go in the surgeons' lounge (they dress there) and it is not always comfortable to spend on-call nights sleeping in a long row of beds fully dressed between several undressed males. We have no place to leave purses and coats and, unlike the men, no place to shower. We were stalled and stalled and we never got the lounge.

> Female restrooms for students and house staff are nonexistent in our hospital.

ATHLETIC FACILITIES The principal examples of discrimination fall in the general category of "forgetting" that there are women students, or of counting the women's needs as less important than the men's. Lack of equipment for women, inequitable access to facilities, and absence of showers and locker rooms are the problems most frequently described.

HEALTH SERVICES: GYNECOLOGICAL CARE The student health service provides more than health care: for medical students it is one of the few examples they see, during their years of medical education, of physicians in action, the "real world' of clinic practice as opposed to the theoretical or ideal taught about in school and in the hospitals. For this reason, the quality of health care provided by the health service is of special importance.

Our first question is whether the female sexual-reproductive system is included within the range of general medical care. Alternatively, are women told by implication that this part of their bodies is exceptional and aberrant, and must receive medical care under unusual (often more inconvenient and expensive) circumstances?

Most departments of medicine argue and teach that examination of the female sexual-reproductive system is part of a general physical examination, and that care of "routine, uncomplicated" health problems in this area falls within the province of the generalist physician. In the real world, internists, family physicians, and other generalist physicians often do not consider themselves to be responsible even for simple matters relating to the female sexual-reproductive system. Although they will examine eyes and offer advice and treatment for simple ophthalmologic problems—sending a patient to a "specialist" only when the problem is complex or otherwise warrants additional expertise—they may refer all matters relating to the female sexual-reproductive tract to the gynecologist. (The reasons for this refusal to care for "female problems" as part of general medical care are complex and probably include such personal dynamics as disgust about female genitals, sexual anxiety, and denigration of the importance of the special health care needs of women.) The effect is to tell the women patient that her genital system is not part of her body in the ordinary sense, but a special, bothersome (offensive?) part of her that has to be shipped out for special care.

If complete general health care is offered to men, but women must go outside the health service (physically, financially, or by delayed appointment) for care for uncomplicated medical problems of the sexual-reproductive system, this is discriminatory.

HEALTH SERVICES: PSYCHOTHERAPY All women in our society live in "special circumstances," different from those of men. These special factors include (1) a socialization that rewards dependency and passivity and discourages autonomy, (2) a cyclic physiology and the ability to bear children, and (3) a social expectation that they will be subservient to men. Women training in a "man's" profession (by traditional definition) may well have many questions and some anxiety about the conflict between the professional role and the stereotypic female role. While many women find support from each other or from individual faculty members to be adequate in managing these questions and anxieties, some may wish to seek regular counseling or therapy. A health service that provides psychotherapy "appropriate to individual needs" will recognize these needs of women students.

DAY CARE Institutional "support" for day care means financial support, since no high-quality day-care arrangements can be paid for by parents—except the wealthy—if caretakers are to be paid an adequate wage. While day care is a problem for parents (and not for women alone), some medical-student parents are single-parent women, so the matter has been included here as an instance of discrimination against some women. I believe that the need for institutionally supported day care is great, and hope that men and women together will work for this cause as an acknowledgment of their responsibility as (current or potential) parents.

AFFIRMATIVE ACTION PLANS The executive orders of 1965 and 1967 and the 1972 law that bar federal contractors and educational institutions from discrimination on the basis of sex require all institutions that receive substantial federal funds (including all medical schools or the universities of which they are a part) to (1) describe the discrimination that presently exists and (2) outline the affirmative steps they will take to reduce discrimination.

That few medical-student respondents know what an AAP [affirmative action plan] is reflects the institutional and governmental apathy surrounding this possible remedy to existing discrimination. While an AAP is no panacea, it does signify that the institution has responded formally to the executive orders rather than exhibiting open defiance or simply ignoring the presence of minorities and women.

Working to help one's school develop an AAP offers a focus for energies and an opportunity for a group of women from diverse backgrounds to share a common set of goals. In addition, the information collected to fulfill the first part of the requirement (the documentation of present discrimination) is enormously revealing, and the entire project has high publicity value. We must, however, be cautious in hoping that the existence of an AAP will bring significant and sweeping changes in the near future.

REPRESENTATION OF WOMEN ON FACULTY AND ADMINISTRATION The AAMC lists information about minority faculty and administrators by school but without denominators so that one could calculate proportions. No such listing is provided for women faculty and administrators.

Students generally remark that they see very few women faculty or administrators: only statements that include some numerical information (or estimate) are included here—again, without denominators it is difficult to calculate the precise significance of these numbers.

The number of senior women at an institution is of course important information for the senior women themselves. For women medical students, these statistics have two kinds of significance: (1) senior women serve as "role models" and counselors for students, and (2) the proportions of women hired by the institution instruct students about the breadth of possibilities for their own future careers.

> There are two women pediatricians who are attending staff. We have no women who are full professors, administrators or advisers. Our hospital has one female intern out of 50 spaces and somewhat more female residents.

> The majority of the teaching staff is male (80 percent).

MISCELLANY There are other instances of institutional discrimination that do not fit neatly into categories.

> Social activities are geared to the single men—like inviting nursing students to parties.

> Surgeons' lounge—with a sign on the door saying "Surgeons and Medical Students Only"—is off-limits to female students, in spite of the fact that a certain amount of relaxed, informal teaching is done there.

> All parties and social events require a woman student to sign up for refreshments—however, some of us refuse to volunteer before each of the other [male] classmates do K.P. (kitchen patrol) first. The number of class parties has declined.

OVERT DISCRIMINATION

The "culture' of the medical schools apparently promotes certain (traditionally) "male" attitudes and behaviors and often is supported by a men's club atmosphere. Open discrimination against women (serious and "in fun") is encouraged by this atmosphere and promoted in the process of professional enculturation. The varieties of overt discrimination against women can be described as baiting, belittling, hostility, and backlashing.

BAITING The occurrence of baiting conveys the men's sense of social support for and approval of discrimination against women: it may, of course, also signify a deep and uncomfortable personal insecurity that can be slightly assuaged by denigrating others.

> "Because of you a man probably went into chiropractic school."
> On one ward a resident called his male students "Dr." and his female students "Ms."

BELITTLING The largest number of overtly discriminatory comments cited by students seemed to fall in this category. The belittling comments noted here are only those with reference to professional women or women physicians; see the section on "Women as Patients" for comments demeaning of all women as patients.

Quote of our new dean: "I don't think women belong in medicine anyway." This sums it up.

"A woman doesn't belong in the OR except as a nurse."—chief of ob-gyn.

A cardiologist said, "It will be interesting to go to your twenty-fifth reunion and see how many of the women have done a full day's work."

HOSTILITY While baiting remarks seem designed to evoke a reaction from the women to whom the remarks are directed, hostile comments appear to be undisguised and open expressions of free-floating anger against woman-as-colleagues. As is always true with discriminatory attitudes and behaviors against any group, a contagion develops that thrives on group support. The interaction between male students and faculty in this regard is apparent. Some women believe that discriminatory remarks are more often made in large lectures because of supports and approval from male students; others (perhaps in more "liberal" areas of the country) say that discriminatory remarks are more frequently made in small groups, especially by instructors who have the power to give grades and comments on the student's performance and personality.

In the first two years of medical school, when large lectures were the rule, it was very common for lecturers to begin sessions with little jokes, invariably with woman as the butts, in an attempt to gain rapport. This, of course, encouraged the men in my class to adopt a similar attitude toward women, and whenever any attempt was made by women in the class to point out these humiliations, they were further belittled.

An example of the private remarks, from a student: "Well, if the women don't like it [the use of "nudie" slides in required lectures], they don't have to come to class."

The head of the ob-gyn department tells obscene degrading jokes while performing surgery and considers it his right to tease Black nurses about bizarre sexual habits in front of 10 other people during surgery.

BACKLASHING In medical schools, as in almost every other social environment, the recent surge of feminism has brought out a particularly nasty kind of male anger, apparently as a reaction to a sense of threat. To a degree this backlash may only offer men an excuse or justification for doing what they would have done anyway, but it is also possible that backlash may promote even more overt (and covert) discrimination than might otherwise have occurred. In medicine, of course, men are reacting to feminism in the general sense (which may, for instance, affect their marriages) but also to the specific changes that are bound to come to their profession as a direct result of the admission of more women students.

> A dean advised several women in our class not to "band together," since there are now so many of us (12 women out of 125) that we don't need each other for support and protection. We were told that we must learn to work with our male colleagues.

SUBTLE DISCRIMINATION

OSTRACIZING Women physicians are often viewed as "fake men," and therefore as imposters. The message conveyed by ostracizing forms of subtle discrimination is that women really do not belong in the profession of medicine and that our very presence is jarring. Both ostracizing and forgetting (see below) must require a fair amount of energy in defense of the delusion that medicine is an all-male profession, since there have been successful and visible women in medicine (about 10 percent) for many decades. One of the ways women are ostracized from membership in a profession is by treating them— and expecting them to act—like dependent daughters, pampered sisters, nurturing mothers, help-meet wives or seductive playmates. It is apparently very difficult for many men to relate to a woman as a colleague; it may also be difficult for women to assume the relationship of colleague, because we have been trained to fill the familial roles.

> When residents talk with male students they talk about diseases, patients, and other medical subjects, but when women students are around, conversation is always slanted toward "women in medicine" and "women's lib."

> On several different occasions of small-group discussions led by several different obstetricians, I'm repeatedly excluded from the group—no one-to-one eye contact, referred to as "honey" (like a patient, all of whom are referred to as "gals" or "girls"), excluded from the camaraderie of the "fellows, who hang their stethoscopes around their necks to impress the chicks" with their prowess and status as docs.

> One woman student was requested to wear a lab coat while making rounds with her tutor (three other male students were not) so that she would "look more like a doctor" to patients.

FORGETTING Even more frequently, the presence of women students in the medical school environment seems to be totally overlooked or forgotten. Even in classes in which the proportion of women is as high as 25 percent, instructors and administrators "forget' that there are any women present.

Activities of the wives' club always exclude the women of the class, married or not, but special invitations are sent to the single men.

Professors have refused to call on women students raising their hands for questions in class and have neglected answering women's questions after class.

SPOTLIGHTING It is nearly equally uncomfortable to be constantly spotlighted as it is to be forgotten. One way to deal with what is perceived as an aberration is to call attention to the phenomenon with a vigor that may reflect kindly interest, amusement or anger. Some men in the medical school atmosphere are apparently so puzzled, or discomfited, by the notion of a *woman* medical student that they always remark on the presence of a woman in this role.

STEREOTYPING I Attribution to women as a group of the traits of dependency, lack of intellectual interest, lack of competence and ambition, and all of the traditional stereotypic characteristics of femininity constitutes the first variant of stereotyping. This "social shorthand" disregards individual talents, interests, and traits by setting a mindlessly rigid standard for appropriately "womanly" behavior: if the object-person is of the female sex she must fit the appropriate mold, and if she does not fit the predictable mold she is not feminine.

This first form of stereotyping is exercised against women medical students either by the expectation that they are all alike (and like all other women) in their interests and capabilities, or by the implication that since they have chosen to come to medical school they cannot be like other women and must therefore be deviant and unfeminine. The alternative sex-role options available to women medical students are a neuter role, denying femininity, or a pseudomasculinity ("being more like the men than the men themselves"). The sum and substance is a denial of the wonderful variations of humanity that occur in female form.

In one class, all analogies were directed to the men, and if a woman asked a question he related it to baking bread or milk cartons.

Female classmate being told by a male colleague after she gave a tutorial report, "You'd make a good fourth-grade teacher."

The most common is a very confused male asking how I will ever be able to be a good mother and a good doctor.

I have often been asked, "Why would a girl go into medicine?"

STEREOTYPING II The second form of stereotyping is based on assumptions about the "proper" roles of women in relationship to men. A woman is expected to be (in some combination) servile, seductive, grateful, admiring, tolerant and patient, respectful, a comfort for wounded pride, and an external super-ego and keeper of morality. If she does not "keep to her place" in her relationships with men but is independent, positive, even argumentative, and refuses to acknowledge and take part in seductive and flirtatious sexual games, she is looked upon as "inappropriate," "abrasive," or "bitchy"; by a process of escalation she may be described as "castrating." Admissions interview questions often reflect these attitudes.

> [In an admissions interview] I was asked repeatedly if I could perform in a class of all boys [sic], if I was looking for a husband, and if I was "really" serious.

> One administrative higher-up talked with a female prospective applicant for 15 minutes and asked nothing about her interests and career plans, only whether her husband knew she was there and wasn't this just a passing fancy.

MALE SEXUAL PRURIENCE The "men's club" atmosphere of medical school is never so apparent as in the laugh-getting comments and pictures about female sexuality. Comments about female sexual practices, habits, and preferences are given as embroidery overlaid on factual material related to the clinical practice of medicine. It is assumed that any man has the right to regard any woman—colleague or patient—as an object of sexual interest.

> The slide of a nude female with arms outstretched was used to illustrate the shape of an IgG molecule.

> "The only significant difference between a woman and a cow is that a cow has more spigots."—lecturer.

> Every description of pathology [in ob-gyn lectures] is accompanied by graphic descriptions of the sex life of a woman with that particular pathology.

HOW DO WE COPE?

There are three broad patterns of response. One may deny the very evidence of discrimination; react with anger; or seek, and give, constructive support to and from other women. These three are not mutually exclusive, and probably all of us use all of these coping mechanisms from one time to another.

Thirty of the 76 questionnaires were completed by students who said that there was virtually no discrimination against women at their school. Nineteen of these then described three or more incidents (many of them quoted in the preceding sections) that have in this analysis been counted as discriminatory. Of the remaining 11 students who said there was little or no discrimination against women at their school, 9 were countered by other respondents from the same schools who reported three or more discriminatory incidents and believed that discrimination against women was a general pattern; the remaining two were the only respondents from their schools.

Women medical students who utilized the energy-conserving adaptation of protective denial were most certainly in the majority in the recent past, and may still be the majority today. There may be a trend over time, however, for first-year student respondents were much less likely than students from upper classes to describe their experiences in this fashion.

Those who feel that there is essentially no discrimination against women in medical school, or who agree with the premises of the discrimination they perceive, often believe that women who react differently are "immature" or expect special favors. They often do not understand the questions in the questionnaire about "self-support," deny that they need support with respect to their status as women medical students, and may be angered by the implications of the questionnaire.

It is usually the reverse: a department chairman will be carefully explaining the mechanism of X in the care of the patient, and I find myself thinking: I'm just a girl and he's taking all this time to explain it to me!

The first step in seeking support during the process of a medical school education is usually among status-peers—other women medical students and older woman physicians. The comments quoted here reflect some of the anger and frustration of these students, and some sense of loneliness. When status-peer groups work well, the sense of strength derived therefrom is also evident.

The women in the freshman and sophomore classes got together on their own twice this year and invited women M.D.s from the [city] community. One was a pediatrician who is married and has three children. The other is a gynecologist who has not married (age about 42). We felt that we learned much from speaking to these women especially in the realm of what to expect and not expect from our colleagues in later years.

[We have] great support for women by other women of all classes—great ombudswomen. Several married women, some with children. Pretty good place for women, actually, though much improvement is needed.

Students who described a reaction of constructive support usually declared themselves as openly concerned with the matter of social equity for all women. They believed that they gained more strength by declaring their devotion to the cause of all women than from trying to please a group of men who seemed never to be pleased by their very presence as real persons. Concern for other women was often expressed by this group as concern for the medical care that women patients receive. Several students indicated that women— often, but not only, women who were declared feminists—were effective class leaders, especially in the role of organizers rather than as elected class officers. Some noted that consequent peer cohesiveness and support served to temper the process of "professionalization" by reducing students' dependence on teachers for support.

WORKING FOR CHANGE

We shall consider four ways to work for change: private negotiations, public "displays," organizing as an action group, and school-endorsed committees or task forces.

PRIVATE NEGOTIATIONS Most student respondents believe that judicious, politic, and carefully planned "confrontations" with persons who have acted in a discriminatory manner can be useful in bringing change. Some commented that one should never go alone—that the male-female, student-teacher dynamics were so well established that even polite protest was likely to back-fire if one were alone. Students who felt confident that two women together more than doubled their strength were not disturbed by remarks about the "timidity" inferred by their support for each other.

Many noted that discriminators confronted in private were most likely to change if their discriminatory behavior had been unplanned, and if the discriminator had some reason to alter his/her behavior (incidents that we have categorized as subtle discrimination). In instances of overt discrimination, some students wonder if the slim chance of bringing change is worth the risk of being scolded, criticized, or formally reprimanded, as by a poor grade. Others feel that the registration of protest accomplishes some purpose in and of itself, and in some instances private negotiations with instructors and administrators have clearly brought changes in behavior, and perhaps even in attitudes.

> We have just begun to speak to the doctor using [nudic slides] to explain that we think it is dehumanizing and that it makes us uncomfortable.

> Sometimes we feel comfortable answering back, depending on how receptive we feel the lecturer is to criticism. Most of the time we feel that answering back will only reinforce their view of us as "women's libbers."

PUBLIC "DISPLAYS" Public "displays" are not "ladylike" and so have a kind of shock value that can be both very informative to witnesses and very gratifying to those who carry them out. While most women medical students are hesitant to use this method of urging change, it is apparent that it can have tremendous psychological impact. Those at whom a "display" is directed may be angry or hurt by the performance; others who observe are often surprised and in some way depressed; and those who perform (especially in a group) can be exhilarated by the sense of group solidarity, the audacity of their performance, and the strength of their statement for a cause.

Most "displays" described by students seem to result from careful political calculation, taking into account the instructor, the mood of the class, and concurrent events in the school.

> The women [students] also now have, of their own, a library of male nude slides [made up from a homosexual magazine]; although the idea is to have no confrontation, if the need be, we will slip some of the slides into the lecturer's carousel of slides.

> We have in response to [discriminatory comments about women as medical students and as patients] (1) walked out of one class (2) confronted several teachers and presented our position (in one instance a professor harassed a woman in front of the class as a result of this).

ORGANIZING: GETTING OURSELVES TOGETHER A unified program to promote change comes most easily through an organized group. The energy derived from anger about discrimination (directed at one's self or at other women) provides a massive impetus for such an organized effort. Why is it so hard? So many of the women medical students tell of fledgling efforts to get together with each other, with older women physicians, and with other women, efforts that are not sustained. There are special skills of organizing that are often unfamiliar to women and to professionals. We are also terribly busy: Medical students and physicians have very heavy demands on their time, and employed or student wives have been shown to have little time for their own personal interests.

As women and as professionals we are brought up to mistrust other women; we learn in the preprofessional years to be individualistic and competitive with our peers; we are urged during professional training to act autonomously; and as women are forced to compete with each other for "scarce-resource" jobs, research grants, and the favor or approval of our male colleagues. Thus it is difficult for all women professionals, students and graduates alike, to work in a sustained cooperative and sharing fashion toward a common set of goals.

It is typical of women in medicine that they are unwilling to stay long enough—much less give the kind of time and energy needed to make the group work. Perhaps if we as individuals understood what we hoped to get from belonging to a group, we could undertake group membership with a greater sense of its value.

SCHOOL-SPONSORED GROUPS Committees, task forces, and caucuses that have the official blessing of the institution usually have simultaneous positive and negative effects. Some changes are likely to come about through the actions or recommendations of an officially designated body mandated to study the status of women at the institution; it is not clear, however, that this is ever the best or only mechanism to bring such changes. School-sponsored groups often have a built-in conservative drag, either by virtue of membership—the inclusion of persons known to be conservative or not overly sympathetic to women, in order to give the group "credibility"—or by virtue of an agenda established by the institution. While small changes (on the order of increasing the number of ladies' restrooms) can be effected, it is less probable that major changes (such as objectifying and publishing admissions criteria or publishing salaries and salary criteria) will come through the efforts of such a group.

There is the further hazard that committee members will be co-opted by the philosophy of the institution. Appointment to the group is something of an honor as well as a chance to "do good" through established channels, and is difficult to refuse. One then becomes privy to the reasoning of the institutions about priorities, as expressed by masters (male or female) of persuasion. It is easy to forget our own goals and priorities. I believe that all institutions must develop such committees; unless they are totally co-opted they serve to raise the consciousness of the institutional community. The very existence of the group is an admission that some matters may need change. But one should be cautious in the belief that school-sponsored groups can be effective in bringing the kind of root-level changes that are necessary. And such groups are much more likely to function effectively both in their internal dynamics and in their communication with the community if they are made up of persons who begin by seeing the problems in a similar light.

WOMEN AS PATIENTS

It is widely believed that there is pervasive discrimination by professional health workers against women as patients. While some of this discrimination is expressed as inappropriate medical care (unnecessary hysterectomies, missed diagnoses because of assumed "psychogenic" or "hysterical" etiology, and so on), an equally serious and more widespread form of discrimination arises from assumptions about women that restrict them (more severely than male patients are restricted) to roles of dependency and uninformed reliance on the physician's authority. We are only beginning to document the extent and consequences of this discrimination against women patients.

It is clear that there is a direct interrelationship between discrimination against women as medical students and as patients: the one supports the other. We have seen that the medical school environment permits or encourages some kinds of blatantly discriminatory attitudes, behaviors, and policies to a degree that would not be considered permissible in other areas of life. Women medical students themselves are often aware of the relationship between their teachers' attitudes toward them, and attitudes toward women patients.

It seems likely that women physicians might be the best advocates for women patients; it seems unlikely, considering the prevailing views about women in medical schools, that very many men will be able to comprehend the force of those discriminatory attitudes and their damaging consequences. If women medical students learn to accept those attitudes (probably excluding themselves as "special" women) they will be less able to work for change in the care of patients, or even to conduct their own practices with women patients in a significantly different manner than that directed by their medical school teachers.

SELECTING A MEDICAL SCHOOL

It should be apparent that no clear differentiation can be made between the various medical schools with regard to discrimination against women medical students. The data collected here are neither sufficiently extensive nor complete (school-by-school) to rank schools as better or worse for women to attend.

One chooses a medical school for reasons of excellence of instruction, curricular emphasis on aspects of medical research or practice of particular interest to the individual student, and geographical considerations; one chooses to apply to schools at least partly because admission seems probable. Discriminatory attitudes and behaviors toward women must be at best a secondary criterion.

SURVIVING (AND THRIVING) AS A MEDICAL STUDENT

Only 6 of the 146 students completing questionnaires failed to encourage and invite other women to join them at their schools. The message, I believe, is that we feel a deep need for the support of other women, a strong hope that the presence of more women at medical schools will help bring change, and a belief that initiation into the profession of medicine is exciting, satisfying and worthwhile.

> It's probably no worse than most med schools. Be prepared for a very ingrown atmosphere and some antiwoman feeling. It's not as bad as I had expected (believe it or not). Come if you can find out how many women there are—and only come if there are 10 or more because otherwise your chances for a good friend are slim…. If my experience is any guide, you will find good and true male friends.

> Academically it is fine and the prevalent attitude toward women medical students is tolerable even though we are such a deplorable minority.

> Please come. We need more women. The only way to change things is to have a larger number of women visible everywhere: in lecture halls, hospital corridors, labs, etc.

Be aware that discrimination exists and that you will run into it, both from your peers and faculty members. Don't let this discourage you. Also be aware that pronouncements or declarations from the administration aren't always the last word and can often be worked around.

A Woman in Residence

MICHELLE HARRISON

Excerpted from Michelle Harrison, *A Woman in Residence*, New York, Ballantine, 1993. Originally published by Random House in 1982. Reprinted by permission.

I am a 39-year-old physician. I graduated from medical school in 1967. As a feminist, family physician, and medical-school faculty member, I was one of many people in the late seventies who were challenging the way in which women were being treated by the health-care system. Attending home births, writing and lecturing, presenting testimony in Washington for HEW, the FDA, and consumer groups, I still felt limited by my lack of specific expertise and training in obstetrics and gynecology—even though I had my board certification in family practice.

At the age of 35, when my daughter was 5 years old, I left teaching and practice to become a resident in obstetrics and gynecology at Doctor's Hospital, a prestigious teaching institution in Everytown, USA. I had sought and found a part-time position, which required my working up to 70 hours a week for half salary, or $8,000 a year. Part-time residencies had been developed to help physicians who were mothers obtain further training and still take care of their children.

Irv Warren likes to challenge me, I think. This morning scrubbing at the sinks before a delivery, he asked, "You don't approve of what I'm doing, do you?"

He's right, I don't. He had been screaming at the woman in the delivery room, yelling, "Push! Push!" then, "You lazy female, push!" When she whimpered, "I'm trying, " he yelled, "You're not trying hard enough. Now push!" and his large round face became red and his belly puffed out, making him a fearsome figure.

At the sinks I responded to his question, "Well, that's not how I would do it," and shrugged, trying not to show how strongly I felt.

He stopped scrubbing for a moment and in a patronizing way said, "Michelle, when people are in a subservient position, sometimes you just have to tell them what to do."

"A 12-week-size uterus is about the size of a grapefruit, " I was telling Caroline, the medical student also scrubbed in on the hysterectomy with Dr. MacDougal.

He was teaching me as we did the hysterectomy, and I was passing on what I knew to the medical student. This woman had a fibroid tumor which had enlarged her uterus to the size of a 12-week pregnancy. The three of us were busily working at tying off vessels, probing, chatting, when Dr. MacDougal, holding one ovary gently in his hand, showed us a small cyst on the surface and said, "I just might take it out. She doesn't need two."

Suddenly worried that this woman's ovary was being so easily discarded, I tried an oblique way to argue for its being left in place. "Dr. MacDougal, I've heard of women's having hormonal problems after a hysterectomy even when both ovaries are left in. What causes that?"

"I don't really know, Michelle, but it happens. I personally think that even if we are careful there is still a cutting off of some of the blood supply to the ovaries when we take out the uterus. They just don't always work as well as before."

Glancing at Caroline, hoping she understood what I was trying to so, I said to MacDougal, "But if it's possible that this surgery will hurt her ovary, then if we take one out, she is more vulnerable to any damage done to the one left in."

Just then Johnson, the fertility expert, walked in and said, "Mac?"

"Yeah," Dr. MacDougal answered. "Hi there. What's up?"

"I was just wondering if you were planning to take out any ovaries this morning. I need some for culture."

"Well, I was thinking about it. Let me think about it some more," he said and turned to me. "You know they don't work as well after hysterectomy."

"Yes, but if you take the one out with the cyst, she might end up with none working."

"Maybe you're right."

"She's only 32, and I think she still wants them," I added.

Johnson shrugged and said, "I don't want to push you. I was just asking," and left.

Later Caroline and I overheard Johnson taking with Enders out in the hall. "I see you have a hysterectomy later today. Are you taking out the ovaries on her?"

"Well, I hadn't made up my mind yet, John. Why?"

"I'm looking for ovaries. I need some."

"Well, I guess I could." Enders paused as though to say more.

"Don't do it for my sake," Johnson interjected, but he had his arm on Enders' shoulder, their closeness making evident the danger to Enders' patient's ovaries.

This last day on OB was 14 hours long, spent primarily with Jackie, my chief, and Hilda Cameron, the attending for the majority of women in labor throughout the day. Jackie, Hilda, and I spent much of this 14-hour day talking.

During the day Esther, a 17-year-old Puerto Rican, tall and massively obese, arrived on the floor. She said, "I'm here to have my baby today. My baby was due last week and I want it now."

She'd had no recent prenatal care, and didn't plan to return after today. She was adamant that she would have her baby today and that we were to make it happen. After asking her some questions, I tried to examine her, but she was terrified and would not let me touch her. I said I had to examine her, and the nurse backed me up. "When Esther let herself be uncovered, I could see huge warts covering her labia; it was difficult even to finger her vaginal opening. As I tried to insert the speculum she pulled her whole body away from me, up toward the head of the bed. When I tried to reach her, she pulled farther away, her eyes bulging. She looked like a cornered caged animal, and I stopped.

I called Jackie, who I knew would want to examine her anyway, so my exam would have been superfluous. I also expected Jackie to do better than I because people, like veins, sometimes know who has more authority and respond differently.

When Jackie tried to examine the girl, however, she had no more success. Esther, still terrified, pulled back, drew her legs together, and would not let herself be touched. Jackie was obviously getting angry, and after two tries, ripped off her gloves and left the room. Once outside, she turned to me and to the nurse and said, "Women like that prove that no woman can be raped unless she wants to."

Realizing how shocked the nurse and I were, she qualified that by saying, "Well, maybe with a gun or a knife.... " Jackie calls herself a feminist. She is known as a feminist physician. Women will come to her because they believe she is different from men.

I wanted especially to do well with Hilda today, since she was the attending with me on my first day on OB. Today I delivered a patient of hers with an episiotomy, then did the repair as Hilda wanted it. She complemented me on my skills and then went on to tease me about my trouble doing an episiotomy the first day.

I have finally mastered running the pH analyzer as well as calibrating it for accuracy, something I've been working on for a while in spite of Richard's insistence that I didn't need to know how, since he could run all the samples.

Hilda had a woman in labor today who had a questionable monitor tracing, so she tried to get a pH sample. The woman was in heavy labor and kept moving onto her side, trying to find a more comfortable position, but Hilda had to keep moving her onto her back. Using the disposable pH kit, Hilda took the long tube, shaped like a megaphone and about 8 inches long, and inserted the narrower end into the woman's vagina. She tried to get it through the slightly dilated cervix, which was especially difficult because the woman moved a lot whenever she had a contraction.

Hilda was unable twice to get the tube set right on the baby's head. After her second attempt she handed the tube to me while she got ready to do it for a third time. When Jackie happened to walk into the room, Hilda turned to her and asked if she would try. As Jackie opened a new kit, and got ready to try, she said to me, "Michelle, the reason you had so much trouble getting a sample,…" thinking because I was holding the tube I was the one that had failed. Hilda did not set her straight.

It wasn't until the day was over that I realized it had been a day spent mostly with women doctors, and yet it had been no different from other days at the hospital.

Last year, teaching at the medical school, I was on a panel about women's health. I was asked by an angry obstetrician, "Are you trying to say that OB-GYN should only be practiced by women?"

"No, I'm not saying that, " I responded, much to his surprise, "because the women in the field are not unlike the men. The problem is with some of the basic practices and basic assumptions about women that are an integral part of the profession. The same system, with women replacing the men, would not change it significantly."

Although I said those words, I had not been without some hope that it really would be different if the doctors were women.

Chapter 50

Race, Class, and Reproduction

I n 1970 at the Senate hearings on the birth control pill, Dr. Louis Hellman was one of the most anticipated and authoritative witnesses. A famous ob/gyn professor, he chaired the FDA evaluations that found the Pill "not unsafe" in 1966 and "safe within the intent of the legislation" in 1969. What would he say now?

A senator pressed the doctor to explain exactly what factors he put into his equation of benefit vs. risk. Dr. Hellman acknowledged he put population and not simply the health of the patient.

Many males in the hearing room found this an enlightened and reasonable statement. Most females did not. From that day on, distrust of population controllers came to characterize the burgeoning women's health movement, which pushed for the development of proposals for curbing population by advancing the status of women *with measures such as literacy programs; loans to help women start their own businesses; public health and pediatric assistance.*

It turns out that feminists were far more on target than the population controllers who pushed risky drugs and devices. Statistics show that as the status of women rises—just about anywhere in the world—the birth rates rapidly decline.—B. S.

Racism, Birth Control and Reproductive Rights

ANGELA DAVIS

Adapted from Angela Davis, "Racism, Birth Control and Reproductive Rights," *Women, Race & Class,* Vintage Books, 1983, pp. 202–221. Originally published by Random House, 1981. Reprinted by permission.

B irth control—individual choice, safe contraceptive methods, as well as abortions when necessary—is a fundamental prerequisite for the emancipation of women. Since the right of birth control is obviously advantageous to women of all classes and races, it would appear that even vastly dissimilar women's groups would have attempted to unite around this issue. In reality, however, the birth control movement has seldom succeeded in uniting women of different social backgrounds, and the movement's leaders have rarely popularized the genuine concerns of working-class women. Moreover, arguments advanced by birth control advocates have sometimes been based on blatantly racist premises. The progressive potential of birth control remains indisputable. But in actuality, the historical record of this movement leaves much to be desired in the realm of challenges to racism and class exploitation.

The most important victory of the contemporary birth control movement was won during the early 1970s, when abortions were at last declared legal.... But in 1973 when the U.S. Supreme Court ruled in *Roe v. Wade* (410 U.S.) and *Doe v. Bolton* (410 U.S.) that a woman's right to personal privacy implied her right to decide whether or not to have an abortion, the ranks of the abortion rights campaign did not include substantial numbers of women of color. Given the racial composition of the larger women's liberation movement, this was not at all surprising. When questions were raised about the absence of racially oppressed women, in both the larger movement and in the abortion rights campaign, two explanations were commonly proposed: women of color were overburdened by their people's fight against racism; and/or they had not yet become conscious of the centrality of sexism. But the real meaning of the almost lily-white complexion of the abortion rights campaign was not to be found in an ostensibly myopic or underdeveloped consciousness among women of color. The truth lay buried in the ideological underpinnings of the birth control movement itself.

The failure of the abortion rights campaign to conduct a historical self-evaluation led to a dangerously superficial appraisal of Black people's [generally] suspicious attitudes toward birth control.... Granted, when some Black people unhesitatingly equated birth control with genocide, it did appear to be an exaggerated, even paranoiac, reaction. Yet white abortion rights activists missed a profound message, for underlying these cries of genocide were important clues about the history of the birth control movement, [which includes] for example, [the advocacy of]... involuntary sterilization—a racist form of mass "birth control."

...As for the abortion rights campaign itself,... women of color [certainly did not] fail to grasp its urgency. They were far more familiar than their white sisters with the murderously clumsy scalpels of inept abortionists seeking profit in illegality. In New York, for instance, during the several years preceding the decriminalization of abortions in that state, some 80 percent of the deaths caused by illegal abortions involved Black and Puerto Rican women. Immediately afterward, women of color received close to half of all the legal abortions.... When Black and Latina women resort to abortions in such large numbers, the stories they tell are not so much about their desire to be free of their pregnancy, but rather about the miserable social conditions which dissuade them from bringing new lives into the world. They were in favor of *abortion rights,* which did not mean that they were proponents of abortion, a distinction missed by those within the abortion rights campaign.

Black women have been aborting themselves since the earliest days of slavery. Many slave women refused to bring children into a world of interminable forced labor, where chains and floggings and sexual abuse for women were the everyday conditions of life. A doctor practicing in Georgia around the middle of the last century noticed that abortions and miscarriages were far more common among his slave patients than among the white women he treated. According to the physician, either Black women worked too hard, or

> ...As the planters believe, the blacks are possessed of a secret by which they destroy the fetus at an early stage of gestation.... All country practitioners are aware of the frequent complaints of planters (about the)... unnatural tendency in the African female to destroy her offspring.[1]

Expressing shock that "...whole families of women fail to have any children,"[2] this doctor never considered how "unnatural" it was to raise children under the slave system. The [position taken by] Margaret Garner, a fugitive slave who killed her own daughter and attempted suicide herself when she was captured by slave snatchers, is a case in point:

> She rejoiced that the girl was dead—"now she would never know what a woman suffers as a slave"—and pleaded to be tried for murder. "I will go singing to the gallows rather than be returned to slavery!"[3]

Why were self-imposed abortions and reluctant acts of infanticide such common occurrences during slavery? Not because Black women had discovered solutions to their predicament, but rather because abortions and infanticides were acts of desperation, motivated not by the biological birth process but by the oppressive conditions of slavery. Most of these women, no doubt, would have expressed their deepest resentment had someone hailed their abortions as a stepping stone toward freedom.

During the early abortion rights campaign it was too frequently assumed that legal abortions provided a viable alternative to the myriad problems posed by poverty, as if having fewer children could create more jobs, higher wages, better schools, etc., etc. This assumption reflected the tendency to blur the distinction between *abortion rights* and the general advocacy of *abortions*. The campaign often failed to provide a voice for women who wanted the *right* to legal abortions while deploring the social conditions that prohibited them from bearing more children.

...It was not until the issue of women's rights in general became the focus of an organized movement that reproductive rights...emerge[d] as a legitimate demand. In an essay entitled "Marriage," written during the 1850s, Sarah Grimke argued for a "...right on the part of a woman decide when she shall become a mother, how often and under what circumstances." But, as she insists, "the right to decide this matter has been almost wholly denied to women."[4]

...Grimke advocated women's right to sexual abstinence. Around the same time the well-known "emancipated marriage" of Lucy Stone and Henry Blackwell took place. These abolitionists and women's rights activists were married in a ceremony that protested women's traditional relinquishment of their rights to their persons, names, and property. In agreeing that as husband, he had no right to the "custody of the wife's person," Blackwell promised that he would not attempt to impose the dictates of his sexual desires upon his wife.

The notion that women could refuse to submit to their husbands' sexual demands eventually became the central idea of the call for "voluntary motherhood." By the 1870s, when the woman suffrage movement had reached its peak, feminists were publicly advocating voluntary motherhood. ...It was not a coincidence that women's consciousness of their reproductive rights was born within the organized movement for women's political equality. Indeed, if women remained forever burdened by incessant childbirths and frequent miscarriages, they would hardly be able to exercise the political rights they might win. Moreover, women's new dreams of pursuing careers and other paths of self-development outside marriage and motherhood could only be realized if they could limit and plan their pregnancies.

In this sense, the slogan "voluntary motherhood" contained a new and genuinely progressive vision of womanhood. At the same time, however, this vision was rigidly bound to the lifestyle enjoyed by the middle classes and the bourgeoisie. The aspirations underlying the demand for "voluntary motherhood" did not reflect the conditions of working-class women, engaged as they were in a far more fundamental fight for economic survival. Since this first call for birth control was associated with goals that could only be achieved by women possessing material wealth, vast numbers of poor and working-class women would find it rather difficult to identify with the embryonic birth control movement.

Toward the end of the nineteenth century the white birth rate in the United

States suffered a significant decline. Since no contraceptive innovations had been publicly introduced, the drop in the birth rate implied that women were substantially curtailing their sexual activity. By 1890 the typical native-born white woman was bearing no more than four children. Since U.S. society was becoming increasingly urban, this new birth pattern should not have been a surprise. While farm life demanded large families, they became dysfunctional within the context of city life. Yet this phenomenon was publicly interpreted in a racist and anti-working-class fashion by the ideologues of rising monopoly capitalism. Since native-born white women were bearing fewer children, the specter of "race suicide" was raised in official circles.

In 1905 President Theodore Roosevelt concluded his Lincoln Day Dinner speech with the proclamation that "race purity must be maintained."[5] By 1906 he blatantly equated the falling birth rate among native-born whites with the impending threat of "race suicide." In his State of the Union message that year, Roosevelt admonished the well-born white women who engaged in "willful sterility—the one sin for which the penalty is national death, race suicide."[6] These comments were made during a period of accelerating racist ideology and of great waves of race riots and lynchings on the domestic scene. Moreover, President Roosevelt himself was attempting to muster support for the U.S. seizure of the Philippines, the country's most recent imperialist venture.

How did the birth control movement respond to Roosevelt's accusation that their cause was promoting race suicide?.... Linda Gordon maintains that this controversy "...brought to the forefront those issues that most separated feminists from the working class and the poor."[7]

...In the context of the whole feminist movement, the race-suicide episode was an additional factor identifying feminism almost exclusively with the aspirations of the more privileged women of the society. First, the feminists were increasingly emphasizing birth control as a route to careers and higher education—goals out of reach of the poor with or without birth control. Second, the pro-birth control feminists began to popularize the idea that poor people had a moral obligation to restrict the size of their families, because large families create a drain on the taxes and charity expenditures of the wealthy and because poor children were less likely to be "superior."

The acceptance of the race-suicide thesis, to a greater or lesser extent, by women such as Julia Ward Howe and Ida Husted Harper reflected the suffrage movement's capitulation to the racist posture of Southern women. If the suffragists acquiesced to arguments invoking the extension of the ballot to women as the saving grace of white supremacy, then birth control advocates either acquiesced to or supported the new arguments invoking birth control as a means of preventing the proliferation of the "lower classes" and as an antidote to race suicide. Race suicide could be prevented by the introduction of birth control among Black people, immigrants, and the poor in general. In this way, the prosperous whites of solid Yankee stock could maintain their superior numbers within the population. Thus class-bias and racism crept into the birth control movement when it was still in its infancy. More and more, it was assumed within birth control circles that poor women, Black and immigrant alike, had a "moral obligation to restrict the size of their families."[8] What was demanded as a "right" for the privileged came to be interpreted as a "duty" for the poor.

When Margaret Sanger embarked upon her lifelong crusade for birth control—a term she coined and popularized—it appeared as though the racist and anti-working-class overtones of the previous period might be overcome. For Sanger came from a working-class background herself and was well acquainted with the devastating pressures of poverty. When her mother died, at the age of 48, she had borne no less than 11 children. Sanger's later memories of her own family's troubles would confirm her belief that working-class women had a special need for the right to plan and space their pregnancies autonomously. Her affiliation, as an adult, with the socialist movement was a further cause for hope that the birth control campaign would move in a more progressive direction.

When Sanger joined the Socialist Party in 1912, she assumed the responsibility of recruiting women from New York's working women's clubs into the party. *The Call*—the party's paper—carried her articles on the women's page. She wrote a series entitled "What Every Mother Should Know," another called "What Every Girl Should Know," and she did on-the-spot coverage of strikes involving women. Sanger's familiarity with New York's working-class districts was a result of her numerous visits as a trained nurse to the poor sections of the city. During these visits, she points out in her autobiography, she met countless numbers of women who desperately desired knowledge about birth control.

According to Sanger's autobiographical reflections, one of the many visits she made as a nurse to New York's Lower East Side convinced her to undertake a personal crusade for birth control. Answering one of her routine calls, she discovered that 28-year-old Sadie Sachs had attempted to abort herself. Once the crisis had passed, the young woman asked the attending physician to give her advice on birth prevention. As Sanger relates the story, the doctor recommended that she "tell (her husband) Jake to sleep on the roof."[9]

…Three months later Sadie Sachs died from another self-induced abortion. That night, Sanger says, she vowed to devote all her energy toward the acquisition and dissemination of contraceptive measures.…

During the first phase of Sanger's birth control crusade, she maintained her affiliation with the Socialist Party—and the campaign itself was closely associated with the rising militancy of the working class.… Personally, she continued to march on picket lines with striking workers and publicly condemned the outrageous assaults on striking workers. In 1914, for example, when the National Guard massacred scores of Chicano miners in Ludlow, Colorado,

Sanger joined the labor movement in exposing John D. Rockefeller's role in this attack.

Unfortunately, the alliance between the birth control campaign and the radical labor movement did not enjoy a long life. While Socialists and other working-class activists continued to support the demand for birth control, it did not occupy a central place in their overall strategy. And Sanger herself began to underestimate the centrality of capitalist exploitation in her analysis of poverty, arguing that too many children caused workers to fall into their miserable predicament. Moreover, "women were inadvertently perpetuating the exploitation of the working class," she believed, "by continually flooding the labor market with new workers."[10] Ironically, Sanger may have been encouraged to adopt this position by the neo-Malthusian ideas embraced in some socialist circles. Such outstanding figures of the European socialist movement as Anatole France and Rosa Luxemburg had proposed a "birth strike" to prevent the continued flow of labor into the capitalist market.

When Margaret Sanger severed her ties with the Socialist Party for the purpose of building an independent birth control campaign, she and her followers became more susceptible than ever before to the anti-Black and anti-immigrant propaganda of the times. Like their predecessors, who had been deceived by the "race suicide" propaganda, the advocates of birth control began to embrace the prevailing racist ideology. The fatal influence of the eugenics movement would soon destroy the progressive potential of the birth control campaign....

Eugenic ideas were perfectly suited to the ideological needs of the young monopoly capitalists. Imperialist incursions in Latin America and in the Pacific needed to be justified, as did the intensified exploitation of Black workers in the South and immigrant workers in the North and West. The pseudo-scientific racial theories associated with the eugenics campaign furnished dramatic apologies for the conduct of the young monopolies. As a result, this movement won the unhesitating support of such leading capitalists as the Carnegies, the Harrimans, and the Kelloggs

By 1919 the eugenic influence on the birth control movement was unmistakably clear. In an article published by Margaret Sanger in the American Birth Control League's journal, she defined "the chief issue of birth control" as "more children from the fit, less from the unfit."[11] Around this time the ABCL offered Lothrop Stoddard, Harvard professor and the author of *The Rising Tide of Color Against White World Supremacy*, a seat on [its] board of directors. In the pages of the ABCL's journal, articles by Guy Irving Birch, director of the American Eugenics Society, began to appear. Birch advocated birth control as a weapon to, "prevent the American people from being replaced by alien or Negro stock, whether it be by immigration or by overly high birth rates among others in this country."[12]

By 1932 the Eugenics Society could boast that at least 26 states had passed compulsory sterilization laws and that thousands of "unfit" persons had already been surgically prevented from reproducing. Margaret Sanger offered her public approval of this development. "Morons, mental defectives, epileptics, illiterates, paupers, unemployables, criminals, prostitutes, and dope fiends," ought to be surgically sterilized, she argued in a radio talk.[13] She did not wish to be so intransigent as to leave them with no choice in the matter; if they wished, she said, they should be able to choose a lifelong segregated existence in labor camps.

Within the American Birth Control League, the call for birth control among Black people acquired the same racist edge as the call for compulsory sterilization. In 1939 its successor, the Birth Control Federation of America, planned a "Negro project." In the federation's words,

> The mass of Negroes, particularly in the South, still breed carelessly and disastrously, with the result that the increase among Negroes, even more than among whites, is from that portion of the population least fit, and least able, to rear children properly.[14]

Calling for the recruitment of Black ministers to lead local birth control committees. ...Margaret Sanger wrote in a letter to a colleague, "We do not want word to get out,"

> ...that we want to exterminate the Negro population and the minister is the man who can straighten out that idea if it ever occurs to any of their more rebellious members.[15]

This episode in the birth control movement confirmed the ideological victory of the racism associated with eugenic ideas. It had been robbed of its progressive potential, advocating for people of color not the individual right to *birth control,* but rather the racist strategy of *population control.* The birth control campaign would be called upon to serve in an essential capacity in the execution of the U.S. government's imperialist and racist population policy.

The abortion rights activists of the early 1970s should have examined the history of their movement. Had they done so, they might have understood why so many of their Black sisters adopted a posture of suspicion toward their cause. They might have understood how important it was to undo the racist deeds of their predecessors, who had advocated birth control as well as compulsory sterilization as a means of eliminating the "unfit" sectors of the population. Consequently, the young white feminists might have been more receptive to the suggestion that their campaign for abortion rights include a vigorous condemnation of sterilization abuse, which had become more widespread than ever.

It was not until the media decided that the casual sterilization of two Black girls in Montgomery, Alabama, was a scandal worth reporting that the Pandora's box of sterilization abuse was finally flung open. But by the time the case of the Relf sisters broke, it was practically too late to influence the politics of the abortion rights movement. It was the summer of 1973 and the Supreme Court decision legalizing abortions had already been announced in January. Nevertheless, the urgent need for mass opposition to sterilization abuse became tragically clear. The facts surrounding the Relf sisters' story were horrifyingly simple. Minnie Lee, who was 12 years old, and Mary Alice, who was 14, had been unsuspectingly carted into an operating room, where surgeons irrevocably robbed them of their capacity to bear children. The surgery had been ordered by the HEW-funded Montgomery Community Action Committee after it was discovered that Depo-Provera, a drug previously administered to the girls as a birth prevention measure, caused cancer in test animals.

After the Southern Poverty Law Center filed suit on behalf of the Relf sisters, the girls' mother revealed that she had unknowingly "consented" to the operation, having been deceived by the social workers that handled her daughters' case. They had asked Mrs. Relf, who was unable to read, to put her "X" on a document, the contents of which were not described to her. She assumed, she said, that it authorized the continued Depo-Provera injections. As she subsequently learned, she had authorized the surgical sterilization of her daughters.

In the aftermath of the publicity exposing the Relf sisters' case, similar episodes were brought to light. In Montgomery alone, 11 girls, also in their teens, had been similarly sterilized. HEW-funded birth control clinics in other states, as it turned out, had also subjected young girls to sterilization abuse. Moreover, individual women came forth with equally outrageous stories. Nial Ruth Cox, for example, filed suit against the state of North Carolina. At the age of 18—eight years before the suit—officials had threatened to discontinue her family's welfare payments if she refused to submit to surgical sterilization. Before she assented to the operation, she was assured that her infertility would be temporary.

Nial Ruth Cox's lawsuit was aimed at a state that had diligently practiced the theory of eugenics. Under the auspices of the Eugenics Commission of North Carolina, so it was learned, 7,686 sterilizations had been carried out since 1933. Although the operations were justified as measures to prevent the reproduction of "mentally deficient persons," about 5,000 of the sterilized persons had been Black.

...As the flurry of publicity exposing sterilization abuse revealed, the neighboring state of South Carolina had been the site of further atrocities. Eighteen women from Aiken, South Carolina, charged that a Dr. Clovis Pierce had sterilized them during the early 1970s. The sole obstetrician in that small town, Pierce had consistently sterilized Medicaid recipients with two or more children. According to a nurse in his office, Dr. Pierce insisted that pregnant welfare women "will have to submit (sic!) to voluntary sterilization,"[16] if they wanted him to deliver their babies. While he was "...tired of people running around and having babies and paying for them with my taxes,"[17] Dr. Pierce received some

$60,000 in taxpayers' money for the sterilizations he performed. During his trial he was supported by the South Carolina Medical Association, whose members declared that doctors "...have a moral and legal right to insist on sterilization permission before accepting a patient, if it is done on the initial visit."[18]

Revelations of sterilization abuse during that time exposed the complicity of the federal government. At first the Department of Health, Education and Welfare claimed that approximately 16,000 women and 8,000 men had been sterilized in 1972 under the auspices of federal programs. Later, however, these figures underwent a drastic revision. Carl Shultz, director of HEW's Population Affairs Office, estimated that between 100,000 and 200,000 sterilizations had actually been funded that year by the federal government. During Hitler's Germany, incidentally, 250,000 sterilizations were carried out under the Nazis' Hereditary Health Law. Is it possible that the record of the Nazis, throughout the years of their reign, may have been almost equaled by the U.S. government-funded sterilizations in the space of a single year?

Given the historical genocide inflicted on the native population of the United States, one would assume that Native American Indians would be exempted from the government's sterilization campaign. But according to Dr. Connie Uri's testimony in the Senate committee hearing, by 1976 some 24 percent of all Indian women of childbearing age had been sterilized. "Our blood lines are being stopped," the Choctaw physician told the Senate committee, "our unborn will not be born.... This is genocidal to our people."[19] According to Dr. Uri, the Indian Health Services Hospital in Claremore, Oklahoma, had been sterilizing one out of every four women giving birth in that federal facility.

...The domestic population policy of the U.S. government has an undeniably racist edge. Native American, Chicana, Puerto Rican, and Black women continue to be sterilized in disproportionate numbers. According to a national fertility study conducted in 1970 by Princeton University's Office of Population Control, 20 percent of all married Black women have been permanently sterilized. Approximately the same percentage of Chicana women had been rendered surgically infertile. Moreover, 43 percent of the women sterilized through federally subsidized programs were Black.

The astonishing number of Puerto Rican women who have been sterilized reflects a special government policy that can be traced back to 1939. In that year President Roosevelt's Interdepartmental Committee on Puerto Rico issued a statement attributing the island's economic problems to the phenomenon of overpopulation. This committee proposed that efforts be undertaken to reduce the birth rate to no more than the level of the death rate. Soon afterward an experimental sterilization campaign was undertaken in Puerto Rico. Although the Catholic Church initially opposed this experiment and forced the cessation of the program in 1946, it was converted during the early 1950s to the teachings and practice of population control. In this period over 150 birth control clinics were opened, resulting in a 20 percent decline in population growth by the mid-1960s. By the 1970s, over 35 percent of all Puerto Rican women of childbearing age had been surgically sterilized.

...During the 1970s, the devastating implications of the Puerto Rican experiment began to emerge with unmistakable clarity. In Puerto Rico the presence of corporations in the highly automated metallurgical and pharmaceutical industries had exacerbated the problem of unemployment. The prospect of an ever-larger army of unemployed workers was one of the main incentives for the mass sterilization program. Inside the United States today, enormous numbers of people of color—and especially racially oppressed youth—have become part of a pool of permanently unemployed workers. It is hardly coincidental, considering the Puerto Rican example, that the increasing incidence of sterilization has kept pace with the high rates of unemployment. As growing numbers of white people suffer the brutal consequences of unemployment, they can also expect to become targets of the official sterilization propaganda.

...The 1977 Hyde Amendment has added yet another dimension to coercive sterilization practices. As a result of this law passed by Congress, federal funds for abortions were eliminated in all cases but those involving rape and the risk of death or severe illness, and many state legislatures followed suit. Black, Puerto Rican, Chicana, and Native American Indian women, together with their impoverished white sisters, were thus effectively divested of the right to legal abortions. Since surgical sterilizations, funded by the Department of Health, Education and Welfare, remained free on demand, more and more poor women have been forced to opt for permanent infertility. According to Sandra Salazar of the California Department of Public Health, the first victim of the Hyde Amendment was a 27-year-old Chicana woman from Texas. She died as a result of an illegal abortion in Mexico shortly after Texas discontinued government-funded abortions. There have been many more victims—women for whom sterilization has become the only alternative to abortions, which are currently beyond their reach.

...Over the last decade the struggle against sterilization abuse has been waged primarily by Puerto Rican, Black, Chicana, and Native American women. Their cause has not yet been embraced by the women's movement as a whole. Within organizations representing the interests of middle-class white women, there has been a certain reluctance to support the demands of the campaign against sterilization abuse. ...While women of color are urged, at every turn, to become permanently infertile, white women enjoying prosperous economic conditions are urged, by the same forces, to reproduce themselves. They therefore sometimes consider the "waiting period" and other details of the demand for "informed consent" to sterilization as further inconveniences for women like themselves. Yet whatever the inconveniences for white middle-class women, a fundamental reproductive right of racially oppressed and poor women is at stake. ...What is urgently required is a broad campaign to defend the reproductive rights of all women—and especially those women whose economic circumstances often compel them to relinquish the right to reproduction itself.

ENDNOTES

1. Herbert Gutman, *The Black Family in Slavery and Freedom, 1750–1925,* New York, Pantheon, 1976, pp. 80–81 (note)

2. Ibid.

3. Herbert Aptheker, "The Negro Woman," *Masses and Mainstream,* 11(2): 12, 1948.

4. Gerda Lerner, *The Female Experience* , Indianapolis, Bobbs-Merrill, 1977, p. 91.

5. Melvin Steinfeld, *Our Racist Presidents,* San Ramon, Calif., Consensus Publishers, 1972, p. 212.

6. Bonnie Mass, *Population Target: The Political Economy of Population Control in Latin America,* Toronto, Women's Educational Press, 1977, p. 20.

7. Linda Gordon, *Woman's Body, Woman's Right: Birth Control in America,* New York, Penguin, 1976, p. 157.

8. Ibid., p. 158.

9. Margaret Sanger, *An Autobiography,* New York, Dover Press, 1971, p. 75.

10. Bruce Dancis, "Socialism and Women in the United States, 1900–1912," *Socialist Revolution,* No. 27, 6(1): 96, 1976.

11. Gordon, op. cit., p. 281.

12. Ibid., p. 283.

13. Gena Corea, *The Hidden Malpractice,* New York, A Jove/HBJ Book, 1977, p. 149.

14. Gordon, op. cit., p. 332.

15. Ibid.

16. Les Payne, "Forced Sterilization for the Poor?" *San Francisco Chronicle,* February 26, 1974.

17. Ibid.

18. Ibid.

19. Arlene Eisen, "They're Trying to Take Our Future: Native American Women and Sterilization," *The Guardian,* March 23, 1972.

The Population Bomb

JEANNE HIRSCH (INGRESS)

Jeanne Hirsch, "The Population Bomb," *Women—To, By, Of, For, and About,* 1(1), 1970. Reprinted by permission.

The "science" of biology has traditionally been used as a tool to keep women in a subservient role and to legitimatize racial bias. The inference that "overpopulation is overcopulation" is used as a scientific cause for all social ills. Historically, overpopulation has been made into a "crisis" issue at times of greatest social upheaval and is spoken of in the same breath as war, famine, pollution, and environmental destruction. Today, with worldwide social and political unrest, the cry of overpopulation again arises. And all the propagandist literature which decries the "population crisis" is accompanied by photographs or inferences that the major offenders of overbreeding are the poor, the uneducated, nonwhites and non-Americans. The pictures are *always* of women and children, the easiest targets of a corrupt and destructive system.

Some of the proponents of Optimum Human Population Levels estimate that there are as many people alive on earth today as have lived here collectively from the beginning of the human species to the year 1850. They call for a U.S. Optimum Population Level well below the present 200 million, or a maximum of 2.3 children per family. Others say that unless there is a total halt on all births for the next 10 years—an obvious impossibility—there is no chance of reviving the rapidly deteriorating ecology. However, ads supporting this type of rhetoric have stated that the government could make "an enormous contribution to world peace," by meeting the population crisis. This implies that overpopulation is a major cause of war and that parents, particularly the mothers, who make too many babies, are to blame not only for overpopulation, but for war as well.

But these women, children, and infants are the victims of war and famine rather than the cause, just as they are the victims of the deterioration of the ecology rather than the cause.

Women are particularly vulnerable to such discussions of the "population bomb" (a term conceived to make the natural birthing processes seem warlike and destructive). The blame for these social ills has been put on overpopulation, but all of the easy solutions for overpopulation have been systematically denied us by the state. When state governments violate the federal constitution by allowing the church to interfere with legislation on birth control education, the free distribution of birth control devices, and free and legal abortions, women are daily violated at the hands of illegal and unsafe abortion practitioners.

Just as we must be very careful in all discussions of biological differences between men and women, which are commonly interpreted as "inferiorities" rather than "differences," so must we be very careful in our approach to the reasons for the need of birth control. If we shall it up here would need for population control, we are denying ourselves the personal dignity of free choice, we are denying our sisters a like choice, and we are perpetuating a racist and misogynistic attitude which is detrimental to our very existence. If we must have a political excuse for wanting—or not wanting—to conceive, carry, deliver, and raise a child, then we must choose a valid political excuse, and not one that has been handed to us by the very structure that we challenge. We must demand equality under the law and 100 percent free choice of how we want to spend our lives and our bodies. We must agree with those population control groups that demand federal laws permitting all methods of voluntary birth control (pills, diaphragms, condoms, intrauterine devices, free abortions, and voluntary sterilization) and the education that must necessarily accompany it. But we must fight those suggested programs which threaten to enforce, by law, strict regulations on family size, because these programs are specifically designed to the detriment of all women.

At the moment, the burden of childbearing and child care is almost totally a female occupation. Until this responsibility is shared by both men and women, it is the woman who must gain control over her birthing (or non-birthing) processes. Most women would be happy, individually or collectively, to have control over the time, place, and number of children they bear, thus diminishing whatever threat of overpopulation there may be. Most women would be happy to contribute to society in additional or alternate ways than just breeding; and those women who choose to breed would be happy to be accepted on an equal basis with those men and women who do not.

Until it is clearly understood that war, poverty, and destruction of the ecology is a very profitable venture for those large corporations which support them, while health, education, and welfare are not, women and children will continue to be the natural martyrs!

In the meantime, we must heighten our own consciousness to the point where we can demand our rightful place in society and find for ourselves alternates and additions to the traditionally sole role of breeding.

Chapter 51

Activists Speak

N ow it can be told: We wouldn't have had a women's health movement without Phil Corfman. He was our mole. He was our inside contact. When we needed to get reliable information we could always get it from him. When we needed to object to something, he saw that we were heard." I spoke those words at Dr. Philip Corfman's retirement luncheon, where I was one of many speakers recalling his career.

Thanks to Phil the FDA was opened to consumer participation; NIH sponsored research on male contraception; the Surgeon General held a task force on diethylstilbestrol (DES) and put in follow-up programs for the afflicted families; the high-dose birth control pills were removed from the market; the RU-486 was made more available; and, through his efforts, numerous women scientists and administrators were promoted to the jobs they deserved.

The magic day that Phil first stood up for activist health consumers was January 23, 1970. Alice Wolfson and her colleagues from D.C. Women's Liberation had interrupted his testimony at the Nelson Pill Hearings, and were dragged away by the Senate guards. Told to resume, he paused... to declare—fearlessly and with conviction, in front of rolling network TV cameras and scores of print reporters—that the demonstrators had raised "important" questions.—B. S.

Philip Corfman

INTERVIEW BY TANIA KETENJIAN

Philip Corfman, M.D., OB-GYN, was a member of the National Institutes of Health, the World Health Organization, and the Food and Drug Administration. This interview was conducted in June 1999.

TK: In its Tenth Anniversary Issue in 1982, *Ms.* magazine voted you one of forty male heroes of the women's movement. You were nominated for your "sensitive response to feminist health activists." *Ms.* lauded your "efforts to change the direction of birth control research so that male methods were included and safe methods for women were emphasized." What made you take paths that diverged from those of your male peers? Why do you have an interest in women's issues?

PC: It's hard to be objective about the reasons for your own interests, but I'll try to respond. Perhaps it started early in my life with my grandmother, Minnie Corfman, who told me that she could drive a team of horses "like a man," or my mother—a housewife—who told me that she earned half of my father's income. My father was a good model for me in that he shared in the housework and enjoyed it, as I do. Going to Oberlin, the first co-educational college, helped, and my wife, Eunice, whom I met there, was a feminist but didn't know it. She played on Oberlin's women's basketball team, and really hated having to play by "women's rules"—only three dribbles, for instance. And I remember her telling me just a few months before she died how she stopped her car to watch some kids playing soccer, and when she saw that they were girls she was so happy that she burst into tears.

TK: So a feminist perspective was ingrained in you very early on?

PC: Yes, I'd say so. And it's certainly enhanced by my partner, Harriet Presser, the demographer, who is a true feminist in that she not only believes in women's rights, but works aggressively for them.

TK: Tell me a little bit about what your aspirations were when you first became an obstetrician and gynecologist.

PC: After Oberlin, I went to medical school at Harvard and took all my specialty training in Boston. I chose obstetrics and gynecology because of the interesting combination of medicine and surgery that the specialty provides, and because even then I was interested in the population problem and the attendant reproductive health issues, particularly the need for better contraceptives.

After our nine years in Boston—during which time we had four children, built a house ourselves, and Eunice published several short stories and had a TV drama produced—I entered a clinical practice in upstate New York. I loved it. My patients were ex-urbanites from New York and farmers. I particularly liked obstetrics. Childbirth is usually a happy time, and I was often able to involve the husband in the delivery.

TK: Why did you leave clinical practice?

PC: I left after four years—during which time we built another house—because I simply didn't want to be only a clinician the rest of my career. I was offered a Macy Fellowship in New York to do cancer research, and took it.

Then, after less than two years, I was asked to join NIH [National Institutes of Health] as a "consultant in Obstetrics and Gynecology." It was clear that I would work on reproductive health issues—including contraceptives—but at first the responsibility couldn't be alluded to in my title.

TK: How long were you at NIH?

PC: I was at NIH for twenty years, from 1964 to 1984. I became the first director of the Center for Population Research in 1968. The Center originated from growing concern and recognition of the "population problem" in the U.S. and world-wide. It also originated out of concern for the safety of the Pill. The Institute was given three million dollars to study this problem in 1965 and I was put in charge, so we started our research work on contraception even before the Center was established.

We originated and supported a large prospective study in California, called the "Walnut Creek Oral Contraceptive Drug Study," somewhat similar to studies underway at the time in the U.K. Ours was a ten year study that monitored the health of women who elected to take the Pill and to see if anything bad happened to them. Fortunately, no unexpected adverse effects of note were discovered. Another major Pill study was a retrospective study by the Centers for Disease Control which demonstrated that the Pill protects women against ovarian and endometrial cancer.

TK: As I remember there were problems with the Walnut Creek Study at the end. I understand that Dr. [Savriti] Ramcharan—who was the principal investor near the end of the project—is thought to have accepted drug company money to promote the Pill and later went to Canada. All this lead the women's health movement to have some doubts about the study. Do you think their doubts are justified?

PC: Certainly not. Only the general practice study in the UK equaled the Walnut Creek Study for it design and scope, and Dr. Ramcharan's didn't work with the project long enough to have an effect on the quality or significance of the published findings. I'd say that Dr. Diana Petitti, a world-class epidemiologist who's now research director at Kaiser of Southern California, and Dr. Susan Harlap, another world-class epidemiologist—both of whom worked on the project much longer that Ramcharan—had a far greater effect on the quality of the work.

TK: Could you mention some of the other work that was done at the Center?

PC: The Center's program covered four very broad areas: basic reproductive biology research in humans and experimental animals; the development of new contraceptives; ascertaining the safety of contraceptives in use; and social science research in the population sciences. Since this involves an incredibly wide range of subjects over a twenty year period it would take a book to describe the work and the findings in a meaningful way.

TK: What led up to your becoming involved in activities at the Food and Drug Administration in 1968, when you were the director of the Center, and working at the National Institutes of Health?

PC: In 1966, before becoming Director, I was appointed by the FDA to its Obstetrics and Gynecology Advisory Committee, first as a consultant then as a Member. This committee was the first formally constituted Advisory Committee at the Agency. It was formed initially to deal with the safety of the birth control pill, but then was asked to address many other ob-gyn issues, such as the IUD, drugs for obstetrics, and hormone replacement therapy.

The Committee was appointed at a very active time in reproductive health issues. It was at the time that I testified at the Nelson hearings on the safety of the Pill about the work that NIH was doing on this problem. That's when I first met Barbara Seaman. I met her again soon after that when she and her colleagues, who were sitting in the corridor outside the Committee meeting, were invited into the meeting by the members so that they could express their views. The FDA staff didn't want them to attend because up to that time, at least, such meetings were closed. Now, of course, most meetings like this are open to the public, in part because of the activism of Barbara are her colleagues.

This was also at the time that Barbara Seaman and others established the National Women's Health Network. I recognized very early that it was essential that Network staff participate in the Committee's meetings and would call them as soon as I knew that a meeting was scheduled.

I continued to attend Committee meetings either as a member or as an NIH Consultant until I was sent by NIH to work at the World Health Organization in 1984. When I returned from Geneva in 1987, I was asked by the FDA to become a medical officer to review new drugs for obstetrics and gynecology, and to be the executive secretary of the very committee that I had been on for many years. Its name had been changed by then to the Fertility and Maternal Health Drugs Advisory Committee, and more recently it was changed again to the Reproductive Health Drugs Advisory Committee.

TK: Why were you recruited to these two quite different positions at the FDA?

PC: I was recruited to the medical officer job because of my training and experience, particularly in reproductive health. As for being the Committee's executive secretary, the original intention when the committee system was set up was to have physicians as executive secretaries, since they were expected to know both the science involved and the scientists who worked in the field. I believe that this applied to me.

I very much enjoyed being executive secretary, because the Committee provided a forum to discuss issues such as the safety of the Pill, or the value of hormone replacement therapy before the public, and it often became possible to take action on such issues rather rapidly.

TK: On January 23, 1970, during Senator Gaylord Nelson's hearings on the birth control pill, Alice Wolfson and her associates from D.C. Women's Liberation interrupted your testimony. The Wolfson women were cleared from the room by guards, as usual. The many other expert witnesses who were interrupted during those weeks of hearings and demonstrations seemed indignant, impatient, neutral, sometimes amused, but, the record shows, even those who most deplored the Pill, didn't want to hear about it from mere patients. Only you, of all the scores of witnesses, took the occasion to speak up in the demonstrators' defense. When Senator Nelson said, "Doctor, go ahead, you may proceed," you veered off from your prepared testimony to exclaim, "Some of the questions placed by people who interrupted our hearings were quite important." What were you feeling and thinking when you said this?

PC: Well, the questions were and are important; no one can deny it. The activists were women worried about the safety of the Pill, and had a right to be heard. They also had a right to be wary of the predominance of men on the Committee and the fact that almost all of those giving expert testimony were also men.

TK: What made you decide to let Alice and Barbara listen in on the advisory committee meetings?

PC: The committee was taking a break when we saw Alice and Barbara waiting in the corridor outside the room. When we asked them what they were doing there, they said they wanted to attend the meeting because we were talking about the safety of the Pill. The committee caucused, and, against the wishes of FDA staff, asked Alice and Barbara to join us and tell us what they had in mind. As I remember, the most important thing they said was that women should be better informed about Pill safety. This lead in time to the patient package insert [PPI] for the Pill—a really big step for which Alice and Barbara deserve much credit.

TK: Why do you think PPIs on the Pill and estrogen are so important?

PC: Simply because patients should know just as much as possible about the pills their doctors prescribe. This applies to all drugs, not just the Pill and other drugs for women.

TK: So why aren't patient package inserts applied for all drugs?

PC: It's primarily a political problem. At the end of the Carter administration, the FDA had in the works a plan to provide inserts for most drugs, but one of the first thing the Reagan administration did was to stop it. Later, when I was at the FDA, we tried to resurrect this plan, but it's bogged down someplace. Advocates must apply political pressure if they want to see some action on this issue.

TK: Years later you took your work to a global scale at the World Health Organization.

PC: After 20 years at NIH, I thought I'd like a new challenge, so I requested a detail by NIH to WHO to help manage the "Human Reproduction Programme." This was an activity quite similar in some ways to what we were doing at the Center, except that it was international in scope, and directed to the interests of developing countries. I very much enjoyed this work, and believe that I made a meaningful contribution. Of particular note was the research then underway at WHO which lead to the availability of RU-486 in three European countries.

TK: And then you returned to the FDA?

PC: My detail to WHO ended in 1987, and I was fortunate to be offered a medical officer position at the FDA, where I worked until I left the public health service in 1998.

I had ten super years at the FDA. In some ways I enjoyed the FDA more than other assignments because what I did was so close to actual clinical practice. We did practical things when I was there, such as bringing the Pill label up to date. Labels may seem unimportant, but I assure you that they are not: a label is the government's record of what a drug is for, what its safety has been determined to be, and how it is to be used. We updated all the scientific information in the label, and added a health benefit section which notes that the Pill prevents anemia, promotes regular cycles, prevents endometrial and ovarian cancers, as well as prevents pregnancy. Some of these findings were based on work that was done when I was still at NIH.

At another time we changed the label to say that a physical exam doesn't have to be done before the woman goes on the Pill. Indeed, I think that the Pill should be available without prescription, but that's another issue. We also removed from the market the higher dose pills which had been shown to be no more effective and somewhat more hazardous than lower dose pills.

Other contraceptive issues that came up during my watch were the approval of Norplant and Depo-Provera. We also were faced with issues relating to drugs for obstetrics and hormone replacement therapy.

TK: Looking back on all these changes in the health and the drug industries, what do you see as the effect of there now being more women in medicine?

PC: It's been great for patients. Women patients, at least, really prefer female doctors, and some men do too. A recent article in the *New England Journal of Medicine* attests to this. Barbara Seaman said some time ago that my specialty, at least, should have predominantly female practitioners, and that's happening:

more than half the residents of obstetrics and gynecology are now women. The old boys are fading away.

Alice Wolfson

INTERVIEW BY TANIA KETENJIAN

Alice Wolfson is a founding member of the National Women's Health Network. This interview was conducted in May 1999.

TK: What gave you the confidence, in 1969, to stand up in such a male-dominated arena as a Senate committee to protest the lack of women's involvement in the birth control pill hearings?

AW: When we first stood up at the Senate hearings we really had no idea that we were doing something that was going to have so much importance. We went as five women from a small group in Washington, D.C., concerned with health issues. Someone told us that there were going to be hearings on the Hill about the birth control pill. After we heard about the hearings we all sat around and talked about our own experiences with the Pill. It turned out that all of us in this small group had had some side effect or another. None of us had been warned that there might be side effects. Not only that, but half of the time, when you complained of a side effect to doctors, the doctors themselves didn't know that the Pill caused side effects. For instance, in my case, when I stopped taking the Pill, I started to lose a lot of hair. I went to a dermatologist who didn't know anything about the connection of hair loss to the Pill, and my gynecologist didn't connect it at all. I was terrified that I was going bald and I had no idea why. So we went to the hearings where we started to hear some very frightening information about the Pill. We were also shocked to see that there wasn't a single woman testifying, no women researchers, no women who had taken the Pill. We had so many questions that we just started to raise our hands asking to be called on, wanting to be heard. It was such an outrageous thing to do that the TV cameras and the newspaper photographers all swiveled around from the senators to focus on the women in the audience!

We really had not planned a demonstration but then, when we saw the kind of reception we got, we understood that the most important issue was not the fact that the Pill had been recklessly marketed and had been approved way before there was enough information about safety, but that women who were taking it, who were dying from a "safe and effective" contraceptive, weren't told anything about the side effects. So the issue grew from our individual outrage at what was happening to an understanding of how important our outrage was, and how much we—meaning all women—had suffered from not having had informed consent when we were given the Pill.

TK: What were some of the more serious known side effects that you had not been told about?

AW: It was hard for us to believe that the FDA was not on the side of women. They held secret meetings about the birth control pill and its side effects. There was data coming over from research done in England; which they were trying to keep secret. We were getting fed different pieces of information by Barbara Seaman, who was in New York. I was in Washington, D.C., and Barbara would call and say, "They're meeting today, they're at the FDA"; and we would go there with some excuse or other, and break into the meeting room. We felt very powerful, like, "Alright, fine, arrest us. We're the people taking the Pill, and if that's what you want, fine, you can arrest us." We were fearless; we would put ten dollars in our boots and go off. If we were arrested, we'd bail ourselves out. They never did, actually, arrest any of us but they threatened us a lot. Senator Dole had us into his office and basically begged us to stop the demonstrations:

"We can't continue if you don't stop." He said something like that. It's not an exact quote. I think we made some kind of deal with him at that point. We agreed that we would stop the demonstrations if they would stop the hearings and bring women back into the next round of hearings.

TK: Tell me about the April 1, 1970 secret FDA meeting. How did you get in? How did Barbara Seaman find out about it and let you know?

AW: Barbara was a health writer in New York. She had many mainstream contacts, and she was very interested in the side effects of the Pill; so she became aware, through her own contacts, of things that were happening in Washington. There was a meeting that was held in secret. Barbara told me who to ask for at the meeting, so I knocked on the door. I think there were three of us there. We were told, "Sorry, this meeting is private; you can't come in." So we pushed open the door, and said to them, "Alright, call the police. We'll call the paper, you call the police."

So doctors were sitting around discussing whether or not to tell women to call them if they got a headache and they were on the birth control pill. There was an argument between a short patient package insert and a longer, more informative patient package insert, and the doctors sat around and said things like, "If you tell a woman she's going to get a headache, she'll get the headache. I'll be beleaguered by calls; my wife will kill me; people will be calling me in the middle of the night about all of these side effects; we can't do it."

Meanwhile, they had data that was definitely showing that women were dying from taking these pills. It's important to remember that it was healthy women who were taking the Pill. This wasn't a pill that was being given to somebody who was sick to make them better, this was something that was being given to women who started out healthy and who were dying. I think one of our signs once said, "Must we die for love?" along with "Feed your pills to the rats at the FDA."

TK: Did you find that you had to hide your radical appearance to be effective in the hearings?

AW: For the first Pill hearing, we dressed for the occasion. We knew we were going to the Senate, so all of us dressed to fit in, not to stand out. We wore dresses, skirts, high-heels, and felt that it would be much more important to have our message heard for what it is, than to be judged for something that would create an immediate kind of knee-jerk reaction to who we were. So for every demonstration that I ever participated in, I dressed up. Just like I do for court today.

TK: What was the D.C. Women's Liberation?

AW: D.C. Women's Liberation coalesced at a particular moment in history. There were a lot of great women who were living in Washington, D.C. at that time—around 1969—early feminists who managed to obtain enough money to actually open an office. We had a humming, vibrant movement. We had day-care and a health group, and we had a newspaper, and the office was active. It seemed like, day and night, we had retreats; we had demonstrations at the drop of a hat. I think people don't know much about what birth control pills were like at the time. Abortion was still illegal, so it was very radical to say that the safest method of birth control was a barrier method followed up by safe, legal abortion. That was basically what the feminists were saying in those days, and it just wasn't said.

Another thing that people don't know much about is that there was a very large population control movement headed by the biggest names in the ruling class—the Duponts, the Mellons, and the Rockefellers—who had a vested interest in marketing population control abroad, and the Pill was one of the tools with which it was marketed. I remember one guerilla theater event where we went into a very large population control meeting of maybe 500 people. There was something called the Women's International Terrorist Conspiracy from Hell (WITCH). We had our hats and our capes stuffed into our purses and at a certain point, we jumped up, put on our hats and capes, ran to the stage, grabbed the microphone, and did a skit, and—I don't remember the skit—but I remember the refrain was, "You think you can cure all the world's ills / by making poor women take your unhealthy pills." And then we would throw the pills out into the audience. We were really making connections to very large issues after starting with small issues—or what we thought was small at the time—that was the birth control pill.

There is a difference between a single issue and a broad spectrum of issues. If the birth control pill or abortion as a single issue are broadened out, they become a whole spectrum of issues called reproductive rights or reproductive choice. Part of being able to choose to have a child is to have the systems in place that make it possible: day care, after school care. When my kids were little, after school care was awful, you couldn't find it anywhere, and it was really hard to figure out what to do with your kids when school was out. Today we're seeing all sorts of cuts in welfare, but we're not seeing a growth in the kinds of systems that we need to support working parents. So, no true choice.

TK: What was the Hyde Amendment and how was it discriminatory?

AW: The Hyde Amendment was the first congressional effort to cut off public funding for abortions for poor women: it actually discontinued Medicaid funding for abortions, discriminating against poor women by not allowing them to have access to the same kind of health care as middle-class women. A group that I belonged to in California, called the Committee to Defend Reproductive Rights, was successful in bringing a law suit and in maintaining MediCal funding for abortion, even though there wasn't any federal funding. The Committee to Defend Reproductive Rights was successful in maintaining MediCal funding, which is California's public funding, on an issue of equal access. The California Supreme Court could be convinced in a way that obviously Congress could not, that poor women had to have equal access to every kind of health care. If, for instance, no health plans offered abortion, it would be acceptable in the eyes of the law for MediCal not to offer it. But if other health plans offered abortion, then MediCal had to.

TK: Can you tell me about the Vancouver conference?

AW: That convened during the Vietnam war and it had two parts. There was one meeting in Vancouver, B.C., and one in Toronto. I was still on the East Coast at the time, so I was one of the planners of the Toronto conference. In addition to being on the two coasts, there were two parts to each conference. One was for women's liberation, and one was led, I think, by Women's Strike for Peace. They were held back to back; first the one, then the other. The women's liberation movement at that time, around 1971, was beginning to be pulled apart by its own internal politics, forces that we didn't realize we had set in motion because of a faulty or an incomplete analysis. I don't know what allowed some of the things that happened to emerge, but there was a great rift between lesbian women and straight women. This was very apparent at the Toronto conference, where there were groups of lesbian women who were interrupting meetings and basically scolding the Vietnamese, Laotian, and Cambodian women who were there and telling them that the war was their fault because they were heterosexual and slept with men. It was truly bizarre. Some of the women had walked weeks and weeks to meet the plane to take them to the conference. Their countries were being blown apart, their children killed—it was too much for me. That was around the time that I moved away from that part of the feminist movement.

TK: Because?

AW: Because I don't think that you can make a revolution by leaving out half the world, and—as it happened—I then went on to have boy children. I didn't know at the time that my children were going to be boys, but I felt, thank goodness, in my gut, that you cannot expect to build a women's movement which makes men its victims. Instead of a woman being valued for giving birth to boys, suddenly having girls was what was important, but it was the same thing. It was oppression based on your body, whether focused on boys or girls, and I just felt that was a mistake.

TK: I know that you became a radical because of anti-war protests and related issues, and then, as a feminist, you began to focus on health. Was it specifically the birth control pill hearings that caused you to focus on health?

AW: I began to focus on health when I began to focus on legalizing abortion. Part of my analysis was that as women, we weren't really going to be able to talk about being free if we couldn't control our own bodies. I saw abortion as a keystone issue for the whole women's movement. I lived in Washington, D.C. at the time, and Washington, D.C. is a majority Black city; back then, it was seventy-six percent black, and you couldn't really talk about abortion without talking about sterilization abuse. So we very early on had an analysis that said you had to think of abortion as larger than a single issue. I always saw the health care system as a microcosm of what was happening in the larger world, and I saw it from the top down. I saw the doctor as the ruling class, which we could put next to a senator, and you could just go right on down to the woman who was the patient.

TK: What was the focus of pre-movement feminist health groups?

AW: I always saw the women's health movement as having two wings: a service-oriented, clinic-based wing, which was composed of the feminist women's health centers and other clinics that women would set up to try and receive the kind of care they wanted: birth control counseling, abortion, humane and respectful medical care, which was so hard to obtain; and the other wing being the community-based, more legislative impact–oriented wing of the women's health movement. There were, of course, many occasions on which they would join together to change a system. There were often times when feminist women's health center issues would end up in court. I always found the work that I did was in what I call the impact-based groups, but many times—for instance, in the early days of the National Women's Health Network—the feminist women's health centers were an integral part of all of that.

TK: So after D.C. Women's Liberation you became one of the founders of the National Women's Health Network.

AW: Yes, that was a direct outgrowth of the Pill hearings. With Barbara Seaman, Belita Cowan, Mary Howell, Phyllis Chesler, we started a little group, which grew into the National Women's Health Network. The purpose of the network was to bring a feminist voice to health issues in Congress.

TK: Tell me more about the founding of the National Woman's Health Network.

AW: In 1975, this small group that I talked of before, Barbara Seaman, Mary Howell, Phyllis Chesler, Belita Cowan, and I led a kick-off demonstration for what then became the National Women's Health Network. Lots more women were involved as well, women like Judy Norsigian and Norma Swensen from Boston and Joanne Fisher from Philadelphia. We were in touch with James Luggen, whose wife, Dona Jean Walter, had died from a pulmonary embolism associated with the Pill. We had a demonstration in honor of her memory outside of the FDA and it got a lot of press coverage. By then, most of the things we did seemed to get a lot of press coverage. But I remember my house in Washington, D.C. was filled with women the night before, making signs such as "Feed your pills to the rats at the FDA" and "Must we die for love?"

You can now see it in history books, which is hard to believe. I remember Barbara's children carrying my baby Eric, in their arms, and from there the National Women's Health Network has become a major and powerful political organization.

Belita Cowan

INTERVIEW BY TANIA KETENJIAN

Belita Cowan is president of the Lymphoma Foundation of America and a founder and former executive director (1978-83) of the National Women's Health Network. This interview was conducted in September 1999.

TK: What made you decide to start the National Women's Health Network?

BC: In 1974, women had very little say when it came to making medical care decisions. Everyone but the patient herself made decisions—doctors, drug companies, hospitals, law makers. I wanted to change that. I envisioned a lobby in Washington to serve as a counter-force to the AMA and the drug industry, a strong voice for women's health rights. I telephoned my friend Barbara Seaman in September of that year to tell her about my idea. I will never forget the encouragement and support she gave. It meant a lot to me. By the end of our conversation, the Women's Health Lobby was born. (We changed the name from Lobby to Network when the organization was incorporated in 1976.)

TK: What were you doing before that?

BC: I was on the faculty of the local community college in Ann Arbor, Michigan, teaching three courses in women's health care, and writing a book on the women's health movement. I worked part-time at the University of Michigan Hospital, a big teaching research facility; I volunteered as a crisis counselor for the largest teen runaway shelter in the midwest, and served as a patient advocate for the local free clinic. In 1970 my lawsuit against the city of Ann Arbor opened up the city's sports programs to girls. I later joined a group of faculty at the U of M and did research on labor law and sex discrimination, which helped us file the first affirmative action complaint in the United States against an institution of higher learning. I credit those early years in Ann Arbor with giving me the experience and confidence to later challenge the health care system.

TK: In Ann Arbor, you uncovered a medical experiment on campus. Tell me about that.

BC: I'd come to the university as a graduate student in 1969 and at orientation we were told about a "morning-after-pill." Actually it was ten pills. You could take them for five days to prevent a pregnancy after having unprotected sex. I had friends who took the "morning-after-pill." I listened to their stories how they were so nauseous, they were vomiting, then quitting the pills after only two days. I wondered at that time: How can these pills be effective? How can they work if they make you so sick that you stop taking them?

After I earned my degree, I started a newspaper in 1972 called *her-self*. There were other feminist papers of course, in Denver, Los Angeles, New York. But none reported primarily on health news. So I published her-self to meet this need. In September, I asked one of our reporters, Kay Weiss, to write an article on what was then an obscure drug—DES diethylstilbestrol, a synthetic estrogen. Earlier, Kay's husband Rick had come across an alarming report in the *New England Journal of Medicine* describing eight cases of a very rare form of cancer in young , otherwise healthy women. All eight were exposed to the drug DES when their mothers were pregnant. This was shocking news. The "morning-after pill" dispensed by The U of M student health service was the very same drug—DES. A cancer-causing drug was being given to college student and the student health service wasn't warning student about the potential danger. So you can imagine what a bombshell it was when I published Kay's article in her-self newspaper.

TK: Why was the university dispensing DES?

BC: A gynecologist at the university, Lucille Kuchera, was testing DES as a "morning-after" contraceptive, and published her results in the *Journal of the American Medical Association* (JAMA) in 1971. She claimed one hundred percent effectiveness in preventing pregnancy among one thousand students, and that the side effects were minimal and insignificant. Common sense told me that this could not be right. I was working at the University of Michigan Hospital then and mentioned this to others. I suspected that with a thousand people, you can't get one hundred percent efficacy, no matter what drug you're testing. I was concerned because the DES had not been approved by the Food and Drug Administration as a contraceptive, and yet it was being tested on students, some of whom were friends of mine. And they had no idea they were participating in an experiment. I had to get to the bottom of this.

TK: How did you do that?

BC: I started a student organization called Advocates for Medical Information, and placed an ad in the University of Michigan student newspaper, asking anyone who took the "morning-after pill" to contact me. I developed a survey and interviewed by telephone more than a hundred students: what they took, the side effects, how they got the pills, the results, and the circumstance for which they took the DES. I found more than minor side effects, and virtually all of the responders were unaware that they had been involved in an experiment.

I organized the survey results and Kay and I flew to Washington to meet with Ralph Nader, Harrison Welford, Dr. Sidney Wolfe (who headed Ralph Nader's Health Research Group), and attorney Anita Johnson. I explained the DES survey and told them what was happening at the University of Michigan. I said we had information that contradicted the JAMA article on DES.

TK: Why Ralph Nader?

BC: We needed national publicity, and who better than Ralph Nader to get it? He was Mr. Consumer, and so well respected. This was two years before we started the Network. The women's health movement had no national voice. So we went to Washington to see if Ralph Nader could help.

Nader's Health Research Group had a press conference and they got a lot of publicity. They also sent a letter to every major college in the United States, informing them that if DES was used on campus, it was not an FDA-approved contraceptive and there might be risks associated with it. Both Sidney Wolfe and Anita Johnson did a superb job with the media.

TK: What lessons did you learn from the Nader group?

BC: The clout and effectiveness of the Nader organization made a strong impression on me. I thought, if Ralph Nader can do this, so can I. I felt that we needed a woman's voice to speak out and stand up for our health rights. That's another reason why starting the National Women's Health Network was so important to me—I needed a strong feminist organization to back up my DES efforts.

TK: Did you meet Dr. Kuchera?

BC: In 1973, Kay and I went on a syndicated TV talk show with Dr. Kuchera and confronted her with the survey results. I said that her research couldn't be true because there must have been some drug failures. If the morning-after pill didn't work in all cases, then children might be born who were at risk for cancer. A surprising thing happened. Some time after the show, Dr. Kuchera wrote a letter to the editor of JAMA, a short letter, retracting her claim off one hundred percent efficacy and admitting that there had been some pregnancies after all.

TK: Was that the end of it or did national interest keep growing?

BC: We convinced reporter Harry Reasoner at NBC to come to the U of M campus to do an exposé on DES for the evening news. That segment helped a lot. Almost instantly, my work became easier because people now took the DES issue seriously.

Then, in 1974 I was asked by Senator Ted Kennedy to testify as an expert witness at his Senate subcommittee hearings on DES and the morning-after pill. I flew to Washington in February 1975 to present my survey results, to expose the DES experiment that had recruited unsuspecting students at the U of M, and to say that there were no reliable safety and efficacy studies on DES. I testified that FDA approval of DES would be a mistake because there was no adequate evidence of safety. I said that DES was being dispensed to young, healthy women at college campuses all over the country, and I asked the senator to stop the FDA from moving forward with its plan to approve the DES as a contraceptive.

A number of cancer experts, including Dr. Peter Greenwald, testified that DES should be banned for use in pregnancy because it had caused an epidemic of cancer in the offspring. [By 1975, there were more than 3,000 documented cases of cancer in DES daughters.] The commissioner of the FDA and two FDA medical officers were brought before the subcommittee, under subpoena. The medical officers said that they had never before seen such a circumvention of FDA procedures as in this case [approval of DES as a contraceptive].

In December 1975, I testified before the U.S. House of Representatives, and arranged for Doris Haire, a childbirth advocate, and two DES daughters to tell their story to Congress. That same month, I helped organize a public demonstration on the doorstep of the FDA, to protest the indiscriminate use of DES, birth control bills, and estrogen replacement therapy in menopause—drugs known to cause cancer, blood clots, and death. This demonstration resulted in publicity for the National Women's Health Network, and we gained many new supporters.

I spent the next eight years fighting the FDA, and also publicizing the need for DES children, both male and female, to seek medical attention because of their increased risk of vaginal and testicular cancer. Years later, it became evident that mothers who took DES during pregnancy had higher rates of breast cancer.

To this day, the FDA has never approved DES as a morning-after pill, and I am very happy for that. I have always believed that one person, acting with passion, can make a difference.

TK: How did you recruit the Network's first members?

BC: In my mind, we needed not only a strong lobby in Washington to influence public health polic, but. a large, grassroots constituency. So I used the her-self newspaper mailing list to get the Network off the ground. There were 2,000 community-based women' health groups, consumer organizations, and individual artists who were subscribers. I sent them each a letter announcing the new organization. The first 1,000 member of the National Women's health Network came directly from my newspaper's mailing list.

TK: How did the other co-founders come to join you?

BC: Barbara Seaman suggested that the visibility and credibility of the Women's Health Lobby would be enhanced if a doctor was on board. She suggested feminist physician Mary Howell, Dean of Student s at Harvard Medical School. Barbara also felt it was important that we include the mental health side of medicine, and suggested psychologist Phyllis Chelser who had written *Women and Madness*. By the beginning of 1975, there were 4 of us listed as co-founders.

But I was in Michigan, Mary was in Massachusetts, and Barbara and Phyllis were in New York City. How could we keep on top of laws and regulations in Washington when none of us lived there? Barbara had been talking with Alice Wolfson, who lived in D.C. and had been involved in the birth control pill hearings years earlier. When I went to Senator Kennedy's hearings in 1975 to testify on DES, I met Alice and felt we could work together, so she joined us. I continued to oversee the Network's activities and provide direction to the many volunteers until 1977, when I moved to Washington D.C. to become the Network's first executive director (1978-1983).

TK: What were some of the other issues the Network was dealing with at the beginning—aside from DES?

BC:➤Menopause. We participated in a lawsuit on estrogen replacement therapy that resulted in the FDA requiring all companies making estrogen drugs to print patient warning labels about the link between those drugs and endometrial cancer.

➤Childbirth. We participated in a Congressional effort that successfully expanded Medicaid coverage to include nurse-midwives.

➤Sterilization (NWHN helped publicize the problem of forced sterilization of poor and minority women, and worked with other groups to help draft federal rules to prohibit this practice).

➤Birth Control. We pressured the FDA to approve the cervical cap as a barrier method of birth control and led a successful campaign from 1979–81 to block approval of the controversial birth control shot, Depo-provera.

➤Abortion .We participated in Congressional letter-writing campaigns and statewide marches to keep abortions safe and legal.

►Self-help. We supported the formation of local, autonomous self-help groups around the country, as well as feminist women's health centers.

►Sterilization. We worked closely with the Breast Cancer Advisory Center to end the radical mastectomy and give women more humane options for breast cancer treatment.

One of the most difficult issues the Network faced in the beginning was its own survival. When I was hired as executive director, we had no office, not even a telephone, and very little money. My job included fundraising, and during my five-year tenure, I raised from direct mail and foundation grants more than one million dollars.

TK: What was Anita Johnson's role in your work ?

BC: She introduced me to Senator Kennedy and his staff, making it possible for me to be invited to testify as an expert witness at the senator's DES hearings. As chair of the Network's board and later as executive director, I consulted with Sidney Wolfe and Anita Johnson on many health issues, and our two organizations often joined with other consumer groups to file petitions or take legal action.

TK: Can you tell me about the case you were involved in with Marcia Greenberger

BC: Marcia Greenberger was a lawyer with the Center for Law and Social Policy in Washington D.C. She asked me if I would agree to have the Network become an intervenor in a lawsuit brought by the Pharmaceutical Manufacturers Association (PMA) against the Food and Drug Administration. At issue was FDA's regulatory authority to require drug companies to provide patients with written cancer groups who intervened (including the Network) against the PMA and the American College of Obstetricians and Gynecologists. The Court's ruling set a precedent for requiring drug companies to print patient warning labeling for all estrogen drugs.

Chapter 52

On Being a Woman

These three articles are all a little bit outrageous and in-your-face, shocking to some readers, delightul to others. Note that "A My Name is Alice," which has roots in the 1950s, was published in 1998. "Femininity 2000," which takes place on January 2, 2000, was published in 1974.

These pieces cry out to be experienced, not discussed, so I'll stop....—B. S..

The Female Eunuch

GERMAINE GREER

Germaine Greer, *The Female Eunuch*, New York, Bantam Books, 1972. Originally published in Great Britain by MacGibbon and Kee, 1970. Reprinted by permission.

THE WICKED WOMB

Women who adhere to the Moslem, Hindu, or Mosaic faiths must regard themselves as unclean in their time of menstruation and seclude themselves for a period. Medieval Catholicism made the stipulation that menstruating women were not to come into the church. Although enlightenment is creeping into this field at its usual pace, we still have a marked revulsion for menstruation, principally evinced by our efforts to keep it secret. The success of the tampon is partly due to the fact that it is hidden. The arrival of the menarche is more significant than any birthday, but in the Anglo-Saxon households it is ignored and carefully concealed from general awareness. For six months while I was waiting for my first menstruation I toted a paper bag with diapers and pins in my school satchel. When it finally came, I suffered agonies lest anyone should guess or smell it or anything. My diapers were made of harsh toweling, and I used to creep into the laundry and crouch over a bucket of foul rags, hoping that my brother would not catch me at my revolting labors. It is not surprising that well-bred, dainty little girls find it difficult to adapt to menstruation, when our society does no more than explain it and leave them to get on with it. Among the aborigines who lived along the Pennefather river in Queensland the little girl used to be buried up to her waist in warm sand to aid the first contractions, and fed and cared for by her mother in a secret place, to be led in triumph to the camp where she joined a feast to celebrate her entry into the company of marriageable maidens; it seems likely that menstruation was much less traumatic. Women still buy sanitary towels with enormous discretion, and carry their handbags to the loo when they only need to carry a napkin. They still recoil at the idea of intercourse during menstruation and feel that the blood they shed is a special kind, although perhaps not so special as was thought when it was the liquid presented to the devil in witches' loving cups. If you think you are emancipated, you might consider the idea of tasting your menstrual blood—if it makes you sick, you've a long way to go, baby.

Menstruation, we are told, is unique among the natural bodily processes in that it involves a loss of blood. It is assumed that nature is a triumph of design and that none of her processes is wasteful or in need of reversal, especially when it only inconveniences women, and therefore it is thought extremely unlikely that there is any "real" pain associated with menstruation. In fact, no little girl who finds herself bleeding from an organ which she didn't know she had until it began to incommode her feels that nature is a triumph of design and that whatever is, is right. When she discovers that the pain attending this horror is in some way her *fault*, the result of improper adaptation to her female role, she really feels like the victim of a bad joke. Doctors admit that most women suffer "discomfort" during menstruation, but disagree very much about what proportion of women suffer "real" pain. Whether the contractions of the women are painful in some absolute sense or could be rendered comfortable by some psychotherapy or other is immaterial. The fact is that no woman would menstruate if she did not have to. Why should women not resent an inconvenience which causes tension before, after, and during; unpleasantness, odor, staining; which takes up anything from a seventh to a fifth of her adult life until the menopause; which makes her fertile thirteen times a year when she only expects to bear twice in a lifetime; when the cessation of menstruation may mean several years of endocrine derangement and the gradual atrophy of her sexual organs? The fact is that nature is not a triumph of design, and every battle against illness is an interference with her design, so that there is no rational ground for assuming that menstruation as we know it must be or ought to be irreversible.

The contradiction in the attitude that regards menstruation as divinely ordained and yet unmentionable leads to the intensification of the female revolt against it, which can be traced in all the common words for it, like the *curse,* and male disgust expressed in terms like *having the rag on.* We have only the choice of three kinds of expression: the vulgar resentful, the genteel ("I've got my period," "I am indisposed"), and the scientific jargon of the *menses.* Girls are irrepressible though: in our Sydney girls' school napkins are affectionately referred to as *daisies*; Italian girls call their periods *il marchese* and German girls *der rote König.* One might envy the means adopted by *La Dame aux Camélias* to signify her condition to her gentlemen friends, but if it were adopted on a large scale it might look like a mark of proscription, a sort of leper's bell. There have been some moves to bring menstruation out into the open in an unprejudiced way, like Sylvia Plath's menstruation poem. Perhaps we need a film to be made by an artist about the onset of menstruation, in which the implications emerge in some nonacademic way, if we cannot manage a public celebration of a child's entry into womanhood by any other means.

Menstruation has been used a good deal in argument about women's fitness to undertake certain jobs: where women's comfort is concerned the effects are minimized—where the convenience of our masters is threatened they are magnified. Women are not more incapacitated by menstruation than men are by their drinking habits, their hypertension, their ulcers, and their virility fears. It is not necessary to give menstruation holidays. It may be that women commit crimes during the premenstrual and menstrual period, but it is still true that women commit far fewer crimes than men. Women must be aware of this enlistment of menstruation in the antifeminist argument, and counteract it by their own statements of the situation. Menstruation does not turn us into raving maniacs or complete invalids; it is just that we would rather do without it.

FAMILY

If women could regard childbearing not as a duty or an inescapable destiny but as a privilege to be worked for, the way a man might work for the right to have a family, children might grow up without the burden of gratitude for the gift of life which they never asked for. Brilliant women are not reproducing themselves because childbearing has been regarded as a full-time job; genetically they might be thought to be being bred out. In a situation where a woman might contribute a child to a household which engages her attention for part of the time while leaving her free to frequent other spheres of influence, brilliant women might be more inclined to reproduce. For some time now I have pondered the problem of having a child which would not suffer from my neuroses and the difficulties I would have in adjusting to a husband and the demands of domesticity. A plan, by no means a blueprint, evolved which has become a sort of dream. No child ought, I opine, to grow up in the claustro-phobic atmosphere of a city flat, where he has little chance of exercising his limbs or his lungs; I must work in a city where the materials for my work and its market are available. No child ought to grow up alone with a single resent-ful girl who is struggling to work hard enough to provide for herself and him. I… hit upon the plan to buy, with the help of some friends with similar prob-lems, a farmhouse in Italy where we could stay when circumstances permit-ted, and where our children would be born. Their fathers and other people would also visit the house as often as they could, to rest and enjoy the children and even work a bit. Perhaps some of us might live there for quite long peri-ods, as long as we wanted to. The house and garden would be worked by a local family who lived in the house. The children would have a region to explore and dominate, and different skills to learn from all of us. It would not be paradise, but it would be a little community with a chance of survival, with parents of both sexes and a multitude of roles to choose from. The worst aspect of kib-butz living could be avoided, especially as the children would not have to be strictly persuaded out of sexual experimentation with their peers, an unnatur-al restriction which has had serious consequences for the children of kibbutz-im. Being able to be with my child and his friends would be a privilege and a delight that I could work for. If necessary the child need not even know that I was his womb mother and I could have relationships with the other children as well. If my child expressed a wish to try London and New York or go to for-mal school somewhere, that could also be tried without committal.

Any new arrangement which a woman might devise will have the disad-vantage of being peculiar: the children would not have been brought up like other children in an age of uniformity. There are the problems of legitimacy and nationality to be faced. Our society has created the myth of the *broken home* which is the source of so many ills, and yet the unbroken home which ought to have broken is an even greater source of tension as I can attest from bitter experience. The rambling organic structure of my ersatz household would have the advantage of being an unbreakable home in that it did not rest on the frail shoulders of two bewildered individuals trying to apply a contra-dictory blueprint. This little society would confer its own normality, and other contacts with civilization would be encouraged, but it may well be that such children would find it impossible to integrate with society and become dropouts or schizophrenics. As such they would not be very different from other children I have known. The notion of integrating with society as if soci-ety were in some way homogeneous is itself a false one. There are enough eccentrics carving out various lifestyles for my children to feel that they are no more isolated than any other minority group within the fictitious majority. In the computer age disintegration may well appear to be a higher value than integration. Cynics might argue that the children of my household would be anxious to set up "normal" families as part of the natural counterreaction.

Perhaps. When faced with such dubious possibilities, there is only empiricism to fall back on. I could not, physically, have a child any other way, except by accident and under protest in a hand-to-mouth sort of way in which case I could not accept any responsibility for the consequences. I should like to be able to think that I had done my best.

The point of an organic family is to release the children from the disadvantages of being the extensions of their parents so that they can belong primarily to themselves. They may accept the services that adults perform for them naturally without establishing dependencies. There could be scope for them to initiate their own activities and define the mode and extent of their own learning. They might come to resent their own strangeness, but in other circumstances they might resent normality; faced with difficulties of adjustment, children seize upon their parents and their upbringing to serve as scapegoats. Parents have no option but to enjoy their children if they want to avoid the cycle of exploitation and recrimination. If they want to enjoy them, they must construct a situation in which such enjoyment is possible.

A My Name Is Alice

JENNIFER BAUMGARDNER

Jennifer Baumgardner, "My Name Is Alice: The Story of the Feminist Playmate," *MAMM* Vol. 7 Oct./Nov. 1998. Reprinted by permission.

THE TIME: THE EARLY FIFTIES.
THE PLACE: NEW YORK CITY'S GREENWICH VILLAGE

Alice Denham, a fiercely independent and dazzling redhead with a master's degree in English and a Phi Beta Kappa from the University of North Carolina, comes to the Big Apple to make it as a writer. From a poor but genteel Southern family, the pert but steely gamine applies for job after job in publishing. Within a few days of pounding the pavement in her pumps, Alice's innocence is shattered: There aren't any jobs for women in publishing in 1953. There might as well be a sign that says "Girls Keep Out!" hanging over the city rather than the promising glitter of the New York skyline at night. "Screw the bastards!" Alice declares as she pours herself a teacup full of whiskey and tries to work out plan B: the one where she can get the respect she deserves in this macho town. Or so Alice Denham's story might begin if it was a novel written by Alice Denham herself. Still petite and red-haired with a drawl that suspends her words in honey and belies her Jacksonville, Florida upbringing, Denham really did move to New York City in the bohemian fifties to find that she couldn't even get interviewed. "All they wanted was secretaries," she says, doll-sized and grinning, dwarfed by the average-sized table of a West Village tea salon. "And I had purposefully not taken shorthand to avoid that fate." Denham decided to focus on writing full-time. No one needed to give her permission to do that. "Writing was the only thing I ever wanted to be or to do, so I decided I would be a writer if it killed me." All she needed in order to get started was a job that paid well and didn't require a lot of time.

CHAPTER 2: ALICE BECOMES A PINUP MODEL

"I was living with a friend who was an actress, and she introduced me to a model. People had asked me to pose for photos from time to time, and soon I started to be sent out for doing romance novel covers," she says, as matter-of-factly as she had mentioned her undeserved reputation as a slut in college (the president of a powerful fraternity sought retribution after she refused to date him) and her breast cancer 10 years ago (lying on her back, she noticed her breast was at a 90-degree angle) during the first few moments upon arriving. Modeling a few hours a week to pay the bills, she taught herself to write a novel during the rest of the week by observation, fiction technique books, and "trial and error." Poring over Dostoyevsky in her Village apartment, Denham gleaned the magic of a strong lead, the art of withholding information, the importance of characterization. Still, "it took me a very long time to write my first novel." She did, indeed, finish her novel, and a few more, but first came a serendipitous piece of fiction called "The Deal." Originally published in the then-prestigious literary magazine *Discovery*, the story centers on a rich man who is so taken with a beautiful woman that he offers her $1,000 to sleep with him once. At that time (the mid-fifties) another magazine was printing serious (read: male) fiction: *Playboy*. Given her day job, our uppity heroine had an idea. "I told my literary agent to say that if *Playboy* would reprint the story, I would be the centerfold." Soon Denham found herself at the Chicago airport, destined to be Miss July 1956, the only playmate to have a piece and be a piece in the same issue. "Hef met me at the airport. I thought he was the limo driver. He was so stiff and formal in his black suit that I got into the backseat of the car. He said, 'Sit up front.' I said, 'What?' He said, 'I'm Hugh Hefner.'" Denham pauses for a moment and then dishes about the man responsible for acmmlining the girl next door. "He was a really silly man, running around in pajamas, and he never grew up," she says, digging into her baked chicken breast. "Ultimately, we had sex," she continues, with a sigh. "It was all right, though he had to watch dirty movies. All of this is in my novel *Amo*—except I changed the names. I called the magazine "Meat" and I called the Playmates "Tidbits of the Month" and I called him "Pelth Pedlar." "The Deal" was her break. Still, Denham admits her family was horrified by her national exposure, despite how tame the shots were back in the early days of girlie mags. That is, except for her brother, an Episcopal preacher, who assured Denham that she looked very cute. "The only thing I cared about modeling was would it pay enough to cover my monthly expenses," says the 66-year-old. "The thing is, I wouldn't have to resort to *Playboy* nowadays," says Denham. "I could have been an assistant editor or a freelance writer."

CHAPTER 3: OUR HEROINE DISCOVERS THE WOMEN'S LIBERATION MOVEMENT

"I think all of my work has largely been about discrimination," says Denham. "Social, gender, all that stuff, one way or another." There was a thriving bohemian literary scene at the time of her arrival in New York, and Denham soon found herself amid the swirl. According to a piece in the *New York Observer* by Darius James, she dated James Jones, Philip Roth, spent a couple of "casual" evenings with Norman Mailer, and enjoyed a close "sexual friendship" with that fey icon of early-sixties cool, James Dean. But when it came time to blurb her book, these scribes of the masculine experience made themselves scarce. One assumes that Denham's memoir-in-progress entitled *Sleeping with the Boys* will do a little toward righting that slight, but it just so happened that she had discovered another downtown intellectual scene—one more interested in her body of work than in her body. As an early second wave feminist, Denham came to the movement as part of the campaign to legalize abortion (which occurred in 1970 in New York and 1973 nationally) and was part of the original National Organization for Women chapter. As an associate professor at John Jay College at the City University of New York during the seventies, Denham handled an Equal Employment Opportunity Commission discrimination case that was settled in the faculty women's favor for $3.5 million. Always an independent, her work became even more confidently pro-woman. *My Darling from the Lions* concerned a feminist centerfold from outer space, and *Amo* chronicled a feminist's mad passion for her tragically sexist husband. Meanwhile, a movie, *Quizas,* was made from the *Playboy* story.

CHAPTER 4: CANCER

Then, 10 years ago, when Denham was 56 and married for eight years to an accountant she had met in her part-time home of San Miguel de Allende, Mexico, she discovered breast cancer. "I think diagnosis refocuses your head," she says. "You no longer think so much about physical beauty or the beauty of your breasts. It's whether you're going to live or not." The former model didn't find that the mastectomy changed her body image so much; cancer affected her desire to create. "My work habits were always good, but I started working harder and faster. I wanted to complete all of these things that were halfway done." Her current regimen is an hour of exercise upon waking, breakfast—"If my husband is home and doesn't have work, he makes breakfast, washes the dishes, and then gets out of the house"—and then she writes all day.

CHAPTER 5: THE FUTURE

Alice Denham is working on a family saga called *Shabby Genteel: A Southern Girlhood* and the aforementioned memoir of her days in the Boho/prefeminist fifties and sixties. She spends summers in Mexico and the rest of the year in New York and writes and publishes in both locales. As for her cancer, there is no act 2, but her last mammogram showed a burst of calcium which her doctors are watching for bad signs. Typically, Denham is candid about her mammography appointment. "They were going to do something awful called a mammotone where they lay you down on a table with your breast hanging down through a hole and they clamp it like a mammogram," she says, eyes rolling. "After taking my breast photos in about a thousand different ways they decided they couldn't do it because [the calcifications were] too close to the skin." She snorts. "Have you ever had a mammogram?" she inquires, peering across the table with a half smile on her face. "You wait."

Femininity 2000
CAROL RINZLER

Carol Rinzler, "Femininity: 2000," in Maggie Tripp, ed., *Woman in the Year 2000*, New York, Arbor House, 1974. Reprinted by permission.

At five o'clock in the afternoon of January 2, 2000, Nora Hones-Cohen, 25 and in her second year as a lawyer with the venerable firm Abzug, Chisholm Holtzman, throws several briefs into her Vuitton briefcase (some things will endure) and takes the helitrain up from Forty-second and Third to her one-bedroom apartment on East Sixty-first Street. She wearily taps the heat-sensitive patternboard of her apartment door with her index finger: one short, two long, three short, one long, one short, one long. Nobody carries keys anymore—and robberies are infrequent—but, since the night when she came home bombed at two in the morning and struggled for two hours unable to remember any combination other than that to her parents' brownstone, she has carried the combination in code right next to her Completecreditcard (the only credit card she, or anyone for that matter, carries).

The door closes gently behind her and she goes to the bar-console in the living room, sets the controls for vodka-martini-straight-up-with-a-twist-on-the-side (some things never change), and pushes a button. With her drinks, the console is also programmed to deliver three pills: weight control, beauty complex I, and brain stimulator.

Nora eschews tranquilizers, mood elevators, and hallucinogens, and so it isn't surprising that she settles down into her overstuffed D/R sofa (an antique inherited from her grandmother) feeling somewhat depressed. It has been a long day.

This is a new year, a new millennium… and did she begin it well by telling George on New Year's Eve that she didn't want to consider Marriage I? Perhaps she is heading for a lonely life. After all, she certainly likes him; they get on awfully well in bed—that is, since she's gotten him to attend sex counseling with her—and at age 28 George shows every sign of rising to the top of his field—advertising, with the Wells Trahey agency. They are both not only passionately involved in their careers, but they also share outside interests: Mozart, Midler (now middle-aged and still electrically vital), and Doc Watson (whose music has become wildly popular 26 years after his death); horseback riding, sky-diving, and ultraviolet apartment gardening; antiquing and traveling (and when they'd gone off for that long weekend to the Moon, there was no question that they were compatible under the worst circumstances—for three days, the air-conditioning in their room was off and the depressurization was down to 60 percent).

Still, at the risk of loneliness, she has no intention of getting seriously involved in a "cemented" relationship. At this point, all that truly consumes her is cementing her career, and that's what she'll concentrate on for the next several months. Perhaps it will be best for the two of them if they wait. (An old cliché that Nora rather likes.)

Enough philosophizing; it's been a long day. Nora settles down to more practical matters. Like hunger. She dials herself a shrimp cocktail, a rare steak, salad (with vinegar and oil on the side), and a dish of pink-bubblegum ice cream. Thank God for weight control pills, she thinks for the ten thousandth time. Until they'd come along five years ago, she'd had to fight an awful tendency to run 10 pounds overweight.

Too bad that the console isn't programmed for anything other than steak; she's getting very bored with it. But programs cost money, and she'd rather save it for a trip or buy more *Ms.* magazine stock. She'd bought in last year just before the news that they were going to acquire Hearst broke, and she saw it triple in five months.

While waiting for dinner, Nora sits down to read the new issue of *Vogue*. Apparently, designers have rediscovered the seventies, and the clothes are loose and flowing, softly colored, and tend to run to ruffles and long skirts. This definitely appeals to the romantic in Nora, who's awfully sick of the straight, practical lines so prevalent for the last five or so years. And she's really had it with vinyl, ultrasuede, and sisal. There is also a feature on the "one-piece"—a new method of dressing up in only a single piece of fabric that need not be sewn: the trick, the art in fact, is in knotting, and the variety of styles is practically infinite. Both men and women are able to use the "one-piece," and the *Vogue* feature presents the Kennedys modeling—Senator John F. Kennedy, Jr., is shown posing in some undeniably masculine, conservative styles, and Caroline is quoted as saying that even her mother is taken with the notion.

In this mood, Nora decides now is as good a time as any to give the house the three-weeks-overdue, thorough monthly cleaning. She goes to the service board in the kitchen and starts to program the buttons that will remove all dust from the house, defrost the refrigerator, scour the bathtub, clean the medicine chest, linen closet, and cabinets. While the surfaces are being dusted, Nora hangs up all her clothes, puts books back on their shelves, unpacks laundry, and makes her bed. Within two hours all is neat and thoroughly clean, and Nora feels terrific. She only wishes she could get it together to do this once a month. She only wishes she had a maid.

At eleven o'clock, Nora removes her makeup with Revlon's "facial duster" (which works on the simple principle of the vacuum cleaner and also includes a moisturizer), jumps into the sauna/shower, and then watches a bit of the *Mason Reese Tonight Show* on the life-size TV screen in her bedroom. At midnight, 25-year-old Nora Jones-Cohen turns off TV and lights, flips on the vibrator, and falls asleep.

Body Parts

"All things, counter, original, spare, strange;
Whatever is fickle, freckled (who knows how?)"
—from Pied Beauty
by Gerard Manley Hopkins

I t might seem odd to introduce a collection of intimate women's writings
about our body parts with lines from a poem by a 19th-century Jesuit priest,
but what language could be more appropriate? Whenever we attempt to
describe ourselves, some man tells us that we got it wrong, and ... If perceptions
are counter... strange... fickle, i.e. we here express our Pied Beauty.

In our recent struggles to describe and define our own experiences of our
bodies (after 5,000 years of being required to let men speak for us), some of our self-
revelations are hilarious, some beautiful, some heart wrenching, some common
sensical, some perplexing.

Body Parts is divided into three areas. The first, which could be called "Up
Top," includes chapters on hair, face, skin, and mouth. The contents of "Skin"
may surprise you. It's a highly political section featuring interviews with leading
health activists for minority women—Patsy Mink, Byllye Avery, Helen Rodriguez-
Trias, and Charon Asetoyer—as well as Rebecca Walker's essay "Higher Yellow"
and Our Bodies, Our Voices, Our Choices from the National Black Women's

Health Project. If you didn't already know it, you'll learn that a woman's skin color is a major determinant of her health care.

The second area, which we'll call "Out Front," conists of torso, heart, breasts, and muscle.

Finally, "Down There" contains just what you may be thinking, the unmentionables... ovaries, womb, fruits of the womb (i.e. pregnancy, motherhood, and childrearing), vagina, and clitoris. "Down There" includes two extraordinary short stories, Lynne Sharon Schwartz's "So You're Going to Have a New Body!" which is about a hysterectomy, and Laura Yaeger's "Having Anne," about a pregnant woman who must take a furlough from her psychiatric medication.

You may wonder how "Fruits of the Womb" differs from the "Motherhood" chapters in Taking Our Bodies Back, and in Still Taking Our Bodies Back. The "Motherhood" chapters deal with the big picture, with political, scientific, and legal issues that could affect any woman. The selections in "Fruits of the Womb" are generally more personal, more specific, in some cases more literary, in others more offbeat or 'cranky.'" We love them!—B. S.

Chapter 53

Hair

*I*n *many ways, women have made astonishing progress in the past 30 years—
medicine, law, Wall Street, Hollywood.... We're far from equal yet, but overall
we're earning more and gaining more self-reliance in the world faster than
we ever dreamed it could happen. Sadly, we've learned that women can no
longer count on men to take care of them. But fortunately, we now know that, if
we must, we can usually gather the strength to take care of ourselves.*

*So why do we have so many unresolved issues surrounding our grooming
and looks? In the first four chapters of this "Body Parts" section, we focus on
matters "Up Top" and discuss issues of physical appearance as they relate to hair,
face, skin, and mouth (eating).—B. S.*

All Hair the Conquering Heroine

LOIS GOULD

Lois Gould, *Not Responsible for Personal Articles,* New York, Warner Books, 1973. Reprinted by permission.

Kimberley Ann, nine, has just decided what she wants to be when she grows up: a part-time cocktail waitress with frosted blond streaks. It is probably just a coincidence that Kimberley Ann's mother recently graduated from law school and lopped off her two-tone gold ringlets right at the dark roots.

Kim's classmate Janice, who is still 8, has her heart set on becoming a file clerk who ties up her hair in a severe bun that can be shaken free, with a single lightning stroke, into a quivering mass of raven tendrils. (Janice's mother is a securities analyst, with a naturally frizzled pepper-and-salt pageboy.)

Nina, 10½, plans to be a schoolteacher with a firm grip and frosted blond highlights. And 12-year-old Stephanie, the cynic, intends to become a frosted blond highlight, period.

Clearly, a fair number of feminists' daughters are having "role model" trouble. The cause seems to be a sudden and widespread cultural confusion about the difference—if any—between a role model and a hair model. As I understand it, a role model is an adult person of your own gender whom you admire and want to be like: a president, an astronaut, a nuclear physicist, a private eye. Whereas a hair model is a stunning, raven-haired president; a luscious red-headed astronaut; a blond bombshell of a nuclear physicist; a frost-streaked poster pinup of a private eye.

It would be easy to blame the confusion on television's newest rage—the female "action-adventure" star who can either ride a motorcycle, toe-tap on a skateboard, shoot straight, do heavy lifting or figure out how to trap a criminal while wearing a dripping wet Bunny costume. After all, no matter what else these new wonder women do besides wonders—and part-time file clerking, school teaching, cocktail waitressing—the thing they all do *best* is their hair.

So it would be easy to blame TV, but, as one of our stunning, raven-haired ex-presidents used to say, "It would be wrong." The truth is, we have always had a little trouble spotting the subtle line between a heroine and a hairdo. In a highly unscientific recent survey, mothers of 9- to 12-year-olds, selected solely on the basis of shampoo, color tint and permanent wave length, were asked the following question: When you were between 9 and 12, who was your "role model," and why?

> ➤ 17 percent answered "Esther Williams, the swimming star, because she could do fifteen minutes of flawless underwater sidestroke with gorgeous flowers twined in her braided coronet."

> ➤ 5 percent named Brenda Starr, the comic-strip girl reporter, on the

basis of her sensational headline set in bold-type curls the color of "a five-alarm fire," an "Irish setter," or a "*saumon fumé.* "

➤ 12 percent had idolized Sonja Henie, the Goldilocks of the ice, because she skated like a wind-up Christmas angel; her hair and feet set off "matching sparks of white light"; she was an "animated gold sequin."

➤ The remainder chose a wide assortment of heroines ranging from the Dragon Lady (dangerous mastermind set in a black curtain of silk hair) to Amelia Earhart and Dale, Flash Gordon's dauntless copilot, both of whom had their heads in clouds of wispy gold tendrils escaping from under their flying helmets.

Nobody had a role model with nonterrific hair.

Film historian Molly Haskell has noted that the long, sexy tresses of movie queens in the hard-boiled dramas of the 1940s was the female equivalent of a gun—an ultimate woman's weapon in a tough man's world of crime and carnality. The new "action" heroines of the seventies, operating in the same man's world, actually get to wield both weapons—the hair and the gun. But it's the same old game: Everything, including the girls, is still owned and operated by the fellow who runs the beauty parlor. Body, soul, gun and frost job, they are strictly *Charlie's Angels.*

Armed with this valuable knowledge, I recently watched my first episode of the TV series *Charlie's Angels,* accompanied by two hard-core 9-year-old fans, Nicole and Sandy. Here's how it went:

Me: Tell me about the "angels."

Nicole: Well, first off you have to know which is which. Sabrina is the smart one, Kelly is strong, and Jill is beautiful. Mostly her hair.

Me: But they're *all* beautiful.

Sandy (patiently): Of *course.* But Sabrina is beautiful *and* smart. Kelly is beautiful *and* strong. Jill is *just* beautiful. Mostly her hair.

Me: Oh. (Pause. On the screen, three women are flashing guns, hair, sexy clothes, and dazzling smiles, like armed stewardesses serving plastic filet mignon.) Which would you rather be—the smart one, the strong one, or the beautiful one, with the hair?

Nicole: Definitely not the beautiful one.

Sandy: Obviously.

Me: Why obviously?

Nicole: Because even if she has the most hair, she has the smallest part. (Sandy nods solemnly.)

Me: What if you had a choice, I mean in real life? You could be smart and strong—or you could be beautiful. Which would you choose?

Sandy: Why couldn't we be all three?

Me: Well, first off, because hardly anybody gets to be all three. And hardly anybody even gets to have a choice. So I'm giving you a choice. Beautiful, but dumb and weak. Or smart and strong, but ugly. Ugly *hair,* especially.

Sandy (frowning): Hmmm.

Nicole (cocking her head so that her long mane of naturally frosty curls tumbles gently around her shoulders): *How* ugly?

Femininity

SUSAN BROWNMILLER AND CARRIE CARMICHAEL

Reprinted with the permission of Simon and Schuster from Femininity by Susan Brownmiller, copyright ©1984. Interview with Carrie Carmichael, May 1999.

From time immemorial, hair has been used to make a visual statement, for the body's most versatile raw material can be cut, plucked, shaved, curled, straightened, braided, greased, bleached, tinted, dyed, and decorated with precious ornaments and totemic fancies. A change in the way one wears one's hair can affect the look of the face and alter a mood. A uniform hairstyle can set a group of people apart from others and signify a conformity or rebellion, devotion to God or indulgence in sensual pleasures. Hair worn in a polarized manner has served to indicate the masculine and the feminine, the slave and the ruler, the young, the old, the virgin, the married, the widowed, the mourning.

There was a time that stretched over many years when I placed myself in permanent bondage to Elizabeth Arden. There, two lunch hours a week, I was shampooed and curled with setting lotion, winding papers, plastic rollers, and metal clips, gently cushioned around the ears and forehead with absorbent cotton, tied in a pink hairnet and placed under a hot dryer for 35 minutes. Mercifully released, I was unpinned, unwound, brushed out, teased, and fluffed into fair approximation of the season's latest fashion. After a blast of noxious spray I was sent out the door in a forged state of feminine chic that lasted for the rest of the day—that is, if it didn't rain. I always felt like a poseur at Arden's. Not once did I let them shape and polish my nails, not once did I submit to the ritual of the pedicure, the waxing of the legs, or the mysterious rites of the Full-Day Treatment. They must have sensed my lack of commitment. But they had a powerful hold on my hair. They tugged at the roots of my deepest insecurity.

SB: I would say one of the biggest problems women have is the obsession with the hair on their heads. Of course, I fall for it too.

CC: We've been obsessed as a nation with Hillary Clinton's hair.

SB: I've never seen such a demonstration of feminine insecurity, due to trying to break the mold in so many ways, as Hillary Clinton. Because she cannot be comfortable with one image. She's been in such agony over "the look" of her hair, and indeed also "the look" of her clothes. And she seems to have no idea how she might look good. Because otherwise she would say, "Hey, this looks good on me. That doesn't. No, I won't do that." But she seems constantly at the mercy of other people's idea of her image in hair and clothes.

CC: I think your point about her insecurity is key. In her politics, no one tells her how to think or what to do.

SB: Unbelievable the get-ups that have been foisted on her, or that she chose, thinking that, "This looks like power. This looks like efficiency. This looks like femininity." She's got all of these advisers. When I was reading the George Stephanopoulos book that shows the role of all these advisers and how the President triangulates, I was trying to think of Hilary Clinton in the White House with the access that she must have to very good fashion advisers, and how it still comes out wrong all of the time. Now I know basically underneath it's not just simply that she is a woman who is trying to break codes of femininity and be a very serious and efficient person who transforms the world. I know that she has real body image issues. I think that secretly, these issues obsess her.

Memoirs of a (Sorta) Ex-Shaver

CAROLYN MACKLER

Excerpted from Carolyn Mackler, "Memoirs of a (Sorta) Ex-Shaver," in Ophira Edut, ed. *Adios, Barbie: Young Women Write about Body Image and Identity*, Seattle, Wash., Seal Press, 1998. Reprinted by permission.

During the winter of seventh grade, the other girls in my gym class suddenly had legs as smooth as an infant and I celebrated the birth of every new underarm hair by grabbing a pair of scissors and trimming it down. Feeling inexplicably weird about the soft blond peach fuzz coating my legs, I pounded my mom with questions about shaving: "When could I? How do you? Could I get my own razor?"

"Wait," she cautioned. "Shave once and you'll have black stubble for the rest of your life."

Heeding no warning, I crouched in the tub with a bottle of Johnson & Johnson's baby oil and my dad's old black Gillette. I was focused, driven. Through hell or greasy water, I would have smooth legs. This experimental style (which resulted in awful itching) was eventually eclipsed by more conventional methods: my own pastel disposable 10-pack, a can of Barbosal shaving cream, and, a few hours later, a smear of Nivea cream to ease chafing. When I shaved at night, I would lie in bed rejoicing in gloriously silky legs, feeling like a real woman.

Oh, I was quite the shaver. I indulged daily, careful not to omit a patch, not even down near my ankles. I bent my knees to scrape them clean and only rarely sliced off some skin in that difficult place in the front where the bone touches so close to the surface. An impressed family friend once joked she would hire me to shave her legs. The guys at school routinely swiped their hands across girls' legs to patrol their shaving prowess and then taunt them if they were slacking off. If I were running late, I'd protect myself by faux shaving—just doing the strip between the bottom of my jeans and the top of my cotton socks.

And here I lived, in this world of plastic legs, where moms and daughters, teachers and coaches, shaved without a bat of the eye. It was all any of us saw; every woman had smooth legs. It was hygienic, like brushing your teeth or clipping your toenails. I tremble to think of what would have happened if I, a vaguely insecure, overly tall, 16-year-old, had paraded into homeroom one morning sporting furry legs and an ample bush under each arm. In a town of conformity (where the gossip of the school was that Marta dared to have "flat hair"—meaning no perm, no hairspray, no poofed bangs), this would have been instant death by humiliation.

Desperately suffocated by this clone-ishness (but seeing no way out from within), I jetted off to college at 18, with aspirations of hobnobbing among the potpourri of people boasted on the promotional fliers. I imagined a borderless territory for etching out exactly who one was, in the absence of relentless peer police. Granted, things were different. The word was that the college years were a time to get all the nose rings, crimson hair, and bottomed-out Birkenstocks out of your system, to quick-get-it-over-with and dabble in bisexuality and menages á trois (or at least talk about it), because you'd probably never get another go. So the parameters of conformity had widened, but ultimately, people still navigated within the confines of what was cool and acceptable. And other than on those marginal take-no-shit women, leg and armpit hair was still uncool. Shaving was still the undisputed norm. And the guys were still on hand to check for stubble.

The summer after my sophomore year, something happened that rocked my closely shaven world forever. I took a month-long mountain trek, and with only enough space for essentials, no forecast of running water, and no one to impress, I left my razor on the shower ledge at home. And for the first time since I had any hair to speak of, my leg and underarm hair began to grow. And grow. And grow. And the strangest thing was that I actually liked it. Not only did it feel good to be free of that constant bristle, it looked healthy and fuzzy and strong— somehow the way a woman's leg should look, not all bald and vulnerable like a little girl's. On the other hand, it felt so bizarre and unfamiliar, like I was this androgynous Bigfoot with hairy legs and pits. The second I reemerged into civilization, I shaved away the evidence, but my perceptions had been altered. In other words, I had dipped my hand in the cookie jar and I liked what I tasted.

In the midst of all this, I had been wading through months of dorm-room body-image rap sessions. It was becoming painfully clear that in our high-powered, image-focused environment, eating disorders ran rampant. To be young and white and female was to have "body issues," as we tenderly referred to them. We all had been afflicted by the bug, in varying ways. We freaked out about our bodies. We paid homage to the Stairmaster and hated it. We opted for salad bar, no dressing, instead of cheesy dining hall pizza. We gained the freshman 15 and struggled to lose the sophomore 20 or 30. Analyzing it ad nauseam was our way of reacting, fighting back, and learning to overcome this pressure for physical perfection. Meanwhile, as we shaved/plucked/waxed our body hair away, a dialogue on body hair lay dormant. We didn't see anything political in it.

But isn't body hair yet another image issue dumped in the exhausted laps of women? My mind begins to reel when I ponder the whole de-hairing ordeal:

Eyebrows: Pluck into symmetrical arches, or at least interrupt the unibrow over the bridge of the nose.

Moustache (more genteely referred to as upper lip hair): Bleach, wax, or zap it with electrolysis.

Chin hair: Tweeze out ASAP, even if it means using the rearview mirror at an intersection.

Random very long arm hairs: Yank.

Rest of arm hair: Bleach if too dark.

Nipple hair: Tweeze or fry with electrolysis.

Underarm hair: Shave, of course.

"Bikini line" hair (deemed so vile, only a euphemism can be used): Shave (and get a lovely rash), fantasize about being able to afford electrolysis, wear granny-style skirted bathing suits or shorts to the beach.

Leg hair: See Underarm hair.

Toe hair. Pull out while talking on the phone. whatever!

Sound familiar? Women's body hair is apparently so dirty, gross, and vulgar that it elicits queasiness in people. It's "excess," meaning it shouldn't be there in the first place. But it is. I'll bypass lugging down the hair-as-fur-for-warmth path, because clothes do that trick—but hair has always been there, and it will always be there. It's easy to forget that women have hairy legs and armpits because we never see them in their natural state. In this society, our eyes have actually been retrained to believe that a woman doesn't have body hair. Our memory omits the razors, waxes, creams, and bleaches that went into making her hairless. In fact, we expect a woman to have smooth legs et cetera and are surprised and often repulsed if she doesn't.

Why has body hair become such a nemesis for women? It poses no health risks. It is not hygienic to remove; it is not cleansing to shave. Rather, the complications arise during the eradication: cuts, infections, rashes, ingrown hairs, dry skin, burning. Is this hairless ideal yet another variation on the tune of "Let's take the best (boobs, curves in some places, hair in very few places) and leave the rest (hips, curves in other places, hair in *lots* of other places)"? Or is it a "Let's make women look like 8-year-olds so we can treat them as such"? Or is it a "If women can fill up their extra hours shaving and obsessing about their bodies then they won't have spare time to plot a world takeover"? Or maybe it's a "Women are *so* grossly overpaid and just don't spend enough on pads, tampons, pantyliners, Ibuprofen, shampoos, conditioners, deodorants, that we should coax them to buy razors, waxes, creams, and bleaches"? A-ha, it's probably a "How about setting another unattainable ideal for women so they will always fall short of the mark." I mean, what are women if they're not feeling insecure about something or another?

Chewing on all these questions, I returned to campus in the fall and began to test-drive not shaving. I would make a firm decision to quit cold turkey, toss all my razors, and let the hair do its thing. For the first few weeks, I could pass on the bad shaver-stubble ticket. Okay, fine. But after month or so, I found myself eager to answer a question in class, yet halted in my tracks by the horror of exposing my tank-topped hairy underarms to the cute guy across from me! Ay! I would settle for wagging my hand around on my desk and vow to stick to T-shirts from then on. But I love tank tops! And here began the eternal debate: Should I shave or should I let it go and feel awkward?

I've finally hit a point where I can hold out through fall, a hairy winter and well into spring. But come summer (lying on bikini-laden beaches, going to the office in a sleeveless dress without stockings, riding a crowded subway and having to reach up to grip the handrail), I start losing steam. At crunchy folk festivals I'm a card-carrying member, but traipsing to a corporate office in midtown Manhattan? Short of bundling up in wool tights and turtlenecks in 90-degree weather, I feel awfully strange about having hairy legs. I start out by rehearsing witty comebacks. I feel bold and strong for about a day and a half. Then I invent outfits to disguise my hairy legs and underarms. Then the debate rekindles. Finally, I lose my chutzpah and shave in defeat.

It's throwing in the towel on all accounts: Besides the strength I derive from rebelling against yet another implicit body pressure, hair feels good. Who could have ever imagined the erotic potential in riding a bike or swimming with hairy legs? The breeze ruffles it, the water swishes through it, wow! And sex? Ever sent someone flying out of bed by rubbing your bristly legs against them? Quite the opposite with hairy legs, as it is ultrastimulating to entwine your furry legs with your lover's. This completely uncharted aphrodisiac is scarily reminiscent of women not being encouraged to experience full sexual pleasure (guys get the hairy leg turn-on). Add to that, body hair looks incredibly sexy and healthy. We're just not used to seeing it on women.

What body hair needs is more visibility. It needs a publicity agent and a marketing campaign. It needs models and actresses to flounce around with hairy legs and pits. When those trailblazing, unshaven singers and songwriters like Ani DiFranco and Dar Williams stomp onto stage, it sends a loud and clear holler into the hairless vacuum. It propels us to see it, to think about it, to actually make the connection that this is a real woman, not the reverse. It cracks open a door that will eventually lead to women having the choice (not the compulsory burden) of whether they want to shave. Maybe someday I'll become a poster child for body hair. For now, I'm just revving up to go an entire summer without shaving, to storm the office in a sundress and sandals, to wear whatever the hell I want to the beach, to not feel ashamed to show my hairy armpits to the world. Every summer I get a little closer. Maybe this time I'll make it.

Body Hair: The Last Frontier

HARRIET LYONS AND REBECCA ROSENBLATT

Harriet Lyons and Rebecca Rosenblatt, *Ms.* July 1972. Reprinted by permission.

Actress Faye Dunaway boldly reveals her unshaven armpits for a photograph in a national magazine, and says that that's the way she will appear in all future film roles.

Eunice Lipton, an art historian in her thirties, strokes the growth on her legs and says, "It may seem ugly, but it's me."

Graduate student Grace Boynton, 23, explains that she has thrown away her razor because "I got insulted that my natural body processes were considered disgusting by society.…"

While cosmetics imply the real woman is not enough, shaving says that the real woman is too much. There is probably nothing more tedious, messy, or Indian for the feminine beauty regimen than the removal of hair from underarms, legs, eyebrows, lips, chin, and breasts.…

An emerging feminist consciousness tells us that all this punishing depilation reflects the depth of our socialized distaste for our bodies. We slavishly remove body hair and substitute artificial scents for natural body odors because we dare not expect approval if we look or smell as we really are.

Despite the all too familiar bother and pain—as well as the new feminist mandate to let it all hang out—the custom of depilating is still alive and well. Those who do vastly outnumber those who don't, but discussions of female body hair reveal disquieting associations.

In psychoanalytic parlance, hair is the accepted symbol of the genitals, so sexual behavior and hair-removal rituals are closely associated. Hairiness, in this lexicon, is translated as unrestrained animal sexuality. Conversely,

extremes of haircutting and shaving are symbolic of castration or the repudia-
tion of the very existence of sex. Anthropological evidence linking shaving customs to celibacy and ceremonial mutilation rites (such as the cutting off of finger joints) supports this symbology.

With hairiness equated to animal sexuality, the unchecked or uncovered
appearance of hair in the armpits and on the legs of women collides with the
culture's premise of female sexuality as passive. The implication that a
woman's underarm and leg hair are superfluous, and therefore unwanted, is
but one embodiment of our culture's preoccupation with keeping women in a
kind of state of innocence, and denying their visceral selves. Some women will
even shave pubic hair, thereby emulating the infantile sexlessness of a little
girl. And only within the last year has the men's magazine *Playboy* conceded
that adult women have pubic hair at all.

The acceptance of hairiness in men, like its suppression in women, is connected to animality, but, ironically the association is misguided, Man/woman
is the only animal sexually active beyond the need to reproduce; the only animal that can experience orgasm at times when conception is impossible. We
are both the most sex-driven and the least hairy of the animal kingdom, yet we
persist in equating sexuality with furriness. The bald or non-hairy-chested
man suffers a minor discrimination all his own.

While our puritanical attitude makes the hairless female body the quintes-
sence of femininity, our obsession with cleanliness works to modify the acceptance of hairiness even in men. Long hair and beards are for dirty hippies. The
clean-shaven and the crew cuts satisfy the American ideal.

Hair shares with feces, urine, semen, menstrual blood, spittle, and sweat a
centuries-old association with impurity. As a result, fastidious women
throughout history have felt obliged to remove hair that appeared anywhere
but on the head or pubis. In the 1850s, women were so devoted to their hygienic images that they inflicted skin ulcers upon themselves by reckless use of
depilatories made from lime, arsenic, and potash....

Race and class, with their attendant prejudices, determine special cultural
attitudes toward body hair. The connotation of dirty foreigner vs. clean
American has always been evident in our national thoughts on hair. A young
woman involved in a bicycle accident was asked by a New York policeman
examining her injured, unshaven leg, "You've not Puerto Rican, are you?"

It's true that, in Puerto Rico, women do not remove body hair unless they are
upwardly mobile or mainland-oriented. In France, only lower-class or provincial
women remain hairy. Even the supposedly earthy Italian women have begun
shaving underarms to conform with standards of chic-ness. In Spain, a mus-
tache on a woman is considered sexy, but not necessarily well bred.

Hair underscores the various myths and mysteries which have arisen from
our different skin colors. Intimidated racial groups try to lose their identity by
adopting the hair texture and styles of the majority or ruling class. The kinky

hair of American-born Blacks has been obscured for generations by straighteners, pomades, and pageboy wigs. In Sweden, where most women are fair enough to make shaving a nonissue, dark-complexioned women shave to be less conspicuous in the homogeneous population.

The Afro-coifed Black and the unshaven woman, regardless of her color, nationality, and class, make of their personal grooming a political statement. They reject an image of beauty and acceptability imposed by the society and risk the censure reserved for the rebel.

In America in the seventies, the hirsute woman is not yet an idea whose time has come. The shaving of body hair by women stubbornly defies extinction. Given the convoluted symbolism of the ritual and the repellent stares directed at the unshaven woman, we are not surprised to discover that even the most liberated women backslide when beach weather arrives.

But more and more individual women are risking those stares to affirm their natural femaleness. Eventually, this small but intimate tyranny will be resisted, so that one more oppressive hang-up can be retired forever and the hirsute will live happily with the hairless.

Browbeating

HAGAR SCHER

Hagar Scher, "Browbeating," *Ms.* magazine, July/August 1998. Reprinted by permission.

While most people barely bat an eyelash at the "news" that hard-core plucking is out for now and big eyebrows in, I confess that I'm absolutely thrilled. This trend makes my heart expand, my fist clench, my mind yell Woman Power! The untamed brows du jour are strong and bold. They remind me of my personal superheroes. Frida Kahlo and Golda Meir, though otherwise unrelated, share the funny brow bond. Their unwieldy forehead locks stand for what has always inspired me—the courage to live outside the lines and march to an original, booming drumbeat. Respect my eyebrows, respect me.

More than 25 years ago in this magazine, writers Harriet Lyons and Rebecca Rosenblatt argued that removing any sort of body hair says that "the real woman is too much." Let it be said that I am not toeing such a fuzzy-equals-feminist line, but I do have a knee-jerk aversion to plucking, even though some of my best friends are devotees. As I recently discovered, my dislike of skinny eyebrows stems from personal, emotional, and, well, fuzzy reasons.

A few months ago, I was feeling really low (a dreaded combination of writer's block, winter blahs, and unwashed-dish syndrome). In one of those moments when core beliefs are abandoned for petty concerns, I went to the drugstore to buy myself some tweezers. I was convinced that taming my Oscaresque (as in *Sesame Street*) brows would help me get it together. Poised to do the deed, I suddenly lost my resolve. Ten little hairs lay sink-side. Yet already I felt like Samson. I was scared that by losing my muss I might also lose my muscle. Once I plucked, might I not feel the need to mince words, bite my tongue, make nice with the world?

My big brows are, undoubtedly, an element of my Middle Eastern heritage, like my poor table manners and my low bullshit threshold. Like straightening kinky hair or dying dark locks blond, going for the minibrow look can be an attempt to hide one's ethnicity.

If the eyes are the windows to the soul, then the eyebrows are, at different times, the shield, the curtain, the dark cloud. Evolutionarily speaking, those hairs are there to stop sweat from irritating our peepers, and depleting them plays into the idea that women don't pounce, kick, compete—or perspire. Metaphorically speaking, they're even more commanding. Think Einstein. Maxibrows like his connote deep thought and determination. When thick eyebrows come together, they can express disgust and rage. Genius, drive, anger—misogynistically speaking, these are unfeminine traits. Thin, immobile brows seem less threatening. As a makeup artist would say, they open up the eyes and beckon, "Come on in. It's safe in here."

Ed Christie, art director of the *Sesame Street* Muppets, regretfully admits that despite the show's egalitarian spirit, eyebrows are used to quickly identify whether an "abstract" critter is female or male. Whereas girl puppets have felt brows that give them "a pencil-line, manicured look that prettifies," manly puppets like Oscar, the Count, and Bert have prominent ones that shout "eccentric, wily, wise, Merlin-like, very intellectual," and also "wild man, Neanderthal, untamed spirit."

So did Frida Kahlo's, but I'm pretty sure she heard that nagging voice asking, "Why don't you do something about those things?" I imagine her at a New York City cocktail party, suffering some clueless guy hitting on her with "You've got a pretty face. If you did something about that unibrow, you'd be a knock-out." Kahlo probably had her private moments of self-doubt when she reached for Diego's nose-hair clippers. But in the end, those dramatic brows were a constant in her life, a reminder, perhaps, of who she was. They made her appear moody, remote, unapologetically artistic.

Golda Meir, my grandpa once told me, was unapologetic in every way. They were members of the Israeli parliament together and although they were at odds politically, he was awed by her. A peacenik like him, I nonetheless am drawn to Meir because of her unflinching resolve, her sharp tongue, her ability to command the attention of a group of men steeped in macho Mediterranean idealism. When I think of Golda, I see two messy brows that sit above two piercing eyes, sending a message: *You'll have to look beneath these furry beasts to find me.*

A few weeks after my near-pluck experience, I flew to London to be with my mother. It was only our second chunk of together-time since she'd been diagnosed with colon cancer last summer. Apart from the bulging red scar that cut from her pubic mound to her chest, she seemed the same to me: calm, brilliant, charming, warm, honest, goofy, with a refreshing disregard for what other people think. One thing was new to me, though. As weird as it seems, I had never before noticed how amazingly bushy my mother's eyebrows are, stray hairs jumping out every which way. In my vision, tousled brows connote a productive life—like my mother's—in which trivial details fall by the wayside and societal constraints play second fiddle to self-realization. An existence like the one I aspire to.

Dreading It... Or How I Learned to Stop Fighting My Hair and Love My Nappy Roots

VERONICA CHAMBERS

Veronica Chambers, "Dreading It... Roots," *Vogue,* June 1999. Excerpted from Sharon Sloan Fiffer and Steve Fiffer, eds., in *Body,* Bard Press, 1999. Reprinted by permission.

There are two relationships I have with the outside world—one is with my hair, and the other is with the rest of me. Sure, I have concerns and points of pride with my body. I like the curve of my butt but dislike my powerhouse thighs. My nose suited me fine for the past 28 years. Then last week, for some strange reason, my nose seemed too big and I started to wonder about a nose job. My breasts, once considered too small, have been proclaimed perfect so often that not only am I starting to believe the hype but I'm booking my next vacation to a topless resort in Greece. But my hair. Oh, my hair.

I have reddish-brown dreadlocks that fall just below shoulder length. I like my hair—a lot. But over the past eight years that I have worn dreadlocks, my hair has conferred upon me the following roles: rebel child, Rasta mama, Nubian princess, drug dealer, unemployed artist, rock star, world-famous comedienne, and nature chick. None of which is really true. It has occurred to me on more than one occasion that my hair is a whole lot more interesting than I am.

Because I am a Black woman, I have always had a complicated relationship with my hair. For those who don't know the history, here's a quick primer on the politics of hair and beauty aesthetics in the Black community, vis-á-vis race and class in the late twentieth century. "Good" hair is straight and, preferably, long. Think Naomi Campbell. Think Whitney Houston. For that matter, think RuPaul. "Bad" hair is thick and coarse, a.k.a. "nappy," and often short. Think Buckwheat of the *Little Rascals*. Not the more recent, politically correct version, but the old one, in which Buckwheat looked like Don King's grandson.

Understand that these are stereotypes: broad and imprecise. Some will say that "good" hair versus "bad" hair is outdated. And it's true, it's much less prevalent than it was in the seventies, when I was growing up. Sometimes I see little girls, with their hair in braids and Senegalese twists, sporting cute little T-shirts that read Happy to Be Nappy and I get teary-eyed. I was born in the sandwich generation between Black Power Afros of the sixties and the blue contact lenses and weaves of the eighties. In my childhood, no one seemed very happy to be nappy at all.

I knew from the age of four that I had "bad" hair because my relatives and family friends discussed my hair with all the gravity that one might use to discuss a rare blood disease. "Something must be done," they would cluck sadly. "I think I know someone," an aunt would murmur. Some of my earliest memories are of Brooklyn apartments where women did hair for extra money. These makeshift beauty parlors were lively and loud, the air thick with the smell of lye from harsh relaxer, the smell of hair burning as the hot straightening comb did its job. To this day, the sound of a hot comb crackling as it makes its way through a thick head of hair makes me feel at home; the smell of hair burning is the smell of black beauty emerging like a phoenix from metaphorical ashes: transformation.

My hair was so thick that the perms never lasted through the end of the month. Hairdressers despaired like cowardly lion tamers at the thought of training my kinky hair. "This is some hard hair," they would say. As a child, I knew that I was not beautiful and I blamed it on my hair.

The night I began to twist my hair into dreads, I was 19 years old and a junior in college. It was New Year's Eve, and the boy that I had longed for had not called. "We'll all meet at a club," he had said. "I'll call and tell you where." But the phone never rang. A few months before, Alice Walker had appeared on the cover of *Essence,* her locks flowing with all the majesty of a Southern American Cleopatra. I was inspired. It was my family's superstition that the hours between New Year's Eve and New Year's Day were the time to cast spells. "However New Year's catches you is how you'll spend the year," my mother reminded me my whole life long. We spent the days before New Year's cleaning our room, watching as our mother put clean sheets on the bed and stocked the house with groceries. On New Year's Eve, my mother tucked dollar bills into my training bra and into my brother's pants pocket so that the New Year would find us flush. The important thing on New Year's Eve was to set the stage, to make sure you kept close everything you needed and wanted.

Jilted on New Year's Eve, I decided to use the hours that remained to transform myself into the vision that I'd seen on the cover of *Essence.* Unsure of how to begin, I washed my hair, carefully and lovingly. I dried it with a towel, then opened a jar of hair grease. Using a comb to part the sections, I began to twist each section into baby dreads. My hair, at the time, couldn't have been longer than an inch. I twisted for two hours, and in the end was far from smitten with what I saw—my full cheeks dominated my face, now that my hair lay in flat twists around my head. I did not look like the African goddess that I had imagined, but it was a start. I emerged from the bathroom and ran into my Aunt Diana, whose headful of luxuriously long, straight black hair always reminded me of Diahann Carroll on *Dynasty*. "Well, Vickie," she said, shaking her head. "Well, well." I knew that night my life would begin to change. I started my dreadlocks and I began the process of seeing beauty where no one had ever seen beauty before. Like Rapunzel, I grew my hair and it freed me, not only from perms that could never quite tame my kinky hair down but from a past in which my crowning glory was anything but.

There are, of course, those who see my hair and still consider it "bad." I have been asked by more than one potential suitor if I had pictures of myself before "you did that to your hair." One friend was so insistent that I must have been prettier without dreadlocks that I wore a wig to meet him one day. Not only did he not like me in the straight black bob that I wore, he didn't recognize me. "I get it," he said. "Those dreads are really you." I have occasionally thought that I carry all of my personality around on my head. A failure at small talk and countless other social graces, I sometimes walk into a cocktail party and let my hair do the talking for me. I stroll through the room, silently, and watch my hair tell white lies. In literary circles, my hair brands me as "interesting, adventurous." In Black middle-class circles, my hair brands me as "rebellious" or "Afrocentric." In predominantly White circles, my hair doubles my level of exotica. My hair says, "Unlike the Black woman who reads you the evening news, I'm not even trying to blend in."

That said, it is important to remember that at the end of the day, my hair is just hair. "Do you think this could work out?" a man said to me recently. Mind you, it was only our second date and I was pretty convinced that I didn't want there to be a third. "What do you mean?" I asked him, sweetly, even dumbly. "I'm very traditional and you're so wild," he said, reaching out for my hair. "I'm not wild. You only think I'm wild," I wanted to scream. For those who are ignorant enough to think that they can read hair follicles like tea leaves, my hair says a lot of things that it doesn't mean. Taken to the extreme, my hair says that I am a pot-smoking Rastafarian wannabe who in her off-hours strolls through her house in an African dashiki, lighting incense and listening to Bob Marley.

I have been asked to score or smoke pot so often that it doesn't even faze me anymore. Once after a dinner party in Beverly Hills, a white colleague of mine lit up a joint. Everyone at the table passed and when I passed too, the man proceeded to cajole me relentlessly. "Come on," he kept saying. "Of all people, I thought you'd indulge." I shrugged and said nothing. As we left the party for the night, he kissed me good-bye. "Boy, you were a disappointment," he said as if I had been a bad lay. But I guess I had denied him a certain sort of pleasure. It must have been his dream to smoke a big, fat spliff with a real, live Rastafarian.

Similarly, it's such hair judgments that make me a magnet for airport security. I loathe connecting international flights in Miami and London, for I am sure to be stopped and stopped again. On a recent trip from Panama, I was stopped by five officers in one hour; each took his time poking through my suitcases. Finally, imprudently, I let the last officer have it. "I know what this is," I told him. "This is harassment. And it's because of my hair." He didn't even blink an eye. "We stopped them too," he said, pointing to a group of white missionaries. "Nothing wrong with their hair." In the Bahamas, a friend and I weren't allowed into a local nightclub because, as the bouncer pointed out, the sign said No Jeans. No Sneakers. No Dreadlocks. I would have laughed if I didn't want to cry. You can change what you're wearing. How do you change the hair on your head? And why should you have to?

I have thought, intermittently, of changing my hairstyle. My hair is too big for me to wear hats, and I sometimes envy women with close-cropped cuts and stylish headgear. The other night, I watched one of my favorite movies, *La Femme Nikita,* and I admired Nikita's no-nonsense bob. "I couldn't be a female assassin with hair like this!" I said, jumping up out of my chair. Even pulled back, my hair is too voluminous to be stark. Then I remembered how, in the movie *Foxy Brown,* Pam Grier pulls a gun out of her Afro, and I was comforted that should I choose the career path of professional ass-kicker, my hair would not be an obstacle. Once, after the end of a great love affair, I watched a man cut all of his dreadlocks off and then burn them in the backyard. This is perhaps the only reason I would ever cut my hair. After all, a broken heart is what started this journey of twisting hair. A broken heart may find me at a new hair road. Because I do not cut my hair, I carry nine years of history on my head. One day, I may tire of this history and start anew. But one thing is for sure, whatever style I wear my hair in, I will live happily—and nappily—ever after.

Chapter 54

Face

Aging (balm for a 27th birthday)

ERICA JONG

Erica Jong, "Aging (balm for a 27th birthday)," from *Fruits & Vegetables: Poems by Erica Jong,* Hopewell, N.J., Ecco Press, 1997, originally published by Holt, Rinehart & Winston, 1968. Used by permission from the poet.

Hooked for two years now on wrinkle creams   creams for
crowsfeet   ugly lines (if only there were one!)
any perfumed grease   which promises   youth   beauty
not truth   but all I need on earth
        I've been studying   how women age

                        how

it starts around the eyes   so you can tell
a woman of 22 from one of 28 merely by
a faint scribbling near the lids   a subtle crinkle
      a fine line
extending from the fields of vision

  this

in itself is not unbeautiful   promising
                    as it often does
insights which clear-eyed 22 has no inkling of
promising   certain sure-thighed things in bed
certain fingers on your spine & lids

                                                        but

it's only the beginning   as ruin proceeds downward
lingering for a while around the mouth   hardening the smile
into prearranged patterns (irreversible!)   writing furrows
from the wings of the nose   (oh nothing much at first
              but "showing promise"   like your early poems

                                                        of deepening)

The No-Nonsense Approach to Cleaning Your Face

DEBORAH CHASE

Deborah Chase, "The No-Nonsense Approach to Cleaning Your Face," *Ms.* ,
November 1974, with a new introduction by the author, 1999. Reprinted by
permission.

When the medically based *No-Nonsense Beauty Book* was first published in 1976, the formulas for beauty products had changed little in over 100 years. Although researchers were beginning to learn more about the causes of a wide range of skin and hair problems, cosmetic companies seemed reluctant to use this new knowledge to develop truly helpful products.

This lack of progress did not inhibit manufacturers from making grandiose claims of performance. These would range from the literary ("turn back the hands of time") to the mystical ("channels the spirit of a legendary Hungarian beauty"). In a regulatory climate diplomatically described as lax, such claims went unchallenged. When I brought insupportable claims for turtle oil, royal bee jelly, and sea salts to consumer agencies I found that they were considered "harmless puffery." The prevailing attitude was that if a woman was dumb enough to believe such promises, then she deserved to buy useless products.

Claims substantiation was made difficult by lack of ingredient labeling. An advertisement promised to cure acne or eliminate lines and wrinkles but would not provide a list of ingredients by which a woman could judge its effectiveness. Up to 1976, one could only guess at ingredients in skin and hair products. I had to help a reader figure out the formulation by its name, feel, and directions on the package.

In 1976, several months after the book's publication, Senator Thomas Eagleton of Missouri successfully introduced a bill requiring all beauty care products to print their entire list of ingredients on the back of each label. Women were now able to search for ingredients to deliver promises or, equally important, to avoid substances to which they were allergic. For the first time, women could make an informed choice about ingredients and price in skin and hair care products.

THE SMALL CHANGE THAT HAS MADE A BIG DIFFERENCE

Looking back over 20 years of writing about beauty, I am especially delighted at the sea change in a woman's relationship to the sun. In 1976 a deep dark suntan was the ultimate beauty treatment. The fact that getting such a tan was arguably the worst thing that one could do to the skin seemed too unfair to accept. While women who read my book accepted most of the advice, they drew the line at tanning. In fact, a large cosmetic company approached me to design a line of No-Nonsense skin care products. In addition to developing formulations that contained the most effective active ingredients, I insisted that they be enhanced with sunscreens. We took the concept out on the road in focus groups through the Midwest. It totally bombed. Women completely rejected anything that would interfere with their relationship to the sun.

Today women of all ages now routinely use powerful sunscreens with SPF of 30 to 60. Sunblocks are now a common ingredient in day creams and moisturizers and viewed as a value-added benefit in foundations, eye make-up and lipstick. It is exactly the kind of lifestyle change that the women's health movement believes can result from a bit of basic beauty science and a list of useful ingredients so that women can make informed choices that were once unimaginable.

Despite the enormous advances made in the fields of biology and medicine in the past 50 years, cosmetics manufacturers, on the whole, have been unwilling to invest the time and money in the research required to come up with a truly revolutionary soap or facial skin care product. Still, there are many safe commercial products that can really help the skin. The trick is knowing which to buy and how to interpret the labels.

CLEANSING

Of the huge array of products offered for cleansing, each has different properties and should be applied to different types of skin.

SOAP

Basic toilet soap consists of a mixture of fat, alkali salt, and water.

Superfatted soap, containing extra amounts of oil and fat, is good for people with normal or slightly dry skin.

Castile soap contains olive oil as its main fat. It is no less drying or richer than basic toilet soap.

Transparent soap, made with glycerin and alcohol—both of which draw water from the skin—is best for people with normal skin.

Deodorant soap contains antibacterial chemicals that kill the bacteria present on the skin's surface. Since there are no apocrine glands on the face, these soaps serve no special purpose for that part of the body.

French milled soap has been specially processed to reduce alkalinity. A low alkalinity makes the soap less drying.

Floating soap floats because it contains extra water and has air trapped in it. It has no special properties for the skin.

Detergent soap is synthetic or "soapless" soap. The cosmetic chemist can adjust the properties of a detergent soap to make it less alkaline, less dehydrating, and less irritating than plain soap to sensitive skin.

Soap with fruit, vegetable, or herb extracts: whatever vitamins or enzymes these ingredients may possess in the raw state are usually destroyed in the manufacturing process.

Cocoa butter soap: cocoa, while not giving any special property to the soap has sometimes been associated with skin allergies.

CREAM AND LOTION CLEANSERS

Cold cream is made up of mineral oil, wax, and borax. When the cream is taken off with tissues, an oil film that contains some dirt may remain.

Cleansing cream is made of wax, mineral oil, alcohol, water, and some kind of soap or detergent. The soap remains in a film that coats the skin, damaging it and drying it out.

Cleansing lotion is made of the same ingredients, but contains more water. It has the same drawbacks.

Washable cream and lotion are made of ingredients similar to those described above. They do a thorough but gentle job of cleansing and are best for normal and dry skins. They do not have enough degreasing power for oily skin.

Milky cleanser is made of soap, water, alcohol, and mineral oil and contains more soap and less oil than washable creams or lotions. Since they are primarily soaps, they are good for normal and slightly oily skin, but are too harsh for dry skin.

Scrubbing cleanser is soap with tiny, hard grains that rub off the surface of the skin. It should be used daily on oily skin, weekly on normal skin, and monthly on dry skin.

OIL-BALANCE CONTROL

Day cream is made of wax, water, oil, and soap, or soaplike chemicals—to make the cream less greasy so that it does not dissolve makeup. The soap in these products makes them bad for dry skin.

Daytime lotion, frequently called moisturizer, is healthier for the skin. It contains more water and much less soap. Excellent products for dry skin, they should be used judiciously on normal skin and avoided for oily skin.

All-purpose hand, body, and face lotion is made with four basic ingredients: water, wax, oil, and glycerin. Although somewhat oilier, they usually do not contain chemicals that encourage the skin to hold water. An important question to ask is what oil it contains.

There are three categories of oils, all of which are meant to coat the skin and delay the evaporation of water. None have any special power to delay aging or prevent lines and wrinkles:

Of all the oils, *animal fat*—particularly lanolin—most closely resembles the natural human oil. The most expensive animal fats, mink and turtle oil, do the same job as cheaper ones. *Vegetable oil* protects the skin well enough, but it is not as good as animal oil. *Mineral oil* has a tendency to dissolve the skin's own natural oil, and can thereby increase dehydration.

Night cream: More nonsense has been written about night cream than any other beauty product. A night cream merely helps the skin to retain a better supply of water. It does not rejuvenate the skin, prevent lines or wrinkles, reach deep down into the pores, or wake up sleepy complexions. Some night creams, containing estrogens and other water-holding substances, do a better job of retaining water in the skin. Night creams are good for dry skin, not necessarily helpful for normal skin, and not needed for oily skin.

TONING

A *toning lotion* can temporarily shrink facial pores, make the skin look firmer, and reinforce a healthy coloring.

A *skin freshener* is an alcohol compound with various additives, such as herb extracts and camphor or menthol. It can be irritating to normal and dry skin.

An *astringent* contains water, less alcohol than skin fresheners, and, most importantly, aluminum or zinc salts. The salts, by causing a slight puffiness or swelling of the skin around the pores, makes them seem smaller. Beware of astringents that cause sharp, stinging sensations. These products probably contain only camphor or menthol

A *clarifying lotion,* also known as an exfoliating lotion, contains water, alcohol, glycerin, and a chemical that dissolves the keratin that makes up most of the skin's top layer of dry, dead cells. The skin looks brighter and cleaner after using a clarifying lotion. These lotions include salicylic acid, resorcinol, and benzoyl peroxide, which presently must by law be listed on the label. Papain, an enzyme extracted from papayas, and bromelin, an enzyme extracted from pineapples, can also dissolve keratin, but neither has to be listed on the label. Both are very powerful agents and have been associated with allergies and chemical burns.

Masks come in two basic forms—clay and gel. A *clay mask* picks up the cellular debris and gives the skin a smooth, even texture. The tightening action stimulates circulation and makes the skin glow. The clay contains mild bleaching agents that cause a gentle lightening of the skin. Clay also soothes the skin, reducing any inflammation and soreness. A *gel mask* is especially good for restoring water or rehydrating normal, normal to dry, and dry skin. Most of the value of a mask is based on the clay or gel base that forms the mask itself. Although certain ingredients are useful, like mint or vitamin A, many commercial masks have other exotic ingredients that do not perform any function.

Saunas: These are marvelous for every type of skin.

Beauty 911

JOEL BLEIFUSS

Joel Bleifuss, "Beauty 911," *MAMM,* June 1999. Reprinted by permission.

Every day, millions of Americans dye their hair, wash their hands, and powder their bodies with products that may add to their risk of contracting a variety of cancers, including ovarian cancer. Ingredients or contaminants that either cause cancer in laboratory animals or have been linked to human cancer by epidemiological studies can be found in dark hair dyes, shampoo, and liquid skin washes, among others. A recently published study of talc blames the substance for at least 10 percent of the cases of ovarian cancer each year. Under federal law, the safety of these products has been left largely in the hands of the manufacturers and their trade group, the Cosmetics, Toiletry & Fragrance Association (CTFA). That organization, and manufacturers such as Johnson & Johnson, steadfastly maintain that there is no proof that use of the products has actually caused cancer in human beings.

Strange as it may seem, the law does not require that cosmetic manufacturers perform any safety testing before putting an ingredient in a product. The Food and Drug Administration (FDA), the only federal agency with authority over the safety of cosmetics and toiletries, can remove a product from the market if it is deemed hazardous, or can require warning labels. The agency has made scant use of these powers, however, and has failed to respond to a two-year-old petition by a Chicago-based activist group asking for warning labels on talcum powder.

Long-time FDA and industry critic Samuel Epstein, M.D., charges that "the FDA bears a very heavy responsibility for escalating cancer rates, for failing to take action on those consumer products under its jurisdiction." FDA spokesperson Ruth Welch told *MAMM,* "We've worked closely with the industry to reduce these contaminants in cosmetic and toiletry products. Once it has been established by sound scientific data that a risk is caused by an FDA-regulated product, the agency will take appropriate action." Ironically, the FDA was established in 1938 because of concern about a coal-tar eyelash dye called Lash Lure that blinded some women. Over the years it has banned six ingredients in cosmetics, including mercury compounds, chloroform, and hexachlorophene.

The new talc study raises questions about the FDA's scrutiny of cosmetics and toiletries. To help readers decide for themselves, here is a review of the evidence.

THE TALC-OVARIAN CANCER CONNECTION

Ten epidemiological studies, the first done in 1982 and the latest published this spring, have connected the use of talc in the genital area to ovarian cancer. The new study concludes that at least 10 percent of the deaths each year from ovarian cancer are the result of talc use. Ovarian cancer is the fifth leading cause of cancer death for American women.

The latest study, funded by the National Cancer Institute, examined the history of talc use by 563 women diagnosed with ovarian cancer between 1992 and 1997 and compared them to a control group of 523 disease-free women. The team found that women who regularly applied talcum powder to the genital area increased their risk of contracting ovarian cancer by 60 percent.

Calling for "formal public health warnings," the research team concluded that the "avoidance of talc in genital hygiene might reduce the occurrence of a highly lethal form of cancer [ovarian] by at least 10 percent. Appropriate warnings should be provided to women about the potential risks of regular use of talc in the genital area."

HOW TALC COULD CAUSE CANCER

Talc is a mineral related to asbestos and can contain microscopic, sharp, asbestos-like fibers. In 1971, researchers discovered talc fibers deeply embedded in 75 percent of ovarian tumors studied, leading to the theory that the fibers had somehow reached there by entering the vagina after the women had dusted themselves with powder.

In 1973, the FDA drafted a resolution that would have limited the amount of asbestos-like fibers in cosmetic-grade talc. But no ruling was ever made. The cosmetics industry claims to have reduced the volume of asbestos-like fibers. But in 1993, the National Toxicology Program, an agency of the National Institutes of Health, conducted an animal study of talc that does not contain asbestos-like fibers and concluded that when inhaled, it was carcinogenic to rats.

Dr. Daniel Cramer, who headed the new study, says that providing direct evidence that talc causes ovarian cancer is virtually impossible. "You are never going to be able to randomly assign women to use talc in their genital area and wait for 20 years. From the perspective of having multiple epidemiologic studies, all pointing to a statistically significant association, there is enough evidence to say that exposure to talc should be avoided."

SHAMPOOS, LIQUID SOAPS, BODY WASHES, SHAVE AND SHOWER GELS

As anyone who has ever looked at a cosmetic label knows, the ingredients list is usually a long tongue twister of chemical names. On cleansing products like shampoos and liquid soaps, the list includes a group of foaming agents and emulsifiers, including cocamide DEA [diethanolamine], soyamide DEA, lauramide DEA, and oleamide DEA, that concern consumer health advocates. When these substances are manufactured, some of the DEA can be left in a separate state and is considered a contaminant. According to Dr. Epstein "lifelong use of [contaminated] products clearly poses major avoidable cancer risks to the great majority of U.S. consumers, particularly infants and young children."

The FDA says that the agency does not believe consumers should be alarmed but adds, "Consumers wishing to avoid DEA may do so by reviewing the ingredient statement" on cosmetics and toiletries. The agency has not taken any action since the statement was issued.

NITROSAMINES IN COSMETICS

Besides being suspect itself, DEA can also turn into a potent class of carcinogens called nitrosamines when it comes into contact with chemicals called nitrites during the production process. From 1985 to 1996, the FDA analyzed only 47 cosmetic products for NDELA [nitrosodiethanolamine], nearly half of which—23—were found to be contaminated with the nitrosamine. In 1992, the agency found one product (the FDA keeps brand names confidential) that contained NDELA at a concentration of 2,960 parts per billion. Two years ago the FDA stopped testing cosmetic products for NDELA altogether. Agency spokesperson Ruth Welch cites budget constraints.

The evidence against NDELA includes a 1995 article in the journal Carcinogenesis in which National Cancer Institute scientists William Lijinsky and Robert Kovatch said the substance is readily absorbed through the skin and concluded, "Not only does NDELA induce tumors over a wide range of doses, but it is a multipotent carcinogen, inducing [cancers in rats] in a number of different organs." Lijinsky, former director of the Chemical Carcinogenesis Program at the National Cancer Institute, believes the FDA is not doing enough to ensure that cosmetics are free of nitrosamines, which he describes as "the most potent carcinogens we know." The fewer tests that are done, the fewer problems there will be to find, he says. "They are evading the problem," he concludes.

Definitive proof of the dangers of DEA and nitrosamines in cosmetics and toiletries will probably never be obtained. Reputable researchers would never deliberately expose human beings to substances known to cause cancer in animals, and epidemiological studies are made impossible by the ubiquity of the substances in consumer products.

HAIR DYES

An estimated 20 to 40 percent of American women dye their hair. For years, controversy has surrounded the safety of coal-tar dyes widely found in hair-coloring products. The FDA's official statement on hair dyes, which it has not updated since 1993, advises: "Compounds suspected of causing cancer are found in temporary, semi-permanent, and permanent dyes."

Research studies of coal-tar dyes have produced contradictory findings. In 1992, a National Cancer Institute study found that women who dye their hair run a 50 percent higher risk of developing non-Hodgkin's lymphoma, a cancer of the lymph system, than women who don't. That research estimated that up to 20 percent of all American women who have non-Hodgkin's lymphoma got their cancer from exposure to hair dyes. A 1994 survey by the American Cancer Society, however, implicated only dark hair dyes, finding that women who used them for two decades or more had a 400 percent greater risk of dying from non-Hodgkin's lymphoma and multiple myeloma, a malignancy of the bone-marrow cells that produce antibodies. Other studies, however, found no increased risk at all.

READ THE FINE PRINT

Dr. Samuel Epstein of the Cancer Prevention Coalition, coauthor of *The Safe Shopper's Bible: A Consumer's Guide to Nontoxic Household Products, Cosmetics, and Food* (Macmillan, 1995), says that at the very least the FDA should institute a system of label warnings for cosmetics. "Industry voluntarily discloses ingredients, but these ingredients mean nothing to the overwhelming majority of experts in carcinogenesis or toxicology, let alone the public," he says. "What is needed is a red-flag warning where any carcinogenic ingredient, contaminant, or precursor would be marked in red."

The incidence of many types of cancer has been increasing. Research by National Cancer Institute epidemiologist Susan Devesa details mysterious increases in the incidence of non-Hodgkin's lymphoma, kidney cancer, testicular cancer, certain types of breast cancer, brain cancer among people under 25, and childhood leukemia. Her report concludes that these unexplained increases "may reflect changing exposures to carcinogens yet to be identified and clarified."

Could these exposures be coming from the cosmetics and toiletries consumers use every day? With no regulatory action by the FDA in the works or expected, consumers have no choice but to read the fine print on labels and make their own decisions.

Susan Brownmiller on Appearance and Makeup

INTERVIEW BY CARRIE CARMICHAEL

Susan Brownmiller is... This interview was conducted in May 1999.

CC: You have chosen a makeup-less life. How did you decide that? When did you decide that?

SB: I never looked good in makeup, and I never was handy at it. I'm less artistic and more verbal, so I was never good at painting my face. In the mid- to late 1960s, when feminism was starting, I used to wear lipstick. Then lipstick color lightened. First they did the white thing, and then the pink thing, and then it was just gloss, so it was very easy to me to get rid of the one thing that I did do, which was put on lipstick. When I had my book jacket photo taken the other day, I decided to err on the side of caution—I had a makeup person do the whole number. Her pictures are very nice, but it's me made up. It's me facing the public under a mask. So I was nervous. I was nervous to go before the camera without makeup. That's dangerous. It's not as though you want to hide and be something else for the photo, but you know what the camera sees, what the camera picks up. I was terrified.

CC: Is that about age?

SB: Certainly it's about age.

CC: Did that experience with the makeup for your photo ease your mind about it?

SB: No. But I'll tell you a funny experience. I went from the photo shoot to visit a sick friend, and when I got there, she had no food, so I had to go out to the local grocery store. We decided we'd make a meal of spaghetti and meatballs. So I was ordering from the guy behind the deli counter, and I asked for some meatballs, and the guy said to me, "Is that all I can do for you?" I said, "Yeah, I just need the meatballs." And he said, "Are you sure? You are so appealing." And I said, "Sir, it's the makeup." I mean this was a full-dress makeup. I guess women don't walk into the grocery store like that—I certainly never walk into the grocery store like that. It reminded me of the time I was on the road for *Against Our Will*. I'd go from city to city, and in the course of the day, every television station would slap on more of the stuff and I was bright orange it seemed to me, totally exaggerated, by the time I got on the plane at night to go to the next city. I'd get on that plane, and guys from other rows would be fighting each other to sit next to me. Their feeling must have been, "She knocks herself out so much for us. She is sending out all of these signals. Wow! I want to be near her." And I had forgotten that totally until I had this experience of walking into the grocery store in full makeup a couple of weeks ago.

CC: Do you choose not to wear makeup because you really don't want that kind of invasion?

SB: No, that's not the reason. I just felt that it didn't add anything to my face when I was young. And there was a time when you didn't have to do any of it, thanks to feminism. I didn't care for any of the procedures. In fact, when this professional makeup person did put on the makeup, she came at me with the eyelash curler, and I practically screamed. I hated to go through that torture, which I remembered full well. I let her tweeze my eyebrows though. So it just depends on what you are willing to endure or not endure. And I was always willing to endure a minimum amount. I just didn't have the capacity to endure a lot. Same thing with shoes. I just don't have the capacity to hobble on high-heeled shoes and risk corns and damaging my toes.

CC: As a city person I call them cab shoes. I can't walk very far in them, and they're too expensive, and it's crippling.

SB: But you know how many people do struggle with it all of their lives, and then they have foot pains.

CC: Do you think that one of the benefits of the women's movement in its current incarnation is that we are able to combine the image of femininity, femaleness, and power? Where are we when it comes to those qualities all in the same woman?

SB: I don't think that you can speak for a "we." I urge you to look at *Bust* magazine. They are kind of neofeminists at *Bust* magazine, and they have an article that a young woman wrote, a little chart about all of the things that she must buy, she must do, in order to present herself to the world. And they're still grappling with it, and they don't get it. They don't know why it costs them more to be a woman in society than it costs men to be men.

CC: There was a time when we felt that the only way that you could present yourself as a strong, serious, thinking woman was to not have any of the trappings of the former Barbie doll image. It's different now.

SB: Yes, that's right. There was a lot of excess. Everything was thrown out. And then they came back.

CC: Do you think concern with appearance has come back and taken over? Where do you think we are in terms of things being in some kind of balance?

SB: Well it's not that it's taken over. It's that our movement raised many, many issues. The ones I concentrated on were violence against women and the right to reproductive freedom, and there has been no retreat on those fronts, although the problems are still with us. But around appearance, saying, "God damn it, I won't do the thousand things I'm supposed to do to feminize my body," there's been a total retreat.

CC: But there are those who would quarrel with your statement.

SB: Oh, sure they would. They'd say it's done now for fun. You can do it or not do it. And that's true. There's a lot more freedom out there: to wear pants, to wear jeans, to go makeup-less. There's a lot more freedom than there was in the 1950s and the early 1960s.

CC: To be seen as female, as feminine, is not just defined as manipulation and being false.

SB: Well, it still is. But there are options. You don't have to be that way all the time, but it should be in your wardrobe.

Chapter 55

Skin

Higher Yellow

REBECCA WALKER

Adapted from Ophira Edut, ed., *Adiós, Barbie: Young Women Write About Body Image and Identity*, Seattle, Seal Press, 1998. Another version of this piece appeared in Kevin Young, ed., *Giant steps: The New Generation of African American Writers*, New York, William Morrow. Reprinted by permission.

I am a woman obsessed with skin, others and especially my own. I squint into mirrors, trying not to see the scars left from my bout with the chicken pox, the wrinkles appearing branchlike across my once satiny forehead, the dark spots reminding me of all the times I was too weak to practice restraint. I turn this way and that in carefully modulated lighting, keeping a fair distance from the looking glass, not wanting to know what it cannot help but say: My skin is not flawless. It ages, chafes, erupts angrily. It sags where I would like it to be taut, pebbles where I want it to be smooth. Ultimately I aqcuiesce, accept the unacceptable—I am human, a mere mortal like everyboody else—and turn out the light.

But there is something else, a remnant of self-hatred that does not go away so easily, that does not fade when the light dims. This other thing is what makes me cringe when my lover pulls my jeans over my hips in the half-light of our bedroom. It is what makes me burn myself in the sun year after year, and idolize Naomi Campbell no matter how much I commit to honoring my own beauty instead of someone else's. Spots, scars, bumps, and keloids just skim the surface of my neurosis. The depth of my obsession with skin revolves around color, and what I perceive to be my lack thereof.

I have always been light. Pale. Honey-colored. Yellow. Near white. Olive. Neon. Sallow. Jaundiced. Pasty. And I have, for most of my adult life, hated being so. While aunts and cousins told me I had good hair and was lucky to be light, I felt gypped, like my mother didn't do her part while I was in utero, like her melanin gene was no match for my father's hearty Slavic-Jewish stock. Sure, there were moments when light wasn't light enough and I wanted to have straight hair and a mom named Jane, but for the most part I have wanted to be darker, with full lips and thicker, more chocolatey thighs. Darker is what my mother is, what my lovers often are. Though I am ashamed to admit to privileging any color over another, darkness is where I have located the beauty that moves me, the beauty that sets my stomach twitching and my mind dreaming. Darkeness is graceful, mellifluous, haunting. Darkness is deeper, smarter, more lovable.

This narrative I've attributed to darkness goes on and on, as obsessive fantasy projections often do. It includes words like community, belonging, stability, justice, righteousness, and moral superiority. In weak moments my mind construes dark skin as a passport that facilitates admittance to cultures that do not disown, that never fail to claim. I imagine that the darkness provides a ready-made identity, a neat sense of knowing as clear and pure and self-evident as skin itself. I think that to be darker is to be on the right side of the powerless-powerful, oppressed-oppressor equation. To be black is to be part of the solution. Black Is Beautiful, remember? But what about beige? I wonder. Is beige beautiful, too? Or am I only half of the thing itself, muddied, watered down, and eternally ambivalent?

I am not the only one reading more into the surface of the body than meets the eye. In our North American culture, and indeed in cultures around the world, the body is a sign, a text to be read and interpreted. For each body part there is at least one widely accepted script already written, a bit of subtext that fleshes out, so to speak, the extremity in question. Long fingers foretell musical agility (and sexual prowess). Big hands and big feet promise a great big juicy you-know-what. Big breasts bespeak fertility. A long neck is elegant. Full lips are sexy. Fat is slothful. A big nose is awkward. Nappy is unhappy. Bald women are unfeminine.

While these scripts purport to be objective observations, they are more often propagandistic narratives, self-serving tracts that operate primarily in the construction of community, be it based on ideology, race, vocation, or class, on a local, national or international level. As long as there is a standard of beauty, a set of positive attributes assigned arbitrarily to a particular set of body parts, there are two camps locked in a xenophobic embrace: those who have the good parts, and those who do not; those who are on the inside of the community, and those who are relegated to its margins.

Enter the civil rights and feminist movements, the gay, lesbian, bisexual, and transgender movement, the Chicano student movement. Enter dyke, hip-hop, *cholo*, biker, skater, tribal, punk, and neo-Nubian aesthetics. Whether its multiple piercings, femme girls with no hair, two-foot-high head wraps, or skin so covered with tats that the whole idea of clear and blemish-free seems hopelessly naive, finally it is clear that as a result of artistic and political movements, new and different scripts are being written. The body, a blank page waiting for words, and beauty, a subjective idea looking for a location, have been liberated to meet up in a variety of unique and often surprising ways. Barbie, with her pert nose and shoulder-length blond hair, no longer reigns supreme.

Yet as we stand at the millennium, patting ourselves on the back for making it this far, why is it that so many of us still struggle to claim our shape and size, color and hue. What compels us to even consider ads exhorting us to reshape, resculpt, redesign, and remake aspects of ourselves that our parents made just fine in the first place? It would be foolish to minimize the power of societal pressure, the waifish models screaming out from every newsstand and supermarket checkout line; nor can we ignore the self-esteem crisis permeating every cell of our culture. But I think there is something else, too, an overlooked by-product of the hysteria to control and commodify an image of ideal beauty: a crisis of the imagination, a dearth of stories, a shocking lack of alternative narratives.

Where are the stories that challenge the notion that perfect happiness can be found in a perfect body? Where are the anecdotes about learning to love parts of ourselves not because of how they look or how they measure up to supermodels, but because of how they feel to us, or how they tell a unique part of our personal history? Where, in this ongoing cultural discourse on body image, is the story of the lover who celebrated the hips we found too narrow or too wide, and caused us to see ourselves anew; the story of the Jewish nose that connects us to an ancestral past; the testimony about that extra 30 pounds that make us feel solid and abundant rather than sloppy or unattractive?

Recently, an article on body shapes caught my eye. "Death to Diets!" the headline caroled. "Figure out which of these four types you are, then follow this strategy for your best body ever." Apparently the more than 2 billion females on the planet fall into four neat but definitive categories. Forget genes, socioeconomic status, and individual soul destiny. According to this article, character, diet, and even career are indicated by the size and placement of your hips, breasts, and thighs. Wow! I thought, scanning to find a celebrity body that matched my own. Think of all the money I could have saved on therapy!

The fact is that we say a lot about how the standard of beauty needs to change, and even find some creative ways to re-vision it, but I know that in my own life, and I presume in the lives of many others, that abstract and theoretical discussion simply has not done the trick. Rigorous deconstruction may lay the new foundation for personal change, but it does not rebuild the house. That work calls for new materials; we need to do more than articulate what is wrong with the standard, we need to document and tell our very personal stories of confronting that standard. I want to read new scripts based not on what the culture dictates, but on what we have come to know and experience in the intimate moments of our day-to-day lives. The body tells its own story, and it is usually not the one you expect. We need to listen for and nurture those stories, the stories that are true.

Until recently I, too, have been decidedly without vision when it comes to accepting, rather than outright hating, my color. For most of my life I have been unable to love my honey thighs, to smile back into my fair-skinned face because I lacked a story I could live with, a story that made sense to me. I have hated my proximity to whiteness, the colonizing tinge that taints and marks me as an outsider, and pushes me to the periphery of brown and black worlds I have longed to call my own. Looking down the length of my barely brown body, I have felt revulsion, a horrifying lack that runs deep. Years of comparing myself to brown-skinned sisters with bangles and curves, abundant head wraps and well-shaped thighs, has left me disatisfied in my angularity and running a constant critique of the sharpness of my profile and the unwillingness of my flesh.

But I have finally begun to tell a better story. It is far from a complete or cohesive narrative, but it begins and ends with my maternal grandmother, her beloved place in her Southern rural community, my grandfather's abiding love for her, the upright way she walked, her wide and easy smile. By the time I knew her, she was already a woman's woman, not slight but solid, and with an air of experience so profound that when she spoke her mind—which was often—everyone present listened with their full attention, even as their eyes turned toward the television, or their hands moved busily over the stove.

She was a woman of appetite and could, even paralyzed by stroke, cruise through a plate of chicken legs and collard greens with grace and appreciation. Even though I have always, my whole life since I was a little girl and holding her hand in the Kingdom Hall, loved and admired her, I have of late begun to notice and prize our similarities. We share full pinkish brown lips and what is called yellow skin but which is more like a light light oak. We both turn our heads to the side in photographs, a gesture which highlights our high, well-defined cheekbones. We both love the natural beauty of the earth and turn our dark eyes to it as often as we can, not letting any little creature go unnoticed, unseen, unappreciated. When I look at her photgraph, which hangs above my desk, I see fullness, a life lived and enjoyed. I do not see a lack. I see a haunting, regal beauty. I recognize a smoldering intensity that sparks, too, behind my own eyes.

And there are other women, too. Lena Horne is in the story too, also staring down from a photo above my desk with an awesome fearlessness. In this Carl van Vechten photo, she is in her early twenties, not much older than I was when

I found the postcard in a Vermont bookstore. I imagine she is out for a day in the country, her glowing, well-scrubbed face facing forward, her small brown eyes smiling honestly and shamelessly into the camera. There is an uprightness, a sad, hard-won pride in her bearing, a moving wistfulness in her startingly direct stare that I find familiar and reassuring: My path has been walked before. I am not alone. I am kin to these striking, self-made women, and because of this, granted a new and fragile pride before the looking glass, a surety of belonging I have never known. My lover is in the story, too, tender and attentive, telling me again and again, as many times as it takes, that I am sexy and beautiful and perfectly complete, my beloved who likes my color and the fact that I am neither black nor white, but both, some land in the middle that is, miraculously, not too threatening to love. And there are others: the striking light-skinned sisters on the subway who move with an awkward grace, the wiry-haired and olive-skinned brother/friend who wraps his strong arms around me enveloping me in a musky and powerful but culturally undefined masculinity, the playful and self-possessed biracial children of dear and daring friends.

These affirming bits are puncuated by moments I have more and more often, when I look down the length of my body and feel not disgust but a tender gratitude for what I do have: skin that covers and protects, that loves to be lotioned and stroked, that is responsive to touch and fundamentally resilient. Skin that is a record, a kind of testimony to who I am, and what my history is. I am the child of a black mother and white father, I fell from my bicycle when I was four and got this scar; this mark came from a trip to Cuba, and this one from a fight with some girls in the Bronx. My body is its own kind of camera, and what it records reminds me that I am constanly changing, moving from day to day and year to year, toward the final physical change of this life, when my body finally falls away, when my body speaks for itself the final chapter.

I know I have a long way to go before I can unequivocally groove on my paleness, but I consider getting this far to be a major accomplishment. To look at the ways we judge and contort ourselves is a radical and self-affirming act in a culture where altering oneself for admission and approval is the norm. To do the actual work of reprogramming, rewriting the words that we have been taught go with the picture, is a much more strenuous and exacting task. That journey to survival is mapped on the body's surface and begins as we extend to our most hated features the first tremblings of compassion.

Our Bodies, Our Voices, Our Choices

NATIONAL BLACK WOMEN'S HEALTH PROJECT

Excerpted from National Black Women's Health Project, *Our Bodies, Our Voices, Our Choices: A Black Woman's Primer on Reproductive Health and Rights,* Washington, DC, 1998. Reprinted by permission.

FOREWORD

Since its inception in 1981, the National Black Women's Health Project has worked to bring together women to talk about our experiences, hopes, and dreams—and to share information that will enhance our lives and health. This primer is designed for Black women to use as an introductory policy reference on reproductive health issues. It contains historical background, the contemporary context, and NBWHP policy statements. We hope it will stimulate greater interest and understanding of reproductive health issues as well as encourage women to take positive action for themselves, their families, and their communities. There is much to learn and much to do.

The principle of self-help guides our fundamental belief that every women—whether heterosexual, bisexual, or lesbian—may substantially increase her chances of achieving overall health and well-being if:

> ➤ She is knowledgeable about her body
> ➤ She is aware of her rights and empowered to ask necessary questions
> ➤ She knows that she is entitled to information and services that are delivered with dignity and respect

We also believe that when women appreciate how history and contemporary events combine to impact our ability to make decisions and to have choices, they will want to get politically involved on matters close to home, across the nation, or around the world.

Historically, all women in the United States have struggled to achieve reproductive health and reproductive rights. While this struggle has been most challenging for poor women and women of color, the fact that Blacks were brought to this country in chains, sold as slaves, and held in bondage for generations has had a deep and enduring impact on our lives.

For 244 years, Black women in America suffered the harsh realities of slave labor, forced breeding, and the wrenching separation of children from mothers and other loved ones. Since Emancipation, we have been burdened by a racist mythology that distorts our sexuality and paints us as loose, immoral, and unfit to be mothers. Over time, we have borne the brunt of a dizzying array of racist policies and programs aimed at controlling our reproduction. In the past 30 years alone, we have dealt with forced or involuntary sterilization, court-ordered insertion of long-acting contraceptives, deadly illegal abortions, punitive welfare policies, and arrest and prosecution instead of treatment and compassion for using drugs while pregnant... the list goes on.

Out of this dismal experience, Black women have grasped a fundamental truth: unless and until we are free to control our own fertility, we will never be able to take care of ourselves or our families, or take full advantage of opportunities in education, employment, and society at large.

Spurred on by this truth, Black women have been involved in the movement for "voluntary motherhood" and reproductive rights since the turn of the century. Racism and discrimination meant that our efforts were largely within our own community, although over time, a number of Black women have played prominent roles in the national reproductive rights movement.

Today, most people think of the phrase "reproductive rights" as the right to choose and abortion. Black women have always understood that the correct phrase is "reproductive *health* and rights"—that our struggle goes beyond our ability to decide whether, when, and how to have a child.

Black women understand that genuine reproductive health and rights are possible *only* when society allows healthy mothers and healthy babies to flourish. Genuine reproductive *health* will be achieved when society ensures that young girls and women have access to all necessary information and basic services, from health care and housing to education and employment. Genuine reproductive *rights* will be achieved when women can make decisions about their sexuality and reproduction that are free from coercion, actual or threatened violence, soul-crushing addictions, and despair—and when society ensures that the resources necessary to support those decisions are readily available.

There are many compelling ways to bring this expansive view of reproductive health and rights into reality. Black women put creative energy and volunteer time into the prevention of violence and homelessness, the promotion of prenatal care and mammography screening, and much more.

Those of us who have been active in the reproductive rights movement have been vital partners in the effort to expand these rights and broaden women's choices. But we have also been vocal critics of options that present problems for many women, such as technologies that have negative side effects or do not provide protection against sexually transmitted diseases, as well as programs that do not offer an ongoing support system for women.

Our historical experience has taught us to examine any new reproductive technology or social program through our triple screen: race, class, and gender. As a result, our view often diverges from the mainstream. Unless we are convinced that a new technology or program will genuinely add to a woman's choices and enhance her health and well-being, we voice our opposition and urge all Black women to consider seriously the facts before accepting that technology or program.

As women of the African diaspora, we have traveled great distances, literally and figuratively. We have survived and often thrived. Let us celebrate our lives as Black women—vital, vibrant, and strong—and move forward to secure genuine reproductive health and rights for ourselves, our daughters, and all our sisters.

Julia R. Scott, RN
President & CEO

SEXUAL HEALTH AND EDUCATION

HISTORICAL EXPERIENCE: RACIST MYTHOLOGY

Racist mythology has defined African-American sexuality and childbearing since slavery. Both African-American women and men were labeled "naturally immoral" and considered sexually irresponsible. After slavery, African-American women were referred to as "Jezebels" and portrayed as promiscuous, "bad" mothers who, unrestrained in their childbearing, passed these same traits on to their children. At the same time, African-American women were involved extensively in child care and rearing of white children as wet nurses and nannies.

For centuries, Black women were caught in a vicious catch-22. First, whites claimed we were sexually "loose" and therefore fair game for white rapists and sexual predators. Then, our sexuality was blamed for helping to "cause" Black men to rape white women, an alleged act which led to brutal, often fatal consequences for many of our men.

CONTEMPORARY CONTEXT: SEXUALITY, SHAME, AND SILENCE

One consequence of our legacy from slavery and the continuing public mythologies about African-American sexuality is that many of us have deeply buried the interconnectedness of our emotional, sexual, and reproductive experiences. Our sexuality is often associated with feelings of shame. Problems related to our reproductive health—from unwanted pregnancies or infertility to cancers of the breast or reproductive organs—are usually kept private.

In addition, mainstream cultural taboos tend to prevent discussion of healthy sexuality among all women. Attacks on public school, family life, and sex education programs by some conservative and religious fundamentalists have severely limited opportunities to help adolescent girls (and boys) at a crucial time in their sexual development to understand and practice decision-making and negotiation skills. Oftentimes, the premises of these attacks are accepted without in-depth examination of cause and effect.

This "conspiracy of silence" has an invisible yet potent impact on the overall health and well-being of Black women. When we are discouraged from asking questions and when we cannot discuss important issues related to our reproductive health and sexuality, our health and that of future generations is jeopardized. Lack of knowledge about sexuality and reproduction is often cited as a major reason that young women engage in irresponsible sexual practices, resulting in high rates of unintended pregnancies and sexually transmitted infections. However, knowledge alone is not the answer either. Confidence, self-respect, and awareness of the benefits of delayed gratification are essential elements as well.

NBWHP POLICY STATEMENT: HEALTHY SEXUALITY BEGINS WITH EDUCATION

A vital component of sexual health is access to age-appropriate family life and sex education programs. All humans are sexual beings from the moment of birth, so it makes sense that attention to our sexual health should begin at the earliest possible age.

African-American girls and adolescents have a critical need for adequate knowledge and understanding of sexuality for two reasons: they are vulnerable to internalizing the negative stereotypes about Black female sexuality; and they are likely to be subjected to sexual abuse or violence. In fact, one in three Black women report sexual abuse at some point in their lives.

Programs for boys are equally important for factual knowledge and under-standing about responsible sexuality, respect for self, and others. We must teach all children appropriate ways to show love and affection and encourage them to disclose and negative incidents in order to reduce their potential for sexual abuse.

NBWHP, supports age-appropriate sex education in multiple settings, including public and private schools, as well as efforts to help families and caregivers to provide accurate information regarding sex and sexuality to their children. Sex education and family life skills should be taught in schools, churches, community centers—as well as in the home—by caring adults. This is the first challenge, and often the most critical one, for achieving a life of good health.

African-American women must take the lead in fostering sexual health for today's young girls and for the generations to come. As adults, we can play an essential role in helping young girls and adolescents to develop healthy atti-tudes and feelings about their bodies and their sexuality. We can do this by willingly and openly discussing any or all topics related to sexuality, by model-ing respectful and loving relationships with others, and by demonstrating love for ourselves through healthy behaviors.

PREGNANCY AND PRENATAL CARE

HISTORICAL EXPERIENCE: FORCED BREEDING

During slavery, Black women in America had no control over their reproduc-tive lives. We were subjected to forced breeding, rape and sexual abuse, and our families were torn apart on the auction block. As slaves, we were valuable for our field labor and as reproducers. Our babies were the "new stock" for slave owners who depended on a continual supply of infants after the import of new slaves was banned in 1808.

Centuries before modern medicine was able to define and treat the fetus separately from the mother, slave owners saw the fetus as a distinct piece of property with great potential value. When a slave owner would punish a pregnant slave, he had to balance his interest in disciplining his worker with his interest in gaining a healthy new infant. The solution became a common practice throughout the South: the pregnant slave was forced to lie down in a depression in the ground so that her fetus would not be injured while she was bullwhipped.

Babies are our hopes and wishes for the future, symbolizing love for our partner, for our families—for life itself. Having a baby that you want is one of life's most glorious gifts. There is a delicious excitement and sense of wonder.

The most powerful act of "resistance" by slave women was ensuring the survival of their children. An enduring legacy from our days in slavery is the strong African-American tradition of forging communal bonds among nonrelated individuals, of taking in children without parents, of caring for one another in the face of extreme odds. This spirit of life-affirming "resistance" continues in our community today.

CONTEMPORARY CONTEXT:
HEALTHY MOTHERS = HEALTHY BABIES

The intergenerational cycle of poverty and near poverty makes it difficult for many African-American families to build and maintain preventive health care habits. An estimated 25–30 percent of inner-city African-American women receive little or no prenatal care during their pregnancies. This is oftentimes due to lack of access to health care services, inadequate care when health care is delivered, language barriers, and/or a lack of information, especially among pregnant adolescents.

Prenatal care is essential for a safe pregnancy and a healthy, full-term infant. In addition to monitoring the pregnant woman's diet and encouraging her to quit smoking, prenatal care includes screening for sexually transmitted diseases, high blood pressure, gestational diabetes, abuse of alcohol and illegal drugs, and domestic violence. When the health care needs of childbearing African-American women are not met, there are grave consequences.

Scientists at the Centers for Disease Control and Prevention (CDC) report that African-American women are four times more likely to die from pregnancy-related causes than white women. On average, an African-American woman dies every 2½ days in the United States from pregnancy-related causes. Many of them could be saved by regular checkups during pregnancy.

Infant mortality rates in African-American communities resemble those in developing nations. Black babies die at the rate of 6,000 more per year than white babies in the same geographical area.

The primary contributing factor to infant mortality is low birth weight. Surprisingly, the frequency of low-birthweight babies is not limited just to poor women in medically underserved areas. Middle-class Black women have more low-birthweight babies than white women of the same socioeconomic class. And, approximately one-quarter of all pregnancies in women of every socioeconomic class and race end in miscarriage.

The fact that high rates of infant morbidity and mortality span all economic classes suggests that elements other than poverty are to blame. Women who are happy to be pregnant are more likely to seek and get medical care before their baby is born (prenatal care). But when our pregnancies are unplanned or unwanted, we often experience mixed feelings and denial—both of which can cause a delay in seeking appropriate medical care for ourselves and the developing child.

NBWHP POLICY STATEMENT: UNIVERSAL PRENATAL CARE IS ESSENTIAL

It is a simple formula: Healthy mothers have healthy babies. Prenatal care truly begins with the health of the mother when she is a child. NBWHP supports lifelong access to adequate medical care, decent housing, and educational opportunities, as well as efforts to promote good nutrition and exercise and opportunities to develop healthy behaviors.

NBWHP opposes mandatory drug testing of pregnant women. Such testing is not an appropriate component of maternal care. However, voluntary drug screening, when accompanied by appropriate counseling and referral to professional treatment, is critical for the health of mother and infant. For women who are willing to seek treatment, there must be adequate access to treatment programs and facilities for pregnant women and women with children.

CHILDBIRTH

HISTORICAL EXPERIENCE: "VOLUNTARY MOTHERHOOD" PROMOTED

Black people have always recognized the value of spaced and well-timed births as a way to reduce high maternal and infant mortality rates and strengthen family life. At the turn of the century, Black women were controlling their own fertility, chiefly by marrying late, having fewer children, and using contraception and abortion. The Black women's club movement had emerged as a dominant force in promoting new social and family values among African-American women. The clubs supported "voluntary motherhood" and shared information about contraceptives.

Historically, babies in this country were delivered at home. The vast majority of babies born in the United States were delivered by midwives during home births. The "granny" midwife was a respected figure in the Black community, especially in rural Southern states where she was the only person who could help mothers—Black and white—to deliver their babies. Grannies would often stay for several days with a mother, helping to care for other children and the house until the mother regained her strength. Many Grannies were illiterate; their traditions and knowledge of herbal remedies and medi cines were shared and passed along to the next generation through oral stories and apprenticeships. However, by the middle of this century, doctors succeeded in taking control of childbirth by banning midwives and prohibiting women from attending medical school.

CONTEMPORARY CONTEXT: BIRTHS TO OLDER WOMEN INCREASE, TEEN PREGNANCIES DECLINE

Between 1980 and 1994, the birth rates for all women remained fairly stable, at an average of 21 per 1,000 for Black women, and 15 per 1,000 white women. However, increasing numbers of Black women are choosing to give birth at later ages. The number of births for African-American women ages 30–44 increased from 1980 to 1996, while births to African-American women ages 29 and younger decreased. The percentage of intended births increases with the age of the mother. In 1995, only 23.4 percent of births to Black women under 20 were intended, compared to 51.8 percent for women ages 20–29, and 70.2 percent for women ages 30–44.

Teenage pregnancy rates—although declining during the 1990s—still remain high, especially for young Black women. Half a million adolescents give birth each year. In 1996, births among girls aged 15 through 17 were more than twice as likely among African-American teenage girls and white teenage girls. Birth rates among African-American girls younger than 15 were 4.5 times higher than for white girls.

Among Black teenagers, 75 percent of pregnancies are "unwanted" or "mistimed." This is a major concern because of the potential social and economic consequences as well as the health effects. Indirectly, patterns of poverty and low educational attainment often become solidified as a result of early childbearing.

NBWHP POLICY STATEMENT: WOMEN HAVE THE RIGHT TO GIVE BIRTH

NBWHP supports the availability of wide options for childbirth, as well as the education of women about these options in advance. In some areas, women have a choice of settings for delivery, ranging from hospital operating rooms or birthing centers to their own homes. Many women are asking nurse-midwives to help them prepare for childbirth and to assist during labor and delivery. Some women prepare for natural childbirth by taking birthing classes where they learn breathing and relaxation exercises; at the time of delivery, some women choose to have little or no pain medication. Others opt for a stronger pain reliever. Pregnant women have a right to participated in the decision about where and how they will have their babies.

In the United States, one in four babies is delivered by cesarean section. It is the most frequently performed major surgical procedure among reproductive-age women. There are several medical conditions that lead to c-sections; however, nonmedical factors also influence the decision. Women who have private medical insurance, who are patients at private (rather than public) clinics, and who are married, older, and/or in a higher socioeconomic bracket are more likely to have c-sections. Nonmedical reasons include the avoidance of pain, convenience, financial incentives for providers (c-sections cost nearly twice as much as vaginal births), and fear of being sued for delivering an infant with a poor outcome after prolonged labor.

A c-section is major surgery and can result in infections, hemorrhage, injury to other organs, and other physical and psychological complications. The maternal mortality rate for c-sections is two to four times greater than that for vaginal deliveries. C-sections not necessitated by medical reasons increase the risk to the infant of premature birth and breathing problems. C-sections can also interfere with breast-feeding and the establishment of the mother-child bond. For all of there reasons, NBWHP opposes the use of c-sections for nonmedical purposes.

NBWHP also opposes efforts to limit reproductive choice, such as recently passed welfare reform legislation that includes "child exclusion" provisions to discourage women receiving welfare from having children. Instead of providing the necessary services, job-training opportunities, education, child support enforcement, and transitional benefits to poor families, the "child exclusion" provisions deny increases in benefits that are needed to raise an additional child. This punishes welfare recipients for choosing childbirth. Ironically, Medicaid covers pregnancy, childbirth, and sterilization but does not provide funds for abortion.

Not only are fertility rates of welfare recipients lower than those of the general population, but the longer a woman remains on welfare, the less likely she is to give birth. Furthermore, the great majority of pregnancies among women on welfare are unintended.

There is no evidence to support the assumption that poor people's child-bearing decisions are motivated by minimal grant increases or incentives. There is evidence, however, that teens are more likely to have children when other life options—such as education and jobs—are unavailable.

As the discussion of welfare reform inevitably turns to "individual responsibility," NBWHP insists that the federal, state, and local governments also act "responsibly" and be held accountable for their failures in providing the economic and social conditions that allow all citizens to have a decent standard of living.

CONTRACEPTION AND DISEASE PREVENTION

HISTORICAL EXPERIENCE: SUPPORT OF BIRTH CONTROL, DISTRUST OF MEDICAL COMMUNITY

By the end of the nineteenth century, Black fertility rates had plummeted by one-third. This was often blamed on racial discrimination, inadequate wages, poor nutrition, substandard housing, and lack of medical care for most African

Americans. While these circumstances did in fact exist, ample evidence also indicates that many African Americans were using "folk" contraceptives and abortion.

The fledgling birth control movement of the early twentieth century drew initial interest and support among Black women and men. As Margaret Sanger's birth control movement grew, many Black women insisted on expanding birth control services in their communities; they were enthusiastic users of the few clinics across the country that were available to them. Because most clinics were operated by whites, some Blacks were suspicious that birth control would be used for genocide or that Blacks would be subject to reproductive medical experiments. Despite such opposition and fear, Black women generally supported family planning and organized to promote it in their communities throughout the first half of the twentieth century.

As part of the 1960s "war on poverty," the federal government began to establish family planning clinics in predominantly Black urban areas. Black nationalists (mostly men) attacked these programs as genocide-suicide—but Black women once more affirmed their right to make their own reproductive choices and resisted efforts to shut down these clinics.

The most notable historical event with regard to African Americans and sexually transmitted diseases is the notorious Tuskegee study. In 1972, the U.S. Public Health Service admitted that for the prior 40 years, it had been studying the course of untreated latent syphilis in hundreds of poor Black sharecroppers in Tuskegee, Alabama. The physicians conducting the study deceived the men about their condition and deliberately withheld effective treatment for the disease, even after penicillin became available.

Published medical reports estimate that 28 out of 100 men died as a result of their syphilis. The wives and families of these men also were affected. Studies later showed that 27 of 50 wives tested positive for syphilis. As a consequence of the research study in Tuskegee, many African Americans continue to distrust the medical and public health authorities.

CONTEMPORARY CONTEXT: UNINTENDED PREGNANCIES, STDS, AND HIV/AIDS AFFECT BLACK WOMEN DISPROPORTIONATELY

High rates of unintended pregnancy, abortion, and teenage childbearing among Black women speak to the great need for better access to and use of effective contraceptives. In addition, with skyrocketing rates of HIV/AIDS and other infections, it is urgent that Black women protect themselves from unwanted pregnancy and *sexually transmitted diseases* (STDs) at the same time.

In 1996, African Americans accounted for 78 percent of all reported cases of *gonorrhea*. African-American teenagers aged 15–19 have infection rates that are 24 times higher than whites. Among young Black adults aged 20–24, the rate is 30 times higher than whites.

The highest rates of *chlamydia* infection are found in individuals aged 15–19 and 20–24 for all racial and ethnic groups. Blacks are infected at much higher rates than whites.

Up to 20–30 percent of sexually active Americans of all races are thought to be infected with *human papillomavirus* (HPV), which causes genital warts.

It is estimated that 45–60 million Americans are infected with *herpes genitalis.* About 80 percent of African-American women and 60 percent of African-American men will be infected with herpes at some time in their lives.

Rates of *syphilis* infection are 62 percent higher for African Americans than whites. Between 1985–1990, this disease increased by 230 percent among African-American women.

In 1995, 10.6 percent of all Black women were treated for *pelvic inflammatory disease (PID)*, compared to 7.2 percent of white women.

The fastest-growing group of persons infected by HIV—the virus that causes AIDS (*acquired immune deficiency syndrome*)—are heterosexual women. In 1996, African-American women comprised 56 percent of AIDS cases among women in the United States. In the majority of cases, they were infected as adolescents or young girls.

Women are at greater risk than men of contracting sexually transmitted diseases and HIV/AIDS because of our anatomical differences. The risks are even higher for adolescent women due to age-related physiological changes in the cervix. Lesbian and bisexual women are also at risk of spreading STDs and HIV/AIDS through the exchange of bodily fluids.

STDs are more difficult to diagnose and less likely to be treated in women. If undiagnosed and untreated, STDs can do great long-term damage to a woman's health, causing premature delivery, stillbirth, infertility, and genital cancers. The presence of an STD—whether it has open, visible sores or is invisible and asymptomatic—will increase a woman's risk of contracting HIV/AIDS.

A wide range of contraceptive methods are available that can greatly reduce the risk of pregnancy; however, few also protect against STDs.

Barrier methods — including the *male condom, female condom, diaphragm,* and *cervical cap*—prevent sperm from reaching the egg and protect against STDs. Used correctly, latex male condoms (not those made from animal tissue) offer the best protection against STDs and HIV/AIDS and are most effective when used with a spermicide containing nonoxynol-9. Unfortunately, spermicides may irritate the vaginal lining of some sensitive women, making them more susceptible to HIV/AIDS infection through the broken skin.

Hormonal contraceptives—including the *pill, intrauterine device (IUD)*, *Depo-Provera* ("the shot"), and *Norplant*—are an effective way to prevent pregnancy. However, they may not be appropriate for women with certain health conditions, such as high blood pressure or a history of cancer or diabetes—and they do not protect against STDs or HIV/AIDS.

"Emergency" contraception (ECP, or the "morning-after pill") is used in the event of unprotected sex, contraceptive failure, rape, or incest. The Food and Drug Administration (FDA) has approved a product for emergency contraception called Preven. The Preven contraceptive kit is currently available by prescription from doctors and other health care professionals.

The only 100 percent guarantee a women has against unwanted pregnancy and STDs is celibacy (no sexual activity), a practice often encouraged by religious groups for unmarried people.

NBWHP POLICY STATEMENT: CHOOSE BIRTH CONTROL,
DISEASE PREVENTION, AND HEALTH CARE

NBWHP supports universal access to health care and family planning services for all women. Black women should insist on full and accurate information from their health care providers about all contraceptive options, including side effects, health risks and benefits, costs to obtain the method, procedures, and costs necessary to have a method removed.

Much attention has recently been placed on new hormonal contraceptive technologies that provide long-term protection from pregnancy without the need to "think about it." It has been argued that these methods are "liberating" for women. NBWHP believes that if ever there was a time for women to think carefully about sexual activity, it is now. Women need to own the fact that sexuality is a natural and normal part of adult life. We need to think carefully—and ahead of time—about whether and when we will engage in sex and how we will prevent unwanted pregnancies and the spread of infections. All women must become comfortable with their bodies and their sexuality so that we can take control of our decision making around the issues of sexual health and reproduction.

NBWHP believes that barrier methods—used properly and every time—should be considered as the first choice for contraception as well as disease prevention. Barrier methods can be integrated into sexual foreplay, and the rewards include increased intimacy with one's sex partner and greater comfort and familiarity with one's own body and sexuality. Family planning programs and health care providers must invest necessary time and resources to ensure that women are encouraged to use barrier methods to reduce their risk of STDs and HIV/AIDS.

Sexually active African-American women of all ages—whether heterosexual, bisexual, or lesbian—need a strong foundation of accurate information as well as support for practicing safer sex if we are going to win the battle against HIV/AIDS and STDs. NBWHP supports HIV/AIDS education and STD prevention programs as the best weapons against the continuing spread of STDs and HIV/AIDS throughout all segments of the population.

NBWHP is also a strong advocate of efforts to ensure that AIDS diagnosis and treatment services are available for early HIV detection within geographic and fiscal reach of at-risk populations such as low-income women and their families, rural dwellers, and the homeless. Outpatient care must entitle patients to receive services appropriate to their needs; including mental health care, housing assistance, and family services—as well as clinical and hospice care.

Early detection and medical intervention are now providing many HIV-infected women a greater life expectancy. Unfortunately, women and adolescent girls infected with HIV receive fewer medical services, such as medication, hospital admissions, and outpatient visits, than similarly diagnosed men. An asymptomatic, HIV-infected female is 20 percent less likely to receive azidothymidine (AZT) than an asymptomatic, HIV-infected male. A female with AIDS is also 20 percent less likely than a male injection drug user to be hospitalized for AIDS-related conditions.

Statistics demonstrate that African Americans do not receive enough early, routine, and preventative health care. Hospital emergency rooms and clinics are a much more common source of medical care for African Americans than for whites, and 20 percent of African Americans (compared to 13 percent of whites) report no usual source of medical care. NBWHP calls for improvements in the health care delivery system to ensure that women of color have access to quality, affordable preventative services, early detection and treatment, and appropriate follow-up care and counseling.

There is currently a debate about making the pill—which is now a prescription drug—available as an over-the-counter drug. NBWHP supports keeping oral contraceptives as prescription drugs because the annual health care visit for birth control pills is the only time many Black women have access to medical services. Furthermore, the side effects of nausea, weight gain, and depression may cause a woman on the pill to need more frequent checkups. Black women have high rates of obesity, diabetes, and high blood pressure and therefore require adequate screening before using the pill. NBWHP is not confident that pharmacists are sufficiently trained to screen customers who would buy the pill over the counter. In addition, pharmacists may not have the time to thoroughly counsel customers.

A seminal issue for the reproductive health and rights of African-American women has been the marketing of long-acting contraceptives. Norplant and Depo-Provera function as short-term or temporary sterilizations, and their potential for abuse was quickly realized. Prior to its approval for use as a contraceptive (in addition to its use as cancer therapy), Depo-Provera had been regularly administered as birth control to women in developing countries, and to Southern Black and Native American women in clinical trials.

In 1982, the National Women's Health Network and its new program, the Black Women's Health Project, announced a class action suit against the Upjohn Pharmaceutical Company. The media focused on the use of the drug at Grady Hospital in Atlanta, where women were not fully informed of the adverse effects of the drug. While the use of Depo-Provera caused many problems, the suit was dropped because the drug did not cause any deaths.

NBWHP and other advocacy groups still oppose the use of Depo-Provera due to the possible increased risk of breast cancer in women under age 35. This may be especially dangerous for Black women, who are more likely to develop this cancer at younger ages. Weight gain of up to 20–70 pounds is not unusual, and this poses a threat to the health of many Black women—50 percent of whom are already overweight and may suffer from diabetes or hypertension. Loss of bone density is another serious risk, especially to adolescent girls whose bones are still growing, and to women who may be susceptible to osteoporosis. Depression is a side effect with a greater negative impact on the health of poor and Black women, many of whom have high levels of psychological stress in their daily lives due to racism, sexism, and economic struggles.

NBWHP also opposes any "incentives" for poor women and women of color to use Norplant or any other long-acting contraceptive, as well as any efforts to restrict choice among forms of contraception. In 1990, Norplant was on the market for just one month when judges began to order it inserted in women. An editorial in a major newspaper suggested that welfare recipients should be given financial incentives to take the drug and reduce their childbearing. Black activists were outraged that legislators would propose laws that would effectively sterilize women for years, simply because they were poor. Furthermore, there was mounting evidence that women having trouble with the drug's side effects were having difficulty obtaining necessary medical assistance to remove the capsules from their arms.

NBWHP supports efforts to develop female-controlled barrier methods of prevention, such as an inexpensive microbicide or virucide. Microbicides and virucides are chemical compounds that women could put in their vaginas before intercourse to block HIV. A women could protect herself against STDs and HIV/AIDS without having to negotiate condom use with her partner. Ideally, microbicides would be made with and without spermicides so that women who want to get pregnant could do so without worrying about contracting a disease.

Scientists are also pursuing several other options, including hormone-releasing vaginal rings that would be placed in the vagina for several weeks or months, skin patches, and vaccines/anti-fertility drugs that generate a temporary immune system reaction against eggs or sperm. Researchers are examining two options for a "male contraceptive," an implant and a vaccine.

The single most urgent concern of all health advocates regarding vaccines is how to prevent their abuse, on both individual and mass scales. An agent that could be secretly combined with other vaccinations or injections, or added to food and water supplies, poses a chilling threat to reproductive rights of women around the world. NBWHP urges the public, press, and legislators to demand answers to critical questions surrounding how these drugs will be used in studies and then used with the public.

STERILIZATION

HISTORICAL EXPERIENCE: STERILIZATION WITHOUT CONSENT

At the turn of the twentieth century, the so-called science of eugenics emerged, teaching that intelligence and other traits were "genetically determined" and if society were to improve, control over reproduction must be exercised. Proponents of eugenics played to White race suicide fears by encouraging "positive eugenics" (more births by White women) and the practice of "negative eugenics" (preventing births by "inferior" people). Compulsory sterilization was advocated by eugenicists to eliminate the "socially inadequate" members of society: the mentally retarded; the mentally ill, epileptics, criminals, prostitutes, and the poor.

Between 1907–1913, a dozen states passed involuntary sterilization laws, but constitutional challenges kept them on hold. However, in 1927, the U.S. Supreme Court upheld the sterilization of a "feeble-minded" White girl in Virginia, and the floodgates opened. In short order, 30 states enacted compulsory sterilization laws. State governments initially focused on sterilizing institutionalized young women who were deemed unfit to be mothers. Women who were deemed promiscuous or who had children out of wedlock were often declared "feeble-minded" and institutionalized simply to be sterilized. The economic crisis in the 1930s prompted sterilization proponents to turn their attention to poor Southern Blacks. As the Depression deepened, whites were concerned that a larger number of Black children would require more public funding.

When Nazi atrocities and their systematic destruction of "undesirable" people came to light in the 1940s, eugenics was discredited as a science, and mandatory sterilization laws were repealed. But the "population bomb" theory of the 1950s triggered racist fears of Black and Brown people overwhelming the White world. White fears were particularly sparked by images of a growing "welfare class" in U.S. cities.

By World War II, more sterilizations were being performed on institutionalized Blacks than whites. In 1973, a legal case involving two teenaged sisters uncovered the widespread practice of government-funded sterilization of women without their knowledge or consent. The case of the Relf sisters revealed the fact that 100,000 to 150,000 poor women—one-half of them Black—were being sterilized each year under the auspices of the U.S. Department of Health, Education, and Welfare.

The scope of the abuse was terrifying. Women of color with no choice among health care providers often had to submit to "voluntary" sterilization to have their babies delivered. Many women were sterilized without their knowledge or permission: they would undergo gynecological procedures only to later discover that they had been sterilized. This was so widespread in the South that these operations came to be known as "Mississippi appendectomies." Physicians routinely performed more complicated surgical hysterectomies rather than simpler tubal ligations because their reimbursement fee was higher, and teaching hospitals permitted unnecessary hysterectomies as "practice" for their medical residents.

CONTEMPORARY CONTEXT: VOLUNTARY STERILIZATION IS AN OPTION, INVOLUNTARY STERILIZATION REMAINS A PROBLEM

Current research suggests that women, by and large, desire to control their family size. Most low-income Black women want and have a small number of children, and spend most of their reproductive lives trying to avoid pregnancy. Although Black women do outweigh their white counterparts in rates of unintended pregnancy, Black women with higher educational and income levels have fewer children. Overall birth trends in the United States exemplify this, with family sizes decreasing from an average of six children in the 1960s to approximately three in 1995.

Sterilization as a means of contraception can be the right choice for individuals who are certain that they do not wish to have any (or any more) children. Today, women are usually sterilized by open (mini-laparotomy) tubal ligation or laparoscopic tubal cauterization, or clip placement. These are operations in which the fallopian tubes are cut, blocked, or clipped to prevent the egg from joining the sperm. Men are sterilized by vasectomy, an operation in which the vas deferens (the tubes that carry sperm) are cut or blocked.

For women over the age of 30, voluntary sterilization via tubal ligation is more commonly used than any other method of birth control. There is usually a high one-time cost for tubal ligation or vasectomy, and these operations are considered permanent, although reversal is sometimes possible. When one partner is sterilized, there is a rate of 99 percent effectiveness in preventing pregnancy. However, *sterilization does not protect against STDs and HIV/AIDS.*

Involuntary sterilization, primarily via hysterectomy to treat gynecological problems, remains a problem today. Hysterectomy—the removal of the uterus—is the second most frequently performed major surgical procedure among reproductive-age women. More than one-fourth of women in the United States will undergo a hysterectomy before their sixtieth birthday. The Centers for Disease Control and Prevention (CDC) report that the number of hysterectomies has stabilized at 600,000 per year with no difference in the rate of hysterectomies based on race.

Although most hysterectomies involve the removal of only the uterus and the cervix, there has been an increase in hysterectomies in which the ovaries are also removed. Surgical removal of the ovaries can result in a need for hormonal treatment for some women.

The most frequent reason for Black women having hysterectomies is fibroid tumors, a condition that disproportionately affects African-American women. However, treatments that provide alternatives to hysterectomies have always been available to certain women. These include laser and other ablative therapies, surgical excision (myomectomy), and medications that, at least, temporarily shrink fibroid tumors.

NBWHP POLICY STATEMENT: BALANCE ISSUES OF ACCESS WITH SAFEGUARDS AGAINST ABUSE

The historical use of involuntary sterilization reflects a societal misconception that Black women have too many children, and this is the cause of our social problems. This belief disregards issues of equity with respect to education and employment, and essentially overshadows the political, social, and economic issues that impact women's quality of life. These ideas are actually contrary to the beliefs that women hold about their won reproductive goals.

NBWHP believes that reproductive freedom is a right of all women regardless of race or socioeconomic status. Current data illustrates that when knowledge and access are increased, women can and do make reproductive decisions that will ultimately have a positive impact on their sexual status. NBWHP supports all voluntary and informed decisions about sterilization. Further, these decisions must be made without coercion. The focus of intervention should not be dictated by stereotypes and inaccurate beliefs, but rather an acknowledgment and effort to address the disparities in education, health care, and opportunities facing Black women.

Because Black women and other women of color were sterilized against their will or without their knowledge through federally supported programs as recently as 25 years ago, safeguards have been put in place to prevent such abuse. NBWHP believes it is possible to balance safeguards against sterilization abuse with a woman's right to choose sterilization without undue bureau cratic red tape or delays.

Involuntary sterilization presents another set of issues. NBWHP believes that hysterectomy should not be considered as the first and only option for the treatment of fibroids. Only after alternatives have been explored—and it has been determined that this procedure is medically warranted—should a hysterectomy be considered. Black women must be presented with options and opportunities to make educated choices about this and all procedures affecting their reproductive abilities. Through appropriate education and exploration of options, a woman can decide, in conjunction with her physician, which choice is best for her. Always seek a second opinion when a hysterectomy is recommended.

NBWHP also advocates for the continued research on alternatives to hysterectomies in the treatment of gynecological problems. Because there is no universally adopted medical standard for hysterectomy, a vast opportunity is created for non-medical factors such as race, age, religion, and socioeconomic status to become part of the decision-making process. Further research into the appropriateness and impact of this and other treatments as they relate to Black women is needed.

Black women must also become savvy self-advocates when exploring options of care. We need to exercise our patient rights and feel empowered to question and/or challenge the medical community in order to make decisions that are right for us.

ABORTION

HISTORICAL EXPERIENCE: A LONGSTANDING PRACTICE

There is evidence that some Black women refused to bear children as slaves—and therefore used contraceptives and abortion, in addition to outright refusing to be mated or raped. It is impossible to determine what percentage of the recorded instances of miscarriage and stillbirth among slave women were self-induced or the result of harsh living conditions and forced labor. The same is true with recorded cases of infanticide.

When "modern" contraceptives first became available at the turn of the century, African-American women were quick to understand the clear need to have access to contraception: illegal abortion was a major method for controlling fertility by African-American women desperate to limit their childbearing. The high rates of illegal abortion translated into tragically high rates of septic abortion and death.

In the 1950s, the medical establishment began to crack down on illegal abortion providers. African-American women who were underground providers were targeted more often than their white counterparts. As access to these generally safe but illegal providers decreased, more and more Black women suffered the deadly consequences of self-induced abortion.

An "underground railroad" offered women access to illegal abortion providers throughout the 1960s. Groups of women learned how to perform abortions and then offered their services at low cost to poor women of color. Black women played important roles in these efforts across the country.

The 1973 Supreme Court decision to legalize abortion was critically important for all women and widely welcomed by the many Black women who had struggled for this basic right. In 1976, Congress passed the Hyde Amendment which eliminated Medicaid funding of abortions for poor women, the majority of whom are African American. Many Black activists were troubled by the failure of the predominantly white, middle-class abortion rights movement to fight harder to prevent passage of the Hyde Amendment.

CONTEMPORARY CONTEXT: ABORTION RIGHTS THREATENED

Abortion is a highly politicized medical procedure in the United States. In 1998, more restrictions on abortions exist than at any time in the past 25 years. Legislation ranging from parental consent/notification and waiting periods to "informed consent" and "gag rules" has virtually succeeded in limiting poor women and adolescents to either have a child or submit to temporary and/or permanent sterilization. The requirement in some states that a teenager obtain the consent and/or notify both parents is a serious impediment to many more African-American teens whose fathers are not available or whose pregnancy is a result of incest.

There is well-organized opposition to women making their own choices about abortion. Opponents' tactics range from fake abortion clinics to "sidewalk counseling" and spreading false information—such as a link between breast cancer and abortion, a claim that has been scientifically debunked. Fanatics have killed health care providers at clinics; even their homes are no longer safe! Many of the targeted clinics are private, nonprofit clinics that provide low-cost services to Black women and adolescents; this threatens young women's access to health care as well as places their lives in jeopardy.

According to estimates based on the National Survey of Family Growth, contraceptive failure is responsible for about half of the 3.5 million unintended pregnancies—approximately 1.7 million. Many women become pregnant even while using contraception because no method is 100 percent effective. Additionally, some women have limited power in negotiations with their partners about whether and when to have children or about the use of a specific contraceptive method.

When faced with an unintended pregnancy, the ratio of Black women who choose abortion is about equal to that of white women. However, Black women experience unintended pregnancies 2.5 times more often than white women, so we are twice as likely to have abortions.

Having an abortion is oftentimes a painful choice for women, but it may be the right choice at the particular time. Many women struggle with the decision to have an abortion and see it only as a last resort. Too often, they delay their decisions and thus require abortions later in their pregnancies.

Currently, there are two forms of abortion: *surgical* and *medical.*

The majority of *surgical abortions* are performed in the first trimester (three months of pregnancy). Early surgical abortion is a low-risk and relatively simple procedure. Surgical abortions in the second trimester are more complex and require two days.

Late-term abortions (24–26 weeks) are complicated surgical procedures usually requiring general anesthesia. Most late-term abortions are performed to save the life or health of the mother, but they are subject to intense legal controversy. Opponents of the procedure have been succeeding in their attempts to limit or ban the procedure.

Medical abortion is a two-step procedure in which a woman takes one drug and then returns two days later to take another drug, which brings on uterine contractions. This regimen must be undertaken within the first seven weeks of pregnancy to be effective. Two drugs currently being used for medical abortions are mifepristone (the abortion pill RU486) and methotrexate.

The advantages of medical abortion include the privacy of taking the drugs in one's own home and lower risks of infection or damage. Some women have said that they feel "in charge" of the medical abortion process, but women should be forewarned that heavy bleeding and cramping—similar to that experienced with a miscarriage—will occur.

NBWHP POLICY STATEMENT: KEEP ABORTION SAFE AND LEGAL

NBWHP unequivocally supports:

➤ The right of all women—regardless of age, income, or education—to make their own decisions regarding whether, when, and under what conditions she will bear children. We firmly believe that each woman, in consultation with her health care provider, is capable of deciding whether or not to carry a pregnancy to term.

➤ Access to complete information and safe, legal, and accessible abortion services for all women, including young and poor women. We encourage young women to consult with parents or other responsible adults in making this decision.

➤ Mandatory requirements that all medical school curricula include surgical abortion procedure training.

➤ The speedy regulation and release process of drugs for medical abortion, and increased training of health care professionals in their use.

➤ Demand for research to determine what, if any, specific side effects there are for Black women undergoing medical abortion.

NBWHP opposes:

➤ Mandatory parental consent or notification laws and regulations.

➤ Restrictive or prohibitive laws or regulations that limit access to abortion services or information, such as the Hyde Amendment and child exclusion policies.

➤ Policies that limit or ban certain medical procedures determined necessary by health professionals. We believe that every woman in consultation with her health care provider, can determine which abortion procedure is best for her.

DISEASES AND CONDITIONS OF THE REPRODUCTIVE SYSTEM

HISTORICAL EXPERIENCE

Historically, tension has existed between the medical community and the African-American community. One hundred years before Nazi atrocities led to the adoption of ethical guidelines for human medical experimentation, Black women were used as medical subjects in studies of reproductive health. Surgical techniques in gynecology were developed in the nineteenth century through countless operations performed without anesthesia on Black women purchased expressly for these experiments.

Based on these and other violations of trust by the medical community, many African Americans remain apprehensive about professional medical care. This problem is particularly disturbing because Black women continue to face conditions that result in poor health and increase the need for competent medical care.

CONTEMPORARY CONTEXT: AFRICAN-AMERICAN WOMEN AT GREATER RISK.

All women face health risks related to their reproductive system, but certain diseases and conditions tend to be either more prevalent or more deadly in the African-American community. These include cancer, fibroids, pelvic inflammatory disease (PID), and infertility.

CANCER is defined by the American Cancer Society as "a group of diseases characterized by uncontrolled growth and spread of abnormal cells." Advanced cancer, the condition in which the disease has spread throughout the body, usually results in death. Cancers of the reproductive organs are a serious health concern for African-American women.

Breast cancer is the leading cause of cancer deaths among African-American women between the ages of 30 and 54. Compared to white women, African-American women have a lower incidence but higher death rate from breast cancer. Detection at an early stage strongly influences the success of treatment. Some health professionals believe that Black women should have a baseline mammogram at age 30 (rather than at age 40) because breast cancer strikes many Black women at earlier ages.

Cancer of the uterus, which includes cervical cancer, is the second largest cause of cancer deaths among African-American women ages 15–34. African-American women are 2.3 times more likely to have cervical cancer than white women. Risk factors for cervical cancer include multiple sexual partners, early age at first intercourse, a history of STDs (particularly the human papillomavirus), and oral contraception use.

Little is known about the causes of ovarian cancer. Age is listed as the highest risk factor especially for women over 60, yet ovarian cancer appears as one of the five leading cancer sites for African-American females ages 35–54. Furthermore, for women with breast cancer, the chance of developing ovarian cancer doubles. Incidence rates for ovarian cancer are slightly lower for African-American women than for white women, but as with breast cancer, our survival rates are also slightly lower.

If detected early enough, there is an almost 100 percent survival rate for all three of these cancers. However, because a disproportionate number of

African-American women live in poverty, have inadequate or no health education, and encounter obstacles to quality health care, most are diagnosed too late to save their lives.

FIBROIDS are benign (noncancerous) tumors that occur in the uterine wall. Fibroids often go undetected because they do not always produce symptoms. More than 50 percent of Black women have fibroids, and fibroids are 3 to 5 times more prevalent among African-American women than white women. Most fibroids are small and harmless. However, if fibroids grow unchecked, health problems may result, including heavy or prolonged menstrual bleeding, abdominal bloating, lower-back pain, fatigue due to iron deficiency, painful sexual intercourse, difficulty becoming pregnant, and recurrent miscarriage.

There are several treatments for fibroids. Injections of hormone (GnRH) Lupron shrinks fibroids temporarily. Also available in a nasal spray, these medications induce a menopausal state in a woman's body, causing the ovaries to cease hormone (estrogen/progesterone/testosterone) production. Small fibroids can also be removed surgically by burning away with a laser or by being scraped off. For larger tumors, a small incision is made in the abdomen for removal by laser or other medical instruments. Another procedure involves cutting off the estrogen and blood supply to the fibroid, which causes it to wither and die. Women who choose removal of fibroids must be made aware of a 30 to 50 percent recurrence rate when multiple tumors are present (within five years). Hysterectomy—complete removal of uterus—is still the most common treatment for fibroids, but it is often unnecessary.

INFERTILITY affects African Americans at a rate up to 1.5 times higher than for whites. The causes most often cited include untreated sexually transmitted infections (particularly chlamydia and gonorrhea) which cause pelvic inflammatory disease (PID); endometriosis (the growth of intrauterine [endometrial] tissue outside of the uterus); nutritional deficiencies; complications from childbirth and abortion; and environmental and workplace hazards.

NBWHP POLICY STATEMENT: GREATER ACCESS TO HEALTH CARE IS NEEDED

Stronger preventive health care and early detection are important steps to protect our health from cancer. Cancer survival hinges on early detection. The sooner the disease is diagnosed and treatment begun, the higher the chances are that the spread of abnormal cells will be stopped before invading other areas of the body. Therefore, women of color must have access to quality, affordable preventive screening (including regular gynecological checkups, breast exams, Pap smears, and mammograms), education regarding prevention as well as warning signals, and follow-up counseling for all types of cancer. Our efforts at prevention must include knowing the importance of nutrition, exercise, regular stress reduction techniques, and the importance of controlling modifiable habits, such as smoking, alcohol, and/or drug use.

There is evidence that many African-American women do not participate in cancer screening programs because they do not know about them. In one study, nearly 60 percent of women of color stated that their reason for not complying with screening guidelines was a lack of appreciation of the importance of screening. Another reason for the continued higher cancer death rate among African-American women may be a less complete follow-up of positive tests, particularly if they do not have a regular source of care.

NBWHP also supports the development of new tests to detect breast cancer in its early stages. Mammograms are not effective in detecting breast cancer in women under 35 years of age because of denser breast tissue. Only 25 percent of early cases are caught by mammograms in this age group. However, mammography remains a very important tool in breast cancer detection, as improved technology is devised.

NBWHP calls for an end to the barriers faced by African Americans seeking treatment for infertility. These barriers include the high cost of infertility treatment; advertising by infertility treatment centers that feature only white infants and fuel the unspoken assumption that white babies are more highly valued by society; and the continued portrayal of Black women as overly fertile, which generates a lesser sense of urgency for treatment of our infertility. Attention must be focused on improving the basic conditions that contribute to infertility, and on improving access to preventive health care and prompt diagnosis and treatment of STDs. Taking these steps might reduce the infertility rate and allow Black women to achieve greater overall health.

Both private and public health care programs have looked at managed care as a way to improve the quality and control the costs of health care. Although managed-care programs have the potential for providing high-quality health care, they have been largely used as vehicle to control costs among the insured, particularly with federal health programs. Managed-care programs have been widely criticized for limiting patient choice of physicians and for lack of quality assurance mechanisms.

NBWHP believes that comprehensive health care reform is crucial to provide all Americans with equal access to quality health care.

MENOPAUSE

HISTORICAL EXPERIENCE: A TABOO TOPIC

Before the turn of the century, any discussion of menopause was considered taboo. In fact, women whose childbearing years were over were widely looked upon as old and sexually unattractive. Menopause itself was viewed as an unpleasant condition to be dreaded and feared, much like a disease.

These attitudes can be attributed, in part, to the fact that until the early 1900s, most women did not live to see menopause. Due to disease, physical labor, and complications related to childbirth, the average life span for a woman was about 45 years. Those who lived into their 50s were considered elderly.

Fortunately, things are changing. Approximately 40 million female "baby boomers" will reach menopause around the decade of the 1990s. As a result of this demographic trend as well as dramatically increasing life expectancies, menopause has become much more of a topic for study and discussion.

CURRENT CONTEXT: THE MEDICALIZATION OF MENOPAUSE

Menopause is the process in which ovarian hormone levels diminish, signaling the end of a woman's reproductive years and cessation of menstrual periods (or flow). Menopause has three phases: premenopause (active menstruation), perimenopause (noticeable changes), and postmenopause (after periods have ended). A woman will know she has reached menopause when she has completed one year without menstruation. A health care provider can confirm this by measuring hormone levels.

Perimenopause is the 2- to 10-year period before the end of menstrual periods, occurring between the ages of about 35 to 48. During this phase, the length, amount, and frequency of menstrual flow may change. Pregnancy and the spread of sexually transmitted diseases can still occur at this time, so precautions must be taken.

Many women pass through menopause with few discomforting signs. Other women who experience a sharp decline in hormone levels may suffer more discomfort. The most common discomforts associated with menopause are hot flashes, insomnia, mood swings, vaginal dryness leading to painful intercourse, weight gain, forgetfulness, waning libido, and irregular vaginal bleeding.

Heavy periods are common during this time, but often subside as estrogen levels drop. Prolonged menstrual bleeding, especially after periods have begun to diminish, may be a sign of abnormal growths in the uterus or an overgrowth of the uterine lining. These problems may lead to cancer. Thus, regular gynecological checkups are important for early detection and obtaining treatment as early as possible.

There are few scientific data regarding how menopause affects African-American women differently than other women. However, anecdotal information indicates that Black women may view this change of life more positively than white women. Many African-American women see menopause as a natural part of life and look forward to the end of their childbearing years. Those who suffer discomforts may turn to home remedies, natural herbs, vitamins, and spirituality rather than, or in addition to, Western medicine for relief.

As a result of widespread media campaigns by pharmaceutical companies that urge women to combat the signs of menopause and aging, many midlife women utilize hormone replacement therapy (HRT). Premarin (a brand of estrogen) has become one of the largest-selling prescription drugs in the United States. However, this drug is primarily used by middle-class women, while poorer women—including those who need the drug after a hysterectomy—are unable to obtain it.

Any decision about using HRT should be made individually, based on complete and accurate information regarding the risks and benefits. HRT is generally inadvisable for women who have had a stroke or heart attack; have had breast or uterine cancer; suffer from impairment of liver function; have unexplained vaginal bleeding; are pregnant; or face a variety of other health conditions. HRT is known to increase the risk of breast cancer after long-term use; increase the risk of endometrial cancer (if estrogen is used alone); and cause (in some women) nausea, weight gain, breast tenderness, uterine bleeding, fluid retention, and/or depression. However, estrogen may reduce the risk of heart disease and osteoporosis.

NBWHP POLICY STATEMENT: MENOPAUSE SHOULD BE TREATED AS A NATURAL CONDITION

NBWHP opposes the medicalization of menopause. It is not a disease, but a natural stage in a woman's life. Because pharmaceutical companies have promoted the medical treatment of "estrogen deficiency disease," many women have been cut off from seeking the advice and wisdom of elder women who have dealt already with this life transition. Furthermore, the ad campaign has contributed to the problem of some in the medical community mistakenly attributing health concerns reported by midlife women to menopause when the actual cause may be serious conditions such as gallbladder disease, hypertension, or clinical depression.

NBWHP supports the management of any uncomfortable signs of menopause with natural, self-help methods, including a diet rich in fresh fruits and vegetables, soy products, plenty of exercise, and stress-reduction activities. however, when signs are severe or women desire a medical approach, access to appropriate medical treatment of menopause must be available. Furthermore, all African-American women approaching menopause must have access to annual medical exams that include a mammogram, Pap smear, and bone density test.

EMPOWERMENT THROUGH SELF-HELP

NBWHP is firmly committed to the conviction that self-help—on both personal and community levels—is the foundation on which African-American women will shape the future for themselves and their families.

Black women simultaneously face racism, sexism, classism, and heterosexism. This umbrella of oppression affects us in all areas of our lives, even when we believe ourselves to be surviving and thriving. By better understanding the ways in which these interlocking oppressions affect our health status, we can examine our wellness within the broader social/political/economic context that is our reality. In this way, efforts to promote our health are clearly political in nature as we take control of our lives and support each other to do the same.

Through self-help, many of us have been able to achieve personal empowerment and make changes in our lives to make ourselves healthier. However, those of us who promote self-help and practice it daily recognize that such activities alone cannot secure democratic rights and freedom. No one can "self-help" her way to employment, housing, education, or health care when basic access is blocked by the discriminatory practices of employers, lenders, service providers, and governments.

We must make the connection between personal empowerment and community empowerment in order to advocate collectively for the public policy changes necessary to improve the quality of life for Black women, our children, families, and community.

THE PROCESS OF SELF-HELP

Self-help begins when we are willing to confront our reluctance to discuss our sexual and reproductive health issues, and when we commit to breaking the "conspiracy of silence" and to taking good care of ourselves.

Self-help continues when we remember that a woman's sexual and reproductive health cannot be separated from the political, social, and economic context in which she lives.

Self-help is strengthened when we understand that true choice is possible only when women have adequate nutrition, health care, education, employment, and housing—and enjoy full and equal access to economic and political power.

Self-help grows when we challenge discrimination in the form of racism, sexism, or heterosexism—all of which kill African-American women—and when we are willing to face our own classism that divides African-American women into "haves" and "have-nots."

Self-help is rooted in our awareness that if the rights of one women are limited, then the rights of all women are threatened—and a commitment to positive action to ensure that women achieve genuine reproductive health and rights.

SELF-HELP: PERSONAL EMPOWERMENT

The effects of racism and internalized oppression—combined with the effects of poverty and violence—cause much of the stress in our lives and contribute to our poor physical, emotional and economic health. NBWHP urges you to adopt the following self-help activities that lead to good health and personal empowerment.

> ➤ *Take positive steps toward your own good health.* Seek appropriate, competent, thorough medical care on a regular basis. Learn about self-examination, and become familiar and comfortable with your own body.

➤ *Discover what works to lift your spirits and cheer your mind* — music, meditation, talking with friends, bubble baths, reading, yoga, laughing with children—and then nourish yourself everyday in at least one special way.

➤ *Share information.* Ask the women in your life—mother, aunts, grandmothers, sisters, cousins, close family friends—to talk about their sexual and reproductive health experiences. Uncover secrets. Get to know your personal history.

➤ *Learn about principles of sexual responsibility.* Apply them to your own life, and help friends and family to do the same. Have the courage to ask for and receive accurate information about sex and sexuality.

➤ *Protect yourself and others from sexual abuse or exploitation.* Value your ability to control your decision making around sex. Create respectful, mutually satisfying relationships that may or may not include sex.

➤ *Commit to achieving a healthy weight,* to selecting and eating more nutritious foods, and to engaging in regular exercise such as Walking for Wellness, the fitness component of NBWHP's self-help groups that involves sisters walking individually and in groups.

➤ *If you choose to drink alcohol, do so in moderation.* Avoid illegal drugs and do not abuse over-the-counter or prescription medications.

➤ *Do your homework on the women's issues in your community.* Decide to become personally involved in community groups or volunteer organizations.

➤ *Exercise your rights!* Register to vote, and be sure to vote in all elections.

SELF-HELP: COMMUNITY EMPOWERMENT

Once you have started to empower yourself, you can help others to do the same. Whether your community is a small town, an inner-city housing project, or a college campus, there are many opportunities to help African-American women achieve better health for themselves and their families. Wherever people are, you can get involved:

➤ Join the local chapter of NBWHP. If there isn't one, start one!

➤ Encourage all women in your life to schedule medical checkups and any necessary screenings. Offer to accompany them and hold their hands for mammograms or medical appointments. Make this part of birthday gifts: after the appointments, take them to lunch!

➤ Volunteer in reproductive health clinics that serve women of color.

➤ Volunteer in schools. Get involved in the PTA, and work for effective sex education for students from the elementary grades through high school.

➤ Volunteer with church groups that are serving the homeless and hungry.

➤ Sponsor walkathons or other health-promoting events for Black women.

➤ Support nonprofit advocacy organizations working on reproductive health and rights issues with either your money, your time, or both.

➤ Join local civic or social organizations and put reproductive health and rights on their agenda. Volunteer to get speakers.

➤ Encourage your family and friends to register and vote. Help get people to the polls on election day.

➤ Write or call elected officials to express your views on political issues affecting the lives and health of African-American women.

➤ Become familiar and involved with local and state politics on reproductive health and rights issues. Organize voter registration drives, circulate, petitions, sponsor educational forums, and promote reproductive health care services.

➤ Let us know what community self-help actions you are undertaking. And remember, NBWHP is available to help with information and assistance.

Patsy Mink on Health Issues for Asian Women

INTERVIEW BY TANIA KETENJIAN

Congresswoman Patsy Mink (D, Hawaii) currently serves on the Education and Workforce Committee and on the Budget Committee. This interview was conducted in June 1999.

TK: What would you say are some of the most prominent health issues facing Asian women?

PM: The statistics with reference to Asian health are shocking and startling in terms of lack of access to typical health facilities. We have to do a lot more to get our health care system to be more aware of the difficulties of getting health information to Asian women. They're not going for mammograms in many cases until they're very, very terminally ill. They're not accustomed to the typical invasive methodologies of the regular health care system and, as a consequence, they withdraw from it. The system doesn't allow things that are culturally comfortable for the Asian population, for example, acupuncture and herbal medicines are not covered services. The two systems do not come together, but diverge, and the quality of life for Asian communities is therefore greatly diminished. President Clinton recently established the President's Advisory Commission on Asian American Health and other concerns. The National Institutes of Health is supposed to make studies and recommendations and to see how these discrepancies can be resolved. The President and the departments of government recognize that the quality of life for Asian Americans is being severely impacted by the failure of the regular health care system.

Breast cancer rates increase dramatically for Japanese women when they move to the United States. This can be attributed to diet or other circumstances of their changed life, but those statistics are really quite alarming. There is a large incidence of cancer and heart disease among all Asian population categories—male and female—as they move to the United States and become second- and third-generation Americans.

TK: What would you like to see changed or developed in health care for Asian women?

PM: Asian women are not very receptive to the calls that traditionally are made to the rest of the population to have annual mammograms, and Pap tests, and so forth. One study showed that only 18 percent of Vietnamese women have ever had a Pap smear. A random sample of 157 Chinese-American women in California showed that 68 percent did not know what a Pap smear was; they had never heard of it! Hepatitis B is 13 times more common in the Asian population than in other American populations. Native Hawaiian women have the highest incidence of breast cancer of all minority women. This is the population group within our country that is suffering and we need to pay attention. We need to find out what it is that we aren't doing right.

TK: Why do you think this situation exists?

PM: If I knew, I would already have begun to implement the solution. We're trying to figure out what we can do to reach out to this population and get them health care services—whether it's the regular variety or alternative medicine—whatever can bring them up to normal health levels.

TK: In *The Conversation Begins,* you say that the women's movement still focuses on middle-class white women. What do you think can be done to change that?

PM: Very little. I don't think that there are enough minority Asian women who participate, who think it's worthwhile to express themselves on behalf of the minority population. As a result, years go by with people paying no attention to anything other than what the middle-class White population is concerned about. There is even less attention to minority women's issues now than there was 10 or 20 years ago.

PM: I think it's mainly that there's no exposure, there's no sensitivity training, there's no one there to keep poking at the White majority when they make a mistake, or forget a certain population, or gear their message to white populations while leaving out the minorities. The absence of even Black women in these groups is quite astounding, so I don't know how we can get Asian women to participate. It's very tough. When we all started the efforts to organize the National Organization for Women and the Women's Caucus, I tried very hard to bring in Asian communities, but they wouldn't participate. Even in my state of Hawaii, neither organization is in existence. I can't even say that in my own circumstances I've been able to create an awareness of the importance of political participation.

TK: Because of the absence of Black women in health organizations, Byllye Avery founded the National Black Women's Health Project. Are there corresponding Asian groups?

PM: We have a lot of Asian health groups. But that doesn't make up for the absence of attention or insensitivity toward our concerns from groups like NOW and the Women's Caucus. They will acknowledge each other as groups, but that's very different from having the population sitting right there in your executive committee and at your conventions, pounding away about exclusions.

TK: What should be done to increase participation?

PM: I don't know how you can get populations to *want* to participate. Even in our own exclusively Asian groups, there are not large numbers participating. A few people in leadership positions have to speak for the many that are silent.

TK: Would you call yourself one of those people?

PM: Yes.

TK: Would you call yourself an activist?

PM: Of course, always.
TK: And how did you get involved in activism?

PM: I think it's just in my nature to run into a problem and to fix it rather than to simply say, "Well, that's a problem; that's the way things are and always will be." I have a personality that says, "Let's go see if we can fix it."

TK: So that's what activism is?

PM: Yes; that's all it is. It is to believe that things can be better, that you don't have to accept the status quo.

TK: How did you decide to become a lawyer?

PM: Well, that was quite accidental. Actually, I was trying to become a medical doctor, but I couldn't get into medical school because women were excluded. I wrote to a dozen or more medical schools and each wrote back saying, "I'm sorry, but we don't take women." So I was very disenchanted. I got my bachelor's degree and I started working as a clerk out in the private, nonprofit sector. One of the women I ran into who was the director of a program said, "Well, why don't you try for just any professional school; it doesn't have to be medicine; if you have the talent, you can direct your professional education into doing other things." She persuaded me to write an application to law school.

By some great magic, I got into law school the first time I tried without knowing what the study of law really was. I went as an experiment, and I found it fascinating, very engrossing. So I stuck with it for three years, got my law degree, came home, and really felt better equipped to challenge the status quo because I had that fantastic educational background.

TK: What do you feel is lacking in the political sector; what needs more focus regarding women?

PM: More women need to be part of the process. I think we could make much greater headway if more women were active instead of just sort of background participants—making coffee, serving whatever, not engaging in the stream of political ideas and immediate change. We need women to get to the forefront and become part of policy making.

TK: How can that happen?

PM: One by one. One by one.

TK: What issues would you like to work on in the future?

PM: We are working very hard on education right now. We want to find ways to improve education because that is the source of the strength of our country and our ability to keep up with global scientific and technological advances. If our educational prowess falls, we're going to diminish our ability to be competitive; so I think that education is terribly important. While it is important for the individual, it is even more important for the nation as a whole; so that's my number one issue. My number two issue is all the health issues: the ability to maintain Medicare, for instance, to provide enough for families to take care of the medical needs of their elderly and sick. And finally, I am concerned about Social Security and the needs of the Asian population. I would say that those three are at the top of my list.

Byllye Avery

INTERVIEW BY TANIA KETENJIAN

Byllye Avery is the founder of the National Black Women's Health Project. This interview was conducted in April 1999.

TK: How did you come to join the National Women's Health Network?

BA: Back in the 1970s we were all working at the Gainesville Women's Health Center, and I remember they sent a letter around saying they were looking for people to serve on their board. So I joined and applied to be on their board and became a member.

TK: When did you decide that a Black women's health project needed to be started?

BA: The project first became an idea in my head in 1980, when I had been at the network for about five years. Black women were not attending the conferences and programs that the network was putting on. They were all good programs with good information, but there were very few Black women participating. So I became concerned with how we could increase participation of Black women in the organization.

TK: Why do you think the NWHN was so dominated by White middle-class women?

BA: It doesn't really have anything to do with "domination." It's just that those were the women on the board and that was the perspective they were teaching. What you have to understand is the way racism affects us. Unless something speaks specifically to Black women, Asian women, Native American women, if you just say "women," then the assumption is "white women." That's what that was about. It wasn't that people were not interested in having Black women be in the organization, that they weren't trying to reach out. They just were not the ones to do it.

TK: What was your vision for the NWHN? What did you want it to accomplish? What were the many problems Black women were facing at the time?

BA: The way I came to understand the MWHN—which might not be the NWHN's vision of itself—was that I saw it as a place where women of all ethnic groups could come together to work collectively for the health of all women. For instance, maybe the board would have an Asian woman organizing Asian women, a Native American organizing Native American women, so that you'd have representatives of hundreds of thousands of women organizing around ethnicity and health issues. I understood that Black women needed to come together to decide what our health issues were. We could look at health statistics and see what we were dying from, but more important to me was what other things we were living with, and that needed to come from a Black women's perspective. That's what was missing for me in the NWHN—the Black woman's perspective. Later I came to understand that all women down that color line, due to class and other such factors, develop their own perspective about their health. Some of the health problems we identified, once we came together, had to do with psychological well-being—not mental illness, but psychological well-being: What are the things that get in the way of your life every day? A lot of people live in a lot of psychological distress. How will we come together and talk about this? A lot of it comes from painful experiences. Women would talk about being victims of domestic violence, rape, incest—all these things kind of gnaw, they really rob us of our power and keep us from being all of who we are. So back in the early 1980s when women really started coming together, we declared that violence was the number one health issue for Black women, just before the CDC and all the rest of them determined that violence was a health issue. Once you got this psychological stuff straight, and got the message that you are a good and whole person just because you were born, then you could start to deal with some of the other issues. Cardiovascular diseases, heart problems, hypertension, cancer, diabetes are all things people are living with, but sometimes they really can't get to them until they become chronic.

TK: The pamphlet *Our Voices, Our Choices* talks about the reproductive and sexual diseases that Black women were facing then and are still facing relative to white women.

BA: Yes, women still have trouble getting prenatal care. Lack of access can mean many things. It could be the bad clinic in my neighborhood or my head telling me not to go in and get the care. A lot of women aren't getting prenatal care early enough. Many are denying their pregnancies because of their situations. In this country we have such a high level of technologically advanced health care systems, but there are very basic things that don't get to all of the people. See, I think they're using the wrong yardstick. We say our health care system is special because we have all these technological advances, but if you can't get them to the people, you really don't have them as far as I'm concerned. There are 47 million people right now without health insurance, and health insurance is your entree. A lot of people get left out of a lot of preventive services, so they get things that could be avoided. Then you see Black women not having preventive care, not having an attitude that every year you need to get your breasts examined, get a mammogram, get a Pap smear, that there are certain routine things that you need to do every single year. And people go for years without doing these things even when they are available. To me that's one of the greatest factors that leads to us having a disproportionate amount of disease. So we work on the access and on the mind: certainly you are worthy of these things, certainly you are good enough for them, certainly you deserve to have them. Most of what we're trying to do is educate women about health.

Overall health means psychological well-being as well as physical and spiritual well-being, and it's the combination of these three that make a whole and healthy being. We're not telling women, "You should weigh 125 pounds," and laying that guilt trip on, because Black women don't have those self-esteem issues around weight. As a matter of fact, it's pretty much the opposite in the Black community, so that strategy doesn't work. We don't have great numbers of women feeling guilty that they wear a size 10. So we try to stress to people to think more about their health problems: What's your blood pressure? What's your cholesterol count? How are your indicators that you're a healthy person?

TK: The other point you're making, if I understand you correctly, is that self-worth is the major issue, because if you feel like you deserve it, you'll make yourself go. How much has the past affected women's feelings about themselves today?

BA: We all come with our history, and it takes a long time to get rid of it, but you have to always examine the history so as to know what's happened. Then you know how to think about things. We can't be too trusting, we must get information ourselves. I know people are tired of hearing about slavery and they're tired of hearing about the Holocaust, but these were horrendous things that happened to people. They not only scarred that generation, they scarred generations to come because they became a part of people's inherent past. The history of slavery told you that you were nothing but a workhorse, from the moment you opened your eyes until, for many people, the moment you died. These things take a long time to overcome. They become ingrained and are passed on as part of our social differences, and different ethnic groups act upon them, so they don't just go away. Then you see bits of them being repeated, such as sterilizations done on poor women and retarded women and women of color. And the sterilization abuse of Puerto Rican women. The history of what we do to each other, the legacy that comes from those actions, lasts many years, for many generations.

TK: What are some of the techniques or skills or attitudes that the National Black Women's Health Project tries to infuse in its members?

BA: We have what we call self-help, which is akin to the consciousness-raising that white women did. Through these self-help groups, we bring the women together to talk about the realities of their lives, to do the analysis, to share, because mostly when you hear the story of someone else's life, you sort of relive your own life and you come to understand why you made decisions or why other people made decisions. You get to claim what was yours and understand the process of discarding that which is not yours. You learn how to discard the pain from the internalized oppression and how to move these oppressive elements out of the midst of your life. We bring women together to sit in a circle to talk openly about their lives and what's going on with them. Through that talking and self-examination, people are able to then make decisions about where they want to go with their lives and get direction and support while they do it. That's the crux of our whole work. People come to understand that no matter what the problem is, somebody else has had that problem and has solved it before them.

TK: What are the main problems a Black woman faces now when she's going out to seek health care as compared to a white woman?

BA: First she has to have the resources—not only the financial resources, she has to have insurance. Only about 38 percent of people have really good coverage or have access to discretionary funds that can pay for things their insurance won't pay for. Then there's a bunch of us who use HMOs, who don't necessarily get doctors we want to see or have to wait a long time. The Black woman's plight is being part of those who are excluded, which means people on Medicaid and all the uninsured and the working poor. They absolutely don't get the best care, they get whatever they can get. So a woman with breast cancer, for instance, needs an advocate with her, someone to help her navigate the system. I have a friend who got breast cancer, and—as much as we all know—it took every single little thing we had to make sure she actually got the three or four opinions, and when they didn't make sense, to find out where else to go to get information. It's very difficult to navigate the system. So you get Ms. Jones who goes right to the clinic, she does whatever the doctor says, and things don't necessarily get better. But she plugs along with it, considering it her lot in life. Whereas if a white woman doesn't like the care, she's got means, so she goes to somebody else and then somebody else until she gets someone who makes sense and who can give her a level of care that she knows she needs to have.

TK: How do doctors affect the process of childbirth for women now and before?

BA: Sometimes they make decisions—not based on information and certainly not based on consultation with their clients—about what treatment people should get, and these decisions are forced on women. Unempowered patients are very accepting, for there are just so many other difficulties in their lives. Take a pregnant woman who's among the "working poor." She works on a line in a factory where there might not be any health insurance. She knows she needs to go in for care, but she doesn't have the ability to take off half a day to go to a doctor appointment. If she leaves for half a day she might lose her job, 'cause there's somebody waiting to take it over, and missing half a day definitely means she'll miss the money from the job. So that's one way women are discriminated against right from the beginning around childbirthing. The women get blamed for not being compliant, not coming in for care, but nobody is looking at the reasons behind that. If doctors had night hours, if employers were required to give pregnant women paid time off to get health care and prenatal care, if we valued our women and our children—there are many ways, with the new laws, to make sure women get what they need. Those are just the simple ways.

TK: What are some of the most prominent health issues facing Black women today?

BA: High blood pressure and cardiovascular disease. A lot of Black women have heart problems. Something like 42 or 43 percent of women over 40 have hypertension. When I'm speaking to audiences and I ask how many people have breast cancer, I might get a few hands. When I ask how many people have problems with their heart, I get so many hands, all the time. Diabetes is another problem. A lot of this stems from being hypertensive, and that has a lot to do with weight and with inactivity. You know how difficult it is to keep yourself active. People have the attitude that they don't have time to go to the gym, they look at it as playing or leisure. Our whole mindset is: that's what you do when you play basketball or football. Breast cancer is maybe third or fourth on the list, even though most women don't die from breast cancer; they die from cardiovascular diseases. Another issue, for a lot of women, is lack of access to abortions. These are women who feel disempowered, who are left out, who are on Medicare and can't have their abortions paid for and are forced to have children that they can't really afford.

TK: So you wouldn't put sexually transmitted diseases up there?

BA: I would put sexual *activity* there. A lot of women are having problems with AIDS, HIV, STDs. Unprotected sex is an issue and leads to a lot of diseases.

TK: Do you think the problem is lack of information or resources to get protection?

BA: I think it's both, but it's also not having a way to present this issue to the man. A lot of women out there are desperate to have men in their lives, desperate to be held, desperate for male companionship, so they'll risk almost anything to have that, and this is the basis for many other problems.

TK: What role have men played in the movement and the project?

BA: They didn't have a presence because we didn't allow them to, but there were men who supported our work all the way from the beginning. Men supported their wives, who came to our meetings—a lot of the women wouldn't have been able to just take off from home and leave their children unless someone was supportive at home. And most of the women, once they found they could see, didn't stop seeing. They took the work home and were able to convince the men in their lives to start to make changes.

TK: What changes have you seen since 1981 when the project started?

BA: Oh, lots! Black women have just absolutely blossomed in the nineties. We first changed our attitude about ourselves, which is probably the most important, how we see ourselves. We see ourselves very differently in the world and a lot of things came together to make that happen. Then we changed our attitude toward each other and once we started doing that, we could start being in the world in a very different way, and being more accepting of our peers in a different way. What I mean is that they're accepting our questioning, forging new horizons, doing different things, being all of who we want to be. A lot of barriers have been removed.

Helen Rodriguez-Trias

INTERVIEW BY TANIA KETENJIAN

Helen Rodriguez-Trias, M.D. was a board member of the National Women's Health Network and was the first Latina president of the American Public Health Association in 1993. This interview was conducted in June 1999.

TK: What are the most serious and prevalent health problems facing Latina women today?

HRT: Latinas, like African-American women and all ethnic groups we tend to lump together are very diverse. Here in California there are many Latino nationalities, organizations and groups. I am on the Policy Committee of one called the Latino Coalition for a Healthy California, a public policy advocacy organization. One of its projects was put together by Latinas organizing around better health. Their report on health access for Latinas reveals that of seven million uninsured Californians, 1.4 million are Latina. That is a serious health issue. But apart from that terrible reality we need to address, I try not to talk just in terms of narrow health issues or, just about health care and lack of access to health care. I try to emphasize the need to improve health conditions: where we work, where we live, what our environment is like, what are the chances of you or someone in your family being victimized by violence, traumatized by violence? What are your chances of tranquillity unless your kids are safe in school and at home? All of these elements in life are determinants and definers of our health. Yes, we have some groups of Latinos who are better off than others in all of the above and their health indicators such as life expectancy and infant mortality are very good. But the fact is that, overall Latinas are among the ranks of the working poor and therefore less likely to have health coverage, more likely to be living poor quality housing and environments and to be working in hazardous conditions. Basically, it all goes together. Having low-income means living in poor environments and reduced access to life's necessities.

TK: What would you suggest to Latina women who want to improve the condition of their health care? Should they go to a local clinic, should they turn to larger institutions? Should they connect with patient's rights and women's organizations?

HRT: Be informed, read all you can, talk to others, know your rights, and speak up. We all need better health information, particularly for folks who have low literacy levels who are not going to read these pamphlets made for college graduates or above. We need to have more commitment on the part of the media that reaches Latina women—radio, television—to give appropriate health messages, to be very proactive about the rights people have to certain services. The previous governor of California, Pete Wilson, was loudly anti-immigrant. He became very aggressive in denying services to immigrants and a lead in denying prenatal care to undocumented women, a right secured by law in California. Public Advocates, the Latino Coalition for a Healthy California and others immediately challenged the denial in the courts. In effect, he could not implement his policies. Nevertheless, the impression that immigrants are not entitled to care still remains and many are afraid. Many, who clearly have a right to enter clinics and receive care, are afraid they are going to be deported or afraid they won't get citizenship. The fear that has been created is keeping people away. People need information; they need to know about their rights; they need to know about available services; they need to know about what in California is known as the Healthy Families Program and nationally as the Child Health Insurance Program (CHIP) so that they can register their kids. They need to have information about how to keep themselves healthy. But I also think that people have to know that they need to organize and that they need to actually advocate for coverage. The California Senate is going to debate a proposal introduced by Senator Hilda Solis to come up with a plan for California to cover all uninsured people. We need to look at how we can move the richest state in the Union to provide universal access to health care. We need to look at what's happening to peoples' working conditions. These are issues that I think Latinos and Latinas need to get involved in. Above all, getting people to vote, getting people together and getting out the vote.

TK: As I was reading through the Reid Memorial lecture, a speech you presented to Barnard students in 1976, I learned that, during the late 1950's, while you were in medical school as a student, you realized that there was a very powerful dual system of health care. Do you feel that any of this has changed since more women have entered the health care profession?

HRT: Yes, I think there have been some changes because the health care profession has recognized the value of primary care—the care that people access immediately. I also think there's been more recognition of people skills in the health professions. Women have had a lot to do with that. Nevertheless there are still major gaps. Although, since the 1960s, there have been more government programs and more support for public health, the fact of the matter is that we still have a system that excludes, under-serves, and even mis-serves all too many people. The latest census tells us that there are over 44 million Americans without health insurance. That is inexcusable!

TK: Would you agree that the majority of this disservice occurs with low-income women rather than with higher status groups?

HRT: Most certainly! There is no doubt that money can buy you good things, good medicine included, although good medicine requires more than money; it also takes a system that has quality controls and well trained people who are compassionate; it takes more than just money but definitely, money does buy better services.

TK: One issue that really came to the fore in your speech was the sterilization abuse of low-income women. Can you discuss the different ways and forms in which coerced sterilization has shown up among different ethnic groups?

HRT: You have to take an historical perspective to understand the phenomena. Sterilization has now become very popular as a means for people to end their fertility and their worries. Sterilization now is not the same as sterilization in the early '60s or late '50s in Puerto Rico, or even in the early '70s in the United States, which was the period I was speaking of. During those earlier decades we already had a procedure—vasectomy—for men that was never very popular among them. Men did not go in any large numbers to get vasectomies although the surgery itself was relatively simple. Prior to 1970 in the United States sterilization of women was relatively infrequent. Voluntary sterilization for women was pretty much restricted by the "rule of 120." That is, if a woman went to an OBGYN and wanted a sterilization, she would be asked how old she was and how many children she had and the rule was that, unless her age multiplied by the number of children was 120 or more, a woman was not a good candidate for sterilization. In other words, a 30-year-old woman would have to have four children to be a candidate. So this meant that sterilization as a voluntary procedure was restricted for certain women, but perversely it was being promoted, if not downright pushed or coerced, for others—women of low-income, women of color, women whom, for whatever reason, the provider decided should not have more children. I think that is the context that we talked about when describing how sterilization abuse manifested itself in many places in the world. And in many places, such as India and Bangladesh, it was the only birth control offered to women

But the point is that now sterilization has become something relatively common among married couples and among couples and individuals who may not be married but have decided they have as many children as they want or that they don't want any children at all. So now we're talking about the more subtle kinds of incentives or coercion for sterilization that may operate in the context of women's lives. For instance, take welfare reform and the pressure not to have additional children. That is a not-so-subtle coercion for women to be sterilized saying, "Let me get this over and done with"—whether or not that's really what they want to do—because it gives them the security that they won't get pregnant. Lack of access to abortion services may also push women to get sterilized. Restrictions on abortions have been going on ever since the 1973 *Roe v. Wade* decision. After a few years of burgeoning services, a backlash has created tremendous hardship for women in accessing abortion services. Currently over 80 percent of the counties in the United States don't have abortion clinics and there are all kinds of restrictions at state levels. We stopped funding abortion services for low-income women recipients of Medicaid. I think there are only five or six states that still use public funds to fund abortion services. All the others stopped funding them in the '70s following the Hyde amendment to the appropriations bill. All of this means that sterilization is a more contextual and complex phenomenon as it now applies to lower-income women and women of color. We always have to look at things in an historical perspective. By the way, the guidelines on sterilization and informed consent that we succeeded in getting into HEW in 1976 applied only to sterilizations funded by public money. They were not necessarily accepted guidelines within private practice.

TK: You are one of the pioneers who initiated an end of sterilization abuse for Latina women....

HRT: I have worked within a collective context from the very beginning. In the early 70s the Committee for Puerto Rican De-Colonization was holding an event at NYU where they were showing the movie Blood of the Condor. It presented a fictionalized version of a Quechua Indian uprising in Bolivia because the women were being sterilized without their knowledge. The organizers of the event asked me to give a talk about how this applied to Puerto Rico. I wasn't sure how it applied to Puerto Rico, so I read some books and talked to people to prepare. That was when I first personally began to understand what had been happening in Puerto Rico during the time I was there as a medical student, as a young mother, and as a practicing pediatrician. During those years of 1956 to 1970 I had been totally oblivious to the campaign to sterilize women that was social policy. I began to understand that social policy could creep up on you without it being explicit public policy. The example today of non-explicit social policy is welfare reform. No one has actually said that women were going to be thrown off welfare and wouldn't have any health insurance, nor that they were going to be put into low-income jobs, be without child care, and there would be pressure on them not to have more children. Yet when we begin to examine the effects on women, it certainly seems that much of this happens to them. It is just that the policies are not explicit in their intent and implementation.

TK: So how did you start things going as an activist and organizer?

HRT: During the question and answer period following my talk on what had happened in Puerto Rico mainly in the '50s and '60s, several people in the audience spoke about similar things going on in the United States. One was a psychiatrist working in a Brooklyn hospital who said that he saw all kinds of things—such as people having unnecessary operations, and women being sterilized without first being told about other kinds of contraception. A young woman, a writer for one of the left Puerto Rican papers, also became very interested and we formed a small group along with several people who started talking after that meeting. Later we met and created the Committee to End Sterilization Abuse. That was in 1974 when a series of abuses were being exposed. The Relf case, about the two black girls in Alabama—two sisters, one twelve and the other fourteen, who were surgically, irrevocably, and illegally sterilized—had come to light at the end of 1973. There was a huge outcry in the African American press and some organization around issues raised by the Relf case and eventually a court suit. There were others among them 10 women in Los Angeles who were suing the County Hospital. The suit, known as the Madrigal case was brought by women who were mainly not English-but Spanish speaking, who had been coerced into sterilization in some way, or lied to.

For me, telling this story as a story of individuals and their organizations is important. I think that individuals and leadership are crucial, but we should never deny the need for organizations and movements because they shape individuals. Some of the distress we of the progressive communities feel comes from the fact that we don't currently have a unifying movement.

TK: What do you think it takes to have a unified movement?

HRT: I think it takes a lot of hard work and organization but it requires other conditions too. There has to be a climate or event that wakes people up to an issue and gives them a vision of change. For health care reform, I think we were closer to having these conditions at the beginning of the Clinton administration. But, having lost those opportunities, to put it mildly, it is now a lot more difficult to re-group around universal health care. It takes a lot of hard work and organization and some force driving people to move toward a vision to get us to a better place.

TK: What are the steps that an individual should take to become an effective activist?
HRT: I think you have to have the heart to say, "I care a lot about this issue." That's the first thing: feeling committed. The second thing is to look around to see who else feels like you do and thinks like you do, or if there's something going on already that you can become part of. I would say single-issue activism more than anything else has united people effectively. Let's take MADD, Mothers Against Drunk Driving, an organization that I really like and that I think is really effective. Mothers anguished by their kids getting killed created it. Or take the women who felt strongly about breast cancer and breast cancer visibility because they had it or someone in their family did. I do think that, for me, the feeling of outrage comes first.

TK: While challenging these sterilization abuses, you experienced obstacles both at local and national, or federal levels. Could you compare the two?

HRT: I saw several things: one was just the capacity that we all have to organize locally. By and large, you're talking about organizing people who are working—most of us actually working full time. For us, local organization is more doable. Another is that whenever you start organizing around a given issue, you will find people out there who are very affected by the issue you are addressing. If you are working locally it is easier to help them find resources and to recruit them for continuing work. In our case, the moment we started doing public things—speaking to colleagues, in churches, organizing workshops in youth clubs, reaching out to social groups, we started hearing from people who wanted direct help. In those years there was some very effective organizing by women's groups at the community level. We did a number of radio shows and, invariably, people called in and wanted help. It wasn't about political analysis. Someone would call in and say, "Three years ago, I was told I had something wrong with my uterus and they took it out and I don't have any children and I'm only twenty two years old and I don't know what's happening." They wanted something concrete, they wanted help, and they wanted information. What I learned is that when you are organizing around an issue, you should be prepared to have some concrete services available for people. You need to know where people can get help. Do not assume that all others will be interested in your issue as you may be, as a political issue, or as an issue of public policy, or as human rights or whatever it is that is your driving ideal. I remember one radio show, when we had at least twenty calls and at least half of them were people calling for help, and we weren't ready for it. It was a painful experience for me.

TK: How about the challenges of organizing nationally?

HRT: Whether organizing locally or nationally, the organizers always have to let people know what they can concretely do. But national organizing does create new challenges. As example, we had a strange hearing in one of those organizing drives around the national guidelines on informed consent for sterilization procedures for HEW, Health and Human Services, now HHS, Health and Human Services. Joseph Califano was the head of it at that time. He was basically anti-choice. And there were some other anti-choice people who were very much in favor of restrictions if not downright prohibitions against sterilization. Many also did not like contraception and opposed any measures that made contraception more accessible. Going national created these kinds of contradictions because in that larger arena we found people who would take up our cause for very different reasons. At the local level it was much easier to keep focused on one issue and work with people whose thinking was somewhat more alike. There are greater hazards of forced compromises and undesirable partners when we go national.

TK: You worked at Lincoln Hospital.

HRT: Yes, from 1970 to 1978. I graduated from medical school in 1960, and I did my residency at the University Hospital in Puerto Rico. Then in 1970 I relocated to New York and became the Director of Pediatrics at Lincoln Hospital.

It was very interesting and maybe more exciting than I had wished. It was a sanctuary of fascinating people, who tried to work together in some way. It was a challenge to try and run a department comprised mainly of young people who supported things I thought were innovative, progressive, and worthy of support while at the same time trying to tone down some of the wilder manifestations of individuals wanting to dress as they wished, even though the community didn't like it, or who wanted to wear their hair or beards long when the community found that disrespectful. It was challenging and there was a lot of opposition from the medical school staff about all that was going on. There were periods when people would organize demonstrations to protest about those uptown institutions, meaning the medical school. Once, the police came into the department of pediatrics conference room because there had been an injunction against the Young Lords and I had allowed some to show a film there. They even arrested one of our doctors for protesting the police violence. Working there was fascinating and complex.

TK: You were also a board member of the National Women's Health Network and the president of the American Public Health Association in 1993. How did it feel to be the first Latina president of the American Public Health Association?

HRT: I enjoyed it tremendously. There is a wonderful Latino leadership in the American Public Health Association, the result of a Latino Caucus formed in the early '70s. I was at the birth of that Latino Caucus, so I remember the contributions to its organization of my wonderful colleagues, great researchers, teachers, activists for public health many of whom who are still active. The Latino Caucus has become a very important structure that young Latino public health folks attach to and where they have an opportunity to grow in leadership skills. It felt very good to preside over that great organization that APHA is for a year.

TK: So you never felt you had to compromise your beliefs or "tone it down?"

HRT: I have toned it down, I think; we all tone it down as we get older. First of all, I realized that a lot of times I wasn't communicating well when I wouldn't tone it down. I just wasn't communicating. I had more than a bit of a confrontational style in those days when it wasn't always worthwhile to be confrontational. There were times you could actually find better points of unity when you were less confrontational and more reasonable and actually listened to other people more and not just see them as being off the deep end, or evil. That was part of what I learned that toned me down. It is less about compromise than it is about being effective. Even with the issue of sterilization abuse that seemed so clear cut to us we needed to use analysis and be more self-critical. When we first devised the draft guidelines for the Health and Hospitals

Corporation, we got to every single hospital in the system, there were fifteen of them, each with an OBGYN department director. I recall that there was not one of the directors who was willing to listen about the guidelines. In part their antagonism was because the document we prepared trying to justify why guidelines were needed actually started out with a list of all the abuses. If you tell people that under their service, their command, their watch, these terrible things are going on, they stop listening right there. You just are not going to make your point, and so we ended up with this infuriated bunch of doctors. After reflection, we realized that we could have said things differently and gotten a more attentive audience. We might have started by stating that there have been a series of lawsuits around issues of inadequate consent processes and here are the guidelines to guard against lawsuits and ensure that patients' rights are being respected. It would have gone much better. As it was, we won anyway, but after a longer and bitterer struggle than was necessary. I certainly have calmed down. But its not been as much about consciously saying, "Well let me compromise on this or on that." It's more about saying, "How can I be more effective in getting from point A to point B? How can I be more effective about persuading this group of people to look at what the outcome of their health care should be, or that they want to be including others at this table. How can I be more effective?"

Charon Asetoyer

INTERVIEW BY TANIA KETENJIAN

Charon Asetoyer is the founder of the Native American Women's Health Education Resource Center. This interview was conducted in June 1999.

TK: What do you think are some of the most prominent reproductive health issues for indigenous women?
CA: The lack of delivery services within communities—Women have to travel long distances to deliver their babies and get prenatal care. And reproductive tract infections are at an all-time high. The Indian Health Service doesn't offer education in prevention and that causes these problems. Too many nonbarrier contraceptives are promoted.

We have people who are working on issues of boarding school survivors, people who were going to boarding schools where there was sexual abuse committed against our children by the Catholic Church. People are just now starting to talk about it. This information is surfacing, and it has had a devastating effect on our reproductive health and will continue to do so until these issues are addressed.

The social problems in our community create situations in which our young women feel that starting their families at an early age is the right thing. In reality, a 14-year-old should still be in school, should be looking at how she can have fun and be a 14-year-old and not at how to be a mother. We need to look at why this is happening to our young people, why they feel that their options are so limited that they start a family. We need to look at what can go on within our communities that will support our young people in staying in school. They need to realize that they have a future and choices. There are very few services that look at improving the status of our young women and that would have a very profound, integrating effect on our reproductive health and rights.

Development, any kind of development, affects the status of health and our families. We need to look at why we haven't made the same forward moves in community development as other people. When you start uncovering all of these issues, you are going to come up with the same answer. We're talking about 500 years of contact—we call it "a.c." instead of "a.d."—500 years after contact, that's how we look at things, 500 years after Columbus. For us, that has had a very profound impact on our current existence and people seem to forget that. People whose culture is completely devoid of origins want us to assimilate into the mainstream. They do not respect cultural differences. There are light-years of difference between that and a people who still feels proud of its culture. I think it is very important that people stop to think, that people respect differences, even if they have lost their knowledge of their traditional ways because they are no longer in their homeland, no longer in Europe. They are here in this country where we lived and flourished long before they came. They need to stop trying to take away very important fundamental human rights that make cultures cultures, and to acknowledge our autonomy, our sovereignty. When that happens, then you will see an increase in the status of health of indigenous patients. We're just so busy trying to fight off corporate America and trying to maintain who we are and to fight the assimilation and fight the mainstreaming. It's very difficult to have time in your day to pay attention to your health like other people do. We don't have the same access as other people and it is fundamentally important to recognize that.

TK: Can you tell me some specific pros and cons of the Indian Health Service?

CA: The Indian Health Service is our primary health care provider and we have to do everything we can to make it a good provider, to improve its services. The Indian Health Service needs to look at community response in order to improve its services. It needs to make more information about sexually transmitted diseases and reproductive tract infections accessible and available to the community. It needs to improve on its preventive services; it needs to establish better informed-consent. The Indian Health Service headquarters has established informed consent but it's amazing that it is not uniformly mandated. This means that every Indian Health Service clinic does not have to use the same informed-consent procedures. In some instances, when you walk in the door, that's considered consent; that's not acceptable. So they have to have more continuity and consistency within their services. They also need to have more culturally sensitive practitioners who are aware of our traditional practices. They need to respect them so that both approaches can work together. There may be patients who are using both—the biomedical approach as well as the traditional, spiritual approaches—for treating their problems. So the physicians need to realize that they are on a reservation, that they are functioning within a different culture, and that it is unacceptable to force a person into complying with all of their procedures. Practitioners need to become more familiar with indigenous practices and, through that, will achieve much better outcomes.

TK: Do issues of self-worth play a role in the difficulties indigenous women have in seeking health care?

CA: I don't think that we don't feel worthy enough to seek health care. The problem is more one of fear. Because of our history, we're dealing with fear of the Western health care provider. There is not a lot of trust within the community for the Indian Health Service. Too many of our women have been sterilized, too many of our babies have died, our midwifery practices have almost been lost because of our being forced to use IHS services, so there is a mistrust of the services the government provides. A lot of people don't want to go to IHS clinics, and will turn to our traditional spirituality and medical practices, or to what remains of them after they were outlawed. For us, it has to do with trust, or lack of it.

TK: What kind of involvement does the Native American Women's Health Education Resource Center have with other women's groups and minority groups?

CA: We try very hard to do as much networking as we can, to network with other indigenous organizations, to network and work with other women of color, and to also work with mainstream women's organizations because, when it comes right down to it, we have to if we're all to survive. Many of us are victims of the same perpetrator: pharmaceutical companies and capitalism—multinational corporations trying to turn a buck on our gender. So its very important that we work together and respect each others' philosophies, communities, and cultures. Together we can make changes; fragmented and working against each other, we can't.

TK: What changes would you like most to see in the next few years?

CA: I would like to see more indigenous women and more women of color sitting on boards of mainstream organizations. I would like to see more foundations and philanthropic efforts directed at women of color and indigenous women so that we can address the kinds of issues in our communities that need to be addressed. We need to develop programs that assist our young women in being able to have better reproductive health and that provide services to improve the status of young women. I'm sure that would create a turnaround in childbearing. I'd like to see healthier women; I'd like to see a reduction in diabetes within our community. I'd like to see respect for indigenous women from the biomedical community; and I would like to see the government back off from so much control and acknowledge the policies that we would like to see implemented in our health care system.

TK: Can you tell me a little bit about your experiences in the National Women's Health Network?

CA: I still feel that the National Women's Health Network is a very important organization and that it's a voice in Washington for all women. They have been incredible advocates, and have impacted policy in Washington for women's reproductive health. I think that the organization needs to continue its existence. I served on the board of directors of the National Women's Health Network for eight years, and I support the organization wholeheartedly. In fact, the NWHN, and the National Latina Health Project and the National Black Women's Health Project, helped us to develop the Native American Women's Health Education and Resource Center fourteen years ago. So I have very high respect for the National Women's Health Network.

TK: Let's say an indigenous woman wanted to turn to someone or someplace for superior care, better care than what is normally available to them, where would you send them?

CA: Well, I would send them to a woman's clinic in Sioux Falls. That is 150 miles away from us. We are in the Yankton Sioux Reservation in Lake Andes, South Dakota. If a woman does not have an automobile, or does not have money to buy gas or hire someone to take her 300 miles round trip, she's out of luck. Most indigenous women on reservations in this country live in very rural, isolated communities. We not only lack access to services within our own community, but we also lack resources that could provide us with other kinds of services.
TK: I know you did some reports on Norplant. Why did you do them and what did you discover?

CA: We did reports on the impact of Depo-Provera and the impact of Norplant in the Native American communities because they seemed to be the Indian Health Service's contraceptives of choice as opposed to the contraceptives of choice of the women in the community. Women were not getting all of the information about these contraceptives, or about the impact they would have on their health, both in the long and short terms. On the surface, Depo or Norplant look like the best things since sliced bread; but that couldn't be more wrong. So it was important that we examine the situation and publish documented reports that would bring all of these issues to the fore. We found that in the case of Norplant, when women realized, "This isn't the right kind of contraceptive for me because I'm having some kind of side effect; I want to have it removed," their request was being denied. Women were being forced to lose their reproductive health, and their reproductive rights were being violated.

Women no longer had choice or control. They were at the mercy of the health care provider. In terms of Depo-Provera, it was and still is the form of contraceptive women are being encouraged to use. After they use it for a while and realize the side effects related to the drug, it's too late to do something about it. Again, it's a provider-controlled contraceptive.

TK: What can indigenous women do to overcome and change all the obstacles they face?

CA: It's not a matter of overcoming these kinds of reproductive health problems; it is one, rather, of being able to organize ourselves in order to move policies forward to prevent these kinds of things from continuing to happen. We have been organizing women for over ten years now. We have seen some changes, positive changes, because of the work that we're doing, both at local and national levels in the form of policy changes and service improvements. I really think that a lot of that is because women are organizing and getting more involved and bringing our day-to-day reality into the policy arena. It's important for indigenous women, for *all* women for that matter, to continue to organize and work on issues of reproductive health.

Chapter 56

Mouth

Fat Is a Feminist Issue

SUSIE ORBACH

Excerpted from Susie Orbach, *Fat Is a Feminist Issue,* New York, Berkeley, 1978. Reprinted by permission

PREFACE

In March 1970, I went to the Alternate U on Sixth Avenue and 14th Street in New York City to register for a course on compulsive eating and self-image— women only. I walked into a room jammed with 40 women of various sizes talking about their bodies and their eating habits. It was the first time since the beginning of the women's liberation movement that women had dared to come forward for discussion groups specifically dealing with body image. The call for the course had seemed to me almost like a travesty—feminists concerned about how they looked! At the time we were used to rejecting male ideals of how we should look as projected in advertisements and movies. We were ostensibly happy in our blue jeans and work shirts. We were not used to discussing clothes or body size with our female friends; there was, in fact, a widespread feeling of relief that we could relax in our bodies and not worry about what was especially fashionable, provocative, or appealing. We wore the clothes of rebellion and did not care what others thought. Or did we?...

I was hesitant to explore the topic of compulsive eating outside the context of a political vocabulary—a vocabulary that looked at the relationship between patriarchy and Western society with the family as the linchpin. I was uneasy but held on to the slogan that the personal is political.

I would not have gone back but for one thing. Despite my discomfort, I also experienced a relief to be in a group with women, fat and thin, who were all compulsive eaters. The problem had been named, and perhaps I did not have to feel quite so ashamed. In the last year or so I had become quite used to talking about very personal topics in consciousness-raising groups, and I was quite excited that we [were going to] discuss in the same way a subject that had been so hidden and so private.

We had taken the formula of a women's group, and one by one we shared how we felt about our bodies, being attractive, food, eating, thinness, fatness, and clothes. We detailed our previous diet histories and traded horror stories of doctors, psychiatrists, diet organizations, health farms, and fasting. We knew enough to know that all our previous attempts at getting our bodies the right weight and shape had not worked. We wondered *why* we had wanted them so right, *what* was so powerful about looking a particular way that we had all tried and succeeded in losing weight dozens of times. We did not understand why we could not keep "it" off, why every time we neared the goal "it" would creep up, or why we always broke our diets. Why were we so plagued by our body size and shape?

We began asking new questions and coming up with new answers. We were a self-help group at the time when energy from the women's liberation movement sparked us all into rethinking many previously held assumptions. The creativity of the movement prepared a fertile soil in which feminist ideas, nurtured and developed in countless consciousness-raising groups, in mass marches and demonstrations, in organized political campaigns, found new applications and usefulness. Compulsive eating was one such area.

Compulsive eating is a very painful and, on the surface, self-destructive activity. But feminism has taught us to be wary of this label. Feminism has taught us that activities that appear to be self-destructive are invariably adaptations, attempts to cope with the world. In our group, we turned our strongly held ideas about dieting and thinness upside down. Slowly and unsurely we stopped dieting. Nothing terrible happened. My world did not collapse. Maybe we did not want to be thin. I developed a new political reason for not being thin—I was not going to be like the fashion magazines wanted me to be; I was a Jewish beatnik, and I would be *zaftig*. I relaxed, ate what I wanted, and wore clothes that were expressive of me. But why was I afraid of being thin? The things I was frightened of came into vision. I confronted them, always asking myself—how would it help to be fat in this situation? *What* would be more troublesome if I were thin? As the image of my fat and thin personality conflated, I began to lose weight. I felt a deep satisfaction that I could be a size that felt good for me and no longer obsessed with food. I promised myself I would not be responsible for depriving myself of the food I liked. I had learned a crucial lesson—that I could be the same person thin as I was fat. Satisfied, I left the group six months later. I no longer defined myself as a compulsive eater, and I had stabilized at a weight I found acceptable. It turned out to be rather higher than my previous Twiggy-like fantasies. Food no longer terrified me, and I could live in my body.

Obesity and overeating have joined sex as central issues in the lives of many women today. In the United States, 50 percent of women are estimated to be overweight. Every women's magazine has a diet column. Diet doctors and clinics flourish. The names of diet foods are now part of our general vocabulary. Physical fitness and beauty are every woman's goals. While this preoccupation with fat and food has become so common that we tend to take it for granted, being fat, feeling fat, and the compulsion to overeat are, in fact, serious and painful experiences for the women involved. Being fat isolates and invalidates a woman. Almost inevitably, the explanations offered for fatness point a finger at the failure of women themselves to control their weight, control their appetites, and control their impulses. Women suffering from the problem of compulsive eating endure a double anguish: feeling out of step with the rest of society and believing that it is all their own fault.

The number of women who have problems with weight and compulsive eating is large and growing. Owing to the emotional distress involved and the fact that the many varied solutions offered to women in the past have not worked, a new psychotherapy to deal with compulsive eating has had to evolve within the context of the movement for women's liberation. This new psychotherapy represents a feminist rethinking of traditional psychoanalysis. A feminist perspective to the problem of women's compulsive eating is essential if we are to move on from the ineffective blame-the-victim approach and the unsatisfactory adjustment model of treatment. While psychoanalysis gives us useful tools to discover the deepest sources of emotional distress, feminism insists that those painful personal experiences derive from the social context into which female babies are born and within which they develop to become adult women. The fact that compulsive eating is overwhelmingly a women's problem suggests that it has something to do with the experience of being female in our society. Feminism argues that being fat represents an attempt to break free of society's sex stereotypes. Getting fat can thus be understood as a definite and purposeful act; it is a directed, conscious or unconscious challenge to sex-role stereotyping and the culturally defined experience of womanhood.

Fat is a social disease, and fat is a feminist issue. Fat is not about lack of self-control or lack of willpower. Fat is about protection, sex, nurturance, strength, boundaries, mothering, substance, assertion, and rage. It is a response to the inequality of the sexes. Fat expresses experiences of women today in ways that are seldom examined and even more seldom treated. While becoming fat does not alter the roots of sexual oppression, an examination of the underlying causes of unconscious motivation that lead women to compulsive eating suggests new treatment possibilities. A new therapeutic approach does not reinforce the oppressive social roles that lead women into compulsive eating in the first place. What is it about the social position of women that leads them to respond to it by getting fat?

The relegation of women to the social roles of wife and mother has several significant consequences that contribute to the problem of fat. An emphasis on presentation as the central aspect of a woman's existence makes her extremely self-conscious. It demands that she occupy herself with a self-image that others will find pleasing and attractive—an image that will immediately convey what kind of woman she is. She must observe and evaluate herself, scrutinizing every detail as though she were an outside judge. She attempts to make herself in the image of womanhood presented by billboards, newspapers, magazines, and television. The media present women either in a sexual context or within the family, reflecting a woman's two prescribed roles, first as a sex object and then as a mother. She is brought up to catch a man with her good looks and pleasing manner. To do this she much look appealing, earthy, sensual, sexual, virginal, innocent, reliable, daring, mysterious, coquettish, and thin. In other words, she offers her self-image on the marriage marketplace. As a married woman, her sexuality will be sanctioned and her economic needs will be looked after. She will have achieved the first step of womanhood.

Since women are taught to see themselves from the outside, they become prey to the huge fashion and diet industries that first set up the ideal images and then exhort women to meet them. The message is loud and clear: the woman's body is not her own. The woman's body is not satisfactory as it is. It must be thin, free of "unwanted hair," deodorized, perfumed, and clothed. It must conform to an ideal physical type. Family and school socialization teaches girls to groom themselves properly.

Furthermore, the job is never-ending, for the image changes from year to year. In the early 1960s, the only way to feel acceptable was to be skinny and flat chested with long straight hair. The first of these was achieved by near starvation, the second, by binding one's breasts with an Ace bandage, and the third, by ironing one's hair. Then, in the early 1970s, the look was curly hair and full breasts. Just as styles in clothes change seasonally, so women's bodies are expected to change to fit these fashions. Long and skinny one year, petite and demure the next, women are continually manipulated by images of proper womanhood, which are extremely powerful because they are presented as the only reality. To ignore them means to risk being an outcast. Women are urged to conform, to help out the economy by continuous consumption of goods and clothing that are quickly made unwearable by the next season's fashion styles in clothes and body shapes. In the background, a ten-billion-dollar industry waits to remold bodies to the latest fashion. In this way, women are caught in an attempt to conform to a standard that is externally defined and constantly changing.

But these models of femininity are experienced by women as unreal, frightening, and unattainable. They produce a picture that is far removed from the reality of women's day-to-day lives. The one constant in these images is that a woman must be thin. For many women, compulsive eating and being fat have become one way to avoid being marketed or seen as the ideal women: "My fat says 'screw you' to all who want me to the be perfect mom, sweetheart, maid, and whore. Take me for who I am, not for who I'm supposed to be. If you are really interested in me, you can wade through the layers and find out who I am." In this way, fat expresses a rebellion against the powerlessness of the woman, against the pressure to look and act in a certain way and against being evaluated on her ability to create an image of herself. Becoming fat is, thus, a woman's response to the first step in the process of fulfilling a prescribed social role which requires her to shape herself to an externally imposed image in order to catch a man. A second stage in this process takes place after she achieves that goal, after she has become a wife and mother.

For the compulsive eater, fat has much symbolic meaning which makes sense within a feminist context. Fat is a response to the many oppressive manifestations of a sexist culture. Fat is a way of saying no to powerlessness and self-denial, to a limiting sexual expression which demands that females look and act a certain way, and to an image of womanhood that defines a specific social role. Fat offends Western ideals of female beauty, and, as such, every "overweight" woman creates a crack in the popular culture's ability to make us mere products. Fat also expresses the tension in the mother-daughter relationship, the relationship which has been allocated the feminization of the female. This relationship is bound to be difficult in a patriarchal society because it demands that the already oppressed mothers become the teachers, preparers, and enforcers of the oppression that society will visit on their daughters. A woman's psychological development is structured in such a way as to prepare her for a life of inequality, but this straitjacket is not accepted lightly and invariably causes a "reaction." Psychological disturbance often distorts a person's physiological capacity: ability to eat, sleep, talk, or enjoy sexual activity.

I suggest that one of the reasons we find so many women suffering from eating disorders is because the social relationship between feeder and fed, between mother and daughter, fraught as it is with ambivalence and hostility, becomes a suitable mechanism for distortion and rebellion. An examination of the symbolic meanings of fat provides insight into individual woman's experience in patriarchal culture. Fat is an adaptation to the oppression of women, and as such, it may be an unsatisfying personal solution and an ineffectual political attack. It is to this problem that our compulsive-eating therapy speaks within a feminist context.

Sacrificing Ourselves for Love

JANE WEGSCHEIDER HYMAN AND ESTHER R. ROME

Jane Wegscheider Hyman and Esther R. Rome, *Sacrificing Ourselves for Love: Why Women Compromise Health and Self-Esteem... and How to Stop,* Freedom, California, The Crossing Press, 1996. Reprinted by permission.

THE CULTURAL IDEAL

Changes in the beauty ideal for women often mirror social changes; ironically, when social rights are expanded, the ideal image tends to become unhealthfully slim. The shift in ideal from plump to slender began around 1920, at about the same time that the woman's suffrage movement triumphed and the First International Birth Control Congress was held. Elizabeth Taylor's figure was considered the ideal in the 1960s, but by 1976 the 91-pound Twiggy had taken her place. The angular fashions of the 1970s suggested that only males—or male impersonators—could enter the world of professional workers and pursue the traditional male goals of independence, personal achievement, and self-control. In the 1980s, muscles became stylish. The "new woman" was not only thin but had firm, shapely muscles, like those of professional dancers or athletes. Thus, the fashion in body shape and clothes became increasingly at odds with the general biological shape of female bodies. In the 1990s, the basic message remains the same: We could all become as straight and lean as athletic boys with breasts if we only tried hard enough.

As the ideal has shrunk, the actual average weight of women under 30 in the general U.S. population has increased. The average U.S. woman is 5 feet, 3.7 inches tall and weighs 144 pounds, a far cry from the average 5 feet, 8 inches, 123 pounds, of fashion models.

LEARNING ABOUT LOOKS AND FOOD

Girls tend to become increasingly sensitive to social expectations and to the opinions of others. At puberty, many are proud of their developing breasts and other signs of womanhood, but are dismayed at a normal increase in fat, especially the fuller hips and thighs so characteristic of women's bodies. Some adolescent girls develop eating disorders when they lose weight through dance, gymnastics, or sports and try to maintain the lower weight; some are told to lose weight for these activities The majority of adolescent girls and high school and college women want to lose weight regardless of what they actually weigh.

Boarding schools and colleges often breed dysfunctional eating. A school environment can be competitive academically and socially, and living in close quarters may encourage a woman to compare her body with those of her housemates. In the close quarters of a college campus or boarding school, we often teach each other how to starve, binge, and purge.

THE EXPERIENCE OF STARVATION

Undernutrition can change body chemistry and affect physical and psychological functioning. Low-calorie diets can alter the functioning of the hypothalamus, which helps control sensations of hunger and fullness. As a result, the brain may lose some of its normal control of hunger and satiety: some women who have starved never feel hungry; some feel constantly hungry even if they have resumed eating meals that would have been filling in the past; some begin eating in uncontrollable binges.

When the cells do not receive enough fuel to burn from food, they feed on both body fat and other sources of calories, such as muscles. Even in moderate undernutrition there is a loss of muscle tissue—including heartmuscle—and a loss of tissue in all organs except the brain.

THE ROLE OF BODY FAT

Body fat is not a useless mass that we can add or carve off without consequences. Fat stores energy, protects organs, and may be crucial to our ability to bear children. Body fat also helps produce and store the sex hormones that control our fertility. In addition to its effects on our reproductive organs, estrogen produced by fat tissue regulates bone metabolism, the synthesis of vital proteins in the liver, and to some extent, even behavior. How the hypothalamus receives its signal is unclear; it may be through estrogen. Estrogen levels gradually rise along with body fat during puberty. And the estrogen in body fat accelerates the secretion of other hormones necessary for a fertile menstrual cycle.

ANOREXIA NERVOSA

Women who tend toward highly obsessive thoughts and compulsive actions are particularly at risk when they diet. Women who are starving during a food shortage become increasingly fatigued, weak, and listless; in contrast, women with anorexia nervosa are extremely active because of their fear of fat. They often have intense exercise regimens, such as running 5 to 10 miles a day or doing lengthy aerobic activities. Some women with anorexia nervosa become reluctant to sit down, fearing that the inactivity of sitting will cause weight gain. In extreme cases, the intensity of her fear can cause a starving woman to pace ceaselessly.

BULIMIA NERVOSA

Some women with a tendency to obsessive behavior develop an extreme form of bulimia—eating in compulsive and uncontrollable binges, then vomiting and purging. They fear that they will be unable to stop eating and actually feel unable to stop. Often they are anxious or depressed and consider suicide.

Virtually all who suffer from this type of binge eating are obsessively preoccu-pied with food and with body shape and weight, and all were once stringent dieters.

Those of us with bulimia nervosa like the sensations associated with dehy-dration. These sensations include feeling washed out, drained, or empty; hav-ing loose clothes; having a flat abdomen; having protruding bones (especially cheek or hip bones); and feeling light or lightheaded.... Many of us who have bulimia nervosa abhor any sensation of food in the stomach—for us starvation is the ideal state.

THE HAZARDS OF ANOREXIA AND BULIMIA

Women who suffer from anorexia or bulimia face the same health risks as women on self-starvation diets, but some of the risks are intensified. They are more likely to have trouble with dehydration, diabetes insipidus, vulnerability to heat and cold, bone loss, and fertility. Cycles of binge eating and purging can cause tooth erosion and tooth loss, disruption of the body's metabolism, spasmodic seizures of the jaw muscles, inflammation of the salivary glands, kidney damage, and, in rare cases, rupture of the stomach and esophagus. Large doses of laxatives and diuretics can deplete the body of potassium and sodium.

FIGHTING BACK

As more women and researchers realize that dieting is not a trivial problem and that unhealthful food restriction can cause a lifetime of problems, more of us are actively opposing thinness and body "control" as requirements for social acceptance.

Ideally, prevention should begin in elementary school, with educational programs that reveal the social influences behind our unrealistic and unhealthy weight and body image goals Unfortunately, many professionals still have misconceptions about what factors actually determine a woman's fatness and leanness. Therefore, it is important for those of us concerned and informed to organize programs on our own or create individual projects for the sake of our health and the health of our daughters.

Chapter 57

Torso

The next four chapters represent what I am calling the "Out Front" portion of this Body Parts section. In "Torso," Louise Bernikow documents that we have, indeed, come a long way toward more comfortable clothes, while Ophira Edut updates the body-image crisis raised in the "Mouth" chapter. Maybe the tight corsets and other concealing under and outerwear of the past spared us from having to obsess about the perfection of our bodies.

"Heart" helps introduce the topic of gender medicine, which is further described in Still Taking Our Bodies Back. As Jen Baumgardner explicates, potential conflict of interest has already invaded this important new scientific turf.

"Breasts." You will meet them from a new perspective in these consciousness-raising selections, and, through her disciple Anne Kasper, you will learn about Rose Kushner, a key foremother of breast cancer activism. Marta Drury's short piece on breast reduction raises many big questions in my mind, such as: Why are women whose breasts are made smaller more likely to be pleased with the outcome than those whose breasts are enlarged?

"Muscle." It's amazing that Lucinda Franks's "Women in Motion" was merely her fantasy for the year 2000 when it was first published in 1974. Few expected that much of it might actually come true. But one who did was Congresswoman Patsy Mink, advocate for Title IX, which opened the world of sports to women by the power of the purse. Very simply, educational institutions that failed to give girls equal training in athletics would lose their funds.—B. S.

Clothing the Body

LOUISE BERNIKOW

Excerpted from Louise Bernikow, *The American Women's Almanac: An Inspiring and Irreverent Women's History*, New York, Berkley Books, 1997. Reprinted by permission.

DRESS/REDRESS

> Let men be compelled to wear our dress for awhile and we should soon hear them advocating a change.
>
> —Amelia Bloomer, *The Lily*, March 1851

> Some say the Turkish costume is not graceful. Grant it. For parlor dolls, who loll on crimson velvet couches and study attitudes before tall mirrors—for those who have no part to perform in the great drama of life, for whose heads, hearts and hands there is no work to do the drapery is all well.... But for us commonplace, everyday, working characters, who wash and iron, bake and brew, carry water and fat babies up stairs and down, bring potatoes, apples and pans of milk from the cellar, run our own errands through mud or snow, shovel paths and work in the garden, why "the drapery" is quite too much—one might as well work with a ball and chain.
>
> —Elizabeth Cady Stanton, *The Lily*, April 1851

In the 1890s, the average skirt, worn over several layers of petticoats, was 13½ feet around the hem and the average waist measurement was 20 inches. This meant 15 pounds of clothing hanging from a constricted waist. By the beginning of World War I, skirts were higher and narrower and waist size had increased by 40 percent. Women's health improved immeasurably.

> The man did not have to please the woman by the small size of his feet, but by the large size of his bank account. His feet were organs of locomotion, hers of sex attraction.

> This corset is as idiotic as a snug rubber band around a pair of shears.
>
> —Charlotte Perkins Gilman, *The Forerunner*, 1915

Adiós, Barbie

OPHIRA EDUT

Excerpted from Ophira Edut, ed., *Adiós, Barbie: Young Women Write about Body Image and Identity,* Seattle, Seal Press, 1998. Reprinted by permission.

Ah, Barbie. Hard to believe the old girl's pushing 40. I mean, look at her. She has thighs like number-two pencils. Her tan lasts all winter. And that pink Corvette has dropped some serious mileage. Then there's the fancy wardrobe, the town house, the swimming pool... and she hasn't worked a day in her life.

Okay, I know she has problems like the rest of us. Her boyfriend, I hear, can't perform too well. She had to have two ribs removed back in the seventies in order to retain that trademark hourglass figure. And she hasn't used the bathroom once in four decades.

But you're busted, Babs. You've been found guilty of inspiring fourth-grade girls to diet, of modeling an impossible beauty standard, of clinging to homogeneity in a diverse new world. Welcome to the dollhouse, honey. Your time is up. Pack your bags and be outta the Dreamhouse by noon.

At the turn of the millennium, body image is a national crisis among young women. Until now, there hasn't been a forum where women of diverse cultures and identities could gather to chronicle their experiences, to usher out the Barbie era with pink champagne and a triumphant "adiós."

And the current national discussion of body image reflects this. To date, most literature continues to popularize the myth that distorted body image is merely a symptom of vanity suffered by bored, middle-class white girls. In 1995, *Newsweek* published results from a University of Arizona study that compared the body satisfaction of Black and white adolescent girls. The gap in results was wider than the one between Barbie's thighs: 70 percent of the African-American subjects reportedly liked their bodies, while 90 percent of their white peers did not. While the Black girls in the study described an ideal body as "full hips and thick thighs," perfection, according to the white girls, came in waifishly impossible dimensions: 5-foot-7 and 100 to 110 pounds. The study's implied conclusion? Black girls have better body image than white girls do.

That didn't sit right with many women I knew. We wondered what would have happened if the study had polled subjects on whether they liked their hair texture, their skin and eye color, their facial features. Moreover, what if the study had asked girls whether they felt safe or powerful in their bodies? The focus on weight failed to connect body image to racism and sexism—to power. Class differences were not mentioned, nor was the history that may have shaped the subjects' varying ideals.

But women's struggle with body image is about power. Body image goes far beyond weight, and it runs deeper than skin color. Our bodies have become arenas for feelings we don't deal with, for unresolved traumas and injustices. Scratch away the surface of "I'm so fat" and "I hate my hair," and you'll find a sister treading water in a melting pot simmering with every "ism" imaginable.

This is difficult to articulate today, at a time when society has taken on the rosy blush of progressiveness. Are we empowered young women, or aren't we? Our inability to answer this question definitively is a natural offshoot of a capitalist, media-driven society that serves young people a daily diet of mixed messages. Society adopts the "girl power" mantra but refuses to arm girls with the tools to achieve it. Textbooks glorify violence and war, but schools won't properly educate students about safe sex, reproductive health, self-defense, and abuse. Multiculturalism is the new media buzzword, but laws upholding it are dismantled while we watch *Yo! MTV Raps* and read *Vibe* magazine. Young women are encouraged to follow rather than to lead, to become passive consumers rather than active creators of our culture and our destinies.

Our bodies—and our convoluted relationships with them—tell the real story. In a world that offers women challenges along with choices, compromise along with control, our bodies may seem the only realm where we can claim sovereignty. So we focus our power there. We start with what we can control—sorta. Our bodies. Our hair. Our weight. Our breasts. Our clothes. When this control inevitably eludes us, our feelings of powerlessness solidify.

Too often, the endless body chase becomes a distraction from a painful reality. Trauma survivors talk about "leaving their bodies" as a survival tactic during violation. For some women, feeling like we're "in our bodies" convinces us we exist. In a twisted way, intense body focus is the one thin thread connecting us to the material world. But gaining a sense of place in our bodies should ultimately build our sense of place in the world. It should be a means of healing rather than escaping from pain. We need to feel connected to our bodies, to understand what they can do. Sometimes, this even means pushing them to new comfort zones. Can we do this with balance? That's the big question.

Young women are attempting to answer this question with a resounding yes by showing that our bodies can be our allies. Rather than simply shun the idea of being defined by our appearances, young women today include our bodies as part of our multilayered self-definitions. In a world that still tries to assume our identities, we rebel with an outward expression of self. Our passion for the truth, in all its messy complexity, compels us to visibly defy easy categories and sweeping labels, even if they were created from within. Rather, we rush to show the world who we are, instead of allowing it to paint us as one-dimensional characters. So instead of declaring "Black is beautiful," a young African-American woman today is more likely to ask, *Why does this world assume I'm "too black" or "not black enough"? Who defines blackness anyway?*

Everything is up for questioning today—the media, our identities, each other, the very concept of beauty. The answer to the body image dilemma can't simply be to allow all women a place in the beauty structure. Sure, it's important to tell women of every size and color that they're beautiful and worthwhile people. But it's also fundamental to offer them a world where they are safe, valued, and free from oppression. A world that values healing more than destruction, that seeks balance over domination.

So take an about-face, if you will, and confront head-on whatever you're running from. Start at the mirror. Take a good, hard look at the part of your body you fear the most and tell it who's boss. Then give it all the love you've got. Instead of putting all your resistance into the leg press machine, focus some on the culture that directs our best energies into body-hating pursuits. Life is an opportunity for joy and celebration. How can our lives be full if our stomachs aren't? How can we understand life's gift when we're too blinded by our own perceived inadequacies to appreciate them?

Hasta la vista, Barbie

Chapter 58

Heart

Science + Corporate Bucks = Health Revolution?

JENNIFER BAUMGARDNER

Jennifer Baumgardner, "Science + Corporate Bucks = Health Revolution?" *Ms.,* May/June 1998. Reprinted by permission.

The medical profession has not traditionally shone on the gender-equity front. During a century that has brought us great technological leaps in the treatment of disease, women have been ignored, fed Valium, told it's all in their heads, and routinely dispensed birth control methods laden with side effects. Health activists, therefore, have rightly focused on liberating women from the medical establishment. Speculums in hand, feminists have fought back via *Our Bodies, Ourselves,* package inserts on birth control pills, and the creation of women's health centers.

But finding women-friendly physicians or making yogurt douches doesn't address one enormous impediment to women's health: research, or the lack of it. Since Hippocrates, medical testing has been done almost solely on men. In 1988, Congresswoman Pat Schroeder caught wind of the medical gynephobia—she wisecracks that researchers wouldn't even use female rats for fear the rodents' hormonal fluctuations would skew results. Schroeder wrote and pushed through the Clinical Trials Fairness Act, legislation that requires women to be included in government sponsored research.

The newest and perhaps most comprehensive effort to study our health is the year-old Partnership of Women's Health at Columbia University. The partnership's director, Marianne Legato, M.D., is a proponent of what she calls "gender specific medicine"—health care based on the understanding of how women's and men's unique biologies play out in the manifestation and treatment of disease—a discipline that she believes will incite the next women's health revolution. Legato's dream is to lead the way to a time when every doctor, beginning at medical school, employs and understands both female and male models of disease—whether that doctor is a heart surgeon or a general practitioner.

To that end, the ambitious mission of the partnership is to gather all existing data on the relationship between gender and biology, to identify gender-specific health issues that need further research, and to initiate and fund studies that will shed light on the differences in female and male biology and health.

"I began," says Legato, "by asking, 'Are there enough differences between men and women, apart from reproductive biology, to really justify our doing a systematic exploration of women? Or are men and women interchangeable?'" Some of the many gender-specific differences that trip off Legato's tongue:

➤Diabetes and hypertension, two common ailments in midlife women, can have a strangely protective effect on their bones that is not shared by men with either disease. One theory derived from this observation is that since women who are diabetic or hypertensive are often also heavy, perhaps it's the estrogen stored in fat that, in turn, prevents bone loss.
➤While men's brains are bigger, women's brains have more neurons.
➤Women complain of heart palpitations much more frequently than men do, and thus far, there are no known, safe preventive drugs for the female heart. Aspirin, for example, was recommended across the board as preventive cardiac care after an influential study of 22,071 subjects in 1988 indicated its beneficial effects. Zero women were included in the study, and it's still unknown whether aspirin has any benefit for them.

"We treat women as if they are small men," says Legato. "And they're not."

The first step in creating female disease protocols is to figure out what is already known. "The data about gender and its impact both on normal human function and on the physiology of disease is scattered throughout the whole of medical literature," says Legato. "No one has ever gotten it together in one cohesive, accessible mass or database."

Until now. The heart of the partnership's work is the creation of a computer-based medical archive called GenCite, which will gather together the aforementioned studies. It will be housed at Columbia University but will be publicly accessible via the Web by this fall. The partnership's researchers have almost finished assembling the data on bone and they have begun to tackle nutrition. They will continue to gather data indefinitely, and the information they get will, in turn, help them identify new areas of research to pursue.

Which leads to the other major project of the partnership: working with scientists and doctors at other esteemed research universities. In the year since the partnership was formed, Legato has focused on developing relationships with researchers at Georgetown, Harvard, Yale, the University of Colorado, and the University of California at San Diego. These scientists will consult, perform research, write papers, and develop education programs for the partnership. At this point, only two projects are off the ground (one at Columbia is looking at the influence of gender on normal heart function, and at UCSD researchers are working on ways to teach gender-specific medicine to doctors and nurses working in hospitals).

A mandate this expansive requires a lot of money—and you find pockets that deep on the pants of corporate giants. Therefore, the partnership was created as a marriage of Columbia University's scientists and Procter & Gamble's money.

Dr. Legato is a 62-year-old researcher who has practiced internal medicine in New York City for 12 years, before which she was a full-time academic researcher. While she was studying the treatment of coronary artery disease at Columbia, where she also teaches, she discovered research showing that the gold standard indicators for heart disease in men—the cardiac stress test—often elicited incorrect results from women. Further, she noticed that men were treated aggressively to ward off an attack while women were treated less aggressively, or "protected." These insights became the basis of her award-winning 1991 book, *The Female Heart,* which not only raised national consciousness about cardiovascular disease as the number one killer of women but revealed the sometimes fatal inequities in health care between the sexes.

The book launched Legato into the spotlight, and soon her work caught the eye of T. George Harris, a San Diego–based health journalist. Harris was a consultant for Procter & Gamble, and he introduced Legato to Craig Wynett, the young innovative director of P&G's Corporate New Ventures. Loath to be just another highly paid consultant, Legato pitched the Cincinnati-based multinational corporation her hypothesis—that gender-specific treatment protocols were most likely needed not just for heart disease but for every disease. She also stressed that the ways in which disease and drugs played out in the female body were an untapped commercial resource; whoever had the information would be ahead of the game in designing effective products for whatever ailed women. Wynett was the right man to pitch this huge idea to; he sets as a goal for the company the creation of at least one new "megabrand"—top sellers such as Crest toothpaste, Tide detergent, and Pampers diapers—a year. The frontier of women's health products was fresh territory for megabrands. After three years of meetings, the partnership was born—ostensibly, a win-win relationship.

In one sense, the partnership is built on the legacy of women's health activism—from the rebellious seventies' collectives to the eighties' legislative muscle. In another sense, the partnership is the result of aggressive corporations zeroing in on the next big market. Attempting to please these strange bedfellows makes Legato, the brilliant front-woman, responsible for maintaining credibility with activists while delivering product-oriented data to P&G.

Legato emphasizes that P&G is supportive of her visions: without even insisting on a contract, P&G CEO John Pepper wrote Legato a one-million-dollar check, thus sealing her fealty. Then he invited the pharmaceutical company Pfizer, the cereal company Kellogg's, and other corporations to put their trust and money into the partnership. While Pfizer's role is yet to be determined, Kellogg's and P&G each have a say in the partnership's research agenda, and each has "adopted" a part of the database, For instance, Kellogg's is funding the "Nutrition" section and will have first dibs and a 90-day embargo on any proposals or data that come out of that part of GenCite. "I think that this is an idea that is so compelling that the big companies are getting behind it," says Legato.

Agreed, but why is the idea of amassing gender-specific health information compelling? Because knowing about the unique aspects of the functions of women's bodies is, as Legato asserts, an intellectual imperative, or because GenCite will be the largest focus group ever created and P&G (and corporate friends) will have first look at any proposals and breakthroughs that come out of this medical archive?

Given its obligation to assist product development, could the partnership be primarily about targeting women as consumers for osteoporosis medicines and hormones? "There is no question that women's health is a rapidly emerging marker and that that fact is fueling much of the current research," says Susan Love, M.D., a feminist breast cancer researcher and author of *Dr. Susan Love's Breast Book* and *Dr. Susan Love's Hormone Book*, "Women make most of the medical decisions, and they are being marketed to by HMOs and pharmaceutical companies."

Legato firmly believes that it's possible to use corporate dough to get the research done without getting baked in the P&G pie. "New idea here: pharmaceutical companies are facing the correctness of the idea that to focus on women is to develop better and more focused therapies for the treatment of disease. They're not simply courting the women customers for propaganda," says Legato, and she freely admits that products are the carrot keeping the companies behind the research. But where does the benefit end and the exploitation begin? "I have no idea," says Dr. Love. "A difficult question—and one that needs open discussion."

Cindy Pearson, executive director of the National Women's Health Network (a group known for having an extremely strict policy about accepting corporate money), acknowledges that, thus far, the partnership seems to be walking the benefit-exploitation line adroitly. "But I question whether [the partnership] is going to break the mold and look at women's health with race and class in mind," says Parson. "The partnership is still looking at women in order to find something that is marketable."

"One of the biggest dangers in this endeavor is in not correcting the feminist fear of it," said Legato, when I mentioned the concerns of feminist health activists. "Women have to be part of the solution to these questions. We are functioning on 6 cylinders when there could be 12. Our purpose is to show the importance of women to better health for everyone. That's my aim," she says. "That and not having the women's health movement blow up in our face." Rather than shooting new projects down, Legato believes women need to get involved, participate in studies, and, in general, grab the medical profession by the horns. Yet she's careful to acknowledge the work of health activists. "I wouldn't be sitting in this chair if it wasn't for their vision and courage to demand something better. The partnership is providing the intellectual paradigm for that spirit."

So then, what is Procter & Gamble and how much can we trust its commitment to women's health? P&G is a 120-year-old company that does $35.8 billion in sales per year from products as diverse as Crisco and Cover Girl, Ivory Soap and Pepto-Bismol. P&G is currently developing a bisphosphonate (a substance that inhibits bone loss) for treatment of osteoporosis that will compete, they hope, with Merck's best-selling Fosamax. P&G also makes at least two hormone replacement patches—Alora, an estrogen, and a testosterone patch currently in development.

The big products on the roster, however, is Olean (aka olestra), P&G's nondigestible "fat-free" fat, which, once it's added to greasy snack foods, may just be the company's next megabrand. The side effect of Olean is gastrointestinal distress, including "abdominal cramping and loose stools"—surely the most unfortunate words ever to adorn a bag of chips.

Olean is clearly not a health food—it simply addresses Americans' decidedly unhealthy desire to eat tons of crap and not gain weight. Americans are getting fatter, and the advent of nonfat foods hasn't changed this. I asked Legato to weigh in on olestra's health effects, especially given women's complicated issues with food. "I think Americans are, in general, overweight," she began, hesitantly. "Strategies to control the diet include Olean—in reasonable amounts." Then she said, "Look, it puts me in a very bad position—I really try to keep away from saying that P&G products are good or bad." Legato is mapping the terrain of women's health, but clearly this corporate alliance does limit her ability to comment candidly, as a physician, on products that affect women.

Olestra, a fat that doesn't add to your fat intake, reminds me of the position that the partnership is in if it fails to retain autonomy—moving a mass of knowledge through the bowels of medicine with no substantive effect on women's health. The side effects of the partnership going awry exceed that of olestra's gastrointestinal distress: a misstep with this alliance could condemn a woman's heart, breasts, brain, and bones to having dollar signs stamped on them before they're deemed worthy of study. Whether the partnership is the site of a revolution in health care, or women's health is the next megabrand, rests on Legato's shoulders.

Women's Hearts at Risk

CHARLOTTE LIBOV

Charlotte Libov, *The Woman's Heart Book,* New York, Plume, 1994. Reprinted by permission.

When I was 40 years old, I was stunned to learn I'd been born with a congenital heart defect, a "hole" in my heart. Since I had never heard of women having anything go wrong with their hearts, I was shocked. I learned the hard way that women do indeed develop heart disease. This is true, despite the stubborn myth that women's hearts are immune.

In fact, heart disease is the biggest killer of women. About 235,000 women die annually from heart attacks. When you add in the deaths from all types of heart problems, the figure mushrooms to over half of a million female deaths a year. These statistics not only involve elderly women; an estimated 74,000 women between the ages of 45 and 64 suffer heart attacks annually, according to the American Heart Association. Heart disease is also a major risk factor for stroke, the third leading killer and greatest crippler of women.

But the problem of heart disease in women is one that has been overlooked for years. "Clear evidence exists that women are not being treated aggressively to prevent heart disease," according to a 1999 statement issued by the American Heart Association and the American College of Cardiology.

This myth that "women don't get heart disease" persists among doctors as well. A 1995 Gallup survey found that nearly two-thirds of the internists and family practitioners queried know that there are important differences in the symptoms of heart attacks and in diagnostic tests for women.

Studies were done on the assumption that only men developed heart disease. These included the 1982 Multiple Risk Factor Intervention Trial, aptly dubbed "Mr. Fit," which looked at lifestyle factors related to cholesterol and heart disease. Later, the Physicians Health Study looked at the preventative powers of aspirin on heart disease in male doctors.

GENDER BIAS AND WOMEN'S HEARTS

"Gender bias" refers to the concern that because it is believed that women are less likely to get heart disease, they are less likely to be properly treated.

WHAT IS CORONARY HEART DISEASE?

Although all types of heart problems are encompassed in the umbrella term of "heart disease," it is coronary heart disease that leads most often to heart attack and death. A heart attack is usually the result of a disease process known as atherosclerosis, which causes the coronary arteries to become narrowed and clogged, shutting off the vital blood supply to the heart.

As we age, our risk of heart disease rises. As women, though, we are generally diagnosed with heart disease 10 to 15 years later than men, when we're in our 1950s and 1960s. This difference, known as "gender protection," is ascribed to estrogen, the so-called female sex hormone.

FAMILY MEDICAL HISTORY

Your risk of heart disease is increased if you have a parent who developed early-onset heart disease. This refers to fathers who developed heart disease before the age of 55 or mothers before age 65. The more close relatives you have with early-onset heart disease, the greater the possibility of this genetic link.

RACE Heart disease is the biggest killer of American women, no matter what their race or ethnicity. However, more African-American women develop it at a younger age, most likely because they develop high blood pressure, diabetes, and high cholesterol earlier as well.

HIGH BLOOD PRESSURE After the age of 50, women develop high blood pressure, or hypertension, twice as often as do men. High blood pressure usually occurs in the absence of symptoms and can cause damage years before being diagnosed.

DIABETES Diabetes, a metabolic disorder, is a powerful risk factor that erases a woman's normal gender protection, meaning she may develop heart disease earlier. Diabetes also causes neuropathy, a nerve disorder that can mask symptoms of chest pain, so a diabetic may not recognize this key warning sign of an impending heart attack.

HIGH CHOLESTEROL When it comes to coronary heart disease, there are three types of lipoproteins that are emphasized. Low-density lipoprotein, or LDL, cholesterol, is the so-called bad cholesterol that builds up within the walls of coronary arteries. Triglycerides are another important type and contain most of the fats in the blood. These are the two types of lipoproteins that contribute to coronary heart disease. A third type of cholesterol, high-density cholesterol, or HDL cholesterol, is known as good cholesterol because it blocks the accumulation of LDL cholesterol by transferring it away from the arteries.

Prior to menopause, women tend to have high levels of the beneficial HDL, cholesterol, so it's not enough to focus on your total cholesterol number. Women need to have their total cholesterol profile done to compare the ratio of the HDL cholesterol to LDL cholesterol and triglycerides.

Traditionally, cholesterol screening has involved just checking these three lipid levels. However, up to half of those who suffer heart attacks have normal cholesterol levels. Because of this, research is ongoing into more than a dozen more cholesterol patterns to learn how the molecules that make up these cholesterol patterns are arranged. Currently, most interest centers on three patterns: LDL pattern A, lipoprotein (a), and LDL pattern B. If you come from a family with a history of heart disease but not high cholesterol, you might want to ask your doctor about being tested for these additional patterns.

SMOKING Female smokers have nearly double the heart attack rate and are more likely to suffer from advanced heart disease than nonsmokers. Smoking also has been found to contribute to the development of heart disease earlier. Even smoking just four cigarettes a day increases heart disease risk. Also, although oral contraceptives alone do not cause heart attacks in women under the age of 35, they do increase the risk for women over that age.

OBESITY Weighing 20 percent or more than ideal increases the probability of coronary heart disease, although the telling factor seems to be in what manner the excess weight is distributed. The risk is higher for women who are "apple"-shaped, women who accumulate excess weight in their stomach, than for those who are "pear"-shaped and carry the excess weight in their hips.

INACTIVITY In the past, being inactive has been associated with heart disease because, if you're inactive, it is more likely you'll develop other risk factors, such as high blood pressure and diabetes. But studies have found that, even in the absence of these other risk factors, being inactive increases the risk of heart disease.

EMERGING RISK FACTORS

HOMOCYSTEINE Homocysteine, an amino acid in the blood, can build up, damage the coronary arteries, and set the stage for coronary heart disease. Not all studies have linked homocysteine risk with increased heart disease, leading to speculation that the amino acid may not be the risk factor but only a marker —the culprit may possibly be low levels of B vitamins.

There is a blood test you can take to check your homocysteine level, but because all the research isn't yet in, it isn't generally recommended. However, if hyperhomocysteinemia, a rare genetic condition that causes too-high homocysteine levels, runs in your family, or if you have family members who developed heart disease in the absence of other risk factors, ask your doctor about it.

STRESS Exactly how stress harms our coronary arteries isn't fully understood, but it is apparently related to the physiological changes that occur. When we are under stress, our nervous system releases hormones that cause our coronary blood vessels to constrict, and our heart rate to increase and even the cells that line our blood vessels to undergo changes.

DEPRESSION Several studies find that clinical depression, the type of hopeless despair that is impossible to shake, may increase heart disease risk.

HOW WOMEN CAN PREVENT HEART DISEASE

QUIT SMOKING Once you quit smoking, your risk of suffering a heart attack immediately diminishes; some studies show that you can decrease the added risk by up to 70 percent.

LOSE WEIGHT If you're overweight, losing weight will reduce your risk. If you're very overweight, you don't necessarily need to lose all those pounds. Research finds that even a modest weight loss 5 to 10 percent of body weight—can significantly lower your heart disease risk.

EAT SMART The American Heart Association recommends that you get no more than 30 percent of daily calories from fat. Saturated fat, which generally comes from animal products, raises blood cholesterol more than any other type, so you should eat no more than 10 percent within that 30 percent figure. Instead, choose liquid vegetable fats, such olive oil.

The possibility that vitamins may help prevent heart disease is a tantalizing one, and the research involving the antioxidant vitamin E is the most hopeful. But not all the research has been consistent.

EXERCISE REGULARLY Regular exercise, such as brisk walking, aerobics, biking, or other types that raise your heart rate for at least 30 minutes three times a week, helps to prevent heart disease. When you exercise, you burn calories, which helps control weight. This, in turn, helps prevent high blood pressure. Exercise also helps you metabolize glucose more efficiently, reduce the risk of diabetes, and improve cholesterol levels.

CONSIDER HORMONE REPLACEMENT THERAPY Numerous studies demonstrate that women who take estrogen after menopause have about a 40 percent decreased risk of heart disease. Estrogen appears to lower heart disease risk in three ways. First, estrogen modulates the manufacturing of cholesterol in the liver, lowering the amounts of the "bad" LDL cholesterol while boosting the production of plaque-fighting HDL cholesterol by up to 20 percent. In addition, estrogen helps keep the blood vessels smooth, elastic, and flexible. Furthermore, estrogen lowers blood levels of fibrinogen, a substance involved in the formation of blood clots that can cause heart attacks. Most of the studies showing this benefit have been done using estrogen alone, known as estrogen replacement therapy (ERT).

In recent years, a new type of hormone replacement, selective estrogen receptor modulators, or SERMs, has developed. They are designed to protect against osteoporosis and heart disease without increasing cancer risk. The first of these drugs, raloxifene (Evista) was approved in 1996. A 1998 study in the *Journal of the American Medical Association* found that, although raloxifene does increase bone density, its ability to prevent coronary heart disease risk is not as strong.

Although the benefits of estrogen are well-documented, not all the answers are in. Most of the studies have been observational ones, and more randomized studies, where some women are put on hormones and others take a placebo, need to be done. Also, although many doctors advocate hormone replacement therapy, there are also nondrug alternatives to reduce the risk of heart disease, including losing weight, diet, and exercise.

HEART ATTACKS IN WOMEN You're probably aware that chest pain is often a warning sign of an impending heart attack. However, this appears to be less true for women. Although some women do suffer chest pain, it is often more subtle and is better characterized as discomfort. Also, unlike chest pain in men, which is acute, such discomfort in women can last for hours. In addition, women may more typically suffer pain elsewhere, like the jaw, back, or even the stomach, as well as symptoms such as shortness of breath, fatigue or weakness, nausea, dizziness, or indigestion.

DIAGNOSING HEART DISEASE IN WOMEN

When it comes to heart disease, women are at a disadvantage because heart disease is more difficult to diagnose. First, heart disease symptoms in women are more subtle and because, when women are younger, they are more likely than men to experience chest pain from nonheart-related causes, such as muscle pain, gallbladder disease, heartburn, and even anxiety.

Another problem is that the most common test for coronary heart disease, known as exercise stress testing, or sometimes treadmill testing, is more accurate when used on men. In women, however, this test too often results in a "false positive" reading that indicates heart disease is present when none exists.

Although this test is not adequate for screening, there are tests that are used to investigate the possibility of heart disease in women who are experiencing symptoms. One technique is to improve the accuracy of this test by combining it with an imaging agent that also provides pictures of the blood flow to the heart. Another alternative is to combine the exercise stress test with echocardiogram that furnishes ultrasound images of the heart.

Women are not referred as often as men for diagnostic tests. This is a particular concern relating to the test known as cardiac arteriography, or cardiac catheterization. This test is required in deciding such interventional techniques as balloon angioplasty and coronary bypass surgery should be considered.

TREATING HEART DISEASE IN WOMEN

Treating coronary heart disease usually involves ways to widen arteries narrowed by atherosclerosis to result in more blood to the heart and prevent heart attack. The main techniques to do this are percutaneous transluminal coronary angioplasty, commonly known as balloon angioplasty and coronary artery bypass grafting, or bypass surgery. In both of these areas, statistics show that women are far less likely to be offered these treatments.

In balloon angioplasty, a catheter-tipped balloon is used to widen the narrowed coronary arteries. Because this technique can replace the need for open-heart surgery, it's not surprising that it is extremely popular. But, according to the American Heart Association's latest figures, only one-third of the 482,000 angioplasties done annually are performed on women. This may be in part because, years ago, when this technique was first devised, it was riskier in women because the instruments used were too large for a woman's more delicate arteries. However, this is no longer true; studies show this is a safe and effective technique for women. Bypass surgery is open-heart surgery performed to reroute, or "bypass," blood around clogged arteries and improve the supply of blood and oxygen to the heart. According to the American Heart Association's most recent figures, only 29 percent of the 598,000 surgeries were done on women. This may be due to the fact that although bypass surgery is safe and effective, it is riskier for women. This is usually attributed to the fact that women have smaller, delicate arteries that make the surgery more technically difficult. Minimally invasive bypass surgery, a new technique that minimize the trauma to the body of bypass surgery, is raising great interest. There are two approaches commonly used: port-access coronary artery bypass, also referred to as PACAB or PortCAB, and minimally invasive coronary artery bypass (also called MinCAB). But research needs to be done to learn what extent this will prove as an alternative to traditional bypass surgery. Rarely, the heart is so weakened as to require a heart transplant. Although an estimated 40,000 individuals could benefit from transplants, the most recent figures show that only 2,290 were done and, of those, only about 25 percent were done on women.

Chapter 59

Breasts

The Anatomy of Your Breasts

MARVIN S. EIGER AND SALLY WENDKOS OLDS

Excerpted from Marvin S. Eiger and Sally Wendkos Olds, *The Complete Book of Breastfeeding*, 3d ed., New York, Workman, 1999. Originally published in 1972. Reprinted by permission.

No matter what the size and shape of your breasts, you can have a gratifying breast-feeding experience. Whether your breasts are broad or narrow, high or sloping, small or large, you can happily nurse your baby. Just as women differ in height, general body build, and facial characteristics, they very considerably with regard to the size and shape of their breasts. Furthermore, most women have one breast that's larger than the other. None of these characteristics are important for feeding a baby.

This is because the milk-producing glands are just one of the four types of tissue that make up the breasts. These four types are the *glands* that secrete milk, the *ducts* that carry it, the *connective tissue* that supports and attaches the breasts to the muscles of the chest, and the *fatty tissue* that encases and protects these other structures.

The size of your breasts is determined by the amount of fatty tissue they contain, and since the only purpose of this tissue is to encase and protect the more functional elements, it has no bearing at all on your ability to produce and give milk. You can be an excellent breast-feeder no matter what the size or shape of your breasts.

THE NIPPLE

Let's look at the breasts with a baby's-eye view. The nipple is the handle by which the infant grabs hold of the breast and also the spout through which she receives her milk.

The size of the nipple is usually as unimportant for nursing as is the size of the breast itself. Nipples come in different shapes. They are cylindrical in some women and conical in others.

The nipples of some women look flat or folded in and do not become erect when cold or when stimulated. Most often, however, by the end of pregnancy such "pseudo-inverted" nipples protrude normally and come out fully when the baby starts to suckle. In very rare cases, a woman has truly inverted nipples, which do not protrude enough for the baby's mouth to grasp them and which do not protrude with the baby's suckling. Fortunately, this condition is almost always correctable during pregnancy.

You have probably noticed that your nipples become erect when they're cold or when you become sexually excited. The erect nipple becomes two to three times longer than in its softer state. The same thing will happen when your baby nurses.

Each of your nipples has 15 to 20 tiny openings through which milk is excreted. As the nursing baby stimulates the many nerve endings in the nipple, this causes uterine contractions that help return the uterus to its prepregnancy size.

THE AREOLA

Surrounding the nipple is a darker-colored circle called the *areola*. In most women the areola is between 1 and 2 inches in diameter, but it can be considerably larger. The areola and nipple are darker than the rest of the breast, ranging from a light pink in very fair-skinned women to a very dark brown in others.

The areolar pigmentation deepens in pregnancy and remains darker during lactation, after which the color fades somewhat; it never reverts, however, to the lighter shade it was before pregnancy. (This is one way doctors sometimes determine whether a woman has ever borne a child.) The darker color of the areola may be some sort of visual signal to newborns, since they must close their mouths upon the areola, not upon the nipple alone, if they are to obtain milk.

You may have noticed little bumps on your areola. These are called *Montgomery's glands*. They become enlarged and quite noticeable during pregnancy and lactation, because they secrete a substance that cleanses, lubricates, and protects the nipple during nursing. The antibacterial properties in this substance also help to prevent infection in both mother and baby. After lactation, these glands recede to their former unobtrusive state.

HOW YOUR BODY MAKES MILK

Directly beneath and behind your areola is a group of *milk pools* (known scientifically as *lactiferous sinuses*). These pools are widened parts of the milk-carrying canals (*lactiferous ducts*), which transport the milk from the place in the breast where it is made to the nipples, where your baby can obtain it.

Each of your breasts has from 15 to 20 ducts, each of which ends at the tip of the nipple. These ducts branch off into smaller canals within the breast toward the chest wall; these canals are called *ductules* . At the end of each ductule is a grapelike cluster of tiny rounded sacs called *alveoli*. The milk is made in these alveoli. Each cluster of alveoli is referred to as a *lobule* (a small rounded complex); a cluster of lobules is called a *lobe*. The lobes, each of which is a miniature gland, are situated at the base of the breast next to the chest wall. There are from 15 to 20 lobes in each breast, each lobe connected to one duct, each duct emptying into one nipple opening, or milk pore.

Both the ducts and the alveoli are covered with smooth-muscle cells. Under the influence of the hormone *oxytocin* (more later about this important hormone), these smooth-muscle cells squeeze the milk out from the alveoli into the duct system. Then the cells in the alveoli burst and extrude fat cells to form the *hind milk* (the fatty milk released at the end of a feeding session).

THE SUPPORTING STRUCTURE

In some cultures, women deliberately pull at their breasts to make them longer so that it will be easier to nurse a baby strapped to their backs. Since this is probably not your aim, you'll want to give your breasts as much support as possible.

Nature provides some support—through the muscles attached to the ribs, the collarbone, and the bones of the upper arm near the shoulder. You can help Mother Nature along by wearing a good, supportive bra, even during sleep, during the latter part of your pregnancy and during lactation.

Although wearing a bra or going without one has no effect at all upon the breast-feeding function, the force of gravity will tend to pull down the heavier breasts of the pregnant or nursing woman. A supportive bra helps to prevent undue stretching of the suspensory ligaments of the upper part of the breast. Some doctors feels that a woman whose breasts are wide at the base will retain her figure whether or not she wears a bra.

THE LET-DOWN REFLEX: HOW YOUR BABY GETS YOUR MILK

When your *let-down reflex* is operating well, you are overjoyed, not "let down" in the sense of feeling disappointed. Also known as the *milk-ejection reflex*

(*MER*) and, in England, the "draught" (pronounced "draft"), the let-down reflex lets down your milk from your breast to your baby. The let-down reflex is automatic, and in almost all cases it does operate well, as it has for millions of years for almost all women (see below).

In the early stage of lactation, it takes anywhere form several seconds to several minutes of your baby's suckling to produce a let-down reflex. After lactation is well established, you may find that hearing your baby cry or even just thinking about your baby will bring it on....

As your baby suckles, she stimulates thc nerve endings in your nipples, which then send signals to your pituitary gland, directing it to produce more of the hormone prolactin. The prolactin stimulates the alveoli to produce milk. As long as your breasts are suckled or otherwise stimulated (as with a breast pump or with manual manipulation), they will continue to make milk.

Your baby's suckling also causes your pituitary to release oxytocin, another very important hormone for lactation. Oxytocin travels through your bloodstream to your breast, where it causes the smooth-muscle cells surrounding the alveoli to contract. As they contract, they squeeze the milk from the alveoli into the ducts. The walls of the ducts also contract, sending the milk out to the milk pools beneath the areolae.

While prolactin makes the milk, oxytocin makes it available to your baby. Animal research suggests that oxytocin also plays a part in stimulating the release of prolactin. In addition, oxytocin released into the brain promotes calming and positive social behaviors. Oxytocin has been called "the quintessential mammalian hormone," "the satisfactional hormone," and the "hormone of love." Besides its role in fostering bonds between parents and offspring, it also causes the uterus to contract during childbirth, orgasm, and lactation.

The Renaissance artist Jacopo Tintoretto portrayed a beautiful representation of the let-down reflex in his work *The Origin of the Milky Way*. The painting tells the story of Hercules, Zeus's son by a mortal woman, whom Zeus put to the breast of the sleeping goddess Hera to make him immortal. After the infant had stopped drinking of Hera's milk, the milk continued to flow from the goddess's breasts. Some went up into the sky, forming the galaxy, and the rest dropped on the ground, forming a garden of lilies.

The British scientist S. J. Folley points out that this picture illustrates two important attributes of the milk-ejection reflex: first, that the stimulus of suckling creates an increased pressure of the milk inside the breasts, causing it to spurt from the nipples, a second, that even though only one breast may be suckled, milk will flow from both.

Although the let-down reflex operates like a clockwork in almost all women, occasionally some women need a little help to "oil the mechanism." Problems with let-down can usually be resolved quite easily. The let-down reflex has a strong psychological basis. The pituitary gland, which controls the release of oxytocin, is itself controlled by the *hypothalamus*. This walnut-sized organ in the brain is often referred to as the "seat of emotion," since it receives messages about the individual's psychological state and, acting on these messages, sends it s own orders to the glands, translating emotions into physiological reactions. The emotions, therefore, exert a powerful influence on such hormone-regulated functions as the menstrual cycle, childbirth, and lactation.

When you have the confidence that you will have milk for your baby, even major stresses like war or natural disasters will not dam up the flow. But when you live in a society like ours, in which women often worry about their ability to provide milk, the slightest of emotions can interfere with your milk production. Pain, embarrassment, fear, fatigue, illness, or distraction can inhibit the let-down reflex and hold your milk back from your baby. If your nipples hurt you, your let-down may not work right. If you are distressed by the disparaging remarks of relatives and friends, your let-down may let you down. If you overtire yourself, don't eat properly, don't respect your own needs for privacy and for relaxation, your let-down reflex may be affected.

SIGNS OF AN ACTIVE LET-DOWN REFLEX

Some of the most common signs that your let-down reflex is functioning are:

➤ A tingling sensation in your breasts
➤ A feeling of warmth and/or fullness in your breasts
➤ Dripping of milk before your baby starts to nurse
➤ Release of milk from the nipple other than the one your baby is sucking
➤ Cramps caused by the contractions of your uterus
➤ The relief of nipple or breast discomfort as your baby nurses

Some women with very powerful let-down do not experience many of these sensations, and some feel a brief period of pain in the early days when their milk lets down. Another way to check your let-down reflex is to look at your baby for signs of active swallowing; if she's swallowing, you're getting milk to her!

Breast-Feeding Revisited

MARGOT SLADE

Margot Slade, "Breastfeeding Revisited," *Child,* September 1998. Reprinted by permission.

When the American Academy of Pediatrics gave its definitive word [in 1997] on how long women should breast-feed, the message was hardly aimed at undermining American mothers.

But that's precisely the way many people interpreted the statement, which recommended that women nurse their children for a minimum of one year, preferably well into the second year of life.

"That sounds like a long time to me!" says Julie O'Shea, a mother of two and an attorney in New York City. O'Shea took pride in the fact that she had surpassed the AAP's earlier recommendation that mothers breast-feed for at least six months and ideally for a year after a child's birth.

Heather King, a regional trainer for Home Box Office in Amesbury, Massachusetts, considers herself a breast-feeding devotee, but she didn't reach the one-year mark with any of her three children. "I could see how some women could freak. A new mom might say, 'I can't make it through a full year, so why do it at all?'"

Interestingly, the AAP statement that shook up so many women was directed at a different audience. It was part of a larger paper, printed in a pediatric medical journal, that documented newfound benefits of breast-feeding and outlined the vital supporting role pediatricians can play in the lives of nursing women.

"Rather than put pressure on women, we hoped our recommendation would give them a mandate to breast-feed by showing there are reasons to do it for a few days, a few weeks, and even beyond a year," says Ruth Lawrence, M.D., a professor of pediatrics and obstetrics and gynecology at the University of Rochester School of Medicine in Rochester, New York, who worked on the AAP policy statement.

The AAP revised its recommendation in response to growing proof that the benefits of nursing are cumulative. That is, the incidence of disease decreases among women the longer they breast-feed and among children the longer they are breast-fed. The more time a woman devoted to breast-feeding over her life, the less her risk of breast cancer, osteoporosis, hip fractures, and ovarian cancer, according to Lawrence M. Gartner, M.D., a professor of pediatrics and obstetrics/gynecology at the University of Chicago and head of the AAP's breast-feeding policy committee.

Benefits for kinds include lower risk of ear infections, digestive problems, some cancers, and chronic illnesses like asthma and juvenile diabetes, and possibly better intellectual performance.

An equally important part of the AAP recommendation—one that many overlooked—is the qualification that nursing should continue *as long as the mother and infant desire.* And part of the problem with breast-feeding in this country is that what mother and child want has long been beside the point.

On one side of the issue have been breast-feeding proponents so ardent that, mothers complain, they care only that women nurse, regardless of overriding health concerns or personal issues. "Women call me in tears and in pain, asking for permission to stop," says Fern Drillings, a lactation consultant in New York City. "They're having a bad time, but to quit would seem like they failed."

On the other side, women say, are individuals and institutions who don't necessarily oppose breast-feeding but don't support it either. Among them are mothers and in-laws who harp on the fact that "we bottle-fed our children and they turned out just fine" and employers who make provisions for smoking and coffee breaks but not for pumping milk.

AMERICANS LAG IN BREAST-FEEDING

This combination of pressure on mothers has left the United States lagging behind when it comes to breast-feeding. In 1997, studies found that America had one of the lowest breast-feeding rates and one of the highest infant mortality rates in the developed world.

In 1995, the AAP reported that 59 percent of women in the United States were breast-feeding exclusively or in combination with formula at the time of hospital discharge. At six months postpartum, only 22 percent of mothers were still nursing.

Though breast-feeding rates in the United States are up (only 23 percent of new moms nursed in 1970), experts attribute the comparatively low rate to the following factors: the continued increase in the number of women in the workforce, the lack of support for the practice from employers, physician apathy, lack of prenatal education, and the aggressive promotion of infant formula through hospitals and advertising.

It hasn't helped breast-feeding's cause that many people still consider the practice to be vulgar, even obscene. In 1996, Dina Tantimonaco was nursing her infant daughter in her car in the rear parking lot of a Connecticut restaurant when a policeman said he'd charge her with breach of peace if anyone complained. But it was Tantimonaco who did the complaining, eventually leading state legislators to pass a law that "no person may restrict or limit the right of a mother to breast-feed her child."

Similar laws have been enacted in 16 states, and more have bills pending, according to Elizabeth N. Baldwin, a legal adviser to La Leche League International, based in Schaumburg, Illinois. "These laws clarify that breast-feeding is not criminal and that women have the right to nurse anyplace they have the right to be with their baby," she says.

BIGGER ROLE FOR PEDIATRICIANS

If more women are going to meet the AAP's minimum one-year recommendation, it will take more than laws that, in effect, decriminalize breast-feeding. It will take proactive support, starting with the medical community.

"Our new recommendations state that a woman's ability to breastfeed is intimately linked to a child's health, and that it is therefore up to pediatricians to learn about breastfeeding so we can encourage mothers to nurse their children and to do so longer," says Dr. Gartner.

This doesn't mean pediatricians will become lactation experts. "I'd rather have a pediatrician who can deal expertly with my kids' asthma," says Ellen Kadden, an international board-certified lactation consultant in Fairfield, Connecticut. "But the pediatrician should be able to tell me where to go for lactation expertise or provide such expertise through his or her office," she adds.

Kadden advises women to beware of pediatricians who seem uncomfortable watching women breast-feed or who recommend formula as a supplement too soon when a breast-feeding problem arises.

WHAT NURSING LONGER MEANS FOR MOMS

Certainly, the AAP's intention is not to make mothers nurse out of guilt. But the academy's statement regarding the benefits of breast milk makes the argument in favor of nursing more compelling than before, Drillings says.

Nursing women tend to agree. Kathy Hayden, mother of an 18-month-old in Detroit, says nursing through a child's second year is probably impractical for a lot of women, "but the AAP information makes a strong statement about nursing as long as you can."

What would help ease the way for women who want to nurse is realistic information about what breast-feeding will entail, say lactation consultants, especially when a mother also wants to resume some of her prebaby activities.

Drillings, who breast-fed her son for 14 months, explains that how much a nursing mother needs to adjust her behavior depends on what her lifestyle was like before she became pregnant.

"For example, I always ate healthfully, so that wasn't a concern," Drillings says. Nor was she chronically ill or on medication—factors that can affect how long, if at all, a mother can nurse. And when she went to a wedding and drank a lot of wine? "I pumped when I got home and tossed out the milk," she says.

Women should also keep in mind that nursing isn't an all-or-nothing proposition. A mother can breast-feed in the morning and evening and pump during the day so that her child is bottle-fed breast milk in her absence. Heather King altered her routine from full-time nursing during her 12-week maternity leave, to part-time nursing and pumping at work, to eventually nursing only at night and supplementing with formula during the day.

Susan Danaher, a senior vice president at MTV Networks in Los Angeles, breast-fed each of her two children for eight weeks. "I couldn't see continuing in the context of my schedule," she says. Rather than offer apologies, Danaher focuses on the benefits her kids reaped from when they were breast-fed.

MORE SUPPORT FOR NURSING ON THE JOB

The new recommendations on breast-feeding have particular significance when it comes to the workplace, where obstacles and negative attitudes toward the practice are legion.

"But demographics are destiny," says Ellen Galinsky, president of the Families and Work Institute in New York City, noting that the American workforce is now 48 percent female. "So-called female issues like breast-feeding are becoming work issues that employers dare not ignore," she states.

Supporting mothers who breast-feed isn't just socially responsible, it's smart business. Data show that because breast-fed babies are less likely to get sick, absenteeism among mothers and general health care costs can decline. Companies that offer lactation support—and this can be simply a quiet, comfortable space in which women can privately express milk—have reported reductions in turnover and in the loss of workers who decide not to return from maternity leave.

Congresswoman Carolyn Maloney, Democrat of New York, is trying to foster more corporate support through legislation making clear that the Pregnancy Discrimination Act of 1978 covers breast-feeding and related activities on the job. Among other provisions, the law would give tax credits to companies that set up lactation facilities and would ensure that nursing mothers be given a year's worth of "milk breaks"—up to an hour a day to nurse or pump.

The message that must be spread is that "breast-feeding is the right thing to do and makes sense from a societal perspective," says Rona Cohen, M.N., head of the Los Angeles Department of Water and Power's lactation program, perhaps the oldest and most comprehensive of its kind in the country.

"How parents feed their babies should be their choice," Cohen says. "It is up to corporations, doctors, health professionals, family, and friends to offer mothers accurate information and options so they can make informed decisions about what is right for them."

Anne Kasper

INTERVIEW BY TANIA KETENJIAN

Anne S. Kasper, Ph.D. is a senior research scientist at the Center for Research on Women and Gender at the University of Illinois at Chicago and the coeditor of *Breast Cancer: Society Constructs an Epidemic.* This interview was conducted in April 1999.

TK: In Rose Kushner's book entitled *Why Me?*, she raises some serious issues about breast cancer and its effects on feminine identity. How do you think these issues manifested in her? How did her cancer affect her identity as a woman and as a person?

AK: Having breast cancer totally fired her up to be a public advocate on behalf of women with breast cancer and, in fact, I think it's reasonable to say that she was the first breast cancer advocate.

TK: After her mastectomy, Rose decided to get breast implants, and unfortunately they burst. What do you think led her to make that decision?

AK: Don't forget that at the time that Rose Kushner had breast cancer, and it's still true today, physicians would tell women that they really wouldn't be able to recover, appropriately return to normal, feel like themselves as women, so forth and so on, without breast reconstruction or breast implants. Although we know that it's not part of breast cancer treatment per se, it's often billed as such and it was probably even more so when Rose was diagnosed. Also, don't forget that these were basically prefeminist days when not only women took seriously everything their doctors told them, but a lot of women were still subjected to pretty precise oppressive and finite definitions of what it meant to be a woman. Today, it's a different story. There are lots of ways to be a woman. Even though doctors today will frequently tell women that they must have breast implants or breast reconstruction to return to normal or feel like a woman, a lot of women today have their own definitions about what it means to be a woman and will reject that outright or simply say, "Yeah, sure, I mean I'm interested in breast reconstruction, but that's not what's going to make me feel like a woman again."

TK: How did Rose's personality incorporate itself into her cause. Did she already have activist tendencies?

AK: Yes, she did. She told me this wonderful story about when she was a little girl, it was during the Depression, and her parents had been small-shop owners in Baltimore and I think they both died within a few years of each other when she was very young and she was sent to live with some aunts. She remembered social workers coming every Saturday with bags of clothing and food for the family because everybody was suffering at the time, unless they were very well-to-do, and Rose Kushner's family was not. She remembered these social workers very vividly, and she said that what she was doing was being a social worker on behalf of breast cancer. For her, it was a way of repaying the care and kindness that she had as a young child from these social workers. Much of what she did was in fact a form of social work in the arena of breast cancer.

TK: You mentioned the reaction of women toward doctors, their seemingly unrelenting trust, prior to the movement. How did Rose Kushner's reactions to doctors reflect the sentiments of the women of her time? She seemed to be constantly challenging her doctors and yet at the same time she did feel a kind of safety with them....

AK: I think you hit the nail on the head. She was very assertive and even aggressive and her feelings were so strong on this subject that even as she put a lot of faith in her doctors—which was pretty much the rule at the time, you don't question your doctors, you put your health in their hands—she was also willing to challenge them up to a point, even challenge prevailing medical notions. That was how she came to fight for other women in the women's health movement around the issue of DES, because she believed that her breast cancer was a direct result of her taking DES when she was pregnant with her children. In the 1940s, 1950s, and 1960s, doctors told women that DES was perfectly safe for use in pregnancy. But Rose came to the conclusion that it was anything but, that in fact it had caused her breast cancer, and this led to her subsequent role as a breast cancer advocate. So there were lots of places where she stood up and said, "Wait a minute, guys, this isn't right."

A classic example of what we owe her—the one she's best known for—involves the fact that when women receive a biopsy and the diagnosis is positive, they now have the option to go home and think about this and meet with their doctors or read up and become informed and begin to make some choices that are consonant with their needs and desires. Whereas, in the past when women were biopsied and it was positive, right there on the operating room table their breasts were taken off. She said, "This is just appalling. You doctors can't continue doing this kind of thing. Women need to have some say in it. We know that timely breast cancer treatment is important, but there's nothing to indicate that a woman can't go home for a week, two weeks, a month and make decisions that are consonant with her well-being before she has a mastectomy." And we really owe that to Rose Kushner, she made clear not only that it was important for women's well-being, but that it wasn't in any way going to impair their health any further. And it really changed medical practice.

TK: What do you think of early-detection claims? Do you think it has improved survival rates?

AK: Well, I certainly don't think it's all that it's been touted to be by any stretch of the imagination and I'm very disturbed that a lot of women think not only that early detection is the be-all and end-all, but also that it's entirely in their hands—that they are somehow responsible for this early detection, and that if they don't find anything and then get breast cancer, it's all their fault. If only they had been more diligent in practicing breast self-examination for however long, they might have found this breast cancer and now they wouldn't be "victimized" by this disease. Another thing that really disturbs me is that we have been so overly diligent about the message of early detection that we have actually cast it as a preventative, so there are women who actually believe that early detection is prevention. And no small wonder—essentially that's the message, hidden or overt, of many of our public education messages about breast cancer. During my research for my current study of poor and low-income women with breast cancer, people in Chicago told me they were really puzzled when they noted a lot of young Latina women coming to breast cancer screening clinics or other clinics asking for mammograms. These women were 17, 18, 19. After a while the clinics asked them, "Why are you here? You're basically too young to have breast cancer. Why are you requesting mammograms?" Many of these women were recent immigrants to this country and perhaps they weren't fully acculturated yet. They answered, "We understand that a mammogram prevents breast cancer. I'm here to have my mammogram, so that I won't come down with breast cancer." That's really an overzealous message.

TK: Since we don't know exactly how many women die of breast cancer, can the statistics be accurate?

AK: There are a certain number of women, perhaps older women, who are diagnosed who will not die from breast cancer because, especially in older women, it's much more slow-growing. As a result the curative rate, or the success rate in treating breast cancer, or maybe even preventing it, has been exaggerated. A lot of women who get breast cancer don't get treated or even diagnosed with breast cancer, and they don't die from it, they die of something else—heart attack, stroke, or any other disease. I don't know the accurate statistics in breast cancer and I don't know if anybody does. One thing that concerns me about poor and low-income women is that they present with much more advanced disease and their survival rate is much lower than for low- and middle-class women. I often wonder if there are women out there who literally don't get seen and don't get treated for their breast cancer and who wind up dying of something else. Since an autopsy is never done, we just don't know if it was breast cancer that killed them or if it was something else. I honestly don't know what the accurate statistics on breast cancer would look like even if we were able to collect them, and I certainly don't think anybody is collecting really accurate ones. I think part of the problem is that the National Cancer Institute has a vested interest in collecting statistics that reflect well on this so-called war on cancer.

TK: Let's talk about the war on cancer. Some say that many latter-day activists don't attribute the fight against cancer to Rose. They attribute their fame and in part the strength of their cause to AIDS groups.

AK: I think the difference is that AIDS had a lot of visibility, in part because at the time there was no chance of a cure—everybody would die—so it had an element of drama that breast cancer and other diseases didn't have. And we mustn't forget that the majority of people with AIDS in the early days were men, and you know men are the power holders. Many who became AIDS activists became easily vocal and powerful because power came naturally to them as men. The breast cancer movement certainly learned something from the AIDS movement, but it also was a natural consequence of the women's health movement that had developed in the late sixties and early seventies, and like a lot of things it just took its time to coalesce. I think we have ignored the fact, to some degree, that Rose Kushner played a pivotal role in the formation of the breast cancer movement. Some attention has been paid to her but certainly not enough. The other problem is that Rose died at a time when there was a mainstream resurgence of the women's health movement. During this so-called rebirth in the early 1990s, when it gained a lot of popularity, a lot of people claimed that they had just simply invented it—the drug companies, high-powered women in Washington, or other people who thought this women's health stuff was their creation. Not only was the previous women's health movement instantly erased, but so was Rose Kushner.

TK: How important was Rose's husband Harvey, not only as a partner but also as an affluent companion who could support her?

AK: Harvey was very supportive of her work with breast cancer; he really stood by her. I imagine it couldn't have always been easy because she ate, slept, drank, breathed the thing.

TK: Can you tell me about your own research?

AK: I have a Ph.D. in sociology and a masters in women's studies, and I've been a member of the women's health movement for more than 20 years. My doctoral dissertation was a study of middle-class women who'd had breast cancer. I wanted to understand how they coped with that diagnosis. My current study, which is funded by a federal agency that's part of the public health service, is a study of poor and low-income women with breast cancer. My basic question is: Is breast cancer different for poor and low-income women than for other women? The unequivical answer is yes, it certainly is. There are lots of social factors in these women's lives which have deep and abiding consequences for their health and their survival from breast cancer.

TK: How do you feel Rose influenced you?

AK: I think there's a little bit of the social worker in me just like there was in Rose. Her passion was very visible and moving, and I think it was infectious. I think my own activism predates knowing Rose, but there's no question that because she lived in the same city—and would drive me crazy with phone calls at midnight—she was influential. I know she had a reputation for being very aggressive and very assertive and she was going to do something about breast cancer if it was the last damn thing she ever did. And in fact she did. She did leave this quite remakable legacy, but while she was alive she was quite rampant about it and I think she infected me with a bit of her passion and her deep concern for women with breast cancer. When I was defending my doctoral dissertation in 1988, at the end I said very nervously to all the professors sitting in the room that I thought breast cancer had such power to it as an issue that soon it would have a political movement of its own, in some degree like the AIDS movement. And I was right. So Rose Kushner was a major influence on me, and I am sure far beyond me.

The Oral History of Rose Kushner

INTERVIEW BY ANNE KASPER

Excerpted from Anne Kasper, "The Oral History of Rose Kushner," for the Schlesinger Library of Women's History, Radcliffe College, April 1983.

RK: My major interest since 1979 when I was on the NIH Consensus Development Conference that recommended the two-stage proceeding… has been to do something in that period between the biopsy and mastectomy or whatever is done—I call it the definitive treatment—to tell women about the availability of options in primary treatment.

The big area where there is a huge information gap is in the newly diagnosed woman. Now let me add that it's also the newly diagnosed cancer patient, period. But I am sticking to breast cancer because that is, as they told me on the board, my "organ site." So, I see no point in giving a woman two weeks between diagnoses and treatment if all she is going to during those two weeks is sit and sweat.

And I consider and have always considered the giving of information to be the first step of rehabilitation. I do think the first thing that any agency or individual can do to help newly diagnosed women is to immediately inundate them with things to do—go to the library, read this or that, and let them know—not just think—that they have a finger in choosing their own destinies.

They've got to know. I will refer women to the National Cancer Institute if they are local, where they are doing clinical trials on comparing mastectomy with lumpectomy and radiation because I think that the people there give the most even-handed, balanced presentation of the risks and benefits, the advantages and disadvantages of both forms of treatment. Out in the real world, if a woman goes to a radiation therapist, no matter how much that person may want to be objective, there will be a bias toward radiation therapy and away from surgery. And the same is true of surgeons; no matter how fair they might try to be, they'll be biased in favor of mastectomy because that's what they were trained to do.

And there are disadvantages and risks attached to radiation therapy and these are rarely spelled out—I'm not talking about the long-term risks of radiation. I'm talking about having to take five days off from work to run to the hospital every day for treatment. Not all women can do that or are temperamentally suited to do that. I don't think I could. Of course, there is the worry about the side effects of radiation: burnt lungs, burnt heart, lymphaedema as a result of the radiation burning off the capillaries, and so on.

AK: Go back to the beginning of the Breast Cancer Advisory Center. When that started, how it started, who are the women that you've served in the past, who are you serving now, the mechanics of doing it…

RK: The Breast Cancer Advisory Center was officially incorporated in late 1974, but it did not get rolling until September 1975, when my first book, *Breast Cancer*, was published. It was going to be temporary but it didn't turn out that way. The first people who contacted me were people who heard about the center as I went around promoting the book. Harcourt, Brace, Jovanovich sent me to 16 cities and I had enormous amounts of media coverage—radio, magazines, and newspapers. I never really appreciated their efforts probably until I got hung up with other publishers. And I would always put out the number. At that time, there was no working cancer information center. So, at that time, the Breast Cancer Advisory Center was the only place anybody had to go.

Breast Reduction

MARTA DRURY

© 1999 by Marta Drury. Original for this publication.

I wish I had had my breast reduction surgery when I was 16 years old. In every photograph of me from the age of 11 on, I am wearing an oversized jacket or cardigan—even in the Badlands of South Dakota in sweltering midsummer heat—standing with my arms crossed over my chest. When I graduated from high school, I wore a size 42 DD bra. Now I wear a 38 B.

Thirty-one years later, when I was 47, I was finally ready for the surgery. My mother had recently died, so there was no fear of "offending" her, and I could afford it; I thought it would be considered a "cosmetic" procedure and therefore not covered by insurance, but as it turned out, I was wrong. The surgery would be covered because I had all the classic problems associated with large breasts: forward neck, indentations in my shoulders from the weight of my breasts, tingling and numbness in my arms and hands, and recurring rashes and infections under my breasts.

None of my friends had had breast reduction surgery—or at least none who had talked about it—so I had to do my own research. I interviewed four surgeons. One doctor spent an hour and a half showing me photos and examining me before he told me he wouldn't consider operating unless I lost 50 pounds. But then I met a female surgeon who told me that she liked doing the breast reduction surgery because she had never had a patient who wasn't happy with the results.

Breast reduction surgery is a major operation. It is performed under general anesthesia and requires an overnight stay in the hospital. I have a low tolerance for physical pain, but from the moment I awoke, whatever discomfort I experienced from the incisions and drainage tubes was overshadowed by my delight. I had what I wanted: reasonably sized breasts that looked good. I came through the surgery without any complications, and eventually the sensation in my nipples returned. (I understand that some women lose it.)

Now, nine years later, I have only the scars to remind me of the surgery, and I rather like them—they are like bridges to my past. I feel taller and lighter than before, and finding clothes that fit is no longer a problem. This surgery enabled me to start the process of accepting my body as it is. My only regret is that I didn't do it when I was 16.

Chapter 60

Muscle

Women in Motion

LUCINDA FRANKS

Excerpted from Lucinda Franks, "Women in Motion," in Maggie Tripp, ed., *Woman in the Year 2000*, New York, Arbor, 1974. Reprinted by permission.

Turn your thoughts back about 25 years. When the Total Human had not yet been born and the average body was just a neglected dormitory for the mind. Try to remember those sedentary days when the finely tuned work of art called the human anatomy was pounding and screaming to get out from under dimpled scalloped layers of fat, sagging muscles, and aching bones entering the final and fatal stages of benign neglect. Who would have thought then that society would rediscover a secret as old as civilization, a secret that would intensify a human's joy in life, that would cleanse the brain and turn agitation and unrest into peace of mind.

Now that we are in the Year of Our Lord 2000, with modern technology and a rebirth of the age of reason having joined forces to put a world hurtling toward catastrophe back on course, it is hard to move back in time—to recall a period when there were no integrated golf and baseball teams, when women athletes were not vying for football scholarships, when indeed it was not known that women are capable of being as strong pound for pound as men and, with equally strenuous training, can match or surpass them in many sports.

Lest we forget, however, there *was* a time when Little League and high-school ball teams were all-male, with coaches swearing they'd dynamite the field before letting girls in and actively defying court orders for integration. There *was* a time when women were regarded, in the words of one sports philosopher of the seventies, as "truncated males, which should be permitted to engage in such sports as men do—but in foreshortened versions."

Somewhere around the mid-eighties, sports finally became an "in" thing. Suddenly the concept of sports had changed, and the very word shifted in its connotations. Just as in the seventies good nutrition suddenly became fad-dish with "natural and health foods," so did exercise and games skyrocket in status. They no longer evoked images of smelly locker rooms, tile floors, exhaustion, and former 99-pound weaklings with muscles the size of water-melons. And female athletes all at once were transformed from "Amazon Lesbos" to "goddesses," thanks to the appearance of Billy Jean King and other coolly feminine tennis pros, who started Americans down the road to female sports-star worship.

At the heart of this change was a realization of what coordinated bodily movements, as expressed in a sport, could do for a sense of well-being. The idea was as old as man. The Greeks had known that a sound mind is inside a sound body. People began to examine the generally well-balanced state of mind that many athletes seem to have. Statistics were taken, polls and studies were made, and the reasons were sought. Athletes came forth with personal descriptions of the almost religious feeling that came upon them after they had stretched their bodies to the limit.

It could not be denied that exercise improve clarity of thinking, alertness, ability to absorb complex ideas; it increased blood flow to the brain, strength-ened the cells, and without a doubt acted on the regions of the brain to decrease anxiety and induce confidence and inner harmony.

And then "gamesmanship" was redefined. In the seventies, the need to win, and the need to have one's favorite team win, was crucial—so crucial, in fact, that the means used, the art of the game itself, was secondary. Now the conquering of one's opponent is not the prime mover in games; it is conquering *one's self.*

Both spectators and participants have now come to place less emphasis on winning or losing than on the way the game is played. Older children's games are structured in a way that lets everybody win. The Harris Games, named after Dr. Dorothy V. Harris of Penn State, are designed to reverse two traditional but still disquieting facts about sports: there are many more losers than winners, and the ones who need to win most generally lose. The Harris Games are intri-cately structured so they do not discriminate against the weak, the fat, the clumsy, or the slow. Instead, the complicated series of games favors each play-er and brings out the one particular thing each can do better than anyone else: the fat child wins the game where weight is important; the small boy, where smallness is crucial.

In the old days, people used to pass the time having parties, drinking liquor, and watching television. If they did venture outdoors, it was to rest on park benches and on beaches. Only the kids, sometimes with their fathers, played games. Now, of course, people celebrate their bodies. School gymnasiums, neighborhood baseball diamonds, and playing fields have replaced the corner cafés and "singles bars" as adult hangouts.

Much of the credit for all these changes belongs to women. Their full and equal entry into the sports arena, after years of chipping away at this narrow and selective male-dominated field, expanded it into a healthful and consciousness-raising pastime for everyone. It is ironic that women should be at the forefront of the "body movement," having launched their modern liberation campaign in the sixties and seventies with a demand for men to stop ogling the female body and start paying attention to the female mind. Once it was generally accepted that the female mind was as sound as the male mind, the battle turned back to the body—to prove that it was more than just a pleasure trove for man.

The array of myths about women and sports fell like dominoes. It was proven that, up until menopause, a woman's bones, though smaller, were no more fragile than a man's, that a woman was *not* more likely to be injured while playing than a man, and that in fact the injury rate per participant was generally lower for girls than boys—in both contact and noncontact sports—because of the girls' extra padding of fat. Breast pads were soon devised for women athletes, similar to men's jock straps. Coaches were convinced by medical testimony that the well-guarded uterus was one of the most shock-resistant internal organs in the body and that strenuous activity actually increased muscular support around the pelvis. Similarly, it was accepted that vigorous exercise helped both menstruation and pregnancy (the U.S. Olympic Committee stopped advising its swimmers and other athletes to use the Pill to prevent menstruation from coming during their contests). The scientific discovery that men also enjoy monthly cycles, with attending emotional highs and lows, also helped to dash the legend of the "female curse." The widely held belief that women athletes developed bulging muscles turned out to be scientifically unprovable—a woman's physique is genetically determined at birth, and no amount of exercise and training can radically change it. When women began to train strenuously for serious athletics in the eighties, it turned out that with the same amount of training they developed less musculature than men and instead used a higher percentage of already-existing fiber. Those shot-putters with bowling-ball shoulders turned out to have had the basic bulges in the first place.

Centuries of ignorance about and lack of research on the female physiology were overcome. Women, exhilarated with this new sense of physical power, began the slow process through the seventies and eighties of throwing over the "femininity game"—luring, baiting, and netting a husband—for the far simpler and honest games that men had enjoyed for years.

After long research into the female physiology, there now appear to be only a few sex-linked differences between the male and female performance in the sports arena. The average female is still born smaller than the average male and thus is at a disadvantage when a random sample women are pitted against a random sample of men. Moreover, she is at a disadvantage when performing in a climate where heat and humidity are high, since the body temperature of a woman must rise two to three degrees higher than that of a man before she begins to perspire and cool off. It was this discovery that led to the successful movement to have lacrosse and field hockey meets postponed form the traditional spring and summer season to late fall and winter.

Women athletes who have undergone steady and rigorous training also have overcome the historical heat dissipation handicap of the average female—that is, that the female has fewer functional sweat glands than the male. It was definitively established that women in fact had, in earlier times, not exercised as much as men had and had thus lost the use of a high percentage of their sweat glands; these needed to be reactivated, and were, by rigorous exercise. The change in conditioning has not altered a basic difference in the female frame, however, and her wider hips and lower center of gravity still place her at a disadvantage in some sports. Nevertheless, women keep closing the gap between men's and women's world records.

Back in 1974, when the bulk of research on the female physiology could barely have filled one small library shelf, it was recognized that the trained woman athlete could always beat the untrained man. But given a man and a woman of the exact same build and training, it was believed that the man would always win because of his greater muscle mass, larger maximal oxygen uptake—or aerobic power—and proportionately bigger heart and lungs. Women were believed to have less stamina and less potential for reaching the heights of male athletes. It took a long time, but eventually it was recognized and accepted by coaches—who had long been as movable as the Pyramids on the issue—that women's physical inferiority was the result less of physiology than of a lifetime of deprivation. It had been so socially unacceptable for a woman to engage in strenuous activities, and she had been encouraged so often to depend on others to defend her—to act as her arms and legs—that she did not know she was capable, for instance, of even lifting a television set.

At first it was thought that even if this conditioning were removed and woman given opportunities to develop in the same way as man, her innate biological inferiority would prevent her form ever being able to compete with the male athlete. It took research by physical education scientists at Penn State, the University of California, and others to finally break the last ball and chain of opinion that was holding sportswomen down.

Until the late seventies, an athlete's maximum aerobic power (the capacity to extract oxygen from the air and deliver it to the working muscles) had been measured relative to his total body weight and was considered the best indication of his endurance capabilities. According to tests, the aerobic power of the female was only 70 to 75 percent of that of the male.

A number of scientists decided that it would be fairer to measure aerobic power in relation to fat-free body weight—in other words, the working muscle. It was found that square inch for square inch of muscle, women are as efficient as men in the use of oxygen. The discovery that at least in the laboratory women had as great an aerobic work capacity as men led to other tests to see if women's muscle power pound for pound was also as great. Not only were women found to be as strong as men in relation to lean body weight (total weight minus the weight of fat), in many tests their muscles proved to be stronger.

The fact that men have about twice the muscle mass of women was finally discovered to be meaningless. Just as men and women utilize only a small percentage of brain cells, so they use only about a quarter of their muscle fiber. This discovery put an end to the practice in the sixties and seventies of feeding female athletes, especially in the eastern European countries, steroids. Women athletes who trained as strenuously as men were found to slowly increase use of muscle fiber and reduce fat. Today, there is virtually no difference in strength between the average-trained male athlete and the average-trained female of the same body weight. It appears that the sedentary lifestyle of women has been largely responsible for the long-standing belief that nature meant her to be weaker.

Little League teams now generally have a preponderance of girls. At the high-school level, all sports are integrated and there are no longer "boys" and "girls" squads.

On the college and university scene, the passage of the Education Amendments of 1972 forced educational institutions receiving federal assistance—virtually every college in the nation—to give early equal treatment to men and women.... The universities, after much rancor and protest, were forced to cut back their men's athletic budgets and skimp on the revenue-producing sports such as football and basketball to give the women a greater share. Women, freed from having to throw bake sales to raise funds for their travel, spent more time in rigorous training and eventually reached levels in which they could compete with men.

On the professional circuit, there used to be a vicious circle in the seventies whereby tournaments of women's golf, tennis, and bowling would not get television coverage unless there was a big purse offered, but sponsors wouldn't provide the big purse unless the tournament was televised. That Catch-22 of women's sports was soon ended, and by the eighties men and women were earning equal prize money.

Women have come a long way in 25 years. Perhaps that is why all this uproar is happening now. Men are frightened by the sight of all these lean compact women—most young girls today do look like they stepped out of an

Egyptian fresco. It is not that women no longer look like women—their muscles, though more outlined, are no bigger, and the sloping feminine lines are sill there. It is the uniform absence of a *traditional* thickness in the female form that seems to be disquieting to the people making the most noise. "You can't pinch women anymore, you can't even get hold of them," grumbled one of the leaders of the new male chauvinism movement recently. And it is true that flesh seems to be the sole province of the over-40 these days. The NMC complains that women have usurped every last asset unique to males: "First, women have a stronger constitution and a longer life—their survivability is superior to ours. Then they equal us mentally, and moreover claim they have the secret of the universe stashed somewhere in their consciousness. They give birth to life, and now they're saying they're just as strong as, if not stronger than we are." One of the more legitimate concerns of the NMC movement is the fear that with the decreasing fatty tissue in active, exercising young women today, a danger is being posed to the species. If the female fat layer is not there to protect sex tissue and the stomach during pregnancy, they ask, are we not raising a generation of female bodies that will be unable to protect their unborn babies? Are we gradually making female fat obsolete, and will the reproductive organs be the next to go? NMC sportswriters are calling sportswomen puppets, charging that they are mimicking males instead of being what they are best at. They are demanding that women quit competing with men. The hue and cry is great. You would sometimes think we were back in the seventies.

The Athletic Triad: A Dangerous Triangle

LILA A. WALLIS

From *The Whole Woman: Take Charge of Your Health in Every Phase of Your Life,* by Lila A. Wallis, M.D., with Marian Betancourt, (Avon, 1999). Copyright ©1999 by Lila A. Wallis and Marian Betancourt. Reprinted by permission.

The "athletic triad" is the combination of excessive athletic activity, weight loss, and menstrual abnormalities. With continued excessive exercise and excessive weight loss, the estrogen level drops, causing menstruation to stop and leading to bone loss. Young ballet dancers and other athletes often get what we call march fractures in the feet and ignore them until pain becomes insufferable. These are hairline fractures that usually cannot be detected without an X-ray. The healthy physiologic limit that should be imposed on the vigorous exercising of young women should be absence of side effects. Young women who exercise excessively might experience several side effects.

Intense physical activity leads to injuries of the musculoskeletal system. Thirty-five to 65 percent of runners are injured per year; the risk of injury increases with the total distance run per week. The critical level varies from one individual to another. Exercise that leads to injury is too much exercise.

The pleasant mood associated with physical activity is a great benefit, but a dangerous point is reached when an athlete's "high" makes her disregard physical discomfort and drives her to increasing amounts of exercise. Watch out for these feelings and behavior.

All in all, the dangerous athletic triad occurs in only a small fraction of young girls, while the malignant "pentad" of physical inactivity/overeating/ obesity/accelerated chronic illness/premature death affects millions of people in our country—between a third and a half of the female population. Physical inactivity and obesity constitute a far more serious public health problem than the athletic triad.

Patsy Mink on Title IX

INTERVIEW BY TANIA KETENJIAN

Congresswoman Patsy Mink (D, Hawaii) currently serves on the Education and Workforce Committee and on the Budget Committee. This interview was conducted in June 1999.

TK: In *The Conversation Begins,* you discuss other issues you were working on when you were first elected. As a politician, what are the things that you've tackled that you're the most proud of?

PM: I was one of the principal advocates for Title IX, the provision in our education laws that says that all educational institutions—from universities all the way down to kindergarten—cannot discriminate against females in their selection of participants for programs, scholarships, fellowships, postdoctorates, and so on. Title IX has probably transformed all educational opportunities for women in the United States. It has opened up law schools, medical schools, all of the professions; certainly it has had a major impact in sports, as young women now typically star in all of our Olympics programs. That's probably been the most phenomenal piece of legislation that I helped to get through. We're still making sure it isn't watered down or changed in any way.

TK: Do you feel Congress now has a greater female presence?

PM: Oh no, we certainly can use many more women. At the moment, we're somewhere around 58 or 59 of the total number and, while that's a lot more than when I started many years ago, this still falls short of our representational entitlement in the country; many, many more women need to consider politics as a tremendous opportunity for participating in our society.

TK: Has there been a failure to address women's issues as a result of that lack of presence?

PM: Definitely, for example, five years ago, we passed the Brady law, which said that a licensed gun dealer had to do a background check on customers with a waiting period of five days. The gun shows were never included in the Brady law, so we were trying to include them because, as the Brady law went into effect, the criminals who didn't go to the gun dealers were going to the gun shows to purchase their illegal weapons. So we felt it was really critical to close that loophole in the sales traffic. But unfortunately, we lost this very simple amendment. Although all of the women of the House literally stood up together—we were all there on the floor at precisely the same moment to make our statement—the amendment was lost. So, yes, the presence of more women would be critical, I think, in a close fight like the one we had last night.

A Mother's Story

PATSY MINK

Adapted from Patsy Mink, "A Mother's Story," Christina Looper Baker and Christina Baker Kline, eds., *The Conversation Begins*, New York, Bantam Books, 1996. Reprinted by permission.

While I was pregnant with my daughter, Wendy, in 1951 and 1952, I was administered a drug that dramatically affected both our lives. My doctor was participating in a University of Chicago experiment to test whether diethylstilbestrol (DES), a form of estrogen, prevents miscarriages. Years later, dust-covered records in a Chicago basement revealed that the blind study had created tremendous health hazards for 1,000 women involved in the experiment and their offspring. For years Wendy had puzzling physical symptoms, the cause of which remained a mystery. In 1976, on her 24th birthday, I received a letter saying, "You were in this test, and our records show that you were given DES. Are you alive? Are you sick? What happened to your child?" They even requested we participate in a follow-up experiment to track the effects of the drug on offspring.

In 1978, I and two others won a significant settlement from the University of Chicago and DES manufacturer Eli Lilly because they had not informed us that we were part of an experiment. Our daughters have been less successful in court. Wendy sued, but since she didn't have cancer at the time, she was awarded nothing. A two-year statute of limitations prevented her from recovering for any DES-related medical problems that developed since 1976.

There was no women's movement in the mid-1950s, when the DES experiment took place, nor when I first entered politics. In my youth I didn't understand that there was such a thing as discrimination against women. I lived my life as I felt inclined, never considering myself a lesser being because I was female. I attribute this to the influence of my parents, who treated me and my brother with absolute equality.

From childhood I had been preoccupied with the idea of becoming a doctor. All my studies were directed toward that end, and in 1948 I graduated from the University of Hawaii with a major in zoology and chemistry and a minor in physics. At the appropriate time I applied to 25 medical schools—my parents willingly paying the application fees. But my dream never materialized. Had I been male I would have been accepted because of good grades, but medical schools across the country simply were not accepting women. The reasons may have been ethnic as well. In any case, I was shattered, and I was left with nothing to do. The jobs I qualified for were unrelated to my goal.

One day my boss said, "Don't be so depressed; life doesn't end just because you didn't go to medical school. Surely there are other ways to express your individuality and your desire to serve people." I asked, "What can I do?" and she enumerated possible careers. "Why don't you go to law school?" she said. "You like to talk." I had no idea what the study of law entailed, but I took her up on it, and in 1950 the University of Chicago accepted me as a "foreign student." I didn't bother to say they were wrong to think me foreign.

I became interested in Democratic politics through friends who pulled me into party workshops and seminars. One thing led to another, and soon I was elected to the state legislature. Campaigning took a lot of time, and much of my political activity in those early years I did alone. Equal pay for equal work was one of my early achievements. Male legislators got up on the floor and ridiculed the legislation ("Equal pay?"), but in 1957 they voted for it. We took pleasure in the fact that Hawaii adopted the bill six years sooner than the nation. As a representative, I helped open up state government after noticing that it was always the same people who served on important commissions. "A lot of talented people want to serve," I said. "Give them an opportunity." In all, I served three terms in the Hawaii legislature.

When I first ran for national office in 1959, I lost by 8 percent. Losing felt awful. It's terrible enough to be rejected by just one person, but to be rejected by thousands you thought were in love with you is devastating. That's why most people don't run for office. You can run again only if you believe strongly that you have something to contribute. After losing I said, "Never again," but soon I reentered local politics and was elected to the Hawaii state senate in 1962.

In 1964 a seat opened in the U.S. House of Representatives, and I decided to seek national office. This time I campaigned for federal aid to education, which became law my first year in Congress. As a representative, I pushed for equity in education. We held hearings to determine how textbooks were demeaning to Black people and looked at gender discrimination in the handling of federal funding. When we wrote Title IX, out of a belief that federally funded institutions should treat girls and boys equally, I had no idea how far-reaching it would be and how it would withstand all the court tests. Though just 20 words long, Title IX has produced stunning results in prohibiting sex discrimination.

I am a feminist—one who cares about the role of women in society—but I do not believe the women's movement is broadly enough based. In limiting itself to a certain segment of society, it leaves out the rest. Millions of women, such as those on welfare, are not connected to it, but I don't see the feminist movement getting involved in welfare reform; women of color are the only ones who care about this issue. I would like to see preschool child care become part of the official educational program so that child-care workers' pay is comparable to that of teachers. Child-care workers are currently paid less than animal-shelter employees. Why aren't feminists campaigning for better salaries for child-care workers? Is an animal more precious than a child?

The women's movement still focuses on middle-class white women, which I don't see changing. The "glass ceiling" is an upper-class ceiling for those aspiring to be bank presidents and executives, not those who can never rise above the minimum wage. The majority of people working at minimum-wage jobs in the United States are women. That's the glass ceiling I am committed to doing something about. American women must stand up and be counted. The new women in Congress have absolutely made a difference—49 is better than 29—but to get more women into office, it must be easier for women to run. If we could just persuade women to support more women candidates, more would win.

HOW WE WON TITLE IX

When I came to Congress in 1965, I was on the Education and Labor Committee chaired by Adam Clayton Powell. From the moment I sat in my chair as a freshman member down in the lower tier, he began hearings on discrimination and textbooks, and we hauled in all the textbooks to show that women were really being discarded. We hauled in the Department of Education because they were issuing films on vocational education which showed women as nurses, teachers, social workers, but not of occupations like scientist, doctor, or engineer or anything of that kind. Finally, with the enactment of Public Law 8910, which was the first federal aid to elementary and secondary schools, we wanted to make sure that women and girls would have an equal opportunity and that was all we were trying to say.

Edith Green, chairperson of the Higher Education Committee, convened a hearing in June of 1970 to add protections for women to the Civil Rights Act. This was all going on at the same time that women in the country were getting excited about the Equal Rights Amendment. But the Justice Department intervened and said we cannot support an amendment of the Civil Rights Act; why not put this measure in the education bill? When the education amendments came up in November of 1971, we were able to argue all of this.

In 1975, opponents tried to exclude college and university athletics from Title IX regulation. They paraded a number of college and professional athletes to testify that Title IX hurt men's sports. The only well-known woman athlete we had to testify was Billie Jean King. The fact that there were virtually no prominent women athletes in our country was a testament in itself of the necessity of the legislation.

Just a minute or so before the critical vote, I got word that my daughter had gotten into a car accident. I rushed off to Ithaca to see how she was. In my absence, the devastating amendment passed by one vote. The newspapers reported that I had left the floor "crying" in the face of defeat. But in reality I was facing a tremendous family crisis. The next day, the Speaker explained the circumstances of my departure and a new vote was taken, preserving the regulations and Title IX's application to athletes.

On July 26, 1999, the *Congressional Record* recorded that: no person in the United States shall, on the basis of sex, be excluded from partipation in, be denied the benefits of, or be subjected to discrimination under any educational program or activity receiving Federal financial assistance. These are the achievements of Title IX.

> ➤When President Nixon signed this bill, about 31,000 women were involved in college sports. Today that number has more than tripled.
> ➤Spending on athletic scholarships for women has grown from less than $100,000 to almost $200 million.
> ➤In 1972, women received 9 percent of the medical degrees and 7 percent of the law degrees in this country; in 1994, the numbers were 38 percent and 43 percent, respectively.
> ➤In 1994, 44 percent of all doctoral degrees were granted to women.

On July 10, 1999, the American team's victory in the Women's World Cup soccer competition reminded us how important it is to have the protections for women that we now have. These young women are the products of Title IX. But this victory was about more than the game and the win. It was about female athletes, sports, and equality.

Chapter 61

Ovaries

O ur "Down There" segment begins here, encompassing the next five chapters and closing out our Body Parts section.

Gloria Steinem's "If Men Could Menstruate" was one of feminism's most persuasive essays of the 1970s, written in a time when, in the face of efforts to elect more women to political office, cockamamie but well credentialed doctors came forth to pronounce that our menstrual cycles rendered us unstable and unfit to lead. Margaret Thatcher was elected prime minister of England, but still a decade later, the selling of premenstrual syndrome became big business, as Andrea Eagan reports.

In the United States, we have not been notably successful in reducing the traffic in unnecessary hysterectomies, nor any questionable surgeries on the female organs, because accurate information on the benefits and risks (not to mention patient satisfaction vs. regret) is still concealed from us. In European countries where surgeons can't get rich by piling on operations (medicine is more socialized), hysterectomy rates are much lower (less than half), and women remain at least equally healthy.

The chapter titled "Fruits of the Womb" deals with mothers and children, adoptive mothers as well as birth mothers, sons as well as daughters, and also with our changing concept of families.

"A Circle of Women" shows how patients, sharing information together, can succeed in developing treatments when their doctors fail.

*The "Clitoris" chapter concludes with Dr. Susan Vaughn's amusing specula-
tions on Viagra for women, which follows a consideration of female genital mutilation; it may be less politically correct than many such discussions, but perhaps
it's more truthful. Germaine Greer, our controversial lioness in winter, continues
to shock some readers with her original, eccentric views on our body parts.—B. S.*

Fertility Awareness in North America

KATIE SINGER

Katie Singer, "Cycles of Hot and Cold: Trying to Learn Fertility Awareness in
North America." © 1999, original for this publication. Reprinted by permission.

Several years ago, my boyfriend and I drove from Santa Fe toward a cabin
north of town to celebrate my birthday. "I've got another yeast infection,"
I said quietly.

The traffic had thinned. Our views of northern New Mexico's mesas and
spring wildflowers were now unobstructed. "Well, that's lousy," he said.

The lousiness wasn't that I was sick but that we wouldn't be able to make
love. Already that year I'd had several yeast infections because of irritation
from the spermicide I used with my cervical cap.

How do I get out of here? I wondered. Out of feeling like my birthday celebration is only about sex, out of birth control that makes me sick?

Sex, fertility, love. Like the burning in my groin, they made a tangle too hot
to touch.

A few years later, I heard about fertility awareness (FA), also called the
sympto-thermal method or natural family planning (NFP), and decided to
learn it. By daily charting her basal (waking) temperature, the secretions from
and changes in her cervix, a woman can tell when she's fertile. If they want to
conceive, couples who chart know the best time to try. To avoid pregnancy,
they postpone intercourse on fertile days.

Fertility awareness is not the same as the (ineffective) rhythm method,
which determines fertility by past cycles' patterns. FA gauges fertility as the
woman's daily chart evolves. According to the World Health Organization,
when used properly for birth control, it's virtually as effective as the Pill.

I began learning fertility awareness primarily by taking classes and reading
literature put out by Catholic organizations. Many statements in the literature
didn't suit me. Despite my discomfort, I started to observe and record my fertility signals. I began to experience explosions of awe: I had never conceived or
tried to, but now I could see bona-fide proof of my fertility. My cycles had often
been erratic, but now (from knowing when I ovulated), I could predict when
my period would come. I was with a new man while I learned the method, and
his interest in my cycles helped both of us appreciate my femaleness. As

awareness of my fertility patterns emerged, they gently took the lead in our relating.

I began to see that while the rhythm of masculine sexuality is often on all the time—men are fertile all the time—feminine cycles invite periodic rest from sexual intimacy. Women are fertile, on average, only one-third of each cycle. Despite my feminist perspective, I came of age expecting that I should be available for sex all the time. I remember one three- or four-month period when I was physically able and wanting to have sex every day. Surely, I thought, my boyfriend and I would stay together if I could keep this up. And how did my access to artificial birth control contribute to such thinking?

Indeed, sterilization, the pill, the IUD, the diaphragm, the cervical cap, and condoms give women the option of having fewer children than earlier generations. These methods allow choice about the course of our lives. Usually, however, these methods are distributed without substantial information about how our bodies or the methods work. Artificial birth control allows people to explore sex without awareness of their fertility.

I began to wonder what price we pay when we don't know this basic information about ourselves.

In the first part of her menstrual cycle, while she's maturing an egg, a woman's body is cooler. Men's testicles, where sperm are produced, hang outside their trunks for the same reason: human eggs prefer cooler temperatures during production. Women heat up after ovulation, during the cycle's second phase, to support an embryo's gestation; they cool down when a new cycle begins. These patterns can be seen when a woman charts her waking temperature.

Cervical fluid (CF) typically cycles through the following pattern: after the period (which some FA teachers assume to be fertile, since CF can't be discerned through blood), a woman will experience several "dry" days. The CF samples she takes with toilet tissue or a clean finger from just inside her vagina will not feel slippery or textured. Then the CF (which, when fertile, can keep sperm alive in the cervix for up to five days) will build up, beginning with a moist sensation and/or a sticky texture. Near ovulation, her CF tends to become slippery and clear—like raw egg white. After ovulation, it typically becomes dry again. A woman who charts can identify her days as infertile or fertile.

Women are like the earth, whose surface continues to develop through processes of heating and cooling and moistening and drying.

Charting began to feel like spiritual practice. I felt much more connected to myself and to other women who understood their own cycles. And as we learned and practiced fertility awareness, my partner began to realize, "I used to wake up and ask myself, 'When was the last time I masturbated? Have I had intercourse in the last 24 hours?'" With FA as our birth control, he wondered instead if I was fertile or infertile.

Why hadn't we learned this method before?

Because of my passion for the method, I began writing a story about its availability in northern New Mexico. I called Shirley Hoeffler, the director of a natural family planning clinic at St. Joseph's Hospital in Albuquerque. Her program teaches a cervical fluid–only method. Just from looking at a woman's charts, Hoeffler told me, she can tell if the woman is prone to miscarriage, ovarian cysts, and other gynecological problems.

When she said she would be offering a course to train people to teach the method, I asked for an application.

"I could send you one," Hoeffler said, "but I couldn't accept you."

I was stunned. "Why?" I asked.

"Because you have genital contact."

"Because I'm not married?" I asked, groping for clarity.

"No," she said. "Because you're single and you have genital contact." If I was celibate or married, then her program could accept me.

This was June 1997.

Hoeffler's policy propelled me onto a tour of conversations with nurse practitioners in women's clinics, the director of medical affairs for Planned Parenthood, the medical journalist Nona Aguilar, and finally Suzannah Doyle, who writes about the method for *Our Bodies, Ourselves*.

Laurie Holmes, a highly esteemed certified nurse-midwife in Santa Fe. She dispenses birth control, primarily to low-income women. "I've seen too many unwanted pregnancies with fertility awareness to feel entirely comfortable endorsing it," she said. "I bring it up, but people need time to learn it and stay with the daily charting. I think you need to be open to failure if you use it. I also find that people don't want abstinence."

I told Laurie (who, like most health care practitioners, is not trained to use or teach FA) about the first woman I met who used it. She'd had two abortions by the time she was 21, then vowed never again to have an unwanted pregnancy. After her second abortion, she chose FA for birth control, and 115 cycles later, she hasn't conceived again.

Laurie Holmes found it exceptional that a woman would have the discipline to take her temperature every morning all these years.

I began to wonder if fertility awareness is not taught as well in the women's community as it is among Catholics (certainly it's less available), and how this figures into practitioners' lack of faith in the method and people's capacity to commit to daily charting. Are the teaching methods, commitments, and self-control expressed in the Catholic community not available to others?

Kara Anderson, Planned Parenthood's director of medical affairs explained that their practitioners rarely have more than 20 minutes with each client. "Most of the people who come to us have been sexually active for six months— without any birth control."… If a client asks to learn fertility awareness (which is unusual), she's usually referred elsewhere—often to a teacher affiliated with a Catholic organization. "To learn this method well," Anderson said, "a woman needs to be in close touch with a teacher for three or four months. In many areas, Catholic organizations seem to provide the method's only teachers."

But how to administer such time-intensive classes? Who would pay for them?

The Couple to Couple League is staffed primarily by volunteer, married couples who perceive teaching as "service," and it's therefore able to offer classes at a nominal fee. Indeed, the CCL admirably meets the needs of religious Catholics. Their classes last for four months, and couples new to the method are encouraged to stay in touch by phone with their teachers.

Currently, there are 525 volunteer couples who teach NFP through the CCL. These teachers are required to sign a principle statement advocating, for example, rejection of abortion, homosexual behavior, marriage and breast-feeding as necessary ingredients in healthy families.

While I appreciate CCL's clear outlaying of their beliefs, their style discourages individual decision making around very personal issues. For me, this makes learning fertility awareness with them awkward at best.

Nona Aguilar's book *The New, No-Pill, No-Risk Birth Control* presents thorough, accurate information on how to chart fertility signals. It also includes inspiring testimony from couples who switched to this method and found it significantly enriched their intimacy. Her book was a treasure, one of only two books I found on the subject after a year of scouting Santa Fe stores, and it didn't come with a moral bias. Aguilar was my heroine.

I told her so when I reached her, then described my frustration that I was not acceptable to the Albuquerque training program.

"Well," she said respectfully, "I agree with that policy."

I leaned back in my chair. "Okay," I said. "I don't understand this. Please explain."

"Properly used, prayerfully used," she began, "sex is about emotional and psychological union. In our culture, artificial birth control—which feminists have strongly advocated—has made sex a recreational activity. But it's meant to be a transcendent one. Sex is the life-bearing force of humankind. When lovemaking is turned into something recreational, it's a little like being color blind during sunset over the Grand Canyon. Union becomes harder to experience, and that's a loss."

Aguilar's thoughts stirred me deeply and encouraged me to revere fertility awareness more than before. Our conversations also clarified my desire for classes that teach people how our bodies work, how various kinds of birth control affect reproductive systems and risk the transfer of sexually transmitted diseases, and that offer opportunity for individuals to differentiate between their personal inhibitions around sexual issues and the prohibitions suggested by society. And still, I felt qualified to teach such classes despite my not being celibate, despite my never having felt moved to marry.

Finally, I called the Boston Women's Health Book Collective. I was given the number of Suzannah Doyle, who's written about the method for the last several issues of *Our Bodies, Ourselves*.

Like Shirley Hoeffler, Suzannah can read a woman's charts and tell if she's prone to miscarriages or ovarian cysts. "That's not hard to learn," she said.

Indeed, charting speaks to a tradition (before male doctors took over the delivering of babies, distributed the Pill, and provided abortions) when women were in charge of their own health care.

Doyle explained that fertility awareness teachers usually tell their clients that they have choices during their fertile times: they can use barrier methods to prevent pregnancy, sexual expression that doesn't include genital-genital contact or postponing intercourse. "In either case," Doyle said, "since women are fertile only one-third of their cycle, using birth control for two-thirds of it is a waste."

Doyle also confirmed that most of the scientists who've done research in this field have been male, Catholic M.D.'s. Until the 1980s, fertility awareness was only available from a Catholic perspective. Since then, nonreligious teachers (who usually learned the method through Catholic organizations) have offered classes.

Now, the fertility awareness community is often divided between those who are pro-choice and pro-life. I like to call myself "*pre*-choice," Doyle said.

Currently, there is no national group that advocates fertility awareness and informed choice. There are several organizations—including the Ovulation Method Teachers Association, the L.A. Regional Family Planning Council, and the Fertility Awareness Network—which, however small, conduct classes in using the method and trainings for teachers. But usually, those who teach fertility awareness in their own communities are in touch with each other informally, without institutional support.

I'm dreaming now: of adolescents knowing how their reproductive systems work before they become sexually active and before they choose a birth control method; of women and men being as aware of our fertility as we are about our sexuality; of fertility awareness classes as available as the Pill; of alliances between those who provide health care education in women's and Catholic communities; of alternative and allopathic medical students learning how to diagnose and treat women's imbalances based on charting of fertility signals,* of medical researchers making use of women's fertility awareness charts; of every person knowing, intimately, the sacredness of their procreative powers.

---

*In China, charts of women's basal body temperatures (BBTs) are routinely used to diagnose gynecological health, as the pulse and the tongue are used to gauge overall health. Like approximately 30 acupuncturists in the United States who have special training in gynecology, mine uses the BBT as a diagnostic tool to treat gynecological imbalances.

Chapter 62

Womb

If Men Could Menstruate

GLORIA STEINEM

Gloria Steinem, "If Men Could Menstruate: A Political Fantasy," *Ms.*, ISSUE, 1978. Reprinted by permission.

A white minority of the world has spent centuries conning us into thinking that a white skin makes people superior—even though the only thing it really does is make them more subject to ultraviolet rays and to wrinkles. Male human beings have built whole cultures around the idea that penis envy is "natural" to women—though having such an unprotected organ might be said to make men vulnerable, and the power to give birth makes womb envy at least as logical.

In short, the characteristics of the powerful, whatever they may be, are thought to be better than the characteristics of the powerless—and logic has nothing to do with it.

What would happen, for instance, if suddenly, magically, men could menstruate and women could not?

The answer is clear—menstruation would become an enviable, boastworthy, masculine event:

Men would brag about how long and how much.

Boys would mark the onset of menses, that longed-for proof of manhood, with religious ritual and stag parties.

Congress would fund a National Institute of Dysmenorrhea to help stamp out monthly discomforts.

Sanitary supplies would be federally funded and free. (Of course, some men would still pay for the prestige of commercial brands such as John Wayne Tampons, Muhammad Ali's Rope-a-Dope Pads, Joe Namath Jock Shields—"For Those Light Bachelor Days," and Robert "Baretta" Blake Maxi-Pads.)

Military men, right-wing politicians, and religious fundamentalists would cite menstruation ("men-struation") as proof that only men could serve in the army ("you have to give blood to take blood"), occupy political office ("can women be aggressive without that steadfast cycle governed by the planet Mars?"), be priests and ministers ("how could a woman give her blood for our sins?"), or rabbis ("without the monthly loss of impurities, women remain unclean").

Male radicals, left-wing politicians, mystics, however, would insist that women are equal, just different, and that any woman could enter their ranks if only she were willing to self-inflict a major wound every month ("you must give blood for the revolution"), recognize the preeminence of menstrual issues, or subordinate her selfness to all men in their Cycle of Enlightenment.

Street guys would brag ("I'm a three-pad man") or answer praise from a buddy ("Man, you lookin' good!") by giving fives and saying, "Yeah, man, I'm on the rag!"

TV shows would treat the subject at length. (*Happy Days*: Richie and Potsie try to convince Fonzie that he is still "the Fonz," though he has missed two periods in a row.) So would newspapers. (Shark Scare Threatens Menstruating Men. Judge Cites Monthly Stress in Pardoning Rapist.) And movies. (Newman and Redford in *Blood Brothers!*)

Men would convince women that intercourse was more pleasurable at "that time of the month." Lesbians would be said to fear blood and therefore life itself—though probably only because they needed a good menstruating man.

Of course, male intellectuals would offer the most moral and logical arguments. How could a woman master any discipline that demanded a sense of time, space, mathematics, or measurement, for instance, without that in-built gift for measuring anything at all? In the rarefied fields of philosophy and religion, could women compensate for missing the rhythm of the universe? Or for their lack of symbolic death and resurrection every month?

Liberal males in every field would try to be kind: the fact that "these people" have no gift for measuring life or connecting to the universe, the liberals would explain, should be punishment enough.

And how would women be trained to react? One can imagine traditional women agreeing to all these arguments with a staunch and smiling masochism. ("The ERA would force housewives to wound themselves every month": Phyllis Schlafly. "Your husband's blood is as sacred as that of Jesus—and so sexy, too!": Marabel Morgan.) Reformers and Queen Bees would try to imitate men and pretend to have a monthly cycle. All feminists would explain endlessly that men, too, needed to be liberated from the false idea of Martian aggressiveness, just as women needed to escape the bonds of menses envy. Radical feminists would add that the oppression of the nonmenstrual was the pattern for all other oppressions. ("Vampires were our first freedom fighters!") Cultural feminists would develop a bloodless imagery in art and literature. Socialist feminists would insist that only under capitalism would men be able to monopolize menstrual blood....

In fact, if men could menstruate, the power justifications could probably go on forever.

If we let them.

The Selling of Premenstrual Syndrome

ANDREA EAGAN

Andrea Eagan, "The Selling of Premenstrual Syndrome: Who Profits from Making PMS 'The Disease of the '80s'?" *Ms.,* October 1983. Reprinted by permission.

In the summer of 1961, I was working as a laboratory assistant at a major pharmaceutical firm. Seminars were regularly given on recent scientific developments, and that summer there was one on oral contraceptives. As a rule, only the scientists went to the seminars. But for this one, every woman in the place showed up. Oral contraception sounded like a miracle, a dream come true.

During the discussion, someone asked whether the drug was safe. Yes, we were assured, it was perfectly safe. It had been thoroughly tested, and besides you were only adjusting the proportions of naturally occurring substances in the body, putting in a little estrogen and progesterone to fool the body into thinking that it was "just a little bit pregnant." The dream, we now know, was much too good to be true. But we learned that only after years of using the Pill, after we had already become a generation of guinea pigs.

Since then, we have presumably learned something: we have become cautious about medical miracles and scientific breakthroughs. To suddenly discover, then, that thousands of women are rushing to get an untested drug to cure a suspected but entirely unproved hormone deficiency which manifests itself as a condition with a startling variety of symptoms—known by the catchall name *premenstrual syndrome* (*PMS*)—is a little shocking.

When I began seeing articles about PMS and progesterone treatment, I immediately had some questions. Why was PMS suddenly "news"? What do we really know about progesterone? And who are the advocates of this treatment?

PMS itself was not news. It was first mentioned in the medical literature in the 1930s, and women presumably had it before then. Estimates on the numbers of women affected by PMS vary wildly. Some claim that as many as 80 percent are affected, while others place estimates at 20 percent. Similarly, the doctors' opinions vary on the number and type of symptoms that may indicate PMS. They cite from 20 up to 150 physical and psychological symptoms, ranging from bloating to rage. The key to recognizing PMS and differentiating it from anything else that might cause some or all of a woman's symptoms is timing. The symptoms appear at some point after ovulation (midcycle) and disappear at the beginning of the menstrual period. (It should not be confused with dysmenorrhea or menstrual discomfort, about which much is known, and for which several effective, safe treatments have been developed.)

While PMS is generally acknowledged to be a physical, as well as a psychological, disorder, there is little agreement on what causes it or how it should be treated. There are at least half a dozen theories as to its cause ranging from an alteration in the way that the body uses glucose to excessive estrogen levels—none of which have been convincingly demonstrated.

One of the most vocal proponents of PMS treatment is Katharina Dalton, a British physician who has been treating the condition for more than thirty years. Dalton believes that PMS results from a deficiency of progesterone, a hormone that is normally present at high levels during the second half of the menstrual cycle and during pregnancy. Her treatment, and that of her followers, relies on the administration of progesterone during the premenstrual phase of the cycle.

Although she promotes the progesterone treatment, Dalton has no direct evidence of a hormone deficiency in PMS sufferers. Because progesterone is secreted cyclically in irregular bursts, and testing of blood levels of progesterone is complicated and expensive, studies have been unable to show conclusively that women with PMS symptoms have lower levels of progesterone than other women. Dalton's evidence is indirect: the symptoms of PMS are relieved by the administration of progesterone.

Upon learning about Dalton's diagnosis-and-cure, many women concluded that they had the symptoms she was talking about. But when they asked their doctors for progesterone treatment, they generally got nowhere. Progesterone is not approved by the FDA for treatment of PMS, there is nothing in the medical literature showing clearly what causes PMS; and there has never been a well-designed, controlled study here or in England of the effect of progesterone on PMS.

Despite some doctors' reluctance to prescribe progesterone, self-help groups began springing up, and special clinics were established to treat PMS. Women who had any of the reported symptoms (cyclical or not) headed en masse for the clinics or flew thousands of miles to doctors whose willingness to prescribe progesterone had become known through the PMS network. And a few pharmacists began putting progesterone powder in suppository form and doing a thriving business.

How did PMS suddenly become the rage? At least part of the publicity can be traced to an enterprising young man named James Hovey. He met

Katharina Dalton in Holland several years ago at a conference on the biological basis of violent behavior. Returning to the United States, he started the National Center for Premenstrual Syndrome and Menstrual Distress in New York City, Boston, Memphis, and Los Angeles—each with a local doctor as medical director.

For $265 (paid in advance), you got three visits. The initial visit consisted of a physical exam and interview and a lengthy questionnaire on symptoms. During the second visit, the clinic dispensed advice on diet and vitamins and reviewed a monthly record the patient was asked to keep. On the third visit, if symptoms still persisted, most patients received a prescription for progesterone.

Last year, James Hovey's wife, Donna, a nurse who was working in his New York clinic, told me that they were participating in an FDA-approved study of progesterone, in conjunction with a doctor from the University of Tennessee. In fact, to date the FDA has approved only one study in progesterone treatment of PMS, which is conducted at the National Institute of Child Health and Human Development, an organization unrelated to James Hovey.

Similar contradictions and misrepresentations, as well as Hovey's lack of qualifications to be conducting research or running a medical facility, were exposed by two journalists last year. Hovey left New York and gave up his interest in the New York and Boston clinics. He is currently running a nationwide PMS referral service out of New Hampshire.

In a recent interview, Hovey said that the clinic business is too time-consuming, and that he is getting out. His "only interest is research" he says. At last report, Hovey still headed H and K Pharmaceuticals, a company founded in 1981 for the manufacture of progesterone suppositories.

Hovey's involvement in PMS treatment seems to have centered on the commercial opportunities. Others, such as Virginia Cassara, became interested for more personal reasons.

Cassara, a social worker from Wisconsin, went to England in 1979 to be treated by Dalton for severe PMS. The treatment was successful and Cassara returned to spread the good news. Cassara began counseling and speaking, selling Dalton's books and other literature. Her national group, PMS Action, now has a budget of $650,000, 17 paid staff members, and 40 volunteers. Cassara spends most of her time traveling and speaking.

Cassara's argument is compelling, at least initially. She describes the misery of PMS sufferers, and the variety of ineffective medical treatments they have been subjected to for relief. For anyone who is sensitive to women's health issues, it is a familiar tale: a condition that afflicts perhaps millions of women has never been studied; a treatment that gives relief is ignored. Women, says Cassara, are pushed into diet-and-exercise regimens that are difficult to maintain and don't always work. One valid solution, she feels, lies in progesterone.

According to FDA spokesperson Roger Eastep, initial studies have yet to be done for progesterone. But in the meantime, more and more doctors are prescribing the hormone for PMS.

Dr. Michelle Harrison, a gynecologist practicing in Cambridge, Massachusetts, is one physician who does prescribe progesterone to some women, with mixed feelings. "I've seen it dramatically temper women's reactions," she says. "For those women whose lives are shattered by PMS, who've made repeated suicide attempts or who are unable to keep a job, you have to do something. But I have a very frightening consent form that they have to sign before I'll give progesterone to them." Harrison also stresses that a lot of PMS is iatrogenic; that is, it is caused by medical treatment. It often appears for the first time after a woman has stopped taking birth control pills, after tubal ligation, or even after a hysterectomy, in which the ovaries have been removed.

When doctors do prescribe progesterone, their ideas of the appropriate dosage can vary from 50 to 2,400 mg per day. Some women are symptom-free as long as they are taking the drug, but the symptoms reappear as soon as they stop, regardless of where they are in their menstrual cycle.

For all these reasons, some women are taking much higher doses than their doctors prescribe. Michelle Harrison had heard of women taking 2,400 mg per day; Dalton had heard about 3,000; Cassara knows women who take 4,000. Because PMS symptoms tend to occur when progesterone is not being taken, some women take it every day, instead of only during the premenstrual phase. Some bleed all the time; others don't menstruate at all. Vaginal and rectal swelling are common. Animal studies have shown increased rates of breast tumors and cervical cancer.

Reminding her of the history of the Pill, DES, and ERT, I asked Virginia Cassara whether she was concerned about the long-term effects of progesterone on women. "I guess I don't think there could be anything worse than serious PMS," she responded. "Even cancer?" I asked. "Absolutely. Even cancer." Later, she said, "I think it's very paternalistic of the FDA to make those choices for us, to tell us what we can and cannot put into our bodies. Women with PMS are competent beings, capable of making their own choices."

I don't have severe PMS, and I don't think I fully understand the desperation of women who do and who see help at last within reach. But given our limited knowledge of how progesterone works, I do not understand why women like Cassara are echoing drug company complaints of overregulation by the FDA. I'm alarmed to see women flocking to use an untested substance about which there is substantial suspicion, whose mode of action is not known, to treat a condition whose very cause is a mystery. And I fear that, somewhere down the line, we will finally learn all about progesterone treatment, and it won't be what we want to know.

One doctor, who refused to be quoted by name, cheerfully assured me that progesterone was safe. "Even if a woman is taking 1,600 milligrams per day, the amount of circulating progesterone is still only a quarter of what is normally circulating during pregnancy." And I couldn't help but think of the doctor at the seminar more than 20 years ago: "Of course it's safe. It's just like being a little pregnant."

So You're Going to Have a New Body!

LYNNE SHARON SCHWARTZ

Lynne Sharon Schwartz, "So You're Going to Have a New Body!" from *The Melting Pot and Other Subversive Stories*. New York, Harper and Row, 1987. Reprinted by permission.

I

Take good care of yourself beforehand to be sure of a healthy, bouncing new body. Ask your doctor all about it. He can help.

Your doctor says: "Six weeks and you'll be feeling like a new person. No one will ever know."

Your doctor says: "Don't worry about the scar. We'll make it real low where no one can see. We call it a bikini cut."

He says: "Any symptoms you have afterward, we'll fix with hormones. We follow nature's way. There is some danger of these hormones causing cancer in the lining of the uterus. But since you won't have a uterus, you won't have anything to worry about."

He says: "There is this myth some women believe, connecting their reproductive organs with their femininity. But you're much too intelligent and sophisticated for that."

Intelligently, you regard a painting hanging on the wall above his diplomas; it is modern in aspect, showing an assortment of common tools—a hammer, screwdrivers, wrenches, and several others you cannot name, not being conversant with the mechanical arts. A sort of all-purpose handyman's kit. You think a sophisticated thought: *Chacun son goût.*

You are not even sure you need a new body, but your doctor says there is something inside your old one like a grapefruit, and though it is not really dangerous, it should go. It could block the view of the rest of you. You cannot see it or feel it. Trust your doctor. You have never been a runner, but six weeks before your surgery you start to run in the lonely park early each morning. Not quite awake, half dreaming, you imagine you are running from a mugger with a knife. Fast, fast. You are going to give them the healthiest body they have ever cut. You run a quarter of a mile the first day, half a mile the second. By the end of two weeks you are running a mile in nine minutes. From the neck down you are looking splendid. Perhaps when you present your body they will say, Oh no, this body is too splendid to cut.

II

You will have one very important decision to make before the big day. Be sure to consult with your doctor. He can help.

He says: "The decision is entirely up to you. However, I like to take the ovaries out whenever I can, as long as I'm in there. That way there is no danger of ovarian cancer, which strikes one in a hundred women in your age group. There is really nothing you need ovaries for. You have had three children and don't intend to have any more. Ovarian cancer is incurable and a terrible death. I've seen women your age.... However, the decision is entirely up to you."

You think: No, for with the same logic he could cut off my head to avert a brain tumor.

Just before he ushers you out of his office he shows you a color snapshot of some woman's benign fibroid tumors, larger than yours, he says, but otherwise comparable, lying in a big metal bowl wider than it is deep, the sort of bowl you often use to prepare chopped meat for meat loaf. You nod appreciatively and go into the bathroom to throw up.

III

Your hospital stay. One evening, in the company of your husband, you check in at the hospital and are shown to your room, which is not bad, only the walls are a bit bare and it is a bit expensive—several hundred dollars a night. Perhaps the service will be worth it. Its large window overlooks a high school, the very high school, coincidentally, that your teenaged daughter attends. She has promised to visit often. Your husband stays until a staff member asks that he leave, and he leaves you with a copy of *People* magazine featuring an article called "Good Sex with Dr. Ruth." This is a joke and is meant well. Accept it in that spirit. He is trying to say what he would otherwise find difficult to express, that your new body will be lovable and capable of love.

Your reading of *People* magazine is interrupted by your doctor, who invites you for a chat in the visitors' lounge, empty now. He says: "You don't have to make your decision about the ovaries till the last minute. However, ovarian cancer strikes one in a hundred women in your age group." Hard to detect until too late, a terrible death, etc., etc.

As he goes on, a pregnant woman in a white hospital gown enters the visitors' lounge, shuffles to the window, and stares out at the night sky. She has a beautiful olive-skinned face with high cheekbones, green eyes, and full lips. Her hair is thick and dark. Her arms and legs are very bony; her feet, in paper slippers, are as bony and arched as a dancer's. Take another look at her face: the cheekbones seem abnormally prominent, the eyes abnormally prominent, the hollows beneath them abnormally deep. She seems somewhat old to be pregnant, around 45. When she leaves, shuffling on her beautiful dancer's feet, your doctor says: "That woman has ovarian cancer."

The next morning, lying flat on your back in a Demerol haze, when he says, "Well?" you say, "Take them, they're yours."

You have anticipated this moment of waking and have promised to let yourself scream if the pain is bad enough. Happily, you discover screaming will not be necessary; quiet moaning will do. If this is the worst, you think, I can take it. In a roomful of screamers and moaners like yourself, baritones and sopranos together, you feel pleased even though you have only a minor choral part. Relieved. The worst is this, probably, and it will be over soon.

A day or two and you will be simply amazed at how much better you feel. Amazed, too, at how many strangers, men and women both, are curious to see your new bikini cut, so curious that you even feel some interest yourself. You peer down, then up into the face of the young man peering along with you, and say, "I know it sounds weird, but those actually look like staples in there."

"They are," he says.

You imagine a stapler of the kind you use at home for papers. Your doctor is holding it while you lie sleeping. Another man crimps the two layers of skin together, folds one over the other just above where your pubic hair used to be, and your doctor squeezes the stapler, moving along horizontally, again and again. Men and women are different in this, if you can generalize from personal experience: at home, you place the stapler flat on the desk, slide the papers between its jaws, and press down gently. Your husband holds the stapler in one hand, slides the corner of the papers in with the other, and squeezes the jaws of the stapler together. What strong hands they have! You think of throwing up, but this is more of an intellectual than a physical reaction since your entire upper abdomen is numb; moreover, you have had almost nothing to eat for three days. Your new body, when it returns to active life, will be quite thin.

No one can pretend that a postsurgical hospital stay is pleasant, but a cheerful outlook should take you far. The trouble is, you cry a good deal of the time. In one sense these tears seem uncontrollable, gushing at irregular intervals during the day and night. In another sense they are quite controllable: if your doctor or strange men on the staff drop in to look at your bikini cut or chat about your body functions, you are able to stop crying at will and act cheerful. But when women doctors or nurses drop in, you keep right on with your crying, even though this causes them to say, "What are you crying about?" You also do not cry in front of visitors, male or female, especially your teenaged daughter, since you noticed that when she visited you immediately after the surgery her face turned white and she left the room quickly, walking backwards and staring. She has visited often, as she promised. She makes sure to let you know she has terrible menstrual cramps this week, in fact asks you to write a note so she can be excused from gym. Your sons do not visit—they are too young, 12 and 9—but you talk to them on the phone, cheerfully. They tell you about the junk food they have been eating in your absence and about sports events at school. They sound wistful and eager to have you returned to them.

IV

At last the day you've been waiting for arrives: taking your new body home! You may be surprised to learn this, but in many ways your new body is just like your old one. For instance, it walks. Slowly. And if you clasp your hands and support your stomach from below, you feel less as though it will rip away from the strain inside. At home, in the mirror, except for the bikini cut and the fact that your stomach is round and puffy, this body even looks remarkably like your old one, but thinner. Your ankles are thinner than you have ever seen them. That is because with your reproductive system gone, you no longer tend to retain fluids. An unexpected plus, slim ankles! How good to be home and climb into your own bed. How good to see your children and how good they are, scurrying around to bring you tea and chocolates and magazines. Why is it that the sight of the children, which should bring you pleasure, also brings you grief? It might be that their physical presence reminds you of the place they came from, which no longer exists, at least in you. This leads you to wonder idly what becomes of the many reproductive organs, both healthy and unhealthy, removed daily: buried, burned, or trashed? Do right-to-lifers mourn them?

You sleep in your own bed with your husband, who wants to hold you close, but this does not feel very comfortable. You move his arms and hands to permissible places, the way you did with boys as a teenager, except of course the places are different now. Breasts are permissible, thighs are permissible, but not the expanse between. A clever fellow, over the next few nights he learns, even in his sleep, what is permissible.

Although you are more tired than you ever thought possible, you force yourself to walk from room to room three times a day, perhaps to show this new body who is in control. During one such forced walk.... Don't laugh, now! A wave of heat swirls up and encircles you, making you sway dizzily, and the odd thing, no one has mentioned this—it pulsates. Pulses of heat. Once long ago and with great concentration, you counted the pulses of an orgasm, something you are not sure you will ever experience again, and now you count this. Thirty pulses. You cannot compare since you have forgotten the orgasm number; anyhow, the two events have nothing in common except that they pulse and that they are totally overpowering. But this can't be happening; you are far too young for this little joke. Over the next few days it is happening, though, and whenever it happens you feel foolish, you feel something very like shame. Call your doctor. He can help.

A woman's voice says he is extremely busy and could you call back later, honey. Or would you like an appointment, honey? Are you sure she can't help you, honey? You say yes, she can help enormously by not calling you honey. Don't give me any of your lip, you menopausal bitch, she mutters. No, no, she most certainly does not mutter that; it must have been the tone of her gasp. Very well, please hold on while she fetches your folder. While holding, you are treated to a little telephone concert: Frank Sinatra singing "My Way." Repeatedly, you hear Frank Sinatra explain that no matter what has happened or will happen, he is gratified to feel that he did it his way. Your doctor's voice is abrupt and booming in contrast. When you state your problem he replies, "Oh, sweats." You are not sure you have heard correctly. Could he have said, "Oh, sweets," as in affectionate commiseration? Hardly. Always strictly business. You were misled by remembering, subliminally, "honey." "Sweats" it was and, in the plural, a very hideous word you do not wish to have associated with you or your new body. Sweat, a universal phenomenon, you have no quarrel with. Sweats, no.

Your doctor says he—or "they"—will take care of everything. For again he uses the plural, the royal "we." When you visit for a six-week checkup, "they" will give you the miraculous hormones, nature's way. In the meantime you begin to spend more time out of bed. You may find, during this convalescent period, that you enjoy reading, listening to music, even light activity such as jigsaw puzzles. Your 12-year-old son brings you a jigsaw puzzle of a Mary Cassatt painting—a woman dressed in pale blue, holding a baby who is like a peach. It looks like a peach and would smell and taste like a peach too. At a glance you know you can never do this puzzle. It is not that you want another baby, for you do not, nor is it the knowledge that you could not have one even if you wanted it, since that is academic. Simply the whole cluster of associations—mothers and babies, conception, gestation, birth—is something you do not wish to be reminded of. The facts of life. You seem to be an artificial exception to the facts of life, a mutation existing outside the facts of life that apply to every other living creature. However, you can't reject the gift your son chose so carefully, obviously proud that he has intuited your tastes—Impressionist paintings, the work of women artists, peachy colors. You thank him warmly and undo the cellophane wrapping on the box as if you intended to work on the puzzle soon. You ask your husband to bring you a puzzle of an abstract painting. He brings a Jackson Pollack puzzle which you set to work at, sitting on pillows on the living room floor. Your son comes home from school and lets his knapsack slide off his back. "Why aren't you doing my puzzle?" "Well, it looked a little hard. I thought I'd save it for later." He looks at the picture on the Jackson Pollack box. "Hard!" he exclaims.

V

Your first visit to the doctor. You get dressed in real clothes and appraise yourself in the mirror—what admirable ankles. With a shudder you realize you are echoing a thought now terrible in its implications: No one would ever know.

Out on the city streets you hail a taxi, since you cannot risk your new body's being jostled or having to stand up all the way on a bus. The receptionist in your doctor's waiting room is noticeably cool—no honeying today—as she asks you to take a seat and wait. When your name is finally called, a woman in a white coat leads you into a cubicle just off the waiting room and loudly asks your symptoms. Quite often in the past you have, while waiting, overheard the symptoms of many women, and now no doubt many women hear yours. As usual, you are directed to an examining room and instructed to undress and don a white paper robe. On the way you count the examining rooms. Three. One woman—you—is preexamination, one no doubt midexamination, one is post.

When your doctor at last enters, he utters a cheery greeting and then the usual: "Slide your lower body to the edge of the table. Feet up in the stirrups, please." You close your eyes, practicing indifference. It cannot be worse than the worst you have already known. You study certain cracks in the ceiling that you know well and he does not even know exist. You continue to meditate on procedural matters, namely, that your doctor's initial impression in each of his three examining rooms is of a woman naked except for a white paper robe, sitting or leaning on an examining table in an attitude of waiting. He, needless to say, is fully dressed. You contemplate him going from one examining room to the next; the devil will not have to make work for his hands. After the examination you will be invited, clothed, to speak with him in his office, and while you dress for this encounter, he will visit another examining room. It strikes you that this maximum efficiency setup might serve equally well for a brothel and perhaps already does. This is a brothel realized.

Your doctor says you may resume most normal activities and even do some very mild exercise if you wish, but no baths and no "intercourse." "Intercourse," you are well aware, stands for sex, although if you stop to consider, sex is the more inclusive term. Does he say "intercourse" because he is unable to say "sex," or thinks the word "sex" would be too provocative in this antiseptic little room, unleashing torrents of libido, or is it an indirect way of saying that you can do sexual things as long as you don't fuck? This is not something you can ask your doctor.

The last item of business is the prescription for the hormones. He explains how to take them—three weeks on and one week off, in imitation of nature's way. He gives you several small sample packets for starters. At home, standing at the bathroom sink, you extricate a pill from its tight childproof cardboard-and-plastic niche, feverishly, like a junkie pouncing on her fix. Nature's way. Now no more "sweats," no more tears. Your new body is complete. What is this little piece of paper in the sample packet? Not so little when you open it up, just impeccably folded. In diabolically tiny print it explains the pills' side effects or "contraindications," a word reminiscent of "intercourse." Most of them you already know from reading books, but there is something new. The pills may have a damaging effect on your eyes. Fancy that. Nature's way? You settle down on the edge of the bathtub and go back to the beginning and read more attentively. First, a list of situations for which the pills are prescribed. Funny, you do not find "hysterectomy." Reading on, you do find "female castration." That must be it. Yes indeed, that's you. You try to read on, but the print is terribly small, perhaps the pills are affecting your eyes already, for there is a shimmering film over the fine letters. Rather than simply rolling over into the tub, go back to bed, fully dressed, face in the pillows. No, first close the door in case the children come in. Many times over the past weeks you have lain awake pinched by questions, pulling and squeezing back as if the questions were clay, weighing the threat of the bony-footed woman pregnant with her own death—an actress summoned and stuffed for the occasion? part of a terrorist scheme?—against your own undrugged sense of the fitness of things. Now you have grasped that the questions are moot. This is not like cutting your hair, and you have never even had a tooth pulled. The only other physically irreversible things you have done are lose your virginity and bear children. Yes, shut the door tight. It would not do to have them hear you, hysteric, *castrata*.

But of course the sun continues to rise, your center is hardly the center of the universe. Over the next few weeks you get acquainted with your new body. A peculiar thing—though it does not look very different, it does things differently. It responds to temperature differently and it sleeps differently, finding different positions comfortable and different hours propitious. It eats differently, shits differently and pisses differently. You suspect it will fuck differently but that you will not know for a while. Its pubic hair has not grown back in quite the same design or density, so that you look shorn or childlike or, feeling optimistic, like a chorus girl or a Renaissance painting. It doesn't menstruate, naturally. You can't truthfully say you miss menstruation, but how will you learn to keep track of time, the seasons of the month? A wall calendar? But how will you know inside? Can it be that time will feel all the same, no coming to fruition and dropping the fruit, no filling and subsiding, moist and dry, moving towards and moving away from?

VI

At nine weeks, although your new body can walk and move almost naturally, it persists in lying around the house whenever possible. And so you lie around the living room with your loved ones as your daughter, wearing an old sweater of yours, scans the local newspaper in search of part-time work. Music blares, Madonna singing "Like a Virgin," describing how she felt touched as though for the very first time. Were you not disconcerted by the whole cluster of associations, you might tell your daughter that the premise of the song is mistaken: the very first time is usually not so terrific. Perhaps some other evening. Your daughter reads aloud amusing job opportunities. A dental school wants research subjects who have never had a cavity. Aerobics instructor at a reform school. "Hey, Mom, here's something you could do. A nutrition experiment, five dollars an hour. Women past childbearing age or surgically sterile."

A complex message, but no response is really required since her laughter fills the space. Your older son, bent over the Mary Cassatt puzzle, chuckles. Your husband smirks faintly over his newspaper. He means no harm, you suppose. (Then why the fuck is he smirking?) Maybe those to whom the facts of life still apply can't help it, just as children can't help smirking at the facts of life themselves. Only your younger son, building a space station out of Lego parts, is not amused. Unknowing, he senses some primitive vibration in the air and looks up at you apprehensively, then gives you a loving punch in the knee. You decide that he is your favorite, that one day you may run away with him, abandoning the others.

VII

The tenth week, and a most important day in the life of your new body. Your doctor says you are permitted by have "intercourse." If your husband is like most men, he can hardly wait. Proceed with caution, like walking on eggs, except that you, eggless, are the eggs on which he proceeds with caution. Touched for the very first time! Well, just do to it and see if it works; passion will come later, replacing fear. That is the lesson of behavioral science as opposed to classical psychology. But what's this? Technical difficulties, like a virgin. This can't be happening, not to you with that hot little geyser, that little creamery you had up there. Come now, when there's a will…. Spit, not to mention a thousand drugstore remedies. Even tears will do. Before long things are wet enough, thank you very much. Remember for next time there's still that old spermicidal jelly, but you can throw away the diaphragm. That is not the sort of thing you can hand down to your daughter like a sweater.

VIII

Over the next month or two you may find your new body has strange responses to your husband's embraces. Don't be alarmed: it feels desire and it feels pleasure, only it feels them in a wholly unfamiliar way. In bed your new body is most different from your old, so different that you have the eerie sensation that another woman, a stranger, is making love to your husband while your mind, your same old mind, looks on in amazement. All your body's nerve endings have been replaced by this strange woman; she moves and caresses the way you used to, and the sounds of pleasure she makes are the same, only her apparatus of sensation is altogether alien. There are some things you cannot discuss with your husband because you are too closely twined; just as if, kissing, your tongues in each other's mouths, you were to attempt to speak. But you cannot rest easy in this strangeness; it must be exposed, and so you light on an experiment.

You call an old friend, someone you almost married, except that you managed in time to distinguish your feeling for each other from love. It was sex, one of those rare affinities that would not withstand daily life. Now and then, at long intervals, a year or more, you have met for several hours with surprisingly little guilt. This is no time for fine moral distinctions. He has often pledged that you may ask him for any kind of help, so you call him and explain the kind of help you need. He grins, you can see this over the telephone, and says he would be more than happy to help you overcome the mystery of the sexual stranger in your body. Like Nancy Drew's faithful Ned.

You have to acknowledge the man has a genuine gift as regards women. From the gods? Or could it be because he is a doctor and knows his physiology? No, your knowledge of doctors would not bear out that correlation, and besides, this one is only an eye doctor. In any case, in his arms, in a motel room, you do rediscover yourself buried deep deep deep in the crevices of hidden tissues and disconnected circuits. It takes some time and coaxing to bring you forth, you have simply been so traumatized by the knife that you have been in hiding underground for months, paralyzed by any kind of penetration. But you are still there, in your new body, and gradually, you feel sure, you will emerge again and replace the impostors in the conjugal bed. You feel enormous gratitude and tell him so, and he says, grinning, "No trouble at all. My pleasure." Perhaps you will even ask him about the effects of the pills on your eyes, but not just now.

"Do I feel any different inside?" you ask. He says no, and describes in exquisite terms how you feel inside, which is very nice to listen to. This is not in your husband's line or perhaps any husband's—you wouldn't know. After the exquisite description, he says, "But it is different, you know." You don't know. How?

He explains that in the absence of the cervix, which is the opening of the uterus, the back wall of the vagina is sewn up so that in effect what you have there now is a dead end. As he explains, it seems obvious and inevitable, but strange to say, you have never figured this out before or even thought about it. (It is something your doctor neglected to mention.) Nor have you poked around on your own, having preferred to remain ignorant. So it is rather a shock, this realization that you have a dead end. You always imagined yourself, along with all women, as having an easy passage from inside to out, a constant trafficking between the heart of the world and the heart of yourself. This was what distinguished you from men. They were the walled ones, barricaded, the ones with such difficulty receiving and transmitting the current running between the heart of the world and the heart of themselves. It is so great a shock that you believe you cannot bear to live with it.

Watching you, he says, "It makes no difference. You feel wonderful, the same as always. You really do. Here, feel with your hand, so you'll know." With his help you feel around your new body. Different, not so different. Yet you know. Of course, with his help it became an amusing and piquant thing to be doing in a motel room, and then it becomes more love, wonderful love, but you cry all the way through it. A new sensation: like some *Kamasutra* position, you wouldn't have thought it possible.

"At least you don't have to worry about ovarian cancer," he says afterward. "It's very hard to detect in time and a terrible way—"

"Please," you say. "Please stop." You cannot bear hearing those words from this man.

"I'm sorry. I know it's hard. I can't imagine how I would feel if I had my balls cut off."

With a leap you are out of bed and into your clothes, while he looks on aghast. How fortunate that you did not marry him, for had you married him, after those words you would have had to leave him. As you leave him, naked and baffled, now, not bothering to inquire about the effects of the pills on your eyes yet thanking him because he has done precisely what you needed done. It will be a very long time before you see him again, though, before the blade of his words grows dull from repetition.

IX

Months pass and you accept that this new body, its torso ever so slightly different in shape from the old one, is yours to keep. Not all women, remember, love their new bodies instinctively; some have to learn to love them. Through the thousands of little acts of personal care, an intimacy develops. By the sixth month you will feel not quite as teary, not quite as tired—the anesthetic sloshing around in your cells must be evaporating. You resolve to ignore the minor nuisance symptoms—mild backaches, a recurrent vaginal infection, lowered resistance to colds and viruses.... Now that the sample packets of hormone pills are used up, you are spending about $15 a month at the drugstore, something your doctor neglected to mention in advance. Would he have told you this, you wonder, if you were a very poor woman? How does he know you are not a very poor woman? Foolish question. Because you have purchased his services. The pills cause you to gain weight, jeopardizing this thin new body and the ankles, so you run faster every morning (yes, it runs! it runs!), racing nature's way. One very positive improvement is that now you can sleep on your stomach. Your husband can touch you anywhere without pain. When he makes love to you, you feel the strange woman and her alien nervous system retreating and yourself emerging in her place. You will eventually overcome her.

And before you know it, it's time for your six-month checkup. You do not respond to your doctor's hearty greeting, but you comply when he says, "Slide your lower body to the edge of the table. Feet up in the stirrups, please." He does not know it, but this is the last time he will be seeing—no, seeing is wrong since he doesn't look, he looks at the wall behind your head—the last time he or any man will be examining your body. There is nothing he can tell you about how you feel, for the simple reason that he does not know. How can he? Suddenly this is utterly obvious, and as you glance again at the painting of assorted tools, the fact of his being in an advisory capacity on any matter concerning your body is both an atrocity, which you blame yourself for having permitted, and an absurdity, such an ancient social absurdity that you laugh aloud, a crude, assertive, resuscitated laugh, making him look warily from the wall to your face, which very possibly he has never looked at before. How can he know what you feel? He has never attempted to find out by the empirical method; his tone is not inquisitive but declarative. He knows only what men like himself have written in books, and just now he looks puzzled.

Why not tell your doctor? That might help. In his office after the examination you tell him—quite mildly, compared to what you feel—that he might have informed you more realistically of what this operation would entail. Quite mild and limited, but even so it takes a great summoning of strength. He is the one with the social position, the money, and the knife. You, despite your laugh, are the *castrata*. Your heart goes pit-a-pat as you speak, and you have a lump in your throat. To your surprise, he looks directly at your face with interest.

He says: "Thank you for telling me that. But not everyone reacts the same way. We try to anticipate the bright side, but some people take it harder than others. Some people are special cases."

X

A few months later, you read a strange, small item in the newspaper: a lone marauder, on what is presented as a berserk midnight spree, has ransacked the office of a local gynecologist. She tore diplomas from the walls and broke equipment. She emptied sample packets of medication and packages of rubber fingers and gloves, which she strewed everywhere, creating a battlefield of massacred hands. She wrote abusive epithets on the walls; she dumped file folders on the floor and daubed them with menstrual blood. As you read these details you feel the uncanny sensation of déjà vu, and your heart beats with a bizarre fear. Calm down; you have an alibi, you were deep in your law-abiding sleep. Anyhow, you would have done quite differently—not under cover of darkness, first of all, but in broad daylight when the doctor was there. You would have forced him into a white paper robe and onto the examining table, saying, "Slide your lower body to the edge of the table. Feet up in the stirrups, please." Not being built for such a position, he would have found it extremely uncomfortable. While he lay terrorized, facing the painting of common tools, you would simply have looked. Armed only with force of will, you would have looked for what would seem to him an endless time at his genitals until he himself, mesmerized by your gaze, began to look at them as some freakish growth, a barrier to himself, between the world and himself. After a while you would have let him climb down untouched, but he would never again have looked at or touched himself without remembering his terror and his inkling that his body was his cage and all his intercourse with the world was a wild and pitiable attempt to cut his way free.

XI

A year after your operation, you will be feeling much much better. You have your strength back, or about 80 percent of it anyway. You are hardly tired at all; the anesthetic must be nearly evaporated. You can walk erect without conscious effort, and you have grown genuinely fond of your new body, accepting its hollowness with, if not equanimity, at least tolerance. One or two symptoms, or rather habits, persist: for instance, when you get out of bed, you still hold your hands clasped around your lower abdomen for support, as if it might rip away from the strain inside, even though there is no longer any strain. At times you lie awake blaming yourself for participating in an ancient social absurdity, but eventually you will cease to blame as you have ceased to participate.

Most odd, and most obscure, you retain the tenuous sense of waiting. With effort you can localize it to a sense of waiting for something to end. A holdover, a vague habit of memory or memory of habit. Right after he cut, you waited for that worst pain to end. Then for the tears, the tiredness, and all the rest. Maybe it is a memory of habit or a habit of memory, or maybe the blade in the flesh brought you to one of life's many edges and now you are waiting, like a woman who after much travel has come to the edge of a cliff and, for no reason and under no compulsion, lingers there too long. You are waiting for something to end, you feel closer than ever before to the end, but of what, you do not push further to ask.

Needless Hysterectomies

MARCIA COHEN

Excerpted from Marcia Cohen, "Needless Hysterectomies," *Ladies' Home Journal,* March 1976. Reprinted by permission.

In the United States in 1973, the most recent year for which statistics are available, hysterectomies were performed on 716,000 women. Only one other major surgical procedure—tonsillectomy—was performed more often. The number of hysterectomies performed increased by 25 percent in only eight years, between 1965 and 1973.

As the number of hysterectomies performed escalates, so does the controversy surrounding them. Women's groups, consumerists, and even many physicians are asking: How much of this surgery is really necessary? Are hysterectomies performed when less radical procedures would suffice? Are women fully informed of what a hysterectomy involves, and what other choices they may have?

WOMEN UNDER 45

Most of us think of cancer when we hear the word "hysterectomy." But in fact, only 20 percent of all hysterectomies are performed to eliminate malignancies involving the cervix, the body of the uterus, or adjacent organs.

But what about the other 80 percent of hysterectomies, those that don't involve cancer? Why are they performed? Some of the most common reasons are fibroid tumors, prolonged or irregular vaginal bleeding or discharge, pre-cancerous lesions (cell changes which may signal impending malignancy), "excessive" menstrual bleeding, uterine polyps, and sterilization. It is in these cases that controversy develops; here is where doctors themselves may disagree about the need for a hysterectomy.

FIBROID TUMORS

In usual practice, most gynecologists recommend hysterectomy when fibroid tumors have expanded the uterus to the size of a 10- to 12-week pregnancy. But many women do not realize that fibroids do not *always* grow to such size, and that they *almost always* shrink after menopause. Elmer Kramer, M.D., professor of gynecology and obstetrics at Cornell University Medical College, is an outspoken critic of the frequent use of hysterectomy for women who have fibroid tumors.

"WORK" A PATIENT

"A doctor can 'work' a patient," contends Dr. Kramer. "He knows she'll get suspicious if he mentions an operation on the first visit, so he just says she has fibroids and gains her confidence. Then, by the third visit, he says: 'Your fibroids are growing. They should come out.' By that time, she figures he's very conservative. Of course her fibroids are growing. But by how much? Two percent a year? The patient could be just about to enter menopause—when the fibroids will suddenly shrink by themselves—and the doctor could talk her into surgery she doesn't really need."

Dr. Kramer's suspicions were given some statistical credence in a study published recently by Dr. Eugene McCarthy, associate clinical professor of public health at Cornell Medical College. In this study, 32 percent of the hysterectomies recommended by the original physician were declared unnecessary by a second, consulting physician. (Dr. Kramer served as one of the "consulting physicians" on the study.) The results—which Dr. McCarthy admits are preliminary—agree almost exactly with the Trussell report, a study made 13 years ago of 239 Teamsters Union members and their dependents. The Trussell report also disputed the need for hysterectomies in one-third of the 60 recommended cases and concluded that "the grave suspicion of patient exploitation could be raised."

Both the Cornell study and the Trussell report have been challenged. The Medical Society of the County of New York countered the Trussell report with a study of its own members' practices showing only 3.2 percent of recommended hysterectomies to be unnecessary and 7 percent questionable, out of a total sample of 504 women in the study.

But Dr. Kramer remains convinced that physicians recommend surgery too quickly, partly because of the relative safely of surgical procedures today and because "they have to make a living." According to him, virtually all the women in the Cornell group whose recommended hysterectomies were disputed by other doctors had fibroid tumors. According to the "second-opinion" doctors, those tumors were not sufficiently symptom-producing to require surgery in those patients.

Hysterectomy is, of course, not only a therapeutic measure but a totally effective method of sterilization. The Health Research Group in Washington, D.C., claims that some physicians are "selling" hysterectomies to patients (particularly minority groups) without informing them that the process is irreversible.

The group's report also documents pressure on hospital interns and residents to secure patients for "training" operations. "Let's face it," one physician admits, "we've all talked women into hysterectomies they didn't need while we were residents and needed to learn."

CAVALIER ATTITUDE

Such a cavalier attitude might seem to suggest that doctors consider the uterus as dispensable an organ as say, an appendix—and some feminists have accused the medical profession of just such callousness toward female patients. But if needless hysterectomies are being performed, the blame must be shared by patient and doctor alike.

"It never ceases to amaze me," said a doctor on the CBS program *Magazine*, "when a patient comes in who has never seen me before—they've picked my name out of the phone book—and after I've examined them and concluded that they would benefit from a surgical operation, they say, 'Okay, when do we do it?'"

Patients—particularly women, according to some physicians—simply don't ask questions. Whether this throne room atmosphere is created by the sexist power delusions of gynecologists, as some feminists claim, or by the timid dependency and undue modesty of women, as some physicians insist, the fact remains that it's unhealthy....

UNQUESTIONING WOMEN

Given the seriousness of this surgery, it is amazing that so many physicians report that many women do not question their doctors closely regarding either the severity of the operation or what other options may be available.

A woman's own informed choice is the best protection against an unnecessary hysterectomy. That means ask questions about your condition, about its severity, about the consequences of a hysterectomy compared to other forms of treatment.

FIND ANOTHER DOCTOR

And if the answers are withheld or given grudgingly, find another doctor. And, most important, every patient facing surgery has the right to a second consulting opinion. Honest disagreement can be just that—honest disagreement. If that happens, she may want a third opinion.

Every one of the gynecologists who were interviewed for this article agreed that a physician who bristles at the suggestion of a second opinion is "not worth his salt."

And finally, the checkups. Every woman should have a yearly pelvic examination and Pap smear. For there is no controversy about the lifesaving value of hysterectomies where malignancy is involved. Any woman who neglects her checkups is not worth *her* salt.

Chapter 63

Fruits of
the Womb

Preface to With Child

ARIEL CHESLER

Preface to *With Child: A Diary of Motherhood* by Phyllis Chesler, ed., New York, Four Walls Eight Windows, 1997. Reprinted by permission.

W*ith Child* is more than just a book to me. It is a very personal account of the beginning of my life. It carries me to pasts that I could never have seen on my own and allows me to understand my mother in a much deeper way. I am able to see her not just in relation to me, but as her own person. A book written for me and about me is the most welcoming gift that I could have received from my mother upon entering this world.

With child is not fiction but a fierce reality. It charts the time of my mother's pregnancy, my own birth, and our relationship, which began long before I was conceived and will last until forever. I am the fetus, the growing clump of cells, the newborn baby in every line of this book, and have been given insight into the reality of my creation, and all mothers' histories.

This book is not only important for women, or young mothers, to read. I think that children can learn from this book. It can help them to see the importance of a strong bond with their own mother. It has shown me the beauty of that bond and the real reasons that we all should deeply respect our mothers.

I think that men should be aware of what the pregnancy process is really about. This will help all men to think about their own roles in the process. We should neither be terrified by nor ambivalent toward pregnant women. We should see the beauty in pregnancy, in that earth-round belly that holds a child.

My mother has given me life and love. I am flesh of her flesh, bone of her bone. I was born of her body, linked to her by nature. Thus, is she not my Adam, am I not her Eve? Must Adam really be male? Or is she my Eve since she has nourished me with forbidden fruit? Yes! She gave me knowledge of good and evil. The only difference is that she valued and praised the "forbidden" knowledge that she gave me. If we have sinned, by her sharing of knowledge, then at least we are exiled together.

My mother writes poetically and beautifully. She writes with passion, bravery, and strength. At certain moments, in the book, I can envision her singing the book. It is her warrior's tale and she is an ancient bard. She sings a prayer that is her *Sh'ma*; her motherly prayer. She writes: "Hear, O Israel, I am one. Mother and Child. Male and Female. Past and Future. My belly warms the sun-glown stones." The *Sh'ma* is the most important prayer in Judaism. I can also hear a fairytale-like sound to her story when she writes: "In colors of blood and air I spin without stopping: colon, foot, eye. By day, by night, for nine months. I weave you: precisely. Faithfully." This is so witch-like, her spinning me into gold, into body. She recites her thoughts throughout this book in song, with a pulsing rhythm and a graceful melody.

My mother does not begin with the beauty of children or family, or even her ideals of motherhood. She begins with the fact of her vomiting. This is her truth, the pure physical reality of pregnancy. Her voice is an honest, helpful, and questioning voice, which she maintains throughout the book.

When I read this book, I feel my mother talking to me. I see her eyes, smell her cappuccino, and hear her voice. I can always pick this book up if I want to converse with my mother. Her questions force me to ask her questions too. I want to ask about her childhood, about her past. I want to learn more about my childhood, and how she dealt with bringing up a male child. I wonder too how she brought me up in a feminist manner and why our relationship is so unique.

I always thought of my mother as "macho" when it came to work. She never took breaks, never relaxed her mind, but I guess she just couldn't (and still can't) allow herself to. This of course is due to the importance of her work as well as the time she devotes to it. However, when she had the additional responsibility of caring for a child, she realized that she could not handle all of her jobs on her own.

In some ways this book can be seen as quite comical. Here was a Ph.D., an intelligent woman, who was naive when it came to being a mother. She only knew how to ask questions of other mothers, and the more she asked the less she comprehended.

With Child is not only both a personal account of motherhood. It is of the utmost political importance for everyone. It signifies a radical revisioning of motherhood for the coming generations.

This book clarifies that, contrary to myth, women do not exist only to give birth to children. They all have their own lives, desires, and needs. In my mother's case, motherhood really hit her hard and shocked her. I brought her back to earth from wherever she was.

The book you are holding is as precious as a newborn child. In fact, imagine that you are actually holding an infant when you pick this book up. Imagine that this infant is still as small as I was when this book was first published. Imagine how difficult it would be for you to carry this book around with you everywhere you go. Then add about 6 pounds. Think about the time it would take to feed the book, clothe it, put it to sleep, change it, entertain it, and still have your own life and career remain intact.

Now, imagine that the book is alive and cannot survive without you. If every time you left the room, the book looked at you, would you leave as quickly? If you loved the book would you be able to leave at all? If you helped to create the book and loved every bit of it could you let anyone else take responsibility for it? Could you even handle the responsibility yourself? Would your nerves shake every time you held the book, since dropping it could mean death?

My mother's office door is shut, but that means nothing to me, I am her one and only son. A mother can always be taken for granted, a mother can always be counted on. I knock calmly on her door and enter before she can reply. Her books surround her as usual and she sits with a pen in hand. "I'm off duty!" she informs me. I do not comprehend that phrase and reply, "You are not a taxi, Mom, I need to talk to you."

This scene was quite common throughout my childhood. I would upset my mother daily, by trying to interrupt her. Although I found her work interesting and was proud, I was jealous of the time and attention it took away from me. In a sense, despite being an only child technically, feminism was my baby sister, the one who got all the attention, it seemed to me, because she was cuter and more important.

However, feminism has had a profound and positive effect on my life. I was thrust into a world of feminism by birth. Ironically, I never became truly involved with feminism throughout most of my youth, despite my exposure to thousands of books, articles, and events. I was surrounded by feminist leaders, including my own mother; so I took the movement for granted. It was only when I ventured out on my own to college, that, without my mother's encouragement, I began to take women's studies courses. I loved them instantly, and discovered my affinity for my mother's work.

It is often quite frightening for me when I compare my political views to those of my peers. Although my friends are intelligent, liberal, and even pro-gressive, that doesn't always mean they are feminist. I have come to realize that like my mother, I, too, am a radical feminist. It's not as easy as I assumed. I am constantly forced to defend all of my views, to enemies as well as my best friends. It becomes quite taxing and I only pray for the strength to voice my opinion in public, especially to other men.

Over the years, many of my friends have asked me what it's like to have a book written about my birth. "Is it weird?" they asked. "Does it cover your con-ception?" I guess the answer to both questions is yes, but I don't usually think of it that way. Who else has a gift like this? What better birthday gift could I have received? That is exactly what this book is—my birthday present. It is a tangi-ble, never-ending gift to celebrate my life. I feel so blessed, so lucky to have this book. I can't believe that I didn't even read it until I was about 14. Perhaps I wasn't ready for it until then.

In fact, I was quite embarrassed by this book when I was younger. I hated the attention I often got because of it. I remember being ashamed when my mother read to my fourth-grade class, and described my strong bond with her as a marriage. "Because of you, I'll return to Earth, transformed: no longer a vir-gin, but a mother, married to a child." I was so embarrassed by this book that I wrote a parody of it. Oh, if I only knew! My piece was entitled "With Mother" and it was hilarious, at least to a fourth-grade sense of humor. Apparently even then I was attempting to come to terms with this book in my life.

I wonder what I would be like if I didn't have this book or if my mother was a traditional mother. I wasn't aware that my childhood was that different from many of my friends. To me, the way I grew up was normal, although my house-hold was quite different from the people I knew. For example, in my house one would be more likely to see me cooking eggs for my mother, rather than her cooking anything for me. I had sophisticated concepts and "adult" issues thrown at me daily from a very young age. I learned how to travel around New York City on my own. I took care of myself quite often. I spent time alone in our house, when my mother had business. I learned to rely on friends and others for help that my mother could not always give me. I had to learn not to rely on my father. I had to redefine "family" for myself. I was in contact with brilliant, even revolutionary people whom I regarded as simply my mother's friends. I also had to deal with attempts to exclude me from feminist events specifically because I was male. I was forced into becoming responsible, independent, and free of the usual stereotypes. That's why I've become who I am today. I think that the freedom I had growing up was the most important and helpful part of my maturation.

I received respect as an individual from the time that I was born. Although this respect quickly brought responsibility (mental, spiritual, and physical) and maturity to me, it was worth it. In fact, my mother seemed to consider my wishes even before I was born. Like most parents, she and my father discussed my name at length. I could have been named Daniel at one point. Not that Daniel isn't a fine name. I even know some very nice people named Daniel. But it's just not for me.

When my mother was about six months pregnant, I visited her in a dream. I told her, from the womb, what I wanted, what I felt, and she listened. I requested a name that began with the letter A. A name that belonged to me, not just given to me, one that I chose. My mother writes, "I dream a wonderful dream. I give birth to a little blond boy.... Have you really visited me in a dream? Are you requesting a name that begins with A?"

I love my name, what it means, how it sounds. This seems extremely important because my name is a big part of who I am. I am glad to be a Shakespearian spirit, a lion of God, a secret nickname for the city of Jerusalem, a small city in Israel, and even a little mermaid if people must insist on it. My name is Israeli, and it means "Lion of God." At times my name is my only path to my roots, my origins, a past that I yearn to know. It is at times my only connection to my father, who is Israeli. It is only when I say my name properly that I feel truly visible. When I say "Arriael," using that rolling R that I love, in that sweet, rolling Israeli way, I feel like me.

So ever since my mother's dream that mind-melding night, we shared the truth in great detail, until we understood one another.

Jan. 4, 1978. My mother writes: "Tonight I descend, tonight I rise. Tonight I am halved, tonight I am doubled. Tonight I lose you forever, tonight I meet you for the first time. Tonight I cheat death. Tonight I die."

Jan. 6, 1997. It is 5:17 A.M. I am tired but my body wakes me up. I look outside to see cold winter waiting for me. Even my windows shivered with the wind. I do not want to leave the warmth of my bed to be born again, not even on my birthday. That comfortable, healing, mother-warmth that one's bed has for them keeps me under the covers. I roll over and go back to sleep.

Jan. 6, 1985. It is 5:17 A.M. and I crawl out of bed to be with my mommy. I stumble into her bed to cuddle with her on my birthday. I am born anew to you Mother, just like I was that first day. Your bed is special and it relaxes me more than anywhere else in the world. It is my earth-womb, the replacement for my first sleeping quarters, your stomach. You also awoke at this time in the morning and we smile at one another, knowing that this is a rare and wonderful occurrence. Soon we fall asleep, with my head resting on your belly, attempting to return to my first world.

Jan. 6, 1978. It is 5:17 A.M. Today I am born, today I am ended. I am wide awake. I am completely exhausted. I am freed from my mother's body, but enslaved by mine. I see everything around me, I am blind. I feel alone, I am surrounded by too many bodies. Everything is new to me, but I've seen it all before. I am cold, I am warmed by my mother's body. I have my entire life ahead of me, and my last one behind me.

My mother's last line of the book asks, "And who could be closer than we two?" To which I reply to her, No one, Mother. No one.

Having Anne

LAURA YEAGER

Laura Yeager, "Having Anne," *The Missouri Review* 21(3), December 1998.

I have stopped taking lithium so that I can have a child. It's that or heart birth defects. My psychiatrist says that I may not get high if I stay on the drug, but we're not taking any chances. We've hired a "sitter," someone to stay with me for nine months during the day. Her name is Penelope, and she wants to be an actress, but she fully understands that she must stay here with me from 9:00 to 5:30 until Richard gets home. I've informed her that until I start having symptoms, she can take an occasional audition if it is all that important. And if she gets a show, we'll just have to find someone else.

This baby-sitting idea is Richard's. He's seen how I speak in half sentences, how I can't sleep for days, how I have direct communications with God. I'm not sure he would have married me if I'd had manic depression when we met.

I was 24, a perfect innocent who designed children's activities for the art museum. Once, he wandered into my finger-painting exercise, looking for the john. People often did that. The bathrooms were next to the children's room in the basement.

"It's the next door on your right," I said, my fingers smeared in yellow, blue, and red. I was teaching the joys of color combinations. I pointed.

He stood there in a beige raincoat that was a little wet and said, "Thank you."

That was the first time I saw him. I remember he walked directly over to the table and looked at the children's paintings. Over one child's purples and greens, he said, "Beautiful."

"We're learning how to mix color."

He was neither tall, nor short, nor fat, nor thin, nor blond, nor brown.

What stood out about him was his face, which seemed to burst into the world.

"Color," he said. He had a paper under his arm, and the museum booklet for the visiting exhibit upstairs.

I remember he looked at me, and I know I must have looked small to him, in a turtleneck and—oh, God—I think, a tartan skirt—my hair in a ponytail, my face covered by the huge, round black glasses I was wearing in those days. Over my clothes, I had on a white lab coat, which was covered in paint smudges.

"What do blue and yellow make?" he asked one child. At the time, he was

32—eight years older than I. "Do they make green?" he said when the child refused to answer. The child ignored him. Another kid, a boy, spoke up. "Yes, green. They make green."

"What is this?" he asked, looking around.

"This is the children's room."

I began to wonder when he was going to go to the bathroom. He was making me nervous. I admired Stacey's ability to not speak to the handsome stranger. She, at 4, knew how to behave around men. As he walked away, I thought of my grandmother's fear at meeting my grandfather. They'd met under an awning in a rainstorm in Akron, Ohio. He had offered her a ride in the taxi. She had not spoken to him, simply followed, petrified.

As the color ran off our fingers into the tiny sinks on the far wall of the room, I wondered who he was and if I'd see him again.

Five years ago, I was perfect. I had a small apartment near the museum, with white furniture and sheets on the windows bunched up into knots to let the sun in. I drank the right teas with honey, served scones on the right-textured dishes, watered my plants, fed my cat. I listened to the right classical station and had friends in. Oh yes, I bought fresh flowers and sat them in blood-red vases on my glass coffee table. I dated occasionally. One guy, Rex, was a part-time museum guard, full-time graduate student in American History. We did things like see movies at the museum, visit my family or his, go for walks, and cook things out of our mutual gourmet cookbooks. Rex's only problem was that he worshiped me. I began to feel unreal around him.

I'd also go to restaurants occasionally with a guitar player who repaired watches. My boyfriends at the time were, compared to Richard, marginal, and they were also young. Richard, whom I did see again—this time when I was eating grapes in the cafeteria—had arrived. He cleaned up hazardous-waste dumps.

The cafeteria, like all of the museum, is white. Richard stood out because that day he was wearing a black jacket and pants. Still carrying a paper, he filled a cup with coffee and proceeded to pay for it.

Eating the grapes was more of a pastime than anything. I had 20 minutes of lunch hour to kill. That was one of the rare days I had forgotten a book. I had, by this time, grapes on all five fingers.

Richard sat down at a table where he could watch me. Recognizing him, I took the grapes off my fingers and ate each one with a fork.

Richard emptied three creams into his coffee and stirred. He smiled at me. He waved.

I waved back, a 24-year-old woman who'd never been to the hospital before for anything. Six months after our wedding, I broke. Richard, who was used to disasters, handled it logically.

At 8:00, I wake up when Richard grabs my toe. "She'll be here in an hour," he says. This is Penelope's first day. I have spent the last two days cleaning the house so that Penelope will be reassured that this is a nice place to work. She has asked Richard about health insurance, but he's declined to pay for it. He's upped her salary to $275 a week—not bad for simply being my companion. Although, if I get bad, she may have to come looking for me in the car, or God knows what.

I lie here for a few minutes, remembering the weight of Richard on me, his even, reasoned thrusts, his patter of kisses.

As Richard ties his tie, I force myself out of bed and into the bathroom that smells like cleanser—into a tub which Richard has politely left as spotless as it was yesterday. I wait while the water warms, looking at him, with his one-day-old haircut. I like him best like this—trim and neat. He looks, in this hairstyle, capable of making and sticking to an earth-shattering, possibly billion-dollar (if money enters into it) decision.

Standing naked in my first trimester, I can see that my nipples have darkened. My breasts are tender, and I'm craving apple juice and cream cheese with scallions. I look around the porcelain bathroom and see that I have gotten everything I wanted. I do not feel guilty that my husband provided it for me. But I do feel a twinge at trying to carry this baby with this disease. I know that I'm putting myself and the baby in danger. I know that at three months, my psychiatrist will demand (because it's procedural in cases of manic depression) that I go back on lithium. I know that I won't. I know that I may go months without sleep. I comfort myself with the fact that we've done some digging and have discovered that ocean-wave music helps manics sleep.

I'm in the shower when Richard says, "Bye. I'll defrost your muffin. It'll be in the microwave."

"Thanks."

In the hot steam, I allow myself, amidst all my worries, to remember the night of our first date.

He must have been taken with me because he came back to the children's room when we where making prints with apples. This was an older group who could use butter knives to carve designs into their apple halves.

"Don't you work?" I asked. I know I must have been fearless then, and I'm sure this attracted him to me.

"Would you like to go roller skating with me?" he said, half smiling, not waiting for a private moment.

Boys went, "Wooooo."

The girls giggled.

"I get off at five."

He was sly in the activities he chose for us to do—they all reeked of adolescence—innocence. He must have thought I was a virgin. I wasn't. I'm sure all along the courtship titillated him because he saw me as a small, young woman in a plaid skirt, yet he did not worship me. This I was grateful for.

His palm sweated as we spun around with seventh-graders.

"This is corny." I closed my eyes and imagined what it would be like to be blind and doing this. Men terrified me for that reason. I was afraid they wanted to lead me. His first kiss was cool and airy. A guy in junior high said, "Look at that."

Penelope comes when I'm just about to eat my muffin. Wanting to make a good impression, I've dressed in a pink lamb's-wool sweater and skirt. As I open the door, I realize we're peers. I can see lines around her eyes. She has to be 27 or 28, maybe even 29, the same age as I.

"God, I couldn't find it," she says. "Am I late?"

"No."

Penelope takes off her long red coat. She has a bag with her, full of scripts, books, and knitting. "Good. I brought some stuff with me."

"That's fine. I'll be working in the upstairs office. Come on in."

She follows me into the kitchen.

"This is a great place," she says. I don't tell her that *Better Homes and Gardens* has approached us for a story. We're considering it. A magazine pictorial of my home almost frightens me—it's too public. Richard agrees.

"Would you like a muffin?"

"That would be great. I didn't have time to eat."

Penelope, I can tell already, is very dramatic. She opens her eyes wide and smiles as if for a camera. She looks good—trim and supple from all kinds of dance classes.

"How old are you?" I ask.

"Twenty-eight."

"I'm 29."

"I'm trying to make a go of theater," she says. "I'm giving myself till 30. Then it's time for a real job."

"I had a real job."

"What did you do?"

"Children's activities coordinator for the museum."

"Neat," she says, showing her teeth again. She has beautiful blond hair, which she swings to one side like Julia Roberts.

"Now I do newsletters on a computer upstairs. Freelance—churches, plumbers. It's not too exciting."

I hand Penelope a warm muffin and a cup of coffee.

"Thank you."

"You can do whatever you want," I say. "Watch TV, use the StairMaster, read, talk on the phone. If you're going out, tell me."

"Okay."

"Maybe we can do something together every day."

"Sure."

"Take a walk or go shopping, go to a matinee. This is going to be a long eight months."

Penelope wipes her nose. She seems appreciative. I suddenly become worried that she might be a kleptomaniac.

Switching on the computer upstairs, I look at our wedding picture we've framed in gold. I remember our wedding day. Penelope is downstairs reading lines from some show.

We got married at St. Anthony's (the patron saint of lost items) with a Baptist minister cocelebrating the ceremony. The two men on the altar seemed to like each other and practically made small talk during the service. Father Nick, who'd confirmed me, swung his arms wildly when he talked. The minister kept saying, "I agree with you. I agree with you," during Father's sermon. For some reason, everyone cried, even the men. The minister, Richard's father's friend, kept saying, "Marriage is a lot of cleaning up after meals."

Father Nick said, "Yes, and a whole lot more."

We held our reception in the art museum—hors d'oeuvres and drinks. We had enough chairs for everyone, but most people stood, gazing up occasionally at an 8-foot by 8-foot Madonna and child or at a portrait or two of a nobleman. It was a cool summer night, and we had both doors of the gallery open so that a wind blew through the place. The wind kept blowing out the Sterno underneath the hors d'oeuvres, and Richard kept pausing to light the cans. Eventually, we let all of them go out, and people still ate every single one of the tidbits. Richard had one beer, and water with lemon all night because he said he wanted to be awake when we got to the hotel. I'd guzzled down 7-Up and grenadine—Shirley Temples with cherries in them. By this time, our priest and minister had decided to run some joint seminars on God. We promised to attend. I felt married, even more married than the first time I saw him.

When we were finally alone, he unzipped my gown, which had cloth-covered buttons sewn on top of the zipper. I was down to one of those white bustiers and a slip. We had, I don't know how, managed to wait. After five minutes in bed with him, I said, "Something has got to happen. Something has got to happen." It did.

Placing our wedding picture back in its place on the desk, I bring up the masthead of the newsletter I'm working on. *Notary News,* for notary publics in the area. With the title comes preset margins. This is a template—something I find very reassuring. For all I know, Penelope could be downstairs robbing us blind. She is unpredictable still; yet no matter how well we get to know each other, she'll never be fully predictable, not like this template before me.

I type in the first article about a new notary in the area—Rod Owens, on 24th Street. Rod has full power to witness any kind of signature, to process titles and registrations.

"Penelope," I yell.

"Yes." She hears me.

"Are you all right down there?"

"Yes. Are you?"

"I'm fine." With the article typed in, I press a button, and it filters into its proper place on the page. "Fine." I get up to take a pee, something I do all the time these days.

I watch Penelope make herself lunch—wheat crackers, slices of cheese and strawberries. She has brought this food and asks if she can leave it in the refrigerator.

"Of course."

She's dieting. I have six newsletters before me, and I'm trying to edit them. I always edit on the kitchen table. It goes back to college days, when all I had was a kitchen table to edit on.

Penelope doesn't eat. She nibbles. "How are you doing?" she asks in a tone that suggests she sees this question is part of her duty. I suddenly feel like a small child.

"No flights of fancy yet."

"What's it like?" She bites into half a strawberry. "If you don't mind talking about it."

"Pregnancy or mania?"

"Mania."

I circle a spelling error in a mortuary-science newsletter. "You feel as if you're communicating with everyone. I feel sometimes that I can read minds."

"Do you think the baby will have it?"

Penelope, I can see, does not mince words. "How should I know?"

Penelope smiles, appearing to be happy in my confession that we are con-trolled by larger forces.

"Anything else?" she asks.

"About the illness?"

"Yes."

"I travel a lot, spend a lot of money. And everything is so colorful. I hear messages on the radio."

"Am I supposed to restrain you if you get like this?"

"There's a straitjacket in the closet."

Penelope drops a piece of cheese.

"I'm only kidding. You're supposed to take me into a dark, quiet room, turn on the ocean-wave music, rub my back, and tell me things are normal, but we might not even have to resort to that."

"I'm an alcoholic," Penelope says.

She seems too proper to be an alcoholic.

"I've been sober for two years."

"Congratulations."

"I have admitted that I'm powerless over my life. I could break down and have a drink any minute. Sometimes I feel like something is following me, or worse yet, like I'm inside of something, and I can't get out. At those times I have to make the bed, take the garbage out, and scrub the toilet."

"I know what that feels like. I feel like my head isn't attached to my body. Like people I love are trying to harm me. Richard isn't like this at all." I look down at page 5 of *Mortuary News,* the page that publicizes new morticians. "Richard doesn't seem to have anything big hanging over him except heaven. Maybe that's why I married him."

"How long have you been married?"

"Three years."

"How did you meet?"

"He was looking for the bathroom at the art museum. He took me roller-skating."

"That's cute." Penelope eats a strawberry. She seems to be eating now with more vigor.

"Are you seeing anyone?"

"I see a few men occasionally, nothing serious. I'm working on my career. My AA group doesn't recommend dating anyone at the meetings. It's hard to find men who want a commitment."

"Do you?"

"Part of me would love to get married and have a man support me, but then I realize it's completely unrealistic of me. I'm perfectly capable of supporting myself. The work isn't steady, but I can't have a full-time job and act, too. Plus, I can't find anyone. I go to these happy hours, and I can't drink, so I drink this lime soda water and sometimes I talk to men. I recognize some of them because I've temped a lot. Do you know what it's like to answer the phone for eight hours a day?"

"I've done it."

"When?"

"In college. I temped."

"Sometimes I crave alcohol. I was drinking eight drinks a day. I quit the day my kitty got lost, and I was trying to find him in the rain. It was pouring outside, and there I was staggering around yelling, 'Tony, Tony.' The police picked me up, asked me who I was looking for. I said, "My husband. I'm looking for my fucking husband." They didn't arrest me. They got me to confess that I was searching for my cat. I never found him. When I woke up, I had bruised kneecaps from falling down so much. The whole thing was pathetic."

While Penelope talks, I remember how what my psychiatrist calls "the break" happened. We were on vacation at Jekyll Island in Georgia. We'd been married two years. I can see myself jumping off the pier, feeling the fall, not knowing if I'd live or die.

"Excuse me, Penelope," I say, picking up my newsletters.

"Are you all right?"

"Fine. I'll be upstairs."

In the bathroom I splash water on my face and decide to get in the tub.

The jump off the pier terrified Richard. He leaped in after me, off a 20-foot pier, all the way to the bottom.

"What the hell is wrong with you?" he asked as we dog-paddled.

Little did we know, I was breaking.

"We never do anything fun," I said. "Want to do it again?" I knew I wouldn't die. I had no fear.

Later that evening, we joined two couples we had never seen in our lives.

"Hello," I said. "We made it. We're here."

"Who are you?" asked one of the wives.

"Excuse us," Richard said. "We thought you were someone else."

"Let's sit with them," I said. I thought we were famous, that everyone would want to sit with us.

This craziness hadn't just appeared out of nowhere. A month prior, I hadn't slept well. I thought two pigeons at the park were God. They were perfectly white.

In the tub, remembering, I take a bar of lemon soap and soap my neck. And then, when I was in the hospital, Richard visited me every night. Every day it was a different flower delivered to the locked doors.

"Hello." Penelope knocks on the door. "Taking a bath?"

"Yes."

"Did I upset you?"

"No."

"Come down when you get out."

"Okay."

"Where are you going?" asks Penelope.

I have been reclining in Richard's chair for the past two hours, playing off and on with an Easter toy, an egg that opens up to reveal a yellow chick when I press a silver button. I can't watch TV. I feel as if they're talking to me, and Penelope gets embarrassed when I talk back. She feels like she's not doing her job. We haven't told my psychiatrist. For all he knows, I'm lucid. She's knitting up a storm out of sheer nervousness. She's frightened of me, but she's sticking this out because she thinks it will inform her acting.

"I need to be near water," I say, patting my five-month baby, who is, at the moment, quiet. I felt the first kick last week.

My mind, now, is always on. The only way I can get to sleep is if Richard rubs my feet in time to the ocean-wave music, but this keeps him up. We're averaging five hours apiece. This isn't good, and I don't imagine Richard is a joy at work. We've stopped having sex.

"I'll come up with you," says Penelope, following me up the stairs.

One thing I so want is privacy. I never get any of it with Penelope and Richard watching me all the time. But Penelope does wash my back, and this does clear my mind. My heart slows down. She washes me in a circular motion, with a washcloth and soap, which seems to center me. When I rinse, I lie on my back and gaze at my stomach. The warm water feels good on my legs and back. My obstetrician has prescribed exercise to relieve the cramps and aches. I like the tub. At this point, Penelope picks up a novel she keeps on the john for this purpose.

I think about our day. We managed to go to the pet store to watch fish. Staring at swimming fish is one of my favorite pastimes now. They seem so orderly and calm.

"Do you have any razors?" I ask Penelope.

She burps. "Razors?"

"Yes, razors."

"What for?"

"I want to shave."

"Richard said you can't have them."

"Look at me, Penelope. I'm covered with hair. I feel gross."

Penelope cranes her neck to see my legs. I raise my arms; a small bush is growing in each armpit.

"What do you need to shave for?" she asks. "Who's going to see you?"

"I'll feel better, Penelope. God, I'm not suicidal."

"Richard thinks you might accidentally cut yourself."

"Oh, shit." I recline in the tub, submerging my head, wondering why I had to be born with this disease. God, what I wouldn't give for some lithium. I don't know how much more of this I can take.

"Penelope, my dear," I say, sitting up.

"Yes."

"Would you shave me?"

She puts her novel down, looking scared.

"I'm not homicidal either."

"This isn't in the job description."

"Neither is breakfast, lunch, and dinner and all that perfume I gave you."

"All right," says Penelope. "What if I cut you?"

"Go slowly. I won't move."

I place my leg on the rim of the tub while Penelope brings the shaving cream and a new razor. With precision, she sprays a long white stripe of cream on my leg. I pat it all over, and she shaves me from ankle to knee. Making slow, smooth strokes, she takes off the first layer of hair. I rinse off, and she repeats until my left leg is smooth. We do the right. This reminds me of when I was hospitalized, except Richard is stricter than the nurses. We were allowed to shave ourselves. They sat themselves next to the tub and listened, picking their fingernails, bored. Their glasses would fog up from the hot water, and their clothes would become damp.

I raise each arm one at a time. Penelope has the poise of a painter gliding a brush along a surface. She does not look at my breasts. When she's finished, I say, "You did it without a nick."

"Beginner's luck." She helps me out of the tub and leaves me to dry off.

With a wet finger, I flick on the radio to station 99.3, a station I believe is in touch with the president of the United States. I feel that these songs reveal what kind of mood the president is in. I feel as if he's set up this system to inform me of his moods because he values my input on world events.

I report back to him by going through station 101.5. I haven't told anyone about this little cataclysmic information-gathering and -relaying device. They'd think I was crazy.

Then, with my clean-shaven limbs, I throw up—morning sickness at 4:35.

"Hi," says Penelope to the owner of the pet shop.

He's taking people's change with a huge snake around his shoulders. "Hi."

"A sign," I say.

"From whom?" says Penelope.

"From God. This man is Adam, only he's getting along with the devil."

"Shhh." Penelope tries to quiet me.

"This is no devil. This is Bob," the owner of the shop says. "He's my pet boa."

"Bless you. You are a chosen one," I say. At this point, I believe slightly that I am Jesus Christ.

"Let's look at the fish," says Penelope. "That always helps you."

We watch the silvery creatures swim in the green water. It's their order that quiets me. They never run into each other, have the ability to glide and turn—like thoughts. I manage to sit down in front of the tank.

The owner wanders back to the fish area, still holding Bob.

"That's a very beautiful snake," I say. "Come out of there."

"Who's she talking to?" the owner says.

"The devil. She's having a bad day."

"That's some bad day."

"She likes to look at the fish."

"I've noticed."

I look very pregnant and funny sitting on the floor, and a total stranger comments on my condition.

"First one?" she asks.

Her attention adds to my other delusion that I am famous.

"Yes," I say.

"Who's your obstetrician?"

"Lucas." Penelope speaks for me.

"She's good."

"My dentist is Jones," I say. "My psychiatrist, Donovan. My podiatrist is Mills. My psychologist is Smith."

The lady backs away when I say this.

"You too will be saved," I tell her.

"What's she talking about?"

"The end of the world," Penelope says. "It's here, by the way. Should be closing up tomorrow."

"Boy, if you could only feel my stomach. My baby knows Morse code."

"Is this lady for real?" the owner asks.

"My baby's kicks have become a full language."

"She has manic depression. We won't come anymore if you don't want us to," Penelope says.

"She likes the fish?" the owner asks.

"They calm her down."

"She can come anytime." He rearranges the snake on his shoulders, as if it were a stole.

I'm getting a glass of water when the exterminator comes in. At seven months without drugs, I believe he's trying to kill me. I'm psychotic. I need some Mellaril too. I freeze and drop the glass.

Penelope comes running in. "We had the service canceled," she says.

"What's wrong with Mrs. Darrow?" the exterminator asks. He has a particularly breezy voice from the chemicals he inhales.

"She's a little tense these days."

I start crying and run out of the room.

"He's the enemy. It's 3:00. He was due here at 2:30." Penelope has me by the shoulders. "He's the exterminator. We canceled him, and he came anyway."

"We did? No, he's tapped our phone."

She hugs me. "It's okay."

"I'm so tired, and I can't sleep. Whenever I lie down, the baby starts kicking, and my mind won't stop racing."

"You poor thing. Let's see if you'll go to sleep. Come on." She talks to me as if I'm a child. We lie down on the bed, and she rubs my back. "Everything is going to be all right."

"For you, but not for the rest of us."

"What?"

"You're going up the mountain soon."

Later in the day, I hear Penelope talking on the phone. "She thinks people are trying to kill her. What if she thinks I'm trying to kill her? Why am I doing this?" She's talking to her sister who has a 1-800 work number. "I don't want to be Dad's secretary. I don't want to sit in that damn garage and talk to truck drivers all day, but this is getting dangerous."

"Penelope," I interrupt. She jumps.

"Yes?"

"I don't love you."

"That's nice."

As usual, she disregards what I say.

"I like being in bed with you better than I do Richard."

"What?" She puts her hand over the receiver.

"You can calm me down better than Richard can."

"Have you told Richard this?"

"No."

"I should start spending the night?"

I can tell Penelope wants the extra money.

"I think you should. I'll ask Richard. Does this mean I'm gay?"

"No. It doesn't mean I'm gay either."

"What's it mean?"

"It means I can bring you down."

Richard and I sit in the waiting room of Dr. Lucas, my obstetrician. He has a wave machine I like to watch. It's a box full of liquid that sloshes back and forth, creating waves. They're never the same twice. "Can Penelope start sleeping with us?" I ask.

People in the waiting room raise their eyebrows. Someone chuckles.

"Why?" Richard asks.

"She gives a good back rub." I know I should save this for later, but I need to know.

"I stay awake for six months to rub your back, and you don't like it?"

"I love it, but Penelope puts me to sleep faster."

"And where would she sleep?"

"With us."

"The three of us in bed?"

"We have a king-size bed."

"Do you feel it's necessary?"

"Yes."

A lady gets up and moves across the room.

It takes extreme concentration to act sane when Dr. Lucas examines me, but I have managed up to eight months to keep her in the dark as to my psychiatric condition. I just don't say anything. I lie on my back and look at the colors in the fluorescent lighting. I can see blue and yellow. I can see a rainbow in the plastic covering the bulbs.

"The baby has turned," she says. "This is good. The baby's head is now in a downward position. How are you feeling?"

"My stomach is itchy."

"That's completely normal."

"I have varicose veins."

"Also completely normal. Everything looks normal."

Before all this happened, Richard and I could go shopping and have fun. Richard would take me to fancy lingerie stores. He'd sit outside the dressing-room door while I'd try on g-strings and push-up brassieres. Richard was usually business-like at these occasions. "Try the peach on again," he'd say. Sometimes he'd come into the dressing room and fondle my nipples so they were hard. He loved navy blue. I must have six navy blue bras.

The colored lingerie has become a sign of my lucidity. When I'm high, I wear nothing but white. The fancy stuff makes me feel unclean, like a hooker.

But then, before all this happened, it was always Christmas.

Richard agrees to Penelope spending the night. This will allow us both to get more sleep. We'll pay her $50 to sleep with us.

"What will she do for $50?" Richard asks.

I'm not too manic to know this is a joke. "Blow us both."

"You're terrible."

"Just think of her as a big child smack dab in the middle of the bed. We're going to have to worry about that soon, anyway."

"What?"

"A baby in the bed."

Richard wears his clothes, his top button buttoned; Penelope, a cotton nightgown. I wear a large T-shirt that says "Baby."

Penelope seems the most attractive she's ever been. I can see she's hot-rollered her hair. She's wearing lipstick. I know she likes Richard, and I'm afraid she'll steal him. "I changed my mind. I can sleep. We don't need you tonight."

"Hush, come on, get in bed. We'll all just sleep," Penelope says.

The way she says "just" makes me wonder what else she wants to do. Richard is snoring in 15 minutes. With one of Penelope's back rubs, I'm down in an hour.

I wake Richard up in the middle of the night. "Do you want her?"

"Who?"

"Penelope. I know you want her."

"I don't want her."

"I'm afraid she'll never leave our house."

"I'll leave," Penelope says sleepily.

Blowing up this orange balloon relaxes me. I take deep breaths and blow, exhaling into the orange rubber. This baby shower was Penelope's idea. I'm afraid it will expose to my family and friends how sick I am. Penelope just says, "Everyone needs a baby shower." We have a few guests—my three sisters, my mother, Richard's mother, two of my girlfriends, and Richard's sister. They've all been briefed as to my condition.

"Why didn't she let the doctor wean her off of the lithium?" my sister Denise asks.

"She thought she'd been on it long enough. She thought she wouldn't have any problems," Penelope says. "Now, we're going to keep this simple. No games, just ice cream and cake and open presents."

"Where's my address book?" I ask.

"It's in your room. Do you want it?" asks Penelope.

"Yes, I do."

"What do you need your address book for?" my mother asks.

"I need to check something."

"Okay, here's the first present," my mother says, with tears in her eyes.

"Why are you crying, Mom?" I ask.

"I hate seeing you like this."

"Like what?"

"Out of your head."

"I'm not out of my head."

"What do you want your address book for?"

"You know."

"It's time to read the names of the chosen," my mother says.

This is what I did when I broke the second time. She was driving me to the hospital, and I was reading the names and the addresses of friends—the chosen ones.

"Here, open this. It's from me. I hope this baby is worth it," my mother says.

"Mom!" my sister Donna says. "How could you say that?"

"I think we should play a game," says my sister Abby.

"No games," says my mother.

"What about that one where you have to remember items on a tray?"

"That's no fun," I say. I hate shower games.

"Okay, here's your address book," Penelope says.

My mom is motioning not to give it to me. "Take that back from her," she says.

"Why?" asks Penelope.

But it's too late. I've begun to read the names. "Henry Dugan, 201 Mordle Avenue, Cuyahoga Falls, Ohio 44221."

"Why is she doing that?" Donna asks.

"These are the chosen. I must read them. Paula Harrington, 6279 Park Road, Stow, Ohio 44224."

"Well, we might as well open the presents," Penelope says. "Who would like to open the presents?"

My friend Dolores volunteers.

"Karen Johnson, 1901 Pullen Drive, Tampa, Florida 33609." She opens a package of receiving blankets.

"Jan Wynn, 54 Riverside Drive, New York, New York 10024."

She opens a baby hamper, a box of diapers, baby T-shirts, footed sleepers, a lamp.

"Michael Gill, 110 West End Avenue, New York, New York 10023."

I need to read loudly, delivering my message. If I can read their names to the universe, they will be saved.

"Oh, look, a rocking horse," my friend Joan says.

They've begun to ignore me. It's their shower now.

"Are you with her all day, dear?" Richard's mother asks Penelope.

"Yes."

"God bless you."

Days later, I'm swimming in cool water. My water has broken.

"We can't go to the hospital," I say.

"Why not?"

"They'll keep the baby." I double over from a contraction.

"They won't keep the baby. The baby is ours."

"They'll get our baby mixed up with someone else's, and we'll raise it for 10 years, and then discover it's not ours. Where's Penelope going?"

"She's going with us."

"Why is she packing?"

"She's packing your clothes."

"She's going to Vegas."

"Penelope is going to the hospital with us. How do you want to do this?" he asks Penelope.

"I think she'd climb out of a car at this point."

"I'll call an ambulance. Lord, why did we do this?"

A contraction grips my back and lower abdomen. "Both of you are going to Vegas, aren't you? You're deserting me."

"God. I've never called 911," Richard says.

"There's a first time for everything."

"Christ, I can't take this. I have to have this baby."

And then I do it. I grab the phone from Richard and say, "249 Pierce Place. Hurry." I start pacing, terrified. I think that God is punishing me for something, for not taking my medicine, for trying to have a baby, for attempting to be normal. Manics should not try to live normal lives. They need their medicine. Their babies will be crazy. I fight back the pain. And then the ambulance comes.

At the birth, I believe not that I'm Christ, but that I'm delivering Christ. I am convinced that the birth is being televised worldwide, a far cry from a stable with farm animals standing around. Each doctor and nurse is an instant saint. The viewing of the miracle cures everyone of anything.

I lift myself off the cart and onto the delivery table. I'm surrounded by stainless steel. I suck on ice chips and hold Richard's hand. My feet are cold, so Richard gives me his socks. I don't want footies from the hospital. Because my mother had an enema and because they shaved her, I ask for these two procedures.

"Times have changed," a nurse says.

"But I want to be as clean as possible."

"We'll get you clean. Don't worry."

I say a Hail Mary and an Our Father. My contractions are two minutes apart. All I want to do is push.

The doctor catches God with both hands, and Richard cuts the cord. I remember now that she is a girl.

Little Christ has a weird-looking pointed head from squeezing through my cervix. Her eyes are blue, and her hair is light brown. She's 8 pounds, 5 ounces. I love to hear her cry. She's crying for the world.

The baby is fine. My psychiatrist meets us here—calm but furious. Twenty-four hours later, I'm on 1,200 milligrams of lithium and 100 milligrams of Mellaril. I can barely speak.

Richard brings flowers and climbs in bed with me. "Are you hearing messages in the TV?"

"No."

"What about from people in the hallway?"

"I thought she was Christ."

"You know she's not, don't you?"

"Yes."

"Well, no harm done."

"Richard, I love you."

"She's the most beautiful baby I've ever seen."

"What should we call her?"

"Penelope?" Richard says.

"I don't like that name."

"Joan."

"What about Anne?"

Saying good-bye to Penelope is hard. We take her to lunch and attempt to give her the recommendations we promised her, yet she doesn't take them, telling us she's landed the part of a waitress in a show. It's a shame because they're good recommendations.

And now, I rely on cool, pink lithium tablets—three a day—to save, preserve, and keep me. After what happened, I love the sound of the pills rattling when I open the bottle. I used to hate this sound. I used to avoid it by sticking my pointer finger inside and pulling out one pill at a time.

Bulletin on Caffeine

MARK PENDERGRAST

Mark Pendergrast, "Bulletin on Caffeine," *Uncommon Grounds*, New York, Basic Books, 1999. Reprinted by permission.

L ike Ritalin, caffeine has a paradoxical effect on hyperactive children with attention-deficit disorder: letting such children drink coffee seems to calm them down.

Surprisingly, there is little evidence that caffeine harms children, despite widespread belief that it stunts growth, ruins health, and so on. Like adults, however, children are subject to withdrawal symptoms—from soft drink deprivation more frequently than from coffee. Many doctors have expressed concern about pregnant and nursing women who drink coffee. Caffeine readily passes through the placental barrier to the fetus, and it turns breast milk into a kind of natural latte. Because premature infants lack the liver enzymes to break down caffeine, it stays in their systems much longer. By the time they are 6 months old, most children eliminate caffeine at the same rate as adults, with a bloodstream half-life of around five hours.

Research has failed to prove that caffeine harms the fetus or breastfed infant, but studies appear to implicate caffeine in lower birthweights.

Take the Blame off Mother

PAULA J. CAPLAN

Paula J. Caplan, "Take the Blame off Mother," *Psychology Today*, October 1986. Reprinted by permission.

B laming mothers for their children's psychological problems has a long and, unfortunately, respected history, particularly among mental-health professionals. Sigmund Freud's work included some such trends, and the more recent coining of such key terms as "overprotective mother," "maternal deprivation," and "schizophrenogenic mother" swelled the mother-blaming tide. So, too, did theorists' obsessional overemphasis on the importance of mother-child "bonding" in the few days—even the first few minutes—after birth. With professionals leading the way, it's not surprising that mother blaming was legitimized in the layperson's mind as well.

Has the women's movement vindicated mothers and stemmed the tide of mother blaming? Critics of the movement say it has, hoping that feminists will pack up and go home, believing their work to be done. A few years ago, however, Ian Hall-McCorquodale, then a graduate student, and I decided not to take this assertion on faith. We studied a wide range of clinical mental-health journals published between 1970—soon after the feminist renaissance began—and 1982, when it was well into flower. During the 12-year span, mother blaming did not abate; indeed, it continued in epidemic proportions.

Professionals have blamed mothers for a wide range of problems. In the 125 articles in our study, mothers were held responsible for 72 different kinds of psychological disorder in their children, ranging from agoraphobia to arson, hyperactivity to schizophrenia, premature mourning to homicidal transsexualism.

In the articles we reviewed, not a single mother was ever described as emotionally healthy, although some fathers were, and no mother-child relationship was said to be healthy, although some father-child ones were described as ideal. Far more space was used in writing about mothers than about fathers. Furthermore, fathers were often described mostly or only in terms of their age and occupation, whereas mothers' emotional functioning was usually analyzed (and nearly always deemed essentially "sick").

This collective portrait of pathogenic mothering, I believe, is not only scientifically implausible but also socially destructive. As long as mothering is assumed to be the only or primary cause of children's psychopathology, then all that remains to be done is to figure out which kind of bad mothering is to blame. This hurts not only mothers and children but also fathers, when we expect too little warmth, humanity, and involvement form them, assuming these to be somehow "unnatural" in men. Mother blaming also hurts psychology and society by preventing us from looking with fully open eyes at the total range of causes for children's unhappiness and psychological problems.

Why, then, does mother blaming by professionals thrive? One reason is that mothers are usually more visible to therapists than are fathers. Since fathers are frequently less involved than mothers in the family, when a child does have a problem, it is almost always the mother who takes the child to the therapist, making mothers—but not fathers—available for study and observation. It's easier to blame the person in the waiting room than to explore arduously what—and who—else might contribute to a child's problems.

Understanding the sources of psychopathology in children requires more than an intellectual knee jerk, because there are many possible causes, and their relative importance varies from case to case. For one child, the mother's behavior may indeed be the major source of trouble; for another, the father's behavior—or perhaps his absence—gives rise to problems. Yet another child may have had disturbing encounters with an adult relative, a caretaker, teacher, siblings, or other children or may be reflecting familial stresses and tensions stemming from difficult social or economic circumstances. Some children—such as those with a high activity level, autistic characteristics, or a genetic predisposition to mental illness—may be so innately vulnerable that they develop mental problems despite the best of parenting. In the studies we reviewed, such individual differences were rarely considered. To leap to the conclusion that flawed mothering made a child mentally ill is simplistic and unjustifiable; other explanations must be explored.

Mother blaming is also perpetuated by blind allegiance to past theories. In the articles we studied, attempts to question earlier mother-blaming theories or reports were distressingly absent. Instead, the authors we studied simply parroted them uncritically to their readers, ignoring the growing body of child-development research that challenges such simplistic interpretations.

Further fuel for mother blaming is the mistaken belief—held by professionals and laypeople alike—that because women give birth and lactate, they are better suited than men for child-rearing. This has had several repercussions. First, it has served to make women—not men—the main caretakers of children, despite the fact that all child-care tasks but lactation can be done by people of either sex and a child can learn from either parent (or from other people, for that matter). Second, it has blinded us to the psychological importance of fathers in children's development and permitted or forced many fathers to be relatively uninvolved emotionally with their families. Third, it has created a vicious cycle of guilt and discomfort for women. Because mothers are made responsible for most child care, they become tense and worried about doing the best possible job and spending as much time as possible with their children. When a child has a problem and a mental-health worker blames the mother, she is likely to take her child's disturbed behavior as proof of her failure, thus reinforcing the professional who blamed her.

What can be done to stop the barrage of blame? First, both mental-health professionals and mothers need to look before they leap to conclusions about why children develop problems. Mothers are unquestionably influential in children's lives, but so are fathers, other members of the child's world, and children themselves—a fact that often eludes both the blamers and the blamed. Mental-health professionals need to face up to the complexity of child development, stop relying on old and often invalid parenting theories, and do the difficult but essential work of searching out and understanding the multiple influences on children's development.

Second, mothers would be less readily scapegoated and more often supported in standing up to professional "experts" who wrongfully berate them if their child-rearing successes were more frequently acknowledged. Our society usually fails to give mothers credit for the good they do, unless they are dead or described in the abstract, as in "apple pie and motherhood." Yet mothers, despite their anxiety and guilt, manage to raise millions of reasonably well-adjusted kids. They deserve far more credit for this than they get.

Third, we need to raise sons in ways that prepare them better emotionally for parenting, and we need to acknowledge the enormous personal and social importance and worth of parenting as a role for both women and men. When both sexes come to understand that there is no biological foundation for assigning child-rearing primarily to women and men are encouraged from childhood to develop and value their own nurturant abilities, we may set the stage for a more equal partnership in child care—and more equal responsibility for children's emotional well-being.

As one of novelist Robertson Davies's characters says: "I'm sick to death of people squealing about their mothers.... What's a perfect mother? We hear too much about loving mothers making homosexuals, and neglectful mothers making crooks, and commonplace mothers stifling intelligence. The whole mother business needs radical re-examination."

Lovely Me

BARBARA SEAMAN

Excerpted from Barbara Seaman, *Lovely Me: The Life of Jacqueline Susann,* New York, Seven Stories Press, 1996. Originally published by Wm. Morrow, 1987. Reprinted by permission.

I t was a strange, divided life Jackie led. They were spending around $2,000 a month on entertaining, making the rounds of Toots Shor's, 21, El Morocco, Sardi's, the Stork Club, the Little Club, Danny's Hideaway, and others. They were out so much at night that Irving figured it cost him close to $1,000 a year to check his hat, yet her days were spent worrying over Guy and dragging him to doctors. And mostly what she got was confusion, contradictions, implications that she had somehow caused his problems, or that she was failing to solve them. Irving's young assistant, a girl named Penny Morgan, recalls: "Guy was the most beautiful baby, and Irving just thought he was different. He had a face like sunshine. Jackie... focused all her energy on getting him well. She never stopped hoping that he would recover; she had constant anguish over it. Outwardly she coped with it well, but she would have traded anything she accomplished in life in return for Guy being normal."

In December of 1949 Guy turned 3, and then his small vocabulary almost disappeared. Friends remember him screaming "Goddammit! Goddammit!" One afternoon the nurse brought him home from the park screaming, as had often happened before, but this time the blood-curdling screeches continued throughout the day and the following night, with breaks only when Guy gave in to exhaustion and slept fitfully. Irving questioned everyone in the park and even hired private detectives, but there was never a clue as to what had provoked the child. The screaming stopped in time, but Guy continued to withdraw. And now his condition was given a name: autism.

The word was used by Dr. Lauretta Bender, to whom Jackie's psychiatric journey had taken her. Dr. Bender was a petite and earthy woman who had originated the Bender Visual Motor Gestalt Test, a tool still in widespread use today as a means of evaluating "maturational levels of children, organic brain defects and deviations in function." She stood somewhat apart from her psychoanalytically oriented colleagues in that she was more inclined to look for physical, neurological bases for such disorders. She thoroughly disagreed with those colleagues who blamed the mother and "poor communication within the home" for autism. "I've had mothers come to me weeping and saying, 'I can't reach my child. I try every way I can but I can't reach my child.' Of course the mothers are very upset," she says, " *because* of the child's behavior. I have never seen one single instance in which I thought the mother's behavior produced autism in the child."

Dr. Bender was interested in Jackie's Uncle Pete, the *meshugge* dentist, and also in Irving's "peculiar" uncle, believing that there was often a pattern of schizophrenia in the family history of the autistic child.* She saw Guy's case as classic in many aspects, including his indifference to affection and his failure to communicate, his fascination with spinning objects, his rhythmic rocking and head banging, and his general withdrawal. She was not very encouraging, but she suggested a controversial approach—a series of shock treatments that might jar him out of his silent world enough so that he could benefit from therapy.

Shock treatments for a 3-year-old? It seemed cruel, yet no one had offered anything hopeful as an alternative. Reluctantly, Jackie and Irving agreed to leave him in the Bellevue children's ward, in Dr. Bender's hands. They compared notes with other parents whose children were there, and were somewhat reassured to find them mostly upper-middle-class people who, like the Mansfields, sought only the best for their kids. One unhappy father, a physician, told her, "This is the last step before putting my little boy away for good."

Irving long regretted the shock treatments. "I think they destroyed him. He came home with no expression, almost lifeless." And now, the doctors advised that Guy be placed in an institution. Perhaps he might have a remission at puberty, Dr. Bender declared, but for now he needed the special care and supervision of an institution.**

They agreed, in the most heart-wrenching decision of their lives, and Guy was taken to his first of many institutions, a Rhode Island facility surrounded by rolling lawns. They left their son there, in one of the red-brick buildings of this strange place where he would be cared for but probably not loved. It was

---

*Others, then and later, are less sure, and in fact so little is really known about autism that experts even now disagree about whether or not it is a form of childhood schizophrenia, from which it differs in several crucial ways.

**Even today, institutionalization is necessary for fully two-thirds of all autistic children, for whom no chemical or psychiatric therapies avail. Behavioral techniques have had limited effectiveness, particularly in cases where some language skills have been developed and retained, but the prognosis for the majority of autistic children is as bleak now as it was in Guy's infancy.

a decision they knew many among their relatives and friends could never understand or accept, so they agreed to keep it from all but a few of the people closest to them. To others, then and for the years that would follow, Guy was said to be attending a special school in Arizona because of a serious asthmatic condition. Jackie's explanation to those who knew the truth was that Guy might recover in his teens, and if so, she didn't want him "stigmatized."

The experience—not only the difficulties with Guy himself, but the grinder she'd been put through by the "experts"—took a harsh toll on Jackie. Autism, which afflicts about 350,000 people in the United States, most of them male, had first been described only a few years earlier, in 1943, by Dr. Leo Kanner of Harvard. At first he and most of his colleagues had blamed the condition on mothers: "refrigerator mothers," "schizophrenogenic mothers," or even—conversely—"smothering mothers." The influential Dr. Bruno Bettelheim had even gone so far as to advocate radical "parentectomy"—the complete and permanent separation of parents and child—as the autistic's only hope. In the intervening decades the tide has turned, and in 1975, a year after Jackie's death, Ruth Sullivan, director of information for the National Society for Autistic Children, would state: "There has probably been no group more crucified by the mental health profession than the mothers of autistic children. It is my own personal belief that it will rank high among the scandals of the twentieth century."

The Madonna's Tears for a Crack in My Heart

AUDREY FLACK

We're closing the house for the summer, leaving for New York. I am in the kitchen loading a huge straw basket, when my husband Bob holds up a picture in the *New York Times Magazine*, a full page black and white photo of a young child.

"Do you think this could be Melissa?" he questions.

I lose my footing and stagger. It's a photograph of my daughter Melissa when she was 5 years old. The photo focuses on her beautiful eyes and nose, the rest of her face partially hidden by the back of a slatted chair, which she presses her lips against. She appears to be behind bars.

Oh those eyes. Extraordinary, beyond belief... wide, green, and unbelievably huge, staring, looking blind yet seeing all, and seeing nothing. Her ethereal beauty was awesome, with delicately arched eyebrows, a finely chiseled nose, and a full mane of chestnut hair. Her eyes gathered the power of her muteness; she would eventually use them to speak for her. I was to find out, years later, that her strange stare was a classic symptom of autism.

The picture was taken at the height of Melissa's autism. Her anger, rage, frustration, and physical pain had run its course. It had ravaged her. She cried incessantly, mercilessly, uncontrollably, during her infancy. I brought her to pediatricians for help and was told I was nervous. After persisting in my cries for help, I was labeled neurotic. They could find nothing wrong—but there *was* something wrong and I knew it! She was in pain, maybe her limbs ached or her head throbbed, she screamed, and all I could do was hold her and watch, nothing alleviated her agony. I begged for help as I watched my beautiful child's body, soul, and mind devoured by a mysterious neurological demon. The next stage of devastation seemed to be a caving in, a giving way, a slide into a world of total bewilderment and confusion. She looked stunned, shocked, stupefied.

Whatever biochemical imbalance had taken place within her small, delicately boned body had affected her comprehension, hearing, depth perception, and motor coordination. She would freeze in panic in the middle of a stairway. Sounds of fear came from her throat, choking sounds, and then she'd collapse in a heap and shake, perched on a too-shallow step.

She would flinch and blink rapidly when my hand came close to her face, to feed her or comb her hair. To strangers it looked like she was an abused child. I learned to move slowly and never approach her peripherally. Her condition seemed much like Helen Keller's, only she was not blind and deaf, she only appeared to be. Just the opposite. Her peripheral vision is amazingly astute, almost like a bird with eyes on either side of its head. Melissa prefers to watch television from the side. Her hearing is uncanny, far exceeding the normal range.

If Melissa's hearing is truly as acute as I know it to be, and sounds, even minor ones, are amplified, it would follow that she had to find a way to turn them off, in order to survive. A bomb could explode in front of her, and she wouldn't blink. Doctors insisted she was deaf, I knew it was just the opposite.

I researched autism, searching out any program available, any information accessible, however pitiful, driving around and dragging Missy from doctor to doctor.

What incredible agony I felt when specialists told me their terrible stories. All were firmly committed to their contradictory diagnosis. She is absolutely deaf! Retarded! Brain damaged! She is incurable! Send her away! Forget her! She's not retarded... just wait until she's 12 years old, she'll straighten out. She's schizophrenic... deviant... mentally ill... hopeless!

Autism was an unknown entity until the late 1950s, when a Dr. Leo Kanner isolated a small group of children who could not be categorized. While their behavior lagged behind the norm, these beautiful and strange children did not appear to be retarded in the classic sense. While some spoke strangely, others stared off into space... even stared right through you. A great many, like my daughter, remained mute, unable to express themselves or make their wants known.

They seemed removed, wanting to be alone, they didn't play with other children and remained isolated, sitting in corners rocking, spinning tops, or mechanically stacking objects. Some stared at bare light bulbs, others covered their ears at the sound of certain noises as if in pain. Melissa did both. Many acted deaf. Some hit, scratched, and kicked. Some mutilated themselves, biting chunks out of their own arms, even gouging out their eyes.

A very few showed extraordinary skills, such as naming what day of the week a certain future date would fall on, photographically memorizing telephone books, and making extraordinarily detailed drawings after just one glance. The term "idiot savant" was changed to "autistic savant." The movie *Rain Man,* starring Dustin Hoffman, exposed the syndrome to the public. The main character was based on an autistic boy who attended Melissa's school. But only one in a million is a savant; the overwhelming majority are severely impaired and far from glamorous.

Most would walk in front of an oncoming car or out the window of a highrise building. The medical establishment said these children wanted to commit suicide in order to get away from their intolerable cold, aloof, destructive mothers. All their abnormal behavior was unconditionally blamed on the mother.

Dr. Bruno Bettleheim, founder of the Orthogenic School associated with the University of Chicago, was the leader of the pack. He labeled us "refrigerator mothers" and unequivocally declared that because we were so cold, removed, and uncaring, our children developed the symptoms of autism.

I can think of no greater nightmare than to have a sick child, a child you have birthed, a child you love with all of your being, a child whom you would (and often did) sacrifice your life for, and be blamed for their condition.

In his book *The Empty Fortress,* Bettleheim compared the homes of autistic children to Nazi concentration camps and suggested that their condition stemmed from extreme frustration in the mother-infant relationship. He said we rarely cuddled or fondled our children, our behavior was mechanical and expressed no feelings of love or parental affection. A substantial body of the medical health profession accepted his position. Mothers were a major "pathogenic" factor in contributing to the disorder.

In an odd way, I almost welcomed the blame. If I was the cause of Melissa's condition, then a change in my behavior could also cure her, and I wanted to cure her desperately. But none of this was true.

I was to find out that Melissa stiffened when being held because her skin was so sensitive. It hurt her to be touched. I had all this love, warmth, and affection for her, which she physically could not accept. She was not rejecting me psychologically, she was in *pain.* She bit and kicked me when I tried to dress her because clothing felt like sandpaper and razor blades scraping her skin. She could not say what she felt.

It is only within the past few years that a few older autistics have been able to describe their feelings. It never occurred to them to commit suicide by walking out a window or stepping in front of oncoming traffic. They tell us that a 10-story-high window can look as if it is on ground level, a car can appear to be miles away one minute or on top of them the next, or not there at all. Stairs can suddenly disappear or wave as they are walking down them. The pattern on an oriental rug can come alive, as if it's moving or jumping up at them. One mother whose child screamed and refused to walk on grass found out years later that he thought he would fall through the spaces between the blades of grass. It is clear that their spatial perceptions are distorted, they go on and off, working sometimes and blurring at other times.

Instead of the "refrigerator mother," the child herself may be doing the rejecting. She may not be able to recognize her own mother's face. How painful not to have your own child recognize you, love you, hug you, or speak to you, but imagine going for help and being systematically tortured and blamed. Most of us stoically took it. There was no other recourse. We learned to say what the doctors and social workers wanted to hear in order to get our children into the only programs available.

After numerous phone calls, researching, and networking, I found out that Lenox Hill Hospital had a special program for autistic children which met for one hour once a week. It was based on Bettelheim as well as Freudian psychogenic doctrine and promoted the theory of blame. The doctors and social workers were instructed not to talk to the mothers in front of our children because we were the cause of their problems and if they saw us talking, the children would not trust the doctors. Melissa was 3 years old and mute at the time.

Everyone (except the other mothers) blamed me. I was an outcast. I could not get help. I had no money. I went to a psychiatrist through a clinic. My behavior was analyzed. Why did I do it? Do what?

Melissa was uncontrollable; I was the only one who could handle her. She did not sleep for four years. She had to be watched every moment. She wandered around the house all night long, throwing everything down, turning on gas jets, taking knives, forks, and scissors out of drawers, putting them in her mouth and walking full speed ahead. I had to protect her from herself.

This meant that I did not sleep for four years... cat naps... one eye open, one eye closed, always in attendance. It got to the point where I didn't know whether I ate or drank. It was only if I felt faint that I realized I had not eaten for the entire day. I was consumed by Melissa. I couldn't bear to tie her to her bed, and there was no other way to keep her still. The 50 minutes I spent in the psychiatrist's office was the only peace I had all day and night. It didn't matter what was said, I could sit still for 50 minutes.

I always put on a smile as I pushed the stroller because Hannah, my younger daughter, needed friends, and if I showed my depression and desperation I was afraid no one would play with her. I kept up a front and maintained some degree of normalcy for Hannah's sake.

It was while waiting in the lobby of Lenox Hill Hospital that I got acquainted with and came to love the other mothers of these sick children. These loving, selfless women not only carried the burden of their sick children, but had to bear the guilt, blame, shame, and accusations heaped on them by the medical profession, including social workers and teachers, as well as an entire society that shows little empathy for those who don't fit in.

Families were destroyed. Husbands left and wives stayed behind, becoming alcoholic or dependent on pills given to them because they were "neurotic." Husbands who remained understandably escaped to their jobs, a relief for them, but not for the wives who were left to care for noncommunicative, mute, and uncontrollable children.

On the rare occasions when we were able to get together, we compared notes and found that we had all started talking to ourselves. Our looks faded, our hair went uncombed. Who had time for lipstick? Who had time for ironing? Food stained our clothing and stuck in our hair.

At least we had each other, as we sat holding or running after our children while waiting our turn, on hard plastic chairs in the cold hospital lobby. We exchanged news about new developments in research, pharmaceutical medicines, and school programs. We understood each other's plight. In those few minutes we could comfort and support each other, offering hope, even if the doctors couldn't.

Our observations and opinions were dismissed as neurotic and therefore invalid, although we knew far more than any doctor about our children's condition, we learned to keep silent or say only what the authorities wanted to hear. We were alone, we didn't even have a group, just these happenstance meetings in the lobby, as we delivered our children and watched them come out of some test or special class, which we were kept unaware of.

Once a child was accepted, the program offered only a small playgroup, which was really for the benefit of the hospital's psychiatric department to conduct psychological studies using our children as specimens. Melissa was accepted and I was instructed to bring her to a private street-level entrance on Lexington Avenue, ring the bell and wait. I followed the instructions, a door opened, a teacher took Melissa's little hand, and without a glance or nod of recognition, proceeded to close the door in my face.

The process of getting Melissa to the hospital was formidable. First there was the ordeal of getting her dressed. She fought, kicked, screamed, and bit. We hear now that the clothing may have hurt her exquisitely sensitive skin. My arms were scarred with bite marks from her desperate attempts to protect her skin, yet I couldn't let her go naked. No one knew the reason or understood the behavior until years later when older verbal autistic adults found ways to express their feelings. We have learned a great deal from people like Temple Grandin, who has written several books about what it's like to be autistic.

Getting Melissa to the program, a simple trip, presented problems of almost insurmountable proportions. I couldn't afford a baby-sitter and had to drag Hannah along with us. I carried one child and held the other. I had to drag Melissa by the hand. Sometimes I tugged so hard, I was afraid I might pull her arm out of its socket. Everyone looked, heads turned. The light turned green, but Melissa refused to walk. Suddenly, in the middle of oncoming Broadway traffic, she would drop, collapse in a heap, and stretch out flat on her back. Panic and terror seized me.

Finally I'd get Melissa up and into my other arm, and we'd get across the street. I now think that Missy must have been disoriented by the moving vehicles and have dropped to the ground for safety, but we still don't know, she can't tell us.

The feat of getting Missy dressed and across town was nothing compared to the stockpile of other problems I had to deal with. Windows had to be locked to prevent her from walking out of them. I had to keep them closed even in the summertime when we had no air-conditioning. I had to keep a constant eye on her. Melissa destroyed the house every day. She turned chairs upside down, pulled cloths off tables, smashed dishes and glassware, unmade beds as fast as they were made. Everything had to be upside down. I now wonder if her retina couldn't reverse vision as normal eyes do, and in her own way she was trying to right things by turning them upside down.

Poor motor coordination made it impossible for her to take food or drink from the refrigerator without disaster. Pouring a glass of milk was traumatic. Sour cream, plop, ketchup, she managed to get the top off, then bang, splatter over the floor and the refrigerator door. She would bite into the cheese with the plastic wrap still on. I'd fight to pry her mouth open to prevent her from swallowing it. I tied a rope around the refrigerator door for sanity, protection, and survival.

One of the few things that kept her attention, and that she enjoyed, was looking down at the cars and passersby on Broadway. We lived on the second floor, and I would hold her for hours while she peered out the window.

I could never leave her alone. She needed to be protected from herself. I even took her into the bathroom with me. I was the basic vehicle for her simple survival. Missy was blessed with good health, but on the few occasions that she did get sick, her temperature shot up from normal to 105–106 degrees in an instant, with no other symptoms. I shook with fear.

Life was unbearable. I could no longer continue. I was forced to make a devastating decision. I sent my child away. I knew she needed help and I had to save the family, which was collapsing under the strain. The Rudolph Steiner School had a residence in Pennsylvania focusing on children with special needs. They followed Steiner's theosophical philosophy and were kind to the children. It was the best option I could find. I couldn't continue alone any longer, and I was very worried about Hannah, who had developed severe asthma. I wasn't about to kill the healthy chicken to make chicken soup for the sick one, and that was the choice.

I mourned for a solid year after Missy went away. What must that have been like for young Hannah? This was the first time my 3-year-old had her mother all to herself… a mother in mourning.

We were not allowed to visit Missy for three months. The theory was that she needed time to adjust to her new surroundings and was not to be reminded of her family.

Can you imagine being 5 years old, in physical distress and mental confusion, unable to communicate, totally dependent on your mother, and having that connection wrenched away? It would have been difficult enough for a normal child, but for an autistic, who also needs to keep the same patterns in order to make sense of life, it must have been devastating. This information was not known at the time; research on the neurological aspects of autism was in its infancy. Melissa became seriously ill, would not eat, would not sleep. I was not told until months later, after she had recovered.

The anguish I felt was unbearable, a large crack had formed in my heart….

I brought Melissa home after a year at the school to institute a program called "patterning" developed by a group that called itself the Institute for Human Potential. The theory was based on improper, missing, or defective brain development. The program involved retracing and reenacting the physical activities of infancy and childhood, such as creeping and crawling. The child was placed face down on a table. It required three people. One moved the child's head, the other two stood on either side moving both an arm and a leg, reproducing the act of crawling.

The procedure itself was simple, but the rules were rigorous. Patterning had to be done for 20 minutes every two hours. This meant finding people who could come to the house, stay for half an hour, and leave. I needed an army, and in fact I found many friends and neighbors who were willing to help. When someone canceled, Hannah handled Missy's head, when she was home from school. But it was a terrible chore to be always scheduling and always in need. I patterned for a year, maybe two. It dominated our lives.

My second husband, Frank, played the cello in pickup orchestras, and I sold a painting here and there. We desperately needed money. When Sid Tillim asked me to take over his drawing class at the Pratt Institute, I grabbed the opportunity. I rearranged my life in order to teach the very next day. It was the start of my teaching career.

It took an hour and fifteen minutes on the subway to get to an early-morning class at Pratt in Brooklyn, and another hour to get back and teach anatomy at New York University, Washington Square. I'd gulp down a cup of coffee and a jelly donut before making a wild dash back to Pratt to teach in the late afternoon. Teaching jobs were hard to come by, particularly for women. Even though I was an excellent teacher and my classes were filled to capacity, I was given the worst time slots and paid the lowest salary. A request for a raise was met with, "You're married, you don't need the job. Be glad for what you've got."

When I finished teaching I returned home to relieve the baby-sitter, clean up Melissa's mess (which was a hundred times worse than a normal child's), calm Hannah, cook supper, and feed the family. Frank would arrive in time to consume a brief dinner, between performances at Radio City Music Hall, where he worked as a cellist. Since there were four to five shows daily, he was rarely home. I washed the dishes, bathed the children, read to Hannah, and prayed that Melissa would fall asleep.

Eventually there came a better time, when Bruno Bettelheim's doctrines were disproven and invalidated, and autism was recognized as a neurobiological disorder that interferes with the functioning of the brain.

How shocked and disgusted I felt when I read *The Creation of Dr. Bettelheim,* a biography by Richard Pollack, whose brother had attended the Orthogenic School. It exposed Bettelheim as a fraud. Bettelheim had invented degrees he never earned. He told of being trained as a psychoanalyst, which he never was, and bragged about his relationship to Freud, whom he never met. He was bordering on psychotic.

The medical establishment backed off, and doctors who had previously blamed the mothers apologized publicly. A feeling of relief and satisfaction came over me when I heard that Bruno Bettelheim had committed suicide. Justice had prevailed, the evil man was dead, and I was, after 40 years of torment, redeemed. Mountains of guilt collapsed like compacted garbage heaps but the emotional trauma remained.

Today I persevere, searching for an answer, but I am no longer alone. A strong body of passionately committed parents, many of them doctors and scientists, is united in their efforts to find the cause and a cure.

Back in the summer house, I look up and see Bob still standing there. He knows that I have been far away and has been waiting for me to return to the present, East Hampton 1986. I must know for sure if it's Melissa's picture in the *Times.*

The next day I call the school where Missy lived 22 years ago, and through them I track down the photographer.

"Are you the person who took the picture of the little girl with the big eyes that was in *The New York Times* this Sunday?"

"Yes, I am."

"Could you tell me the name of the girl?"

"Melissa," he says slowly, "her name was Melissa."

With a heavy sigh of relief, and a flush of excitement, I tell him, proudly yet timidly, that I am her mother. Then, I flood him with questions.

He says he visited the school 22 years ago and noticed this incredibly beautiful child with huge, soulful eyes.

"I shall never forget her," he says. "You are her mother? Tell me, are her eyes the same? How is she doing?"

"Ironically, she is still in Pennsylvania," I reply, "near Paoli. She is doing well. She still cannot speak, but she has found other ways to communicate. And yes, her eyes are still as big. Would you like a picture of her?"

"Yes," he says, "and I will try to find a print for you. I am touched by your call. Several people have called me about that photograph today!"

Is this why I painted Dolores of Cordoba with a torrent of tears pouring down her cheeks, gritting her teeth in a grimace? The statue in Cordoba has an oversized, thick gold heart placed in the dead center of her chest. Twenty-five daggers pierce her heart, and blood gushes, drips, and spurts from the stab wounds. Some find Spanish Baroque passion sculpture extreme. I find it realistic.

The Secret Side of Psychotherapy

THOMAS MAEDER

Excerpted from Thomas Maeder, *Children of Psychiatrists: The Secret Side of Psychotherapy*, New York, Harper & Row, 1989. Reprinted by permission.

Psychoanalysts, Freud asserted, should be like surgeons, concentrating on the skilled performance of their operation without interference from feelings or human sympathy. The theoretical role of conventional psychotherapy is not to teach or direct, but merely to correct by releasing patients from pathological compulsions or constraints that inhibit the natural development of their innate individual selves. Implicit in this belief lies the assumption that psychotherapists are actually able to view the disordered mind with cold, scientific logic, and can tell a normal personality apart from abnormal forces that restrain it. Whatever patients choose to do with themselves afterward are not properly the therapist's concern. Therapists, after all, are trained in techniques, not in philosophy, ethics, or theology.

Today, however, we question even the surgeon's supposed objectivity. Hysterectomy, for example, is far from a purely logical procedure—it involves very human judgments and biases about weighing risks and benefits, deciding what constitutes "disease," and identifying an ideal surgical endpoint. What faith can one have, then, in the detachment of psychotherapists, who labor in far more ambiguous terrain. Therapists bring their own notions of sexuality, morality, duty, quality of life, and sense of a life well lived into the consulting room with them. Not so long ago, the American Psychiatric Association officially classified homosexuality as a mental illness. What therapists elicit from patients is in part a reflection of their own techniques and expectations: it is no coincidence that people in Freudian analysis have Freudian dreams and grapple with childhood sexuality, while those who submit to a Jungian analysis have Jungian dreams and wrestle with archetypes, shadows, and anemia. Therapists wield a tremendous authority over their patients, yet these patients generally do not—and perhaps cannot—view them with the same critical appraisal they would apply to other advisers, even parents or trusted friends.

Who are psychotherapists, and how might their personalities, beliefs, and motivations influence the sort of therapy they deliver? It seems vicious to say that people who help others should be suspected ipso facto of ulterior selfish motives. Nonetheless it is true that the "helping professions" such as nursing, charitable work, the clergy, and psychotherapy attract people for curious and often psychologically suspect reasons. People who proclaim, "I want to help other people," harbor the odd underlying assumption that they are in a position to help and that others want to be helped by them. They may be lured, knowingly or unknowingly, by the position of authority, by the dependence of others, by the image of benevolence, by the promise of adulation, or by a hope of vicariously helping themselves through the process of helping others. Some helping professionals, fortunately, have humbly and realistically perceived that they have something to offer and are willing to take on the responsibility of doing so, but others use the role to manipulate their world in a convenient, simplistic manner, ultimately not taking responsibility in a meaningful way at all, but using authority precisely to avoid it. For these people, psychotherapy is not merely a way to earn a living: it becomes the essence of their lives.

One often hears the accusation that psychotherapists are crazy and that this is probably what led them to their jobs, a simplistic exaggeration built on an element of truth. A president of the American Academy of Psychotherapists once said in an address to his organization, "When I first visited a national psychiatric convention, I was dismayed to find the greatest collection of oddballs, Christ-beards, and psychotics that I had ever seen outside a hospital. Yet this is to be expected: Psychotherapists are those of us who are driven by our own emotional hunger."

"I rarely have found a healthy, well-integrated, happy person seeking this profession," one training analyst told me, while a clinical psychologist remarked, "I question your calling it a myth that therapists are crazy, because the fact is that most of them are. If you needed any proof, let me tell you that every patient who comes into this office who has had a previous experience with some other therapist has some kind of horror story to tell, some major failing on the therapist's part, including, quite often, sexual abuse, verbal abuse, things that cross the boundary of mere bad technique and come pretty damn close to the criminal."

Abundant anecdotal evidence and a smattering of hard research indicate that people drawn to therapy as a profession tend to be troubled people seeking answers to their own problems and a way to feel more at ease in the world. This can, of course, be an enormous advantage. Mythology and religion abound with figures who must learn to heal themselves in order to heal others, and come to recognize and forgive their own sins before earning the humility and compassion necessary to forgive anyone else. The "wounded healer" is a noble heroic figure, and who would not rather be helped by someone who had known pain and suffering, and overcome them, than by someone who had never known troubles at all?

Anger arises when wounded healers fail to resolve or control their own injuries. There is, I believe, a bifurcating path in the helping professional's career. The more arduous, but ultimately more satisfying, road leads to a painful confrontation with one's own problems and weaknesses, and ultimately to self-knowledge. Ideally, therapists overcome their difficulties; at worst, they may be forced to live and cope with insuperable handicaps. In either case, though, the result is a clear perception of their ambitions, needs and potential temptations and task at hand. They can approach others with honesty, compassion, and humility, confident that they are motivated by genuine concern, not by some ulterior motive.

The alternative path is easier and disastrous. Psychotherapists, can come, consciously or unconsciously, to recognize the profession as a way to avoid the need to deal with problems. Authority and power compensate for weakness and vulnerability. Therapists acquire a set of slippery dialectic techniques that enable them to justify their own actions in almost all circumstances, perhaps even to shift blame onto somebody else. The therapeutic relationship is perverted and turned to the service of this hidden purpose. Such therapists are ultimately not there to treat patients, but, via a circuitous and well-concealed route, to treat or protect or comfort themselves. Patients are not objects of empathy and altruism, but unsuspecting victims taken into the therapists' realm of personal needs and subjective impressions, and assigned roles there that they do not recognize or want.

In becoming psychotherapists, such people may even exacerbate their own problems, because they discover a justification for divorcing themselves from emotions that have caused them such pain, consoling themselves with the heady deceit that they have become cold, accurate instruments that can help others at the selfless expense of themselves. The flaw in this logic is that they are not being selfless at all, but seeking, through the very medium of ostentatious self-denial, a perverse gratification of personal needs. For these therapists the wound becomes encapsulated, walled off both from causing pain and from susceptibility to healing. Diverted from the arduous and humbling process of self-examination and personal reconstruction that might otherwise have made them whole, they are forced, continuously and forever, to work just to stay where they are. With this encapsulated problem now forming a foundation stone of their personal and professional lives, the farther along they go, the more difficult and costly it becomes to attempt to correct the mistake. It is an almost Faustian tragedy, in which they have sold their hopes of future redemption for temporary power, comfort, and knowledge.

Several studies have noted a tendency for people with what Ernest Jones called a "god complex"—a sort of narcissistic disorder—to be drawn to the practice of psychotherapy. The daily exercise of their profession can, in such cases, reinforce attitudes that are potentially dangerous for therapist and patients alike. However much therapists may try to play the part of mediator rather than guide, the very therapeutic situation necessarily presses them into a position of superiority where, by whatever direct or subtle means, they assert their notion of what is good for the patient above what the patient believes. In addition, patients themselves force therapists into superior positions through idealization—therapists' marriages must be wonderful, their children perfect, their interests cultured and profound, their grasp of issues clear and correct. Many patients aspire to be like their therapists and begin to mimic some of their tastes and mannerisms. And quite often patients do not simply want dispassionate help or even advice from their therapists: as children they expected magic from their parents, and thanks to the transference, they often entertain similarly unrealistic hopes that the therapist will soothe their fears and miraculously resolve their problems.

A good therapist—which requires an exceptional human being and constant vigilance—resists the temptations that the therapeutic setting and the seductive admiration of patients proffer. The best antidote to self-delusion and grandiosity is a normal life of one's own, complete with genuine human loves and friendships. By dealing with people as equals, in symmetrical relationships where the corners tend to get knocked off of one's fantastic monuments to oneself, one lives as a real, solid human being who takes true pride in genuine strengths and recognizes and deals with genuine weaknesses.

Many therapists, unfortunately, lack such relationships. Several studies have found that therapist marriages are often unusually distant and formal, based on shared intellectual and recreational activities rather than on affectionate personal interaction. Considerable anecdotal evidence suggests that therapists, both men and women, tend to marry troubled, dependent partners who only make things worse through their combined admiration and need. "Therapists marry their patients," it is said—which is sometimes even literally true—and end up in relationships that are anything but equal.

"My father was very shy and insecure," I was told by one woman, the daughter of an analyst, "and he insisted that the family provide him with a lot of reassurance all the time. He stayed very close to the home in every way—his office was in the house—and there was this ritual that my mother had to tell him how wonderful he was even though he wasn't, and how great the things he did were even when they weren't. That seems to be why he needed her."

Close friendships, other healthy influences, are also often lacking. Psychotherapists explain this away as a result of the tremendous demands of their professional lives—long hours, the teaching, society meetings—but such rationalizations seem forced when one looks at the figures and finds that, for example, psychiatrists have more free time than almost any other medical specialist or than many nonmedical professionals. The real reason often may be a disturbing one. Many therapists do not need friends. For people who are uncomfortable with others and with themselves, the therapeutic situation offers an unparalleled opportunity for asymmetrical intimacy. The rules of therapy demand that the patient tell the therapist everything, while the therapist is under no obligation to reveal anything at all and thus open himself to the painful risks incurred in normal human relationships. "My father had an inability to relate with his family or other people," said an analyst who was also the son of an analyst, "and his way of being close was through his patients. It was a way for him to have an interaction, but there was always a wall, or a desk, or a couch to protect him." Life in the office can be exciting—more exciting, socially redeeming, and financially rewarding than watching soap operas.

The therapeutic situation can become a sort of surrogate life, with both therapist and patients enjoying a level of intimacy difficult to replicate in the world outside. "It's a very tricky situation," remarked one psychologist. "It seems as though you've had all this intense personal contact, and then you go out and who are your friends on the outside? Well it turns out you don't have a lot of friends, and this is very surprising, because it *seems* as though you have forty very close friends. But you can't socialize with them, you can't have them over to dinner, you can't go stay at their houses in the mountains."

The particular danger to the patient against which therapists must be vigilant, but often are not, is that therapy begins to settle in as part of the patient's life rather than remaining an active process aimed at reintegrating the patient into a life that happens elsewhere. Some patients look forward to sessions and live life for the unacknowledged purpose of interesting and pleasing the therapist. Problems may be apparently resolved and changes made more for the dramatic value or for the therapist's approval than from a sense of inner need. Patients do not want to leave the idealized therapist, and in the type of relationship outlined above, nor does the therapist want patients to leave. In the worst case, therapy is poisoned by the fact that ultimately, unconsciously, the therapist cannot bear to cure patients because that would entail suffering their loss.

Several teaching analysts and psychotherapists readily agree that what posed as enthusiasm and professional dedication is often at heart a morbid addiction. A training analyst in New York discussed the unwillingness of analysts to leave their practice.

"They may say that they can't give up the income, or offer some other explanation, but what they really miss is feeling needed. Personally I think that it is unethical and immoral for analysts to practice beyond a certain time in life. You can say a word for experience, but how much experience is experience? You can't really say that 70-year-old's experience is better than that of someone who is 55. What is someone like that doing for his patients? He can't see as well, he can't remember as well, he can't hear as well, but he's still in there, and nobody's going to tell him what to do, and since there are no rules or laws or need for operating room privileges, nobody can stop him, and he'll just keep doing it. And, transferential feelings being what they are, the patient doesn't have enough sense to move on."

The 40-year-old son of an analyst remarked:

"I don't know what personal gratification my father derived from helping people—seeing someone come into his office and then go out, 40 years later, better adjusted to the world. He may get some satisfaction out of that, I don't know. What it did do was to give him a world; it gave my father a life. He grew up unhappy, with an awful father—a father so terrible that not a single kind word was said about him even at his funeral. My father's childhood was just dreadful: he was on his own, and he didn't have many people to relate to in life. His patients gave him a world, they were people to relate to, whether emotionally or unemotionally, as the case may be. And even if he was unemotionally involved in their problems—it didn't personally affect him that So-and-so had this terrible sexual problem with her boyfriend—he could still react emotionally to the fact that this person was telling him that, and that he was saying something back. His world was defined by his hours of practice. I don't know whether people who dig ditches find that ditch-digging gives them a world. It gives them a job, makes them some money, but at the end of the day they get out of that ditch. I don't know if my father, when he came home from his world, ever stepped into another world. He may have left that other world behind and stepped into some middle region, but I'm not really sure that he ever stepped into the world where his family lived. I contend that this was all because of the person he was. Being an analyst didn't make him any different, except that perhaps, over the years, it may have dulled his senses, inured him, dulled his ability to deal with his family. He could look forward to tomorrow, when he could go back to the world where he really belonged."

For some patients, the narcissistic therapist's encapsulated wound and secret self-centered agenda may have no discernible effect on a simple program of self-discovery. Just hearing oneself talk is enough help for some. But in cases that demand more from the therapist, or treat close to the therapist's own problems, or issue challenges that his therapeutic persona cannot easily handle, serious difficulties may arise. The patient may innocently enter into an extraordinarily powerful and complex relationship that leads not back toward a normal and independent life, but away.

They Came to Stay

MARJORIE MARGOLIES AND RUTH GRUBER

Excerpted from Marjorie Margolies and Ruth Gruber, *They Came to Stay*, New York, Coward, McCann & Geoghan, 1976. Reprinted by permission.

I n 1970, Marjorie Margolies decided at the age of 25 to adopt a Korean child.
She encountered a variety of responses: her mother told her to get married
and have her own kids, her boyfriend Seth threatened to end their relationship, and adoption agencies rejected her because she was single. *They Came to
Stay* recounts Margolies' experiences navigating the complicated world of
adoption, the relationships she forged with what became two adoptive children—one from Korea and the other from Vietnam—and the difficult moral
and identity issues she and her daughters were forced to confront. The power
of this memoir is not only in Margolies' pioneering redefinition of the
American family and defiance of sexist adoption policy, but in its honest,
unglamorized window into American cultural arrogance, the paradox of
assimilation, and the human need for reconciliation with the past.

The idea exploded in my head.

I would adopt a child.

It was a hot July afternoon. A warm breeze blew the sheer curtains into my
studio apartment.

But I felt chilled.

I would adopt a child no one else wanted. An abandoned child. Perhaps an
orphan from Southeast Asia.

How would my mother and father react?

Like a sleepwalker, I found myself walking down the stairs of the old red
brick house. Three blocks away, across Rittenhouse Square, my parents lived.

My mother looked through the peephole.

"Oh, it's you, Monkey. Come in."

I followed her through the foyer into the kitchen.

"Where's Daddy?" I asked.

"At a meeting in Camden."

It would be easier if he were here. I ought to wait.

"Mom," I heard the words come out "you remember the picnic I covered
for the six o'clock news last week? The picnic of that Open Door Society—those
families that adopt children and get together—"

"Mom," I blurted out, "I want to adopt a child."

"What?" She looked at me. "Repeat that. I don't think I heard right."

"I said I want to adopt a child—a child—like one of those hard-to-place
children at the picnic."

She shook her head unbelievingly.

"You must be out of your mind. Look, Monkey. I'm like any other mother. I
want to see you get married. Then you can have as many kids as you want."

"I may get married some day. But that's in the future. Right now I want to
give a home to some child who's been abandoned or orphaned. When I think
of the suffering some of these children have gone through—the tragedies
they've known—I feel I want to help one of them. What's so wrong about that?"

"It's crazy, Margie. You've got an exciting television job. You're free to get up and go any time you want—anyplace in the world. Once you have a child, that's all finished. You won't be free for the rest of your life."

I was unprepared for the intensity of my mother's reaction.

Her anger made me realize I must have touched a raw nerve, perhaps something out of her background, her own frustrations.

"Look, Mom," I said in a low voice. "I'm sure I can cope. You know how I love kids. Look at the kids I shepherded across the country on bicycle tours. The kids I took on summer trips—to Greece—to the kibbutz in Israel."

"Then have your own."

"I just have this feeling. If there's a child without a home, why wait?"

"You think you're some kind of superwoman—you can work and take care of a child at the same time?"

"Millions of women do. Why can't I?"

Her voice dropped. "I couldn't do both. I had to give up my work as soon as Phylis was born."

Was that the raw nerve I had touched? That she had been forced to stop her creative work as soon as my sister Phylis was born. Until then she had worked full-time as a commercial artist.

She paused. Her voice was softer, less strident. "I didn't resent having a baby. I didn't resent Phylis. I resented giving up my career. Maybe that's why this thing you've thrown at me—out of the blue—maybe that's why it bothers me so much. This isn't the way I see you fulfilling yourself. Just don't mess up your life."

There was a whole landscape of agencies for adopting children. One needed a kind of road map to find one's way. Even then one needed a set of law books to understand the codes.

Their questions on the phone were almost always the same.

"What kind of child do you want to adopt? Name? Husband's name?" No husband. I'm single.

"Sorry, we not place children with single persons."

Some said it bluntly, some with hostility. One agency told me, "You must hate men. You're probably a women's libber. We don't give children to single people who might psychologically feed on children for fulfillment."

At work I rolled film in the darkroom. Pictures of children fleeing down burning streets in Vietnam. A little boy bending over a dead mother. Rows of children lying apathetically in orphanages in Korea. A frightened Korean woman abandoning a baby on the street in Seoul, looking around surreptitiously, then running away. A stranger handing the baby to a policeman.

The commentator was talking:

"Hundreds of thousands of abandoned children in Vietnam and Korea. What becomes of an abandoned girl? If she is mixed race, if her father was an

American or a European, she is the object of ridicule. If she is lucky and can go to school, she will be ridiculed by all the children. If her mother associated with foreigners or was a prostitute, she will probably never go to school. Perhaps by 9 or 10 she may be on the streets as a prostitute herself."

I was more than ever convinced. There were special agencies that brought in children from Korea—the International Social Services, known as ISS; Welcome House, the agency Pearl Buck started in Bucks County, Pennsylvania; the Holt Children's Services in Oregon. I telephoned all of them. I wrote letters. I went to interviews. Always the same answer. The same stone wall.

The single-parent syndrome.

I kept hearing the words in my dreams: No single parent wanted.

The obsession never left me.

Then, one day, visiting my mother, she said, "Daddy and I are planning to visit Japan at the end of May. How about joining us?"

Japan! Japan was a short flight from Korea.

Korea was where the Holt agency had its orphanage.

I called Roberta Andrews [an associate director of the Children's Aid], to tell her I might be going to Korea. Was there a possibility I might find a child and bring her back?

"Who knows?" she said, "We'll try."

Three days later, Holt answered. "You are welcome to look up Jack Theis, our director in Seoul, Korea."

I went back to New York, mulling over the letter from Holt. I telephoned Seth.

"If you really take off and go to Korea," he said angrily, "and if you actually come back with a child, I'll know you've made your decision about us."

My sense of inner direction was spinning like a compass in a magnetic minefield. Was I running away from Seth? Was I incapable of a real commitment? Did the trip to Korea mean I was preparing myself for a new kind of commitment? Should I go? Was I setting myself up for more roadblocks, more heartaches?

The next morning I telephoned Roberta.

"Go," she said. "You know how to get to people. Put yourself across."

How would I feel if I really got a child? Would I go instantaneously from being the child of my parents to the mother of my child?

"On 2/25/70, a child was found by the Buk-ae-dong police box and had been protected for one month until her placement."

"What's a police box?" I asked.

"It's a small police station," [replied Jack Theis]. "Many Korean children are abandoned that way—left in front of a police station. Each year five to six thousand children are abandoned in South Korea. Some are left on the street or in front of a hotel or railway station. Whoever finds them brings them to the local police box. The police keep them in a reception center for a month in case the mother changes her mind or perhaps the child is lost and some relative may come looking for it."

He continued reading:

"Physical history: Fair-complexioned child, with slender build. Walking and running well, she seems to enjoy a normal progress. Social history: Responsive to questions. Gets along nicely with friends and is more of a leader. Tries to excel in everything, keeping her personal effects in good order."

"Bright and quick," I whispered.

He nodded.

I felt my hands begin to tremble. "Nothing negative?" I asked. I had waited so long.

He thumbed the file. "The next report was written a month later. It reinforces the first one. It just adds, 'She loves apples for snacks.'"

I laughed. "Apples. That'll be easy to supply."

His assistant knocked at the door. "Mr. Theis. She has not been assigned. She is available for adoption."

"You're in luck." He handed me a tiny snapshot of a little girl with a round face, pretty bow lips, and almond eyes that looked sad. It seemed to me the face of a child who had known much suffering and learned to contain it. It was a head-and-shoulder shot, like a hospital picture, with a white sign beneath her collar: Lee Heh Kyung, 3-15-63.

This was the little girl—if things worked out—the little girl I would know for the rest of my life.

I was still studying the snapshot when the door opened again. A tiny girl who scarcely reached my hip and who looked about 4 years old entered. She walked straight toward me, put out her hand, and said, "Haw doo yoo doo?"

My first impulse was to pick her up and hug her. Instead I held her hand. Even her hand felt fragile, vulnerable.

She looked at me quizzically and repeated, "Haw doo yoo doo?"

She was graceful as a dancer, amber-skinned, with penetrating eyes. She wore a short white dress with little red flowers and multicolored Korean rubber slippers. Her black hair was cut short with a kind of ponytail standing straight up on the top of her head.

"I'm fine, thank you," I said. "How are you?"

FOUR YEARS LATER, JUNE 1974

My doorbell rang. It was Ruth Gruber, my collaborator on this book.

It was scarcely an hour since Ruth had dropped her bags in her own apartment. She and her daughter had just returned from Korea and Vietnam where they had gone to research the past lives of Lee Heh and Holly [my second adopted daughter from Vietnam].

"Let's start with Lee Heh," Ruth said. "I met her brothers in an orphanage in Inchon—the town where General MacArthur landed during the Korean War."

Ruth handed me the photos of the two boys.

"Margie," Ruth said. "I think I solved the puzzle. The reason Lee Heh blocked out her past so completely, language and all, Lee Heh was warned [that] she must admit to nobody that she had a family. Brainwashed."

"Who brainwashed her?"

"Let me read you my notes. Kyoo Bok, Lee Heh's older brother is speaking."

"'Our little sister was born in Kwangju—it's about 300 miles south of Seoul. Our father was a sergeant in the army. Our sister was 8 months old when he died. We were poor, poor. When our sister was a little over a year, our mother took us to live in Inchon. She worked very hard to feed us. She earned a little money, sewing Korean native dresses and cleaning people's houses. We three children went with her and helped her clean floors.

"'We moved every two or three months because we had no money for rent. Still, we were happy. We played with our little sister. Our mother loved us very much.

"'At last our mother found a job that paid well. Working as a cook in the Sung Rin Orphanage in Inchon. The director let her keep us with her in the orphanage. But one day the director found out that our mother had tuberculosis. He told her she must leave right away. He put her into the Inchon Provincial Tuberculosis Hospital, and she didn't have to pay.'"

I remembered how Lee Heh had described her mother lying on the floor sick. Not permitted to kiss her, she told me, because her mother always had a cold.

So it was TB. The disease of poverty.

"Kyoo Bok told me they had an aunt—their mother's sister. She and their mother talked things over and decided to leave the two boys in the Sung Rin Orphanage and put Lee Heh up for adoption.

"Why would she put only Lee Heh up for adoption?" I asked. "Why would she want to get rid of her one little girl?"

Ruth put her book down. "I asked myself the same question. Korea is a Confucian male-oriented culture. Boys are much more important than girls. Their mother may have thought that her little daughter, with neither father nor mother, might be doomed to living on the street—maybe have to become a prostitute."

She paused. "A girl without a family in Korea is a nonperson."

"Kyoo Bok heard his aunt warn her [little sister], 'You must never tell anybody you have a mother who's living. Or that you have two brothers. You must tell everyone that you are an orphan.'"

I felt my voice constrict.

Ruth went on. "'Our mother cried and we cried. But our little sister was very obedient.'"

"By now their mother was very ill. The aunt took Lee Heh to the police box. The police kept her for a month and when nobody came, they put her in the Star of the Sea Orphanage in Inchon. That was March 20, 1970. The nun in charge decided Lee Heh was bright and pretty, and could be adopted, so after three days they sent her to Il San—the Holt Children's Center where you found her. Her mother died a year after she came to America."

Suddenly her behavior those first months became clear to me. Her refusal to speak any Korean. Her panic when she met my father's Korean friends. Her fear that if she did anything bad I would abandon her, send her back.

"She had to bury these memories. She had to wipe them out of her consciousness in order to survive."

I had scarcely said the words when we heard, "Hi, everybody." Lee Heh rushed into the living room, hugged me, and flung her arms around Ruth. "Welcome home."

"Ruth brought you pictures of your brothers." I handed her the photos.

She shouted, "That's my brother, Kyoo Bok. And my little brother, Kyoo Sik."

She placed the photos on the glass coffee table, knelt beside them, and stared at the faces as though she wanted to imprint them on her brain.

We watched her in silence.

Then Ruth asked, "Would you like to see yourself as a little girl with your mother and father?"

Lee Heh lowered her face to the photo on the table. She looked solemn. "This must be my father because he's wearing a soldier's cap and uniform." She stared at the father whose face she had surely long forgotten.

She drew her index finger gently around her mother's fine, sensitive face, frail and thin, as if TB had begun consuming her lungs.

She took the picture and taped [it] on our living room wall. She seemed to be drawing her mother and father into our home. We were one family.

[After Lee Heh had left, Ruth continued,] "Some of the things I found out about Holly are so painful, it's going to be hard for her to relive some of this."

I was apprehensive. "I know she's been traumatized."

"Our quest began the second we landed in Vietnam. [We went] immediately to the Holt Center. There we met a key person in our search, Loan."

She pronounced it Low-Ann. "Why do I know that name?"

"She signed some of the reports that were sent to you on Holly."

"Loan gave us our first real insights on Holly's life," Ruth said. She knew Holly and... a lot about children with American fathers. She first met Holly in August, 1973."

August.... Eight months before Holly came to me.

I could almost hear Loan speaking as Ruth read her words, "'I was looking for a child to send to my good friend—American colonel in Utah. He want to adopt Vietnamese orphan girl. I hear about a lady who keep children of bar girls. Mrs. Thu. She like a baby-sitter; keep 10 mixed-race children in her house. I saw this child. She was cute. Thu Nga. You call her Thu Nga also? Or she have American name?'

"'We call her Holly,' I told her. She liked that name.

"'Pretty name. From now on, she be Holly to me, too. This lady, Mrs. Thu, say I can take Holly for my friend in America to adopt. Her foster mother very poor; she want to give her away. I take her home. I think I will keep her about 10 days, and get all her papers right, and send her to Utah.'"

Ruth's voice grew muted. "The day she brought her home, Loan noticed deep red scars around her wrists. 'I ask her what are these scars. She says her mother get electricity with sharp ends. She wind the wire around Holly's hands. Tie them together. And shock her.

"'Holly tell me sometimes her mother hung her up by the hands from the ceiling, because Holly did something wrong. She hung Holly over [a] table five or ten minutes until Holly say, "Sorry for that." Sometimes she spanked Holly with a leather belt with a heavy buckle—like a man's belt. Holly show me her back. Big, big bruises.'"

Ruth's voice choked. She stopped talking.

I couldn't sit still. I went into the kitchen where I had prepared iced tea and brought the glasses to the coffee table. Ruth sipped slowly.

"Loan really wanted to help Holly go to America, get away from all the brutality. But there were problems with her own family: 'sorry.'

"'I take her back to baby-sitter, Mrs. Thu. I tell her I can't keep her. She don't want Holly back. Foster mother don't want her back. But I don't know anyplace else.'

"In October, 1973, she went to work for Holt. A month later Holly was brought to the Holt Center by the baby-sitter, Mrs. Thu, and Holly's foster mother, Mrs. Hieu.

"This is the story Mrs. Hieu told:

"'I worked in a bar in Nha Trang. One night my friend came over to me in bar and told me she pregnant. I told her I want the baby. She say okay. But then the baby was born, she said no, she wants to keep baby. Real pretty. Then after 10 days, she come to me and says lots of people want to buy her. Some even pay $200. But I will give her to you because I know you take good care of her.'

"I questioned Mrs. Hieu closely. 'When you brought Holly to Holt you told Loan you found her in a garbage can. Which story is true?'

"'The true one is what I tell you now.'

"'Why did you make the other one up?'

"'Because I don't want Holly to know her real mother is alive.'

"I was stunned," Ruth said. "'So her real mother is alive! Where is she? What's her name?'

"'I don't know her name. I don't know where she live. Maybe far away—in Qui Nhon.'

"'Did you know Holly's father?' I asked her.

"She allowed herself a rare smile. 'I know him very well. He was a contractor.'

"Mrs. Hieu said he was about 40," Ruth explained. "'He very rich but he drink a lot. He like Holly but he didn't pay much attention. I don't know his name,' she said very quickly, lest I ask her.

"I called Loan aside and said, 'I'm beginning to think Mrs. Hieu is Holly's real mother. First she made up the garbage can story; maybe she also made up this story of her friend the bar girl.'"

"Is she really Holly's mother?" I blurted.

Ruth shrugged her shoulders. "Loan insisted she wasn't. She said, 'When Mrs. Hieu bring Holly to Holt, she never once come back to see her. A real mother always come back.'

"I asked Mrs. Hieu if she would allow us to visit her.

"She agreed. 'When you come to my house,' she said, 'I give you a present for Holly.'"

Ruth took out of her tote a brown leather zippered pouch [a picture album].

I unzipped the pouch. There was Holly as a cuddly toddler in a bathing suit with a beautiful seductive woman also in a bathing suit and carrying a parasol.

"That's Mrs. Hieu," Ruth said, "in Nha Trang—before she lost her money and her job."

I heard the key in the door. I slipped [the album] under a pillow.

Holly rushed into the living room, kissed me, and then flung her arms around Ruth.

"I so glad you home again, Ruth."

Her English was improving with astonishing speed. "I miss you. You have a good time Vie'nam? You like Vie'nam?"

"I love Vietnam, Holly," Ruth said.

[Holly asked for permission to watch TV in the bedroom and left the room.]

Ruth lowered her voice. "Two days after we saw Mrs. Hieu I decided to fly to Nha Trang where she said she had lived with Holly.

"Nguyen Minh Chieu Street was a labyrinth of alleys winding into alleys alive with bars and brothels and—in the orphanages—mixed race children born of the bars and brothels.

"We came finally to a two-story wooden house with an outdoor flight of broken stairs and found ourselves in the very room where Holly had lived. Mrs. Thu, the baby-sitter, greeted us. She was one of the smart bar girls. She had saved her money and put it into real estate. Now she lived in one room and rented out the others."

"We had tracked down the very house Holly had lived in. But where was Mrs. Hieu?

"'She leave you present,' Mrs. Thu said. 'She not pay rent many many months. I tell her she not able to lived here if she not pay. She go away just now.

She sleep on floor someplace. I don't know where she go. She very very poor.'

"Honestly, Ruth, what do you think," I whispered. "Do you think Mrs. Hieu was her mother?"

"Let's suspend judgment until we see Holly's face when she looks at the pictures of Mrs. Hieu."

I sighed. "I'm not sure we should show her the pictures right now. She's beginning to make progress now. I'm so afraid these pictures could stir everything up again."

Ruth put her hand on my arm. "I think we ought to show them to her."

I hesitated.

Holly ran into the room. "TV finished."

"Holly, honey." I made up my mind. "Come look at these pictures Ruth brought you."

I held my breath as Ruth handed her the brown leather album.

"That's my ma-ma's picture book," she shouted with amazement. She unzipped it. "Look, Mommy. My ma-ma."

It was Mrs. Hieu.

She began to squeal and coo with pleasure. "Look, Mommy, me and my ma-ma in Nha Trang. On beach. Holly little baby. So cute."

She leafed through the other pictures and then cried out, "My sister Hong. I love her. My brother Phuc. Look, he big soldier. He love me very much."

Holly put the pictures into the album and hugged it to her as if she was embracing a child. Embracing the child she had been in Nha Trang.

There was no hysteria. She nestled in Ruth's arms. "You bring me real good present from Vic'nam, Ruth."

"It was a present from your mother, Holly. She wanted you to have these pictures so you will never forget."

In the end I realized both [Lee Heh's and Holly's] mothers had behaved the way most mothers would behave when faced by death or starvation. Lee Heh's mother gave her up only when she knew she was dying of tuberculosis. Holly's mother gave her up when she could no longer cope with hunger and hopelessness.

Both mothers gave their daughters up, to be adopted in America, in the hope they could live with decency and dignity, without hunger and without fear.

For each of their mothers it was not only an act of desperation, it was an act of love.

An Adopted Daughter Meets Her Natural Mother

BETTY JEAN LIFTON

From *Ms.*, MONTH, 1975, excerpted from Betty Jean Lifton, *Twice Born: Memoirs of an Adopted Daughter*, New York, McGraw-Hill, 1975. Reprinted by permission.

I said, "Who am I?"
Looking into the mirror my eyes
searched for clues.
There were none.
Nor were there likely to be.
For I am adopted.

You wouldn't know it to meet me. To all outward appearances I am a writer, a married woman, a mother, a theater buff, an animal fanatic—yes, I can pass. But locked within me there is an adopted child who stirs guilty and ambivalent even as I write these words. The adopted child can never grow up. Who has ever heard of an *adopted adult?*

For most of my life my adopted state was a secret I kept from everyone, a game I played. But now I'm ready to break the rules.

Just think, I was 30 when I made the unexpected discovery that the parents I had been told were deceased at the time of my adoption had been very much alive—indeed, still might be. I was seized with a longing to know who they were—who, as the Bible puts it, begat me.

And so I started out on that perilous journey that Oedipus took so long ago. I did not expect to be the king's daughter, but I knew I could not refuse that call to adventure, which is the call to self.

I went into the labyrinth and emerged with what I sought—my story.

It took a year to find my natural mother—a year in which I contacted the adoption agency and then, armed only with her maiden name, searched tediously through musty record offices in three cities for birth, marriage, and death certificates, consulted old phone books for previous addresses, and then, in desperation, put a lawyer friend in the role of sleuth.

We finally managed to locate my mother's brother, Oran, who became the go-between. But she was recovering slowly from a glaucoma operation and was startled to hear of my reappearance. I was a painful secret in her past. After a few months of tortured indecision, she agreed to talk with me at her brother's home.

The day I went to meet my mother I dressed all in black. I often wore black, but this darkness was unrelieved by color: a black suit, black hat, black hose, black shoes, black purse. Not even a bright scarf. Although I felt joyous inside, this was not a celebration. This was something dark and secretive to be acted out in shadows. My guilt toward my adoptive parents covered me, making me invisible as I moved toward the execution of this nefarious deed.

My uncle's house in Queens reflected the simplicity of his life as an accountant. It was an unpretentious ranch house, the kind one sees sprawling over all the suburbs of this land. When he had called, he said "weather permitting" he and his wife would not be home. But it was pouring rain, and they were at the door waiting for us. "We've pulled the shades in the living room to protect her eyes," they said. She too needed that darkness.

She was sitting in a chair on the far side of the room with large sunglasses covering her eyes. I could not look into them. She rose as my husband Bob and I entered.

She was much shorter than I had imagined she would be, large hipped and bosomed. We approached each other tentatively. I'm sure the possibility of our rushing into each other's arms must have crossed her mind earlier too, but now the impossibility of it seemed to reach us both at the same time. I put out my arm, and we shook hands indecisively. Her fingers lay cold, limp in mine. Then she returned to her chair, and I perched tensely on the edge of the sofa at the opposite end of the room. Bob sat near me.

My aunt and uncle paced in the doorway like heraldic lions guarding the entrance.

According to Jung, the desire to be reunited with the mother is the desire to be reborn through her. I sat and looked at the woman across from me and knew I would not have recognized her as my mother had we passed each other on the street. Jung says the mother is a symbol of the unconscious to which an individual wishes to return in order to seek a solution for his psychic conflicts. Now here she sat in the flesh, nervously twisting a handkerchief in her lap, as ill at easy as I was. Yet everything in my life seemed to have led irrevocably to this moment. Her voice was gentle and caring as she spoke the first words.

"Betty, I want you to know you are from a good family." She used my adopted name, not Blanche—as she had named me. They she reeled off some of the prominent New York relatives and their various professions, placing herself and me socially so that I need not look down on her, or myself.

"I expected you to look me up some day," she added to fill the silence which followed. "But I did not think it would take this long."

She began to weep at this. It was only later, much later, that I understood the true meaning of her words. She had lived with the hope that she would one day hear her daughter had fared well and was successful—perhaps that would redeem her sin. But she had also been living in fear with this secret—fear that the phone would ring one day, or a knock would come at the door that would expose her to the world.

The phone had rung, and here I was.

She was not the big, strong, all-powerful mother ready to take the frightened child in her arms and dispel the demons. She too was riddled with demons. She too was afraid: afraid of her secret, afraid of that cold, domineering, loveless mother of her own. Afraid of me. She was a disconcerting combination of self-awareness and denial, but she told me the story I had come to hear as best she could. She was brave about that.

My mother was not married to my father. She had had only a few dates with him in Freeport, Rhode Island, when her family moved, according to prior plans, to Brooklyn to be near her rabbi grandfather. When she realized she was pregnant, her wealthy aunt in Freeport tried to persuade my father to marry her. She promised an immediate annulment: all that was wanted was his signature on a piece of paper. He was a few years older, already a man about town. He refused.

A few months before I was born, my mother was shipped off by her family to a shelter for unmarried girls in Staten Island. She went there alone, unaccompanied by a relative or friend. She went in exile to that island, the waters of whose narrow channel would seem to her as wide as the oceans that separated exiled emperors and generals from the shores of their homeland. Her grief and loneliness would be as great as theirs. And she was only 17 years old.

When her time came, my mother went alone in a taxi from the shelter to the hospital. She does not remember the hour I was born. She stayed alone in the hospital with me and then returned to the shelter for five months to nurse me. She had no visitors.

My mother said she was determined not to give me up. She must have been a strong-willed person—then. She hoped to persuade her mother to see me eventually and to allow me into the home. But my grandmother refused to recognize my existence.

My mother admitted there was talk of sitting *shiva* for her, that ceremony of mourning that Orthodox Jews hold for those prodigal children who marry out of the religion or transgress in other equally unforgivable ways and who must forever after be considered dead.

However, there was no *shiva* ceremony necessary for her since everyone soon began acting as if I had never been born. She was finally allowed back into the house, alone. Still she must have gathered strength in her exile, for in spite of the advice of social workers and other family members, she refused to part with her baby. Rather than place me for adoption, she put me in an infants' home in the Bronx and visited me there on weekends for the next year and a half.

Once her father (also afraid of her mother) dared to sneak out secretly to visit me with her. But no one else ever saw me.

"I took a job in a dress firm to support you," my mother said. "And every Sunday during visiting hours I came with a little toy. I called you 'Bubeleh,' and you held out your arms to me. You had such a lovely smile."

Here she began to weep again, and my aunt cautioned her from the doorway that she would hurt her eyes.

"But when you were older and standing up in your crib, I would look at you surrounded by all those other homeless children, and cry. 'My child should have something better than this,' I told myself."

During this period my mother kept hoping my father would call. Once she actually visited Freeport and phoned his house. He was not there. She left her office number in New York, but she did not hear from him.

"I suppose I was hoping he would change his mind and marry me when he saw you," she explained. "Then I would have had a home to take you to.

"When you were two, you had to have a mastoid operation. They told me you would die if you did not get a family of your own. They encouraged me to let you go for adoption if I really loved you. I was afraid you would die or I would never have done it."

Again she wept, and again my aunt poked her head in to caution her.

Another aunt, the wife of one of my mother's successful uncles, knew about the adoption agency run by the Reform rabbi, Stephen Wise.

"She told me you would go to a wealthy family," my mother said. "That the agency knew just the right people for you."

And so my mother, at the age of 19, signed the papers that released her child from her care forever. She was never told where I went or to whom. And in keeping with adoption-agency practice, she was never given a report as to my progress. So does society unconsciously punish women who produce offspring out of wedlock.

Or is it conscious?

Never in this life are they allowed to see or hear of their children again. The agencies say they are protecting the "privacy" of these mothers.

In losing the battle to keep her child, my mother was like the luna moth who lays her eggs and dies. One part of her died, the part that was spirited and had dreams. From that moment she must have begun to change into the conventional, frightened, submissive woman I saw before me now. The only thing she kept of me was her secret: and this secret was to grow in her until it became one of her vital organs.

My mother became docile, even dutiful toward her own mother, who continued to put her down. Two young doctors—not one, but two—wanted to marry her, she said. But she was afraid they would find out her secret. Doctors notice things like that. When she met her first husband, a year after my adoption, she married him because he "pressured" her with kindness.

A businessman wouldn't notice.

During those years of her first marriage, my mother continued currying her mother's favor, as if only this woman could give her absolution for her crime. Then her son was born.

Her husband thought it was her first child.

When my half brother was still in my mother's womb, my father called her at her office.

"When I heard his voice, I began crying hysterically," she said. "I told him it was too late and to leave me alone. To never call me again."

He never did. We'll never know what he wanted.

After her son was born, my mother lived like a well-to-do Jewish matron. She even had a special nurse for her baby. She worked actively in philanthropy.

"One night a whole congregation at the temple stood up to honor my work. But I thought: I am not worthy of this. If they only knew what I have done. Yet I had another thought: If this could happen, couldn't something nice happen too? If only my daughter could know about this honor I am receiving tonight."

Now she knew.

When my half brother was 13, my mother divorced his father and moved in with her mother. She worked in a dress shop on Madison Avenue for a while. Then she married a second time.

"He was a sport like your father," she admitted with a shy smile. He followed the races—but she married him in spite of her mother's strong disapproval. "He had a daughter in her twenties, just the age you would have been. I always felt distant from her. I could never forget that she might have been you, and that *you* might have been living with us instead of her."

Again she daubed her eyes.

"You asked Oran if I was happy," she went on. "I asked him if you had asked that. I knew you would. But I want you to know that I felt I could never be happy after giving you up. There was always something unsatisfied in me that nothing could feed. I would look at other women with their daughters on the street and wonder if any of them could be you."

She didn't see the contradiction as she added: "No one knows you called except Oran and his wife. And they will keep my secret. I must not let my husband know. Or my son until he's graduated."

There was a silence as the room was washed by the waves of that secret.

Now I asked about my father. He was like a presence holding us together and yet standing between us. Who was he? What was he like?

I was unprepared for her response.

She stiffened in her chair, and her voice became tense. "I have spoken to you honestly today," she said, "and told you everything I know. But you must *never* ask your father's name."

Bob interrupted here to help me out. "His name is not important," he said softly. "But maybe you could tell Betty something about him."

I added quickly that now that I had heard her story, I certainly did not feel any kindness toward my father; my sympathy was entirely with her who had been through so much those first years.

She seemed relieved to hear this, and now her nemesis having been brought down to size, she volunteered the information that had been haunting her along with the secret.

"No one must know this," she warned. "He was a… a bootlegger."

"A what?" I asked. I couldn't quite understand the word she muffled in her embarrassment.

"You know… a rumrunner… a *bootlegger*," she repeated nervously, as if federal agents might appear at the door even as she said the word.

I wanted to laugh. A bootlegger! Just like Gatsby. How romantic. How incredible.

"I'm sorry to have to tell you this," she said mournfully.

I tried to explain to her that I did not care what my father was. I had not come to judge either of them, just to learn the truth.

I asked her nothing further about my father, who being the source of me, was the source of her pain. Out of loyalty to this woman who was my mother and had tried to keep me, I closed my heart to that nameless man. It would be many years before I could bring myself to search for this part of my story.

The table in the dining room had been laid with cold cuts and open-faced sandwiches, enough to satisfy all the grown babies in that infants' home had they arrived with me. During our talk my mother would occasionally interrupt to urge Bob and me to eat something. I could not think of food, and even though Bob can always think of it, he was circumspect enough to leave the table untouched.

Now, it being almost evening, it was time to talk of food again—in earnest. Although I was a secret from the past, she insisted on taking us to a restaurant near Oran's house. She wasn't afraid of being seen with me: but then this wasn't *her* neighborhood.

She was flushed and excited, and a bit unrealistic. She spoke of having me meet a favorite aunt of hers, one of those millionaires who seemed abundant in another branch of the family but whose abundance did not spill over into her modest circumstances.

"But how would you introduce me?"

"I could say you were a niece of my husband's."

She spoke of telling my half brother about me—as soon as he graduated. She began listing some other prominent aunts, uncles, cousins.

I said as delicately as I could that I did not want to meet relatives, not now, not disguised as someone else. (I wasn't sure I wanted to meet them at all—perhaps it would make my disloyalty to my adopted family even more official.) We parted promising to see each other again before Bob and I left for Japan.

This time we embraced warmly.

But we were still strangers.

This woman had given birth to me and so she was my mother, but she had separated from me, and so she was a stranger.

Yet her whole life had been retribution for having borne me. I had influenced this stranger's life just as she had influenced mine. She had carried her loss within her longer than she had carried me.

It was all very confusing, but I did not feel disturbed by it—yet.

I was coming to grips with some of the complexities of the human condition. My mother was locked as I was in the intricate tangle of the past: I was the darling baby, the lost child, the ache in her heart; but I was also the dark secret, the one who had almost ruined her life and threatened to again.

And for me this woman was the beautiful lost mother, but she was also the one who had abandoned me.

I kissed her on the cheek as we parted. I promised to write while we were in Japan but to address my letters to her brother, Oran, who would relay them to her, thus preventing her husband and son from ever seeing them.

I promised to help her keep her secret.

It was a light casual kiss I gave her, like the brush of a butterfly's wing.

My Mother's Death: Thoughts on Being a Separate Person

JUDITH ROSSNER

Judith Rossner, "My Mother's Death: Thoughts on Being a Separate Person," *Ms.*, September 1974. Reprinted by permission.

I was born, I grew up. My mother died. She had no place in my everyday life, yet it is generally accepted as reasonable that my mourning should be deep and long. How long and how deep?

"I can't cry," she said in December.

Her face was soft and dry, and her voice was small and dry, and her hands were always cracked and dry—or at least she thought they were—even though she washed few dishes; I have used a huge jar of cream on my hands since January 9.

I cry often, but when I think of that most painful thing she said to me, that she couldn't cry, I cannot cry. Nor could she sleep. The first time that the last doctor gave her the last sleeping pills along with specific instructions for their use (two followed by cocoa, in bed, with a book—not television, which leads to catnaps—but a book), that night she slept for several hours but aside from that she didn't sleep for more than an hour or two each night, and for weeks at a time not even that, but only for a few minutes on the sofa or perhaps on the soft Moroccan rug in my house. My father slept for both of them. She lusted for sleep. She hoarded all the sleeping pills given her by all the doctors who need to get her pain out of their offices and only used them when she had enough to guarantee the kind of sleep she had wanted for so many years.

And the last doctor thought that he observed, when my father called him to the house, that she hadn't used the pills he'd given her, only the ones given her by the previous doctor; but he was wrong. And the previous doctor wanted to know if she'd been taking the antidepressants he'd prescribed during the time when she'd finally taken the others; he was fairly sure she'd stopped taking them or she wouldn't have done it, but he was wrong too. Both of them, finally relieved of her pain, did not want some new one of their own. All of which is irrelevant if I am a separate human being.

Item. I write a novel which I know isn't about me except in the inevitable sense. My mother reads it and says it is about her.

In December she asked me what reason she had to continue living. A literary slave of the truth, I told her that we were the reason. That while it was true it would be easier for her not to, it would be too painful for us to lose her. She watched my son loading cars onto his car carrier and told me she couldn't love him or any of her grandchildren. I said that I understood and didn't mind. I told her that her feelings would return when this depression ended, and she said she was afraid this depression would never end. (I can't cry.) I put my arms around her.

"My God," she said. "Do you know how long it is since you've done that?"

But Mother, I thought, I'm not *supposed* to do it. There is a proper order of things. How could we all be so middle-class and yet never follow the proper order of things? On my wedding morning someone had to remind us that a bride was supposed to have a bouquet. There is a decorum that, when one is willing to subscribe to it, eliminates coarse possibilities like forgetting bridal bouquets and committing suicide.

What she wanted I couldn't give her. I could have tried harder, much harder than I did, and still not have given it to her. I began to withdraw.

Item. At quiet times my left breast hurts. Her left breast was cut off four years before she died.

Before we moved to this house we had a cat that had a litter of which we kept one kitten. When we moved two miles up the road to this house, mother cat and year-old kitten moved with us. Mother cat and kitten were affectionate to each other, licked each other, nestled together, were abused by our children together. After a couple of months here, mother cat decided to return permanently to the other house. Kitten remained with us. If they were to meet now, they wouldn't even know each other.

Item. "I just put in a new bridge for her," said my mother's heartbroken dentist. "She was so pleased with the way she looked." Relevance. The way one looks is really important. You feel better when you feel as if you look good. "They were two beautiful girls," he said, remembering my mother and her sister at the City College fraternity party where he introduced my father to my mother. She was still pretty. Black hair her friends didn't believe she didn't dye until a pure white hair began to appear here and there against the others. Because I did not resemble my mother, I was thought not to take after her, but when closely examined, many of my faults and virtues turn out to be visible symptoms of her inner qualities or negative reflections of her outer ones.

Item. My mother took castor oil to induce my birth because she had struck a bargain with her best friend, who was due at the same time, that whoever gave birth first would have the services of a particularly fine maid who would be available. I took castor oil to induce my daughter's birth because an obstetrician who didn't want to risk being late for his vacation advised that the baby would be very difficult to deliver if it got much bigger. Same action, different reasons. A play instead of a novel. The actions show, the motives are hazy. Interpretations constantly change so that only the action remains.

She wouldn't have taken those pills if she believed in an afterlife. It wasn't life she was after. This is important. Aside from her one wildly symbolic gesture of accidentally sweeping the alarm clock off her night table that morning before my father left for his plant, a touch so obvious that it would be unusable in a work of fiction, there was no sign of disorder or regret in the room. Which I did not see until weeks later. She showered, and folded the towel afterward. She got into bed, the blankets were neat, the phone straight on the table and the receiver secure in its cradle.

Now my husband tells me, "The room was a mess when I first saw it that night. I straightened it up." And seeing my stricken face, adds, "Maybe the cops did it."

The cops don't mess up the bedroom of a middle-class white suicide. Maybe he means when they took her away. I don't ask. There is no way for me to face this new fact. I can only try to digest it by writing it down. My mother had the writer's consciousness without the writer's impulse. If she had been able to write, she might have digested the ironies of her life instead of letting herself be poisoned by them. Writing is my survival kit. My independence.

Item. A dream. I am looking at a hanging painting of a person sitting in a rocking chair. The painting is in a realistic manner but the person is hazy. "Who is that sitting in the rocker?" I ask a servant of the house. "There's no one sitting in the rocker," the servant says. "The rocker is empty." End of dream.

My 2½-year-old son brings me the bright-green ski sweater my mother knitted for him.

"Who brought this?" he asks.

I say, "Grandma made it for you, sweetheart."

He says, "No. Grandpa bought it."

He was always closer to his grandfather, anyway. He is the first in our family to strongly resemble my father, with his blue eyes and fair hair, but there is more to it than that. My mother always seemed remote to him. Never hostile or domineering. Always gentle. But remote. She was a gentle person, but how much of her gentleness was violence rendered ineffectual?

"Grandma was never mean to me. She was *always* nice," says my daughter, who has to live with my temper but is certainly not aware that my mother entered a suicidal depression each time my sister or I became pregnant.

For my daughter, the loss is a serious one. For my daughter, who was born five years earlier in all of our lives than my son, my mother existed. For my son she always had the quality of those few dried-out autumn leaves that contrive to stay on the ground through spring.

"You'll write about me, won't you?" she said in December.

"Everything I write is about you," I said.

How Science Is Redefining Parenthood

BARBARA KATZ ROTHMAN

Barbara Katz Rothman, *Ms.*, July-August 1982. Reprinted by permission.

T he United States has produced its first "test-tube" baby. I read about it in the newspaper. Some woman bore it, of course, but the child, I am told, is a product of medical technology. Doctors put it in, and interestingly, doctors took it out—this baby, like Louise Brown, the first of the test-tube babies, was also removed surgically, born by cesarean section.

All the fanfare that has greeted the birth of these babies, the marvel at their "production," is itself an interesting thing to observe. In vitro fertilization—sperm joining ovum in a test tube (actually on a glass dish, but let's not quibble)—is not just one more treatment for infertility. It is that, certainly, and no small thing—NEW HOPE FOR THE CHILDLESS, the headline read. But it is also a challenge to traditional definitions of parenthood, the latest in a long line of such challenges, and that's where we'd best pay attention.

What does it mean to be a parent in this society? The first thing we do is to separate social from biological parenthood. The modern, anonymous adoption taught us that distinction: a woman who adopts a baby is its social mother. She is not simply a woman raising a child, she is the child's *mother*, with the rights and obligations of motherhood. Women have always done a certain amount of raising one another's kids—taking in a dying sister's child or taking on one twin. In some societies that makes you a mother, and in some it doesn't. Making it formal, legal, and especially *anonymous* clarified the social-biological distinction.

Being a social parent now clearly means being a child-rearer, and is usually but by no means always associated with biological parenthood. But what is biological parenthood? We can now think in terms of "genetic" parents, those who provide half of the genetic material for a child; "physiologic" or biological parents, those who nurture an embryo/fetus in their bodies; and "social" parents, those who rear a child.

Women never before were able to think about genetic motherhood without pregnancy, or pregnancy without genetic motherhood: if we were biological mothers (carrying babies) then we were genetic mothers. But making the inseparable separate is what the technology of reproduction is all about. And it is this issue that we are now facing: women, for the first time, have the potential for genetic parenthood without physiologic motherhood. At all. No pregnancy. No birth. No suckling. Women are about to become fathers.

THE TECHNOLOGY OF BIOLOGICAL FATHERHOOD

Biological fatherhood has meant genetic parenthood: a biological father contributes half of the genetic basis for the child-to-be. Men can make their genetic contribution to conception without mating with the mother, substituting an "artificial" form of insemination. The continued secrecy surrounding artificial insemination is telling. Adoption is discussed openly, and the parents of babies fertilized in vitro are holding press conferences, but very few people who have used artificial insemination with donor sperm, AID, seem ready to come out of the closet. Maybe that is because biological fatherhood still means genetic parenthood, and social fatherhood is so ambiguous. It's not really being a child-rearer—so many fathers do so little child-rearing. What makes a man "really" the father of a child in this society, if not genetics? And a child without a father in a patriarchal society is called illegitimate. Men as social fathers "claim" or name children, legitimate them.

Like in vitro fertilization, "artificial" insemination is a treatment for infertility. An important difference is that AID is a treatment for male infertility. Women do not really need men to have children—we need only their semen. Men, on the other hand, do need women, if they are to have children. Much as we have been taught to think mechanistically about our body "parts," a womb does not live without a woman. When we are pregnant, we are pregnant with our whole bodies—to have children, men need living whole women. Our wombs really cannot themselves alone be rented or sold. But once women have the semen, we do not need the man's body to have our babies. And in a capitalist society, semen, along with blood and with milk, the essential fluids of life, is for sale.

While women without mates have used AID as a route to the socially fatherless child, the most common, and surely the most socially sanctioned, use of AID, is for the fertile woman married to the infertile man. In most of the literature on AID the reader is asked to sympathize with her plight, and to view artificial insemination as the solution.

Historically, when infertility was assumed always to be the "fault" of the wife, husbands were given the recourse of divorce. Now, given the technological sophistication available that can prove beyond all doubt that the male is responsible for the "barren" state of the couple, in this situation maternity is a privilege rather than an obligation of the wife.

Defining artificial insemination as a "gift" for the woman, something a husband "allows," means two things. One is that we gloss over the range of choices the woman in the situation has: she after all can be a mother by taking on a new husband, or simply taking a lover. The second consequence is that in the emphasis on genetic ties as defining fatherhood, the sharing of a pregnancy and birth by the woman's husband is dismissed as meaningless. In some states in the United States, the husband of a woman who has had artificial insemination (even at his written request) must formally adopt the child. He adopts a sperm. Thus the potential of biological fathering is reduced to a single-cell genetic contribution, and trivialized, purchased cheaply.

THE TECHNOLOGY OF BIOLOGICAL MOTHERHOOD

Biological motherhood encompasses both aspects of biological fatherhood, the genetic and the sexual, and a great deal more. Biological motherhood also involves pregnancy, the birth process, and suckling the baby. As the technology has become and continues to become available to make substitutes for one or another of these aspects of motherhood, the problem of defining biological motherhood, defining female infertility, gets more complicated.

Before the advent of the rubber nipple, the pasteurizing process for cow's milk, and the development of formulas to substitute for breast milk, if a woman could not produce milk, she could not be a mother: her babies would die. Her only alternative was to find a substitute, or surrogate mother, a wet nurse. Often that meant the sacrifice of the wet nurse's baby for the purchaser's baby. In modern America we no longer think of the breasts as necessary for fertility.

A woman with a very small pelvis, perhaps deformed from an accident or from rickets in childhood, cannot "give birth"—her baby must be removed surgically. Before the advent of the techniques necessary to do cesarean sections, women with small pelvises were perforce infertile; they could not produce a live baby and survive.

Pregnancy may in fact end quite early, and still produce a live baby. With the advent of the technology for caring for premature babies, it became the rule rather than the exception for premature babies to survive. This particular technology got even more media attention than did the current "test-tube" babies: incubators with preemies were a world's fair exhibit, and an exhibition at Coney Island. A baby in an incubator, fed on formula by a tube, was a "manmade" or "artificial" product. But that too got incorporated into our definitions of motherhood, and an inability to carry a pregnancy to term does not now mean infertility.

So far the test-tube babies like Louise Brown, like all of the previous "artificially created" babies, the artificially incubated, artificially fed, artificially (surgically) born babies, have all been the genetic offspring of their social/biological parents. There is no reason why they should have to be so any longer. Extrauterine or in vitro fertilization might in fact be a lot easier from the technological standpoint if the source of the ova were not a woman who was to host it. Yet the "ethical" guidelines established by the Ethics Advisory Board to the Secretary of the Department of Health, Education, and Welfare, and the current convention, are that in vitro fertilization is to be used only with married couples as the genetic parents.

Closely related to in vitro fertilization is the technology of embryo transplants. Embryo transplants are being done routinely with several species. When embryos, or just ova, can be transplanted from one woman to another, then who is the biological mother: the "donor" or the "host"? How different is the "donor" using this kind of technology from the woman who, in an earlier technology, used a wet nurse? Both are using the reproductive capacities of another woman. But looking at it another way, the donor is not a mother at all. She is a father: she contributes half of the genetic material, her "seed."

Now let us consider it from the perspective of the "host," the woman who carried the pregnancy. For women who cannot conceive, who are currently therefore infertile, a new option opens up: they can enter biological motherhood at the point after conception, carrying and birthing what will be their social children. Such a woman might not be a genetic parent, but social motherhood would begin with a biological tie, with pregnancy. With the new technology, an inability to conceive, or even to ovulate, will not mean infertility, any more than an inability to lactate or to labor now means infertility.

MODELS FOR THE NEW MOTHERHOOD

We used to talk about futuristic, science fiction–sounding things like embryo transplants as 1984 visions. Well, that may be right on target. There is no technological reason why human embryo transplants should not be available by 1984.

In *The Dialectic of Sex,* Shulamith Firestone says that new reproductive technology could free women from motherhood, and that would indeed free women. Not all of us shared that view of the relation between motherhood and feminism then, and even fewer of us share it now. This new technology is not being used to free women from motherhood. Quite the contrary, it is being used to make biological motherhood available to more women.

One of the standard objections made to proceeding with the new technology of reproduction is that it is an unwise and ultimately exploitative use of resources. With all the unwanted babies in the world, with overpopulation and world hunger, why should we invest so much energy in getting a few elite women pregnant? Indeed. Why not adopt? we say. Biology shouldn't matter. People can have the full experience of parenting by adopting. Well, yes. And no. Women do sometimes want simply to be pregnant, to give birth. These too are experiences, like the parenting experience, which a woman, or a woman and her mate, may want to have. But there is an even more serious objection to the why-not-adopt argument.

Adoption has been based on another set of exploitations: the exploitation of biological mothers. Where exactly do people think adoptable babies come from? They used to be available because the demands of a patriarchal system created them. Pregnant women had so few choices.

Because women are no longer so tightly bound by the rules of the patriarchal family in America, we have lost the supply of domestic babies. So we turn to third world women, and cash in on their "surplus" babies, the babies they would have aborted or would have kept, had life offered them choices. Loving, eager parents take these babies home from airports and raise them, accepting the genetic and biological donations of anonymous parents.

Does adoption provide us with a model we can use for managing embryo transplants? Will we come to think of some embryos as "adoptable"? Will a market for embryos develop, like the market for adoptable babies, with those of the whitest, healthiest, best-fed, best-educated women the most prized?

Because elective abortions for nonmedical reasons will be the most readily available source of healthy embryos for transplantation, once the technology is perfected, this may change the very meaning of abortion. When one woman's abortion becomes another woman's pregnancy, and ultimately another woman's child, then just what is an abortion? Can it be some kind of an adoption procedure?

Another meaning of pregnancy, a definition for which feminists have fought, is that it is a condition of women, a state of our bodies, like menstruation, ovulation, or menopause. If pregnancy is an undesired state, abortion is a remedy. That meaning of pregnancy essentially denies the presence of a future or potential child. The argument goes that just as there is a potential for a child with an early pregnancy, so too is there that potential with each ovulation. We will no more mourn the loss of a child with an early abortion than we would a few weeks earlier at the time of menstruation. With this set of meanings, donating an embryo is much like donating an ovum. That should be much like donating semen.

But is it? And do we want it to be? Will women accept this kind of nonresponsible, irresponsible parenthood? If we are going to become fathers, is that the kind of father we want to be?

Neither adoption nor sperm donation provides the model we should be seeking, a way of dealing with biological motherhood that is ethical, feminist, moral, fair. The history of surrogate mothers too has been largely a history of exploitation, in which rich mothers used poor mothers, in which slave mammies and peasant wet nurses sacrificed their own motherhood.

But the potential for nonexploitative surrogates, like the potential for women being good fathers to their genetic children, is really there. The new technology offers us another opportunity to work on the definitions of parenthood, of motherhood, fatherhood, and children. Earlier technologies *could* have revolutionized the family, but were incorporated instead into the existing family. Think of how formula might have changed women's and men's roles in child-rearing.

With this new technology the opportunity once again exists to evolve new relations between parents and children, to ask new questions and rethink old answers. We can now ask, should genetics matter at all for mothers? If we say no, then what are we saying about the meaning of biological fatherhood? Should the biology of motherhood, the carrying and birthing of babies, matter at all for mothers? And again, what does our answer tell us about fatherhood?

Reproductive technology will not make social change; as long as our social definitions remain the same, the technology will be used to support those definitions.

But not if we say no. Not if women want to be good fathers to their genetic children. As fathers we can perhaps be like aunts—aunts too share a genetic tie to their nieces and nephews. Not if we reject being or using "surrogates," reject the idea of one human being substituting for another. Not if we join together to form new families—a reproductive communism, with each giving according to his or her ability. We do not have to be "donors" and "hosts" and "surrogates"—we can be mothers and fathers and aunts and uncles. We can take away the gender assignments and leave the relationships. We are coming to understand this with social parenting, that several people, including fathers and other men, can "mother" a child. Perhaps we will learn the lesson for physical parenthood too.

Misconceptions

GENA COREA

Adapted from Gena Corea, "Preface," *Misconceptions: The Social Construction of Choice and the New Reproductive and Genetic Technologies,* Gwynne Basen, Margrit Eichler, and Abby Lippman, eds., Hull, Quebec, Voyageur, 1994. Reprinted by permission.

An elderly couple walk among the physicians and scientists in the lobby of the Hilton Hotel Convention Center in Jerusalem in 1989 silently handing to each "technodoc" a photocopy of a letter they have written. The couple are afraid. Would these participants of the VI World Congress on In Vitro Fertilization and Alternate Assisted Reproduction call the police? Throw them out? That prospect was terrifying, yet, as the old man, Alexander Werba, 67, told me, that was actually—when he later thought about it—what he wanted: He wanted the police to scream in with sirens, and reporters to rush in with them, notebooks open, cameras rolling, and then he could tell them why he and his wife had come, how these doctors—no, they were not doctors, he said angrily, they were child-production engineers—how they had killed his daughter.

The letter the Werbas distribute states that their daughter, Aliza Eisenberg, died as a result of an egg capture procedure in the in vitro fertilization (IVF) program at Haddasah Hospital. It protests the fact that the physician who performed that egg capture had been named secretary of the congress.

I had spoken with the couple for hours the night before about the death of their daughter and they had shown me the letter they planned to pass out this morning at the congress.

They speak no English. If a technodoc reading the letter addresses them, they fear, they will be unable to understand or reply.

Prima approaches the huge lecture hall to which the technodocs will soon return. She tries to enter but a woman in the red uniform of the congress employees stops her. Prima is not registered for the congress. She has no badge.

Fearing the uniformed woman, Prima waits until she leaves. Then she enters the empty hall and places a letter on each of the seats, always looking to each side to see that no one is coming.

As she is leaving, she looks up, spots a young man, catches a glimpse of the name on his badge: It's him! The man who took her daughter's eggs. The man who left her daughter bleeding to death.

Prima quickly exits. She and Alexander are too upset, too frightened, to continue distributing the letter. Trembling, they leave the convention center.

The Werbas' fear went deeper than a concern that they would not be able to understand the technodocs' English. They explained it to me later when I visited them in their home in Haifa.

Poles, they both survived the Nazi time in Europe. Alexander's parents had been transported in a train in Treblinka. After running away from a work camp and obtaining false identity papers, he lived on the Aryan side of Warsaw, working in the dark room of a photography shop, thankful that he did not have to be out in the dangerous streets. He was afraid all the time. The fear he had felt during that year and a half in Warsaw, before he joined the Resistance, was exactly the fear he felt at the IVF congress, he told me.

Prima "dreams that the Germans are running and shooting," Alexander tells me. "Soldiers and SS men. She sees that in her dreams very often. Now, after this case with our daughter, she dreams more about doctors. Every night."

She told me of her reaction to seeing for the first time the man who had attempted IVF on her daughter. "I was afraid like when I was with the Germans, when they led me to the crematorium in a cargo train."

"There were many people from the conference center to make sure that everything was in order and was going 100 percent smoothly," Alexander explains, "and she saw the Nazis in every such official in the red uniform. All these associations. Maybe they would throw us out. Or arrest us. You understand me? I didn't want it to come to that.

"But now I am sorry I didn't make a big scene where they called the police and arrested me or tried to throw me out. Then someone would have come from the press or television. I could have said in the press everything that was written in the letter. But at that time I was so—that was dumb. They were no Germans. Why was I so afraid? I wanted to go sit in a corner where no one could see me."

The association Prima and Alexander Werba made between life under the Nazis and their daughter's ordeal from reproductive technology experimentation is an association consciously made by a number of feminists. They recognize in these technologies the totalitarian project of controlling who will be allowed to be born into this world; the eugenic attempt to eradicate, even before birth, the lives of those judged "unworthy of life."

The Nazis' "Final Solution" originated within mainstream medicine. More than 70,000 people—patients all—were killed in gas chambers installed in psychiatric hospitals. The doctors and gas chambers were then moved to Poland to kill ("heal," in the Nazi metaphor) on a grander scale. The Nazis called this "the great therapy of Auschwitz."

Many Germans today feel a special responsibility to speak out against and stop the proliferation of new reproductive technologies (NRTs) because, unlike Americans, they well understand what is going on here and where it leads. In fact, it was German women who organized the first international feminist conference in resistance to the new reproductive technologies. I remember that 1985 conference in Bonn, Germany, well since I was invited to address it.

One of my memories from that conference is of Theresia Degener. A young woman in jeans, she delivers a paper to a speaker on stage. She holds the paper in her teeth. She has no arms. She had not been disarmed by her genes. (Genes are responsible for but a small portion—3 to 5 percent—of disabilities.) No. She had been injured by medical treatment, in the form of Thalidamide, administered by well-educated, mainstream physicians.

The first time I met Theresia, in Frankfurt, Germany, she interviewed me for a magazine article. With her toe, she turned on her tape recorder. When the recorder malfunctioned, she impatiently pushed it aside with one foot, and pulled a pen and notebook out from her tote bag with her toes. As I spoke, she scribbled notes with the pen between two toes.

In the following years, we often worked together at conferences of the Feminist International Network of Resistance to Reproductive and Genetic Engineering (FINRRAGE). At one such conference in Spain, she told me at breakfast that she'd toiled much of the night on the paper she was to give that afternoon. She hadn't wanted to disturb her roommate's sleep, so she brought her typewriter to the hall outside her hotel room and typed there, with her feet. Several people had staggered drunk down the hall at 3 A.M. She could just imagine them now at breakfast, she told me, her eyes sparkling in delight, saying they were so drunk last night they thought they saw an armless woman in the hall typing with her feet! We roared laughing.

Imagine Theresia, with her joy, empathy for others, courage, deep intelligence —all qualities she took to law school with her, all qualities that infuse her work in the feminist and the disability rights movement—imagine Theresia, on some prenatal test, judged "life unworthy of life"!

The fascist project of eliminating "unworthy" life through use of reproductive technologies leads feminists like Abby Lippman to pose this question: "Why have efforts to find every fetus with Down's syndrome become so important to us that universal triple screening is entering recommended medical practice, while ensuring early prenatal care for all women [the lack of which is a major cause of disability] is still an unachieved goal?"

It is not only reproduction that is now being engineered. The public discussion of the NRTs and of genetic engineering is also engineered. The forces behind medicine and industry have been largely successful in controlling the kind of information and the kind of interpretation ("stories," in Lippman's phrasing) we receive on the technologies.

The public discussion is framed in a way that excludes any consideration of the risks to women or the community, filmmaker Gwynne Basen points out. What's left out is just what feminists insist on including in the alternative framework we provide: the extraordinarily high failure rate of IVF; the experimental nature of the techniques; the damage of the techniques to women physically, emotionally, and spiritually; the preventable and ignored causes of infertility—including environmental factors and sexually transmitted diseases—some of those diseases, transmitted to the women when they were sexually abused as children; increasing medical and technological control over procreation; the violations of women's integrity, dignity, and freedom involved in the techniques; the unimaginable stress placed on women who suddenly become the mothers of three or four infants following the implantation of multiple embryos; the increasing industrialization of reproduction; the connections between the use and promotion of experimental contraceptives in dominated (third world) countries and the promotion of proceptives, like IVF, in dominating countries; woman's status in a sexual caste system; the increasing use of women as experimental models for other species.

When ethics are publicly discussed, women's experiences are largely absent from consideration. At the IVF congress in Jerusalem where the Werbas passed out their letter, the panel on ethics was entirely composed of men. The men did not notice the omission of women. It occurred to none of them that experimentation on women might be an ethical issue related to IVF. No one spoke of the Nuremberg and Helsinki codes on protection of human experimental subjects, let alone pointed out the many ways IVF violates those codes. (And IVF is experimentation, as feminist analysts have been documenting for years and as the World Health Organization has acknowledged.) Though the moderator of the ethics panel was on the IVF team at Haddaseh Hospital, Aliza Eisenberg's name never passed his lips.

On Becoming a Grandmother

FRANCINE KLAGSBRUN

Francine Klagsbrun, "On Becoming a Grandmother," *The Jewish Week*, February 19, 1999. Reprinted by permission.

As of this writing, my first grandchild, a girl, has turned a week and a half old. Even as I type that sentence, every part of it fills me with amazement: That I have actually become a grandmother, a status I have longed for but cannot yet fathom; that this tiny being has already passed the milestone of a week and a half of life; that I am able to use my fingers for typing when, to paraphrase the psalmist, all my bones cry out in joy, "God, who is like You?"

She was born on a Friday evening, not long after sundown. "Friday's child is loving and giving," the old nursery rhyme says. But a Shabbat eve child is something more, a gift delivered to this world by the Sabbath Queen. I wonder if her parents will remember to tell her that some day.

Right now they cannot stop marveling at the miracle of this person in miniature—the little hands with their surprisingly long fingers, the perfect head with its downy coat of hair, the feet that curl to the touch. "Can you imagine," my son-in-law says in awe, "that just a short time ago, this complete human being was inside her mother?"

I cannot imagine it. In spite of the billions of babies born on this earth, I still cannot imagine how from a microscopic speck of sperm and egg a human being develops. In spite of photographs and sonograms, I cannot picture how that being lives and thrives within its mother's womb. Like my daughter and son-in-law, I can only gaze in astonishment at our newest family member. To look at her is to see God's handiwork. To look at her is to witness Creation.

For me there is also another miracle, one the couple cannot recognize. It is the miracle of their immediate transformation from children to parents themselves. My daughter feeds her baby day and night tenderly, without a moment's impatience, although she's fatigued from childbirth and lack of sleep. My son-in-law reads and talks to the infant, knowing full well that she doesn't understand a word he is saying, yet reveling in every changed expression. In some ways they're like kids playing house.

But in more ways they see themselves fully as parents now.

And as parents have always done, they're ready to place their child's well-being above their own. That is surely the essence and miracle of human parenthood.

I'm not certain what the essence of grandparenthood is. Part of it, I know, is letting go of your grown children so they can exercise their own parental roles without interference.

After my daughter told me she was expecting a child, she went impulsively to her closet and pulled out an album of her baby photos. We looked through the pictures together for more than an hour, holding on tightly to the past before allowing ourselves to venture into the future.

But another part of grandparenthood is being available to help our children in rearing their children. In today's high-pressured world, where mothers and fathers juggle a million obligations, they need all the help and support we can give.

The trick, of course, is to balance being available with letting go, giving with nonmeddling. To a great extent that has always been the hardest challenge of parenthood. The balancing act just becomes more delicate now, when we must be parents to grown children who are parents themselves.

I've said little so far about the grandparent-grandchild relationship itself. That's because it is still a mystery to me.

My granddaughter will grow up in a world I cannot begin to foresee. She will never know a home or classroom devoid of computers. She may have friends who are clones of their relatives and eat genetically powered foods as yet uninvented. Bill Clinton and Monica Lewinsky will be ancient history to her, and my parents and in-laws only distant names on a family tree.

How will I relate to this unknown being? After my daughter was born, my father-in-law, who spoke Yiddish-accented English, took speech lessons because he wanted to communicate clearly with his granddaughter. I, too, will do my best to keep up with the trends and patterns of her world.

But like grandparents throughout time, I will also try to ground her in my world, in the art that I love and the Jewish texts that have been a passion of my existence. People say that grandchildren represent our immortality, our compensation for having given up the tree of life for the tree of knowledge. Our best assurance of that immortality as Jews is passing on our teachings to each new generation. That I hope to do.

Meanwhile, I will love and cuddle the beautiful being who has joined our family. The Midrash says that the soul of every newborn dwells in the Garden of Eden until the moment of conception.

This soul, released into our lives, has touched us with paradise.

Chapter 64

Vagina

A Circle of Women

TARA GREENWAY

Excerpted from Tara Greenway, *A Circle of Women,* 1998. Reprinted by permission.

A circle or women gather in a public high school room in Manhattan every fourth Tuesday evening of the month. We are young, old, and in between; businesswomen and homemakers; single, married, and divorced; mothers and club hoppers. We talk, almost exclusively, about our vaginas.

We are not a consciousness-raising feminist group. We are not in the room to get in touch with our sexual selves. We are here to talk about our pain—our doctors, our drugs, our herbal remedies, our methods of managing or avoiding sex. We are here to confirm that our pain is not in our imaginations. We are here to pull each other through our pain.

For a roomful of women talking about pain, we are having a really great time. We do not have to explain that although our vaginas hurt like the devil almost all the time and have for the past year or five years or ten years, we are still attractive and sexual women. We talk about our doctors' or our lovers' ignorant reactions to our pain, and we laugh uproariously, because when we come to this circle, the whole thing is suddenly... hilarious. When a new woman comes, we let her speak first. We just say, "Tell us your story." Her eyes widen, and she looks a little pale. She begins hesitantly:

"It started when I was 26. There was this burning and stinging down there. I went to the gynecologist; he said I probably had a yeast infection. He gave me Monostat. I used it up, but the burning got worse. My boyfriend and I were really in love, and before all this, we had sex, like, all the time. But after this started, we'd try to have sex, and there was this incredible pain, like… like a knife going up me."

"And the rest of the time it felt like squatting over a blowtorch?" someone asks helpfully.

"Yes!" the new woman says, perking up a little. "I kept changing doctors because the second or third time I'd go in and say it was worse, not better, the gynecologist would always get really mad at me. He'd say, 'Well, if you won't respond to the treatment there's really nothing I can do.' "

"How about, 'You'll just have to learn to live with the pain'?" someone interjects.

By now the new girl's eyes are flashing and her cheeks are pink. "Yeah! One said that to me! And they would run all kinds of tests, for yeast, HIV, AIDS, herpes, and they'd all be negative, and they'd say, 'There's absolutely nothing wrong with you, dear.… ' "

Five or six voices complete the infamous sentence with her: "It's all in your head!"

Chuckles of recognition ripple through the circle, and someone asks, "So who finally diagnosed you?"

"No one. I was searching the Internet one day, and I came across all this stuff about vaginal pain. I found you guys, and I came tonight. Do you know what's wrong with me?"

We have good news and bad news for the new woman. The bad news is she almost certainly has vulvar vestibulitis. When you are finally told that you have this incurable disease, the first feeling you have is relief. It has a name. Only later do you think, Oh, no. What am I going to do? But then there's more good news. There are many treatments for vestibulitis (although they're not cures). Everyone's symptoms and responses vary, and you have to work through each treatment by trial and error, but eventually one of them will probably work for you.

From the time vulvar pain, and the resulting excruciating intercourse, was documented in ancient Egypt through Freud's theories, the medical community has rushed to the curious conclusion that if women complain of pain during sexual intercourse, they are emotionally disturbed. Finally, in 1983, vulvodynia was defined by the International Society for the Study of Vulvar Diseases as "chronic painful vulvar discomfort." (Vulvar vestibulitis is one type of vulvodynia.) Vestibulitis is not an easy diagnosis, since frequently it has no visible symptoms—although often there is significant red inflammation of the vulva.

Vulvar vestibulitis has the reputation of being a "rare" condition, and the commonly reported statistic is that it affects 1 percent of women. However, in a study by Dr. Martha Goetsch in 1990, 37 percent of women visiting gynecologists had some vulvar pain and 15 percent had vulvar vestibulitis. In our monthly meetings we have noted that there are more women with vestibulitis than there are with breast cancer—and breast cancer has a postage stamp!

Even when a doctor knows it is a physical problem, not a psychosomatic one, he or she often will tell a patient that the only treatment for the condition is surgery, but there are dozens of documented treatments that must be tried first. Treatments include blocking the pain with drugs such as tricyclic antidepressants like Elavil and anticonvulsants like Neurontin. Biofeedback, which involves inserting a sensor into the vagina and doing pelvic floor rehabilitation exercises, has helped many women. The low-oxalate calcium citrate diet and the no-yeast diet have also proved helpful. Many have found relief taking combinations of herbs recommended by herbalists and naturopathic-homeopathic doctors, and others find acupuncture valuable. Interferon injected into trigger points is another treatment, as is physical therapy including myofascial release. Some treatments that have proven to do more harm than good are laser surgery, topical or oral antibiotics, and topical steroids. Vestibulectomy (a surgery performed by scalpel, not by laser) has been successful for some women.

Although these treatments are effective in varying degrees, most people with vestibulitis are still living with some pain, and some have found no relief at all. The condition desperately needs the attention of the medical community; it needs funding for research and publicity. Physicians could tell patients about the fact that antibiotics kill off "good bacteria" along with "bad bacteria" and recommend taking acidophillus to replenish the system's natural flora while on antibiotics. Gynecologists could learn that if a woman says her burning is worse after taking Monostat, they should not just ignore her feedback and prescribe more.

What can we do when we sit in overwhelming pain as the fifth doctor in a row looks us straight in the eye and says, "It's all in your head"? For now, we can join together. We can believe each other. We can become members of the nationwide grassroots organizations started by women with vestibulitis—the National Vulvodynia Association and the Vulvar Pain Foundation. We can be part of a "virtual support group" on the Internet, where there are hundreds of articles and many Web pages, including an e-mail list. For now, we can be one of a circle of women meeting across the nation, telling each other of medications and herbs and doctors; sharing our pain and our vagina stories; reminding each other of our grace, our humor, our strength, our hope.

Chapter 65

Clitoris

The Whole Woman

GERMAINE GREER

Excerpted from Germaine Greer, *The Whole Woman*, New York, Knopf, 1999, with an introduction by Jennifer Baumgardner. Reprinted by permission.

Germaine Greer's new book *The Whole Woman*, her 30-years-later follow-up to *The Female Eunuch*, is thoroughly disliked by everyone from the staid stylists at *The New York Times* to the chatty philosophers at salon.com. The consensus is that the book is shrill and disorganized, the work of a past-her-prime second-waver: bitter, batty, and male-bashing.

The fact that her critics, former fans all, find her to be so sour and incompetent points to the central difference between her audience then and now. *The Female Eunuch* spoke to women on the brink of a tumultuous shift in status and consciousness. *The Whole Woman* is written for feminists, women for whom finding the political roots of what appear to be personal problems is a matter of course. Instead of being happy with whatever progress has been made, Greer wants women to be insulted and angry by the scraps now offered us as "feminist emancipation," be it the "privilege" of abortion or "flex" time for overworked mothers.

With *Eunuch*, Greer said that women were castrated, cut off from their sexuality, and tried to get women to assert cunt power when most feminists were focusing on political power. Now that the pro-sex, get-on-top, use-toys, he-better-make-you-come aspect of feminism is ascendant (see *Bust, Minx, Susie Bright*, etc.), Greer is again fighting for the neglected side, turning her attention to politics… analyzing everything from deadbeat dads to transsexualism to girlie culture to female mutilation. And some of Greer's strongest inquiries concern women's health.

"Revolution," the final chapter of *The Female Eunuch*, concludes with the challenge, "What will you do?"; in *The Whole Woman*, Greer renews her question, asking not only what we will do, but what, during a three-decade interim, we actually have done.

I hope that despite the bad reviews, serious students of feminism will still read *The Whole Woman*. So much about what makes an ambitious book become big is timing. Yet the fact that the 34 heavy-hitting essayettes of *The Whole Woman* could be dismissed so easily is evidence that, despite the fragments of feminists' rhetoric in every atom of our culture, the whole of women's liberation that Greer envisions is still as hard for us to picture as the round earth was for Columbus's shipmates. To think that Greer is recanting on her free-your-ass credo from 1970 is to see just half the picture. Greer didn't think women could fuck themselves into liberty, but that we needed to be free to fuck as well as to do anything else. Her definition of *whole* means for women to be sexual and confident at the same time as they are political and conscious, and that's my definition, too.

T his sequel to *The Female Eunuch* is the book I said I would never write. I believed that each generation should produce its own statement of problems and priorities, and that I had no special authority or vocation to speak on behalf of women of any but my own age, class, background, and education. For 30 years I have done my best to champion all the styles of feminism that came to public attention because I wanted it to be clear that lipstick lesbianism and the prostitutes' union and La Leche and the Women's League for Peace and Freedom and pressure for the ordination of women were aspects of the same struggle toward awareness of oppression and triumph over it. Though I disagreed with some of the strategies and was as troubled as I should have been by some of the more fundamental conflicts, it was not until feminists of my own generation began to assert with apparent seriousness that feminism had gone too far that the fire flared up in my belly. When the lifestyle feminists chimed in that feminism had gone just far enough in giving them the right to "have it all," i.e., money, sex, and fashion, it would have been inexcusable to remain silent.

In 1970 the movement was called "women's liberation " or, contemptuously, "women's lib." When the name "libbers" was dropped for "feminists" we were all relieved. What none of us noticed was that the ideal of liberation was fading out with the word. We were settling for equality. Liberation struggles are not about assimilation but about asserting difference, endowing that difference with dignity and prestige, and insisting on it as a condition of self-defin-ition and self-determination. The aim of women's liberation is to do as much for female people as has been done for colonized nations. Women's liberation did not see the female's potential in terms of the male's actual; the visionary feminists of the late sixties and early seventies knew that women could never find freedom by agreeing to live the lives of unfree men. Seekers after equality clamored to be admitted to smoke-filled male haunts. Liberationists sought the world over for clues to what women's lives could be if they were free to define their own values, order their own priorities, and decide their own fate.

The Female Eunuch was one feminist text that did not argue for equality. At a debate in Oxford one William J. Clinton heard me arguing that equality leg-islation could not give me the right to have broad hips or hairy thighs, to be at ease in my woman's body. Thirty years on, femininity is still compulsory for women and has become an option for men, while genuine femaleness remains grotesque to the point of obscenity. Meanwhile the price of the small advances we have made toward sexual equality has been the denial of female-ness as any kind of a distinguishing character. If femaleness is not to be inter-preted as inferiority, it is not to signify anything at all. Even the distinction between the vagina, which only women have, and the rectum, which every-body has, has been declared, as it were, unconstitutional. Nonconsensual bug-gery, which can be inflicted on both sexes, has been nonsensically renamed "male rape." In June 1998 an overwhelming vote of the British House of Commons recognized the right of 16-year-old homosexual men "to have sex," by which they meant, apparently, for it was never explained, the right to pen-etrate and be penetrated anally. This the MPs saw as granting homosexual men the same rights as heterosexuals. For them at least, rectum and vagina were equivalent; in many cultures (and increasingly our own) the most desirable vagina is as tight and narrow as a rectum. Postmodernists are proud and pleased that gender now justifies fewer suppositions about an individual than ever before, but for women still wrestling with the same physical realities this new silence about their visceral experiences is the same old rapist's hand clamped across their mouths. Real women are being phased out; the first step, persuading them to deny their own existence, is almost complete.

In the last 30 years women have come a long, long way; our lives are nobler and richer than they were, but they are also fiendishly difficult. From the beginning feminists have been aware that the causes of female suffering can be grouped under the heading "contradictory expectations." The contradic-tions women face have never been more bruising than they are now. The career woman does not know if she is to do her job like a man or like herself. Is she supposed to change the organization or knuckle under to it? Is she sup-posed to endure harassment or kick ass and take names? Is motherhood a privilege or a punishment? Even if it had been real, equality would have been a poor substitute for liberation; fake equality is leading women into double jeopardy. The rhetoric of equality is being used in the name of political correctness to mask the hammering that women are taking. When *The Female Eunuch* was written our daughters were not cutting or starving themselves. On every side speechless women endure endless hardship, grief, and pain, in a world system that creates billions of losers for every handful of winners.

It's time to get angry again. (pp. 3–5)

The womb rudely awakens the growing girl to its presence by causing her to shed blood through her vagina. The more difficult the process, the more bloated and bilious she feels, the more dragging the pain, the more negative the ideas of a womb will seem to her. As she has heard the womb spoken of as a space inside her, like a room she did not know she had, her menstruation appears like a troublesome tenant after whom she has to clean up…. Though feminists have argued that we should celebrate the menarche as a young woman's coming of age, with a visible rise in status to compensate her for the inconvenience of menstruation and ward off any attempt on her part to cancel the whole process by remaining a skinny child, nothing has happened to endow the cycle with glamour or respect. We call the napkins used to soak up menstrual discharge "sanitary protection" as if the blood was both dirty and dangerous. Sanitary protection may now be advertised on television, not because women's functions are no longer considered shameful or disgusting but because the potential earnings are enormous. High profit margins on napkins that women have no choice but to buy are used to subsidize marketing campaigns for luxury products.

Neither women nor men have a positive attitude to menstruation…. The questions of the exorbitant cost of napkins and tampons has been raised regularly by feminists; feminists were the first to point out the dangers of asbestos in tampons and of toxic shock syndrome…. If women regard their own menstrual fluid as "googoomuck" we are a long way from taking the pride in our femaleness that is a necessary condition of liberation. Hundreds of feminists have tried all kinds of strategies for filling the idea of menstruation with positive significance, but it remains a kind of excretion, the liquefaction of abjection. Advertising of sanitary protection can no more mention blood than advertising of toilet paper can mention shit. When we come to recognize the taste of our menstrual blood on the lips or fingers or penis of a lover, perhaps then we will realize that it is not putrid, not dangerous, not in the least disgusting. One of the latest explanations of the real function of the uniquely human process of menstruation holds that the shedding of the blood is not an excretion but protection of the sloughing womb from infection.

For 30 years feminists have struggled to develop a positive imagery of the womb and ovaries. Feminist artists have painted, modeled, woven, potted, photographed, filmed, videoed, and embroidered sumptuous images of the female genitalia to absolutely no purpose. As far as mainstream culture was concerned, cunt art was no more than a subbranch of gynecology. Though much of the most influential art of the 1990s was focused upon the body as the locus of gender and the modality of socialization, no girl drifted off to sleep at night and dreamed of her mysterious innards under any shape she could recognize. Though women artists devised myriad fabulous boxes, purses lined with satin or fur, and glimmering bottomless caves, ordinary women derived little comfort from a new awareness of themselves as buried treasure. It would take more than a trip through the vagina of sculptor Niki de St. Phalle's 90-foot-long female figure "Hon" to awaken the consciousness of the womb. More memorable perhaps were the artistic experiences of the womb dramatized as bruising encounters with obstetric technology.

Perhaps womb pride was too much to expect. The word "womb" originally meant any hollow space and by extension came to mean "belly" or "abdomen." The use of the word in modern times exclusively to signify the organ of gestation demonstrates our inability to think of the womb as anything but a passive receptacle, a pocket inside a person rather than the person herself. The ideal body is imperforate; the wombed body is grotesque and gaping, like Luna Park. Women's "inner space" implies a negative, an unsoundness, a hollowness, a harbor for otherness. But the term is misleading; there is no more a void inside a woman than there is inside a man. The unpregnant womb is not a space, but closed upon itself. The womb is not a sinus or a sac. The image of the uterus as a void waiting to be filled is an artifact derived from billions of lying diagrams that represent the fabulous baroque biochemistry of the womb as if it were the pocket of a billiard table. Women artists have done their best to counteract this by introducing fiber-optics into their own bodies, to show the quivering liveliness of the cervix's puppy-muzzle and the surging pulse of the fallopian tube amid its dancing fimbriae. Very few are watching, and for those who are there can be no shock of recognition. Consciousness is made of language, and we have no language for this. Cock and balls have a thousand names but uterus and ovaries have only their medical labels. (pp. 40–43)

To justify the dragooning and torturing of women the public health establishment uses the rhetoric of feminism. Screening for cervical cancer was hailed as a woman's right; the taxpayer willingly stumped up for it, convinced that if women just had this itty-bitty test every now and then they would stop dying of cervical cancer. But they didn't. Deaths from cervical cancer, which were already falling, continued to fall, at a rate of about 7 percent a year. Meanwhile the one in six tested women called for retesting suffered agonies of fear and bewilderment, as well as all kinds of surgical interventions from colposcopy to hysterectomy. Women were practiced on with an inefficient diagnostic tool because they were not the point; control was the point. The rest was oversold as an insurance against developing cervical and uterine cancer when it was no such thing. In case this sounds incredible, let me explain.

The current state of our understanding of cervical cancer is that it is in whole or in part a sexually transmitted disease, caused by the human papilloma virus (HVP), which causes genital warts and is carried by male and female.... Between 1960 and 1980 the incidence of cervical cancer in women under the age of thirty-five trebled and the number of deaths from the disease in this age group rose by 72 percent. In the nineties 15 percent of cases occur in this age group. The disease appears to progress slowly, taking about ten years to become manifest, but in general its career is not well understood.

The national cervical cancer screening program is based on the Papanicolaou smear, which has a false-negative rate estimated in 1979 as anywhere between 25 and 40 percent; where invasive cervical cancer is concerned, the rate may be as high as 50 percent. Abnormal Pap smears will also result from common infections. The remains of blood, or sperm, or contraceptive creams and jellies, vaginal douches, and deodorants in the vagina will affect the quality of the sample. Contraceptive pills and medications of other kinds can also distort the cell profile. If the test is not taken twelve to sixteen days after a period, and forty-eight hours or more after the last intercourse, its reliability may be compromised. As the supposedly premalignant changes in cell conformation are quite subtle, the job of evaluating cervical smears is both immensely boring and unremittingly stressful, even without the constant pressure for greater productivity. *The Wall Street Journal* reported in 1988 that a large proportion of U.S. smear tests were read in high-volume cut-rate laboratories where technicians were sometimes given financial incentives to up the number of slides they read in a day to as many as 300, four times the maximum recommended if the human error rate was to be kept to a minimum. Some laboratories paid screeners of a piecework basis, sometimes as little as 45 cents a slide....

The adoption of a simple positive-negative classification conceals seven categories, from minor and almost certainly insignificant changes in the cell structure to changes considered definitely precancerous to actual in situ carcinoma. The difficulty in assessing smears correctly is clearly illustrated by the wide variations in practice between one region and another.... In Britain 5.5. million women a year are given smear tests; an average of 7 in every 100 of their smears will be considered positive, giving a total of 385,000 smears. In fact no more than 4,500 women will develop cervical cancer in any year, so 380,500 will have been frightened needlessly.... In June 1995 an article in *The Lancet* reported that "staff live in fear of being blamed for failing to prevent invasive cases of cancer. The desire to avoid overdiagnosis, which in the past kept the detection rates low, has now been outweighed by the need to avoid any possibility of being held responsible for missing a case." The result is an epidemic of terror....

To be recalled for a second Pap smear is to catch the disease of fear. The test having been oversold in the first place, the woman is sure that there is something terribly wrong. After all, if it is true that atypical cells usually clear up spontaneously, what was the point of going through all the humiliating palaver of the test in the first place? The woman who is recalled may be given the all-clear after another sampling or two, but will she quite believe it? If she keeps being called back, every three months, or every month, she is very likely to make sure that she hasn't got cervical cancer by opting for and actively seeking a hysterectomy. A hysterectomy is a major operation with a long recovery period. The hysterectomized woman will need hormone replacement therapy and be "under the doctor" for a very long time, perhaps the rest of her life....

Every time the newspapers report that a health authority has had to recall-screen women because a second examination of their slides has led to different conclusions about their status, fear stalks the land. Public health consultant Dr. Angela Raffle dared to tell the truth, that cervical screening is "actually expensive, complicated, and relatively ineffective. Only about 50 percent of cases are picked up and there is huge and escalating overdetection and overtreatment." Raffle went on: "Screening has become something of a feminist icon and it is very hard to explain that cervical cancer was a rare and diminishing cause of death before we even began screening." Male-dominated governments are remarkably unaware of "feminist icons" and don't often, if ever, invest huge amounts of money in them. If the American government now spends $4.5 billion on Pap smears every year, it is not because they are being pushed around by a bunch of noisy feminists but because of the power and priorities of the medical establishment....

No pressure group within the medical profession is lobbying for the right to save men's lives by regularly examining the prostate. Occasionally we hear that clinicians regret men's unwillingness to be routinely poked and prodded and x-rayed, but the temptation to set up a screening service for men has so far been successfully resisted, on the same sorts of considerations that should have prevented the setting up of women's screening programs. There is a strong impression that men are no more likely to submit their testicles to official care and attention than they are to wear their muffler when it is cold and keep their feet dry. The service exists for them to avail themselves of if they want to, and that is deemed to be sufficient. Men have the right to take care of themselves or not, as they see fit, but women are to be taken care of whether they like it or not. Screening is many times more likely to destroy a woman's peace of mind than it is to save her life. Women are driven through the health system like sheep through a dip. The disease they are being treated for is womanhood. (pp. 117–123)

You and I need all the mothers we can get. Governments rely for the funds that run our societies on tax on current earnings; the people now in work pay for the care and support of the people who are not in work. As the work force shrinks and life expectancy increases it becomes harder and harder to pay the social security bill. We all need the children being born now and we need them to grow up as well-educated, useful people, not circling aimlessly round the poverty trap. In *The Female Eunuch* I argued that motherhood should not be treated as a substitute career; now I would argue that motherhood should be regarded as a genuine career option, that is to say, as paid work and as such an alternative to other paid work. What this would mean is that every woman who decides to have a child would be paid enough money to raise that child in decent circumstances. The choice, whether to continue in her employment outside the home and use the money to pay for professional help in raising her child, or stay at home and devote her time to doing it herself, should be hers. By investing in motherhood we would inject more money into child care, which is the only way to improve a system that at present relies on the contribution of disenfranchised, low-paid, unresourced, and unqualified women. The sooner we decide that mothers are entitled to state support to use as they wish, the less it will cost us in the long run. We will be told on all sides that we can't afford it. If we weren't paying to send aircraft carriers to the Gulf and any other place Bill Clinton thinks a saber should be rattled, we could afford it. It is a question of priorities. Dignified motherhood is a feminist priority. A permanent seat on the UN Security Council is not. (pp. 215–217)

In *The Female Eunuch* I argued that feminism would have to address the problem of male violence both spontaneous and institutionalized, but I could suggest no way of doing this beyond refusing to act as the warrior's reward. Even then radical women were demanding the right to aggression as a basic human right and women's groups were training in self-defense and martial arts. The assumption seemed to be that all human beings were violent unless they were deprived of the right to aggression by an oppressor. Freedom had to include the right to beat your enemies up. The outcome of a free-for-all seemed to me obvious: if violence is a right the strongest and the cruelest will always tyrannize over the gentle and the loving-kind. Only those women who were strong and cruel enough could join in the butchery. The rest would be butchered.

That was not an outcome that I could tolerate, so I argued feebly that women should devalue violence by refusing to be attracted to it or to reward the victors…. In the years that followed aggression was carefully studied and we began to understand rather more about it. The role of women in fomenting male aggression is, I now believe, marginal, even irrelevant…. Our culture now depicts much more elaborate violence in more media more often than it did 30 years ago. Regardless of official ideologies our culture is therefore, by my judgment, less feminist than it was 30 years ago. Brutality, like other forms of pornography, damages everyone exposed to it. Violence disenfranchises all weaklings, including children, old people—and women.

Children, old people, and women are all short of testosterone. Even 10 years ago, testosterone was a word not often heard; nowadays the presence of testosterone in the environment is often remarked on. When the stands at the football ground are packed with vociferating fans it is described as a testosterone storm. When a driver kills another driver who cut him up at a corner, he does it in a "blind testosterone rage."... By invoking testosterone a man can abdicate responsibility for his own behavior.

Testosterone does seem to be powerful. Women who have been dosed with pharmaceutical testosterone as part of hormone replacement therapy report distinct and unnerving changes in personality, which are, as one might expect, increased tension and irritability, and clitoral sensitivity raised to the point of discomfort. When women began to complain of personality changes as well as irreversible changes in voice and distribution of body hair, HRT preparations containing testosterone were deleted. it would seem that testosterone is the hormone of dominance; a survey from Mount Sinai School of Medicine in New York found that, the higher up the career ladder women had risen, the higher their testosterone levels....

Violent sex offenders have been found, again not consistently, to have the highest testosterone levels of all. The effect of alcohol and drugs is variable; habitual use suppresses testosterone but occasional use can stimulate secretion, possibly as a feedback effect of disinhibition. This raises a further possibility that violent men are not violent because they have more testosterone to cope with, but that they have more testosterone because they are more violent....

Taking courage, then, from the notion of biology as alterable, we can entertain the possibility that ours is a culture in which elevated testosterone levels are sought, prized, and rewarded, no matter how destructive the consequence.... Testosterone converts fear into hostility; fear stimulates secretions of testosterone along with other body chemicals associated with aggression, and off float the pheromones into the surrounding air. Could it be that we enjoy being scared and angry more than we enjoy serenity?...

Pluggers of the "future is female" line like to tell us that women's management skills are different, because women are nonconfrontational and more interested in compromise and settlement than in imposing their will. If aggression is fun and if the biochemistry of aggression can be stimulated by cultural demand, we cannot rule out the possibility that women will gradually become as dangerous to themselves and others as men are. If the nonviolent woman is simply a subservient creature, too repressed to acknowledge her own murderous propensities, war will continue to be the human condition. War will not be rendered obsolete unless feminism and pacifism agree to persist in their historical cohabitation and build a culture of nonviolence. (pp. 161–171)

The propaganda machine that is now aimed at our daughters is more powerful than any form of indoctrination that has ever existed before. Pop is followed by print is followed by video and film, and nothing that a parent generation can do will have any effect other than to increase the desirability of the girlpower way of life. Nobody observing the incitement of little girls to initiate sexual contact with boys can remain unconcerned. Regardless of the dutiful pushing of condoms in the girls' press, the exposure of baby vaginas and cervixes to the penis is more likely to result in pregnancy and infection than orgasm. We know that some of today's young women regard oral sex as little more than a courtesy routinely offered by cool girls to demanding boys, the girls themselves having no expectation that any man would ever do as much for them. The girls' press does not question this iniquity; rather it reinforces the idea that boys are nabobs who can get any kind of sex anywhere and mostly cannot be bothered. To deny a woman's sexuality is certainly to oppress her but to portray her as nothing but a sexual being is equally to oppress her. No one doubts that teenage boys have peremptory sexual urges, but they are never depicted as prepared to accept any humiliation, endure any indignity, just to get close to some, any, girl. Nor are they pushed to spend money on their appearance or to dress revealingly or drink too much in order to attract the attention of the opposite sex. In every color spread the British girls' press trumpets the triumph of misogyny and the hopelessness of the cause of female pride. (pp. 331–332)

The trouble is not that "Sisterhood is powerful," as the title of Robin Morgan's book has it, but that it isn't. Sisterhood does not rule and will never rule, OK? The principle of sisterhood is power-sharing, which is another name for powerlessness. In a society constructed of self-perpetuating elites a grassroots movement exists to be walked on. Elites tumble down but the grass survives to spring again through the thickest pavement. All studies of gender difference agree on one thing, that females are less variable than males. If men and women were poppies, both the tallest and shortest poppies would be men. The women would cluster around the median, the norm. If we look at intelligence or mathematical ability we can see the same phenomenon. Men are, as it were, built for competition, already separated out into winners and losers, while women are built to understand each other, to co-operate, to pull shoulder to shoulder. Indeed, we could see the historic pattern of binding a woman to a man and forcibly separating her from her female peers as a precaution against the development of a female tendency to agglomerate. Men are afraid of women in groups.

One of the advances in the last 30 years has been that women's friendship is now a serious topic, and an entrenched value in women's lives. Girls' magazines treat the vicissitudes of friendship with more seriousness than the endless flummery about boys. Women's "being there for each other" features in soap operas. Women students consider themselves bound to accept each other's word without question, flying in the face of the prejudice that women are incapable of loyalty or trust. Only when sisterhood is real can sisterhood become powerful. We are on the way. (p. 243)

Breakthrough Against Female Genital Mutilation

NOY THRUPKAEW

Noy Thrupkaew, "Senegalese Women Win Ban on Female Genital Cutting," *Sojourner,* March 1999. Reprinted by permission.

In response to a nationwide campaign led by a Senegalese women's group, the Parliament of Senegal banned female circumcision/female genital mutilation (FC/FGM) on January 15. Senegal joins Burkina Faso, Central African Republic, Djibouti, Ghana, Guinea, Togo, and Egypt in their ban on FC/FGM. The success of the Senegalese women's campaign, a grassroots community-based effort, marks a turning point in increasingly global efforts to eradicate FC/FGM. Tactics previously used in attempts to abolished the practice have ranged from government-led top-down legislation to Western imposition—methods that have not been as effective in promoting widespread change. Increased international pressure to ban female genital cutting—in part due to high-profile cases of women seeking political asylum to escape FC/FGM—has also contributed to recent bans on the practice.

The punishment for anyone "having violated or attempting to violate the physical integrity of the genital organs of a person of the female sex" is six months to five years of imprisonment, according to Article 299 bis of Senegalese law. The amendment covers all forms of FC/FGM, and men or women who provoke or demand that FC/FGM be performed are sentenced to the same punishment as those who cut young women's genitalia. The maximum penalty is applied to members of the medical or paramedical fields who condone of perform the practice. If a woman dies from her FC/FGM injuries, those found guilty of her death are sentenced to forced labor for life.

While the terms "female circumcision" and "female genital mutilation" are sometimes used interchangeably, each has distinct and powerful political connotations. "Some African people think that the term FGM attacks their culture and tradition, but by labeling it "female circumcision," you are making it sound equal in severity to male circumcision... you are making it more acceptable," said Rana Badri of Equality Now, a New York–based group that advocates for women's human rights domestically and internationally. Badri, who is the FGM Eradication Campaign director of Equality Now, which publishes an FGM-awareness publication entitled *Awaken,* added that "the term 'Female Genital Mutilation' brings out the ugliness and the severe damage that the practice does to women." The World Health Organization (WHO) calls the practice "FGM" as well.

Seble W. Argaw, women's human rights activist and member of the Boston-based Ethiopian Adbar Women's Alliance, noted, however, that practitioners of female genital cutting who see "FGM" as a foreign label, "can think to themselves—'I don't do that'—and then they dismiss the whole idea." By speaking about FGM in terms of its traditional cultural name female circumcision, Argaw seeks to encourage its eradication through "education and persuasion."

Though performed primarily by the Muslim populations in the Middle East and Africa, FC/FGM knows no boundaries of religion or class. In Mali, for example, where an estimated 93 percent of the female population has undergone FC/FGM, 85 percent of the female Christian population has also had FC/FGM performed on them. WHO estimates that 130 million women have been subjected to FC/FGM and each year, 2 million young women, girls, and infants undergo the ritual of genital cutting. While Egypt, Ethiopia, Kenya, Nigeria, Somalia, and the Sudan account for approximately 75 percent of FC/FGM cases, FC/FGM is also performed in Indonesia, Malaysia, Pakistan, and India. Genital cutting practices range in severity. In Senegal, practitioners generally remove the clitoris and part of the external and internal genital folds, and some may also loosely stitch the parts of the wound together.

GRASSROOTS GROUP TOSTAN BREAKS NEW GROUND

The Senegalese women's group Tostan is remarkable not only for its success in convincing the Senegalese government to pass legislation banning FC/FGM but also—more importantly—for mobilizing widespread community support for the ban. Based in the village of Malicounda Bambara, Tostan—which means "breakthrough" in Wolof, the native language of Senegal—did not originally focus on FC/FGM issues. Begun by Molly Melching, a U.S. citizen who had lived in Senedgal for over 20 years, and supported by UNICEF, the government of Senegal, and the American Jewish World Service, the group initially worked on literacy, women's health, and human rights. After discussions about how to improve prenatal health, women in the group became aware that many Senegalese women's health problems were a direct result of their past FC/FGM.

The women of Tostan then embarked on a villagewide campaign to persuade husbands, village elders, and religious leaders to commit themselves to abolishing the practice. By enlisting men in their cause, the women gave their message more weight and legitimacy within traditional village social structures. As Ethiopian Adbar Women's Alliance member Argaw notes, "You have to visualize the whole pattern, how it works. The men are thought of as the defenders of the nation, the breadwinners. The women are not in the same position as in the West." To bring about change in this society, "you must convince the men, the village elders."

As a result of Tostan's successful organizing, no FC/FGM took place in Malicounda in 1997. Tostan members spoke to a group of 20 Senegalese journalists, and the press coverage led to the first national discussion on FC/FGM. Bolstered by the support of Senegalese President Abdou Diouf, the campaign quickly spread to other villages in Senegal. The women of Nigeria Bambara followed the lead of the Malicounda Bambara women and renounced the practice of FC/FGM within their village.

Male and/or religious spokesmen came to the forefront of the anti-FGM movement when the village of Ker Simbara decided to consult the members of their extended family over a communal decision to ban FC/FGM. Two Bambara men, Cheikh Traore (a Tostan facilitator) and Demba Diaware (an imam or religious leader and former Tostan participant) traveled to the outlying regions where the Der Simbara kin live, and discussed FC/FGM with the villagers. The outlying villages then formulated the Diabougou Declaration, abolishing the practice of FC/FGM and leading a total of 8,000 villagers into the forefront of the FC/FGM eradication movement.

Thirteen members of the Tostan program spoke about their experiences with FC/FGM before deputies of the Senegalese parliament of January 12, 1999, the first time a group of villagers has testified before the National Assembly. They strongly urged the Assembly to pass the law, but recommended that the legislation be tempered with measures that allow for FC/FGM education programs to ease the transition. Most of the members of the assembly supported the eradication of FC/FGM, but based on the testimony of villages of the Diabougou Declaration, attempted to request a delay for the enforcement of the law. Many members were concerned that repressive measures would cause a flurry of FC/FGM activity nationwide, a fear backed up by the actions of at least one village. At the end of December 1998, 120 girls in the Kedougou village were cut by one person, wielding one knife, perhaps in anticipation of the ban. The National Assembly is still conferring over the best way to implement and enforce the law.

NEW MODELS, OLD PROBLEMS

Many activists say that Tostan provides a critical new model for fighting FC/FGM. By beginning with a broad examination of the totality of women's lives, Tostan opened up a forum for women to discover for themselves the far-reaching effects of their past FC/FGM. Argaw commented that native women's leadership in such campaigns was essential, adding, "A grassroots approach is very important." After Senegal's ban was announced, Carol Bellamy, executive director of UNICEF, also commented on the grassroots, women-led campaign. She told The *New York Times* that, "The work of African grassroots organizations seems increasingly to demonstrate that most women would not accept female genital mutilation as a part of tradition if they had the power to change their fate."

Badri noted that the Tostan campaign differs from earlier FC/FGM eradication efforts that tended to focus on ideological opposition to genital cutting. She said that Tostan has shown that "the only way to stop the practice is to raise awareness of the [health] side effects. There is a shift in approach and strategy."

Both Argaw and Badri stressed that organizing against FC/FGM is complicated because the practice is viewed in countries that practice it as a sacred religious ritual or age-old cultural tradition. Reluctant to abandon the practice in the face of increasing Westernization, male and female practitioners defend the tradition as part of their culture. The context behind FC/FGM is further complicated by political and ethnic divisions. Some ethnic groups practice it, and others have no history of the tradition. As so many regions of Africa depend on a delicate balance between such groups, potentially divisive issues such as FC/FGM do not enter public debate.

Western anti-FC/FGM movements are often perceived as heavyhanded colonialist interference. According to Badri, "Some efforts were unsuccessful because they attempted to impose drastic changes upon the natives." Argaw concurred, stating, "Sometimes people feel defensive, like Westerners are looking down or putting down their culture. Some people feel that Westerners also do strange things—breast implants, plastic surgery. They feel it's an assault on the culture. So there's a conflict within the immigrant community here too." Immigrants in the United States who turn against FC/FGM practice are often viewed as "agents of Westernization," who have betrayed their native culture.

Some human rights groups have proposed that Western governments link foreign aid negotiations with abolishment of FC/FGM, but this approach seems counterproductive and ultimately unjust to many grassroots activists. Similarly, repressive, top-down government measures often result in frantic outbursts of FC/FGM activity. The governments of Egypt and Sudan placed bans of FC/FGM but did not meet with much success. In contrast to the current situation in Senegal, the anti-FC/FGM movement in Egypt and the Sudan had not gained sufficient popular momentum before the bans were implemented, "and huge numbers of young girls are still initiated into the painful reality of living with FC/FGM in these countries."

INCREASING WESTERN AWARENESS OF FC/FGM

While much work remains to be done to improve working relations between Westerners and native FC/FGM eradication activists, increased Western awareness has aided the movement greatly. The efforts of grassroots organizations and the increase in Western scrutiny have created an environment that encourages governments to address FC/FGM through education and legislation.

U.S. awareness of FC/FGM issues has grown as immigrants from practicing countries arrived in the United States in increasing numbers. As doctors and other health care providers began to encounter women whose genitals had been cut, "a need emerged to develop policies to address the most appropriate way to respond to the needs of circumcised women," Badri explained. Unaware of the cultural differences between the United States and their respective homelands, "immigrants would go to the hospitals to have their girls circumcised," she said.

Western media coverage of FC/FGM has also intensified in the past 10 years. In 1992, prominent author Alice Walker wrote a fiction book on FC/FGM, entitled *Possessing the Secret of Joy*, and followed that book with a nonfiction account of research into FC/FGM. Of these books, Badri remarked, "They help raise the awareness of the American community, draw attention to circumcised women's needs, help mobilize activities." Argaw expressed another opinion, stating that the books are "good and bad, in a sense. Good because it publicizes FGM, so more people will be aware. On the other hand, it might create a backlash against perceived Westernization. People say it didn't come from the inside. But it's definitely a start."

The case of Fauziya Kassindja also brought FC/FGM practices into the international spotlight. In December of 1994, Kassindja fled to the United States from Togo after learning that her husband-to-be had demanded that she undergo FC/FGM as a prerequisite to marriage. She was imprisoned after U.S. immigration judge Donald V. Ferlise dismissed her case, stating that her story lacked "rationality and internal consistency." She was subsequently placed in the Esmor Detention Center in Elizabeth, New Jersey—shackled and in an isolation cell.

After a cousin enlisted the aid of law student Layli Miller Bashir, Kassindja's case began to gain momentum. Equality Now began a letter-writing campaign to the U.S. Justice Department, and Karen Musal, law professor and acting head of American University's International Human Rights Clinic, handled Kassindja's appeal. On April 5, 1996, the Justice Department filed a 36-page brief supporting her continued incarceration. But The *New York Times* ran an article on her case on April 15, 1996, and she was freed 9 days later. In June 1996, the Board of Immigration Appeals, the highest administrative tribunal in the U.S. immigration system, overturned Ferlise's ruling and granted Kassindja asylum.

Delacorte Press signed Kassindja to a book contract—*Do They Hear You When You Cry?*—which focused on both Kassindja's experiences with FC/FGM and her incarceration in the United States.

FUTURE CAMPAIGNS: HOLISTIC APPROACHES TO HUMAN RIGHTS

Argaw advocates a holistic approach toward organizing against genital cutting based around the internal energy of grassroots initiatives run by native women. Badri agrees, adding that for all determination and vision that these women's groups exhibit, they still need the support of women worldwide. Badri declared, "People should recognize that FC/FGM is a violation of women's reproductive rights." Bellamy of UNICEF also commented, "Women around the world who have the courage to take a stand on female genital mutilation need sustained international support in order to convince their societies to move away from this horrendous practice."

As for how Western feminists can be most helpful, Argaw urged greater involvement in "the big picture of human rights and conditions," saying that only after people "have enough to survive, food on the table," can they begin to talk about FC/FGM. She said, "Western women should work with the grassroots organizations on broad issues like nutrition, motherhood, opening hospital branches." Africans often become defensive about the Western attention to FGM, thinking that "all the American women talk about circumcision when so many other issues are not addressed as a whole. This is not the only thing that happens to women." She added, "It's part of the whole picture of oppression."

THE HISTORY AND PRACTICE OF FC/FGM

The practice of FC/FGM ranges in severity from region to region. As classified by the World Health Organization (WHO), type 1 refers to genital cutting where only the prepuce (skin of the clitoris), and/or parts of the clitoris are removed. Type 2 FC/FGM involves the excision of the clitoris with partial or total excision of the labia minora. Type 3, infibulation, accounts for approximately 15 percent of FC/FGM. Infibulation encompasses the excision of part or all of the external genitalia. The incision is then stitched together, leaving a matchstick-sized opening for urine and menstrual blood to pass out of the body. Most often, countries in the Horn of Africa—Djibouti, Somalia, the Sudan, and parts of Ethiopia—practice infibulation. Type 4 involves a whole host of genital mutilation, ranging from the piercing or burning of the clitoris, scraping or cutting of the vagina, or the insertion of corrosive substances or herbs into the vagina to cause bleeding or to narrow or tighten it.

In all of its forms, FC/FGM affects normal bodily functions, often causing difficult childbirth, hemorrhaging, infection, and sometimes death. Often performed under unsanitary conditions with crude, unsterilized tools such as old razor blades, FC/FGM also severely limits sexual sensation, and subjects women to a host of other long-term physical and mental health complications. Traditional practitioners, usually elderly women who have inherited their role... from their families, often lack medical training and do not have the resources to effectively address medical complications that can arise from FC/FGM. Wealthier families can turn to health care professionals, who can—in many ways—do even greater damage by "medicalizing" and legitimizing the practice of FC/FGM.

The practice of FC/FGM is deeply embedded within cultural traditions. Many practitioners believe that Islam mandates FC/FGM, while others believe in the sanctity of cultural traditions and the rule of their forefathers' way of life. As the WHO FC/FGM Web site notes, "Some Muslim communities... practice FGM in the genuine belief that it is demanded by the Islamic faith." As they also note, however, "the practice predates Islam." In a ruling upholding a ban of FC/FGM, the Egyptian Supreme Court recently ruled that FC/FGM had no place in the Islamic religion.

Often performed as part of a woman's coming-of-age ceremony, or prior to her marriage, FC/FGM is traditionally thought to signal a woman's arrival as a full, mature member of her community. But as the age of the FC/FGM inductees drops every year, WHO argues that FC/FGM's connection to coming-of-age rituals is growing more tenuous. In much of Ethiopia, for example, FC/FGM is performed "very early in childhood, perhaps 40 days after birth," according to Seble W. Argaw of the Ethiopian Adbar Women's Alliance. "It's done so early, you wouldn't know you had it. You don't know if your future sickness comes from that or not."

Issues of control of women's sexuality are also deeply intertwined with the tradition of FC/FGM. Rana Badri, director of the FGM Eradication Campaign of Equality Now, told *Sojourner,* "the reason why people practice this is to curb women's sexual behavior." The WHO FGM home page also states that FC/FGM is thought to "maintain chastity and virginity before marriage and fidelity during marriage, and increase male sexual pleasure." Some men say the artificial tightness of infibulation enhances their pleasure. Others find the smooth scar aesthetically pleasing. But the scar ultimately serves as a chastity belt of a women's own flesh, deadening her sexual pleasure, or even causing severe pain during intercourse.

Badri continued, "Some people think a woman's clitoris has a poisonous discharge, so by removing it, they are protecting her husband and child." An uncut woman is often perceived as unclean, or oversexed, selfishly seeking out her sexual pleasure despite the shame it would bring upon her husband or male relatives. Traditional practitioners of FC/FGM argue that it serves as a manmade safeguard against the social disorder that women's infidelity or sexual promiscuity can cause. In this way, FC/FGM is thought to maintain "social integration and the maintenance of social cohesion," according to WHO.

Intact women are often mocked and ostracized, and their fathers may be forbidden from speaking at village meetings. Men's power and status seem inversely linked to women's sexual freedom—the men gain more respect when the women's power or sexuality is curtailed, or brought in line with social norms. In this way, FC/FGM becomes a powerful indicator of men's status as well. They are rendered socially and politically impotent if their female relatives remain intact. Men often, therefore, put pressure on the women around them to submit to FC/FGM in order to regain or increase their political power.

As for its part in the commodification of women, FC/FGM serves as a status marker of a woman's marriage and social standing and a physical indicator of her future economic well-being. According to WHO, some practitioners believe FC/FGM enhances fertility and promotes child survival—without this ritual, a woman can lose valuable status because she may be perceived as potentially sterile. Because many men perceive intact women as damaged, or flawed, it becomes difficult for these women to marry and gain economic stability. Their families often cannot afford to support them, and the women are left with no choice but to undergo FC/FGM. During the ritual, a young woman's sexual status is also established—if the woman is a virgin, she can earn a larger dowry and her family is honored. According to folklore, nonvirgins bleed profusely during the cutting, while virgins do not. After the ritual cutting, the young woman is feted by hundreds of family members who feast and celebrate for days, and many young girls look forward to the day they will be so honored.

The Viagra Chronicles

SUSAN C. VAUGHAN

Susan C. Vaughan, *Bazaar*, September, 1998. Reprinted by permission.

I was curious," explains Katie, a physician in her mid-thirties who gave Viagra a go just one month after the FDA approved the drug for male impotence. "There's nothing wrong with my sex life, but it's only natural to wonder whether it could be even better." Katie wrote herself a prescription for a 25-milligram, a 50-milligram, and a 100-milligram pill. The results? "At 25, I felt nothing. At 100, I was nauseous, and everything I looked at had a filmy, blue visual effect that made the world look like an old movie. But at 50," Katie says, with a smug smile reminiscent of Goldilocks upon discovering the bear chair that was just right, "at 50 it was great. I was definitely more aroused, and I had lots of orgasms with much less stimulation than usual, and it's unusual for me to have more than one." Would she take it again? "Definitely," she says, "but only on special occasions. It reminds me of trying a recreational drug and liking it a little too much. You have to be careful, or you'll get hooked."

Since Viagra's arrival on the market six months ago, more than 200,000 prescriptions have been written weekly, making it the most prescribed new drug in history. It's clear that many members of the male half of America are already hooked, and it seems likely that the female half won't be far behind. Although the drug hasn't been approved for women, curiosity—as in Katie's case—is leading them into their partner's stash to sample it in hopes of better, quicker, or even multiple orgasms. Even Elizabeth Dole confessed, giggling, "It's a great drug," after husband Bob revealed he had used it in clinical trials.

Carolyn, a 42-year-old nurse who works for a urologist, is no different. "The guys had been getting Viagra for over a month," she says, "and I wanted to know what it was like." She also had a problem she hoped Viagra could help her with: "I don't like to have sex when I have PMS; I'm just not as interested as

I'd like to be." So the next time PMS hit, Carolyn took a 50-milligram pill from the samples that a drug rep had left at the office where she works. "I started to feel this vaginal tingling and got really turned on while my boyfriend and I were watching a movie," she says. "We made love, and it was great." It was so good, in fact, that Carolyn decided to take Viagra again, this time when she wasn't PMSing. But on her second and third tries, the results weren't as good. "It didn't do much, though clearly I had more blood flow," she says. "It was almost like my clitoris was too sensitive, and I couldn't come.

Just as Carolyn's interest stemmed from observing the positive reactions of male patients, other women seem to have become interested after their husbands have taken the drug. As a psychiatrist, I see plenty of women in this situation. Consider the story of a patient of mine in her mid-sixties, whom I'll call Vicky. She requested that I give her a small number of pills of her own after her husband's internist prescribed Viagra for his erectile dysfunction resulting from diabetes. "I want to be able to keep up in bed," she said. "There are some things that I could never do, like have an orgasm during intercourse. It always seemed like it was all over just as I was getting started. Our sex life has slowly dwindled. I'm not sure how I feel about rekindling it, but I do know that if Bob is going to take Viagra himself, I want to be ready. I don't want him running off with some sweet young thing—not that he would." Vicky laughed, but the tension in the room was palpable, particularly since the first Viagra lawsuit has been filed by a woman against her spouse, who took the drug and had an affair four days later.

Vicky's complaint that she'd always had trouble having orgasms during intercourse is common. Although the clitoris is the only organ in the human body devoted purely to pleasure, it is not well-positioned anatomically to be stimulated during intercourse. As the female comedian Reno puts it, "By the time penis-vagina sex really gets going, the clitoris is out in the backyard, banging on the door—'Hey, can I get back in there? I was your most valuable player just three minutes ago and now you're treating me like a pesky little sister.'" And even when the clitoris is stimulated during intercourse, women take three times longer on average to reach orgasm than men do. So a man needn't be a premature ejaculator to finish too quickly for his female partner's enjoyment. If Viagra increases clitoral sensitivity and heightens excitement, women may need less direct clitoral contact and may reach orgasm in a shorter amount of time, making men's and women's sexual responses better suited to each other. And because men who take Viagra often sustain their erections after they ejaculate, women may find that even if they don't take Viagra, partners who do can continue intercourse longer, ensuring their pleasure as well.

"It makes sense that Viagra would work in women too," says Jennifer Berman, a urologist at the University of Maryland. Berman believes that since Viagra can result in increased blood flow to the male sexual organs, it can also trigger orgasm in women by increasing blood flow to the clitoris, which is composed of the same dense clusters of nerve endings and erectile tissue as the penis. And because Viagra also prolongs and boosts smooth-muscle relaxation within the pelvic blood vessels, it can trigger a heightened degree of arousal in response to the same amount of stimulation. In men this translates into a firmer, harder erection that lasts longer. In women, it may mean greater sensitivity to stimulation—perhaps putting them closer to climax—and more vaginal lubrication than usual, setting the stage for more comfortable sex.

The results of early pilot studies by Berman have been promising: Ten women who suffered sexual dysfunction following hysterectomies all reported substantial improvement, with some who were completely unable to achieve orgasm preoperatively finding that Viagra enabled them to have orgasms during intercourse. Berman has also recently received a grant from the American Foundation for Urological Diseases for a study of Viagra that will include postmenopausal women, the group she expects to be most helped by the drug, since a plummeting estrogen level after menopause results in decreased vaginal lubrication. Pfizer, the drug's manufacturer, has also begun trials in postmenopausal women in England and will soon study Viagra in older American women.

Urologist Stanley Bloom is impressed by the prospects of Viagra for sexual dysfunction in women, but he cautions that its safely and efficacy in women have not yet been established. He's decided to wait until more systematic work has been done before prescribing Viagra to his female patients. "I'd expect most side effects in women to be like those in men—flushing of the skin, stomach upset and headaches," Bloom says. "Women of childbearing age should probably avoid the drug completely, since Viagra's effects on fetal development are not yet known."

Jessica, a professional woman in her late forties found out about side effects the hard way. She received a 50-milligram Viagra pill as a gag gift for her birthday from a friend who had cajoled it out of her boyfriend, and took it without telling her husband. "I turned red as a beet and had such a severe headache that I felt like my head would explode," she says. "I finally confessed to my husband so that he'd know what was wrong with me if I fainted. It was scary. And I was just too sick to have sex." Jessica's decision to try Viagra was due partly to curiosity and partly to a sense that she was having a more difficult time reaching orgasm than she did when she was younger. "It's a mixture of things—perhaps the effect of my diet, a lack of exercise, or just thinking about which kid has which after-school activity when I should be focused on sex. And, frankly, my decreased arousal might have something to do with the thrill of sex having worn off after all these years of marriage."

Although Jessica's physiological response to Viagra made her reluctant to try it again, her test-drive still had unexpected benefits. "I think it turned Roger on to realize that I wanted to be more excited in bed. It got us talking and made us realize that if we wanted our sex life to improve, we'd have to work on it, set aside time for it. Viagra's a little like a diet pill. You want it to be the magic bullet, but it isn't. But if taking the pill and thinking about the problem gets you to the gym, then maybe it has worked after all."

As we await the results of studies already under way, some physicians are starting to judiciously prescribe Viagra to their female patients who have sexual dysfunction. But often pharmacies refuse to fill a Viagra prescription written out to a woman, and insurance companies—who are scrambling to decide on monthly limits for men—won't cover it. Clearly, it's going to take time for people to take female potency problems seriously. Already, Viagra seems to be surpassing Lassie as man's best friend. But maybe, like Elizabeth Dole, other women will soon find that these little blue diamonds are a girl's best friend.

VENUS & VIAGRA

Safe for women? Scientists don't yet know the possible long-term effects on women, but they're worried Viagra may affect fertility. Some female studies are being conducted now, but FDA approval for women may take up to two years.

THE MARKET: Up to 60 percent of women experience sexual problems, including difficulty reaching orgasm—a result of such things as stress, anxiety about sex, use of antidepressants, hysterectomy, and diabetes.

GETTING AN RX: Doctors can prescribe the drug for women for "off label" or unapproved use (common in the medical field), as long as patients are informed that Viagra isn't FDA-backed.

OUT-OF-POCKET EXPENSE: At $10 a pill, a woman could spend as much as $1040 a year for just two nights of sex per week.

BETTER SEX: Increased clitoral blood flow and vaginal lubrication can occur less than an hour after taking the drug, translating into quicker orgasms. The effect can last up to four hours.

I'VE GOT A HEADACHE: Side effects of Viagra include headaches, flushing, upset stomach, diarrhea, dizziness, and blue-tinted vision.

Still Taking
Our Bodies Back

Y ou are an activist, says Byllye Avery, if you are "not afraid to speak out, stand up, and challenge the status quo."

When women get in trouble, society plays blame-the-victim. Did her husband beat her up? She provoked him. Did the mammogram bruise her? Her breasts are too big. Did she lose her sex drive on the Pill? It's not the chemicals in the Pill—she's a perverse woman who can't enjoy sex unless she fears pregnancy. Activists try to maintain constant vigilance against such slurs.

The other side of blame-the-victim is credit-the-technology (for the good stuff), which we are often manipulated to do. But, as Alessandra Liberati wrote in the British Medical Journal, August 31, 1997:

"The quality and relevance of much clinical research fall short of patient needs. Although there are many reasons for this, one is that clinical research has been delegated largely to the pharmaceutical industry, whose main motivation is its own economic welfare. Another reason is that research priorities do not flow from a transparent process where the views of all the relevant stakeholders are equally considered."

This is changing. Since the establishment in 1991 of the National Breast Cancer Coalition (NBCC), a grassroots organization formed to end the epidemic through action and advocacy, survivors have demanded a say in research policies and funding. NBCC's science training program, Project LEAD, empowers activists to resist intimidation by professionals, so they can fully participate in the design and execution of clinical trials. Alessandra Liberati predicts that in time the patients will be "equal partners with health professionals, scientists, and policy-makers in preventing the disease, improving treatment, and ensuring better quality of care. Without such a partnership—difficult though it may be—research is unlikely to become more productive or relevant." The National Academy of Sciences/Institute of Medicine in Washington, D.C., endorses this view in a new report.

Obviously the potential for the impact of consumer/patient representatives on medical research is revolutionary. Other areas of notable progress in the 1990s include:

➤ the more sensitive treatment of domestic violence victims, as well as women who are sexually harassed in the workplace or at school, or by authority figures such as doctors and divorce lawyers;
➤ the development of gender medicine research;
➤ greater attention to lesbian and minority health; and
➤ efforts to bring possible conflicts of interest to the attention of the public. For example, some medical journals require contributors to include full disclosure of their funding sources when they publish their research.

Too little effort has gone into relieving the exhaustion of working mothers. This is so widespread that some activists view it as the number one health crisis affecting women today. New York Congresswoman Carolyn Maloney has developed innovative legislation that could bring some relief. Ask her about it, and ask your representatives to support it if you agree.

Most activists find the life rewarding (but not financially) and are prone to exceptional longevity as well. Elizabeth Cady Stanton and most of her colleagues survived into their eighties. Physical exercise helps life extension, but so does getting exorcised (as in incensed). Almost everyone I know who is really old and really interesting finds something she objects to in her morning paper.

Activists cannot be counted on to judge our own progress. An example is the despairing note I sounded in my speech on pelvic autonomy at the 1975 conference on women and health at Harvard Medical School:

"The individuals who determine health care policies are not responsive to the demands of feminists.... In 1974, out of 3,750 obstetrics-gynecology residents, only 96 were women. While the ratio of women in the field is about 1 in 17, the ratio of women entering the field has declined to about 1 in 40."

What I didn't know was that Title IX would soon kick in, and how much the bar of girls' ambitions was being raised by feminism. In 1999-2000, as the millennium turns, female obstetrics-gynecology residents number 3,181, while males number only 1,522.—B. S.

Chapter 66

Breast Cancer Activism

I n the 1990s, when health insurance as we knew it crashed, many individuals and families were unexpectedly dismissed from the care of doctors they had counted on and trusted. Dismay and even panic followed, but soon a plus side began to manifest. Word spread, especially among women, that alternative remedies were more available and cheaper than biomedicine, had fewer side effects, and often seemed to work.

Breast cancer activists were among those who quickly took up the study of complementary and alternative medicine (CAM). They were meeting together in support groups, swapping information, and many were all too knowledgeable about the drawbacks of their regular "biomedical" remedies. By 1997 the Journal of the American Medical Association (JAMA) learned in a survey that since 1990 there'd been a 380 percent increase in the consumer use of herbal remedies, as well as a 130 percent increase in the use of high-dose vitamins. In a speech at a medical school graduation, Harold Varmus, the director of the National Institutes of Health, declared that his top priority for "health improvement" was to "eliminate the divide between alternative and conventional medicine." Trying to play catch-up, in November 1998, JAMA and its nine associated specialty journals published 80 articles about CAM.

A majority of women in the United States are now using some alternative remedies. Breast cancer patients have their favorites, such as Essiac, but they do not always confide this to their regular physicians.—B. S.

Stolen Conflicts: A Feminist Revisioning

SHARON BATT

Adapted from Sharon Batt, *Patient No More: The Politics of Breast Cancer*, Charlottetown, Canada, Gynergy Books/Ragweed Press, 1994.

When I was undergoing treatment for cancer, I often felt disconnected from the medical proceedings. What impressed me about AIDS activists was precisely their personal involvement in the public process. They refused to parcel AIDS into public and private components. When I decided myself to speak out publicly, in a newspaper article, the process was exhilarating. I felt engaged in a personally meaningful struggle, not just as a "woman fighting cancer" but as a citizen taking part in a larger societal battle with the disease.

In the past ten years, increasing numbers of women have decided to "go public" about having breast cancer. Often, they describe their encounter with the medical system in terms of estrangement. They liken medical treatment to being on a conveyer belt. They seek vital information in vain. They don't understand what the doctor is talking about. When they try to articulate their fears, those around them urge a "chin up" attitude.

BREAST CANCER AS PROPERTY

The cancer patient's alienation can be framed in personal terms—you are in shock, facing a new situation, terrified of death—but this is a too-easy out. Of course every woman with breast cancer suffers personal trauma. But equally important, the institutionalization of our "problem" distances us from our lived reality. The state system, designed to "control" cancer, in reality controls the woman—and particularly her conflict with cancer—more effectively than it controls the disease. We are labelled "patients." We are thrust ("no time to waste!") into a medical system governed by undisclosed rules. Here, "compliance" gains approval. Physicians speak to us in the private jargon of medical science, or with an infantalizing "there, there dear" paternalism. "Recovery" programs encourage us to "look normal" and "get on with life." Soon charities descend, urging us to "fight cancer with a check-up and a check." The money goes into "support" programs in which we have no say, or to researchers studying questions unrelated to our own.

From the moment of diagnosis, we are protagonists in a drama which may end in our death. If ever we should feel fully engaged, it is now.

BREAST CANCER TURFS

We live in a society that values expertise. In every sphere, we divide the world into professionals and the lay public. Professionals engage in the work of problem-solving in their own sphere. They own those problems. If we challenge the strict separation of breast cancer into public and private property, we are saying professionals will have to cede some of their ownership of the disease.

As a property, breast cancer is vast. No one agency lays claim to the whole. In the past century, various groups have divided up the turf and set mutually agreed-on boundaries. Treatment is one parcel and the main owners are oncologists. Research is another parcel. Medical researchers stake the largest claim here. Fundraising is a third parcel, owned by the cancer charities and the state. A fourth large chunk, encompassing support and educational services, is owned largely by the cancer charities. The private anguish of breast cancer is a separate turf. That belongs to the woman with the disease and her loved ones.

In the analysis that follows, I examine each of four public turfs to see how the present owners gained title and what the conflict means to them. I examine the reasons activists have ventured onto each section of public property and the reaction they have met on arrival.

THE TREATMENT TURF

A study of oncologists at Harvard teaching hospitals explored the reasons why these physicians chose oncology. The researchers found that the physicians described their commitment to the field in terms of "challenge." A radiation oncologist said, "We have a superb program... it is dangerous... we are right up to what we can get away with. It's exciting...." Another, a medical oncologist, explained, "...I didn't want to deal with zits. Or people who couldn't sleep, or have low back pain and are depressed. *Everyone who walks into my office might die.* And although I don't wish them all to die, I... get more of a buzz out of dealing with something."

Women with breast cancer have entered the treatment turf largely because they question the current treatments. Many are angry to learn that punishing treatments which had been promoted as cures have uncertain and limited benefits. They are shocked to discover how little mortality rates have changed in fifty years. They wonder if other treatments, particularly less toxic ones, might not be just as beneficial as the "slash/burn/poison" trilogy—or more so. Women also seek to expand the definition of treatment into the psycho-social sphere. Medical treatments don't begin to address our subjective experience of cancer, which reaches to every area of our lives.

Women with breast cancer want more than the much-touted partnership of shared decision-making in medical treatments. This would be relatively easy to negotiate. The more contentious ownership questions involve redefining the treatment terrain—moving the boundaries beyond the medical. Oncologists resist because their primacy in the treatment struggle is questioned.

THE RESEARCH TURF

Researchers own the enigma of breast cancer. As custodians of the intellectual conflict with the disease, they engage in the search for understanding that could eventually solve the puzzle. In this struggle with the unknown, they define what questions are important.

In the researcher-driven process, scientific peer review panels explicitly exclude members of the public. A place on the research turf, however, is one of the demands advocates have pressed hardest for. As with treatment, women with breast cancer seek involvement on a changed turf, not the one that currently exists. We ask different questions.

In San Francisco, the group Breast Cancer Action has lobbied for advocacy representatives on breast cancer research committees at all levels. Their goal was "a say in the research process based upon the real life experience of people living with cancer." They were determined to be engaged in the process, ideally in a collaborative relationship with scientists. "We can be adversaries or partners in accelerating research," they said. "We would prefer to be partners." After eight months of negotiations with the head of the local cancer centre, the activists had the beginnings of a working partnership. Dr. Craig Henderson, who described the women as "surprisingly intelligent, bright and verbal," granted a seat for an activist on scientific committees, review of grant proposals for new projects, and input into the research process for large clinical trials groups.

Despite such concessions, many researchers still oppose patients' participation in the research arena, even though breast cancer activists have dramatically increased the amount of money available for breast cancer research. The nub of the resistance is our wish to redefine the puzzle.

THE FUNDRAISING TURF

Cancer fundraising was first "owned" by the American Society for the Control of Cancer (ASCC), precursor of the American Cancer Society. ASCC founders were progressive-thinking physicians and wealthy women in the New York area. From 1913 until the mid-1940s, the ASCC was a relatively small charity that raised most of its money through rich local benefactors.

The first cancer fundraising turf war took place in the mid-1940s when Mary Lasker took over the ASCC and transformed it into the American Cancer Society (ACS). Lasker was the wife of advertising tycoon Albert Lasker who pioneered a campaign urging women to smoke using the slogan, "Reach for a Lucky Instead of a Sweet." She added leading businessmen to the board and applied corporate advertising and fundraising techniques to cancer charity work. Lasker also cultivated links with influential federal politicians and drove the lobby to expand the funded National Cancer Institute (NCI) into a major research institute.

When the tax-funded NCI began to boom in the late 1940s, ACS leaders worried that the American public would let their donations flag. The two agencies agreed to divide the turf: the NCI would use its funds, raised from taxes, for research; the donations-dependent ACS would have jurisdiction over services and education. The plan worked. In the post-war years, the budgets of both organizations expanded exponentially. The public has had scant say in how these funds are disbursed.

In a few short years, breast cancer advocacy has radically transformed cancer fundraising. In late 1992, advocacy pressure sprang $214 million in earmarked breast cancer funds from the American defense budget. Rather than welcoming the new money, however, researchers responded anxiously. Typical was a breast cancer researcher at the Mayo Clinic in Rochester, Minnesota, who complained the increase in funds was "very politically motivated."

In fact, politics are hardly new to research fundraising. The NCI was born of assiduous lobbying by the cancer research community. The difference in this case was that breast cancer activists took the bows and demanded a say in how the monies would be spent.

In many communities, women with breast cancer have formed small grassroots self-help groups which raise funds to finance their own activities. Often the incentive for forming these groups is the women's dissatisfaction with Cancer Society services.

THE SUPPORT AND INFORMATION TURF

Charities have also owned breast cancer support and information services. These activities have long emphasized the importance of early detection and prompt medical care. Appeals for funds are effective because the public backs these goals.

The educational messages of the cancer charities reflect the views of physicians rather than patients. Established services don't begin to meet the emotional and information needs of women with breast cancer. Services may even aggravate, not alleviate, patients' problems. The late Jackie Winnow, who was diagnosed with breast cancer in 1985, described a seven-week ACS support group she attended as "very controlled." At one point, she recalled, "somebody had a lot of complaints about a doctor and I wanted to know who that doctor was. The social worker said, 'You can't ask that question because it's not an objective response.' I was horrified." The incident catalyzed Winnow to start a Women's Cancer Resource Center in San Francisco.

Support-turf owners may respond to survivor-run support services by trying to absorb them. Women should be cautious of agreeing to such takeovers in the area of support, says the Hon. Monique Bégin, for many years Canada's minister of health. Government bureaucracies try to absorb these initiatives into their ways of doing things and, in doing so, may kill what is so special about them, notes Bégin. "While this may be the price of success, it must be opposed."

THE PRIVATE TURF

In the established order, the personal anguish of breast cancer is women's private domain. Paradoxically, the taboos against exposing the lived experience of breast cancer disengage us from our feelings.

Audre Lorde wrote forcibly about the politics of silence. What is important to me, Lorde said, "must be spoken, made verbal and shared." In the harsh light of self-examination following her first breast biopsy, Lorde saw what she regretted most in her life: the occasions when, out of fear, she silenced thoughts she wanted to speak. Her understanding that the ultimate silence—death—might come sooner than expected pushed her to another realization: silence would not protect her from dying. Silence isolated her; speaking her beliefs brought her into contact with women who had the same fears and sparked a collective, strengthening examination of the issues.

Psychologist Ross Gray, an advocate of patients' participation on policy planning committees, surveyed health care professionals' attitudes to having people with cancer sit with them around the board room table. Professionals in the cancer community, he found, resist having people with cancer on their committees because patients raise personal, emotional issues that medical professionals and administrators would rather not discuss. No wonder the medical system deals poorly with our emotional trauma! Removing the artificial barrier between public and private spheres can only improve this glaring weakness in the system.

PATIENT NO MORE

Masculine values define oncology. Characteristics of the field are specialization, hierarchical power structures, heroic intervention, rational-scientific thinking, and high-tech methods of treatment and diagnosis. The popular war metaphor used to describe the fight against cancer creates a military climate that further valorizes macho behavior. From diagnosis to death, oncology veers to the highest cost and the riskiest heroics. Even when the cancer strikes a female organ, male ownership of the struggle seems almost mandatory.

As more women with breast cancer find their voices, the clash between the masculine ideology of the owners and the feminist values of the owned is increasingly obvious. One example is the activist opposition to experiments in hormone manipulation. Another is the pressure for preventive research into environmental toxins. A third is the interest in "soft" alternative treatments that enhance the woman's sense of well-being and control. Women with breast cancer are bargaining for non-interventionist, preventive, and low-tech solutions.

We are saying: it's our conflict. We want it back.

POSTSCRIPT TO A DECADE OF ACTIVISM

The breast cancer movement had, and still has, a radical core. Many of the women who spoke out at the beginning had been involved in activist politics before their diagnosis and I continue to meet politicized women with breast cancer who bring a mature feminist outlook to their current activism. Yet fundamental change remains elusive. One explanation is that many women who wrote and spoke and lobbied had no political analysis. They just had breast cancer. These women were co-opted very early on by vested interests who saw the harnessing of women's energy as a way to leverage more research funds, and to promote mammography, treatments, and genetic testing. Establishment and corporate-sponsored vehicles like National Breast Cancer Awareness Month and the shower card brigade already existed when the movement was defined in the early 1990s. They very quickly got bigger and slicker. By sheer force of marketing, they soon shaped the movement in their own image. With the vast majority of the medical community onside, it wasn't difficult to persuade most women in search of direction that wearing a pink ribbon, handing out shower cards, and Running for The Cure were ways to bring about change. The simplistic idea that breast cancer was an underfunded area of research had enough of a feminist ring that a lot of women bought it without question, along with the corollary that lobbying for more funds would soon turn things around. What about the radicals? A lot of them died. It's easy to underestimate the impact of death as a looming presence for women with breast cancer, compared to, say, women dealing with the birth control issue who had their health and their whole productive lives ahead of them. With breast cancer, you get a group together and within a few years someone will develop metastasis. Some women get scared and pull back. Others become caregivers to the dying women. When she dies, the mourning process changes the energy of the group. And if she was the group's leader, well she's gone. Do you regroup, or do people go back to their families and jobs? I believe we're in for a long struggle, with a lot of redefining of issues and factions within the broad movement, like the women's movement itself. Eventually, people will have to question the adequacy of shower cards and fundraising runs. There will be a defining book or a medical scandal or a critical mass of savvy women and we'll have a second wave.—January 1999

Dr. Samuel Epstein Speaks on the Politics of Breast Cancer Prevention

CARLA MARCELIS

Carla Marcelis, *DES Action Canada Newsletter*, March 25, 1999. Reprinted by permission.

More than 300 women and men gathered in the McGill University Medical Faculty in Montreal on March 25, 19XX, to hear leading American public health and cancer expert Dr. Samuel S. Epstein make his claim that cancer is preventable. Dr. Epstein was invited to Montreal by DES Action Canada, Breast Cancer Action Montreal, and the McGill Centre for Research and Teaching on Women.

Epstein refutes the common claim that breast cancer occurs randomly in women and can only be controlled by early detection and aggressive treatment. According to Epstein, a number of risk factors can be avoided. Among his "Dirty Dozen" are such common medications and interventions as early and prolonged use of the birth control pill; high-dose and prolonged use of estrogen replacement therapy; non-hormonal prescription drugs, such as tranquilizers and antidepressants; silicone breast implants and early and repeated premenopausal mammograms.

Epstein also warned against the risks of carcinogens in our diet, especially in animal fat, in our environment, and in household and cosmetic products. Referring to research, he explained that the significant increase in breast cancer over the past forty years has taken place in estrogen-sensitive breast cancer and not in the non-estrogen-sensitive types. He pointed out that many of the carcinogens in his "Dirty Dozen" mimic the actions of estrogens in the body (as does DES), which is the reason they pose a breast cancer risk.

According to Epstein, prevention is possible if there were a political will to make scientific information public and decision-making processes transparent. He called the strong links that exist between the industry, the major cancer institutions, and the government a threat to democracy and advocated for criminal sanctions for "white collar crime" when scientific evidence is distorted or documents are destroyed or hidden in the bottom of public employees' filing cabinets. Epstein has created six legislative proposals that are intended to reverse the cancer epidemic. He outlined several regulatory means for reduction of harmful products and mechanisms by which consumers and advocates can have access to information, participate in expert committees and make complaints.

The evening's moderator, Dr. Michele Brill-Edwards, agreed with Epstein that the process by which drugs and chemicals are approved is not one that serves the interest of the public. According to Brill-Edwards, the favors paid by industry to bureaucrats and academics unduly influence their decisions about a product's safety. Brill-Edwards, who resigned from her job as a drug reviewer at the Health Protection Branch of Health Canada because of the industry's influence over the drug approval process, said that these favors are standard industry practice.

The evening ended on an optimistic note: Both Epstein and Brill-Edwards believe that we as citizens can make a difference by letting the government know that public safety should be their primary concern for drug and chemical approval processes.

Epstein and Brill-Edwards have each founded public advocacy organizations which campaign, each in their own way, for improved drug regulation. Maybe all of us can rest a little easier, knowing that we have such good allies in the struggle for better health protection.

Fighting the "War" on Breast Cancer: How a Metaphor Has Shaped the Debate on Early Detection and Treatment

BARRON H. LERNER

Adapted from earlier versions that first appeared in *Annals of Internal Medicine*, July 1, 1998, and *The Journal of the College of Physicians and Surgeons of Columbia University*, Winter 1999. Reprinted by permission.

More than twenty years ago, Susan Sontag argued that metaphors interfere with how American society understands and responds to diseases such as cancer. In the case of breast cancer, "war" has been the dominant metaphor, implying that the disease is an actual enemy to be vanquished on a medical battlefield.

Military language has revealed the fierce determination of anticancer organizations, such as the American Cancer Society and the National Cancer Institute, to lower mortality from the disease. The notion of fighting breast cancer has also held great personal appeal for many women with this dreaded disease. But the use of war metaphors also points out how physicians and activists involved in the war effort have at times oversold the value of available screening and treatment modalities.

Although Richard Nixon formally initiated the U.S. government's war on cancer in 1971, that war had been raging since at least 1936 when anticancer activists formed the Women's Field Army. The Army's "war cry" was for "trench warfare with a vengeance against a ruthless killer"—cancer. Since then, it has been almost impossible to discuss breast cancer without using military terminology.

By 1950, the standard strategy for breast cancer was early detection of cancerous lumps, followed by an extensive, deforming surgical procedure known as the radical mastectomy. The operation removed not only the cancerous breast but the underarm lymph nodes and both chest wall muscles on the affected side. By the early 1950s, a small group of physicians and statisticians began to question the value of early detection, and the universal need for radical mastectomies. These critics pointed to data that showed no consistent association between a delayed diagnosis and the extent of the cancer or between the size of the primary lesion and the cancer's spread to other sites. They also noted the failure of radical mastectomies to reduce national mortality rates. They proposed an alternative model of "biological predeterminism," which attributed the fate of patients more to biological factors, such as tumor virulence and immune response, than to early detection.

The data were ambiguous, pointing definitively in neither direction. But the scientific debate reflected none of that. The vitriolic tone of the discussion bespoke an unwillingness to analyze a thorny problem in a rational manner. Limited warfare held little appeal.

Physicians had long identified breast lesions resembling cancer that had not invaded the underlying breast tissue. By the 1930s, pathologists, believing that such lesions were "precancers," began to term them ductal or lobular "carcinoma in situ." Carcinoma in situ raised two questions: (1) Were such lesions inevitably precancerous? and (2) Did detection mandate mastectomy?

A few surgeons favored a conservative approach, advising only observation. However, most physicians, using familiar military metaphors, essentially equated breast cancer predisposition with the actual disease. Viewing lobular carcinoma in situ as a "powder keg," surgeons generally recommended mastectomy.

Treatment of the lobular carcinoma in one breast led to scrutiny of the other breast. Studies had reported that women with lesions of one breast developed cancer in the other breast in as many as 25 percent of cases. Mammography was most often used to find such lesions, but some surgeons recommended a more aggressive approach: random biopsy of the second breast. Such biopsies were of high yield, generating cancer or carcinoma in situ up to 59 percent of the time. In such cases, mastectomy of the second breast usually followed.

Some surgeons pushed early detection and treatment even further. Fearing that biopsies would miss existing lesions, they performed routine prophylactic removal of the second breast in women diagnosed with lobular carcinoma in situ. The war on breast cancer may have reached its pinnacle when a marker of possible future cancer in one breast became a rationale for bilateral prophylactic mastectomy in women without other risk factors.

By the mid-1970s, the use of mastectomy for lobular carcinoma in situ was being challenged. Physicians increasingly concluded that most women treated only with lumpectomy never developed breast cancer, and those who did often developed ductal carcinomas, which could not have emanated from the lobular lesions. Meanwhile, extensive controlled trials demonstrated, as the predeterminists had claimed, that radical mastectomy was almost never necessary for the treatment of actual breast cancer.

In January 1997, angry debate about early detection of breast cancer broke out once again when an NIH panel decided not to recommend routine screening mammograms for women forty to forty-nine years of age. The debate had little to do with the scientific value of mammography; it has been claimed that there was broad agreement on what the data showed. Instead, the antagonism stemmed from political, economic, and legal concerns. Interest groups, ranging from cancer activists to radiologists to the U.S. Senate, had again proven unwilling to declare a truce and discuss the pros and cons of breast cancer screening in a dispassionate manner. As a result, physicians and patients were left without adequate guideposts for applying early detection to clinical practice.

The next front in the war against breast cancer will be the "genetic battlefield." Tests identifying BRCA1 and BRCA2 genetic mutations, which are already being termed "time bombs," represent a powerful new method for obtaining early information about potential breast cancers. Healthy women who test positive for the BRCA1 or BRCA2 genetic marker are at very high risk for the disease. In order to decrease their likelihood of developing breast cancer, some women are choosing to have bilateral prophylactic mastectomy.

Lacking knowledge about the actual value of genetic testing, history warns us not to conflate the *ability* to find these markers with the *need* to find and act on them. In the past, at least, an "all or nothing" wartime mentality has encouraged aggressive intervention for such ambiguous lesions. While prophylactic mastectomy may be the correct choice for some women, careful counseling about the limitations of the operation remains mandatory.

Chapter 67

Further Toward a New Psychology of Women

A *s woman presses onward toward equality, new areas of exploitation and abuse—formerly overlooked, taken for granted, hidden, or minimized— emerge into the open and are addressed. One discovery begets another, the second begets a third. In the 1980s the frequent abuse of patients by psychiatrists and other therapists was documented, but the professions claimed that the perpetrators were "fringy" types. Then it was revealed that Dr. Jules Masserman, one of the world's most eminent living psychiatrists, was himself a perpetrator. In the 1990s families of the perpetrators came forward as "lineal" victims, and organized their own support and activist organizations. What next?—B. S.*

An Interview with Jules Masserman

KATHRYN WATTERSON

Excerpted from Kathryn Watterson, "Afterword: An Interview with Jules Masserman," *You Must Be Dreaming*, Poseidon Press, 1992. Reprinted by permission.

You *Must Be Dreaming* sent shock waves through the professional psychiatric community. Kathryn Watterson tells the story of coauthor and singer Barbara Noël, who battles to bring her world-renowned psychiatrist, Dr. Jules Masserman, to justice for his sexual and ethical betrayals. Watterson also includes the stories of several other patients who brought charges and won out-of-court settlements against Masserman.

Step by painful step, the book details the hidden life of Jules Masserman, past president of the American Psychiatric Association, cochair of psychiatry and neurology at Northwestern University, and author of 411 journal articles and 16 books. It details how the man who was called "psychiatry's ambassador to the world" systematically and ritualistically injected many of his most attractive and vulnerable female patients with Amytal, a barbiturate, and kept them unconscious for six to eight hours at a time in a little room off his main consultation office. Barbara Noël awoke during one of these sessions as she was being raped, and others recounted breakthrough memories of Masserman kissing and fondling them. In addition, Masserman took many of his female patients to his "home office," where he played the violin for them. He took them out on his sailboat *Natad, Nymph of the Lakes*, gave them gifts, and accepted gifts from them.

Neither Masserman's abuse of his patients nor and the failure of his profession to censure him are unique. The best available data indicate that from 6 to 10 percent of psychiatrists and psychologists have had sexual contact with their patients, and that the majority of their colleagues know of such cases but do not intervene. More than half of the psychologists and psychiatrists interviewed in various surveys indicate that they have treated women patients who had been sexually involved with previous therapists.

The American Psychiatric Association responded to *You Must Be Dreaming* by issuing a public apology and undertaking a yearlong review of its ethical policies and procedures for reporting misconduct. The task force recommended that the job of policing and punishing its members is antithetical to the purpose of promoting the profession, and that the job should be turned over to an independent regulating agency.

Dr. Masserman looked at me intently and smiled. "Please sit down," he said, indicating the couch. I sat there, behind a coffee table that held a small black tape recorder, a stack of textbooks, and a copy of *Who's Who in the World*. Dr. Masserman sat in an easy chair next to the couch, and Mrs. Masserman sat in a swivel chair facing us.

They set up the conditions of this interview: I could not tape-record it. Mrs. Masserman said, however, that they planned to tape-record, because Dr. Masserman "has suffered so much injustice" and they didn't want his comments "taken out of context." "I'll tell you what," Dr. Masserman said pleasantly, as if he had just lit upon a solution. "If my lawyer approves, after reviewing the tape, of course, then I'll send you a copy." At the time this book went to press, I still had not received a copy of the tape.

Mrs. Masserman turned on the tape recorder and also took notes on a white pad as we spoke. From time to time during the following two and a half hours, she would scribble notes on her pad, signal Dr. Masserman, and hold up the pad to show him what she had written.

Dr. Masserman picked up some papers and began with statements he had prepared. He enunciated his words carefully and formally, without contractions:

"I will be straightforward and honest and give you demonstrable facts. I am a very ethical practitioner, and so I cannot tell you confidential information about my patients. I took a Hippocratic oath, and even though I have retired, I still abide by that oath.... For the past forty years, under the aegis and supervision for four different universities, I have treated literally thousands of patients. Until Miss Noël's complaint, not a single previous one of my patients—simply not one—ever made one complaint against me." In 1983, one year prior to Barbara Noël's complaint, a patient, Cheryl Russell, sued Dr. Masserman for needlessly injecting her with Amytal and injuring her in the process. Her lawsuit, civil case No. 83L-10063, was settled against Dr. Masserman, by his insurers, for $50,000 not long after Barbara initially filed her complaint.

I started to ask about his use of Amytal, but Dr. Masserman waved his hand toward the stack of reference books, commenting that his own book "is a classic in the field now."* He pointed out the dozens of plaques on his walls that paid homage to him, and invited me to look at his entry in *Who's Who in the World*, saying, "It's an unusual honor... it's a rare honor to be in that book."

Continuing his prepared talk, Dr. Masserman said: "I can say a few things about Barbara Noël's treatment. She profited so greatly from Amytal interviews when necessary. I can't tell you *why* they were necessary, because that would be revealing."

He added, "The only complaint Barbara Noël ever made came on September 24, 1984. Had there been any unethical conduct that morning when she said she was conscious—there were no locked doors in my office. All she had to do was to go into the next office and complain.

---

*In the stack, he had two different editions of *Comprehensive Textbook of Psychiatry* by Freedman, Kaplan, and Saddock; and *The Technique of Psychotherapy* by Louis Wolberg.

"She had been my patient for eighteen years," he said, shaking his head.

"What happened on that day [September 21, 1984] is relevant," Dr. Masserman continued. "She did not call me back and make any complaints. She went to her gynecologist and stated to him that she may have dreamed the whole thing. She went to the police with various allegations.... I can assure you, I would have been arrested like *that* had her complaints been true...." Dr. Masserman also mentioned "a prominent Chicago attorney" who "investigated her allegations and then withdrew from the case." Then he sat back in his chair, folded his hands across his chest, and seemed to relax.

"But what about the other lawsuits?" I asked. "Why do you think they surfaced?"

Dr. Masserman, his eyes bright and friendly, smiled sweetly and comfortably. "You put me at a disadvantage because the two other lawsuits—" he said, "I don't know who you talked to—"

I said, "There were five other lawsuits, not two, but of the two I think you're referring to, I talked to both of them."

"Well, the major one—the principal one under my therapy—resumed the practice of law, joined a prominent firm, married a rich client, invited me to her wedding and publicly proclaimed her gratitude in the presence of her father! Neither woman had made any complaints whatsoever. Both left owing me money, but I had written statements pledging to pay me.... "

"Why do you think their accusations surfaced? Do you think they're based on malice, profit, fantasy?" I asked.

"My attorney advised me to say this.... Please note that there were no criminal charges filed at any time, let alone rape. The only action filed was to obtain money, to secure money."

Asked if he denied all the allegations, he replied, "Absolutely." Raising his voice in irritation, he added, "I never did anything unethical to any patient."

"Then why did you agree to give up your medical license?" I asked. "Why didn't you fight it?"

"I'm glad you asked that," he said, meeting my eyes, "At the time the suit was settled, I had already given notice to the building where I kept my office that I was retiring at the end of that year." Dr. Masserman said he'd planned to retire because he was "taking a great deal of time dashing home to feed my wife, to take her to the toilet, to get her out of bed," because she needed a hip operation. He said he also was having three operations for prostatic cancer during that time.

"What's your reaction to these lawsuits? How do you feel about all these allegations?" I asked.

"Being a very sensitive person—which I have to be to be a psychiatrist—and now this has come up again—it's been seven years of unjustified tension, which I have withstood. Many another might not have." He looked at me with a wounded gaze, not unlike a child who has been refused a treat.

I asked him why he continued to use Amytal regularly, when most psychiatrists say it fell out of use after the early 1950s because it was never very effective.

"With the Amytal, I followed precisely what I wrote in my textbook and what everybody else writes... " he said, pointing again to the textbooks.

I said everybody else seemed to think Amytal should *not* be used regularly... that he himself had written that the Amytal interview "was a preferred treatment only in extreme cases... and that little could be achieved by drug narcosis that could not also be achieved by therapeutic interviews conducted without its use."

He said, "There are many instances in which I only used talk therapy and I always talked afterwards."

I asked him if he had any colleagues who use Amytal on a regular basis, and he said, "Of course I do... many."

I asked, "Who?"

"Among others, Louis Wolberg used it frequently." He gestured to Dr. Wolberg's book.

Referring to my notes, I said, "Well, in fact, Dr. Wolberg writes that Amytal is used only in extreme cases—that it's '*sometimes* employed intravenously as an *emergency* measure in quelling intense excitement.... 'and you yourself say that it's used for 'morose, evasive withdrawn patients in early schizophrenic or depressive reactions.... '" I said it seemed it was normally used only in a hospital under emergency situations.

"No, no. It was used regularly during World War Two and ever since then.... "

I asked him why he used Amytal so regularly.

"I only used it with patients that had serious crises—to prevent suicide when someone was so desperate and needed relief, or to *prevent* a bout of alcoholism.... "

I asked, "Didn't you worry about it being addictive?"

"*It's not addictive,*" he said.

I said, "In the *Physician's Desk Reference*, in *Goodman & Gillman's*, in *Martindale's*, and every other drug reference, it says it's habit-forming and carries warnings to that effect. Even Louis Wolberg writes that 'Short-acting barbiturates, Pentothal, Seconal, and Amytal are particularly addictive. They are truly as addictive as heroin or morphine.... '"

"Amytal is habit-forming only in the sense that they might try to get drugs on the outside," he said, "and naturally I wouldn't give them any... "

I was reeling from the illogic of that statement, but I asked, "What did the people you prescribed Amytal to have in common?"

"They would be people inclined to very severe anxieties, depressions, melancholy, and temptations toward suicide...."

"In references they say that it's given rarely, and yet you used it repeatedly over the years. One patient recently told me there were many periods she got it every week. Why did you do that? Did they have that many crises?"

"There have been years with no Amytal," he said. "But during the past year with Ms. Noël, before September 1984, there were various crises, more frequent than usual. "

"You gave them Amytal to help them through a crisis every time—all that often?" I asked.

"I would have to judge each case. Before I ever gave an Amytal interview, I would call in the family; I would consult the[m]. Sometimes I would give the Amytal instead of hospitalizing the person and sometimes I would hospitalize the person instead… "

"Did you ever recommend that Barbara be hospitalized?"

"I can only say what's positive," he said with an apologetic smile. "I did send her to a friend of mine at Northwestern University who helped her by having her do some music therapy at Northwestern with students…. I did refer her to other physicians, which shows that I did consult other medical doctors when it was called for."

I said, "Saddoff and Freedman's textbook says Amytal is used only in extreme cases, in emergency situations. They also say 'narcotherapy is *infrequently* used in clinical practice' and when it's used, it's for *acute* symptoms.'"

Dr. Masserman waved his hand as if to dismiss all this and said, "There are a great many psychiatrists who are so caught up in analytic thinking that they believe only in talk therapy, without using every known therapy—using drug therapy, diet, behavior therapy—I use them all, whatever is called for."

I asked: "Did you use combined drug therapy and talk therapy with most of your patients, some of them, half of them, or…?

"Less than 1 percent," he said.

"You gave Amytal to *less than 1 percent* of your patients?"

"That's right."

"You mean to say that *all six lawsuits* came from that less than one percent of your patients who had Sodium Amytal?"

"Yes, the six lawsuits were part of that 1 percent… "

I said, "I'm confused about Amytal… From what I understand from talking with others, it's a short-acting barbiturate."

"I never gave barbiturates…"

"But Amytal is a barbiturate!"

"Yes, but not in addition to that. I didn't give drugs in therapy…."

"But I'm confused about something… The patients I talked to—and in your own descriptions—said they were asleep from like 7 A.M. to 2 or 3 P.M. in the afternoon or later, sometimes 4:30 or 5, and then afterwards they were often groggy for the entire evening or into the next day—"

"They're not asleep. They're relaxed, at ease. They were conscious, and just in a relaxed state so they could converse…. "

"But the people I talked to said they never remembered anything afterwards."

"But they *do*," he said, enunciating the words slowly, and meaningfully nodding his head as he looked at me, as if we two knew the truth. "They *do*. Part of the technique is to talk about it afterward."

"Well, I was wondering, since Amytal is a short-acting drug, did you add a sedative to the Amytal or use a continuous IV drip to help them stay out for that long?"

"No, no, absolutely not! I only gave the standard dose of Amytal."

I said, "One woman I talked with told me that you had recommended she take Amytal when she was pregnant, and another told Barbara Noël that she'd had Amytal and subsequently lost her baby. Did you ever give Amytal to a pregnant patient?"

"She never told me she was pregnant," he said. "None of my patients ever told me she was pregnant."

"Do you think it's ever justified for a therapist to have sex with a patient?"

"Of course not!" he said vehemently. "I have sat in on ethics committees in the past and expressed that view unequivocally!!"

"You mention in *Psychiatric Odyssey* that "perverse sexuality has deprecatory meaning only in Western culture...." Do you think it's only Western culture—that maybe Americans are too repressed and overly concerned about these ethical matters? Do you think in another culture or in Biblical times, these things would be considered normal or harmless?"

Dr. Masserman raised his eyebrows in surprise, but then looked rather pleased and amused. "Well, that is true," he said. "In many cultures homosexuality was preferable, for instance. In Greek classic times, homosexuality was not only acceptable, but was considered preferable. Socrates initiated his apostles and that was considered a normal thing. Even cannibalism was accepted in some cultures. But psychiatrists should not make such broad general statements. I deplore this kind of guerre attitude...."

"In *Adolescent Sexuality*, you mention incest can be harmless and can be a non-neurotic experience if it's treated properly. You say, 'Contrary to many current concepts... noninjurious parent-child or intersibling sexual relations, even when verified, usually leave no serious adverse effects, and require only judicious avoidance of social and legal traumata.... ' Is that still your position?"

"Well, that's true if the child isn't dragged through the humiliation of testifying and all," he said. "Certainly, making the child testify can do a great deal of unnecessary harm. There was one example in that book about a girl whose stepfather molested her. The girl didn't want him to go to jail and break up the family... "

I said, "Several of your patients talked about your taking them on boat rides of airplane rides or to your home for home office visits and on trips.... Did you do that to broaden their horizons or for what purposes?"

Dr. Masserman said he had never taken any patient out on his boat. "Let me show you something," he said, asking me to stand up. The three of us stood and looked out the window; Dr. Masserman stood close to me. I remembered Barbara, Daniella, and Annie telling me about their trips out on his boat—being rowed from the dock to the boat and back. "See that house?" he said, pointing out the clubhouse. "And the dock beside it? I keep my boat in the harbor, and I have to row from that dock to my boat…. If I was stupid enough to take anyone else but my wife out to that boat, she'd know it before I got home!"

"Honey, you didn't mention this." Mrs. Masserman said, picking up a pair of binoculars.

"That's right," he said with a little chuckle. "I'm under surveillance at all times…. Not really!" Dr. and Mrs. Masserman both laughed. In depositions, when asked if he had ever taken patients out on his boat, Dr. Masserman had said, under oath, "Yes. Ms. Noël on one occasion."And when he was asked, "Have you taken anyone else on your boat, any of your other patients?" he had answered, "Yes, I have." He had also admitted, under oath, that he had taken female patients flying in his airplane.

"But why would these different people say that they went out on the boat and the airplane with you?" I asked. "Are you saying they were making that up, or having the same delusion or something?"

"See that picture?" Dr. Masserman asked me, pointing out a small oil painting of a gray-blue boat with full white sails listing in rough seas.

"It's nice."

"I have the same picture in my office."

"You do?"

"Yes, and I have a picture of the plane I flew when I was flying, in my office. I have a picture of my playing a violin, in my office. It is one part of one technique called *transference*, which illustrates by personal example that there are many activities in life that can give more satisfactions than drinking or quarreling or competing or seeking revenge. And so people ask me these things:

"Do I sail? What sort of boat? Oh, do you fly? Do you take people up? They can make all sorts of fantasies from their own ends… "

"So you say they're fantasizing this?" I interjected.

"That's exactly what I'm saying."

The interview was over and we all stood up. Dr. Masserman invited me to look around his music room—and showed me his beautiful old Albani violin and viola. I thought he was starting to say he would be glad to play something for me, but his wife cleared her throat and interrupted, so he didn't finish his sentence. After I left, I felt an amazing sadness. I gave a lot of thought to Dr. Masserman's defense—and to his magnetism. I thought it was no wonder he charmed Barbara and his other patients into believing him. He was compelling and appeared so genuine that I had actually liked him, even when I was so vividly aware of his wrong-doing.

Later, I called Dr. David Spiegel, M.D., professor of psychiatry and behavioral sciences at Stanford University and a leading expert in the field. I asked

Dr. Spiegel whether the dose of Amytal Dr. Masserman claimed to have used could possibly have kept anyone out for seven to eight hours. "Not from one dose of Amytal!" he said without pause. "It's a short-acting barbiturate. They might be groggy for an hour or two afterwards, but they wouldn't be that deeply affected by it." When I asked him whether a continuous IV may have been used or a sedative added to the Amytal, he said that would make sense. Dr. Spiegel said he didn't know of anyone who still uses Amytal in the normal practice of psychiatry, and that he had never heard of it being used on a repeated basis, since, of course, it is highly addictive.

Lineal Victims

PHYLLIS L. FINE

Phyllis L. Fine, "Lineal Victims: Family Members of a Perpetrator," Speech adapted for this publication.

With the growing national recognition given to the serious problem regarding abuse by professionals, the therapy community has responded to the needs of the primary victims of the perpetrator, whether they be patient, client, or parishioner. Even the family members of the primary victim are being recognized for the pain they suffer. However, lineal victims—the family members of the perpetrating professional, including the spouse, the children, and the other family members—have until recently been the unrecognized, unacknowledged victims who often suffer for years, if not a lifetime, from the effects of having been connected to the perpetrator.

Just as the patient has been victimized by the perpetrating professional, so have the spouse and the children. Generally, the family has been subjected to years of abuse. Overtly or covertly abused, they have been manipulated and often live in a world filled with deception. The abusive personality one experiences at home and the manipulating personality that was able to seduce the client/patient/parishioner is often not the personality viewed by the outside world.... The Jekyll-Hyde personality of the perpetrating professional is brilliantly masked, bringing further pain and confusion to family members.... Family members suffer tremendous isolation, desperately needing the connection of others who can understand the overwhelming destruction shattering their lives.

Lineal victims often carry within themselves a sense of shame, that—although it does not belong to them—isolates them from the world. They may fear being judged for having been connected to the perpetrator as well as fear angry repercussions from the primary victims and their families. A triangle of fear is created by the perpetrator, a triangle that separates the victims....

Surviving devastation of this magnitude is exceedingly difficult [because of] the many complicating factors impacting the family. It is often the families who are left struggling financially, especially if the professional should lose the ability to practice. As of recent years, insurance companies have restricted their involvement in malpractice suits to paying only for legal costs. Any resulting damage awards or settlements are the responsibility of the perpetrating professional. Although this may appear to be fair, it is the spouse and children who once again are unjustly left struggling, for it is generally the marital assets which are the source of payment for these damages.

For those who have not been abused, it is difficult to understand why these professionals carry so much power, and even more difficult to understand why spouses stay in abusive situations. The skillfulness of the narcissistic personality to be able to manipulate and control vulnerable people cannot be sufficiently emphasized.

There are many spouses and families who choose not to remain in denial, but rather choose to face their greatest fears and break the isolation. It is a most difficult and pain-filled journey, and one that needs to be recognized and made less isolating.

Women and Madness: A Feminist Diagnosis

PHYLLIS CHESLER

Phyllis Chesler, "Women and Madness: A Feminist Diagnosis," *Ms.*, November/ December 1997. Reprinted by permission.

Twenty-five years ago Phyllis Chesler's book *Women and Madness* challenged the psychotherapeutic community's routine pathologizing of women. She documented the patriarchal straitjacketing of women's mental health and urged sweeping reforms in both the theories and the practices. In this excerpt from the introduction to the special anniversary edition of this landmark work, Chesler reflects on what has and has not changed. —The Editors

When I started writing *Women and Madness* I immersed myself in the psycho-analytic literature, and located biographies and autobiographies of women who'd been psychiatrically treated or hospitalized—women who were unable to leave home, or to lead lives outside the family. I read novels and poems about sad, mad, bad women; and devoured mythology and anthropology, especially about goddesses, matriarchies, and Amazon warrior women. I interviewed the real experts: women who had been psychiatric and psychotherapy patients. I interviewed white women and women of color, heterosexual women and lesbians, middle-class women and women on welfare, women who ranged in age from seventeen to seventy women whose experiences in mental asylums and therapy spanned a quarter century.

And so I began to document how patriarchal culture and consciousness had shaped human psychology for thousands of years. I was charting the psychology of human beings who, as a caste, did not control the means of production or reproduction and who were in addition routinely shamed—sexually and in other ways. I was trying to understand what a struggle for freedom might entail, psychologically, when the colonized group was female.

Women and Madness received hundreds of positive reviews, and over the years more than two and a half million copies were sold. However, those in positions of institutional power either ignored the challenge this book posed, or said that, by definition, *any* feminist work was biased, "neurotic," and "hysterical." (Yes, our critics psychiatrically pathologized an entire movement and the work it inspired—much as individual women were pathologized.) Some said my feminist views were "strident" (how they loved that word), "man-hating," and "too angry."

Piffle.

What has really changed since I wrote this book? The answer is too little—and quite a lot. Although there has been enormous progress—a sea change even—the clinical biases I first wrote about in 1972 still exist today. Many clinical judgments remain clouded by classism, racism, anti-Semitism, homophobia, ageism, and sexism. I have reviewed hundreds, possibly thousands, of psychiatric and psychological assessments in matrimonial, criminal, and civil lawsuits. The clinical distrust of mothers, simply because they are women, the eagerness to bend over backward to like fathers, simply because they are men, is mind-numbing. Mother-blaming and woman-hatred fairly sizzle on clinical pages.

Even many of those clinicians who are less likely to gender-stereotype still exhibit (often unconscious) preference for men over women. Their sexism may be sophisticated, subtle. Often, female clinicians are much harder on women than are male clinicians. They may feel they have to be—as a way of distancing themselves from a despised group. One 1990 study confirmed that there was less gender-stereotyping among psychiatrists in 1990 than in 1970. However, more of the female psychiatrists rated "masculine" traits as optimal for female patients while more male psychiatrists chose "undifferentiated, androgynous" traits as optimal for both male and female patients.

Continuing clinical bias affects women in at least five important areas: women (and to a lesser extent, men) with medical illnesses are often, and wrongfully, psychiatrically diagnosed and medicated. Women who allege sex discrimination, harassment, rape, incest, or battery are being ordered into therapy and/or diagnostically pathologized at trial. Women (and men) who have no money and no insurance cannot afford therapy nor are they always respected or understood by therapists who are middle-class in orientation. Women of color, Jewish and other Semitic women (and to a lesser extent, men) still face an extra level of clinical fear and hostility. Psychotherapist-patient sexual abuse still exists.

While society has changed, it also remains the same. For some, family life has changed radically in the last twenty-five years. Nearly half of all marriages end in divorce; many mothers are daring to leave men who abuse them and their children. Lesbians and gay men are creating alternative families and raising children.

Nevertheless, most girls and boys continue to experience childhood in father-dominated, father-absent, and/or mother-blaming families. Sex-role stereotyping still exists in many homes, as does, though to a lesser extent, maternal and paternal child abuse. Incest and family violence remain epidemic but have, increasingly, been depoliticized. First, by women who believe that "going public" might help them. Second, by the media, which are all too happy to capitalize on the entertainment value of their public confessions. And third, by the understandable but misguided belief in the power of individual "therapeutic" solutions as opposed to collective legal or social justice solutions.

The cumulative effect of being forced to lead circumscribed lives is toxic. The psychic toll is measured in anxiety, depression, phobias, suicide attempts, eating disorders, addictions, alcoholism, and such stress-related illnesses as high blood pressure and heart disease. It is therefore not surprising that many women still behave as if they've been colonized.

The image of women as colonized is a useful one. It explains why some women cling to their colonizers the way a child or a hostage clings to an abusive parent or a captor; why many women blame themselves, or other women, when they are captured (she really "wanted" it, she freely "chose" it); and why most women defend their colonizers' right to possess them (God or nature has "ordained" it).

In *Women and Madness,* I described asylums as dangerous patriarchal institutions. Tragically, such snake pits still exist in the United States today, in which patients are wrongfully medicated, utterly neglected, and psychologically and sexually abused.

Women who have been repeatedly raped in childhood—often by authority figures in their own families—are traumatized human beings; as such, they are often diagnosed as borderline personalities. If they are institutionalized, they are rarely treated as the torture victims they really are. On the contrary, in state custody, women are more, not less, likely to be raped again (and each time is more, not less, traumatic). Instead of being trained to understand this, most institutional staff—psychiatrists, psychologists, nurses, and attendants alike—do not believe the rape victims, nor do they think of a rape as a lifelong trauma.

There is no excuse for subjecting institutional inmates to the same awful conditions that existed in the nineteenth century. By this, I am referring to solitary confinement, restraints, unending physical and psychological cruelty, and criminality unrestrained among the inmates by overworked or punitive staff.

Institutional psychiatry may fail us, but madness still exists. I said so in 1972, but I also said that most women were not mad, merely seen as such. My own and other historical accounts of asylums strongly suggest that most women in asylums were not insane; that help was not to be found in doctor-headed, attendant-staffed, and state-run institutions; that what we call "madness" can also be caused or exacerbated by injustice and cruelty, within the family and society; and that freedom, radical legal reform, political struggle, and kindness are crucial to psychological and moral health.

On the other hand, the family members and friends of people who suffer from schizophrenia or manic depression know that something is seriously "wrong" with a relative who can no longer eat or sleep, hears voices, can't work, is afraid to leave the house, has become suicidal, or verbally and physically aggressive. They see they are suffering, learn that they cannot help them or even continue to live with them. Families of the mentally ill often see major improvements with psychiatric medication and psychotherapy and are concerned about the right to treatment.

Obviously, consumer education and legal action remain crucial in the struggle to humanize both institutional and noninstitutional life.

Often those who condemn institutional psychiatric medication, shock therapy—any kind of therapy-for-hire—do not feel responsible for the female casualties of patriarchy. Such critics, even if well-intentioned, may be confusing the fact that quality mental health care is not available to all who want it with the question of whether quality mental health care exists at all.

So what did I mean when I said that quite a lot has changed in the last twenty-five years? For one thing, we've learned more about the genetic and chemical bases of mental illness. We've learned that those suffering from manic depression, depression, or schizophrenia often respond to the right drug at the right dosage level; that all drugs have negative side effects; that we shouldn't prescribe the same drug for everyone, especially without continually monitoring the side effects; and that supportive therapies are often impossible with such medication.

Despite the progress in biological psychiatry, both women and men are still wrongfully or overly medicated—or denied proper medication—by harried psychiatrists and psychopharmacologists. Psychiatric inpatients are often overly medicated for the convenience of staff, who do not always treat the to-be-expected side effects with compassion or expertise.

As bad as many institutions are, turning the mentally ill loose, into the streets, is not the solution; it is merely another unacceptable alternative. People do have a right to treatment, if that treatment exists. I realize this statement is almost laughable today, given how insurance and drug companies, managed care, and government spending cuts have made quality psychotherapy totally out of reach for most people. This means that just when we know what to do for the victims of trauma, there are very few teaching hospitals and clinics that treat poor women in feminist ways.

Medication by itself is never enough. Women who are clinically depressed or anxious also need access to feminist information and support.

What does a feminist therapist do that's different? A feminist therapist tries to *believe* what women say. Given the history of psychiatry and psychoanalysis, this alone is a radical act. When a woman begins to remember being sexually molested as a child, a feminist does not conclude that the woman's flashbacks or "hysteria" prove that she's lying or "crazy."

A feminist therapist *believes* that a woman needs to be told that she's not "crazy"; that it's normal to feel sad or angry about being overworked, underpaid, underloved; that it 's healthy to harbor fantasies of running away when the needs of others (aging parents, needy husbands, demanding children) threaten to overwhelm her.

A feminist therapist believes that women need to hear that men "don't love enough" before they're told that women "love too much"; that fathers are equally responsible for their children's problems; that absolutely no one—not even feminist, self-appointed saviors—can rescue a woman but herself. A feminist therapist *believes* that self-love is the basis for love of others; that it's hard to break free of patriarchy and that the struggle to do so is both miraculous and lifelong; that very few of us know how to support women in flight from, or at war with, internalized self-hatred and violence against women and children.

A feminist therapist tries to listen to women respectfully, and does not minimize the extent to which a woman has been wounded. A feminist therapist remains resolutely optimistic because no woman, no matter now wounded she may be, is beyond the reach of human community and compassion.

A feminist therapist does not label a woman mentally ill because she expresses strong emotions or is at odds with her "feminine" role. Feminists do not view women as mentally ill when they engage in sexual, reproductive, economic, or intellectual activities outside of marriage. We do not pathologize women who have full-time careers, are lesbians, refuse to marry, commit adultery, want divorces, choose to be celibate, have abortions, use birth control, have a child out of wedlock, breast-feed against expert advice, or expect men to be responsible for a full 50 percent of the child care and housework.

Some feminist theorists and therapists have been moved by the radical liberation psychology in *Women and Madness*. They agree that women's control of our bodies is as important as sexual pleasure, and that we must be able to defend "our bodies, ourselves" against violent or unwanted invasions like rape, battery, unwanted pregnancy, or unwanted sterilization.

As feminist clinician Janet Surrey says, "The work of feminist healers is to integrate our minds and our bodies, ourselves and others, human community and the life of our planet. I question our profession's fear of feminism. I practice psychology within a feminist liberation theology."

In *Trauma and Recovery,* psychiatrist Judith Lewis Herman models a new vision of therapy and of human relationships, one in which we are called upon to "bear witness to a crime" and to "affirm a position of solidarity with the victim." Herman's ideal therapist cannot be morally neutral but must make a collaborative commitment, and enter into an "existential engagement" with the traumatized. Such a therapist must listen, solemnly and without haste, to the factual and emotional details of atrocities, without flight or denial, without blaming the victim, identifying with the aggressor, or becoming a detective who "diagnoses" ritual or satanic abuse after a single session, and without "using her power over the patient to gratify her personal needs."

While the love and understanding of relatives, friends, and political movements are necessary, they are not substitutes for the hard psychological work that victims must also undertake with the assistance of trained grassroots professionals; in fact, even enlightened professionals like Herman cannot themselves undertake this work without a strong support system of their own.

Make no mistake: feminists have learned what works, what must be done. Nevertheless, the most important feminist work has been "disappeared" or never made its way into the graduate and medical school canon. This is truly astounding given that contemporary mental health professionals did not learn about incest, rape, sexual harassment, wife-beating, or child abuse from graduate or medical school textbooks but from feminist consciousness-raising and research and from grassroots activism. We all learned from the victims themselves, who had been empowered to speak not by psychoanalytic but by feminist liberation.

When I began writing *Women and Madness,* there were few feminist theories of psychology and virtually no feminist therapists. Now we are everywhere. Feminists have established journals, referral networks, conferences, and workshops—programs that are both psychoanalytic and antipsychoanalytic in orientation. We have served incest and rape survivors, battered women, batterers, mentally ill and homeless women, refugees, alcoholics, drug addicts, the disabled, the elderly—and each other. Feminists have also published many extraordinary books and articles.

Today, there are feminist psychopharmacologists; forensic experts; lesbian therapists; sex therapists, family therapists; experts on recovered memories, race, and ethnicities; and, perhaps the truest sign of having arrived: feminist critics of feminist therapy! Despite such progress, most feminists in mental health understand how much remains to be done. But we have come a long way.

We now understand that women and men are not "crazy" or "defective" when, in response to trauma, they develop post-traumatic symptoms. We recognize that trauma victims may attempt to mask these symptoms with alcohol, drugs, overeating, or extreme forms of dieting.

We now understand more about what trauma is, and what it does. We understand that chronic, hidden family/domestic violence is actually more traumatic than sudden violence at the hands of a stranger, or of an enemy during war. We understand that after even a single act of abuse, physical violence is only infrequently needed to keep one's victim in a constant state of terror, dependent on her captor and tormentor.

We understand that rape is not about love or even lust, but about humiliating another human being through forced or coerced sex and sexual shame. The intended effect of rape is always the same: to utterly break the spirit of the rape victim, to drive the victim out of her (or his) body and to make her incapable of resistance and quite often out of her mind. The effects of terror on men at war and in enemy captivity are equivalent to the trauma suffered by women at home in "domestic captivity."

What do victims of violence need to ensure their survival and to maintain their dignity? Bearing witness is important; being supported instead of punished for doing so, especially by other women, is also important. Putting one's suffering to use, through educating and supporting other victims, is important; drafting, passing, and enforcing laws is important. However, as Judith Herman has written, "The systematic study of psychological trauma… depends on the support of a political movement.… In the absence of strong political movements for human rights, the active process of bearing witness inevitably gives way to the active process of forgetting."

In my view, in addition to therapy and political movement, we also need rape prevention education, i.e., compulsory self-defense training for girls. And more: military training for girls; swift, effective prosecution of rapists; a nonstop series of successful civil suits for monetary remuneration, in addition to criminal prosecution. Perhaps most important, we need to support women who have fought back against their rapists and batterers and who are wasting away in jail for daring to save their own lives.

Despite my own early critique of private patriarchal therapy geared primarily to high-income clients, I have come to believe that women can and do benefit from feminist therapy. Some feminists have questioned whether any therapy, including feminist therapy, is desirable. They have noted, correctly, that "therapism" may indeed siphon activist energies. They are right, but severely traumatized women cannot always rise to the occasion of political action. For example, an incest survivor with insomnia or panic attacks often cannot sit in a room long enough to have her consciousness raised; an anorexic or obese woman who is obsessed with losing weight may not be able to notice others long enough to engage in fund-raising; a woman on a window ledge or in an alcoholic daze may not have the peace of mind to analyze her fate in feminist terms.

Being traumatized does not necessarily make one a noble or productive person. Some women rise above it; others don't. Some women want to be "saved"; others are too damaged to participate in their own "redemption."

A feminist author bell hooks writes: "It had become more than evident that individual black females suffering psychologically were not prepared to go out and lead the feminist revolution.... Working with women, especially black women, I have found that many of us are willing to acknowledge the evils of sexism, the way it wounds and hurts everyone, but are reluctant to make that conversion to feminist thinking that would require substantive changes in habits of being."

This applies to women of all colors. As feminist psychotherapist E. Kitch Childs said: "We need a whole new level of consciousness-raising groups and networks. We must learn how to speak our bitterness about each other to each other. It will liberate our energies to keep on working together."

We need a Feminist Institute of Mental Health that is both local and global, a learning community that lasts beyond our lifetimes, a clinical training program that is not patriarchal, a spiritual retreat with an intellectual agenda, a health club with a political agenda, a place where feminists can come together to both learn and teach in ways that are inspired, rigorous, humane, and healing.

I wanted to create such an institute from the moment *Women and Madness* was on the way. It was too soon. Now, at last, I and many others have begun to do so. For example, the Cambridge Hospital Victims of Violence (VOV) Program was cofounded in Massachusetts in 1984 by psychologist Mary Harvey and Judith Herman. It offers crisis intervention, supportive therapy, and group support to "survivors of rape, incest and childhood sexual abuse, domestic violence, and physical abuse/assault." A multidiciplinary staff develops programs, presents workshops, and conducts in-service trainings. VOV offers support groups in Trauma Information, Parenting for Mothers with Trauma Histories, Time-Limited Rape Survivors Groups, Male Survivors of Childhood Trauma, etc.

We need such programs in every city, every community, worldwide.

I am currently associated with the Choices Mental Health Center, which, as the Women's Medical Center, Inc., started a rape crisis center in 1991, and became a fully licensed mental health clinic in 1995. Since 1971, women had been coming to the Choices Women's Medical Center for abortions and other reproductive health services; they talked about being raped, battered, drug-addicted, and victims of incest. Choices has now begun to offer short-term, crisis-oriented feminist therapy for the adult victims of violence on an HMO, Medicaid, or fee-for-service basis. The center is also beginning to work with children and with batterers who are court-ordered into treatment. We envision creating and consulting on similar programs both nationally and internationally.

Freedom and justice do wonders for one's mental health. So, in response to my brother Sigmund Freud's infamous query, what do women want? For starters, and in no particular order: freedom, food, nature, shelter, leisure, freedom from violence, justice, music, poetry, nonpatriarchal family, community, compassionate support during chronic or life-threatening illness and at the time of death, independence, books, physical/sexual pleasure, education, solitude, the ability to defend ourselves, love, ethical friendships, the arts, health, dignified employment, and political comrades.

Airless Spaces

SHULAMITH FIRESTONE

Shulamith Firestone, *Airless Spaces,* New York, Semiotext(e), 1998. Reprinted by permission

Refusing a career as a professional feminist, Shulamith Firestone has found herself in an "airless space" since the publication of her first book, *The Dialectic of Sex.* Lost women in and out of (mental) hospitals are the lens through which Shulamith Firestone views the cultural shrinking of individuality. Using the small crises in the lives of women who are continually framed inside and outside of institutional walls, Firestone illustrates the limits of experience, consciousness, and space at the end of this century.

PATCHES

When she came out of the hospital, her Levi's no longer fit her. She dug through her hand-me-downs to find a pair of scruffy light blue jeans with big rips at the knees that she had found thrown out in front of an old brownstone. She wore them through the winter with long johns underneath the rip, until at last when spring came, the rip had widened to way beyond fashionable, and it was time to invest in a new pair. Her figure eventually wasn't going to return. After a confusing and fruitless shopping trip to Canal Jeans, where all three used Levi's were incorrectly sized, and she fled the jammed dressing rooms in despair that she no longer was able to shop, she finally settled on the first pair of jeans about her size she saw on an outdoor rack. They had a hole in exactly the same place as the previous jeans, the right knee, but it was a smaller hole, and since the jeans were a little long she figured unless she wore a belt the tension point of the knee would not fall exactly on the hole and widen it to a rip again. There was a long line waiting for the dressing room, and she didn't have the heart to go through all the jeans in the rack to find the one with a less obtrusive hole, and the very handsome salesboy let her know she couldn't tie up the dressing room any longer even if she wanted to. So she plumped down fifteen bucks, which was the lowest sale price for levis anywhere, holes or no holes. Besides, she had already invested $2 in an iron-on patch from Woolworth's for the old pair, but it was the wrong color for the new pair.

Still stiff from the Haldol she was on, she prevailed upon a friend to help her iron the patch on the new jeans before the hole should widen in the wash. Her little ironing board did not hold up, so they had to use a towel on her butcher block kitchen table, unplugging the refrigerator to find a near outlet. But after forty-five minutes the patch began to unpeel around the edges and they had to clumsily sew it on, wrong color, oversized, and scrubby, with no guarantee it wouldn't come out in the wash anyway, since she had neglected to sew together the hole before ironing on the patch.

Thus it was that she went from scruffy fashionable with splits at the knees to pickaninny-in-patches wherever she went.

PASSABLE, NOT PRESENTABLE

She remembered the time before she had gotten sick. When it was a challenge to dress, how good it felt to look just right and be certain of one's appearance. Then came losing her looks in the hospital, and the ghastly difference it made in the way she was received; the way people turned away from her after one glance in the street. And the slow climb back, trying to disguise the stiffness in her gait, and the drooling moronic look on her face that came from the medication. Perhaps this was why the mentally disabled always seemed so bland-looking as a group: they had to strive to look ordinary, to "pass." That little bit of extra aplomb that made one stand out of the crowd was beyond them.

Chapter 68

Sexual and Reproductive Health

T*he point and counterpoint between carefree sex and sexually transmitted diseases (STDs) goes on. The STDs are winning, so it is "back to the barriers" at many student health services and clinics.*

And yes, the contraceptive experimentation on women goes on as well. I still say it isn't fair to leave men out of it. Here's my modest proposal. We should vasectomize all boys at age 13, freeze their sperm, and allow them to unfreeze it when they have saved enough money to provide for a child through age 18. This would serve a double purpose of eliminating deadbeat dads.

Yes, I'm kidding, but maybe the threat of such a measure would at least get men to carry condoms in their wallets.—B. S.

Empowering the Pelvic Exam

LILA A. WALLIS

From *The Whole Woman: Take Charge of Your Health in Every Phase Of Your Life,* by Lila A. Wallis, M.D., with Marian Betancourt (Avon, 1999). Copyright ©1999 by Lila A. Wallis and Marian Betancourt.

Historically, pelvic exams were so unpleasant and hurtful that women avoided them at all costs, even it they had symptoms that needed to be checked. There is no reason for a painful pelvic exam—other then the physician's failure to learn how to make it painless.

Few women know that! They have hated the clinical invasion of their bodies, the sight and cold feel of a steel instrument (the speculum) entering that private space. In addition to the discomfort and pain, women resented the frequently unfeeling, brusque, and condescending attitude of the doctor.

The women's health movement of the 1960s, 1970s, and 1980s exposed the patronizing attitudes of many physicians toward their female patients. The pelvic exam became a symbol of female subjugation and abuse. A call was issued for a more meaningful partnership between the physician and patient regarding her care and the examination of her reproductive organs. What follows are suggestions for women who desire more involvement in their gynecological care as well as freedom from the shame and secrecy historically attached to their own bodies.

The doctor should communicate with you as a partner in your care and let you know what will be happening during each step of the examination. The first pelvic examination for a young woman should include an explanation of the anatomy. Ask if there is a plastic model or detailed illustration of the anatomy available to make the instruction clear. This will give you a better idea of what the doctor is going to do during the examination. Hold the speculum in your hands and ask what part of the instrument actually goes into your vagina.

The doctor should ask you about you sexual experience as well, whether or not you are a virgin, if you have had sex, whether any part of it was painful and if you used contraceptives. The doctor should ask if you have been performing breast self-exams or if you have noticed any changes in your vulva. This lets you know your doctor considers you a partner in your health care.

The physician's hands and instruments must be warm, and he or she should tell you before touching each part of your body. The caring physician should also offer you some choices about how you wish to proceed by asking you some questions.

➤Do you want to be draped during the exam? The drape is used to avoid exposing your body and to create a sense of privacy. However, if you want to watch the examination or see with the aid of a mirror, then you would not have a drape.

➤Would you like to watch? If you would, ask if your head can be elevated, the drape displaced. A mirror and lamp can be arranged so that you can see your own vulva, vagina, and cervix. This is the beginning of empowerment. It involves you in the process.

➤Are you able to relax? It is impossible to be totally relaxed during a pelvic exam, but your physician can teach you some ways to relax your perineal and abdominal muscles. First tighten these muscles, as if you were interrupting urination, and then relax them several times before the instrument or doctor's fingers are inserted. Take deep breaths or a series of painting breaths to relax.

➤Are you comfortable in the foot brackets? These can be shortened to allow your knees to bend. This helps you bear down when necessary, so the cervix moves closer to the vaginal opening. If you had a condition that made your movements difficult, such as arthritis, you should ask for the foot brackets to be lengthened. If you do not like putting your heel into the cold metal foot bracket, keep your socks and shoes on or ask for foam booties.

Above all, the examination should be gentle. No doctor would consider being brusque or squeezing hard on a man's testicles, so expect the same sensitivity from a physician who is palpating your ovaries and uterus.

WHAT THE PELVIC EXAM INCLUDES

A doctor performing a pelvic examination is following a certain procedure designed to provide information. There is usually a nurse present during the examination because assistance is sometimes needed. You always need to empty your bladder before a pelvic exam because a full bladder makes it difficult for the physician to feel the internal organs. There are five parts to the exam.

EXTERNAL GENITALIA First, the doctor will examine the vulva, clitoris, labia, and glandular ducts to look for anything out of the ordinary. After examining the external genitalia some doctors may wish to do a "mini pelvic," using one finger to identify the position and direction of the cervix for the speculum insertion.

SPECULUM EXAM The speculum is an instrument that is inserted into the vagina and pushes the walls of the vagina apart to allow light and other instruments to be inserted. The speculum should be warmed first by holding it under warm water. As long as they are cleaned and sterilized after each use they don't need to remain sterile; the vagina is not sterile. Some doctors use disposable plastic specula. These are thicker than the ones made of steel, they make a loud click when they are opened or locked, and might frighten the patient.

A smaller, narrower speculum is used when a girl's hymen is still intact. If insertion is difficult, the doctor might teach the girl how to gently dilate her hymen and come back for the completion of the exam.

COLLECTIONS OF SPECIMENS

These specimens are taken for routine laboratory studies. While the speculum is inserted, the doctor can insert instruments such as cotton-tipped applicators, cervical brushes, and wooden scrapers and take scrapings and specimens of secretions from the cervix and vagina or endometrium for various tests, such as a Pap smear and sexually transmitted disease cultures.

BIMANUAL VAGINOABDOMINAL EXAM This means the doctor is using both hands, one inside your vagina and one outside your body, pressing on various locations on your abdomen. The uterus, ovaries, and tubes are located, and any abnormalities are detected. The uterine size might alert the doctor to the possibility of pregnancy, an irregular uterine outline to the possibility of fluids. The ovaries and tubes are usually small. Often they are difficult to palpate either because a patient cannot relax her abdominal muscles, or because she is overweight and a layer of fat interferes, or she has intestinal bloating. In that case, a pelvic sonogram would be needed to visualize the ovaries.

BIMANUAL RECTOVAGINAL EXAM Here the doctor inserts his or her middle finger into the rectum and the index finger into the vagina while pressing with the other hand on the abdomen to recheck the findings of the bimanual vagino-abdominal exam. Ovaries are found in the back of the uterus so they are better palpated on the rectovaginal exam. Standard procedure for this examination is to check any fecal matter on the doctor's glove for blood, which could indicate the presence of ulcerative colitis, a bleeding peptic ulcer, polyps, colorectal cancer, hemorrhoids, or fissures and lacerations from rectal intercourse.

FORMULATION: DIALOGUE WITH THE DOCTOR

Once again, get fully dressed after the examination before you talk with the doctor. One woman told me her doctor discussed his findings with her for ten minutes while she sat naked and vulnerable, having just had a breast exam in the examination room.

Once you are dressed and back in your doctor's office, you will hear what the doctor has to say. I call this step "formulation." This is a summary of what has been found on examination. Your doctor should explain the working—or possible—diagnosis as well as other possibilities, and what additional tests might be needed to confirm the diagnosis. If the working diagnosis is correct, then expect a detailed explanation of recommended treatment.

Now is the time to ask some questions. Don't be embarrassed to ask the doctor to repeat things you missed, to define medical jargon, explain your procedures, draw clear pictures for you, or refer to medical diagrams and illustrations.

Listen carefully and take good notes or have your friend or relative take the notes. If medications are prescribed, write down instructions for their use. Ask about side effects and remind your doctor of other drugs you take, including oral contraceptives or hormone therapy, in case there is potential for additional side effects. Find out if a generic drug can be substituted. Some insurance plans will pay only for generic drugs. Some will pay for certain drugs. Often the newest or most expensive drugs are not included.

If the proposed plan of action interferes with your work schedule or other plans, ask the doctor to work out a more convenient timetable, as long as it does not endanger your health.

Find out when results of your blood and urine tests will be available, and ask that a copy be sent to you, or ask if you may call the doctor the next week and ask about the findings. Ask if you should call the doctor with a report of your condition—for better or worse—in a few days or weeks.

Before you go home, make a follow-up appointment if you need one. As soon as you get home, bring your Woman's Health Record up-to-date.

Once you find a competent, compassionate, considerate and thorough physician, take good care of her or him. Even if you see this doctor only for yearly physical checkups, you are building a relationship of trust and mutual respect. Now you have the peace of mind of knowing you have someone to call if you are ill.

Self-Helpless Gynecology

CAEDMON MAGBOO CAHILL

In this exploratory paper Caedmon Magboo Cahill spoke to 10 college-age women to understand how the women's health movement of the 1970s affected their attitudes, growing up in the 1990s, toward the pelvic exam and the role of the doctor.

The majority of women in this ethnography want to take control over their health and their bodies, yet surprisingly look toward the doctor's validation and expertise to gain this control and to feel normal and healthy. Since the vagina is hidden and therefore can not be compared as easily as hips or breasts—there is no cultural norm of what the vagina should look or feel like—instead young women turn to what the gynecologist has accepted as standard....

Many of my informants feel that once they are at the recommended age for the exam, their reproductive organs are now in the domain of the medical authorities, and have difficulty learning the intricacies and details of their own body on their own. There is an understanding among these women that only through a mastery of women's genitalia, something medical professionals assume, can they then self-diagnose or determine what they feel is normal. The responsibility many of these women feel to "take care of themselves" by their yearly gynecological examination in part stems from this feeling that they are in possession of something far more medically important and medically complicated than to trust themselves....

The women interviewed describe themselves as feeling vulnerable and often embarrassed during the exam; vulnerability they attribute to the doctor's presence, and embarrassment due to the exposure of their vagina. Many women expect this vulnerability and embarrassment and accept it as an inherent part to the exam, yet still feel safer under medical authority, rather than in their own hands.

Many women leave the exploration of their vagina up to the gynecologist entirely. Not only do they not feel comfortable deciding what feels normal or healthy, but they also do not feel comfortable learning about their vagina outside of the doctor's office. It is clear that women depend on the doctor to mediate between themselves and their pelvis. When asked whether they performed pelvic self exams all of the women answered no. Most explain that they do not feel capable to perform the exam and some feel uncomfortable to even look into their vaginas....

Visiting the gynecologist allows these women to feel as if they are talking care of themselves and "getting in touch with themselves." Many women, especially those who decided to have a pelvic exam before it is usually recommended, would rather make themselves physically and emotionally uncomfortable so that they may feel satisfied, knowing they are being healthy having a doctor examine them. Some even reserve for the doctor the first touch into their vagina, for the sake of "health" and feeling "normal."

Gynecology, for these young women, is used to sustain the separation between women and their genitalia, and having pelvic exams relieves them of the responsibility of understanding their bodies personally, by their own touch and exploration. What makes gynecology particularly susceptible to this is the fact that women do not yet feel comfortable to understand their genitalia with their own hands, and unlike aches of the stomach, throat, or head, they are reluctant to seek advice outside of the doctor's office either from their mothers or friends. Only when women reclaim themselves and feel a part of their genitalia is complementary gynecological attention most effective. When the separation is diminished between themselves and their reproductive organs during the exam itself and then outside of the exam as well, young women can begin to care for and appreciate their bodies, not as reproductive machines but rather as extensions of themselves.

Norplant: The Contraception You're Stuck With

BARBARA SEAMAN

Excerpted from Barbara Seaman, "Norplant: The Contraceptive You're Stuck With," *The Doctors' Case Against The Pill,* New York, Hunter House, 1995. Reprinted by permission.

G regory Pincus, a father of the pill, was wary of estrogen, uncomfortable with its possible role in the development of cancer. His dream was to create a progestin-only contraceptive, and that is what he intended to test in his historic 1956 Puerto Rican clinical trials. Those were the trials, remember, when hundreds of mostly poor and uneducated Puerto Rican women were given the newly developed pill experimentally. In August 1956, several months into the study, Pincus sent a curious letter to his colleagues in San Juan. He apologized that a recent shipment of experimental pills was "contaminated" with a small amount of estrogen, and he reassured them it would not recur.

There was a problem with progestin contraceptives: they produced irregular and unpredictable spotting, or conversely, a complete absence of menstruation. Cycles ranged from just a few days in length to many months, a condition aptly called *menstrual chaos*. Pincus, after wavering back and forth, eventually put estrogen back into the pill being tested.

How much Pincus wavered is evidenced in his papers, which are now available at the Library of Congress and comprise 213 containers, 85.2 feet of shelf space, and approximately 44,000 items. His records reveal an awesome scientific and entrepreneurial brinkmanship and make one wonder why he didn't burn the evidence.

Evidence of what?

Well, for example, evidence that late in the study, the FDA informed Pincus that he would need a control group, and when the recruiter at the Family Planning Association in Rio Pedras could get no volunteers, Pincus instructed her to relabel the drop out fulds as "controls.

This made the records especially confusing, since it wasn't until May 1959 that the then-final formula, with the final amount of estrogen officially added to the progestin, was fabricated and shipped to the trial participants. Thus, the so-called control group was not only a drop-out group, but it was a drop-out group from a different pill.

It is interesting to note that female medical students and nurses at the University of San Juan were fearful of the study and refused to participate. According to a doctor who corresponded with Pincus, the medical students were punished with lower grades. The letters don't say what happened to the nurses.

THE PROGESTIN-ONLY CONTRACEPTIVE YOU CAN'T QUIT ON YOUR OWN

Since the days of the very first pills, the fatal flaw in progestin-only contraceptives has never been overcome. These products may be safer than those containing estrogen. They may be less associated with cancer, blood clots, and other crippling side effects, though whether or not all progestins are truly less of a cancer risk than estrogens remains unknown. But no scientist has ever been able to make them mimic the normal menstrual cycle in a majority of users.

Despite the menstrual chaos so often precipitated by progestin-only pills, they arrived on the market in the late 1960s, about 10 years after Pincus' first pill, Enovid. Today these brands include Micronor and Nor-Q-D (both of which contain norethindrone, the first orally effective progestin) and Ovrette (which contains norgestrel and which some doctors suggest women might wish to "testdrive" if they are contemplating Norplant).

Norplant is a system of six matchstick-size Silastic capsules, which are implanted in the fleshy underside of a woman's arm, above the elbow. They contain levonorgestrel, a synthetic progestin, which slowly leaks out of the capsules and enters the bloodstream, providing a high degree of protection against pregnancy for up to five years.

Research for the development of Norplant was begun in the 1960s by Drs. Sheldon Segal and Horacio Croxatto of the Population Council, a not-for-profit organization dedicated to global population control. More than 10 compounds were evaluated and discarded.

A troubling fact about Norplant is that although it was tested for decades prior to receiving FDA approval, some of it worst "bugs" have never been corrected, and vital questions about long-term safety remain unanswered.

Norplant has a three-fold effect. About half the time, it suppresses ovulation. However, should ovulation occur, Norplant has thickened the cervical mucus, preventing migration of sperm through the cervical canal to the uterus. Finally, Norplant suppresses the endometrium, so a pregnancy cannot be supported.

THE SELLING OF NORPLANT

In 1983, Finland became the first country to license Norplant, and Leiras Pharmaceuticals became its manufacturer. Although the product is assembled in Finland, its constituent hormone—levonorgestrel—is owned by U.S. manufactured Wyeth-Ayerst, who is also the distributor in the United States.

While Leiras has kept the price to developing countries at $23 per set, the cost in the United States was set much higher. Wyeth-Ayerst obtains its capsules from Leiras, repackages them with a few inexpensive items such as a plastic inserter, and resells the kits for at least $350 wholesale. The health care provider or pharmacy may then add a retail mark-up, which averages $75.

Norplant insertion runs $100 to $250, and removal runs as high as $400 to $500. Thus, the cost for a woman in the United States to try Norplant today can be over $1000.

Price notwithstanding, Norplant's debut in the United States in 1991 was most auspicious, due in part to aggressive promotion by Wyeth-Ayerst and the Population Council.

HOW SAFE IS NORPLANT?

The answer to the question of Norplant's safety, in terms of immediate deaths and disabilities, would seem favorable. Cynthia Pearson of the National Women's Health Network has received reports of only one death, and that was from general anesthesia used during a difficult removal.

Is it all right to insert Norplant immediately after childbirth, or should implantation be deferred? The Population Council warns against giving Norplant to nursing mothers, but this advice is often breached. Traces of Norplant occur in breast milk; how might this hormone exposure effect the nursing baby when she or he grows up?

In addition to unanswered questions, the evidence we do have about Norplant is not entirely unbiased. In large-scale surveillance studies of Norplant, the comparison or control groups tend to be IUD users. IUDs also create a measure of menstrual chaos, as well as pelvic inflammatory disease, so studies cannot tell us how Norplant users fare compared to women with normal, healthy menstruation.

Some women on Norplant may bleed for two to three weeks, then spot for any number of days, then bleed again for another two to three weeks. Other women may go several months without a period, then bleed or spot irregularly.

OTHER SIDE EFFECTS

Besides menstrual chaos, other side effects of Norplant have been reported: gain or loss of more than five pounds (32 percent), headaches, nervousness, or depression (15 to 33 percent); androgenic effects, including acne, growth of facial hair, and loss of scalp hair (up to 15 percent). Less common but also notable side effects include dizziness, breast soreness and nipple discharge, nausea, rashes, and infection or chronic pain at the insertion site.

These side effects, however, don't normally kill. The Norplant manufacturer relays warnings of more crippling or lethal complications, most of which are associated with blood clots. These warnings are based on experience with estrogen-containing contraceptives and may or may not be applicable to Norplant, or, if applicable, may occur much less frequently than with combination estrogen-progestin pills. It is hard to understand why, after decades of development, scientists have not yet determined whether Norplant may be implicated in strokes, heart attacks, birth defects, blood clots, or cancer, and why no solid information about long-term side effects exists. In the blunt words of Native American health advocate Charon Asetoyer, "The manufacturers of Norplant are marketing their product based on an assumption that the drug is not dangerous. There is no proof of this. Such overt negligence is inexcusable on the part of the company."

Wyeth-Ayerst, the U.S. distributor, lists the following as absolute contraindications for Norplant's use:

➤Pregnancy
➤Acute liver disease, noncancerous or cancerous liver tumors
➤Unexplained vaginal bleeding
➤Breast cancer
➤Blood clots in the legs, lungs, or eyes

Patient information pamphlets place other conditions in a "gray zone"— meaning they do not preclude Norplant use, but require medical supervision. These include: breast nodules or other abnormalities; diabetes; elevated blood fats; high blood pressure; headaches; gallbladder, heart or kidney disease; history of scanty or irregular menstruation; and smoking.

Norplant users are advised to expect tenderness and swelling in the upper inner arm for a couple of days, while the insertion site heals. The implication is that, thereafter, the discomfort disappears. For many women, perhaps a majority, this is simply not so: a low to moderate level of tenderness, and sometimes inflammation, persists.

THE IMPACT OF NORPLANT ON A WOMAN'S LIFE

The World Health Organization, the Population Council, and the Norplant manufacturer have all set standards and conditions to be met before Norplant use, including a pregnancy test to assure that the patient is not pregnant, and a complete medical history. In addition, Norplant should not be given to a nursing woman, and no woman should be pressured to use it.

These guidelines, however, are often disregarded. Nursing mothers have routinely been started on Norplant without being advised that hormone residue will appear in their breast milk. Since women cannot remove their capsules without medical intervention, they become captive to them, regardless of worries or side effects. Even satisfied women who keep their implants for five years must in the end have them removed but may not be able to afford the often hefty price for the removal. They have no choice but to leave them in and suffer the consequences.

Providers of Norplant make little or no effort to grasp what the menstrual chaos may mean in a woman's life. In Thailand, on the one hand, pharmacist Judith Richter observed that at one hospital, half of the women provided with Norplant were prostitutes. When bleeding, they were unable to work and were deprived of their livelihood. In Indonesia, on the other hand, social anthropologist Jannemieke Hanhart learned that many Norplant recipients couldn't work because they were devout followers of Islam and, under Islamic law, women cannot pray, cook, wash their hair, fetch rice from the rice barn, plant certain crops, have intercourse, or participate in social ceremonies while they are bleeding. The women in one village lived seven kilometers from a water source; their water was carried on horseback or motorcycle to the village, so the more frequent washing of themselves and their clothing during menstruation was onerous.

If there is a positive outcome from the menstrual chaos caused by Norplant, it is that the most popular argument for omitting barrier methods from population programs has finally been laid to rest. In *The Politics of Contraception,* Dr. Carl Djerassi, the father of modern progestins took issue with this author and other health feminists for suggesting that women in developing countries should be offered barrier contraceptives: "On safety grounds the diaphragm is clearly the best female contraceptive, and... may be ideal... for the motivated American woman willing to use it, but it is totally unsuitable for the impoverished woman living in a hovel lacking running water, toilet and privacy.... How can an affluent American female recommend to her impoverished sister in some Asian country that she use a diaphragm when this woman has not even any storage place for it or the jelly?" Norplant, which requires the most washing up of any contraceptive, opens the door for promoting safer methods.

THE POTENTIAL ABUSE OF WOMEN'S RIGHTS

Norplant presents abundant opportunities for coercion and social control. In Indonesia, where the government is making efforts at population control, the army has been used to scare people into trying implants.

No sooner was Norplant approved in the United States, than some judges, penal authorities, and state legislators moved to use it coercively. They recommended a two-pronged approach: rewards, such as paying welfare mothers to go on it, and punishments, such as sending abusive mothers to jail if they refused it.

A report by the Hastings Center suggests the following guidelines for policy makers and health care providers for "the safe and respectful use of Norplant."

➤ *Fair pricing.* "The current pricing structure of Wyeth-Ayerst is questionable and should be changed.... [Norplant's] development and testing were supported by the federal government and private foundations," so the company can't claim it is only trying to recoup its development expenses.

➤ *Insurance coverage.* When women have public or private insurance coverage for Norplant or IUDs at the time of insertion, they risk being uninsured when they wish its removal. "Financial guarantees of removal should be extended at the time of insertion.... Insurance coverage of removals should be unconditional."

➤*Service delivery systems.* If skillful insertion and removal and appropriate follow-up care are lacking, the method should not be offered.

➤*Availability to adolescents.* As with adults, appropriate access requires adherence to informed consent and confidentiality.

➤*No links to public assistance.* Making Norplant use a requirement for receiving public assistance is inappropriate. "A woman's health may make it dangerous for her to use a hormonal method, or she may be unable to tolerate the side effects.... Her local health care system may lack personnel with adequate training and expertise.... She may be celibate or perfectly happy with her current method and competent in its use."

WHAT DOES THE FUTURE HOLD?

The word is that Norplant is in trouble. Sales are down to the point that the Population Council—which counted on a certain royalty from the sale of the implant—has had to freeze salaries.

Three separate class-action lawsuits seeking damage for hundreds of users have been filed. The plaintiffs assert that they were sorely wounded by Norplant, suffering "severe pain and scarring" when their practitioners attempted to remove the contraceptive. Either large, impenetrable masses of scar tissue, called "fibrous envelopes," formed around the capsules, or the capsules were incorrectly implanted and proved difficult to find, or the capsules broke, or they dislodged from their original location and moved to areas deeper in the body, or the practitioners lacked training and expertise in removal. How much more responsible and productive the introduction of Norplant could have been if these concerns had been taken seriously and the following suggestions thoroughly addressed.

First, no coercion will be used. Second, no practitioner will be licensed to place Norplant until she or he has demonstrated skill at removal. Third, every practitioner inserting Norplant must sign a document agreeing to remove the capsule, free of charge, at the user's request. Fourth, no woman with any of the problems Charon Asetoyer mentions—overweight, diabetic, or a heavy drinker—will be given Norplant until the health concerns about these matters are clarified by the industry. Fifth, veterans of studies in remote places must be located and assisted with contraceptive removal. Sixth, women whose activities, religious or mundane, would be sabotaged by menstrual chaos will be offered Norplant only if they fully understand what might happen. Seventh, along with her $600 Norplant installation kit, a patient will receive a generous supply of condoms—in a variety of colors and textures—and be reminded that, with or without Norplant, sex can kill, and barrier methods must be used as well.

Today, we check the claims for new products. With Norplant, women's health advocates are performing and publishing their own studies, and pooling information at international conferences. In the United States, through such organizations as the National Women's Health Network, the Boston Women's Health Book Collective, the Black Women's Health Project, the Native American Women's Health Education Resource Center, and the Committee on Women, Population and the Environment, we are spreading awareness.

Quinacrine Alert

MARLENE FRIED

Marlene Fried, "Quinacrine Alert: Controversial Sterilization Pellet May Be Used In U.S.," *Sojourner,* March 1999. Reprinted by permission.

A doctor in Ft. Lauderdale, Florida, may soon begin using quinacrine, the "controversial method to sterilize women without surgery," despite the fact that the Food and Drug Administration (FDA) has not approved the drug for sterilization purposes, the *Miami Herald* reported.

Quinacrine, originally developed as an anti-malarial drug, is a form of chemical sterilization for women. It is inserted in pellet form into the uterus. There it discovers, traveling into the fallopian tubes, causing scarring. The resulting scar tissue blocks the tubes, causing irreversible sterilization. Preliminary studies link quinacrine with potential risks of cancer, ectopic pregnancy, fetal damage, and toxicity. Moreover, quinacrine may be less effective than surgical sterilization. Presently, no regulatory body supports the use of quinacrine as a sterilant.

Yet Dr. Michael Benjamin, part of an activist group of doctors who says it believes quinacrine will improve women's health, calls the chemical pellet "a practical answer to one of the world's biggest problems—overpopulation." Benjamin said he would provide quinacrine free to low-income Florida women and for $200 to women who can afford to pay. On his web page, at http://www.drbenjamin.com/QS.htm, Benjamin states that "we are eagerly awaiting the first shipment of Quinacrine in pellet form to be produced in the U.S. We expect no difficulty in making QS [quinacrine sterilization] immediately available to the significant segment of our family planning patients who wish to be sterile but for medical, financial or psychological reasons are not candidates for surgery."

Since the FDA permits approved drugs to be used "off label"—that is, for uses other than the ones for which they were originally licensed—doctors can prescribe quinacrine, an approved antimalarial, for whatever purposes they wish. The FDA told the *Miami Herald* that it has, however, "cracked down on quinacrine self-sterilization kits sold over the Internet."

Use of the drug for sterilization purposes has been debated internationally, with questions raised about its medical hazards and the motives of immigration-control groups promoting and funding its use in developing countries.

Vietnam, Chile, and India have banned the drug, and a Swiss company that made the pellets announced that it would no longer manufacture them. As the *Miami Herald* noted, opponents contend that the use of quinacrine "smacks of eugenics, racism and contraceptive imperialism."

Proponents of the "Q-method" contend that it is "safer and cheaper than surgical sterilization," and anticipate that it will eventually "outpac[e] even the pill." Quinacrine primary distributors are the North Carolina-based Center for Research on Population and Security, headed by Stephen Mumford, and the International Federation for Family Health, headed by Elton Kessel. Mumford and Kessel have distributed quinacrine in 19 countries around the world, including Bangladesh, Chile, China, Costa Rica, Croatia, Egypt, India, Indonesia, Iran, Pakistan, the Philippines, Venezuela, Vietnam, the United States, and possibly in Brazil, Guatemala, Thailand, Malaysia, and Romania. Mumford and Kessel believe that quinacrine is a cost-effective way to reduce population growth, since the quinacrine needed for sterilization costs less than one dollar. They claim that they are saving women's lives by preventing unwanted pregnancies in countries where there is a high risk of dying from childbirth complications.

Mumford and Kessel are now working on bringing the drug to the United States. Mumford said, "I never believed that quinacrine would be limited to the third world." Kessel has stated that official government approval is "desirable but not necessary" in the continued use of quinacrine as a sterilant. With private funding from such organizations as the Turner Foundation and Leland Fykes, Mumford and Kessel have been distributing quinacrine for free to researchers, clinicians, and government health agencies worldwide. (The Turner Foundation has recently stopped funding this work.)

For more information on quinacrine and efforts to monitor its use, contact the Committee on Women, Population and the Environment at the Population and Development Programs/SS, Hampshire College, Amherst, MA 01002. Tel: 413-559-5506; e-mail: cwpe@hampshire.edu

Sexually Transmitted Diseases on College Campuses

LORI BARER

©1999 by Lori Barer. Original for this publication.

In sharp contrast to the steady decline of teenage pregnancy, the epidemic of sexually transmitted diseases (STDs) in young adults is increasing at an alarming rate. Each year, approximately 15.3 million new cases of sexually transmitted diseases are contracted with 65 percent of those cases affecting people under the age of 25. With so many young people affected, college campuses are virtually swarming with infection. For many, college is a time of self-discovery and exploration. As the first time away from home, inhibitions are often silenced under the deafening sounds of fraternity music and drowned in cheap beer. Young adults awaken in unknown dormitory rooms with little or no recollection of the night before, not to mention the person beside them.

Young women have become at particular risk for STDs as date rape drugs become ever more popular. College parties have become sites of these drugs, such as rohypnol and gamma-hydroxy butyrate, which foster the STD epidemic with the incidence of unconsensual, and often unprotected, sex. While date rape does not account for an enormous portion of STD infections, date rape drugs are being used more and more frequently which only increases the number of young women unknowingly infected.

Forty-six percent of female college students are now infected with human papilloma virus (HPV), the same virus that causes both genital warts and cervical cancer. Many of these women will now be plagued with one or both of these ailments for the rest of their lives. Generally, women suffer greater consequences of STDs than men, in part because the infections are so often asymptomatic that care isn't sought until serious complications have developed. These complications may be of great emotional, physical, and monetary cost to the women. The societal cost of these ailments is also huge, costing taxpayers billions of dollars. In 1994 sexually transmitted diseases and their complications, not including HIV, cost the United States almost $10 billion.

Meanwhile, colleges around the country are failing to provide adequate knowledge and distribution of barrier contraception, the only reliable method for preventing STDs. Health care professionals at many colleges and universities may be too quick to prescribe birth control pills. While the pills are one of the most reliable birth control methods when used correctly, they do not provide any protection against STDs. Birth control pills, if prescribed at all, should be meant for women in monogamous relationships that have been tested (along with their partner) for sexually transmitted diseases. Instead, they are handed out faster than fliers on central campus: young people are not being careful enough

At the University of Michigan in Ann Arbor, condoms are freely displayed throughout the University Health Services. Students are often encouraged to take as many, as often, as they want. If a woman does decide she would like to use birth control pills, she must first watch a video explaining the seriousness of the pills. Then, she is given a gynecological examination, after which she can discuss the various options of birth control and the preferred options that she is interested in using with her doctor. Unless there are no medical concerns, the clinician will at that point normally prescribe the requested method. The woman is instructed to wait until the Sunday after her next period before starting the birth control pills. The women usually then have ample time to decide if the pill is the appropriate form of contraception for them. By making the birth control pills more difficult to attain, the spread of STDs is combatted at a faster rate.

Many parents feel that, even at the college level, handing out condoms promotes sexual promiscuity. Although many studies have been performed to prove this correlation, they have never been successful. However, universities often hear only the sound of crisp dollar bills, and since tuition is coming from Mom and Dad, so are the university's policies. Now we have created an environment where it is easier, and perhaps much less embarrassing, to offer medication that could very well be harmful to your health, than it would be make free condoms available at the health clinic. We have also created a lot of new STDs, wasted a lot of money and left a lot of parents wishing their children had used protection.

Chapter 69

More Motherhood

O f these articles, Carrie Carmichael's is hilarious, but some, such as Edith
White's, are deeply disturbing. Mothers are still not being given the facts to
make up their own minds if they want to breast feed. I'm a great admirer
of Susan Jordan's The Baby Contract. She is on to something major, and I look
forward to her book. Erica Jong is brave and brilliant in "Monster Mommies."
Most mothers now work outside the home, and yet society remains judgmental
and harsh. Working mothers with young families are too stressed out and
exhausted to do much advocating for themselves, and are fortunate that Erica is
on their case.—B. S.

Determination

BARBARA KATZ ROTHMAN

Excerpted from Barbara Katz Rothman, "Determination," *Genetic Maps*, New York, W.W. Norton & Co., 1998. Reprinted by permission.

What are the characteristics that we think we can control when we plan our children? As the genetic map is unfolded and read, we expect finer and finer resolution. But we're looking at a map, not a crystal ball, and we're not dealing with three wishes from the blessing fairy. Our choices are limited to those things we believe are genetically determined.

The logic of genetic thinking as Evelyn Fox Keller summed it up is that genes are primary agents of life; to read genes is to predict traits; and to order traits you have to select or construct the genes. Want a blue-eyed kid? Select for the gene that causes blue eyes.

But are genes causes? Ruth Hubbard would have me never use the word "cause" for the action of a gene. A gene does not cause or do something, and it certainly is not "for" something. A gene is associated with, involved in, active in. And while I know she is right, somehow I think that the language of a gene that causes something, like blue eyes or sickle-cell anemia, is a reasonable way to speak. What, after all, ever causes anything in this world?

I fell down the stairs and broke my ankle. But it is perhaps a bit more complicated. How did I come to be on the stairs? My aunt Joan lent us the down payment for this house with its big staircase. I was carrying the Chanukah presents at the time and couldn't see where I was going—Judah Maccabee fought the battle that Chanukah commemorates. American Jews only make such a fuss over Chanukah to compete with the commercialization of Christmas. And besides, some little child who shall remain nameless lest godforbid she get a complex, left a plastic bag on the third-from-bottom step. And how can you break both bones in your ankle by falling three steps? Look at a skeleton some time—the whole weight of the body tapers down to this absurdly thin point right above where the foot twists.

So what was the cause of my broken ankle? Aunt Joan, Judah Maccabee, Jesus Christ, American capitalism, a nameless child and an orthopedic design flaw.

"Causality" in science is basically only a hypothesis you can't disprove (yet). So with the hedging of my bets and all, I'm still ready to use the word "cause" sometimes in connection with a gene. I know that genes only code for the production of proteins. They don't do anything, they don't even produce the protein, but still, in the more-or-less approximate way I use to talk about cause, I feel comfortable saying that a gene causes, say, blue eyes. Sickle-cell anemia. What else?

We make a list of characteristics, qualities, traits, states of being, and then see if we can find a "gene for" the characteristic. Is intelligence, sexual orientation, schizophrenia, the tendency to divorce, depression, the inability to spell, genetic or not? The discussion too often seems to degenerate into "Is too!" and "Is not!"

Probably the most public, vociferous, and politically important of the discussions has been the long-standing one focused on genetic components in intelligence, and the more recent one focused on the "gay gene." The intelligence discussion has been hopelessly mired in the racism that surrounds it. So let's take a look at the "gay gene" discussion: Is there a "gene for" being gay? If an identical twin is gay, the chances of his twin being gay are 50 percent. That is considerably higher than chance, but an awful lot lower than the odds on eye color.

Chandler Burr has helpfully compared male sexual orientation with handedness. For both we have a dominant and a minority orientation. About 92 percent of the population is right-handed. Left-handedness has at various times in history been treated as evil, sick, sinful, or an ordinary variation. Handedness is experienced as a very powerful given: it is not changeable by an act of will, though one can hide or pass if necessary. And so it seems to be with male homosexuality.

But is handedness "genetic"? If an identical twin is left-handed, the chances of his twin being left-handed are 12 percent, or one and a half times chance. That is, the identical twin of a left-handed person is only one and a half times more likely to be left-handed than is the person sitting next to him on the bus. It is not a powerful argument for genetic causality. But it doesn't make handedness a "lifestyle choice."

It seems as if what we are really talking about when we invoke genes is predestination versus free will. Genes seem to function in our language and our thinking as equivalent to inevitability, determination, predestination, fate. Yet what we hear from the geneticists is that genes work as probability factors in a causal equation. They play their part.

If you keep leaving things on the steps (and if I've said this once I've said it a thousand times), someone's going to get hurt. And if people march up and down stairs day after day, year after year, it's no surprise when eventually someone falls. And if you carry packages and can't see where you are going, well, what do you expect? To each of these things, and probably a dozen more, maybe even one or two that are "genetic," having to do with bone structure, clumsiness and distractibility, we can assign a probability rating. What are the odds of falling under each set of circumstances?

Now we're approaching some basic philosophical questions about determinism and inevitability. Was it inevitable that I break my leg? Given everything that happened in the world to that exact second—including the history of architecture, my relationship with Aunt Joan, the world history that brought that nameless little child who shouldn't have a complex about this into my life, the invention of plastic, the evolution of the ankle—given all of it, was it inevitable? Did I have to put my foot there? Was it fate?

That is a fascinating philosophical question, but it is not terribly useful practically. For practical purposes, we focus on one or two of the factors that we think we can control. Don't leave things on the stairs. Watch where you are going. And we act as if—we have to act as if—we have control.

When genes become more and more important in our thinking, we start assigning them greater and greater causal power, moving them to more central positions. Sometimes that has meant giving up, that metaphorical throwing your hands up in the air and saying "it's genetic," meaning "And that's that." The "gay gene" might be useful as a political tool if involving that gene becomes another way of saying, give it up, you have to accept that some people are inevitably, determinedly, gay. But if the question we are looking at is not "Why are some men gay?" but "Why are more black men in prisons than in colleges?" then saying "It's genetic" is quite dangerous.

What complicates it these days is that the way things are going, "It's genetic" might very quickly not be a throwing-up-of-your hands kind of problem, but rolling-up-of-your-sleeves kind of problem. "It's genetic" might be coming to mean, so let's fix it, let's engineer it, let's construct it to order. Let us make the determination and let us predetermine.

Take that highly publicized "gay gene," XQ28, now officially recorded as GAY1. The idea that there is a genetic component to being gay leads pretty quickly to either selecting against that gene or engineering to change it.

Gay is a highly politicized trait. But every day seems to bring some other "gene for" some other quality, characteristic, trait. Can we control all of it? Can we test and select, read and decode and splice our way to what we really want in our children, for our children?

And have we any right to do that? I'm not talking about our legal rights, our rights as citizens. Rather, I am thinking about our rights as parents in our relationships with our children. Do we even want to order them, to have them custom-made? Would we have wanted our parents to have ordered us, chosen our traits, predetermined whatever they could or wanted to about us? Whether it is what you like best or least about yourself, you probably won't like thinking about that as something your parents put on an order form.

Parenthood does not come with guarantees. Motherhood, I've often said, is one more chance for a speeding truck to ruin your life. The world has plans for your children, and your children have plans for themselves: you will not be able to control this.

Motherhood is not about consumer choice, and it's not about guarantees. The Dutch word for midwife, *vroedvrouw*, translates—as it does in many languages—to "wise woman." For wisdom on motherhood, I turn to midwives. The Dutch midwives worry about all of the new testing, and the implicit but false guarantee it seems to offer. Women say they want testing because they could "never raise a retarded child," or "couldn't bear" to have a disabled child. As if these things could be predetermined, as if they were all written in code ahead of time. Test, select, do what you think you can, but remember, as one midwife said,

> You are eager to have a healthy child, but after a chorionic villus sampling, amnio, an ultrasound and birth, your worries are not over yet. When the child is there you still have your concerns. Can he walk along the street on his own, and near the water, I hope he gets no accident, and I hope he doesn't get some wrong friends. It is a process, all life long, isn't it? Somehow or somewhere you have to let it go, you cannot control everything, and maybe you have to start to let it go at the beginning. You should dare to leave some questions without an answer.

And for Breast-feeding, Too, the Band Played On

EDITH WHITE

Adapted from Edith White, *Breastfeeding and HIV/AIDS: The Research, the Politics, the Women's Responses*, North Carolina, McFarland & Co., 1999. Reprinted by permission.

In 1989 the prestigious *New England Journal of Medicine* reported that 83 percent of the babies who were breastfed by HIV-positive French mothers became HIV-infected, compared to only 25 percent of the bottle-fed babies. Numerous reports from other countries confirmed that while HIV-positive women can transmit the virus to their babies before or during birth, breast-feeding significantly increases the risk. The information about breast-feeding and HIV, however, has been downplayed by the leading health agencies, for fear that the information would hurt campaigns to promote breast-feeding for all its benefits to HIV-negative mother-baby pairs. Like Randy Shilts' 1987 book *And The Band Played On*, this section chronicles delays and failures on the part of leading health agencies to respond to the threat of HIV.

African delegates to the May 1997 World Health Assembly expressed their unhappiness at not having been informed about breast-feeding and HIV. Dr. Timothy Stamps, Zimbabwe's Health and Child Welfare, made a joint presentation on behalf of the African countries. Dr. Stamps had long been a harsh critic of the formula companies for their unethical marketing of formula in areas where clean water is lacking. Now Dr. Stamps was critical of UNICEF and the World Health Organization (WHO). He asked: "Are we to accept that our children's survival should be compromised by the risk of infant AIDS in the cruelest sense through the promotion of unlimited, unmodified and unchallenged breast-feeding policies?"

The silence about HIV and breast-feeding was not limited to Africa. Most people in industrialized countries still do not know that breast-feeding can readily transmit HIV. Either the primary research articles about HIV and breast-feeding were not discussed, or the findings were given a better spin when they were mentioned in secondary sources. Looking back now at some of the reports from the 1980s and 1990s gives an overview of what the international agencies were saying about breast-feeding and HIV. Annually published reports such as UNICEF's *State of the World's Children* are particularly revealing.

The early 1980s were the highpoint in worldwide breast-feeding promotion efforts. The 1982–1983 *State of the World's Children* announced that breast-feeding was to be one-fourth of a children's survival revolution—one-fourth of a world revolution being a huge undertaking. But between 1983 and 1987 less and less emphasis was placed on breast-feeding. The 1987 report hardly mentioned breast-feeding.

UNICEF and WHO never discussed why they placed less emphasis on breast-feeding. But others have. Director of the Human Lactation Center Dr. Dana Raphael suggested that UNICEF de-emphasized breast-feeding because of HIV. Leading AIDS researchers Dr. Sophie Le Coeur and Dr. Marc Lallemant suggested that WHO saw doubts about the safety of breast-feeding and HIV as a threat to years of prevention efforts. Dr. Susan E. Holck, a WHO expert on breast-feeding, said that she was "struck by how much denial there was around 1990 of the evidence we had that HIV could be transmitted through breast-feeding." Much of the denial, she claimed, "undoubtedly was fed by people who had invested so much in promoting breast-feeding and feared what confirmation of that transmission might do to the gains that were made in breast-feeding."

The initial de-emphasis on breast-feeding happened just after HIV transmission through breastmilk was first reported in the medical journals. Nor was there much by way of solace in other scientific reports. Researchers already knew that maternal milk was a major mode of transmission for many animal retroviruses. They knew that breastmilk was a major mode of transmission for the first recognized human retrovirus, HTLV-I. Researchers, moreover, had already confirmed that HIV was a retrovirus. In the mid-to-late 1980s, some hoped that the antibodies in breastmilk would protect babies, even though antibodies generally do not stop milk-born transmission of other retroviruses. Also, by the end of 1986, people realized the magnitude of the epidemic in Africa. In short, there was good reason to worry.

It is understandable that UNICEF's strongest promotion of breast-feeding slacked off between 1983 and 1987. Those who had the benefit of scientific advisors must have recognized that HIV transmission via breastmilk was a potentially huge problem. If there was any doubt that HIV/AIDS could devastate breast-feeding programs, it was soon shattered by the early reports from Africa. Take for example the scene in 1988. The report had just come in from

Kinshasa, capital city of Zaire (now renamed Democratic Republic of Congo). A radio broadcaster pointed out the connection between breast-feeding and AIDS. There was an immediate 30 percent drop in breast-feeding initiation rates. That 30 percent drop must have been the most unwelcome news to those who were trying to restore exclusive breast-feeding. And this was just one of many radio reports in Africa, where people get much of their news from radio and by word of mouth.

In 1987 the WHO issued a statement about HIV and infant feeding. It noted that there was insufficient evidence to conclude that breast-feeding was a significant source of HIV transmission, and that in developing countries, breast-feeding was a life-saving intervention. Therefore HIV-positive women should still breast-feed.

The 1988 *State of the World's Children* said that HIV could threaten breast-feeding if misinformation was allowed to affect breast-feeding programs. This report stated that it is theoretically possible that breast-feeding can transmit the AIDS virus and "worldwide there are two cases where this is thought to have happened." It is not clear which are the "two" cases acknowledged in this 1988 report, even if one counts only the reports already published in the medical journals.

LESS AND LESS TALK ABOUT HIV AND BREAST-FEEDING

The 1989, 1990, and 1991 *State of the World's Children* reports each had a full-page panel devoted to AIDS. The 1989 report insisted that "breast-feeding is not a significant means of transmitting AIDS," though it cited no research that corroborated its position. On the contrary, reports published in leading medical journals such as *The Lancet* and Blanche's report in *The New England Journal of Medicine* had already suggested that breast-feeding was a very significant means of transmitting. In the Italian Multicenter Study, of 65 babies who were breast-fed by HIV-positive mothers, 46 became HIV-infected.

UNICEF's 1990 and 1991 full-panel reports on AIDS completely omitted any reference to breast feeding and AIDS. The 1992 *State of the World's Children* report had only one sentence about mother-to-child transmission; it stated that one million children have been "born HIV-positive." Later *State of the World's Children* reports also failed to address the emerging picture of HIV transmission through breast-feeding, even though the medical journals and conferences were continuing to make significant announcements. The large European Collaborative Study, for example, reported in 1991 that 32 percent of babies breast-fed by HIV-positive mothers became infected, compared to only 12 percent of bottle-fed babies.

In 1991 Baker reported that women in Zambia knew that breast-feeding can transmit HIV and many were afraid to breast-feed. Further, health workers in Zambia were accusing authorities of having a double standard for infant feeding in developed and developing counties.

UNICEF's 1992 and 1993 reports did not even mention breast-feeding and HIV. In 1993, UNICEF published a lengthy booklet AIDS: The Second Decade, in which UNICEF executive director James Grant described in detail efforts to reduce HIV infections among adults and adolescents. But this report from a children's organization did not discuss how children become HIV-infected. The one relevant sentence in the long report fails to clarify the role of breast-feeding and HIV: "Approximately 1 of 3 children born to these women is HIV-infected."

In 1993, the WHO published a book called *Breast-feeding: The Technical Basis and Recommendations for Action.* The book referred to discussions about research on the possible transmission of HIV through breastmilk as belonging under the category of spreading false rumors.

UNICEF's 1994 report acknowledged that AIDS was reversing hard-won gains in child mortality, but never discussed the ways by which children get AIDS. It said that children are "born with the virus." The 1995 report mentioned very briefly that HIV was known to have been transmitted in breastmilk in some instances.

UNICEF's 1996 report mentioned HIV/AIDS very briefly, noting only that children become orphaned when their parents die of AIDS. The report never mentioned that children become HIV-infected. The report also discussed the under-5 mortality rate (the rate of child mortality for children up to their fifth birthday). It said that this rate "appears to have increased in several countries, including Madagascar, Zambia and Zimbabwe." It never said why.

UNICEF's 1996 *Promise and Progress: Achieving Goals for Children* also noted that the under-5 mortality rates were up in some areas, but it too failed to explain why. UNICEF, however, did make a recommendation: the countries should readjust their mortality targets.

UNICEF's 1997 report mentioned HIV/AIDS very briefly, and then only to note that the epidemic had pushed more children into the labor market because their parents died. Even though AIDS was the leading cause of death for children in a growing number of countries, the report never mentioned AIDS in children.

UNAIDS (1997) noted that, in Namibia, HIV caused nearly twice as many deaths across all ages as malaria, the next most common killer. In the trading centers of Uganda, nearly nine out of ten deaths are related to AIDS. A report in conjunction with the 1996 International Conference on AIDS noted that AIDS may increase child mortality rates in Zambia nearly threefold by the year 2010.

In 1997 WHO issued a fact sheet called "Reducing Mortality from Major Childhood Killer Diseases." It never even mentioned HIV/AIDS. The section about major childhood killer diseases in Zambia did not mention AIDS, although AIDS is the leading cause of childhood death in Zambia.

Finally, in 1998, UNICEF's *State of the World's Children* report had a section on breast milk and transmission of HIV. It made many of the same recommendations as UNAIDS, suggesting, for instance, that voluntary testing and counseling be made more accessible. It stated that if an HIV-positive mother has access to adequate breast milk substitutes that she can prepare safely, she should consider this or wet-nursing or heat treatment of expressed breast milk.

COMMENTARIES

Various commentators have offered opinions on the responses of the international health agencies. Nicholas Eberstadt, a researcher with the Harvard Center for Population and Development Studies, opined that UNICEF's "blinding ideology" to promoting breast-feeding and boycotting Nestle's had left it particularly ill-equipped to deal with HIV transmission through breast-feeding: "You can think of UNICEF's medical obtuseness as a cruel manifestation of bureaucratic inefficiency, a product of blinding ideology, a simple human tragedy, or some combination of the three."

Elliott Abrams, who had been U.S. assistant secretary of state for international organizations, also accused UNICEF of being addicted to the ideology of breast-feeding declaring that UNICEF was in a state of denial.

Zambian gynecologist Mavis Sianga was critical of the prohibition of free formula for babies of HIV-infected mothers. "It is rather unfair that women in developing countries must risk passing on the infection just because WHO and UNICEF want to keep their programs flying." She feels that a policy of not helping HIV-infected women to formula-feed has chauvinistic overtones. Men are given free condoms, but when it comes to a woman wanting to protect her baby, it is "suddenly political, it is cultural, it is expensive, it is impossible. What nonsense is this?" asks Geloo.

UNAIDS/WHO/UNICEF no longer recommend that HIV-positive women in developing countries should breast-feed. Instead, they recommended that all women be allowed to make an informed choice about how they feed their babies. Most women, however, are still not given any information about HIV.

While UNICEF announced in March 1998 that it would begin pilot projects to distribute generic infant formula to babies of HIV-positive mothers, no HIV-positive mothers had been given any formula as of May 1999. For breast-feeding, the band still seems to be playing on.

Moms in Dark about OTC Drugs, Survey Shows

FRANCES CERRA WHITTELSEY

Frances Cerra Whittelsey, "Moms in Dark about OTC Drugs, Survey Shows." © 1999, original for this publication.

A survey by the Women's Consumer Foundation shows that many inner-city mothers are in the dark about basic aspects of choosing and using non-prescription drugs, exposing them and their children to the possibility of serious illness or death.

The survey showed, in fact, that taking more than the recommended doses of these medicines is far more common than drug manufacturers acknowledge. Further, it showed that many of the women take medicines without knowing what is in them. Specifically, the survey found that less than half of the mothers could identify the active ingredient in the most widely advertised nonprescription drug, Tylenol, or even define the term "active ingredient" itself. (The active ingredient in Tylenol is acetaminophen.)

"We have issues of human life at stake here," commented Dr. John Renner, founder of the Consumer Health Information and Research Institute. "Not knowing the ingredients in common pain killers, with as much publicity as some of these products get, is remarkable. And with the overdosing that was found, can lead to real trouble."

The survey found that one out of eleven of the women knew of an adverse reaction to an over-the-counter (OTC) medicine that had resulted in a trip to an emergency room or doctor. Forty-four percent of the women said they knew people who very often, or somewhat often, take more than the recommended dosages. Twenty-five percent admitted to doing so themselves.

The survey results have been collected into a report called "Brand Loyal But in the Dark about Over-the-Counter Medicines," which includes an analysis and recommendations for action. It has been forwarded to the U.S. Food and Drug Administration, which is finalizing new regulations that will standardize the formats and improve the readability of over-the-counter drug labels.

Asked to comment on the survey findings, the Nonprescription Drug Manufacturers Association said that serious illnesses or deaths due to adverse reactions from OTC medicines are "extremely rare."

In a written statement, the Association said "No drug is without potential toxicity, but OTC's have a very wide margin of safety."

Further, the Association maintained that "dozens of nationally representative independent surveys have found that consumers are responsible in their use of OTC medicines; they do read and understand labels; and do not take more than the recommended daily dosage." The Association noted that the surveys focused on mothers living in New York City.

While deaths and hospitalizations due to mistakes or reactions to prescription drugs have been widely reported, there is evidence that nonprescription drugs can also be dangerous: Gastrointestinal complications caused by aspirin, ibuprofen, naproxin, and other nonsteroidal anti-inflammatory drugs (some of them available only by prescription) result in approximately 76,000 hospitalizations and 7,600 deaths annually, according to the American

Gastroenterological Association. This death rate is comparable to that for asthma, cervical cancer and melanoma. People who consume three or more alcohol-containing drinks a day can suffer liver failure even when taking only the recommended dosage of acetaminophen (two 500 mg tablets four times a day), according to Mike Cohen, president of the Institute for Safe Medication Practices. People with allergies to aspirin may unwittingly take popular pain relievers or sleep aids that contain aspirin, and suffer life-threatening reactions. The institute reported that an 18-year-old woman, for example, had to be resuscitated and admitted to the intensive care unit after taking Excedrin Extra-Strength tablets. She knew she was allergic to aspirin, but did not realize that Excedrin contains aspirin.

"It is not being alarmist at all," commented Cohen, to suggest that ignorance about OTC medicines can result in serious injury or death. Cohen's Institute monitors adverse reactions reported to the U.S. Pharmacopoeia and to the FDA's Med Watch program, and issues advisories about them that are published in medical, nursing, and pharmaceutical journals.

Fred Mayer, whose 1990 petition to the FDA began the process that will soon lead to new regulations for OTC labels, said in an interview that a 1989 federal report on adverse reactions to both prescription and OTC drugs suffered by the elderly put the price tag at $10 billion annually.

"A lot of [the problem] is mixing prescription and OTC medicines," said Mayer, president of Pharmacists Planing Service, Inc. "It's an epidemic and no one's in control."

Barbara Seaman, founder of the National Women's Health Network, also noted that more and more people with chronic diseases like depression, high blood pressure, and high cholesterol are on maintenance regimens of prescription drugs. "They need to be more conscious of possible interactions of prescription drugs with nonprescription drugs," she said.

According to a report prepared for the Nonprescription Drug Manufacturers Association by the research firm Kline Company, Inc., American consumers spent $14 billion a year on OTC medicines in 1997,

By purchasing generic brands and single-ingredient, rather than heavily advertised or combination medicines, consumers could save 50 percent or more on OTC purchases, according to price checks conducted by the Women's Consumer Foundation.

But the survey showed that many of the women questioned are unable to follow thrift advice because they do not understand the meaning of "generic," and the concept of active ingredients. As a result, they unnecessarily spend their limited resources on higher-priced, widely advertised name brands and combination medicines.

Three-quarters of the women surveyed were raising their families in New York City on $35,000 a year or less in total family income.

The survey was a project of the Women's Consumer Foundation, a nonprofit, New York–based organization that also publishes the SIS Web site. It was conducted during the second half of 1997 at a Harlem health center and at a Brooklyn shopping mall. A total of 181 women, who identified themselves as mothers and the primary buyers of over-the-counter medicines for their families, answered 35 questions read to them face-to-face by a surveyor. The study was financed with a grant from the Shelley Donald Rubin Foundation of New York City.

Less than half of the women surveyed—only 43 percent—could correctly define the term "active ingredient." An overwhelming 77 percent did not understand the word *antihistamine*. Nearly half—48 percent—did not know that acetaminophen is the ingredient in Tylenol (they were given four possible answers from which to choose), despite the fact the Tylenol was the drug that the women said they bought most often.

These findings become alarming when viewed in conjunction with the results showing widespread disregard for dosage limits, and that many mothers do not or cannot adequately read and understand OTC drug labels.

What were the consequences of this overdosing and difficulty reading and understanding labels? The survey did not establish cause and effect, but 30 of the women, or nearly 17 percent, said that they or a family member had suffered an adverse reaction from an OTC drug. Fifteen of the women, or 8 percent, said the reaction was severe enough to require medical attention.

The pharmaceutical industry spent $2.03 billion on all forms of OTC drug advertising in 1997, according to Nielsen Media Research. In a pivotal decision in 1983, the Federal Trade Commission chose not to follow the recommendation of an administrative court judge that ads for OTC drugs always disclose the generic names of their active ingredients. Instead, the Commission said such disclosure would be required only under certain limited circumstances.

The response of the pharmaceutical industry ever since has been to avoid those circumstances. Ads promise symptom relief without usually identifying the agents of that relief. This confuses consumers into believing that brand-name products are unique formulations worth their high prices, instead of heavily advertised versions of common, inexpensive drugs.

If consumers understood OTC drugs better, their savings could be significant. For example, store-brand pseudoephedrine HCL can frequently be found for one-half to one-third the price of the name-brand decongestant, Sudafed; generic versions of Nyquil cost 50 percent less. A single dose of TheraFlu, a combination product, costs 83 cents. If the three active ingredients in TheraFlu were, instead, bought separately, a single dose would cost 28 cents.

Among the benefits of smarter self-medication, said the Foundation, are healthier children and adults; fewer absences from school and work; fewer adverse drug reactions; fewer trips to doctors and emergency rooms; more competition among drug manufacturers, and, consequently, lower prices for OTC drugs.

Patenting Life: Are Genes Objects of Commerce?

BARBARA KATZ ROTHMAN AND RUTH HUBBARD

Barbara Katz Rothman and Ruth Hubbard, "Patenting Life: Are Genes Objects of Commerce?" *MAMM,* May 1999. Reprinted by permission.

When people think of patents, they think of patenting inventions—gadgets, tools—a self-wringing mop, the proverbial better mousetrap. They don't think of patenting the better mouse. But in this brave new world, the more profitable patent is likely to be on the mouse rather than on the mousetrap. OncoMouse was, appropriately enough, the first patented animal in the world. OncoMouse can develop all kinds of cancer, but it is for breast cancer that she was primarily designed and patented, and is best known. A mouse produced to order, like the mousetrap designed to specifications, has come to seem like a reasonable thing to patent.

And yet, there is something absurd about the idea of patenting animals or their—or our—genes. You can hold a mouse in your hands and make eye contact with it—can you imagine patenting a living being? And genes: Genes, we're being told, are the essential building blocks of life. So how can you patent life? How can you patent parts not only of mice, but of people? It just doesn't make sense.

Tell that to John Moore. Cancerous cells from his spleen were turned into the "Mo cell line," and used to develop a series of proteins for fighting cancer and bacteria. The cell line was making a lot of money—Moore sued for his share. But Patent No. 4,438,032 stands, and Moore is not getting a cut of the profits. The California Supreme Court ruled that while Moore could sue his doctors for not informing him of what they intended to do with his cells, the cells, once the doctors had them, were no longer Moore's.

HISTORY

Patenting in the United States dates back to the founding of the nation. Thomas Jefferson, himself an inventor, was one of the first patent commissioners. Patenting was designed to give individuals ownership of the fruits of their labors.

Governments issue patents when they recognize an invention as having three qualifications: novelty, nonobviousness, and utility, as they are termed. In other words, first it must be something new under the sun, something that didn't exist before. Second, it must not be an obvious variation on something already existing (Once the black Model T Ford was patented, you couldn't get a patent for a red one). Third, it must have a practical use—you can't patent a painting or sculpture.

The issuing of a patent gives its inventor, or the "holder" of the patent, exclusive rights to that invention for a limited time, during which anyone in that country who wants to use or sell the invention has to buy the rights from the owner, the patent holder. In the United States, most patents last 17 to 20 years. During those years, the inventor can manufacture the object herself, sell the patent to a manufacturer, or license it for a fee or for a royalty, pay-per-use, or per-sale agreement. DuPont collects royalties on OncoMouse in the United States, and may soon in Europe.

How did we get from patenting gadgets and tools to patenting genes and mice? Thomas Jefferson, who patented his own inventions, such as the automatically closing French door, did not consider patenting plants even though he was a farmer and a plant breeder. (And if he could have seen where DNA testing was eventually going to land him—in the most famous and drawn-out paternity suit of all time—he might not have been in favor of DNA patenting at all!) Plant patents did not occur until 1930, when the first Plant Patent Act allowed for the patenting of nonsexually reproducing plants. This marked the beginning of agribusiness and its threats to biodiversity. Seed companies could buy the patent to a strain of crops, or develop and patent their own, setting us on the path to the patented fruits and vegetables that have appeared on our dining tables ever since.

But it was in 1980 that the brave new world of patenting living beings began to take shape. Ranajit Chakraborty, a researcher at the General Electric Co., used the new technology of gene-splicing to create a microorganism, a bacterium that would "eat" oil. The genetically modified bacteria, Chakraborty and GE claimed, thus met the qualifications for patenting: They were new, nonobvious, and useful.

And yet, bacteria are not machines, not things or a process—they are living beings, and so, many argued, patently unpatentable. Chakraborty and GE took the case all the way up to the U.S. Supreme Court. In June 1980, by a five-to-four majority, the court upheld the validity of the patent. Living beings, albeit very small ones, had been patented, and that opened the floodgates. In 1985, the U.S. Patent and Trademark Office declared that plants and seeds were themselves patentable, and in 1987 the patent commissioner announced that the license to patent also encompassed animals.

Europe was slower to go along, but in 1992, five years after the U.S. patent, the European Patent Office granted Harvard a patent for OncoMouse. It opened the door to patenting of animals in all the European member countries. The patent, which will now affect all of the European member countries, hinges on whether there is sufficient medical benefit to justify the animal's suffering. OncoMouse, Donna Haraway says, is a Christ figure, promising us the salvation of a cure for cancer through her suffering.

But whether you think of her as a metaphorical Christ or just another product for better living brought to us by DuPont, OncoMouse is the world's first patented animal: We have gone from patenting the mousetrap to patenting the mouse.

PATENTING HUMAN GENES

What genes do is specify the compositions of proteins. We often talk as if there were a "gene for" something—a gene for being tall, or a gene for breast cancer, but genes are not order forms. By affecting the production of proteins they play a part in a sequence of events that may eventually lead, for example, to a girl growing up tall or a woman developing breast cancer. What is important to remember is that genes are only a part of the sequence of events, and that the genes themselves are not simple packages. Genes vary in their details from one person to another. Think of it as something like a nose: Everyone has one, and they all perform essentially the same functions, but they vary quite a bit. You can't really talk about patenting "the gene for… " any more than you can talk about patenting "the human nose." To patent a functioning gene sequence would mean patenting a whole set of sequences, the details of which may differ, and cannot even be fully predicted.

No one is suggesting that genes are patentable while they function in the body, any more than anyone would try to patent someone's nose. What some scientists are arguing, however—and the courts are finding reasonable—is that once a specific gene sequence has been taken out of a person, then either the scientists who isolated it or the institutions they work for should be able to patent it. It is the separation from the body that turns genes into "inventions."

Scientists have long maintained that they don't "invent" things, don't make things up: They just discover truths, facts, reality. It is ironic now to hear scientists forced by the system of patenting to describe their "discoveries" as "inventions." This is not just an academic distinction. Remember the purpose of patenting: to enable inventors to profit from the fruits of their labors. Patenting human gene sequences means enabling someone to "own" and thereby profit from that sequence.

And it is no longer really some "one." Very few patents of any sort in biotechnology are held by individual scientists, or "inventors," alone. It is corporations and universities—what is called the life science industry—that control patents. That industry includes chemical, pharmaceutical, and agribusiness companies. *Science* magazine identifies them as three interlocking circles—with corporations like DuPont and Monsanto at the center, working in all three spheres.

Patents are about profit: Biotechnology companies are not likely to fund research unless they can profit from it, and scientists rarely work unless they can get funded to do it—there are no lone scientists working weekends in their garages hoping to invent the cure for cancer. Though clothed in statements about intellectual property rights and how to extract the greatest benefits for suffering humanity, a struggle over competing rights to profits is at the heart of the debate about patenting.

PAYING THE COSTS OF PATENTING

And where does profit come from? Consumers. Us. While the United States permitted patents on gene sequences, the United Kingdom fought it. A British briefing paper called "No Patents on Life" was prepared in opposition to legislation making human gene sequences patentable in the European Union. The paper argued that medical costs would rise with patenting. After a 10-year battle, gene patenting legislation did indeed pass in the European Union; since May 1998, human gene sequences have been patentable throughout the member countries.

Most gene sequences have been found with the help of publicly funded research. Furthermore, many of the gene sequences being patented were found only with the voluntary cooperation of affected families. It is wrong that, at the point when the knowledge might produce useful results, its applications should be exploited for private profits. Genes should not be turned into objects of commerce.

Nor is patenting necessary to spur research. Proponents of patenting argue that unless scientists, universities, and private entrepreneurs can patent genes, they will not invest the necessary work and funding to create useful products such as diagnostic tests and therapies. But patents aren't just a way of encouraging research: They are also a way of hampering it. They introduce economic and proprietary barriers into what should be a free exchange of ideas and information. Scientists can no longer freely present their ideas at conferences or publish them in journals. They now must hold them in silence until patents have been applied for. The effort to establish patent rights is more likely to slow down scientific exploration than it is to further it.

Gene patenting is an ethical problem. No one, and no multinational corporation, should hold patents on our genes. As Jonas Salk said in a far-different era when someone suggested he patent his polio vaccine: "It would be like patenting the sun." Our genes are not commercial resources.

Geriatric Obstetrics: Oh, Baby!

CARRIE CARMICHAEL

Carrie Carmichael, "Geriatric Obstetrics: Oh, Baby!" *The East Hampton Star,* July 17, 1997. Reprinted by permission.

In the new medical specialty of geriatric obstetrics (GO for short), you can accurately say the wrinkled newborn looks just like his old mom or old dad. That's some of the good news coming after the birth of a daughter to that 63-year-old Californian who is for now the oldest new mother in the world.

Times have changed and so must the geriatric obstetricians. They must ask a new set of questions, like: "How many decades ago was your last period?"

"Will Medicare reimburse for deliveries?"

"During labor and delivery will the fetal monitor disable the mother's pace-maker?"

"Can I require a lie detector test about a prospective mother's age?"

"HMOs have already cut my income, now I must give a senior citizen discount?"

AARP TWOFERS?

It's not just the doctors who will have to change. The American Association of Retired Persons will have to revamp, too. It will have to add discounts if members are buying a twofer, such as a stroller and a wheelchair in the same week, dentures and teething rings, human eggs and chicken eggs, Ensure and baby formula.

Of course, discounts for diapers—both kinds. Depends and Huggies. The AARP should recommend that members make sure their new kids are out of diapers before they need them.

Can new old parents take their tots on Elderhostel trips?

START-OVER DADS

Not long ago *The New York Times* enshrined men it called Start-Over Dads (SODs). Guys in their sixties, seventies, and eighties. George Plimpton among them, who had no children until they were elderly or who hadn't bothered to take time out of busy career years to raise their first batches of kids.

Male geezers have long fathered babies, to the delight of the tabloids. Wink, wink, nudge, nudge. He can still do it! Tony Randall, a first-time dad at 77, is the most recent example. And he wants another baby right away. Quick, before he can no longer schlep the stroller and the baby bag.

The New York Times did not address the COKs (Cast-Off Kids) or COWs (Cast-Off Wives).

GEEZELLES

Techno-obstetrics evens the reproductive score for post-menopausal women. Now geezelles have equal opportunities to become SAMs (Scientifically Assisted Moms).

The conditions that attract young women to old, wrinkled, wealthy men now exist for old, wrinkled, wealthy women. A rich older woman no longer has to give up a younger man as a mate because he wants a child of his own. With enough money to pay for fertility treatments, she can have her baby boy and boy toy, too. As Oprah says, GO girl!

In fact, retired women can offer something younger women may not. No longer busy with careers, like rich older SODs, rich older moms can either hire young help to run after their kids, or marry it.

CERTAIN BLESSINGS

Being an older parent may be an asset. An elderly parent who needs less sleep now may already be up for the 4 a.m. feeding. Being an extremely old parent of a teenager may bring the blessing of not being able to remember at dinner the insults hurled at breakfast.

Now that science has extended the possibility of giving birth almost to the point of death, what other mind-boggling possibilities are on the horizon?

It seemed fitting when the news broke about the 63-year-old mother that she lives in California, where looking young is coin of the realm and lying about your age common. Movie stars aren't the only ones to shave years. Anyway, 63 isn't as old as it used to be and plastic surgery can keep you from facing your years.

This latest GO mom had to lie about her age to get the fertility treatments. I wonder if GO dads face an age cutoff, too.

MIND-BOGGLING

With GO marching on, an older woman who wants a baby cannot count on breaking the record and becoming the oldest mother on record. She can't trust some tabloid will come along and cover the fertility treatments, finance her child's education, and enhance her retirement portfolio.

That is a long shot. Her older sister may beat her our.

Let's not forget that the all-time geriatric motherhood award goes to Sarah in the Bible.

Margaret Mead wrote about PMZ, postmenopausal zest, the focused energy that women get after childbearing years. GO moms are going to need it.

Now that science has extended the possibility of giving birth almost to the point of death, what other mind-boggling possibilities are on the horizon?

NEVER SAY NEVER

I had my children premenopausally. One is in high school, the other in law school. I assumed my childbearing years were over. Science is now telling me, "Never say never."

Who knows? I may want to have more children when my future grandchildren are old enough to babysit.

I am single now. Maybe a young, offspring-hungry guy will cross my path. GO lets me say to him,"Baby, I want to have your baby."

Come to think of it, GO takes the pressure off the younger generation to produce grandchildren for us. My daughter can say, "Mom, do it yourself."

But not right now. My first batch of children is launched. My complexion is clear.

The Baby Contract

SUSAN JORDAN

Susan Jordan, "The Baby Contract and the Value of Motherhood," from the forthcoming book, *The Baby Contract*. Reprinted by permission.

> *Susan J., and I, Jesse L., as marital partners agree on this 3rd day of June, 1996, to hereby contract to raise our son in a manner that we have determined will be most beneficial for the child and all members of the family and that will not penalize the parent who forgoes working outside the home. Upon mutual agreement....*

M other. Spoken in the 1950s, that word evoked warm and fuzzy images of a smiling woman, holding a pie, surrounded by children. Spoken in the 1990s, the image is vastly different. The once cohesive concept of The Mother has splintered. In her place, we have the working mother, the stay-at-home mother, the divorced mother, the welfare mother, the single mother, the step-mother, the teenage mother, the unwed mother, the soccer mother; each subject to some degree of criticism and scorn. This fractured perception of motherhood is but one small measure of the staggering decline in status and legal rights of all mothers, regardless of their category.

Similarly, our definition of what it means to "mother" children has grown increasingly abstract. Now, mothers who stay at home are more likely to be seen as liabilities for their children—a view that is encouraged by questionable research that claims to show that children of working mothers fare better than those whose mothers don't work outside the home. If you factor in the rapid advances being made in reproductive technology and the spawning of unique surrogacy arrangements, you find not only are mothers poorly regarded and perceived as increasingly unnecessary but, in some cases, it is disturbingly unclear, even to the courts, 'who' the mother is.

With gathering momentum, the devaluation and, perhaps, termination of the active role of the mother has begun. It's looking more and more like Aldous Huxley's *Brave New World*. Ironically, while many readers associate that novel with the description of test tube babies, few recall that the most degraded, despised, and superfluous role in the "new world" was the role of the mother.

There are many reasons for the rapid devaluation of the role of the mother. Anyone who tunes in to the greatest social dilemma of our time—balancing work and family—is familiar with the two most commonly cited co-conspirators: the globalization of the economy forcing real wages into decline, thereby increasing the need for two paychecks, and an American feminist movement that seeks equality through parity in the workplace and reproductive control (primarily access to abortion).

If the yardstick of progress is workforce participation then there can be no question that women have made tremendous advances and feminism deserves much of the credit. But at what price? Workforce participation for women is at an all-time high. By 1990, 75 percent of all women aged 25–44 years old were in the paid labor force. But the majority of working women are not in fast-track, high-paying careers; they are in low-paying service sector jobs that lack adequate health benefits, paid leave, or retirement pensions. And, while it is a generally accepted fact that women have narrowed the wage gap from 59 cents to 73 cents for every dollar men make, it is not so much because women's wages have increased but because men's wages have been on a serious decline; from 1979 to 1991 the average woman earning median income saw her hourly wages increase only 1.3 percent while the equivalent man endured a 14.3 percent plunge.

But it is women with children who pay the worst long-term penalties, particularly if they take time away from their careers to mother their children; estimates are that a woman's earning potential drops by 19 percent with the birth of her first child. And the myth that women can move in and out of the mommy track without consequences is contradicted by a recent study by Professor Schneer of Rider University that suggests that women executives who take time off and then return to work permanently sacrifice career advancement and earning potential. This penalty is echoed in the findings reported by June O'Neill, Director of the Congressional Budget Office, who reported that "among women and men, aged 27–33, who have never had a child, the earnings of women in the National Longitudinal Survey of Youth are close to 98 percent of men's." It is the women who have children who drag the average down to the seventieth percentile.

The modern feminist movement, born in the 1960s, has been remarkably effective in getting society to address the gross inequities to which all women have been subjected. But as Barbara Katz Rothman put it, "Giving women all the rights of men will not accomplish a whole lot for women facing the demands of pregnancy, birth, and lactation." Thus, despite the fact that mothers are one of the most vulnerable segments in today's society, the feminist movement has been disturbingly silent when it comes to defending mother's rights. Feminism's ambivalence has prevented it from, as Christina Looper Baker so eloquently put it, "reinventing motherhood so that it does not eclipse feminism and redefining feminism so that it does not exclude motherhood."

Hamstrung by defining liberation and equality as "sameness" with men and focusing on equality in the workplace and the right not to have children (i.e. abortion and contraception), feminists have been reluctant to fight for the protection of women's differences. By lobbying primarily for remedies that facilitate women's quick return to the workplace (i.e., brief maternity leaves, government and industry-sponsored day care, etc.), feminists have failed to adequately question the viability and impact of programs and policies that separate women from their infants and small children, sometimes arguing to the extreme that day care is actually better for children. By insisting that being able to raise children at home is just a white, middle-to-upper class problem, feminists have missed the precise point that women in lower socioeconomic classes have already unequivocally lost the right to mother their own children. It's gotten to the point where the poorest mothers—those on welfare—can be threatened with a loss of benefits based on the number of children they have and no one raises an eyebrow.

However, the increasing separation of women from their children is not a signpost of liberation and equality but one of the most subtle and far-reaching forms of discrimination and repression affecting women today. In her book, *The Illusion of Equality,* Martha Albertson Fineman, a feminist scholar, painfully details the impact that this gender-blind stance has had on family law and credits feminism with facilitating the removal of gender-specific rules that protected mother's rights, including the "tender years" doctrine. In the early nineteenth century, mothers had essentially no rights when it came to their children; fathers retained an absolute right of ownership and control over their children and had the corresponding duty of supporting them. Court documents routinely depicted women as the "inferior parent." It wasn't until the late nineteenth century when early feminists fought for the rights of mothers and children that family law shifted its emphasis to the "best interests of the child." Though far from perfect, under this construct, women's special skills as nurturers were recognized and the presumption of maternal custody during a child's "tender years" became the norm.

The acceptance of a mother's essential bond to her child was a powerful and radical notion that has been slowly chipped away by reforms in family and divorce law that increasingly emphasize "equality" between the sexes and the rights of fathers and noncustodial parents. So much so that when there is a divorce (a more than 50 percent chance), the law which varies from state to state makes little or no economic allowance for the sacrifices and contributions that women have made for their families.

Most women remain unaware of the economic penalties and risks they face when they become mothers or the extent to which their legal rights have been eroded until their marriage or relationship dissolves and they find themselves in divorce court. By then, it is too late.

For example, if a woman has the misfortune to reside in a separate property state (41 states out of 50), she is entitled only to a minimal child support award and if she is deemed capable of self support by the court, she may receive no alimony or maintenance support whatsoever. Distribution of marital property is at the discretion of the judge and generally mirrors the degree of financial contribution each of the parties has made.

That's not the worst of it. Few women know that if they support their spouse through professional or graduate school they are less likely to receive alimony and, contrary to common lore, may not receive any reimbursement for their spouse's professional advancement or future earnings. And many are shocked to realize that in some states their spouse can petition to reduce maintenance support and child support payments in order to support a new or "second" family.

And despite all this talk about dead-beat dads, if a spouse fails to pay his support obligations consistently over time, he is often in a better position to have his "arrearages" forgiven; the court's logic being that if his family has managed to survive the months or years without it then they must not have needed it after all.

Most working mothers, in particular, think that they will be protected under "equitable distribution." But what the court defines as equitable is usually two-thirds to the higher wage earner and one third to the lower wage earner. If a woman's earned income is substantially less than her husband's, then she will receive substantially less of the assets that they have accumulated together as "partners" during the marriage.

Custody of the children, which most women assume will be granted to them, particularly if they have been the primary caretakers, is now up for grabs. True, women are still more likely to get custody. But when a father wants it, he wins 70 percent of the time. And because the law no longer presumes that mothers should be the legal custodians of children during their "tender years," men have become adept at manipulating pleas for physical custody in return for further reduced financial arrangements. Remember that child support ends at 18 and that, in most states, non-custodial parents do not have to contribute to college education for their children, and it is apparent why so many women trade away their rights to future retirement income for upfront money to pay college tuition.

Why does this inequity prevail? It prevails because the legal system has, as Fineman points out, adopted a gender-blind stance toward women and their children. And while it may sound nondiscriminatory on the surface, it is often disastrous in application. Mirroring society, family law now requires that women and men be viewed as "situationally the same" regardless of the degree to which women have assumed the role of mother/caretaker. In the shuttered eyes of the law, "men and women are equal" and they deserve no more or no less regardless of the way they have functioned in the family over the years. But men and women are not the same. Women have babies and men don't. And while fathers are increasingly involved in their children's lives, it is most often the mother who makes the sacrifices in her career to mother their children.

In the face of a society that refuses to acknowledge the importance of the role of the mother, women must craft their own legal solution. Recognizing that every time a woman marries she signs a contract governed by the state, there is nothing to prevent her from negotiating the parameters of that contract with her partner. In fact, men and women do this all the time. Note the numerous pre-nuptials signed by the wealthy that are designed to shelter their assets and future income from a new and untested spouse.

But if one can shelter assets, one can legally affirm the intention to share them as well. A "baby contract," would offer women (and some men) the opportunity to modify the state-defined marital contract via a binding pre- or post-marital contract. Its purpose would be to explicitly recognize the implicit value of the role of the mother and ensure that individuals who actively mother their children are economically protected from the inequities of a system that penalizes them.

To accomplish this goal, the baby contract would redefine the family as one economic unit comprised of two partners who share equally in the ownership and access to all assets and earned income of the household while legally recognizing that the partner who assumes the role of mother is entitled to equivalent economic compensation in the future should the marriage dissolve. And while the baby contract would call for the valuation of the role of the mother, it need not and should not discriminate based on gender; men who choose to assume the role of the mother are subject to the same penalties and risks that women are and should be protected as well.

Working to correct the economic imbalance within the household while attempting to reform the inequities present in the current state-by-state patchwork of family law, the baby contract represents a major step forward in the continuing struggle for equality for all parents who want 'to mother' their children.

Bold Type: Childbirth Is Powerful

BARBARA FINDLEN

Barbara Findlen, "Childbirth Is Powerful," *Ms.*, January/February 1995. Reprinted by permission.

Outspoken, frank, and decidedly feminist, pregnancy and childbirth expert Sheila Kitzinger makes no bones about her mission: the empowerment of women in the birth process.

"Information is power," says the British author of 18 books and mother of five grown daughters. "It's extremely difficult to act as your own advocate—unless you have the information to challenge doctors who often treat women as if they were irresponsible, selfish, and concerned only with their own emotions."

Thirty years after her first book, *The Experience of Childbirth*, hit the shelves, Kitzinger, a social anthropoligist, has released two new, very different books.

The Year after Childbirth: Surviving and Enjoying the First Year of Motherhood (Scribner's) arose out of Kitzinger's realization that of the hundreds of books available about childbirth, baby care, and child development, "there was nothing that was woman-centered about the year after childbirth. All the books were about the baby, and the woman was marginalized."

By contrast, *The Year after Childbirth* focuses on the experiences and feelings of new mothers—with nods of inclusion to women with disabilities, lesbians, adoptive parents, HIV-positive women, survivors of sexual abuse, and single women. The book is full of practical information—tips on breast-feeding, advice on getting help and support from friends and family, realistic execise guidelines—combined with reassurance about what to expect emotionally.

All of this comes in the context of Kitzinger's lively, unadulterated feminism. For example, she calls episiotomy—an incision to enlarge the birth opening that is performed routinely in industrialized countries— "our Western way of female genital mutilation." She lambastes medical professionals who chalk up postpartum depression to women's hormones: "With all its joys—and these can be vivid and exultant—motherhood is intensely stressful. Research might be more productive and realistic if it examined why some mothers are not depressed."

In *Ourselves As Mothers: The Universal Experience of Motherhood* (Addison-Wesley), Kitzinger compares childbirth and mothering in many different cultures. What emerges is a powerful critique of childbirth practices in industrialized countries, where doctors often induce labor or perform cesarean births for their own convenience, and where the whole process is depersonalized and taken out of women's hands. "Our society sets us up to feel socially isolated, guilty, and as if we are failures as mothers," she says. "In many traditional societies there is much more woman-to-woman support in pregnancy, during the birth, and afterward."

Kitzinger's family lives out a version of this supportive model. She and her husband, Uwe, live outside Oxford, England, with two of their daughters, their son-in-law, and their two young grandchildren. The extended family shares meals, laundry, and child care.

The author also practices what she preaches by running the Birth Crisis Network, a telephone counseling resource for women who have had invasive or humiliating birth experiences. "It's like a rape crisis line," says Kitzinger. "The emotional trauma after a violent childbirth is not unlike the trauma after rape. The woman's body has been forcibly invaded."

Kitzinger has been inspired by her mother—a pacifist and feminist who in the 1930s founded one of the first birth control clinics in southwest England—and her daughters, three of whom are radical lesbian feminists. "They call me a wishy-washy liberal feminist." she says.

"My work is all about women finding a voice, women growing in confidence, women sharing with each other," Kitzinger says. "All my writing has come out of my joy in birth."

What Do You Love about Being a Lesbian Mom?

CATHERINE GUND

Excerpted from Catherine Gund, *Letters of Intent,* New York, Free Press, 1999. Reprinted by permission.

Today, many of my lesbian friends have kids ranging from newborn to 10 years old. When I came out I didn't assume being a lesbian and being a mother were mutually exclusive. I never thought I couldn't or wouldn't have children. And so my lover, Melanie, and I have. Our baby girl Sadie Rain will turn three years old on November 1, 1999.

A few years ago, with four other couples, we had some informal dinners and ongoing conversations about choosing to have children. We talked about adoption, foster care, and pregnancy. Also about how to get pregnant, anonymous or known donors, known donors as daddies or uncles. We discussed using midwives or doctors, our parents' presumed reactions, which one of each couple would carry, how many kids we wanted, whose biological clock was ticking the loudest, whose relationships were solid enough for this calling, and so on. From that group, we now have two girls and at least five more babies twinkling in their mothers' eyes. In our little circle, as in the wider United States society, there is a veritable lesbian baby boom under way.

It's a cliché to say that many aspects of parenting are the same for everyone; we all change diapers, have nursing and feeding routines, bathe the little ones, create spaces and time for them to sleep and play, and consider their health, safety, intelligence, looks, and well-being. A cliché maybe, but all that is true. However, as lesbian moms, we have a good share of unique issues to deal with.

In our case, we have a known donor who lives nearby and will know our daughter and be part of her life. Since most of our friends have used anonymous donors, we didn't have a lot of known-donor role models (maybe the next generation will have that in uol).

Interview with Arlene Eisenberg

TANIA KETENJIAN

Arlene Eisenberg is the author of several bestselling books including *What to Expect When You're Expecting.* This interview was conducted in June 1999.

TK: Dr. Spock's *Baby and Child Care* was the leading book of that genre before your *What to Expect in the First Year.* What do you feel is different in your book, and how does it replace Spock's?

AE: Actually, I used Dr. Spock's book when I was a young mother. But I think one of the big differences is that *What to Expect in the First Year* was written by three mothers. I think that we have more insight into what's going on.

TK: In *Memoirs of an Ex-Prom Queen,* Alix Kates Shulman discusses the contradictory feelings of a young mother when she brings her first child home. She attributes her confusion to Spock's suggestions, which went against her own instincts. So what is it that women as mothers (even first-time mothers) can grasp that male doctors simply cannot?

AE: When you've gone through breast-feeding, for example, you really know what it's like and what the problems are. And that goes for so many other aspects of parenting. I remember listening to a doctor talk about giving a child a healthy diet, and that that's all you have to do. Of course, you can give it to them, but they're not necessarily going to eat it; so therefore, it's a good idea to supplement with vitamins. So there are a lot of things doctors who aren't taking care of children just don't have any idea about. I think that was true about pregnancy.

TK: How did you arrive at that conclusion? What was the impetus that pushed you to write this book?

AE: The first book we wrote was *What to Expect When You're Expecting;* that was when my coauthor Heidi Murkoff was pregnant. She went out and bought a whole lot of books that were either very scary or very inaccurate, or both. Books tended to be written either from the point of view of the woman without full understanding of the medical aspects, or they were written by doctors who didn't understand the families' needs. So I think we were able to combine them both. One of my coauthors, Sandy Hathaway, has been an ob-gyn nurse, and I have a good medical background as well. So we combine medical backgrounds with being mothers, stay-at-home mothers at that. There are doctors who are mothers who go out to work and have somebody else take care of their kids; but we all took care of our kids; we all stayed home with them. So I think we had a big advantage.

TK: Did you find major contradictions when you were following Spock's book?

AE: I didn't have a lot of trouble with that. Actually, I first read Dr. Spock when I was about 12 years old for a Girl Scout badge. I think some his ideas probably stayed with me. But it wasn't a complete guide. His book is a small book that deals with kids from birth through their teen years. Our books are big, fat books that deal with one or two years at a time; they're just much more thorough; we deal with much more.

TK: Your book gained popularity by word of mouth. At that time, it was difficult for women to challenge their doctors. How did your book allowed them to do that with confidence?

AE: Most doctors recommend our books; I think that is why women feel confident to use them from a medical point of view; and the doctors themselves use them. Over and over we hear from both pediatricians and obstetricians that they probably couldn't have gotten through their pregnancy or the first year of their child's life without our books. So they use them and they recommend them; that really has made a big difference.

TK: What do you think are the most potent messages in the book? How does it solve the problem of the contradictions that existed with Spock's book?

AE: Our point of view is that there isn't one answer that will work for every mother and every baby. It just isn't possible. Everybody is different, every baby is different, every mom is different. You have to use your own instincts and feelings and see what works for you and for your baby. There are four things that are invaluable. One is that you have to take care of your baby's health; there are certain things you must do: immunizations, regular checkups. Safety is the second thing. You have to make your house safe for your baby; you always have to use the car seat, that kind of thing. Then you have to love your baby; it's very important. And the other thing is that, along with loving your baby, you have to set limits. Limits are also very important, and different people have different ways of setting them, and different rules. In some households, you can't walk or put your shoes on the sofa; in others, they don't care about that, but there are other rules, like you can't eat sugar. It doesn't matter what they are, but there have to be consistent rules that your kids know they have to follow. Those are the four things that everyone has to be concerned with. Beyond that, there are no rules. You have to do what works for you, and what you're comfortable with, and that's different for each family.

TK: When you wrote *What to Expect When You're Expecting*, what made you so intuitively aware of the questions that mothers had?

AE: It helped that there were three of us because we all had different points of view in certain areas. We had different experiences with our pregnancies and with our doctors, so that started us off with a wide range. But we also did a lot of research and handed out a lot of questionnaires; that was extremely helpful in finding out what people were concerned about.

TK: You were already a writer before you wrote these books. Was it part of your vision to write a book and was *What to Expect When You're Expecting* the ideal one?

AE: I'd written books before that one. In 1975, I did a college textbook on health, which gave me a very good background in medicine. It took me four and a half years and I consider it to be my medical education. My co-author, Sandy, is a nurse and has a DSN, and Heidi was also a writer. So we had expertise, which I think was valuable, because without knowing how to communicate as writers, we probably could not have done as good a job. We had the advantage of medical backgrounds, of being mothers, and also of being writers.

TK: You say expertise; how would you distinguish between professionalism and expertise? What would you say the differences are?

AE: We're not professionals because we don't get paid as medical personnel, but we do have expertise. Somebody told me she went in to ask a question of her doctor and the doctor said, "Excuse me a minute," and they looked up the answer in our book. So we do have a certain amount of expertise from our experience as well as from our research.

TK: What is the focus of the What to Expect Foundation?

AE: The What to Expect Foundation provides materials and programs for low-income and low-literacy moms, and dads as well, of course. We think that's important because the middle class has been able to use our books very successfully, but unfortunately, a lot of people in the lower income brackets either can't afford the books, or really find them overwhelming. We're going to provide books that are easier to read, and that deal with a lot of the ethnic and cultural issues that aren't in our other books.

TK: Until the nineteenth century, it was mothers that were writing books about how to care for children; but then, in the 1830s, it started being doctors, and that lasted until you wrote your ground-breaking book. What allowed that change?

AE: There was a feeling that doctors weren't always meeting the needs of patients because they didn't always understand. Our books have helped because they help doctors to better understand what mothers are going through during pregnancy, or as new parents. When we proposed the book to our publisher, his response was, "A doctor has to write this," and we said, "No, no, no." He was willing to listen to us and to go along with us. A writer knows how to research, how to gather material and make sure it's accurate; I've been doing that for over 40 years.

TK: How much do you think has changed since the 1970s in regards to when a woman decides to have a child and what to do when she has a child? How have those views changed?

AE: A lot has changed. When we first wrote the book, there was an attitude that if you accepted any kind of pain relief during labor, you somehow failed in your job of natural childbirth. We took the position, which was different from that in many books, that if you needed pain medication, then you should have it and be willing to take it. I remember a young woman who cried after she delivered, saying, "I had medication; I failed"; she was really upset. The only thing that's really important is that you and your baby come through that delivery well and healthy; that's what really counts. Anything else is not important. There are women who deliver "naturally" around the world and yet one woman dies every minute in childbirth. "Natural" is not synonymous with healthy or right. I think we changed that attitude and that women now feel that if they need to take medication, it's OK. I think that we've tried to be non-judgmental about what people do. We think breast feeding is by far the best way to feed a baby, but there are some women who just either can't breast feed or don't feel comfortable doing it. If you're not comfortable breast-feeding, your baby's going to get that message anyway; so we tried not to be either judgmental or authoritarian, and we tried to say, "These are your choices; this is what is good about each thing, and you have to decide what's going to work for you." These are some of the things we had some impact on.

TK: Looking back at when you first wrote the book, would you do anything different now?

AE: We have been changing it. When we first wrote *What to Expect*, we actually did not include material about problem pregnancies and complications because we wanted to write a very reassuring book. Then we got letters from people saying, "But you didn't talk about this and you didn't talk about that." So in the revised edition, which came out in 1992, we added all that.

TK: Are there other books that you think are also pretty good?

AE: There are some books that we recommend in our book. One of them is Richard Ferber's book, *Solving Your Child's Sleep Problems*.

TK: The use of midwives seems more popular than it used to be and several people suggest that midwives are the way to go, what do you think of that?

AE: It's a matter of choice, of what you're comfortable with. Midwives are terrific in many cases, but they should be either practicing in a hospital setting or in a setting where you can immediately get emergency care from a physician if it's necessary, for example, if an emergency c-section is needed. In England, they use midwives primarily, but they always have an ambulance standing outside ready to take you to the hospital. Midwives are wonderful because a lot of women are more comfortable with them, and they tell you more and give you more comfort and information, but you also have to be sure you get the best technical medical care as well. That combination is terrific.

TK: Are there any books that you would suggest for men when their wives are expecting?

AE: There are a few out, but I haven't really read them. There's a new one called *Business Dads*, which looks very good, that helps a father who has been working day and night to change his life style in order to be home more with his family.

TK: Would you suggest to a man that he read *What to Expect*?

AE: We do have a section for men in it, and we do recommend that they read the whole thing, and a lot of men do.

TK: So that they understand where their wife is coming from.

AE: Absolutely, it's really valuable, otherwise you don't know. I think it's really important for them to read it.

TK: How quickly did the book become famous?

AE: It was slow. In fact, when it first came out, I think there were 5,600 books ordered, and I think either Barnes and Noble or one of the other big chains didn't even order it because they said they had too many pregnancy books already. It really took a little time for mothers to tell each other about it and then for doctors to start recommending it. It was a gradual, uphill thing. It was a couple of years before it really started to hit the bestseller list.

TK: That isn't too long.

AE: With most publishers, if you don't hit it right away, they stop pushing it. We were very lucky to be with Workman Publishing, which really tries to sell all the books they publish; they made a really good effort. The most important things in our books are not the answers to the questions, but the questions themselves. Because when you find out that everybody has the same questions and worries that you have, you start to think, "Ah-ha, I'm not crazy." A lot of the questions women have they don't want to ask their doctors because they think they're dumb. Our point is that there isn't such a thing as a dumb question. If you're worried about something, then it makes a good question, and when you see that everybody else has the same worries, you're comforted, and I think that is really important.

Monster Mommies

ERICA JONG

> What is home without a mother?
> —Alice Hawthorne

Mommy Guiltiest? So reads the headline in the *New York Daily News*'s rehash of the "Nanny Case," which has riveted the media's public since everybody overdosed on treacly elegies to Diana, Princess of Wales. The *Daily News* has proved once again the old saying "Vox populi is, in the main, a grunt." The *News* is supposed to cater to the downmarket crowd that doesn't read *The New York Times* or *The Wall Street Journal*, but in truth most people in the word biz read all three, as well as *The New York Post* and *The New York Observer.* But without the *News,* you can't possibly know all that's not fit to print. And, of course, that's what tells you about the vacillations of the zeitgeist. And the zeitgeist is currently into blaming mommies for the deaths of their kids.

For this is the lesson of the nanny trial; Louise Woodward may have been nineteen, inexperienced, drowsy in the mornings and moonfaced at night, but Dr. Deborah Eappen was really the one at fault, because she worked three days a week as an ophthalmologist rather than staying at home full-time with her baby. Never mind that she came home at lunch to breast-feed on the days she worked. Never mind that she pumped out breast milk on the other days. Never mind that she was an M.D. working a drastically reduced schedule—a schedule no intern or resident would be permitted to work. She is the one to blame for the heinous crime of baby murder.

In an age when most mothers work because they have to, it is nothing short of astounding that this case resulted in raving callers to talk shows who scream that Dr. Deborah Eappen deserved to have her baby die because she left him with a 19-year-old nanny.

So much for twenty-five years of feminism. So much for smug commentators who say we live in a "postfeminist age." The primitive cry is still "Kill the mommy!" She deserves to be stoned to death for hiring a nanny.

Of course, we Americans already knew that welfare mothers were monsters. Dear Bill Clinton, champion of women and children, signed the most disgusting welfare bill in American history—a bill more appropriate to Dickensian England, a bill basically reinstating the workhouse in millennial America. But, of course, we know the American poor deserve nothing. Poverty is, after all, un-American, America has abolished any definition of the worthy poor (children, mothers, the blind, the lame) and decided that they alone shall pay for the budget deficit run up by male politicians. After all, children have no votes—unlike savings and loan officers. Besides, the latter have lobbyists, and poor children naturally can't afford them. So we have no worthy poor in the country I so lavishly fund with my taxes, but neither have we any child care initiatives—let alone child care.

Even some reactionary countries—La Belle France, for example—have mother care, crèches, kindergartens, but in America we rely on nature red in tooth and claw, so crèches are seen as "creeping socialism," and nobody's allowed to have creeping socialism except the army and the non-tax-paying superrich.

Okay—welfare mommies are monsters, but what about entrepreneurial M.D. mommies? What about women who delayed childbearing to finish school, had babies in their thirties and forties, and work part time? Well, now we learn that they, also, are monsters. Why? Because they don't stay home full time. Apparently all mommies are monsters—the indigent and the highly educated both deserve to watch their babies die.

Wait a minute. What happened here? Is this 1898 or 1998? It doesn't seem to matter. Where motherhood is concerned we might as well be in Dickens's England or Ibsen's Norway or Hammurabi's Persia. Mothers are, by definition, monsters. They're either monsters because they're poor or monsters because they're rich. Where mothers are concerned, everything is a no-win situation.

Poor Louise was nice but somewhat incompetent. Maybe she did shake poor little Matty—the medical evidence is inconclusive. After all, she was a Brit, and Brits love caning kids; shaking is nothing to them. But Deborah was even worse than Louise. She was a doctor's wife (and a doctor, but who cares?) who chose to work.

Both women have been thoroughly trashed. Nobody inveighs against the other Dr. Eappen—the one with a penis—and nobody screams that his baby deserves to die. Nobody talks about Matty either. He's just a dead baby. Dead babies have no votes and no lobbyists. No—what everyone carries on about is which woman is at fault.

The mommy or the nanny? The lady or the tiger? Women, by definition, are always guilty. Either they're guilty of neglect or they're guilty of abuse. Nobody asks about the father's role or the grandparents' role. If it takes a village to raise a child, as Hillary Clinton's bestseller alleges, then that village consists of only two people: monster mother and monster au pair. Everyone else is off the hook. (Including a government that penalizes working moms in its tax policies, its immigration policies, and its lack of day care.)

How must Dr. Deborah Eappen feel, first losing her son and then facing this chorus of harpies (for the women-haters are often women)? Imagine the trauma of losing your baby, the trauma of reliving the pain at the trial, only to face the further trauma of trial by tabloid. Dr. Deborah chose her job because it allowed flexible hours. So did her husband, Dr. Sunil Eappen, but nobody's blaming him. If we have come so far toward the ideal egalitarian marriage, then why does nobody discuss the couple? Only the women are implicated. Both nanny and mommy face death by tabloid firing squad.

If the nanny trial is used as a litmus test for social change, then we must conclude that very little change has occurred. No wonder generation Y is full of young women who want to stay home with their babies! They saw what happened to their weary boomer mothers, and they don't like what they saw. If all feminist progress is dependent on the mother-daughter dialectic (as I believe it is), then we are in for a new generation of stay-at-home moms, whose problems will be closer to our grandmothers' than our own. Betty Friedan's *Feminine Mystique* will be as relevant in 2013 as it was in 1963—and our granddaughters will have to regroup and start feminist reforms all over again.

No wonder feminism has been ebbing and flowing since Mary Wollstonecraft's day. We have never solved the basic problem that afflicts us all—who will help to raise the children?

Chapter 70

Violence Against Women and Girls

*J*udith Herman's Trauma and Recovery *has been described as the most important new psychiatry book since Freud. A compassionate thinker and a lovely
writer, Judy has greatly influenced the thinking of her psychiatric colleagues,
as well as the general public. Several selections in this chapter have been consciousness raising. Norma Fox Mazer's* Out of Control *is a popular young adult
novel. Bernard Lefkowitz's* Our Guys *is the first and only book by a man to be
reviewed on the front page of both the* New York Times Book Review *and the*
Women's Review of Books. *Jennifer Gonnerman has helped change public policy on the incarceration of battered women who kill in self defense.—B. S.*

Trauma and Recovery

JUDITH HERMAN

Excerpted from Judith Herman, *Trauma and Recovery,* New York, Basic Books, 1992. Reprinted by permission.

A single traumatic event can occur almost anywhere. Prolonged, repeated trauma, by contrast, occurs only in circumstances of captivity. When the victim is free to escape, she will not be abused a second time; repeated trauma occurs only when the victim is a prisoner, unable to flee, and under the control of the perpetrator. Such conditions obviously exist in prisons, concentration camps, and slave labor camps. These conditions may also exist in religious cults, in brothels and other institutions of organized sexual exploitation, and in families.

Political captivity is generally recognized, whereas the domestic captivity of women and children is often unseen. A man's home is his castle; rarely is it understood that the same home may be a prison for women and children. In domestic captivity, physical barriers to escape are rare. In most homes, even the most oppressive, there are no bars on the windows, no barbed wire fences. Women and children are not ordinarily chained, though even this occurs more often than one might think. The barriers to escape are generally invisible. They are nonetheless extremely powerful. Children are rendered captive by their condition of dependency. Women are rendered captive by economic, social, psychological, and legal subordination, as well as by physical force.

Captivity, which brings the victim into prolonged contact with the perpetrator, creates a special type of relationship, one of coercive control. This is equally true whether the victim is taken captive entirely by force, as in the case of prisoners and hostages, or by a combination of force, intimidation, and enticement, as in the case of religious cult members, battered women, and abused children. The psychological impact of subordination to coercive control may have many common features, whether that subordination occurs within the public sphere of politics or within the private sphere of sexual and domestic relations.

Former prisoners carry their captors' hatred with them even after release, and sometimes they continue to carry out their captors' destructive purposes with their own hands. Long after their liberation, people who have been subjected to coercive control bear the psychological scars of captivity. They suffer not only from a classic post-traumatic syndrome but also from profound alterations in their relations with God, with other people, and with themselves.

A NEW DIAGNOSIS

Most people have no knowledge or understanding of the psychological changes of captivity. Social judgment of chronically traumatized people therefore tends to be extremely harsh. The chronically abused person's apparent helplessness and passivity, her entrapment in the past, her intractable depression and somatic complaints, and her smoldering anger often frustrate the people closest to her. Moreover, if she had been coerced into betrayal of relationships, community loyalties, or moral values, she is frequently subjected to furious condemnation.

Observers who have never experienced prolonged terror and who have no understanding of coercive methods of control presume that they would show greater courage and resistance than the victim in similar circumstances. Hence the common tendency to account for the victim's behavior by seeking flaws in her personality or moral character. Prisoners of war who succumb to "brainwashing" are often publicly excoriated. Sometimes survivors are treated more harshly than those who abused them. In the notorious case of Patricia Hearst, for instance, the hostage was tried for crimes committed under duress and received a longer prison abusive relationships and those who prostitute themselves or betray their children under duress are subjected to extraordinary censure.

The propensity to fault the character of the victim can be seen even in the case of politically organized mass murder. The aftermath of the Holocaust witnessed a protracted debate regarding the "passivity" of the Jews and their "complicity" in their fate. But the historian Lucy Dawidowicz points out that "complicity" and "cooperation" are terms that apply to situations of free choice. They do not have the same meaning in situations of captivity.

DIAGNOSTIC MISLABELING

This tendency to blame the victim has strongly influenced the direction of psychological inquiry. It has led researchers and clinicians to seek an explanation for the perpetrator's crimes in the character of the victim. In the case of hostages and prisoners of war, numerous attempts to find supposed personality defects that predisposed captives to "brainwashing" have yielded few consistent results. The conclusion is inescapable that ordinary psychologically healthy men can indeed be coerced in unmanly ways. In domestic battering situations, where victims are entrapped by persuasion rather than by capture, research has also focused on the personality traits that might predispose a woman to get involved in an abusive relationship. Here again no consistent profile of the susceptible woman has emerged. While some battered women clearly have major psychological difficulties that render them vulnerable, the majority show no evidence of serious psychopathology before entering into the exploitative relationship. Most become involved with their abusers at a time of temporary life crises or recent loss, when they are feeling unhappy, alienated, or lonely. A survey of the studies of wife-beating concludes: "The search for characteristics of women that contribute to their own victimization is futile. It is sometimes forgotten that men's violence is men's behavior. As such, it is not surprising that the more fruitful efforts to explain this behavior have focused on male characteristics. What is surprising is the enormous effort to explain male behavior by examining characteristics of women."

While it is clear that ordinary, healthy people may become entrapped in prolonged abusive situations, it is equally clear that after their escape they are no longer ordinary or healthy. Chronic abuse causes serious psychological harm. The tendency to blame the victim, however, has interfered with the psychological understanding and diagnosis of a post-traumatic syndrome. Instead of conceptualizing the psychopathology of the victim as a response to an abusive situation, mental health professionals have frequently attributed the abusive situation to the victim's presumed underlying psychopathology.

An egregious example of this sort of thinking is the 1964 study of battered women entitled "The Wife-Beater's Wife." The researchers, who had originally sought to study batterers, found that the men would not talk to them. They thereupon redirected their attention to the more cooperative battered women, whom they found to be "castrating," "frigid," "aggressive," "indecisive," and "passive." They concluded that marital violence fulfilled these women's "masochistic needs." Having identified the women's personality disorders as the source of the problem, these clinicians set out to "treat" them. In one case they managed to persuade the wife that she was provoking the violence, and they showed her how to mend her ways. When she no longer sought help from her teenage son to protect herself from beatings and no longer refused to submit to sex on demand, even when her husband was drunk and aggressive, her treatment was judged a success.

While this unabashed, open sexism is rarely found in psychiatric literature today, the same conceptual errors, with their implicit bias and contempt, still predominate. The clinical picture of a person who has been reduced to elemental concerns of survival is still frequently mistaken for a portrait of the victim's underlying character. Concepts of personality organization developed under ordinary circumstances are applied to victims, without any understanding of the corrosion of personality that occurs under conditions of prolonged terror. Thus, patients who suffer from the complex aftereffects of chronic trauma still commonly risk being misdiagnosed as having personality disorders. They may be described as inherently "dependent," "masochistic," or "self-defeating." In a recent study of emergency room practice in a large urban hospital, clinicians routinely described battered women as "hysterics," "masochistic females," "hypochondriacs," or, more simply, "crocks."

This tendency to misdiagnose victims was at the heart of a controversy that arose in the mid-1980s when the diagnostic manual of the American Psychiatric Association came up for revision. A group of male psychoanalysts proposed that "masochistic personality disorder" be added to the canon. This hypothetical diagnosis applied to any person who "remains in relationships in which others exploit, abuse, or take advantage of him or her, despite opportunities to alter the situation." A number of women's groups were outraged, and a heated public debate ensued. Women insisted on opening up the process of writing the diagnostic canon, which had been the preserve of a small group of men, and for the first time took part in the naming of psychological reality.

I was one of the participants in this process. What struck me most at the time was how little rational argument seemed to matter. The women's representatives came to the discussion prepared with carefully reasoned, extensively documented position papers, which argued that the proposed diagnostic concept had little scientific foundation, ignored recent advances in understanding the psychology of victimization, and was socially regressive and discriminatory in impact, since it would be used to stigmatize disempowered people. The men of the psychiatric establishment persisted in their bland denial. They admitted freely that they were ignorant of the extensive literature of the past decade on psychological trauma, but they did not see why it should concern them. One member of the Board of Trustees of the American Psychiatric Association felt the discussion of battered women was "irrelevant." Another stated simply, "I never see victims."

In the end, because of the outcry from organized women's groups and the widespread publicity engendered by the controversy, some sort of compromise became expedient. The name of the proposed entity was changed to "self-defeating personality disorder." The criteria for diagnosis were changed, so that the label could not be applied to people who were known to be physically, sexually, or psychologically abused. Most important, the disorder was included not in the main body of the test but in an appendix. It was relegated to apocryphal status within the canon, where it languished to this day.

NEED FOR A NEW CONCEPT

Misapplication of the concept of masochistic personality disorder may be one of the most stigmatizing diagnostic mistakes, but it is by no means the only one. In general, the diagnostic categories of the existing psychiatric canon are simply not designed for survivors of extreme situations and do not fit them well. The persistent anxiety, phobias, and panic of survivors are not the same as ordinary anxiety disorders. The somatic symptoms of survivors are not the same as ordinary psychosomatic disorders. Their depression is not the same as ordinary depression. And the degradation of their identity and relational life is not the same as ordinary personality disorder.

The lack of an accurate and comprehensive diagnostic concept has serious consequences for treatment, because the connection between the patient's present symptoms and the traumatic experience is frequently lost. Attempts to fit the patient into the mold of existing diagnostic constructs generally result, at best, in a partial understanding of the problem and a fragmented approach to treatment. All too commonly, chronically traumatized people suffer in silence; but if they complain at all, their complaints are not well understood. They may collect a virtual pharmacopoeia of remedies: one for headaches, another for insomnia, another for anxiety, another for depression. None of these tends to work very well, since the underlying issues of trauma are not addressed. As caregivers tire of these chronically unhappy people who do not seem to improve, the temptation to apply pejorative diagnostic labels becomes overwhelming.

Even the diagnosis of "post-traumatic stress disorder," as it is presently defined, does not fit accurately enough. The existing diagnostic criteria for this disorder are derived mainly from survivors of circumscribed traumatic events. They are based on the prototypes of combat, disaster, and rape. In survivors of prolonged, repeated trauma, the symptom picture is often far more complex. Survivors of prolonged abuse develop characteristic personality changes, including deformations of relatedness and identity. Survivors of abuse in childhood develop similar problems with relationships and identity; in addition, they are particularly vulnerable to repeated harm, both self-inflicted and at the hands of others. The current formulation of post-traumatic stress disorder fails to capture either the protean symptomatic manifestations of prolonged, repeated trauma or the profound deformations of personality that occur in captivity.

The syndrome that follows upon prolonged, repeated trauma needs its own name. I propose to call it "complex post-traumatic stress disorder." The responses to trauma are best understood as a spectrum of conditions rather than as a single disorder. They range from a brief stress reaction that gets better by itself and never qualifies for a diagnosis, to classic or simple post-traumatic stress disorder, to the complex syndrome of prolonged, repeated trauma.

Although the complex traumatic syndrome has never before been outlined systematically, the concept of a spectrum of post-traumatic disorders has been noted, almost in passing, by many experts. Lawrence Kolb remarks on the "heterogeneity" of post-traumatic stress disorder, which "is to psychiatry as syphilis was to medicine. At one time or another [this disorder] may appear to mimic every personality disorder.... It is those threatened over long periods of time who suffer the long-standing severe personality disorganization." Others have also called attention to the personality changes that follow prolonged, repeated trauma. The psychiatrist Emmanuel Tanay, who works with survivors of the Nazi Holocaust, observes: "The psychopathology may be hidden in characterological changes that are manifest only in disturbed object relationships and attitudes towards work, the world, man and God."

Many experienced clinicians have invoked the need for a diagnostic formulation that goes beyond simple post-traumatic stress disorder. William Niederland finds that "the concept of traumatic neurosis does not appear sufficient to cover the multitude and severity of clinical manifestations" of the syndrome observed in survivors of the Nazi Holocaust. Psychiatrists who have treated Southeast Asian refugees also recognize the need for an "expanded concept" of post-traumatic stress disorder that takes into account severe, prolonged, and massive psychological trauma. One authority suggests the concept of a "post-traumatic character disorder." Others speak of "complicated" post-traumatic stress disorder.

Clinicians who work with survivors of childhood abuse have also seen the need for an expanded diagnostic concept. Lenore Terr distinguishes the effects of a single traumatic blow, which she calls "type 1" trauma, from the effects of prolonged, repeated trauma, which she calls "type 2." Her description of the type 2 syndrome includes denial and psychic numbing, self-hypnosis and dissociation, and alternations between extreme passivity and outbursts of rage. The psychiatrist Jean Goodwin has invented the acronyms FEARS for simple post-traumatic stress disorder and BAD FEARS for the severe post-traumatic disorder observed in survivors of childhood abuse.

Thus, observers have often glimpsed the underlying unity of the complex traumatic syndrome and have given it many different names. It is time for the disorder to have an official, recognized name. Currently, the complex post-traumatic stress disorder is under consideration for inclusion in the fourth edition of the diagnostic manual of the American Psychiatric Association, based on seven diagnostic criteria (see box). Empirical field trials are under way to determine whether such a syndrome can be diagnosed reliably in chronically traumatized people. The degree of scientific and intellectual rigor in this process is considerably higher than that which occurred in the pitiable debates over "masochistic personality disorder."

As the concept of a complex traumatic syndrome has gained wider recognition, it has been given several additional names. The working group for the diagnostic manual of the American Psychiatric Association has chosen the designation "disorder of extreme stress not otherwise specified." The International Classification of Diseases is considering a similar entity under the name "personality change from catastrophic experience." These names may be awkward and unwieldy, but practically any name that gives recognition to the syndrome is better than no name at all.

Naming the syndrome of complex post-traumatic stress disorder represents an essential step toward granting those who have endured prolonged exploitation a measure of the recognition they deserve. It is an attempt to find a language that is at once faithful to the traditions of accurate psychological observation and to the moral demands of traumatized people. It is an attempt to learn from survivors, who understand, more profoundly than any investigator, the effects of captivity.

SURVIVORS AS PSYCHIATRIC PATIENTS

The mental health system is filled with survivors of prolonged, repeated childhood trauma. This is true even though most people who have been abused in childhood never come to psychiatric attention. To the extent that these people recover, they do so on their own. While only a small minority of survivors, usually those with the most severe abuse histories, eventually become psychiatric patients, many or even most psychiatric patients are survivors of childhood abuse. The data on this point are beyond contention. On careful questioning, 50 to 60 percent of psychiatric inpatients and 40 to 60 percent of outpatients report childhood histories of physical or sexual abuse or both. In one study of psychiatric emergency room patients, 70 percent had abuse histories. Thus abuse in childhood appears to be one of the main factors that lead a person to seek psychiatric treatment as an adult.

Survivors of child abuse who become patients appear with a bewildering array of symptoms. Their general levels of distress are higher than those of other patients. Perhaps the most impressive finding is the sheer length of the list of symptoms correlated with a history of childhood abuse. The psychologist Jeffrey Bryer and his colleagues report that women with histories of physical or sexual abuse have significantly higher scores than other patients on standardized measures of somatization, depression, general anxiety, phobic anxiety, interpersonal sensitivity, paranoia, and "psychoticism" (probably dissociative symptoms). The psychologist John Briere reports that survivors of childhood abuse display significantly more insomnia, sexual dysfunction, dissociation, anger, suicidality, self-mutilation, drug addiction, and alcoholism than other patients. The symptoms list can be prolonged almost indefinitely.

When survivors of childhood abuse seek treatment, they have what the psychologist Denise Gelinas calls a "disguised presentation." They come for help because of their many symptoms or because of difficulty with relationships: problems in intimacy, excessive responsiveness to the needs of others, and repeated victimization. All too commonly, neither patient nor therapist recognizes the link between the presenting problem and the history of chronic trauma.

Survivors of childhood abuse, like other traumatized people, are frequently misdiagnosed and mistreated in the mental health system. Because of the number and complexity of their symptoms, their treatment is often fragmented and incomplete. Because of their characteristic difficulties in close relationships, they are particularly vulnerable to revictimization by caregivers. They may become engaged in ongoing, destructive interactions, in which the medical or mental health system relicates the behavior of the abusive family.

Survivors of childhood abuse often accumulate many different diagnoses before the underlying problem of a complex post-traumatic syndrome is recognized. They are likely to receive a diagnosis that carries strong negative connotations. Three particularly troublesome diagnoses have often been applied to survivors of childhood abuse: somatization disorder, borderline personality disorder, and multiple personality disorder. All three of these diagnoses were once subsumed under the now obsolete name *hysteria*. Patients, usually women, who received these diagnoses evoke unusually intense reactions in caregivers. Their credibility is often suspect. They are frequently accused of manipulating or malingering. They are often the subject of furious and partisan controversy. Sometimes they are frankly hated.

These three diagnoses are charged with pejorative meaning. The most notorious is the diagnosis of borderline personality disorder. This term is frequently used within the mental health professions as little more than a sophisticated insult. As one psychiatrist candidly confesses, "As a resident, I recalled asking my supervisor how to treat patients with borderline personality disorder, and he answered, sardonically, 'You refer them.'" The psychiatrist Irvin Yalom describes the term "borderline" as "the word that strikes terror into the heart of the middle-aged, comfort-seeking psychiatrist." Some clinicians have argued that the term "borderline" had become so prejudicial that it should be abandoned altogether, just as its predecessor term, *hysteria,* had to be abandoned.

These three diagnoses have many features in common, and often they cluster and overlap with one another. Patients who receive any one of these three diagnoses usually qualify for several other diagnoses as well. For example, the majority of patients with somatization disorder also have major depression, agoraphobia, and panic, in addition to their numerous physical complaints. Over half are given additional diagnoses of "histrionic," "antisocial," or "borderline" personality disorders. Similarly, people with borderline personality disorder often suffer as well from major depression, substance abuse, agoraphobia or panic, and somatization disorder. The majority of patients with multiple personality disorder experience sever depression. Most also meet diagnostic criteria for borderline personality disorder. And they generally have numerous psychosomatic complaints, including headache, unexplained pains, gastrointestinal disturbances, and hysterical conversion symptoms. These patients receive an average of three other psychiatric or neurological diagnoses before the underlying problem of multiple personality disorder is finally recognized.

All three disorders are associated with high levels of hypnotizability or dissociation, but in this respect, multiple personality disorder is in a class by itself. People with multiple personality disorder possess staggering dissociative capabilities. Some of their more bizarre symptoms may be mistaken for symptoms of schizophrenia. For example, they may have "passive influence" experiences of being controlled by another personality, or hallucinations of the voices of quarreling alter personalities. Patients with borderline personality disorder, though they are rarely capable of the same virtuosic feats of dissociation, also have abnormally high levels of dissociative symptoms. And patients with somatization disorder are reported to have high levels of hypnotizability and psychogenic amnesia.

Patients with all three disorders also share characteristic difficulties in close relationships. Interpersonal difficulties have been described most extensively in patients with borderline personality disorder. Indeed, a pattern of intense, unstable relationships is one of the major criteria for making this diagnosis. Borderline patients find it very hard to tolerate being alone but are also exceedingly wary of others. Terrified of abandonment on the one hand and of domination on the other, they oscillate between extremes of clinging and withdrawal, between abject submissiveness and furious rebellion. They tend to form "special" relations with idealized caretakers in which ordinary boundaries are not observed. Psychoanalytic authors attribute this instability to a failure of psychological development in the formative years of early childhood. One authority describes the primary defect in borderline personality disorder as a "failure to achieve object constancy," that is, a failure to form reliable and well-integrated inner representations of trusted people. Another speaks of the "relative developmental failure in formation of introjects that provide to the self a function of holding-soothing security"; that is, people with borderline personality disorder cannot calm or comfort themselves by calling up a mental image of a secure relationship with a caretaker.

Similar patterns of stormy, unstable relationships are found in patients with multiple personality disorder. In this disorder, with its extreme compartmentalization of functions, the highly contradictory patterns of relating may be carried out by dissociated "alter" personalities. Patients with multiple personality disorder also have a tendency to develop intense, highly "special" relationships, ridden with boundary violations, conflict, and the potential for exploitation. Patients with somatization disorder also have difficulties in intimate relationships, including sexual, marital, and parenting problems.

Disturbances in identity formation are also characteristic of patients with borderline and multiple personality disorder (they have not been systematically studied in somatization disorder). Fragmentation of the self into dissociated alters is the central feature of multiple personality disorder. The array of personality fragments usually includes at least one "hateful" or "evil" alter, as well as one socially conforming, submissive, or "good" alter. Patients with borderline personality disorder lack the dissociative capacity to form fragmented alters, but they have similar difficulty developing an integrated identity. Inner images of the self are split into extremes of good and bad. An unstable sense of self is one of the major diagnostic criteria for borderline personality disorder, and the "splitting" of inner representations of self and others is considered by some theorists to be the central underlying pathology of the disorder.

The common denominator of these three disorders is their origin in a history of childhood trauma. The evidence for this link ranges from definitive to suggestive. In the case of multiple personality disorder the etiological role of severe childhood trauma is at this point firmly established. In a study by the psychiatrist Frank Putnam of 100 patients with the disorder, 97 had histories of major childhood trauma, most commonly sexual abuse, physical abuse, or both. Extreme sadism and murderous violence were the rule rather than the exception in these dreadful histories. Almost half the patients had actually witnessed the violent death of someone close to them.

In borderline personality disorder, my investigations have also documented histories of severe childhood trauma in the great majority (81 percent) of cases. The abuse generally began early in life and was severe and prolonged, though it rarely reached the lethal extremes described by patients with multiple personality disorder. The earlier the onset of abuse and the greater its severity, the greater the likelihood that the survivor would develop symptoms of borderline personality disorder. The specific relationship between symptoms of borderline personality disorder and a history of childhood trauma has now been confirmed in numerous other studies.

Evidence for the link between somatization disorder and childhood trauma is not yet complete. Somatization disorder is sometimes also called Briquet's syndrome, after the nineteenth-century French physician Paul Briquet, a predecessor of Charcot. Briquet's observations of patients with the disorder are filled with anecdotal references to domestic violence, childhood trauma, and abuse. In a study of 87 children under twelve, Briquet noted that one-third had been "habitually mistreated or held constantly in fear or had been directed harshly by their parents." In another 10 percent, he attributed the children's symptoms to traumatic experiences other than parental abuse. After the lapse of a century, investigation of the link between somatization disorder and childhood abuse has only lately been resumed. A recent study of women with somatization disorder found that 55 percent had been sexually molested in childhood, usually by relatives. This study, however, focused only on early sexual experiences; patients were not asked about physical abuse or a more general climate of violence in their families. Systematic investigation of the childhood histories of patients with somatization disorder has yet to be undertaken.

These three disorders might perhaps be best understood as variants of complex post-traumatic stress disorder, each deriving its characteristic features from one form of adaptation to the traumatic environment. The physioneurosis of post-traumatic stress disorder is the most prominent feature in somatization disorder, the deformation of consciousness is most prominent in multiple personality disorder, and the disturbance in identity and relationship is most prominent in borderline personality disorder. The overarching concept of a complex post-traumatic syndrome accounts for both the particularity of the three disorders and their interconnection. The formulation also reunites the descriptive fragments of the condition that was once called hysteria and reaffirms their common source in a history of psychological trauma.

Many of the most troubling features of these three disorders become more comprehensible in the light of a history of childhood trauma. More important, survivors become comprehensible to themselves. When survivors recognize the origins of their psychological difficulties in an abusive childhood environment, they no longer need attribute them to an inherent defect in the self. Thus the way is opened to the creation of new meaning in experience and a new, unstigmatized identity.

Understanding the role of childhood trauma in the development of these severe disorders also informs every aspect of treatment. This understanding provides the basis for a cooperative therapeutic alliance that normalizes and validates the survivor's emotional reactions to past events, while recognizing that these reactions may be maladaptive in the present. Moreover, a shared understanding of the survivor's characteristic disturbances of relationship and the consequent risk of repeated victimization offers the best insurance against unwitting reenactments of the original trauma in the therapeutic relationship.

The testimony of patients is eloquent on the point that recognition of the trauma is central to the recovery process. Three survivors who have had long careers in psychiatric treatment can speak here for all patients. Each accumulated numerous mistaken diagnoses and suffered through numerous unsuccessful treatments before finally discovering the source of her psychological problems in her history of severe childhood abuse. And each challenges us to decipher her language and to recognize, behind the multiplicity of disguises, the complex post-traumatic syndrome.

The first survivor, Barbara, manifests the predominant symptoms of somatization disorder:

> I lived in hell on earth without benefit of a doctor or medication.... I could not breathe, I had spasms when I attempted to swallow food, my heart pounded in my chest, I had numbness in my face and St. Vitus dance when I went to bed. I had migraine headaches, and the blood vessels above my right eye were so taut I could not close that eye.

> [My therapist] and I have decided that I have dissociated states. Though they are very similar to personalities, I know that they are part of me. When the horrors first surfaced, I went through a psychological death. I remember floating up on a white cloud with many people inside, but I could not make out the faces. Then two hands came out and pressed on my chest, and a voice said, "Don't go in there."

> Had I gone for help when I had my breakdown, I feel I would have been classified as mentally ill. The diagnosis probably would have been manic depressive with a flavor of schizophrenia, panic disorder, and agoraphobia. At that time no one would have had the diagnostic tools to come up with a diagnosis of [complex] post-traumatic stress disorder.

The second survivor, Tani, was diagnosed with borderline personality disorder:

I know that things are getting better about borderlines and stuff. Having that diagnosis resulted in my getting treated exactly the way I was treated at home. The minute I got that diagnosis people stopped treating me as though what I was doing had a reason. All that psychiatric treatment was just as destructive as what happened before.

Denying the reality of my experience—that was the most harmful. Not being able to trust anyone was the most serious effect.… I knew I acted in ways that were despicable. But I wasn't crazy. Some people go around acting like that because they feel hopeless. Finally I found a few people along the way who have been able to feel OK about me even though I had severe problems. Good therapists were those who really validated my experience.

The third survivor is Hope, who manifests the predominant symptoms of multiple personality disorder:

Long ago, a lovely young child was branded with the term *paranoid schizophrenic.* … The label became a heavy yoke. A Procrustean bed I always fit into so nicely, for I never grew.… I became wrapped, shrouded. No alert, spectacled psychologist had trained a professional mind upon my dull drudgery. No. The diagnosis of paranoid schizophrenic was not offered me where I could look kindly back onto the earnest practitioner and say, "You're wrong. It's really just a lifetime of grief, but it's all right."

Somehow the dreaded words got sprinkled on my cereal, rinsed into my clothes. I felt them in hard looks, and hands that inadvertently pressed down. I saw the words in the averted head, the questions that weren't asked, the careful, repetitious confines of a concept made smaller, simpler for my benefit. The years pass. They go on. The haunting refrain has become a way of life. Expectation is slowed. Progress looks nostalgically backward. And all the time a lurking snake lies hidden in the heart

Finally, chains begin to be unlocking. Spurred on by the fresh, crisp increase of the Still, Small Voice. I begin to see some of what those silent, unspoken words never said. I saw a mask. It looked like me. I took it off and beheld a group of huddled, terrified people who shrank together to hide terrible secrets.…

The words "paranoid schizophrenic" started to fall into place, letter by letter, but it looked like feelings and thoughts and actions that hurt children, and lied, and covered disgrace, and much terror. I began to realize that the label, the diagnosis, had been a handmaid, much like the letter "A" Hester Prynne embroidered upon her breast.… And down all the days and all the embroidered hours, other words kept pushing aside the badge, the label, the diagnosis. "Hurting children." "That which is unseemly." "Women with women, and men with men, doing that which is unseemly.... "

I forsook my paranoid schizophrenia, and packed it up with my troubles, and sent it to Philadelphia.

CHARACTERISTICS OF COMPLEX POST-TRAUMATIC STRESS DISORDER

A history of subjection to totalitarian control over a prolonged period (months to years). Examples include hostages, prisoners of war, concentration camp survivors, and survivors of some religious cults. Examples also include those subjected to totalitarian systems in sexual and domestic life, including survivors of domestic battering, childhood physical or sexual abuse, and organized sexual exploitation.

1. ALTERATIONS IN AFFECT REGULATION

Persistent dysphoria
Chronic suicidal preoccupation
Self-injury
Explosive or extremely inhibited anger (may alternate)
Compulsive or extremely inhibited sexuality (may alternate)

2. ALTERATIONS IN CONSCIOUSNESS

Amnesia or hyperamnesia for traumatic events
Transient dissociative episodes
Depersonalization/derealization
Reliving experiences, either in the form of intrusive post-traumatic stress
disorder symptoms or in the form of ruminative preoccupation

3. ALTERATIONS IN SELF-PERCEPTION

Sense of helplessness or paralysis of initiative
Shame, guilt, and self-blame
Sense of defilement or stigma
Sense of complete difference from others (may include sense of special-
ness, utter aloneness, belief no other person can understand, or non-
human identity)

4. ALTERATIONS IN PERCEPTION OF PERPETRATOR

Preoccupation with relationship with perpetrator (includes preoccupation
with revenge)
Unrealistic attribution of total power to perpetrator (caution: victim's
assessment of power realities may be more realistic than clinician's)
Idealization or paradoxical gratitude
Sense of special or supernatural relationship
Acceptance of belief system or rationalizations of perpetrator

5. ALTERATIONS IN RELATIONS WITH OTHERS

Isolation and withdrawal

Disruption in intimate relationships

Repeated search for rescuer (may alternate with isolation and withdrawal)

Persistent distrust

Repeated failures of self-protection

6. ALTERATIONS IN SYSTEMS OF MEANING

Loss of sustaining faith

Sense of hopelessness and despair

How to Befriend a Battered Woman

BARBARA SEAMAN AND LESLYE E. ORLOFF

Compiled and excerpted from Barbara Seaman, "Domestic Violence: What the Doctor Should Do," *The Lawyer's Manual on Domestic Violence,* Supreme Court of the State of New York, Appellate Division, First Department. Anne D. Lopatto and James Neely, eds. ©1995. Reprinted by permission. Leslye E. Orloff, "Effective Advocacy for Domestic Violence Victims: Role of the Nurse-Midwife," *Journal of Nurse-Midwifery,* 41(6): 473–494, 1996. Reprinted by permission.

BARBARA SEAMAN ON DOMESTIC VIOLENCE:
WHAT THE DOCTOR SHOULD DO

Public health, as well as law enforcement, authorities have come to recognize that "wife beating" is not only a crime, but also a major cause of death and injury to women. Many battered women who fear accessing the police and courts do, of necessity, access health facilities, especially hospital emergency departments. One physician compares sending a domestic violence victim home to "tossing a burn victim back into a fiery house." According to the American Medical Association, "Seventy-five percent of battered women first identified in a medical setting will go on to suffer repeated abuse."

A woman may be safer on the streets at night than at home with her own husband. The AMA accepts the estimate that more than half of female murder victims are killed by current or former partners, that 8 to 12 million women in the United States are at risk of abuse:

"Domestic violence also known as partner-abuse, spouse-abuse, or battering, is one facet of the larger problem of family violence. Family violence occurs among persons within a family or other intimate relationships, and includes child abuse and elder abuse as well as domestic violence. Family violence usually results from the abuse of power or the domination and victimization of a physically less powerful person by a physically more powerful person. Changes in traditional services, including medical care, are needed to meet the needs of abused women."

As these changes, for which the regulatory underpinnings are now in place, come into full expression, the health-care system will likely be recognized as a logical first point of intervention in battery, not as a mere adjunct. Ultimately, health care can do better than legal services at rescuing battered women, because the health provider's duty is solely to the patient, and is unambiguous. Unlike the police and the courts, protective efforts of the doctor or other health provider are not constrained, delayed, or inhibited by "he says/she says" conflicting explanations of the victim and the perpetrator. The AMA's Council on Ethical and Judicial Affairs has concluded that the principal of "beneficence" requires physicians to intervene in cases of domestic violence, and warns that if an injured woman is treated by a physician who does not inquire about abuse or who accepts an unlikely explanation of the injuries and she then returns to the abusive situation and sustains further injuries, the physician could be held liable.

MEASURING THE MEDICAL RESPONSE During the 1980s, a handful of women physicians began to collect evidence that emergency departments and other medical facilities were failing to give appropriate care to most of the battered women who apply for treatment, and that only a fraction of domestic violence victims are correctly identified when they enter the system. At the typical emergency department, no more than 2 to 5 percent of women presenting with injuries are recorded as having had them deliberately inflicted, while the true figure ranges from one-fifth to one-third. A corner was turned in 1985, when then-U.S. Surgeon General Everett Koop, persuaded by the new research, announced his conclusion that more women are injured by battery than by rape, muggings, and accidents combined.

THE TIME FRAME It took a dozen years or more, from the first stirrings of the "battered women's movement" in the early 1970s, until Koop's acknowledgment in 1985, to the identification of "wife beating" as a major source of both morbidity and mortality; the leading single cause of injury to women.

From 1985 to 1992, the government, public health, and organized medical authorities, under the national leadership of Koop and his successor, Antonia Novello, developed a blueprint for sweeping changes in the medical response to domestic violence. Although regulations are insufficiently publicized to lay persons, by 1993 most health care facilities throughout the United States were subject to national, state, and local regulations requiring that suspected victims of both domestic violence and elder abuse receive attention and processing which is quite similar to that afforded to victims of rape and to abused children.

The president of the AMA gives domestic violence education the highest priority, while the American College of Obstetrics and Gynecology is also deeply committed. It is now recognized that: many males first commence battering when their wives or girlfriends are pregnant; 1 in 6 pregnant women is battered; pregnant adolescents are apt to experience multiple beatings, at the hands of parents as well as sex partners.

Our society is now allocating resources to carry out the new requirements. A national objective of the U.S. Public Health Service is that by the year 2000, at least 90 percent of hospital emergency departments have procedures for routinely identifying, treating, and referring victims of spouse abuse. If this goal is met, it will have taken domestic violence from a private sin and sorrow, outside the concern and purview medical practitioners, into as unquestioned a public health responsibility as the requirement that surgeons scrub their hands before performing surgery. And, like the adoption of sterilized operating procedures, the enforcement of laws against drunk driving, and other successful programs in public health, the relative cost of enhanced domestic violence identification will be modest. However, knowing what to do with that information is another matter. Health providers need training in a new set of skills, procedures, and resources, as Dr. Nancy Kathleen Sugg's study of primary care physicians in Seattle clearly demonstrates. Faced with a possible domestic violence situation, the doctors readily acknowledged that discomfort, fear of offending, powerlessness, time constraints, feelings of inadequacy, and above all fear of opening either "Pandora's box" or a "can of worms" (both phrases were used repeatedly), inhibited them from making appropriate interventions. Many pointed to the complexity of the problems and complained that they had "no tools" to help. Sixty-one percent complained that they had had no domestic violence training whatsoever in medical school or residency, or in continuing medical education courses. Thirty-nine percent conceded that identification with patients might blind them from considering the possibility of domestic violence in their own social class.

REGULATIONS In recent years, regulations—state, local, and national—have required emergency departments to identify, treat, and refer battered women, while compiling an evidentiary record and taking steps to secure their safety. In 1990, the American Medical Women's Association became the first major medical group to pass resolutions concerning physician responsibility toward victims of domestic violence. In the same year, the New York State Health Department became one of the first to issue domestic violence protocols for hospital emergency services.

Effective January 1992, the Joint Commission on Accreditation of Healthcare Organizations (JCAHO) revised its *Accreditation Manual for Hospitals* to require that: "standards previously addressed only to the management of child abuse and rape victims be expanded to include victims of spousal and elderly abuse." JCAHO, which has the power to close down a hospital for noncompliance, acknowledges that more than 1 million women every year use emergency departments for treatment of immediate injuries from battery.

The following four-step intervention strategy is suggested for use by all health care providers who treat female patients. It includes specific steps to take if a patient discloses the abuse.

1. IDENTIFY battered women by interviewing all female patients alone and out of earshot of any accompanying partner. Ask directly, for example, "Are you in a relationship where you have been physically hurt or threatened by your partner?"

2. VALIDATE her experience. Believe what the battered woman tells you. Offer positive messages such as "You are not alone" and "You don't deserve this." Document her injuries and symptoms in the medical record.

3. ADVOCATE for her safety and help her expand her options. Assess for safety by asking: "Is it safe for you to go home?" and "Is there somewhere else you can go—a friend or family member?" Be prepared to refer her to domestic violence service providers who can assist her in finding emergency shelter. In all identified cases, offer written and verbal information about local domestic violence services.

4. SUPPORT the battered woman in her choices. Recognize that she is the best judge of what is safe for her. Your intervention is a success if she is talking about the violence and beginning to explore her options. Remember that for most battered women, leaving is a long and difficult process. Most battered women leave and return six to eight times before leaving for good.

RECOGNIZING AND TREATING VICTIMS OF DOMESTIC VIOLENCE

It is important to recognize that the primary goal of all interventions for battered women and their children must be their safety. The following is based on the American Medical Association's Diagnostic and Treatment Guidelines on Domestic Violence.

If you treat women, whether in private practice or in a hospital, you are almost certainly treating some patients who are victims of domestic violence. The following decision tree is designed to help you assess a patient's risk of domestic violence and offer appropriate help to those in need of it.

IDENTIFYING VICTIMS OF DOMESTIC VIOLENCE

Although many women who are victims of abuse will not volunteer any information, they will discuss it if asked simple, direct questions in a nonjudgemental way and in a confidential setting. *The patient should be interviewed alone, without her partner present.* You may want to offer a statement such as: "Because violence is so common in many women's lives, I've begun to ask about it routinely." Then you can ask a direct question, such as "At any time, has your partner hit, kicked, or otherwise hurt or frightened you?" If patient answers yes, the following steps are suggested:

ENCOURAGE HER TO TALK ABOUT IT: "Would you like to talk about what has happened to you?" "How do you feel about it?" "What would you like to do about this?"

LISTEN NONJUDGMENTALLY. This serves to begin the healing process for the woman and to give you an idea of what kind of referrals she needs.

VALIDATE: Victims of domestic violence are frequently not believed, and the fear they report is minimized. The physician can express support through simple statements such as: "You are not alone." "You don't deserve to be treated this way." "You are not to blame." "What happened to you is a crime." "Help is available to you."

DOCUMENT: The patient's complaints and symptoms as well as the results of the observation and assessment (complaints should be described in the patient's own words whenever possible); the patient's complete medical and trauma history and relevant social history; a detailed description of the injuries, including type, number, size, location, resolution, possible causes, and explanations given; an opinion on whether the injuries were consistent with the patent's explanation; results of all pertinent laboratory and other diagnostic procedures; color photographs and imaging studies, if applicable; if the police are called, the name of the investigating officer and any action taken (the police should be called if patient exhibits a reportable injury).

ASSESS THE DANGER TO YOUR PATIENT: Assess your patient's safety *before she leaves the medical setting.* The most important determinants of risk are the woman's level of fear and her appraisal of her immediate and future safety. Discussing the following indicators with the patient can help you determine if she is in escalating danger: an increase in the frequency or severity of the assaults; increasing or new threats of homicide or suicide by the partner; threats to her children; the presence or availability of a firearm.

PROVIDE APPROPRIATE TREATMENT REFERRAL AND SUPPORT: Treat the patient's injuries as indicated. In prescribing medication, keep in mind that medications which hinder the patient's ability to protect herself or to flee from a violent partner may endanger her life. If your patient is in imminent danger, determine if she has friends or family with whom she can stay. If this is not an option, ask if she wants immediate access to a shelter for battered women. If none is available, can she be admitted to the hospital? If she doesn't need immediate access to a shelter, offer written information about shelters and other community resources. Remember that it may be dangerous for the woman to have these in her possession. Don't insist that she take them if she is reluctant to do so. It may be safest for your patient if you write the number on a prescription blank or an appointment card. You may wish to give her the opportunity to call from a private phone in your office.

If the patient answers no, or will not discuss the topic:

BE AWARE OF CLINICAL FINDINGS THAT MAY INDICATE ABUSE: injury to the head, neck, torso, breasts, abdomen, or genitals; bilateral or multiple injuries; delay between onset of injury and seeking treatment; explanation by the patient which is inconsistent with the type of injury; any injury during pregnancy, especially to the abdomen or breasts; prior history of trauma; chronic pain symptoms for which no etiology is apparent; psychological distress, such as depression, suicidal ideation, anxiety, and/or sleep disorders; a partner who seems overly protective or who will not leave the woman's side.

IF ANY OF THE ABOVE CLINICAL SIGNS ARE PRESENT, IT IS APPROPRIATE TO ASK MORE SPECIFIC QUESTIONS. BE SURE THAT THE PATIENT'S PARTNER IS NOT PRESENT. Some examples of questions that may elicit more information about the patient's situation are: "It looks as though someone may have hurt you. Could you tell me how it happened?" "Sometimes when people come for health care with physical symptoms like yours, we find that there may be trouble at home. We are concerned that someone is hurting or abusing you. Is this happening?"

IF THE PATIENT ANSWERS NO: If the patient denies abuse, but you strongly suspect that it is taking place, you can let her know that your office can provide referrals to local programs, should she choose to pursue such options in the future.

DON'T JUDGE THE SUCCESS OF THE INTERVENTION BY THE PATIENT'S ACTION. A woman is most at risk of serious injury or even homicide when she attempts to leave an abusive partner, and it may take her a long time before she can finally do so. It is frustrating for the physician when a patient stays in an abusive situation. Be reassured that if you have acknowledged and validated her situation and offered appropriate referrals, you have done what you can do to help her.

LESLYE ORLOFF ON EFFECTIVE ADVOCACY
FOR DOMESTIC VIOLENCE VICTIMS

Many battered women become trapped in abusive relationships because abusers lower their victims' self-esteem and convince their victims that they deserve the abuse, that it is normal, or that no one will believe them if they seek help.

Nurse-midwives and other health care professionals are uniquely situated to help abuse victims bring an end to the domestic abuse they experience. Health professionals are often the only professionals with whom abuse victims have continuing contact from the time before they learn that they may obtain help leaving their abusers, through failed attempts to leave, and after they survive the abusive relationship.

Health care professionals, particularly midwives, generally establish long-term trusting relationships with their patients. These trusting relationships make battered women more likely to disclose abuse and seek help and support from a midwife long before she might be ready to seek social services or legal relief. The midwife may be the first, and only, source of ongoing support for many abused women and their children. Nurse-midwives, whether they realize it or not, often see women before and after they are abused. Workers in the health care system are perhaps the only professionals who have regular contact with abuse victims at *all* stages of the abuse continuum. Frequently, the midwife or the physician is the only professional with whom the abuser will allow the battered woman to have contact.

It can therefore be seen that health care professionals have a special responsibility to abuse victims to identify abuse early, provide what may be the first message that abuse is not normal or tolerated in our society, treat victims injuries, offer referrals to legal and social services, and support the victim as she goes through what may be a lengthy struggle to leave an abuser. For these abuse victims, the health care provider's office may be the only safe place they can go when they seek a break from ongoing violence. Midwives must be aware of this and make patients aware that their office will always be a place where they can find safety.

The most important roles for the nurse-midwife are identifying the domestic violence, documenting the abuse for subsequent legal proceedings, referring the victim to social and legal services and supporting the victim through the frustrations she may encounter as she turns to police, prosecutors and the courts for help.

BARBARA SEAMAN ON WHAT THE NEIGHBOR SHOULD DO

More American women are injured by battery than by rape, muggings, and accidents combined. Think of that! A woman is safer roaming the streets at night than snuggled up on the couch at home reading a book with her husband stewing in the den.

An American crisis! Yes, because so many of us who are tuned in to the media have heard it all (think of Nicole Brown Simpson and Hedda Nussbaum) but just don't know what to do. Haven't you seen some signs around you? Sunglasses and heavy makeup in the elevator? A cheerful coworker who becomes inexplicably depressed and suffers a limp due to recurring "accidents"? Or it may be thuds on your ceiling. And of course you have doubts ("Frank? He always has those annual barbecues... "). But remember, 82 percent of batterers are Jekyll-and-Hyde types. When acquaintances doubted that a person as likable as my batterer (whose main method of assault was to run at me and knock me down, as in a football tackle) could have broken my ankle and smashed out my teeth, the downstairs neighbors set them straight.

Not wanting to probe in people's "personal" lives, we often gape at the puffy eye and remain silent. But, as Keith Haring put it, "Silence equals death";

we must reach out to these battered women (or men or children) in order to save their lives (and save America). It can feel so hard to do, so awkward, right? Well, here are a few tips on how to befriend a battered woman: Take her aside and quietly ask, "Are you safe at home? or "Did someone hurt you?" If she doesn't acknowledge it, ask again next time. Keep telling her, "No one has the right to hurt you." Many battered women are brainwashed into blaming themselves. Comments such as "He must be crazy" have the power to break through the haze. Don't ask her what she did to provoke him. When a batterer reaches the boiling point in his compulsive cycle, the excuse can be anything…or nothing. My batterer once beat me up after we returned home from the opera because I'd toted a purse that he considered too large and "day-timey." Don't ask why she doesn't leave. She may be well aware that escaping is apt to escalate the danger. Instead, help her devise a safety plan.

So the next time you see a locker mate at the gym with a suspicious black-and-blue handprint on her thigh, start talking. It just may work.

Fifty Ways Not to Leave an Abusive Spouse

ELAINE WEISS

Elaine Weiss, "Fifty Ways Not to Leave an Abusive Spouse," *Hadassah* , December 1998. Reprinted by permission.

D omestic abuse conjures up the image of a bruised, depressed, timid woman tiptoeing through her house while her unemployed husband swigs beer and throws furniture. The full horror of domestic abuse is this: Women in abusive marriages look like everyone else. They look like me.

I am the daughter of a physician father and a college-educated mother. My Judaism was as integral to my identity as my tendency to be picked first for spelling bees and last for volleyball. I had best girlfriends. I also had boyfriends; mostly bespectacled Jewish boys who played chess or clarinet. I fell in love with one during my sophomore year in college. We married in the summer of 1967. Eight years, seven months, and 21 days later I left.

I have spent 20 years trying to unravel the tightly woven threads of physical and verbal abuse that made the fabric of that marriage. Why bother? Why not just be grateful that I found the strength to leave? Because I still have nightmares. Because, beautiful though *Carousel* is, I can't watch Billy Bigelow hit Julie Jordan—and watch her forgive him. Because I cry when I see Charles Boyer methodically driving Ingrid Bergman slowly mad in *Gaslight*. And because after O. J. Simpson's arrest, I overheard a woman in the beauty parlor proclaim, "you know, the women who let themselves be abused are just as sick as the men who abuse them. She should have walked out the very first time he raised a hand to her. That's what I would have done."

She should have—our glib answer to abused women. Miep Gies, who helped hide Anne Frank and her family, heard this in Amsterdam. "If these terrible things are happening to the Jews, they must be doing something very bad." These days we know enough not to blame the woman directly; instead, we say she should have gotten therapy. She should have called the police. She should have been more assertive. She should have been more accommodating. So as if the pain of the relationship weren't enough, we tell women it is their fault. They hear she should—never he should. It's "She should have stood up to him"—which, ideally, she should—but never "He should have stopped being abusive."

I know it's not that simple. I know that men who batter are themselves in pain. I know their behavior is a desperate attempt to feel in control. I know they can't just stop, that they need professional help. And I sympathize, just as I sympathize with alcoholics and drug addicts. I'm no longer angry with my former husband (this took years to accomplish). But I am hotly, fiercely angry when I hear "Why don't these women just leave." To me, this is as meaningless as asking the victim of a train wreck "Why didn't you just drive to work that morning?" Here is my answer.

I didn't leave because abuse wasn't supposed to happen to women like me. In 1967 the term spouse abuse didn't exist. No one thought to join those two words, since no one accepted that it happened. Or if it did, it happened only to uneducated women who were married to unemployed alcoholics. I certainly didn't happen to nice Jewish girls from Westchester County, New York; they went to college, married nice Jewish boys, then started a family. They didn't have to worry about abuse because Jewish men don't beat their wives. So when the abuse started—within a week of the wedding—I had no way to frame what was happening.

I didn't leave because I thought it was my fault. My only experience of marriage was the 17 years in my parents' home, where I saw kindness and love. If my marriage looked nothing like theirs, I assumed I was doing something wrong. My husband would throw me against a wall, then berate me for "egging him on." Lying in bed at night, I would try to pinpoint the moment I had gone wrong. I always found it. I should have laughed when he told me the dinner was disgusting. I should have ignored it when he called me a fat dummy. I shouldn't have cried when he announced he wanted to sleep with other women—and if I didn't like it, I was insecure and possessive.

I didn't leave because I believed I could fix it. During our courtship he was tender and affectionate. He told me I was the most wonderful "girl" in the world. So I held on to the image of the man who was once my loving boyfriend. He told me I had changed, that I was no longer the pure, bright girl he had married—and I imagined he must be right. Since rational people don't suddenly turn violent without provocation, I must be provoking him. I thought that if I could just get it right, he would be nice to me again.

I didn't leave because I told myself I was overreacting. Yes, he would occasionally punch me in the stomach or choke me—but at least he never gave me a black eye or a broken arm. Yes, he would delight in pointing out an obese woman on the street and saying, "your ass is even bigger than hers"—but perhaps I did need to lose weight (I was then as I am now, a size 6). Yes, he would indicate another woman, tall, blond, buxom and leggy, and scold "Why can't you look like that?" But this was the 1960s, when the Beach Boys wished we all could be California girls, and maybe a petite brunette couldn't hope to be seen as attractive. Yes, he would occasionally put a pillow over my face while I slept, then watch with detached interest as I woke up half smothered—but I had to be imagining that, didn't I?

I didn't leave because there was no place I could tell my story and be told "It's not you—it's him. There's no way you can get it right because he desperately needs you to get it wrong." I never confided in a rabbi; since everyone knows Jewish men don't beat their wives. Instead, we saw a psychiatrist. I tried to find the words to pin down my husband's actions: He goes through a door ahead of me and gives it an extra push to make it swing back and hit me. He tells me I'm so ugly that his new nickname for me is uggles. I feel like I'm constantly walking on eggshells. The psychiatrist insisted my husband couldn't function without me, that I must learn to become that sort of wife he would want to treat well. We spent two years in weekly visits to this man. Nothing changed.

I didn't leave because I grew accustomed to living a lie. Maintaining our loving appearance became a conspiracy between us. He called it "not airing our dirty linen" and I agreed. After all, I was to blame for his behavior and he would treat me well if I could make him happy. A wife who doesn't know how to make her husband happy—why would I want that to become public knowledge? I agreed to the charade and played my part well. Which probably explains why, when I left, no one believed I had any reason to escape such a wonderful marriage.

And then one day I left. A total stranger was the catalyst. My husband was working at a prestigious New York law firm and I had started graduate school at Columbia University. One afternoon as we stood at a downtown crosswalk, I spotted a lovely old building with a magnificent garden on its terraced roof. "Isn't that building beautiful? I said. "Which one," he sneered, "you mean the one that looks exactly like every other building on the street?" A woman standing beside us turned abruptly. "She's right, you know. The building is beautiful—and you are a horse's ass." As the light changed and she stalked off, I suddenly realized this man was never going to change. Within a year I announced I was leaving.

Yes, it took more than this one encounter. Fellow students became close friends. With professional and personal successes, it became easier to shrug off my husband's abuse. The day I told him the marriage was over (my twenty-eighth birthday), he cried and begged me to stay. He swore he would change. He painted an idyllic picture of the new life we would build. I barley heard him.

I am one of the lucky ones. He didn't threaten me. He didn't stalk me. He didn't murder me. Some men do. I am one of the lucky ones. I didn't commit suicide. I didn't become homeless. I didn't turn to drugs or alcohol. I didn't enter into a series of abusive relationships. Some women do.

Instead, I earned a doctorate and developed a successful consulting practice. I remarried. My husband and I have a strong marriage and *shalom bayit* —domestic tranquility. Life is good. But I still have nightmares. I still can't watch movies that show violence against women. And I still, and probably always will, feel anguish when I hear someone ask, "Why don't these women just leave?"

Out of Control

NORMA FOX MAZER

Excerpted from Norma Fox Mazer, *Out of Control*, New York, Morrow Junior Books, 1993. Reprinted by permission.

Saturday morning, Rollo, Candy and Brig play cutthroat, two-on-one, switching partners after each game. They play hard for a couple of hours.

Afterward, standing in the showers, Brig analyzes their games and instructs Rollo about his mistakes. "There's such a thing as hitting too hard. You can't hit the ball and not think about the next shot."

Rollo turns off the shower. Okay, he powers the ball, but that's what he has going for him-power and muscle. He loves to let go and smash the ball. He loves the sound of the ball smacking against the racket. He isn't swift and showy like Brig, who likes to run up the walls and kill every ball, and he isn't a precision player like Candy.

"This is a game of strategy, not strength."

"I got strategy," Rollo says.

"Where, in your ass? You see the ball and your muscles start popping and pow, you send it to kingdom come. That's why we lost that third game to Candy." Brig punctuates his words with snaps of the towel. "All you did was set Candy up. You kept sending the ball right back to him."

"Hey, that was my superior playing that won that game," Candy says. He's in front of the mirror, towel knotted at his waist, blow-drying his hair.

Brig zips up his pants. "Why didn't you call me back last night, Rollo? I was waiting."

"Last night?" Rollo dives into his locker for his shirt. "I didn't talk to her," he mumbles. "I'll do it, I'll call her today, you can count on it. Just remind me-"

"I'm not reminding you of anything!" Brig's face twitches, and he walks away toward the washroom.

Rollo looks at Candy. "He wanted me to call Arica for him."

"He's really cut up over her. He got too involved."

A group of men walk in and noisily get their gym bags out of their lockers and walk out again.

"You know how I started going with Arica?" Brig says, coming back from the washroom. "She was hanging around my locker. She was giving me the eye. She was saying cute things." He drops down on a bench. "What am I talking about her for? I don't want to talk about her. It's all over." He punches his leg, and he's crying.

Rollo has never seen Brig cry. It's terrible. Brig is making these hoarse, choking sounds, and Rollo can hardly stand it. He pats his friend's shoulder over and over. "I'm sorry, Brig. I'm really sorry. I should have called her. Brig, I'll do it."

"Forget it, I said. I don't care."

"That's the way," Candy says, hovering over Brig, too. "Just forget her. What do you care about her?"

"I don't. I don't care about her."

"Good. You can get another girl."

"Right," Rollo says. "There's a lot of other girls."

"They're like fish in the ocean," Candy says. "Brig just has to drop his line."

Brig slaps at Candy halfheartedly. "What do you know about it, Candrella? You ever have a girlfriend?"

"Plenty."

"You did?" Rollo says. "When was that?"

"When was that?" Candy mocks, sitting down next to Brig. "You think you know everything about me?"

Rollo lets his mouth drop open and shakes his head like a rube. He's playing dumb, doing it for Brig, to cheer him up. And it seems to be working. Brig is almost smiling.

They sit on the benches facing each other, their knees banged in together, and talk about how many years they've been friends and all the things they've done together. They talk about the other night, how crazy it was the way Brig and Rollo drove down into Union, and the way they faced off with Mark Saddler.

Candy brings up the time he and Rollo broke into the guardhouse near the quarry. And after that they go over the famous night when they all sneaked out of their houses at midnight. "We stayed out until two in the morning," Rollo says.

"No, it was three o'clock," Brig says.

"Don't laugh, you guys," Candy says "I know what I'm going to say is corny, but you know what I'm thinking sitting here listening to all this?" He looks from one to the other of them. "I'm thinking how our friendship is more important than any girl."

Rollo's eyes get damp. He gets his arms around Brig and Candy and sort of hugs them. Then they're all hugging, and their faces are close. Close enough to kiss, Rollo thinks. A weird thought, but maybe Candy has the same weird thought, because suddenly he pounds Rollo on the leg, really pounds him hard, and says, "Hey, cream puff! Hey, you big cream puff!" And they all laugh and break apart.

The hall is empty. The three of them stand still for a moment, then Brig walks quickly to the stairs. Rollo and Candy follow. When they turn the corner, they hear footsteps on the stairs.

"Let's get her," Brig says, and they run up the stairs. They run up the stairs quickly and quietly.

Maybe Brig doesn't say anything. Maybe Rollo only thinks he hears Brig say that. Maybe it goes like this: They hear footsteps on the stairs, and no one says anything, but they run up the stairs anyway. They run up the stairs after her. They are fast, they are quiet. They are taking the stairs two at a time. They are running up the stairs quickly and quietly.

On the second-floor landing, they listen, and they hear the footsteps still going up. Going up to the third floor. They follow. They go up after the footsteps. After Valerie Michon's footsteps. They don't talk about it, they just do it.

It's a game. Fun. They glance at each other, and they take the stairs swiftly, grinning. It's a game, and then, too, it's like a dream. Rollo feels something dreamlike in the way he is running up the stairs, running after Brig so smoothly, so swiftly, and the way Candy is running after him, and the way they are all running up the stairs after the footsteps.

Maybe there is nobody there, Rollo thinks. Just for a moment he thinks that—nobody there, no body, no person, no Valerie Michon. Nobody, just the footsteps leading them on.

Then they are on the third floor and they see her.

Her back is turned to them. She is at the end of the corridor in front of the window that looks out over the woods behind the school.

She doesn't seem aware of them. She's leaning forward, her hands on the windowsill, looking out.

She's like a shadow against the window, like cardboard, a dark cutout against the wintry white light flooding in from outside.

They trot toward her. They are not so quiet now.

She turns and looks at them. She says "What do you want?" Her eyes flicker one way, then the other.

She starts to move around them and Brig grabs her. And then they all grab her. They just do it, all together. It happens fast, so fast. It's like reading each other's minds. Let's get her. Did Brig say it? They don't say anything now, they just grab her, and you can't tell who does what, whose hands are where.

"Stop! Quit! Oh, damn, no—oh—oh—stop—"

Rollo hears panting. Maybe it's himself. He hears grunts, and he's aware of his hot breath. His face and hands are burning, and his hands are on Valerie: he has some part of her in his hand, some soft flesh, some thrilling part of her.

She's twisting around, trying to get away, trying to get free, but they have her.

Rollo's sweating and grinning. He can feel the grin stretched across his face, and he remembers slipping and sliding down the winding road into Union, the car skidding through the snow—dangerous, thrilling—You know you should stop but you keep going, you don't want to stop, you just want that thrill—that thrill—

Valerie is flailing and yelling. She wrenches free, her arms swing wildly, and she stumbles and crashes to her knees. Then Brig is trying to straddle her, trying to get on her back, and she's jerking around frantically.

A bell rings and it shrills into Rollo's brain.

He blinks and stumbles back, breathing hard.

Candy pulls at Brig. Valerie is up on one knee. Her hair is down around her face.

They leave. They walk down the hall, tucking in their shirts.

The auditorium is still dark. The play is still going on. The same characters that were onstage when they left are still onstage, sitting around the laden table: Tiny Tim, Scrooge, the "baby" in the high chair—

Rollo moves quietly toward his seat. He tiptoes, lifting one foot at a time, the way you do when you're entering a room full of people, and you're trying not to disturb anyone. You pick up each foot carefully, put down each foot carefully, and carefully lower yourself into your seat, hoping the floor won't squeak, the seat won't creak.

He sits and looks up at the stage. Denise Dixon is there, her head tilted to one side. Any moment now Tiny Tim will say, God bless us all. Rollo stares at Denise Dixon, and for a moment everything blurs. Nothing is distinct. The stage and everyone on it, the auditorium and everyone in it, collapse into a smear of sound and light. He looks at his friends. Brig is leaning back, legs out, arms crossed over his chest. He catches Rollo's eye and nods soberly. Candy seems absorbed in the play, bent forward, chin in hand.

Rollo's heart slows down, his breath is quiet. He watches the stage.

From the corner of his eye, he sees a door open on the other side of the room. A bar of light appears. Someone leans into the auditorium, someone else rises. All the way across the dark room, Rollo senses whispers, ripples of movement. The door closes again.

"God bless us all!" Tiny Tim cries.

A moment later, a hand taps Rollo on the shoulder, Mr. Maddox's tall and slightly bent form is standing over him. "Come with me," he whispers. He taps Brig on the shoulder, then Candy. The auditorium is clapping. The three of them follow Mr. Maddox into the hall and down the corridor.

"Where are we going?" Rollo says.

Mr. Maddox glances at him. "Principal's office."

It's not much of a walk, just over the bridge into the addition, down three steps, and around the corner, but it seems long, because no one says anything after that. Brig whistles quietly. The only other sound is the muted thump of their feet on the wooden floor.

In the outer office, the secretaries look up when they enter. A printer is spitting out paper. A phone rings. One of the secretaries answers, and another phone rings. Each time, Rollo's stomach lurches a little.

Mrs. Andresson, the one with gold hair and two chins, nods to Mr. Maddox and says, "I'll say you're here." She raps on the door beyond the counter that says *S. Ferranto, Principal*, opens it, and goes in. When she comes out a moment later, she tells the boys to sit down. "Thank you, Mr. Maddox," she adds.

Mr. Maddox bends over Rollo and looks into his face. Like Coach at the end of the season, he goes to each of them and bends close, but, unlike Coach, he makes no speeches. He only stares, as if he's trying to understand something incomprehensible.

He leaves. The door shuts quietly behind him.

Candy, who's sitting between Rollo and Brig, says, "What do you think?"

"Michon must have told," Rollo says.

"Right." Candy glances at the women working behind the counter. "What do you think she said?" he asks quietly.

"A bunch of lies," Brig says.

Rollo can't get comfortable on the wooden bench. He crosses and uncrosses his legs. He's hungry again. He watches the women working behind the counter. He wishes Mrs. Andresson would smile at him. He likes her. She never raises a fuss when he needs a pass or forgets his locker key.

They sit there for a long time. People look at them, but nobody talks to them.

Our Guys

BERNARD LEFKOWITZ

Bernard Lefkowitz, *Our Guys: The Glen Ridge Rape and the Secret Life of the Perfect Suburb*, Berkeley and Los Angeles, University of California Press, 1997. Reprinted by permission.

Bernard Lefkowitz's book *Our Guys* evokes the lives of some high school athletes in an affluent New Jersey suburb and that of a retarded young woman whom they raped with a baseball bat and a broom stick. In this excerpt he recounts his first visit to the town and compares it to what he found when he wrote an earlier book, *Tough Change*, about poor youngsters in Newark, New Jersey.

The sense of social nihilism expressed by many youngsters in Newark was attributable, at least partially, to their economic condition and the social devastation it created. The immutable condition they all shared was poverty. Being poor was the ongoing trauma of their childhoods. You could draw a line from the rubble of the streets to the rubble of their lives.

Of course, Glen Ridge was different. It was a town where almost everybody was pretty well off. If I decided to write about this place, I would have to read-just my perspective. The prosperity of Glen Ridge didn't negate the impact of economics on the values of young people in this suburb. But instead of writing about the sense of impotency arising from generations of poverty I might be writing about how affluence and privilege could inflate the self-importance of otherwise unremarkable young men, not always with good results.

This was all surmise from a distance. Before I decided to write about Glen Ridge, I wanted to take a closer look at the boys involved in the alleged rape, at the residents, and at the town. In the late afternoon of June 23, 1989, I board-ed a number 33 DeCamp line bus from the Port Authority bus terminal in New York City. Forty minutes later, I got off at the intersection of Bloomfield and Ridgewood Avenues in Glen Ridge. I followed the crowd that was walking toward the field behind the high school, where the graduation ceremonies for the Class of '89 were about to begin.

My first mental snapshot: Glen Ridge was a squeaky-clean, manicured town that liked to display its affluence by dressing its high school graduates in dinner jackets and gowns. What impressed me most was the orderliness of the place. The streets, the lawns, the houses—everything seemed in proportion. There were no excesses of bad taste, no evidence of neglect or disrepair.

Although graduation was an emotional ritual, made more intense by the recent arrest of four seniors on rape charges, there were no outbursts of feel-ing, no overt expressions of anger, grief, or remorse. The adults and their prog-eny exercised near-perfect restraint.

It was if these graduates had fulfilled the first requirements of a master plan for their lives. Their parents' success had secured them a place in this charm-ing town. Now they would follow their parents down the same road, passing all the trailmarks that led to achievement, security, and fulfillment. The constrast with Newark was overwhelming. The youngsters I met there had no idea what they would be doing tomorrow, let alone five years from now. The teenagers in Glen Ridge seemed to exude confidence in the future. It was a future that included more years of higher education, then entrance into an occupation or career. After that, marriage, children, and, perhaps, residence in Glen Ridge or a place very much like it.

They were secure in the knowledge that they would be protected as they made their passage into adulthood. Most of them would have their college board and tuition paid by their parents. If they needed to buy new clothes or a car or to pay a doctor's bill, they could depend on a check from home. Most of them had the luxury of easing into independence.

That's what I thought on the first night I visited Glen Ridge. But I also recognize that, even with all these advantages, kids don't always fulfill their parents' expectations. Some people have the benefit of wealth and nurturing parents and a good education, and still wind up morally and financially bankrupt. There are no foolproof master plans for success. I knew that because of what had happened three months before in this town, only a few blocks away from where I was sitting on this warm, humid night in June. What I didn't know was why it happened. If I found that out, I might have an interesting theme for a book.

Later that night I got my first glimpse of some of the boys who had been in the basement. They showed up for one of several parties that the town was holding for the graduates. As these thick-necked, broad-shouldered young men circulated in the crowd of students and chaperones, I felt a surge of recognition. I knew these kids! I had seen them all my life. They were the kids on my block who had developed faster than all the other boys of their age. They were out driving cars and dating and having sex while I was still fussing with my stamp collection. They were the guys in the jock clique of my high school, louder and tanner than the students who never saw sunlight because they were always home studying so they could win the Nobel Prize in chemistry before they turned fifty.

The kids in Newark, black and brown, speaking Spanish, hoods over their heads, wheeling their stolen cars over to the local chop shop—they were aliens in America. Strange, forever separate and separated from the American ideal. But these Glen Ridge kids, they were pure gold, every mother's dream, every father's pride. They were not only Glen Ridge's finest, but in their perfection they belonged to all of us. They were Our Guys.

And that was the way they were being treated that night at the graduation party. Parents and kids collected around them, slapping them on the back and giving them big, wet, smacky kisses. Who would have guessed from this reception that some of them had been charged with rape and more of their pals would soon be arrested? In the bosom of their hometown, they were greeted like returning warriors who had prevailed in a noble crusade. Or, if you prefer, martyred heroes.

It may have all been a bravura show of solidarity by a bunch of scared people who saw their world crashing down on them. But it looked real to me. The accused looked like a bunch of carefree kids who had just wrapped up high school and were heading off to the shore for some sun and fun before they started college. Then I heard a voice next to me saying, "It's such a tragedy. They're such beautiful boys and this will scar them forever." The man who said that drifted away before I could ask him a question, but others I spoke to repeated this sentiment, "It's such a tragedy." Often they identified the victims of the tragedy. It was a short list: the young men who had been arrested, their families, and the good name of Glen Ridge. The list, more often than not, omitted the young woman in the basement and her family.

The Campaign to Free Charline

JENNIFER GONNERMAN

Jennifer Gonnerman, "The Campaign to Free Charline," *The Village Voice*, December 10, 1996. Reprinted by permission.

Marvin Brundidge told his wife repeatedly that he would kill her. Instead, she killed him.

Marvin, 46, and Charline, 37, had been together for seven years. From almost the beginning, he abused her physically, verbally, and sexually. On the night of April 21, 1985, they went out drinking together at a few bars near their Rochester home. Following a familiar pattern, Marvin became paranoid and possessive, accusing his wife of cheating on him. He said he wanted her to "get the fuck out" of their house.

Back in their bedroom, Marvin grabbed Charline by the throat, shoved her down on their bed, and started slapping her face. He called her a "whore" and a "bitch." Charline kicked him off and staggered away. "His eyes and his nostrils were flared," she later said. "It was like he was foaming at the mouth."

Marvin, who weighed 250 pounds and stood 6 feet, 2 inches tall, picked up his wife by the hair and smashed her head against the wall so hard it left a visible dent. Seven inches shorter and only 130 pounds, Charline was at a marked disadvantage. She grabbed on to the dresser to keep from falling.

While Charline slumped bleeding against the dresser, Marvin undressed, wrapped a maroon bathrobe around his naked body, and lay on their bed. Then he called the police. Dialing 911 and pretending to need protection was one of his favorite ploys, according to Charline's attorney. This way, Marvin could beat up his wife until the police arrived and then avoid arrest by blaming her.

"My wife is leaving," Marvin told the dispatcher, according to a police tape of the incident. "I just want them to be here if she come[s] back, 'cause I don't want her."

While Marvin was on the phone, Charline reached into the top drawer of the dresser and pulled his .38 caliber revolver out of its leather holster. From a few feet away, she unloaded five bullets into Marvin's head and chest. His body crumpled. She picked up the phone and found the dispatcher still on the line.

"Send the police here," she said. "I just shot my husband."

Today, Charline Brundidge is one of thousands of battered women across the country who killed their abusers during the 1970s or 1980s and are still incarcerated. She has served 10 years already and, with a 15-years-to-life sentence, will not be eligible for parole until 2001. But much has changed in the 10 years since "domestic violence" became an everyday term.

Many prosecutors now consider a defendant's history of abuse before charging her, thereby increasing the chance she will be charged with a lesser crime—manslaughter, say, instead of murder—that carries a shorter sentence. When cases go to trial, judges are far more likely to allow testimony about past abuse. And the defense now often includes an expert witness on domestic violence.

As a result, jurors are better informed, and more sympathetic, than ever before. For example, a Rockland County grand jury declined last year to indict a woman who had stabbed her husband to death with a fishing knife. And this summer, a Bronx woman who shot her husband in the throat—but didn't kill him—got only probation. If Charline Brundidge—or the many like her—had committed her crime this year, her sentence might have been far less stiff.

There is now a statewide movement to free Charline. More than 50 lawyers, legislators, and antidomestic violence activists, as well as the judge who sentenced her, have written to Governor George Pataki urging him to commute her sentence. Charline even has the support of Libby Pataki, the governor's wife, who met last month with Charline's lawyer. Were the governor to grant clemency, he would probably do so around Christmas.

If Charline is freed, she will be the first victim of domestic violence in New York to benefit from a nationwide movement to release women imprisoned for killing their batterers. Since 1978, governors in 23 states have granted clemency to more that 100 women. In 1990, Ohio's governor commuted the sentences of 25 battered women. Maryland's governor released 8 domestic violence victims in 1991.

Charline's current lawyer, Mary Lynch, has spent more than two years building Charline's case. While Charline refuses to talk to the media, she did let the *Voice* view a 15-minute videotaped interview that she has submitted along with her written petition. The picture that emerges from this videotape—plus interviews with Charline's friends and family, hospital records, police reports, and trial transcripts—is of a woman who is neither bitter nor angry, only eager to be reunited with her family.

When Charline was growing up in Gulfport, Mississippi, in the 1950s, she says, she often saw her father hit her mother. The lesson she learned from the older women around her was that "the man loved you if he beat you," Charline says in her interview. "My mother told me I should be able to take a lick."

Throughout her marriage to Marvin, this is exactly what Charline did.

Charline met Marvin through her sister when she was 30 years old. She'd already been married twice and had a 14-year old daughter, Tyra. The two moved to Rochester in the fall of 1978 to live with Marvin, who ran a local bar. Charline eventually worked as a typist and then a clerk at the state Department of Agriculture, where she collected glowing performance evaluations.

"Everything that first year was beautiful," Charline says in her videotape. But it did not stay that way for long. "I really realized something was changing when Marvin started becoming really physical with me, beating me up," Charline says. "It was like his normal behavior. He wasn't talking to me anymore; he was always hitting me. All that we had in the beginning—all of that openness and him talking—that was gone. His size, [his] legal permit to carry a gun, his temper, and his ability to use it all was very intimidating."

Charline wore sunglasses to hide her bruises, but she could not keep the battering secret. Five former coworkers attested to her abuse in letters they wrote supporting her clemency request.

Like many abusers, Marvin monitored his wife constantly. When Charline attended seminars for work, Marvin came along to watch her from the back of the room. He demanded she return home or to his bar immediately after work each day. And he timed her to make certain she did not make any stops. The drive home from work was about 20 minutes. If Charline took longer, Marvin would accuse her of having an affair.

As the beatings worsened, Charline's confidence crumbled. With violent, controlling behavior, Marvin crushed her sense of self. "I wasn't even me anymore," she says. "He had literally destroyed me. I didn't know who I was."

Charline tried to leave Marvin many times. Sometimes she hid in the attic. Other times she escaped to motels. Once she fled to her family in New Jersey, but Marvin tracked her down and enticed her to return with promises that he would change.

"The times that I did leave him, it was like he could find me anyway," she says in her videotape. "It seemed like I couldn't get away from him no matter where I went."

Marvin's blows sent Charline to the hospital several times. He burned her with cigarettes, held a butcher knife to her face, and raped her. In the two years before Charline shot Marvin, the police were called to their house at least four times. Often, the officers did no more than advise the couple to "stay away from each other." One time, when Charline showed up at the emergency room with a busted lip, a police officer asked who had hit her. "Nobody," Charline said, as Marvin glared at her from nearby.

Today, this scenario is likely to play out differently. Police and hospital workers across the state are trained to interview battered women in private. Moreover, under a policy that went into effect in January, officers are required to make an arrest when they break up a domestic dispute if there is evidence of a crime.

When a case involving a batterer now reaches the district attorney's office in the county where the Brundidges resided, it goes to a prosecutor who specializes in domestic violence. This lawyer contacts victims, urges them to press charges, and offers information about a hot line and shelter. If this program had existed a decade ago, it might have saved Charline, and Marvin.

Charline was first convicted of murder in September 19, 1985. Her defense was that she suffered from an "extreme emotional disturbance." At the time, few attorneys had developed expertise in defending battered women. Charline's lawyer, John Speranza, did not call many witnesses who had seen Marvin abuse his wife. A jury found Charline, who had no prior criminal record, guilty of second-degree murder.

In a rare move, the judge set aside Charline's conviction a few days later because the wife of a juror stepped forward to say her husband could not have been impartial because he too was a batterer.

While waiting to be retried, Charline stumbled across a newspaper story about Charles Ewing, a lawyer and forensic psychologist from Buffalo, who had just written *Battered Women Who Kill*. From Monroe County Jail, Charline wrote to Ewing about her predicament. He agreed to testify for free as an expert witness in her second trial.

Speranza developed a new strategy. He argued the murder was an act of self-defense and emphasized Charline's suffering as a domestic violence victim. A slew of new witnesses testified that they had seen Marvin hit her. Ewing told jurors that Charline had reason to believe her life was in danger. He also explained that she suffered from battered woman's syndrome, which left her feeling so helpless that she no longer viewed leaving as a viable option.

But the jurors, who may have been hearing about domestic violence for the first time, might not have realized how much pain Marvin had inflicted. Moreover, Judge Eugene Bergin refused to let the jurors see portions of hospital records reporting that Charline had said her trips to the emergency room were caused by Marvin's abuse. The prosecutor, Charles Siragusa, claimed that Charline was not a "real" battered woman. "If slaps, pushes, and shoves amount to a basis for a syndrome, then I know sisters at the grammar school I went to, that are in deep trouble," said Siragusa, who is now a judge. Charline's current attorney, May Lynch, says, "It's a characterization that I don't think today would be appealing to a jury."

Despite the new defense, Charline was again convicted of second-degree murder. The judge gave her the minimum sentence of 15 years to life. "Charline didn't fit some of the stereotypes that people had about battered women," Ewing told the *Voice*. "There was a belief that battered women were small physically. That they were unattractive, stay-at-home women—not assertive in any aspect of their life. And that they didn't have careers or interests of their own."

Starting in October 1988, Charline's home was a 6-by-10-foot cell at Bedford Hills Correctional Facility, a maximum security prison in Westchester County. She lived behind a steel door with a Plexiglas window. Wakeup time was 5 A.M. At Bedford Hills, she spent her days working as a typist, clerk, tailor, and kitchen helper.

A model prisoner, Charline eventually landed a coveted job conducting orientation classes for new inmates. "She kept her nose clean, minded her own business, read her Bible," says David McCoach, who ran the prison's skills-assessment program and supervised Charline for more than three years. "She received respect from not only her fellow inmates, but state employees as well."

Behind bars, Charline has earned both an associate degree and a bachelor's degree. "I'm really proud of her," says her daughter Tyra. "She's accomplished a lot of things that she wanted to accomplish when she was married to [Marvin], but wasn't able to."

For many battered women like Charline, prison is the haven they never had. They don't have freedom, but at least they no longer have to worry about being awakened in the night by the punches of an angry boyfriend or husband. "This has been like a shelter for me—a healing period in my life," Charline says in her videotape. "While I have been incarcerated, I have found myself."

Mary Lynch, an Albany Law School professor, first heard about Charline more that two years ago. As director of the school's domestic violence clinic, Lynch had been looking for an ideal battered woman on whose behalf to file a clemency petition. Charline fit the bill.

There are no rules about how to write a clemency plea. Even a note scrawled to the governor on a piece of toilet paper will do. As prepared by Lynch and her interns, Charline's clemency petition runs 337 pages and includes everything from her high school report cart to a photo of a dent in the wall made by her head.

Lynch's team tracked down dozens of Charline's friends, relatives, and former coworkers, who wrote letters testifying to her character and her abuse. Perhaps the most persuasive letter is from Judge Bergin, who presided over Charline's second trial. Writes Bergin: "This, in my view, is the only case I have ever experienced that merits commutation in 32 years as a prosecutor and judge."

Nonetheless, there are people who firmly believe the governor should not free Charline. "I think she should stay in for the rest of her life because she took a life she could have avoided taking," says Archie Brundidge, Marvin's 60-year-old brother. Richard Keenan, first assistant district attorney for Monroe County, says, "We would hope that she would serve out her minimum sentence."

No one knows exactly how many women are incarcerated in New York State for killing their abusers. Estimates range from 30 to 200. One of the goals of Charline's petition is to draw attention to these women. Says Lynch, "We convicted them, sentenced them, and forgot about them."

There is no trace of resentment in Charline's voice as she talks on the videotape, made earlier this year. "I feel the loss of Marvin," she says. "I take full responsibility for my actions. He played a huge part in our marriage that didn't work. And I played a huge part in our marriage." About the night she shot Marvin, Charline says, "It's a day I don't want to remember."

Charline, now 49, grows most excited when she talks about daughter Tyra, now 31, and her grandchildren. Charline has not seen Tyra for 10 years. "I don't like prisons," explains Tyra. And until recently, Tyra and her husband, an Air Force sergeant, lived on the West Coast.

"It would mean a lot to me to be there with my daughter's family," Charline says. "I talk to my [grandchildren] when I call Tyra and they call me 'Grandma Charline.' Have you ever heard a little voice on the telephone say, 'Hi, Grandma'? I just want to be there to hold that little person where that little voice came from."

Charline has never met two of her three grandchildren, who were born after she was jailed. But if Pataki commutes Charline's sentence, she will join them in Delaware, where she plans to work as a counselor for domestic violence victims. If her clemency request is denied, Charline will not be eligible for parole until 2001.

"She was in prison when she was married to Marvin," says Tyra. "I feel now she's being doubly punished. She's done her time."

Governor George Pataki awarded clemency to Charline Brundidge on December 23, 1996. She was released from prison a month later and moved to Delaware to live with her daughter's family.

Chapter 71

Conflict of Interest

How do we measure conflict of interest? What do we include in the term? There is frequently much more to conflict of interest than simple financial greed. It can be the outcome of loyalty to a professor or friend. Here's a tragic example of the complexity:

Dr. William Halsted (1852-1922), father of the radical mastectomy, was also a founding father of Johns Hopkins, and the esteemed professor of many later surgeons who went on to head their own departments at prestigious medical schools. With all his gifts, Halsted was a cocaine and heroin addict who was several times hospitalized for his addictions. His colleague, Dr. William Osler, knew that Halsted never recovered, and kept records to that effect. When Osler left Johns Hopkins he took his records to Canada, where they would not be opened until 50 years after Halsted's death. When they were, Halsted's incorrigible problem was acknowledged in several small-circulation surgery journals, but was not brought to the attention of mainstream doctors, nor the breast cancer community. By 1974, when his addiction had been brought to light, Halsted's theories on the spread of breast cancer had also been discredited. In the Hopkins Medical Journal, *A. McGhee Harvey explained, "Halsted's knowledge of breast cancer and its modes of spread was different from what is now known about the disease. There is no evidence at the present time to support the concept that immediate mastectomy following a positive biopsy of breast cancer is necessary." This also was not communicated to the breast cancer community, so the practice of doing fast mastectomies, without awakening the patient to consult with her, went on.*

No one is likely to have received direct financial benefit from this deception. Perhaps some elderly surgeons did not want the public to disrespect their late once-adulated chief. Perhaps other surgeons were loathe to acknowledge the error of their practice, or the unnecessary cruelty. Still, on some level this surely is a profound conflict of interest—between the authority and prestige of breast surgeons, and the welfare of their patients.

The provocative and illuminating articles in this chapter, as well as Tania Ketenjian's interview with Dr. Diana Petitti, illustrate the many faces of conflict of interest, some of them possibly unintentional or based on ignorance, others deliberate or evil.—B. S.

Pharmaceutical Propaganda in the Nineties

THOMAS PAZ-HARTMAN

D ES, the Dalkon shield, and the pill should have taught the pharmaceutical industry a lesson in humility, but misleading and potentially life-threatening advertising campaigns persist to the present day. Most recently, in response to the concerned lobbying of the National Women's Health Network, the FDA ordered Zeneca Pharmaceuticals to withdraw a magazine advertisement, and a promotional brochure, for the controversial breast cancer drug tamoxifen (Nolvadex). The magazine ad included *no* information on risks, side effects, or contraindications, in clear-cut violation of FDA rules, while the risk information in the promotional brochure lacked "the prominence, readability, scope, and depth… dedicated to the presentation of efficacy information." This lack of fair balance is particularly troubling, as the brochure was actually a reprint of a purportedly impartial scientific abstract. Among other omissions and deceptions, the abstract overreported Zeneca's own findings on efficacy in breast cancer reduction, exaggerated the scope of Zeneca's study, and skipped the fact that healthy women had a 250 percent greater risk of getting endometrial cancer on Nolvadex as compared to placebo. Shortly after pulling the print ad, Zeneca aired a television ad where a series of women make statements reflecting commonly held but inaccurate "facts" about breast cancer (young women don't get breast cancer, women don't get breast cancer unless they have a family history of the disease, etc.) that are then corrected by large graphics. Viewers are told that there *is* something they can do about breast cancer risk (though they are not told specifically what), and encouraged to call Zeneca's toll-free number to get more information. This ad bypassed FDA regulations by not mentioning tamoxifen by name. However, Zeneca is a profit-generating enterprise, and television spots are expensive. Obviously, drumming up tamoxifen sales is the ultimate goal. Tactics have evolved, but greed and misogynistic disinformation remin unchanged. Advocacy groups that hold pharmaceutical companies and government regulators to task play a vital role in women's quest for accurate, impartial information about their bodies and available medical treatments. In an important sense, feminists pioneered the concept of the patient's right-to-know, and they will surely continue to play an important role as watchdogs in years to come.

The Secret Battle for the American Mind

DERRICK JENSEN

Derrick Jensen, "The Secret Battle for the American Mind: An Interview with John Stauber," *The Sun*, March 1999. Reprinted by permission.

A ustralian academic Alex Carey once wrote that "the twentieth century has been characterized by three developments of great political importance: the growth of democracy, the growth of corporate power, and the growth of corporate propaganda as a means of protecting corporate power against democracy."

In societies like ours, corporate propaganda is delivered through advertising and public relations. As editor of the quarterly investigative journal *PR Watch*, John Stauber exposes how public relations works and helps people to understand it. In addition to starting *PR Watch*, Stauber founded the Center for Media and Democracy, the first and only organization dedicated to monitoring and exposing PR propaganda. In 1995, Common Courage Press published a book by Stauber and his colleague Sheldon Rampton titled *Toxic Sludge Is Good for You: Lies, Damn Lies, and the Public Relations Industry*. Their second book, *Mad Cow U.S.A.: Could the Nightmare Happen Here?*, came out in 1997 and examined the public relations coverup of the risk of mad-cow disease in the United States.

DJ: How is a propaganda war waged?

JS: The key is invisibility. Once propaganda becomes visible, it's less effective. Public relations is effective in manipulating opinion—and thus public policy— only if people believe that the message covertly delivered by the PR campaign is not propaganda at all but simply common sense or accepted reality. For instance, there is a consensus within the scientific community that global warming is real and that the burning of fossil fuels is a major cause of the problem. But to the petroleum industry, the automobile industry, the coal industry, and other industries that profit from fossil-fuel consumption, this is merely an inconvenient message that needs to be "debunked" because it could lead to public policies that reduce their profits. So, with the help of PR firms, these vested interests create and fund industry front groups such as the Global Climate Coalition. The coalition then selects, promotes, and publicizes scientists who proclaim global warming a myth and characterize hard evidence of global climate change as "junk science" being pushed by self-serving environmental groups out to scare the public for fund-raising purposes.

In order to confuse the public and manipulate opinion and policy to their advantage, corporations spend billions of dollars a year hiring PR firms to cultivate the press, discredit their critics, spy on and co-opt citizens' groups, and use polls to find out what images and messages will resonate with target audiences.

For obvious reasons, public relations is a secretive industry. PR firms don't like to reveal their clients. Some of them, though, can be identified. Here's a list of just a tiny fraction of the clients represented by Burson-Marsteller, the world's largest PR firm: NBC, Philip Morris, Trump Enterprises, Jonas Savimbi's UNITA rebels in Angola, Occidental Petroleum, American Airlines, the state of Alaska, Genentech, the Ford Motor Company, the Times Mirror company, MCI, the National Restaurant Association, Coca-Cola, the British Columbia timber industry, Dow Corning, General Electric, Hydro-Quebéc, Monsanto, AT&T, British Telecom, Chevron, DuPont, IBM, Reebok, Procter & Gamble, Glaxo, Campbell's Soup, the Olympics, Nestlé, Motorola, Gerber, Eli Lilly, Caterpillar, Sears, Beretta Pfizer, Metropolitan Life, McDonnell Douglas, and the governments of Kenya, Indonesia, Argentina, El Salvador, the Bahamas, Italy, Mexico, [South] Korea, Saudi Arabia, and Nigeria....

Burson-Marsteller alone has 2,200 PR flacks—that's slang for a public relations practitioner—in more than thirty countries. In its promotional materials, the firm says that "the role of communications is to manage perceptions which motivate behaviors that create business results," and that its mission is to help clients "manage issues by influencing—in the right combination—public attitude, public perceptions, public behavior, and public policy."

DJ: Why don't we read more about these hidden manipulations in the news?

JS: Primarily because the mainstream, corporate news media are dependent on public relations. Half of everything in the news actually originates from a PR firm. If you're a lazy journalist, editor, or news director, it's easy to simply regurgitate the dozens of press releases and stories that come in every day for free from PR firms.

Remember, the media's primary source of income is the more that $100 billion a year corporations spend on advertising. The PR firms are owned by advertising agencies, so the same companies that are producing billions of dollars in advertising are the ones pitching stories to the news media, cultivating relationships with reporters, and controlling reporters' access to the executives and companies they represent.

DJ: How does politics figure into this equation?

JS: Public relations is now inseparable from the business of lobbying, creating public policy, and getting candidates elected to public office. The PR industry just might be the single most powerful political institution in the world. It expropriates and exploits the democratic rights of millions on behalf of big business by fooling the public about the issues.

DJ: But if it's not illegal and everyone uses it, what's wrong with public relations?

JS: There's nothing wrong with much of what is done in public relations, like putting out press releases, calling members of the press, arguing a position, or communicating a message. Today, however, public relations has become a huge, powerful, hidden medium available only to wealthy individuals, big corporations, governments, and government agencies because of its high cost. And the purpose of these campaigns is not to facilitate democracy or promote social good, but to increase power and profitability for the clients paying the bills. This overall management of public opinion and policy by the few is completely contrary to and destructive of democracy.

In Washington, D.C., issues are no longer simply lobbied. They are "managed" by a triad composed of (1) public relations experts from firms like Burson-Marsteller; (2) business lobbyists, who bankroll politicians, write legislation, and are often former politicians themselves; and (3) phony grassroots organizations—I call them "astroturf groups"—that the PR industry has created on behalf of its corporate clients to give the appearance of public support for their agendas.

Take the Persian Gulf War of 1991. We now know that the royal family of Kuwait hired as many as twenty public relations, law, and lobbying firms in Washington, D.C., to convince Americans to support that war. It paid one PR firm alone, Hill & Knowlton, $10.8 million. Hill & Knowlton set up an astroturf group called Citizens for a Free Kuwait to make it appear as if there were a large grass-roots constituency in support of the war. It was Hill & Knowlton that arranged the infamous phone congressional hearing at which the daughter of the Kuwaiti ambassador, appearing anonymously, falsely testified to having witnessed Iraqi soldiers pulling scores of babies from incubators in a hospital and leaving them to die. Her testimony was a complete fabrication, but everyone from Amnesty International to President George Bush repeated it over and over as proof of Saddam Hussein's evil. A University of Massachusetts study later showed that the more TV people watched, the fewer facts they actually knew about the situation in the Persian gulf, and the more they supported the war.

Historically, after the Wilson administration succeeded in getting the public behind World War I, public relations practitioners who'd been involved in the campaign—like Ivy Lee and Edward Bernays—began looking for business clients. The tactics of invisible persuasion that they'd honed working for the War Department were put to use on behalf of the tobacco, oil, and other industries. And with each success, the public relations industry grew. Tobacco propaganda has surely been the most successful, longest-running, and deadliest public relations campaign in history.

DJ: Wasn't Bernays central to that?

JS: He was, although, to his credit, he later recognized the deadly effects of tobacco and condemned colleagues who worked for tobacco companies. Prior to the 1950s, the tobacco industry actually hired doctors to promote tobacco's "health benefits." It calms the nerves, soothes the throat, and keeps you thin, they said. We have Bernays, Ivy Lee, and other early PR experts to thank for that. Then, when major news outlets began reporting tobacco's links to cancer—some publications even curtailed tobacco advertising—the tobacco industry launched what's called the "crisis-management campaign," primarily under the leadership of John Hill of Hill & Knowlton. Hill's goal was to fool the public into believing that the tobacco industry could responsibly and scientifically investigate the issue itself and, if it found a problem, somehow correct it and make tobacco products safe. What really happened, we all know, is that tobacco companies spent hundreds of millions of dollars funding and publicizing "research" purporting to prove tobacco doesn't cause cancer, and at the same time created one of the most powerful political lobbies in history to prevent tobacco regulation.

Another proven strategy is polling the public to find what messages will resonate with people's values and desires. If they find, for example, that women have a desire to be free from male domination, the strategy might be to market cigarettes as "torches of liberty," as Bernays did in the '20s, when he arranged for attractive New York City debutantes to walk in the Easter Fashion Parade waving lit cigarettes. That single publicity stunt broke the social taboo against women smoking and doubled the tobacco industry's market overnight.

It's even better if you can put your message in the mouth of someone the public trusts. This is called the "third-party technique" and was also pioneered by Bernays. Surveys show that scientists are widely trusted, so the public relations industry hires "scientific experts" to say things beneficial to the industry's clients.

DJ: How did you get started doing this sort of work?

JS: Ironically, I owe my inspiration to Burson-Marsteller, because it was after I caught them infiltrating and spying on a meeting of public interest activists that I decided to start PR Watch and shine a light on this sordid industry. In 1990, I organized a meeting of citizen groups opposed to the Monsanto company's genetically engineered bovine growth hormone, called rBGH. Shortly before the meeting, I received a call form a woman who identified herself as "Lisa Ellis, a member of the Maryland Citizens Consumer Council." She asked if her organization could send a representative; it wanted to make sure schoolchildren could avoid rBGH-produced milk. I said they were certainly welcome, and a woman named Diane Moser attended our meeting.

A few months later, a reporter told me that Monsanto was bragging about having placed a spy in our meeting. A little sleuthing revealed that both Diane Moser and Lisa Ellis were working for Burson-Marsteller on the Monsanto account. Who was Burson-Marsteller? I found I was up against one of the largest, most effective, best-funded, best-connected public relations campaigns in history. A 1986 survey done for the dairy industry—which has worked hand in hand with Monsanto to promote rBGH—showed that the term "bovine growth hormone" caused consumers to worry, so the industry began calling the drug bovine *somatotropin,* which is Latin for "growth hormone." Then a PR firm that monitors reporters began giving positive marks to those who called it bovine somatotropin, and negative marks to those who referred to it by its proper name, bovine growth hormone.

If you can control the terms of the debate, you'll win every time. If you read something about bovine somatotropin, a "natural protein" used to enhance yields in dairy farming, your response will likely be more positive than if you read about injecting dairy cows with a genetically engineered growth hormone.

DJ: How do PR firms get away with planting these terms in news stories?

JS: Journalism is in drastic decline. It's become a lousy profession. The commercial media are greed-driven enterprises dominated by a dozen transnational companies. Newsroom staffs have been downsized. Much of what you see on national and local TV news is actually video news releases prepared by public relations firms and given free to TV stations and networks. Academics who study public relations report that half or more of what appears in newspapers and magazines is lifted verbatim from press releases generated by public relations firms.

The wheels of media are greased with more than $100 billion a year in corporate advertising. The advertisers' power to dictate the content of what we see as news and entertainment grows every year. After all, the real purpose of the media as a business is to deliver an audience to advertisers.

Not only this, they've become dependent on PR firms for the stories they do write. All journalists know, if you want to investigate a corporation, you eventually have to talk with someone there. Unless you belong to the same country club as the top executives, you're going to pick up the phone and get the "vice-president of communications"—i.e., a public relations flack. You need this person's help. If you write a hard-hitting piece, no one at that corporation will ever speak to you again. What's that going to do to your ability to write about that industry? What's it going to do to your career?

Some PR companies—such as Carma International and Video Monitoring Service—specialize in monitoring news stories and journalists. They can immediately evaluate all print, radio, and television coverage of a subject to determine which stories were favorable or unfavorable to their clients' interests, and cultivate relationships with cooperative reporters while punishing those whose reporting is critical.

DJ: We often hear charitable giving referred to as "good public relations." How does that work?

JS: Corporations want us to believe that they are concerned, moral "corporate citizens"—whatever that means. So businesses pump millions of dollars into charities and nonprofit organizations to deceive us into thinking that they care and are making things better. On top of that, corporate charity can buy the tacit cooperation of organizations that might otherwise be expected to criticize corporate policies. Some PR firms specialize in helping corporations to defeat activists, and co-optation is one of their tools.

DJ: Why does this strategy keep working?

JS: E. Bruce Harrison has made a lucrative career out of helping polluting companies defeat environmental regulations while simultaneously giving the companies a "green" public image. In the industry, they call him the "Dean of Green."

As a longtime opponent of the environmental movement, Harrison has developed some interesting insights into its failures. He says, "The environmental movement is dead. It really died in the last fifteen years, from success." I think he's correct. What he means is that, in the eighties and nineties, environmentalism became a big business, and organizations like the Audubon Society, the Wilderness Society, the National Wildlife Federation, the Environmental Defense Fund, and the Natural Resources Defense Council became competing multi-million-dollar bureaucracies. These organizations, Harrison says, seem much more interested in "the business of greening" than in fighting for fundamental social change. He points out, for instance, that the Environmental Defense Fund (whose executive director makes a quarter of a million dollars a year) sat down and cut a deal with McDonald's that was probably worth hundreds of millions of dollars in publicity to the fast-food giant, because it helped to "greenwash" its public image.

DJ: How so?

JS: After years of being hammered by grass-roots environmentalists for everything from deforestation to inhumane farming practices to contributing to a throwaway culture, McDonald's finally relented on something: it did away with its Styrofoam clamshell hamburger containers.

But before the company did this, it entered into a partnership with the Environmental Defense Fund and gave that group credit for the change. Both sides "won" in the ensuing PR lovefest. McDonald's took one little step in response to grass-roots activists, and the Environmental Defense Fund claimed a major victory.

Another problem is that big green groups have virtually no accountability to the many thousands of individuals who provide them with money. Meanwhile, the grass-roots environmental groups are starved of the hundreds of millions of dollars that are raised every year by these massive bureaucracies. Over the past two decades, they've turned the environmental movement's grass-roots base of support into little more than a list of donors they hustle for money via direct-mail appeals and telemarketing.

It's getting even worse, because now corporations are directly funding groups like the Audubon Society, the Wilderness Society, and the National Wildlife Federation. Corporate executives now sit on the boards of some of these groups. PR executive Leslie Dach, for instance, of the rabidly anti-environmental Edelman PR firm, is on the Audubon Society's board of directors. Meanwhile, his PR firm has helped lead the "wise use" assault on environmental regulation.

DJ: It seems the main thrust of the PR business is to get the public to ignore atrocities.

JS: Tom Buckmaster, the chairman of Hill & Knowlton, once stated explicitly the single most important rule of public relations: "Managing the outrage is more important than managing the hazard." From a corporate perspective, that's absolutely right. A hazard isn't a problem if you're making money off it. It's only when the public becomes aware and active that you have a problem, or rather, a PR crisis in need of management.

DJ: How does your work at PR Watch help?

JS: The propaganda-for-hire industry perverts democracy. We try to help citizens and journalists learn about how they're being lied to, manipulated, and too often defeated by sophisticated PR campaigns. The public relations industry is a little like the invisible man in that old Claude Rains movie: crimes are committed, but no one can see the perpetrator. At PR Watch, we try to paint the invisible manipulators with bright orange paint. citizens in a democracy need to know who and what interests are manipulation public opinion and policy, and how. Democracies work best without invisible men.

How Do You Know It's True?

VICTOR COHN

Victor Cohn, "How Do You Know It's True? Probable Fact and Probable Junk," *NewsBackgrounder*, Los Angeles, Foundation for American Communications, 1994. Reprinted by permission.

A politician says "I don't believe in statistics," then maintains that "most" people or "many" do or think such-and-such. Based on what? A doctor reports a "promising" new treatment. Is the claim justified or based on a biased or unrepresentative sample? A poll says "here's what people think" with a "three point plus or minus margin of error." Believable, when we know polls can be wrong? An environmentalist says a nuclear power plant or toxic dump will cause cancers. An industry spokesman indignantly denies it. Who's right?

What can we believe? What's worth reporting? And the question that must concern us both as reporters and citizens: what's worth doing something about?

Some years ago I set out to try to find some answers, especially answers for a nonmathematician like me, confounded by forbidding formulas. I talked to many statisticians and epidemiologists. I was told that a critical understanding of claims about almost anything requires not so much an understanding of formulas as an understanding of the bases of science and rational evidence. And I found that we reporters could copy the methods of science and try to judge claims of fact, whether by scientists or physicians or others, by the same rules of evidence scientists use. An honest investigator may first form a hypothesis or theory, an attempt to describe truth, then try to disprove it by what is called the null hypothesis: to prove that there is no such truth. To back the hypothesis, a study must reject the null hypothesis. Similarly, a jury is instructed to start with a presumption of innocence and say to the prosecution, prove your case, provide the evidence and disprove innocence. Somewhat similarly, we reporters may say to ourselves, at least, "I don't believe you; show me."

We may ask simple yet revealing questions like:

➤*How do you know?* Are you just telling us something you "know" or have "observed" or "found to be true?" Or have you done or found any studies or experiments?

➤*What are your data, your numbers? Where or how did you get them?*

➤*How sure can you be about them?* What is your degree of certainty or uncertainty by accepted tests? (See "Probability" below.)

➤*How valid (in science, valid means accurate) are they?* How reliable, which means how reproducible? Have results been fairly consistent from study to study?

We can then go a long way toward discerning the probable facts from the probable junk, a long way toward judging claims and statistics that are thrown at us, by learning six basic concepts that apply to all science, all studies and virtually all knowledge of society and the universe. Remembering these can teach us to ask, "How do you know?" with a considerable degree of sophistication.

They are:

UNCERTAINTY

All science is almost always uncertain to a degree. Nature is complex, research is difficult, observation is inexact, all studies have flaws, so science is always an evolving story. Almost all anyone can say about the behavior of atoms or cells or human beings or the biosphere is that there is a strong probability that such-and-such is true, and we may know more tomorrow.

This tells us why things so often seem settled one way today and another tomorrow, and why so much is debated, whether the effects of global warming, a pesticide, a high-fat diet, or a medical treatment.

Why so much uncertainty? There are many reasons: lack of funds to do enough research; the expense and difficulty of much research; the ethical obstacles to using human beings as guinea pigs. But a main reason is the lack of long, continuing observations of large populations to track one possible effect or another, observations that would often be perfectly possible.

It is important to tell all this to the public, including our readers, viewers, and listeners, so they will understand why "they" say one thing today, another tomorrow—and how uncertainty need not impede crucial action if society understands and uses these other principles.

PROBABILITY

Scientists live with uncertainty by measuring probability. An accepted numerical express is the *P value*, determined by a formula that considers the number of subjects or events being compared to decide if a given result could have seemed to occur just by chance, when there actually had been no effect.

A P value of .05 or less is most often regarded as low or desirable, since it means there are probably only five or fewer chances in 100 that this result could have happened by chance. This value is called *statistical significance*. In judging studies, look for both a P value and a high confidence level, another measure.

Do not trust a study that is not statistically significant. By know that this may or may not mean *practical* (or in medicine, *clinical*) significance. Nor does it alone mean there is a cause and effect. Association is not causation without further evidence. Remember the rooster who thought his crowing made the sun rise.

The laws of probability and chance tell us to expect some unusual, even impossible-sounding events. Just as a persistent coin tosser would sometime toss heads or tails several times in a row, nature will randomly produce many alarming clusters of cancers or birth defects that have no cause but nature's coin tossing. These produce striking anecdotes and often striking news stories, but they alone do not constitute reliable information that says, "there *is* a cause."

There is something else to remember when someone says, "how do they know this stuff isn't causing harm?" Science cannot prove a negative. No one can prove that little green men from Mars have not visited Earth. The burden of proof should be on those who say something is true.

POWER

Statistically, power means the likelihood of finding something if it's there, say, an increase in cancer in workers exposed to some substance. The greater the number of cases or subjects studied, the greater a conclusion's power and probable truth.

Be wary of studies with only a small number of cases. Sometimes large numbers indeed are needed. The likelihood that a 30- to 39-year-old woman will suffer a heart attack while taking an oral contraceptive may be about 1 per 18,000 women per year. To be 95 percent sure of finding at least one such event in a one-year trial, researchers would have to observe 54,000 women. This tells us why we so often learn of a drug's harmful side effects only after it has been studied and approved and is being used by many thousands.

There is also a great problem in trying to identify low-level, yet possibly important risks, whether of air pollution, pesticides, low-level radiation, or some other cause. For lack of power (that is, enough cases), a condition that affects one person in hundreds of thousands may never be recognized or associated with a particular cause. It is probable and perhaps inevitable that a large yet scattered number of environmentally or industrially caused illnesses remain forever undetected as "environmental illnesses," because they remain only a fraction of the vastly greater normal case load.

BIAS

Bias in science means introducing spurious associations and reaching unreliable conclusions by failing to consider other influential factors—confounding variables. Among common biases: failing to take account of age, gender, occupation, nationality, race, income, health, or behaviors like smoking.

For years, older age and smoking were largely ignored variables or factors when scientists considered the ill effects of birth control pills. In occupation studies, the workers exposed to some substance often turn out to be healthier than persons without such exposure. The confounding variable: workers are healthier than the general population with its many unhealthy people.

Polls, political and otherwise, as well as medical and environmental studies, are all subject to sampling bias, since every group studied is only a sample of a larger population, and selecting a sample is never foolproof. If you stood on a street corner and asked people whether they had heart disease, you could throw out the result. Too many of the heart diseased were staying home.

Watch for bias by asking, "Are there any other possible explanations?"

VARIABILITY

A common pitfall of science is that everything measured or studied varies from measurement to measurement. Every human experiment, repeated, has at least slightly (and sometimes markedly) different results. Among reasons: our constantly fluctuating physiologies; common errors or limits in measurement or observation; and biologic variations in the same person, between persons and between populations. Persons in different parts of the country often react differently to the same conditions, thinks to differences between persons or environments, or thanks to pure chance. This is a common trap for the environmental observer or reporter.

Ask, too, about any association's statistical strength—in other words, the odds. The greater the odds against an association's being a matter of chance, the greater its strength. If a pollutant seems to be causing a 10 percent increase above background, it may or may not be a meaningful association. If a risk is 10 times greater—the relative risk in cigarette smokers versus non-smokers—the odds are strong that something is happening.

HIERARCHY OF STUDIES

There is a hierarchy of studies—from the least to the generally most believable, starting with simple anecdotes and going on to more systematic observation or "eyeballing," then proceeding to true experiments, comparing one population or sample with another under controlled or known conditions.

Many epidemiologic and medical studies are retrospective, looking back in time at old records or statistics or memories. This is often necessary. It if often unreliable. Far better is the prospective study that follows a selected population for a long period, sometimes years. The famous Framingham (Mass.) study of behaviors and diets that may be associated with heart disease began following more than 6,000 persons in 1948.

When someone tells you, "I've done a study," ask, "What kind? How confident can you be in the results? Were there any possible flaws in the study?" An honest researcher will almost always report flaws. A dishonest one may claim perfection. All we have said also tells us that a single study rarely proves anything. The most believable studies and observations are those repeated among different populations with much the same result, and supported, if possibly, by animal or other biologic evidence.

Understand rates. There is a wide lack of understanding of the difference between a rate—so many per so many per unit of time—and a mere number. A headline in the Washington Post once read, "Airline Accident Rate Is Highest in 13 Years," but the story, like many others misusing the word "rate," merely reported death and crash totals. A correction had to be printed pointing out that the number of accidents per 100,000 departures had been declining year after year.

Similarly, watch risk numbers. Their choice can be someone's decision picked to influence reporters and the public. Someone may use an annual death total, or deaths per thousand or per million, or per thousand persons exposed, or deaths per ton of some substance or per ton released in the air or per facility. There can be lots of choices to make something sound better or worse.

An example. A proposed federal law would have required anti-pollution devices to remove 98 percent of auto tailpipe emissions, compared with a current 96 percent. Industry called that only a 2 percent increase in removal. Environmentalists called it a 50 percent decline in auto pollution. The solution: report both numbers.

All this says: look for evidence, including sound statistics, that make a study or indeed any statement of fact supposedly backed by statistics worth reporting. As, "How do you know?" and other questions. As a doctor at the National Institutes of Health once said while exhibiting a sophisticated body scanning machine to reporters, "Ask to see the numbers, not just the pretty colors."

Dr. Diana Petitti

INTERVIEW BY TANIA KETENJIAN

Diana Petitti, M.D. is a practicing epidemiologist and the director of the Research and Evaluation Department at Kaiser Permanente Medical Program in the Southern California region. This interview was conducted in May 1999.

TK: You have long been attempting to help the public distinguish between sound medical studies and those that leap to premature or misleading conclusions.

DP: Yes. I would like people to be more focused on telling the truth about what research says, free of political or commercial biases. I feel that there are many interests that tend to distort the truth to fit both political and financial ends. This is a source of great frustration to me.

TK: What have you done that has caused controversy in the science, health, and pharmaceutical industries?

DP: My research findings have caused controversy because they are not necessarily in the interests of vested groups. Distortions are not limited to the pharmaceutical industry. When people have a bias about a drug or an intervention, they tend to take the data and interpret it selectively for their own purposes, or to attack the person and the data because it doesn't confirm things in their terms.

TK: How should we interpret the contradictory medical information with which we are bombarded?

DP: First of all, people looking at evidence should understand that no single study ever finds the absolute truth, so there's a red light when a single study is interpreted as being definitive. What is truth today may not be all of the truth tomorrow. In thinking about, for example, oral contraceptives and hormone replacement therapy—fields that I work in—in the early '60s, there was a substantial amount of evidence to show that oral contraceptives used then had a substantially high risk of vascular complications. Now here we are, almost forty years later, and we have new pills and new ways of using oral contraceptives that are safe for most women. There can be problems in using single studies as if those single studies are a definitive answer to a specific question. Take, for example, how the Nurses' Health Study at Harvard and anything that comes out of it is considered to be *the* answer to the question for now and all time. I think that is an oversimplification of the evidence and an unfortunate reliance on a single study.

TK: So how should someone know whether they can really rely on a study? What are the characteristics of a well done study?

DP: Take a topic—for example, does hormone replacement therapy prevent cardiovascular disease—a person who relies on a single study on that topic would really be fooling themselves. I think that when one looks at an individual study and tries to assess its quality, the criteria should be: how well described is the protocol; was this a study that had, depending on the design, a good response rate; has the analysis been conducted appropriately; was there attention to validity and reliability in the primary data collected; have the authors appropriately interpreted the results; and was the study large enough to support whatever conclusions are being made from the data? But again, interpretation of single studies is not really something that concerns me in the science of health today. The problem is more the selection of a single study, and drawing conclusions based on that single study, while ignoring the remainder of the evidence. Even if it is a good study, single studies don't tell the truth.

TK: What answers do we most urgently need?.

DP: I'd like to see us get answers more quickly on some topics where we have fairly definitive evidence for men, but don't have definitive evidence for women. One example is the use of aspirin for the primary prevention of coronary heart disease. That is a topic where we have a lot of data for men and don't have it for women. I wish we could more quickly get a definitive answer to the question of whether or not hormone replacement is effective as the primary prevention of coronary heart disease. That answer will only come from randomized trials and we're going to be stuck with no large randomized trials for probably at least another six years.

However, the Heart and Estrogen/Progestin Replacement study (HERS) has answered one of the questions of hormone replacement therapy and coronary disease for women pretty well. This study was a large—more than 2000 subjects—randomized trial that studied the effect of combined estrogen/progestin replacement therapy on coronary heart disease in women who already had coronary disease. After four years, rates of heart disease and death were identical between the women who took hormone replacement and those who took a placebo.

TK: Can you define a randomized trial?

DP: A randomized trial is a kind of study in which women are assigned to treatment at random… that is, by chance. When there is randomization, subjects in the study are identical in all respects other than treatment and the randomized trial is considered to be the best method for finding out whether drugs and other kinds of medical treatment really work.

TK: The pharmaceutical and medical industries have their own biases and financial needs. How does that affect the work that you do?

DP: The pharmaceutical industry has an enormous amount of money to invest in clinical research and I think that they are, in general, excellent in designing and conducting large-scale randomized trials. The problem is that they are not interested in topics that hold for them no commercial interest. I think the hormone estrogen-progestin replacement study funded by Wyeth-Ayerst (hormone manufacturer–Premarin) is an example of study design being influenced by the company's commercial interest in promoting combination estrogen-progestin replacement therapy. That study should have had an arm that also looked at estrogen alone.

TK: Can you discuss Years of Potential Life Lost—YPLL—and the difference between death of women arising from heart disease, which is more common, versus death arising from breast cancer, where women die at an earlier age?

DP: In the end, it's actually a matter of personal preference more than something that policy makers can dictate. For an individual, it's a question of, "Would I rather get breast cancer when I'm forty in order to prevent heart disease when I'm eighty?" And that is a personal choice. There are a number of measures that attempt to balance adverse effects or positive effects on health at an early-versus-late age and the years of healthy life lost is one of those metrics.

TK: What should a patient know when she is looking into elective drugs? What should she look for; what information should she seek out?

DP: When people are deciding whether or not to do something—to take a drug or make a lifestyle change in order to prevent future death or disability, or to actually prolong healthy life—they have to think very carefully about whether there is an evidence-base for making that lifestyle change or using that drug.

When you're healthy and you do something to enhance health, that intervention should be held, both for individuals and for society, to a very high standard of evidence proven to work in randomized group trials. That should be a standard for individuals and for society. Then, beyond that, obviously there are questions of, "Is this convenient for me; how expensive is it; am I likely to be one of those people who will specifically benefit from this?"

TK: How can a patient figure that out?

DP: Scientists and policy-makers have an obligation to try and make this information available to people in a form that they can understand. Scientists, funding agencies, and policy-makers are obligated to support studies that answer questions definitively and to not promote changes in lifestyle or use of drugs for prevention until they are proven definitively to work.

TK How do you think they can make that happen?

DP: They can get it done through political activism, through organizations like the National Women's Health Network, and through media and the influence of consumers on the media.

TK: What was your experience as an advisor to the Food and Drug Administration?

DP: It was actually fun. I enjoyed participating in the process of deciding what drugs should be allowed onto the market. My experience with the FDA as a member of their advisory committee and as an expert consultant, which I've been doing for almost twenty years now, is that the work done by the FDA is on a very high level scientifically, and that the advisory committee is a group of very hard working people who are doing everything they can to make the right decisions.

TK: So you approve of the way the FDA works?

DP: I like the way the advisory committee that I was on worked; I was impressed with the quality of the work and with the staff.

TK: Do you find that there are some general beliefs about heart disease that are inaccurate and that really need to be changed?

DP: In the last five years there has been a gratifying increased recognition of the contribution of both heart disease and stroke to morbidity and mortality of women. I do think there had previously been a tendency to think of coronary heart disease in particular as being a disease in men and not a disease in women, so that's been a major change. Because of the promotion of hormone replacement therapy as a way to prevent heart disease, women have in general ignored other things that they might do in order to maximize their cardiovascular health including maintaining ideal body weight, getting screened for cholesterol, and use of cholesterol-lowering drugs if they have high cholesterol. Probably someday, if we have the definitive information, we can start thinking about taking aspirin to prevent heart disease and maybe not taking cancer-causing hormones.

TK: Are cholesterol-lowering drugs effective?

DP: In my opinion, there is convincing data that cholesterol-lowering drugs in people who have elevated cholesterol and even in people who have only bor-derline elevated cholesterol, do decrease morbidity and mortality. The data, although very sparse, shows that conclusion also applies to women.

TK: What do you think of estrogen replacement therapy and hormone replace-ment therapy in relation to heart disease?

DP: In my opinion, we do not have the definitive study showing that either estrogen replacement therapy or hormone replacement therapy is useful for primary prevention of coronary disease in women, and that is an extremely important question. We have a large body of observational data which is sort of consistent but which in my opinion all suffers from the same bias.

TK: What same bias does the body of observational data suffer from?

DP: All observational studies of HRT and cardiovascular disease suffer from the possibility of selection of healthier women and women who follow healthy lifestyles for estrogen use. This has been called "compliance bias" - the obser-vation of lower cardiovascular mortality in men and women who are compli-ant with taking the medications. Both "prevention bias", the propensity of women who take hormones to be more likely to engage in other behaviors that might prevent cardiovascular disease, and "compliance bias" have been demonstrated empirically. In other words, these biases are not just theoretical.

TK: There seem to be a number of different sorts of biases that can skew test results. Would you expand a little on them?

DP: Bias is a general term that is used to refer to something that distorts the truth. When people who take and don't take a drug differ for reasons other than drug taking, there is the possiblity of bias—distortion of the truth.

Selection bias, prevention bias, and compliance bias are three categories of ways that ERT/HRT users might differ from non-users and might distort observational studies. Selection bias refers to demographic characteristics such as education and race that differ between users and non-users. Since education and race are related to heart disease, studies could conclude that ERT/HRT use prevents heart dis-ease when the real reason for the lower risk is factors like race and education.

Prevention bias refers to differences between HRT users and non-users in other preventive interventions and behaviors, for example, exercise or a low fat diet. Since these reduce the risk of heart disease, studies could conclude that ERT/HRT use prevents heart disease when the real reason for the lower risk is more exercise and better diet in ERT/HRT users.

Compliance bias is subtle—it has been shown that people who take their pills, even their placebo pills, are less likely to die of heart disease than people who do not take their pills—even placebo pills. Users of ERT/HRT are all, by definition, pill takers. The lower risk of heart disease in non-experimental studies of ERT/HRT may be because ERT/HRT users are pill takers—that is, the studies are subject to distortion because of compliance bias.

TK: What made you decide to become an epidemiologist?

DP: I loved statistics and I wanted to be a researcher because, at the time that I was training to be a physician, it was my opinion that much of what we told people to do and not to do was not based on evidence. I wanted to find the answers before I told people what to do with their lives.

TK: What do you feel has changed since you started working as an epidemiologist?

DP: What we tell people to do and the basis of medicine is much more firmly grounded in high quality evidence now than it was twenty-five years ago when I graduated from medical school and decided to become an epidemiologist.

TK: And there are still changes that need to be realized, one of them being that people don't focus so much on one study?

DP: People are no longer focusing so much on one study: studies are bigger, better, and designed correctly. The whole era of the randomized trial is really a phenomenon of the last two decades.

TK: Do you know of any centers or institutions that provide reliable studies in general?

DP: I think that National Institute of Health-funded studies are very high quality. I have a very hard time finding any randomized trial funded by NIH that is not held to an extremely high standard both in terms of the science and the monitoring of the science, and the publications that come from there. I think we have to be really proud of the industry that we've created through the NIH of getting high quality data.

TK: Of which of your accomplishments are you the most proud?

DP: Well, I am actually proud of my book. I wrote a book entitled *Meta-Analysis, Decision Analysis, and Cost-Effectiveness: Methods for Quantitative Synthesis in Medicine* (Oxford University Press, NY: 1994), which is a methods book about how to synthesize evidence, and the book, which was kind of ahead of its time, has been very successful and very well received. It was a little different than doing an individual study, actually more difficult. I am very pleased with the studies I did on oral contraceptives and vascular disease. I have done quite a lot of work as a member of the World Health Organization's steering committee on reproductive health. I have been on that committee off and on since 1983, and the work that that steering committee oversaw resulted in about 100 different publications related to reproductive health in developing countries. It was a major accomplishment with which my name is not actually associated for anything other than having served on the committee. I am pleased with my membership on the FDA advisory committee because during my tenure, I was on the committee that recommended the approval of emergency contraception and RU-486. Those were incredibly controversial topics for any organization and I think the committee made the right decisions.

TK: What is the most important thing you learned in your work?

DP: The lag time between asking a question and getting an answer is incredibly long and I think that's probably one of the most important things I've learned in the last twenty-five years that I have been working as a researcher: how incredibly long it takes to get an answer. I think the answers to the questions that were posed ten years ago will only be forthcoming in the next five years.

A Different Prescription

ANNE ROCHON FORD

Anne Rochon Ford, *A Different Prescription: Considerations for Women's Health Groups Contemplating Funding from the Pharmaceutical Industry,* Toronto, Institute for Feminist Legal Studies, 1999. Reprinted by permission.

INTRODUCTION

In Canada over the past 10 years, community-based women's health organizations have been experiencing continued government cutbacks.

At the same time, nonprofit organizations in many sectors—not just health—are being strongly encouraged to form "partnerships" with industry. Although it is not always clear exactly what is meant by "partnerships," one thing that is usually implied is the assumption that money should be sought from industry and if money is offered it should not be refused.

For the corporate sector, it is in their best corporate interest to spread some of their wealth and to give generously to community-based organizations and enter into sponsorship arrangements with them.

You may be such an organization struggling with this issue and trying to determine whether you should put your energy into developing such partnerships and, more specifically, whether you should accept money from the pharmaceutical industry.

This booklet may help to shed a little more light on your decision. It has been developed out of strong concerns about the implications of pharmaceutical industry sponsorship of women's health organizations, and what they might mean both to individual groups and to the women's health movement as a whole.

Why just women's health groups? We decided to narrow the focus because women have a particular relationship to pharmaceuticals, which makes some of their issues unique. Women are often the specific target for advertising by pharmaceutical companies, either because of their reproductive needs or because women are most often the ones in their families who make decisions about their family's health care needs. They visit doctors more often than men, either for themselves or for other family members, and therefore are more likely to be prescribed drugs. They are prescribed mood-altering drugs at a higher rate than men. As the sole users of most birth control products—a particularly lucrative market for the pharmaceutical industry—they are often faced with difficult decisions about the safety and efficacy of their choices. As the primary caregivers of sick family members, they are more likely to see the effects—both positive and negative—of other women who have had bad experiences with a particular medication, and are more likely to have read magazine and newspaper articles about medication which has been helpful for particular conditions.

Pharmaceutical companies specifically target women's groups because women's health is becoming increasingly medicalized. It was only a few decades ago that there were no drugs for menopause, menstrual discomforts, irregular menstrual cycles, breast cancer prevention, and fertility problems.

In short, we have a relationship to this issue which is specific to us because we are women. Added to this equation is the fact that drugs and devices that have proven to be harmful to women have appeared on the market in recent decades. Because of the legacy of harmful drugs and devices such as DES, thalidomide, and the Dalkon shield, many North American women in particular have become increasingly wary about the decisions they make in relation to prescription drugs. At the same time, the pharmaceutical industry has increased its efforts to sell its products directly to a public that has become highly dependent on drugs.

A COMMON SCENARIO

A women's health organization in a large Canadian city has been offering useful information and support to women who have been diagnosed with a particular disease or disorder. Users of this service indicate that they are grateful for the help the service offers them in making difficult decisions about treatment options. They appreciate being able to talk to other women with the disease and feel like they can get on with the rest of their lives.

A member of the board of directors of the organization brings a plan to the board and the staff members. She has a good friend who works for drug company X, manufacturers of a drug frequently used by women with this disease. This friend has been telling her that she knows her company would give money to help out the service—they just have to say how much they need. The board member presenting this thinks it is a good idea. The board is divided. Opinions vary widely.

Let's take a closer look at some of the comments made by the board members and staff.

"It's a win-win situation—they get to feel better because they're doing something that makes them look good, and we have money to keep our service running. What can be wrong with that?"

On the surface, this scenario does indeed look like a win-win situation. And some groups will come to the decision to take the money and not only be quite comfortable with that decision but be able to put the money to good use. Their members will benefit and the drug company will be able to say it has done a good deed with their donation.

A representative from a group for women with AIDS who spoke at the panel discussion described their decision to accept pharmaceutical money: The money they have received from the industry has allowed them to offer programs that they feel they could not otherwise offer. She also pointed out that the survival of her group members is partially linked to the drugs they take, so they have always had a close relationship with the drug industry. The money is often used for direct donations to the women in need as opposed to being directly tied to a product line.

On the other hand, others feel that it may look like a win-win situation, but the winning is mostly by the pharmaceutical company. One panelist, who had canvassed representatives from some of the manufacturers of the most commonly prescribed drugs for women's reproductive conditions, learned that most donations to women's health groups (and other non-profit health organizations) come from the marketing budget of a company. In most cases, donations are linked to a product or product line of that particular company. Therefore, you would not likely see a company which does not manufacture, for example, a fertility medication, giving money to an infertility support group, and similarly, companies which manufacture fertility medication would specifically target infertility groups for their donations.

The industry has much to gain from making such donations and forming such links. First, association with a reputable organization can provide a more credible endorsement of their product than if the promotion were coming directly from the industry (i.e., the goodwill associated with a company's name when they are seen to be making contributions to groups can have a direct impact in the public's mind about the value of their products).

Secondly, if a company is in the pre-launch phase of the introduction of a new drug, they can use the captive audience of the group they have funded to spread awareness among the public about their drug and about the disease that the drug is treating. This awareness will generally not extend to prevention and other forms of treatment, specifically not to other drugs made by competitors. Funding an organization to provide educational outreach about a disease such as osteoporosis serves to raise the general public's awareness of this issue and, importantly for the drug company, of drug treatments which are being developed to treat it.

Finally, if a drug company is seeking approval from regulatory bodies for a drug that they have manufactured, they can use their funded groups to help them argue for the need for approval of this drug.

There is, however, one way in which an industry wins and the recipient of their money can lose: Support from the industry dulls criticism. The National Women's Health Network in the United States, for example, has developed a policy not to take money from the pharmaceutical industry. The main reason they offer is that one of the foundations of their educational work is to encourage women to seek alternatives to pills and surgery in dealing with their health problems, and to look at the social and economic reasons behind much ill health.

"I think we should just take the money wherever we can get it. It's the only way we'll keep this service alive. We can't afford to be purists."

This is a commonly held opinion. Many groups are dealing with the sheer logistics of survival and staying alive, and feel they can't afford to look a gift horse in the mouth.

Although hard to look at, it might be worth asking, "Is this really the *only* way you'll keep this service alive?" Frequently the option of pharmaceutical money comes to groups without a lot of effort. The industry is looking to form partnerships such as this, and in the larger scheme of things, offering money to a community-based women's health organization to keep its doors open represents a drop in the bucket of their profits.

Groups are often surprised when after years of hounding philanthropic organizations and individual donors for money, the offer for money from a pharmaceutical company comes to them almost effortlessly. Understandably, this is enormously appealing to anyone who is sick and tired of trying to raise money. But the question then might be, if this came so effortlessly, is it the only money to be had without much struggle?

You may want to consider the local bank where your group does banking, companies which employ your board members or families of consumers who use your service. Is there a member of your group who knows a wealthy individual dealing with the health problem your group is involved in? One patron can often donate as much as an individual company.

"What do you mean?—'It's dirty money?' Isn't all money dirty money?"

The term "dirty money" has been used to describe money which may have been used for less than honorable purposes. Some people have argued that there is no difference between taking money from the pharmaceutical companies and accepting money from banks, insurance companies, or other large corporations. The argument goes that those companies or financial institutions which may appear to have no strings attached to their money may also be funding practices or carrying out activities, particularly in third world countries, which your group would find ethically questionable.

"Isn't this just free publicity for the company?"

If your organization does choose to accept money from a pharmaceutical company which manufactures a product used by members of your group, it is worth keeping in mind that you are indirectly providing endorsement of that company and their product through your action. It is in the company's best interest to have this endorsement of their product from a non-commercial source.

Similarly, if the company funding you is developing a new product for your user group (e.g., a fertility drug in the case of an infertility group) your group may unwittingly become the focus for promotion of this drug by the company. The group may become a conduit of information for the company to the potential users of the drug. In the case of a drug which is badly needed and has been properly tested, this may not be such a bad thing. In the case of a drug which is simply a copy-cat of another product on the market, the relationship becomes a little more questionable.

Some groups may be quite comfortable with this while other may not. Each group must come to its own conclusions about what role they may want to play—either directly or indirectly—in promoting a company and its product. Some groups go as far as outright promotion of a product in exchange for funding.

If you are accepting money, you may want to be very clear from the start what the parameters of that relationship are and get it in writing. At a minimum, the company should be made to understand clearly that it cannot directly attempt to influence the advice a group gives its members, nor can it use the members as targets for promotion of their products. This may be easier said than done. You may need to seek legal advice around the wording of your contract or letter of agreement.

"This same company also manufactures pesticides which have been shown to contribute to this disease. Why would we want to endorse that?"

In part from pressure from environmental and health activists, more research is slowly being done into the links between cancer and toxins in the environment, such as pesticides. As women's health groups probe further into this, we have been disturbed to find that sometimes the very companies which are manufacturing cancer therapy are also producing toxic pesticides which may be contributing to cancer in the first place.

For example, Zeneca, the manufacturers of tamoxifen citrate, earn $470 million each year marketing this cancer therapy drug, at the same time as it earns $300 million each year from sales of the carcinogenic herbicide acetochlor.

The women's health movement and more recently the breast cancer movement has long purported prevention as one of the main tenets of its outreach and advocacy efforts. When links are found between potential funders and the causes of the diseases the groups are fighting, this is often a connection many are not prepared to live with.

When considering funding from a pharmaceutical company, it is always helpful to do some background research on the products the company manufacturers and other aspects of their dealings. You may also want to consider a company's employment practices—how it treats its workers, if women have been allowed to advance equitably in the company, and about its practices in Third World countries.

This information is easily found in public libraries, in the company's annual reports, and on the Internet. Doing this kind of research is generally good advice for accepting *any* corporate donations, not just those from pharmaceutical companies, since corporations can often have disparate holdings you are unaware of.

"If we take their money, we're turning our backs on all the women who object to this type of sponsorship, women who feel they've been harmed more than helped by the pharmaceutical industry."

There is no question that many products of the pharmaceutical industry help countless people worldwide to both stay alive and to live a better quality of life. Nevertheless, in its aim to increase its profits, the industry has *also* manufactured products which have seriously harmed many women, usually due to improper initial testing.

It is wise to keep in mind that a decision of whether or not to be involved with the pharmaceutical industry is a decision which is taken within an historical context. The context is one which has a particularly problematic legacy.

"Most women just want the help. They don't really care where the money comes from."

This may be very true for a number of women and for many organizations. Certainly when we are dealing with diseases such as cancer, it is often the case that people will "do anything" to get help or get access to a new treatment, whatever the emotional or financial cost.

Staff members and members of boards have a duty to make fair and ethical decisions on behalf of their members or clients. A group may choose to use this time of decision-making as an opportunity to raise awareness about a number of related issues: (1) the role the pharmaceutical industry plays in our lives and the extent to which we have become a society dependent on pharmaceutical solutions; (2) discuss the level of transparency and accountability in the regulation of drugs by the federal government; or (3) arrange an evening with speakers from women's health organizations who have developed policies on this issue.

There is no one correct prescription for everyone on this issue. Each group must decide for itself which is the best route to go.

"They've told us there are no strings attached to this money and they seem to be willing to stick to that. Their attitude seems to be 'hands off.' Why should we doubt that?"

One women's health organizer, looking at this issue for her organization, commented, "There are strings, but they are strings of gossamer," meaning there are strings but you can't always see them.

It is important to remember that an industry's motivations for giving money to an organization are not philanthropic in nature. They give money to targeted groups in targeted fields that relate to their product lines.

Groups may find themselves in this situation unwittingly. The original overture from a drug company may have come from a perfectly well-intentioned individual who cared about their group. Companies are made up of individuals, and individuals of all companies would like to feel they work for a business that is a good corporate citizen. As much as companies wish to buy goodwill, staff in drug companies also pressure their employers to make donations to community-based organizations they feel committed to. Although the donation may come from marketing and all that that involves, the original impetus may not.

Similarly, most researchers who work for pharmaceutical companies come directly from university or have been recruited from a research project. Most of them begin their career with good intentions of hoping to "cure" diseases. While the company as an entity is concerned with profit, the individuals lower down the hierarchy are not always so motivated. Contacts between individuals from a pharmaceutical company and a community organization can be made with the best of intentions by the initial individuals. Later the group may be taken by surprise when the company indicates they would like a higher level of public recognition or sponsorship or indicates they don't like the way in which their product or the whole industry is portrayed in the group's literature.

One thing your group can do is talk to other community organizations that have accepted money from or engaged in some sort of partnership with that same company. Find out what their experience has been in working with that company. For example, the Infertility Network (Canada), which has received funds from Organon and Serono, agreed to have their name added to a brochure about infertility produced by Serono. The executive director noted, "This was important to them [the company], but it helped raise our profile and so it suited our purposes to do it." Another group might feel compromised by the same experience. Each organization has their own story to tell.

We can learn from the experience of other organizations who have worked through this issue. The following are some general guidelines culled from the

May 1997 panel discussion and from other groups consulted since then about how to proceed when entering into sponsorship agreements with a pharmaceutical company or in accepting money from them.

1. If you are a newly formed group or one that has not yet dealt with this issue, it is probably best to assume that you will be confronted with it at some point. Most groups find it helpful to develop a written policy on the subject and to make the policy known to their members. The policy may be as formal as being a part of your by-laws or, more commonly, a general policy of the organization. Some treat it as a separate policy while others include it as part of their overall policy on corporate donations.

2. Be very clear with newly-hired or volunteer fundraisers what your group's policy is on this issue. Be as specific as possible with anyone doing this work on your behalf (e.g., "We will not consider funds from individual pharmaceutical companies but will consider accepting funds from pharmaceutical organizations." "We will consider all types of funds, regardless of their source." "We will not take money from any organization that manufactures substances that have been linked to cancer." "We will consider money from companies which have made a strong public statement and put money behind the advancement of women," etc.)

3. When dealing with representatives from a pharmaceutical company who may potentially give your group money, you may want to consider, as some groups have, only meeting on your "turf," i.e., not meeting at their offices, and having a policy not to accept free meals or other freebies as part of the discussion. The point is to maintain control of the discussion and not to be beholden to them, whatever your group's decision may be.

4. Be sure that any arrangements entered into with a pharmaceutical company are documented and copies are kept in your files and sent to the donor. These can take the form of a letter of agreement outlining what your terms are (e.g., "We agree to use this money responsibly but/and agree/do not agree to enter into the promotion of company X's product." "We agree/do not agree to carry the company's logo on our printed materials.") Be as clear as possible about your intent. Possibilities left open to interpretation may not always work in your group's best interest.

RESOURCES FOR RESEARCHING SPECIFIC PHARMACEUTICAL COMPANIES

Rachel's Environment and Health Weekly, available electronically or by mail, covers a wide range of environmental and corporate issues. An electronic search will bring up anything they have published on questions relating to the environmental practices of specific corporations. Available from Environmental Research Foundation, PO Box 5036, Annapolis, MD 21043; fax: 410-263-8944; email: erf@rachel.org; Web site: www.monitor.net/rachel.

Multinational Monitor, published 10 times a year, tracks corporate activity, especially in the third world, focusing on the export of hazardous substances, worker health and safety, labor union issues, and the environment. To contact: *Multinational Monitor,* PO Box 19405, Washington, DC 20036; email: monitor@essential.org; Web site: www.essential.org/monitor/monitor.html.

IF YOUR GROUP DECIDES TO BECOME INVOLVED WITH THE PHARMACEUTICAL INDUSTRY... David Gilbert, in his paper, "Much to Gain, More to Lose," suggests that there are six questions a group can ask itself when considering this issue: (1) Do we need to accept funding from a company? (2) What do we seek to gain from such an arrangement? (3) What are our views on the use of medicines for the patients we purport to represent—what do the patients think (i.e., attitudes to care and treatment choice issues)? (4) What are our views on the nature of the industry? (5) What are the alternatives to company funding? and (6) What are the risks of such arrangements?

The Bitter Pill

LEORA TANENBAUM

Leora Tanenbaum, "The Bitter Pill," *on the issues,* Winter 1998. Reprinted by permission.

B arbara Dworkin, 61, is one of 8 million American women taking Premarin, an estrogen replacement that eases menopausal symptoms such as hot flashes and dry skin. Dworkin started on Premarin 15 years ago and plans to take the drug for the rest of her life. Although studies have shown that Premarin may increase the risk of breast cancer by 30 percent, as well as cause fatal blood clots, the drug also offers protection against osteoporosis and decreases the risk of fatal heart disease by 53 percent. Besides, as a 911 operator living on Long Island, New York, she leads stressful days fielding emergency calls and feels thankful for Premarin because it "makes my life much more pleasant and secure."

But Premarin costs between $15 and $25 a month. If there were a generic version, Suffolk County, New York (which covers Dworkin's drug plan) could cut its costs by 30 percent, more than $3,000 for her lifetime. If you consider that millions of other women lack health insurance or prescription drug coverage, a generic could save them more than $300 million a year.

But economizing isn't the only reason to push for a generic. Premarin is derived from the urine of pregnant horses, a fact that concerns animal rights supporters and repulses many users. People for the Ethical Treatment of Animals (PETA) claims that the collection methods on "urine farms" are barbaric: some 80,000 pregnant mares are confined to stalls for six months out of the year so that their urine can be collected; the 65,000 foals born to them are slaughtered as unusable byproducts of these pregnancies. PETA advises women to switch to an alternative hormone treatment that doesn't harm animals.

An alternative, however, will not be forthcoming. The FDA announced in May 1997 that it will not approve a recently manufactured, affordable, plant-based generic form of Premarin, even though FDA research has shown the generic to be just as effective as the brand-name drug. Rather than heed the recommendation of its own Office of Pharmaceutical Science, the FDA appears to have bowed to political pressure at the expense of women. While there are several plant-derived, FDA-approved estrogen regimens such as Estrace and Estraderm, they have not been proven to offer long-term health benefits. Only those who can afford Premarin or whose insurance will pay will be able to relieve their menopausal symptoms, ward off heart attacks, and avoid bone fractures.

It's no surprise that the commercial interests of Premarin's manufacturer, Wyeth-Ayerst, have superseded health considerations, but the tactics involved are particularly outrageous. Wyeth-Ayerst cultivated influential supporters through financial contributions. Then, when the company needed them, it prodded its beneficiaries to take a stand against their competition. The result? Several highly visible politicians and advocacy groups who knew nothing about the issues involved testified before the FDA against the generic form of Premarin. In the end, the consumer's ability to get the best drugs for the lowest price was sacrificed. The saddest part of this whole incident? Feminist politicians and women's groups were key players.

"DOCTOR, I WANT MY PREMARIN"

You don't have to be menopausal to recognize the brand-name Premarin. No doubt you've seen the drug's fear-inducing magazine ads, which suggest that midlife women who don't take estrogen will be crippled by osteoporosis if they don't die from a heart attack first. The ads also intimate that midlife women who don't take estrogen can never hope to achieve the carefree, wrinkle-free look of the models depicted.

Premarin, of course, is merely one of dozens of prescription drugs aggressively advertised in magazines such as *Newsweek, Redbook, Mirabella,* and *The New Yorker.* In recent years, drug companies have bypassed physicians and marketed their products directly to consumers. Eli Lilly's multimillion dollar campaign for Prozac, for instance, includes ads in more than 20 magazines. Some magazines, like *Good Housekeeping* and *Ladies' Home Journal,* contain so many drug ads you might be tempted to double-check the cover to make sure you're not reading a professional medical journal. Which is precisely the point: Drug manufacturers want consumers to play doctor by asking their physicians to prescribe particular drugs. And 99 percent of physicians do comply with patients' requests, market research confirms. In this era of "managed care," when physicians are pressed to see as many patients as possible in the shortest amount of time, educated patients who know how they want to be treated are a dream come true.

A dream come true, that is, for physicians and drug companies—but not necessarily for the patients. We may believe that by asking our physicians for Premarin or Prozac we are empowering ourselves by becoming more assertive in our relationships with our physicians, because only we really know our bodies and what's best for our health. But in reality, the drug companies are taking advantage of our adherence to this *Our Bodies, Ourselves* credo. We are intermediaries in a loop of influence that originates in magazine ads and culminates in a prescription.

Last year alone, pharmaceutical companies spent nearly $600 million advertising prescription drugs directly to consumers—twice as much as they spent in 1995 and almost 10 times more than they spent in 1991, according to Competitive Media Reporting, a company that tracks ad spending. None of that money, however, seems to be spent on factual research: more than half of the drug ads scrutinized last year by the Consumers' Union advocacy group contained misleading information on risks and benefits, and false claims about efficacy. In the end, the consumer's ability to get the best drugs for the lowest price was sacrificed. Feminist politicians and women's groups were key players.

POLITICS VS. SCIENCE

But as the case of the massively popular Premarin shows, the influence of drug companies goes far beyond false advertising. Wyeth-Ayerst Laboratories is a pharmaceutical Goliath that garners $1 billion a year in revenue from Premarin, the most commonly prescribed drug in America. Owned by American Home Products, Wyeth-Ayerst has maintained a monopoly on Premarin ever since it began manufacturing the estrogen replacement in 1942. Even though the patent expired more than 25 years ago, Wyeth has gotten the FDA to change its guidelines in determining bioequivalence in generics, making it difficult for competitors to match Premarin. A lot is at stake: sales could reach $3 billion within five years, with more than one-third of all women in the United States currently over the age of 50, and another 20 million entering the menopausal years within the next decade.

Because of the size of that market, two small generic drug companies have decided to compete with Wyeth. After the FDA concluded in 1991 that an effective generic requires only two active ingredients (estrone and equilin), Duramed Pharmaceuticals Corp. and Barr Laboratories Inc. teamed up to develop a urine-free generic according to FDA guidelines. In response, Wyeth filed a citizens petition requesting that one of Premarin's ingredients (an obscure estrogen called delta 8,9 dehydroestrone sulfate or DHES) be reclassified as a necessary component. Duramed has not been able to replicate an equivalent of DHES and Wyeth holds the patent on the estrogen. Furthermore, in 1995 the FDA found that based on clinical trials, there was no evidence that DHES was anything other than an impurity.

And so Wyeth shrewdly lined up the support of several influential women's and health groups by making donations to Business and Professional Women/USA, the American Medical Women's Association, the National Consumers League, and the National Osteoporosis Foundation, among others. Representatives of these groups testified before the FDA on the drug company's behalf, saying that they opposed the approval of a generic that lacks DHES, despite the FDA's own contention that the estrogen wasn't essential. The president of the Women's Legal Defense Fund also testified, although this group did not accept money from Wyeth. None of these groups had taken a position on DHES prior to being contacted by Wyeth.

The company also developed close ties to the White House and the Senate. John Stafford, chairman and CEO of Wyeth-Ayerst's parent company, American Home Products, attended an intimate 17-person White House "coffee klatsch" with President Clinton in November 1995. And in June 1996, according to the Federal Elections Commission, American Home Products made a $50,000 contribution to the Democratic National Committee. Several months later, Democratic senators Barbara Mikulski (Md.) and Patty Murray (Wash.) wrote the FDA for assurance that "it has no intention of approving a generic version of Premarin that lacks the 'same' active ingredient as the innovator." According to her press secretary, Murray became involved in this issue after she "was contacted by women's groups. As a result, our office spoke with the manufacturer, who was in contact with the same women's groups."

Lo and behold, the FDA reversed its stance. Janet Woodcock, M.D., director of the FDA's Center for Drug Evaluation and Research, announced on May 5 that "based on currently available data, there is at this time no way to assure that synthetic generic forms of Premarin have the same active ingredients as the [urine-based] drug."

No matter how you look at it, the FDA flip-flop appears to be the result of Wyeth-Ayerst's considerable lobbying muscle. Of course, just because a decision is politically influenced doesn't mean it's wrong. But an internal FDA memo dated May 3 (two days before the decision was announced) supports the generic, saying that DHES is not a necessary component. Even the vice president of Wyeth-Ayerst's regulatory affairs department admitted to The *Wall Street Journal* that there's "probably nothing" special about DHES, and that "it's but one of many components in Premarin."

Consumer health is clearly the last thing on the minds of everyone involved in the Premarin debacle. "This decision is pure politics," fumes Cynthia Pearson, executive director of the National Women's Health Network, the only women's organization that publicly supports the generic. Coincidentally, the network does not accept donations from drug companies. The decision "was not backed up by science," says Pearson. "This never would have happened without political pressure orchestrated by Wyeth-Ayerst."

Duramed has challenged the FDA decision in an administrative appeal; the company intends to file a court appeal if it is turned down. But Wyeth is already a step ahead: it is busily working to ensure that no matter what happens, it will continue to dominate the estrogen replacement market. After all, Wyeth is the sole sponsor of an important "memory study" on Premarin's effectiveness in warding off Alzheimer's disease, a study conducted under the aegis of the government-sponsored Women's Health Initiative. If a correlation is found, physicians and consumers alike will naturally turn to Premarin as a preventative for Alzheimer's.

COMMERCIALLY SPONSORED MEDICINE

Wyeth is hardly the only drug company to use political leverage to protect its turf. In 1997, the *Journal of the American Medical Association* (JAMA) published results of a 1990 study on thyroid medications and reported that the maker of Synthroid, one of the drugs under study, had suppressed for years the fact that three other medications were equally effective. Like Premarin, Synthroid has long enjoyed domination in a lucrative market because its manufacturer falsely claims that its product is superior to the competition.

Ten years ago, in order to establish Synthroid as the most effective drug in its class, Flint Laboratories (then the drug's manufacturer) approached researcher Betty Dong of the University of California, San Francisco. Dong signed a contract with Flint to conduct comparative studies of the bioequivalence of Synthroid and three other preparations. When her research was completed in 1990, Dong submitted the results to Boots Pharmaceuticals (which had since taken over Flint). It turned out that all four drugs were bioequivalent, and that consumers who chose the other drugs over Synthroid could save $356 million annually. Boots became alarmed: After all, it is the leader in a $600 million-a-year market.

With so much revenue at stake, Boots did everything it could to publicly discredit Dong's research. It dishonestly claimed that the research was flawed in design and execution, and that Dong had breached research ethics. It then published Dong's results in a "reanalysis" that reached the opposite conclusion. Conveniently, Boots was able to prevent publication of Dong's own account of her research, since the contract she originally signed stipulated that nothing could be published without written consent from the drug company.

Finally, under pressure from the FDA, Boots (now part of Knoll Pharmaceutical) agreed to allow Dong's results to be published—seven years after the study was completed. Later, Boots/Knoll agreed to pay $98 million in a settlement to consumers who purchased Synthroid between 1990 and 1997.

A MATTER OF TRUST

The growing power of pharmaceutical companies is troubling on a number of levels. It is frightening how poorly we are informed about the appalling treatment of animals in drug manufacturing. It is wasteful to pay for needlessly expensive medications. Forget about President Clinton's 1992 plea to the drug companies to control their prices. In the last few years, big-name drug companies such as Merck and Hoechst have withdrawn from the generics field because they realized they could make far more money selling brand-name drugs. But the real bottom line is that the drug companies have robbed consumers of the ability to trust anyone in the area of drug research: commercialism has infected everyone involved. We can't trust those companies to which we entrust our health to accurately represent their products. We can't assume that the FDA has weighed all of the scientific research fairly. We can't even take for granted that the scientists who perform drug research are working independently.

Savvy consumers, of course, realize that drug companies are motivated by profit. But what about advocacy groups, including women's and health organizations? Aren't they supposed to be looking out for the public good?

"All medical organizations receive money from the pharmaceutical companies," rationalizes Debra R. Judelson, M.D., president of the American Medical Women's Association, one of the organizations that accepted money from Wyeth and testified before the FDA on the same issue. "There are no virgins. We've all been lobbied by the pharmaceuticals on all the issues." The National Women's Health Network, the lone women's advocacy group to support the Premarin generic, must be the only virgin at the orgy.

But perhaps the ever-increasing power and determination of certain drug companies to quash their competition isn't so terrible. Look, if we all just took Prozac, it wouldn't seem so bad.

In 1999, Wyeth-Ayerst finally lost its monopoly of the U.S. market in conjugated estrogrens. Duramed got its product, called Cenestin, approved, though not as generic. As a result, the product is not likely to be as inexpensive as it could have been.

Raloxifene: The New Estrogen

NATIONAL WOMEN'S HEALTH NETWORK PERSPECTIVE

Perspective, bulletin prepared by the National Women's Health Network, 1999. Reprinted by permission.

THE NEW "DESIGNER ESTROGENS"

The newest drug therapy to hit the mainstream women's health market is "new designer estrogens": selective estrogen receptor modulator or SERMs. Targeted at today's baby boomer, fifty-something women, these antiestrogens are intended to be the next generation of estrogen replacement therapy. Their makers hope SERMs will give post-menopausal women all of the gains that estrogen seems to deliver, including a healthy heart and healthy bones, but without the fear of breast cancer. This of course, seems almost too good to be true and unfortunately, there isn't enough research available yet to prove otherwise.

HOW SERMS WORK

It is important to first learn what these SERMs are all about: The SERMs being developed today (raloxifene, from Eli Lilly and Co., was just approved by the FDA, making it the first drug of its kind on the market) are intended to replace current therapies by staving off osteoporosis without any risk of cancer. These drugs are believed to work as "partial" estrogens. Researchers have found that estrogen receptors in the body are divided into at least two types, with Alpha receptors dominant in the breast and uterus and Beta receptors more common in the bone and blood vessel. The SERMs that bond to Beta Receptors such as raloxifene, and an earlier drug, tamoxifen, may prevent osteoporosis without increasing cancer risks.

TAMOXIFEN—THE FIRST SERM

Much of what we already know about hormone blockers is because of the long term studies done on women who have used the drug tamoxifen. Early studies with tamoxifen showed that it could reduce the chance of recurrence in women who had breast cancer by at least 30 percent. This beneficial effect lasts for at least five years. However, two randomized trials have shown that women who take tamoxifen for ten years are more likely to experience a recurrence of breast cancer. Like the new SERM raloxifene, tamoxifen blocks estrogen in the breast while preventing bone loss and reducing cholesterol levels. It is important to to note that it took ten years for the breast cancer promoting effect to appear. The new SERMs being researched and marketed by drug companies like Eli Lilly may have short term evidence that they reduce the risk of breast cancer, but how sure are they when it comes to the long term effect?

KEEP YOUR EYE ON RALOXIFENE

Raloxifene is currently in at least three randomized trials including more than 13,000 post-menopausal women. Results after two years show that women taking raloxifene increased bone mass by about 2 percent while those on calcium lost bone. About one quarter of the women on raloxifene experienced hot flashes, compared to less than one fifth of the women on calcium. Studies have also shown that raloxifene lowers levels of bad cholesterol (LDL), but does not seem to affect "good" cholesterol levels (HDL). Most importantly, it seems that early data on breast cancer in one of the studies suggest a positive protective effect from raloxifene. We believe that it is crucial that Eli Lilly and other drug companies that plan to market similar products follow up with long term studies to determine the ultimate effect of raloxifene on breast and other cancers. In December 1997, only three weeks after the FDA Advisory Committee meeting, raloxifene, under the brand name Evista, was approved for the prevention of osteoporosis in post-menopausal women. We are concerned that Lilly will take advantage of these early results to create an enormous market for raloxifene among women concerned about their chances of developing breast cancer, exposing millions of healthy women to a drug with unknown and potentially harmful long-term effects.

THIS IS WHAT WE KNOW

In a two-year study of 1,800 postmenopausal women:
- ➤Raloxifene has prevented bone loss (2–3 percent).
- ➤Raloxifene has reduced cholesterol levels.
- ➤Uterine cancer rates were not increased.
- ➤About one quarter of women on raloxifene had hot flashes.
- ➤The most serious side effect reported is the increased risk of blood clots.

AND THIS IS WHAT WE DO NOT KNOW
- ➤*If* raloxifene can prevent fractures, as opposed to increasing bone density…
- ➤*If* raloxifene can help lessen instances of heart attack…
- ➤*If* raloxifene can help prevent breast cancer in postmenopausal women…

CONCLUSION

Having SERMs widens the options available to women, that is for sure—but it remains to be seen whether prevention drugs like raloxifene are for everyone. It is worth remembering that a study is only as good as its time frame. As we recall the lessons learned from tamoxifen, that long-term use can be harmful even if short-term use is beneficial; it is necessary that raloxifene and other new designer estrogens be treated with caution.

For more information on SERMs and raloxifene contact the National Women's Health Network. For a copy of the NWHN testimony before the FDA on raloxifene, please write: National Women's Health Network, 524 10th St. NW Suite 400, Washington, DC 20004; 202-347-1140; fax 202-347-1168.

"Should Prescription Drugs Be Advertised?"

MICHAEL CASTLEMAN AND MARYANN NAPOLI

Excerpted from Michael Castleman, "But Wait, There's More," and Maryann Napoli, "The Wrong Rx," *MAMM*, October/November 1998. Reprinted by permission.

BUT WAIT, THERE'S MORE

Open newspapers and magazines these days, and you're likely to see ads that were not there a few years ago—ads for prescription drugs. Known as direct-to-consumer advertising, and formerly reserved for medical journals, prescription drug ads, now take center stage in magazines such as *Glamour.*

However, you can't just trot down to the pharmacy on your own. You have to ask you doctor for a prescription.

And there's the rub. Many doctors don't want people asking for prescription drugs by name and are calling for restrictions on direct-to-consumer ads. According to a survey of 454 family physicians published in the December 1997 issue of the *Journal of Family Practice*, 71 percent said that TV, radio, and print ads "pressure physicians to use drugs they might not ordinarily use."

Doctors also complain that consumer drug advertising can be misleading; more than 75 percent said so in the *Journal of Family Practice* survey.

Finally, some observers fret that direct-to-consumer ads drive up drug prices. Myra Snyder, executive director of the Center for Healthcare Quality Improvement in San Francisco, contends that drug cost increases are one of the leading causes of medical inflation, and that direct-to-consumer ads fan the flames.

This controversy is not a tempest in a medicine chest. One of the biggest changes in the industry has been direct-to-consumer advertising. The pharmaceutical industry spent just $12.3 million on consumer advertising in 1989. Now it spends an estimated $1 billion a year, an 80-fold increase.

Direct-to-consumer drug advertising does represent a change in our health care culture. And it is difficult for doctors to contend with requests for specific brand-name drugs that might not be best. But doctors are trained to handle some very tough discussions, for example, telling people that they have a terminal illness. Compared with such life-and-death exchanges, it's not all that challenging to say: "No, I don't think that brand is best for you. I'm going to prescribe another."

As for the cost issue, has direct-to-consumer advertising really driven drug prices through the roof? Not according to the Consumer Price Index: Lately, drug-price inflation has been running at a 2.5 to 3.5 percent year, about the same as the overall cost of health care.

It's also a stretch to think that prescription ads seriously mislead the public. We live in a culture absolutely inundated by advertising and people understand that ads use a germ of truth to spin a web of half-truths.

Direct-to-consumer drug ads are, arguably, less misleading than many other ads. Their information is regulated by the FDA and thus subject to much more government scrutiny. And consumers can't buy prescription drugs without a doctor's approval.

These ads can also alert people that a product exists. Consider the ads for Sporanox, used to treat fungal infections. Millions of Americans have no idea why their toenails are discolored and deformed. Sporanox ads offer an explanation: Hey, what do you know, I have a fungal infection. Maybe I'll get it treated.

Of course, these ads are not an exercise in public health education. They're trying to sell product. Information gleaned from any advertising, not just direct-to-consumer drugs ads, should always be taken with a prudent dose of skepticism.

THE WRONG RX

At first it seemed like a good idea. Advertising prescription drugs directly to consumers would give us some control over our health care. We could learn about a new drug our doctors might not have thought to prescribe, and read about its side effects for ourselves.

As it turns out, the idea was a fantasy.

Advertising is about selling, not about balanced information. It's about creating demand and brand identity for prescription drugs, and it has been part of an enormously successful effort. Americans spent $78.9 billion in 1997 on prescription drugs, up from $37.7 billion in 1990, and the amount is rising at a rate of about 17 percent a year, according to an analysis in *The New England Journal of Medicine*. The pharmaceutical industry allocated $1.3 billion for direct-to-consumer advertising last year, more than the amount devoted to advertising directed at doctors. The doctors, however, were visited in person by drug company representatives at the incredible cost of $5.3 billion for the first 11 months of 1998, according to *the New York Times*.

The ads, of course, promote new drugs. New always means more expensive but not necessarily better. Cheaper and often equally effective alternatives may already be available. For FDA approval, the manufacturer need only prove its drug performed better than a placebo. No head-to-head comparison with an older competing drug is required, no showing of superior efficacy. These "me-too" medications could be a chemical notch or two away from a competitor's drug, without a significant difference in what they do. Think Valium and Librium, Prozac and Soloft, Pravachol and Mevacor—or Coke and Pepsi.

One peril is inappropriate drug choices.

The slick persuasiveness of some ads may also cause consumers to risk serious side effects to achieve a cosmetic result. Novartis Pharmaceuticals, for example, has heavily advertised Lamisil as a remedy for toenail fungus. A course of treatment costs $500 and carries the rare possibility of liver toxicity. Other ads create worry about medical problems that might never occur. "Is it just forgetfulness… or is it Alzheimer's disease?" asks Pfizer's ad for Aricept, a new drug intended to improve cognition, for example.

In the ubiquitous Claritin TV commercials, the name of the drug is used, but not its purpose. By leaving out either the drug name or its purpose, the companies do not have to meet FDA requirements to provide side-effect information. For print ads, these requirements dictate publication of a page of print

so fine you need a magnifying glass to read it. What percentage of the participants in trials of the drug benefited from it, and what was the benefit? With
rare exceptions, you'll be hard-pressed to find answers to those questions even
if you read every tiny word.

If you have any doubts that drug advertising can result in inappropriate
drug choices, look at its effect on medical professionals.

Today, an aggressively promoted drug family used to treat hypertension,
known as calcium channel blockers (CCBs), stands out as the best documented example of advertising's malevolent influence on physicians. CCBs (like
Cardizem, Procardia, and Adalat) should not be the first-choice drug for people with hypertension because the less-costly diuretics and beta blockers are
the only two drug classes proven to reduce rates of cardiovascular death and
heart attack. Over the years, scathing commentaries in medical journals on the
underuse of the more effective drugs have failed to put a major dent in the
problem. The effect on consumers? An increased risk of death, heart attack,
stroke, and cancer, according to several studies on CCBs.

Doctors have at least some education in pharmacology. If they can be dangerously misled, why can't we?

Dear John Letters

E. JAMES LIEBERMAN, SAMUEL EPSTEIN, JULIE BECKER

Reprinted by permission.

LIEBERMAN V. SLOAN-KETTERING

E. James Lieberman, M.D.
The Family Institute

December 14, 1996
[second mailing 1st sent Oct 6, no response]

John S. Reed, Chairman
Citicorp

Dear Mr. Reed:

As a new Citicorp stockholder I was privileged to vote by proxy at the 1996
Annual Meeting for the first time. But this letter also has to express disappointment and protest. I withheld votes for three directors in the balloting,
including you. The reason: along with Richard Parsons (President, Time
Warner) and Rozanne Ridgway (Co-Chair, The Atlantic Council) you serve on
the boards of tobacco companies. Distinguished business leaders like you
three hardly need such roles, since you hold other important directorships and
doubtless have to turn down many significant invitations.

The situation suggests that you approve of the development and marketing of the cigarette, a product which has only lately begun to achieve the notoriety it deserves. I won't belabor the point, except to say that even the American Medical Association now asks that doctors not invest in tobacco companies.

Nowadays companies such as Philip Morris (Parsons, Reed) and RJR Nabisco (Ridgway) need you more than you need them. Resigning from their boards would be an act of ethical leadership and enhance your reputations among a wide audience. It would decrease your income but surely you have more compelling reasons for staying in those hot seats. I am eager to know your rationale for continuing to participate, if in fact you and your colleagues do, and wonder if others before me have raised this concern.

Yours truly,
James Lieberman

Jan. 13, 1997
Dear Dr. Lieberman:

Thank you for your support. Regarding John Reed not answering your letter of last October, this is a common thing.

Of course, it is a difficult letter to answer but the president or the chairman has to be capable to take care of all situations. As to the matter of the intent of your letter about him and other directors being on boards of tobacco companies and also the question of selling the shares, some companies like American Brands have divested themselves of the tobacco division. Some others, like the ones you mention, are also in the food business and pressure is on the company managements to spin off the food division to the shareholders. Of course, being bankers like John Reed, these tobacco institutions have millions of dollars of bank accounts, plus pension funds in which the banks receive income on your behalf.

Of course, the important thing here is that letters should be answered even though you may not agree with the intent. I shall, of course, mention about answering letters at the stockholders meeting.

Many thanks again for your support and your note. I am enclosing some recent clippings for your enjoyment.

Sincerely,
John J. Gilbert

March 14, 1997
Dear Dr. Lieberman:

Mr. Reed asked me to respond because the press on occasion raises the same issues and I have represented his belief that individuals have the right to pursue actions that are not illegal even though they may be deemed dangerous.

He does recognize that people of good will and sound mind can come to a different position, and he understands your deep feelings on the subject.

We appreciate your taking the time to express your concerns.

Sincerely,
John M. Morris
Director, Media Relations
Corporate Affairs

Paul A. Marks, M.D.
President
Memorial Sloan-Kettering Cancer Center

November 18, 1997
Dear Dr. Marks:

I am in receipt of your fund-raising letter of October 20, and appreciate the good work MSKCC is doing and has done over many years.

It has also come to my attention that at least one trustee of MSKCC, John S. Reed, is a director of Philip Morris, one of the major tobacco companies. Cigarettes are known to be a leading cause of lung cancer, the all-too-prevalent malignancy that you mention first in your letter.

While it is clear that cancer treatment rather than prevention is the focus of your efforts, Mr. Reed's presence in a leadership position with MSKCC leaves me—and others I have informed—breathless with astonishment.

I am sure you can understand that, until this matter is addressed satisfactorily, I and others like me will find it impossible to contribute to your program.

Yours truly,
James Lieberman

Department of Health and Human Services
National Institutes of Health

March 26, 1998
Paul A. Marks, M.D.
President
Memorial Sloan-Kettering Cancer Center

Dear Dr. Marks:

I am enclosing a communication received from E. James Lieberman, M.D., of The Family Institute. He has suggested there is an appearance of conflict of interest created by the joint appointments of John Reed as Trustee for Memorial Sloan Kettering and as Director for Philip Morris. Not only has he raised this issue with the National Cancer Institute (NCI), he has directed his comments to *U.S. News and World Report*.

As you know Public Health Grants Policy requires that all grantee institutions have in place a process for resolving conflict of interest. This process must be applied to members of governing bodies of an institution as well as to investigators. Given the visibility of tobacco as an issue for the American public, I would urge you to formally submit John Reed's appointment as Trustee to your institutional conflict of interest review process.

Sincerely,
Maureen O. Wilson, Ph.D.
Deputy Ethics Counselor
National Cancer Institute
cc: E. James Lieberman

Date: Fri, 24 Oct 1997
From: Jack Morris, jack.morris@citicorp.com
To: "E. James Lieberman," ejl@gwis2.circ.gwu.edu
Subject: Re: John Reed

Dr. E. James Lieberman wrote:
When I tell friends that Mr. Reed is on the board of a tobacco company and a trustee of MSKCC, which prides itself on being the leading cancer treatment center in America, they are shocked. How do you reconcile the matter? Do you see any problem in promoting cancer and trying to cure it at the same time?

Date: Thu, 18 September 1997
From: Jack Morris
To: E. James Lieberman
Subject: Re: John Reed

Dear Dr. Lieberman:
I have nothing to offer you that will satisfy you. John Reed is comfortable in the roles that you find difficult to comprehend. I suspect that you also may take actions and hold convictions that others might feel are at odds. But at any rate, we understand your feelings and ask only that you agree to disagree with Mr. Reed.

Sincerely,
Jack Morris

The American Cancer Society: The World's Wealthiest "Nonprofit" Institution

The American Cancer Society is fixated on damage control—diagnosis and treatment—with indifference or even hostility to cancer prevention. This myopic mindset is compounded by the interlocking conflicts of interest with the cancer drug, mammography, and other industries. The "nonprofit" status of the Society is in sharp conflict with its high overhead and expenses, excessive reserves of assets, and contributions to political parties.

In 1992, the American Cancer Society Foundation was created to allow the ACS to actively solicit contributions of more than $100,000. A close look at the heavy-hitters on the Foundation's board will give an idea of which interests are at play and where the Foundation expects its big contributions to come from. Among them:

➤David R. Bethune, president of Lederle Laboratories, a division of American Cyanamid, which makes chemical fertilizers and herbicides while transforming itself into a full-fledged pharmaceutical company. In 1988, the company introduced Novatrone, an anti-cancer drug.

➤Gordon Binder, CEO of Amgen, the world's foremost biotechnology company, whose success rests almost exlusively on one product, Neupogen, which is administered to chemotherapy patients to stimulate their production of white blood cells.

➤Diane Disney Miller, daughter of the conservative multimillionaire Walt Disney, who died of lung cancer in 1966.

➤George Dessert, famous for his former role as censor on the subject of "family values" during the 1970s and 1980s as CEO of CBS.

➤Alan Gevertzen, chairman of the board at Boeing.

➤Sumner M. Redstone, chairman of the board, at Viacom.

The results of this board's efforts have been a million here, a million there—much of it coming from the very industries instrumental in shaping American Cancer Society policy, or profiting from it.

Of the members of the society's board, about half are clinicians, oncologists, surgeons, radiologists, and basic molecular scientists. The society has close connections to the mammography industry. Promotions of the society continue to lure women of all ages into mammography centers, leading them to believe that mammography is their best hope against breast cancer. These promotions expose premenopausal women to radiation hazards from mammography with little or no evidence of benefits.

Conspicuously absent from the society's National Breast Cancer Awareness month activities every year is any information on environmental and other avoidable causes of breast cancer. This is no accident. Zeneca Pharmaceuticals —the sole manufacturer of tamoxifen, the world's top-selling anticancer and breast cancer "prevention" drug—has been the sole multimillion-dollar funder of National Breast Cancer Awareness Month since its inception in 1984. Imperial Chemical Industries, Zeneca's parent company, manufactures industrial chemicals incriminated as causes of breast cancer. Zeneca profits from treatment of breast cancer, and hopes to profit more from large-scale use of tamoxifen for prevention.

The intimate association between the American Cancer Society and the cancer drug industry is further illustrated by the unbridled aggression that it has directed at potential competitors. Just as Senator Joseph McCarthy had his "blacklist" of suspected communists, the Society maintains a "Committee on Unproven Methods of Cancer Management," which periodically "reviews" unorthodox or alternative therapies. The Committee is comprised of carefully selected proponents of orthodox, expensive, and usually toxic drugs, who naturally oppose cheap, nonpatentable, and minimally toxic alternatives. The committee's statements on "unproven" methods are widely disseminated. Once a clinician becomes associated with "unproven methods," he or she is blackballed by the cancer establishment and funding becomes inaccessible.

HOW TO EVALUATE HEALTH INFORMATION ON THE INTERNET

The Internet is a huge and unwieldy repository of information. With more than 10,000 web sites offering a wide range of health information, how can consumers be assured of the quality and the context of health information in order to make critical, life-changing decisions? Some questions to assess the content of web sites:

➤Who operates the web site? The suffix on the end of the web address provides a big clue: ".edu"—an educational institution; ".com"—a commercial firm; ".gov"—a government site; or ".org"—an organization that is usually non-profit. A reliable site should list a postal address, an e-mail address, and a phone number.

➤Is the site operated by an organization or group that you have heard of? Do you know how careful the group is about the quality of information it distributes? This affects the credibility of the site. If you haven't heard of the group before, it doesn't mean the information is not reliable but you should try to corroborate the information through additional sources.

➤Are there advertisements on the web site? Some organizations and companies permit advertising by "sponsors" and this may affect the content of the information on the web site. Organizations may not present all the pros and cons of health issues or treatments if it might undercut a sponsor.

➤Who wrote the information? Make sure the name of the author, the date it was published or posted, and the credentials and affiliations of the author are listed, and that the research (if mentioned) is cited fully so you can find it.

➤Is the information presented on more than one site? Does the web site present one aspect of a particular problem or issue? Does the author have a limited point of view? Are there testimonials? If the answer is yes, consider other sites that present different points of view for balance. Do not rely upon only one source. Make sure the information can be corroborated on other web sites.

➤How much information should you provide about your condition? The Internet is a transparent way to exchange information between different people whom you do not know. Be cautious about providing personal information over the Net, unless you are clear how that information will be used and interpreted.

➤A healthy dose of skepticism is appropriate! Focus on the quality and the context of web site information. Stay alert to how web sites filter information based upon particular points of view of the organization, or the authors, or the funders. For example, if a non-profit organization's web site is funded by a pharmaceutical company, the information provided on that site may not be critical of the products made by this company. It is imperative to be careful! Educated consumers can access a wealth of information on the Internet—but need to assess the quality and context of web sites and make health care decisions in consultation with professionals and other trusted individuals.

Chapter 72

Gender Medicine

*"It seemed as if the Almighty, in creating the female sex,
had taken the uterus and built up a woman around it."*

*—Professor M. L. Holbrook, 1870
Address to a medical society*

Research into gender medicine seems inevitble. What took it so long? Yet even today, many people have difficulty understanding exactly what it's about. We are pleased to bring you three lucid pieces: from Betty Rothbart in Hadassah; Dianne Hales *author of* Just Like a Woman: How Gender Science is Revealing What Makes Us Female, *here interviewed by Tania Ketenjian; and Charles Mann in* Science *magazine.*

The question remains: Outside of our female organs, why didn't *doctors want to study us—until feminists got the power to force the issue? The answer appears to be that at first they* weren't ready, *and then for a long time, we* weren't.

From the mid-19th century through today, organized medicine has been deeply concerned with its image building—getting and holding power, keeping all alternative practitioners—midwives included—at bay, restricting the number of women doctors to a tiny percent. Organized medicine, as Barbara Ehrenreich and Deirdre English have well demonstrated, was no less than in the service of perpetuating myths of female weakness and inferiority. *What if they performed research and found out they were wrong?*

By the end of World War I the ruling male physicians had succeeded in closing most of the women's medical schools, and getting midwifery banned in many states.

When the second wave of feminism arrived in the 1960s, there were few women in medical research, almost none in positions of power; it was tacitly understood that research on sex differences was premature, and could be used against us, struggling, as we were, to establish our fitness for equal opportunity. It would take another twenty years until we were secure enough to acknowledge, and risk determining the underlying differences in men's and women's bodies that will allow us to more accurately tailor medical and surgical treatments by gender, presumably to the benefit of everyone's health.—B. S.

Venus and the Doctor

BETTY ROTHBART

Betty Rothbart, "Venus and the Doctor," *Hadassah*, June/July 1999. Reprinted by permission.

> I attribute much of our modern tension
> To a misguided striving for intersexual comprehension.
> It's about time to realize, brethren, as best we can,
> That a woman is not just a female man.
> —Ogden Nash

At the dawn of the twenty-first century, medical researchers at last are realizing that woman is indeed not just a female man. The new discipline of gender-specific medicine is the most compelling trend in women's health, as researchers discover a startling array of sex-linked differences in how men and women respond to disease. As society moves steadily toward an ever more enlightened era of equal opportunity in jobs, paychecks and dishwashing duties, the medical community is reminding us that physiologically, equal doesn't mean "the same."

Recent research indicates that women's and men's brains function differently and their feet aren't the same, either; to help women avoid stress on their joints, shoemakers need to rethink women's footwear design. From saliva-flow rates (men's are twice as fast) to motility of food through the digestive tract (three times slower in women) to bone breakdown and buildup (different patterns in men and women) to the behavior of liver cells in tissue culture (different metabolism and responses to medications), the list goes on and on. But the bottom line is the same: "The hormonal influence is more profound than we'd ever thought," says Marianne J. Legato, M.D., director of the Partnership for Women's Health at Columbia University and member of Hadassah's Health Advisory Council.

Why has it taken so long for researchers to address gender differences? Vivian W. Pinn, M.D., director of the Office of Research on Women's Health, National Institutes of Health, cites several reasons:

➤*A unisex mindset.* Researchers believed that any findings about men automatically applied to women, too. This approach has a certain efficient appeal, but it just doesn't work.

➤*Women's distracting baggage.* Researchers regarded women's hormones as mischief-makers that interfered with the purity of data. Take the menstrual cycle, for example. Women's monthly fluctuations are a virtual symphony of rhythmic hormonal play. Instead of taking estrogen's peaks and valleys into account, researchers exasperatedly referred to women's cycles as confounders. Men, in other words, were easy; women were confusing.

➤*Potential complications of pregnancy and childbearing.* Medical disasters such as thalidomide-linked birth defects and the increased incidence of clear-cell carcinomas in the uteri of daughters of women who had taken DES during pregnancy were among the events that led to the establishment in the 1970s of the National Institutes of Health Office of Protection from Research Risk.

WOMEN AS NO-SHOWS

Researchers complained that even when they wanted to include women, they were harder to recruit and retain. Men seemed to have fewer problems with transportation and scheduling; they were more likely to drive and less likely to have family obligations that interfered with their ability to keep appointments.

CHANGING COURSE

By the 1980s many grassroots views of women's health activists had moved into the mainstream. In mid-decade, an NIH task force urged a stronger government focus on women's health, and the NIH enacted a policy recommending inclusion of women in clinical studies it funded. However, a General Accounting Office study in 1990 revealed that researchers often ignored the policy and that compliance could not be ascertained since there was no system in place for documenting how many women participated in studies.

In 1993 Congress passed the NIH Revitalization Act, which mandated inclusion of women and minorities in National Institute of Health-funded studies of conditions that affect both women and men. Dr. Pinn points out that women often didn't participate because they didn't know about the studies and their doctors didn't refer them. The ever-growing popularity of the Internet has alerted more women to clinical trials and led to numerous self-referrals. Researchers also are incorporating more "women-sensitive factors," such as providing or supporting child care and transportation, and establishing support groups that keep women involved and interested. Epidemics of AIDS and breast cancer have given rise to a vigorous advocacy, which has made people more aware of the advantages of participating in clinical trials.

LOOKING AHEAD

Fine-tuning for females. It used to be thought that adapting a drug for women simply meant administering a smaller dose. It is more complicated than that. More research is needed in pharmacokinetics and pharmacodynamics: how the body handles drugs, how drugs affect the body, and how drugs interact with each other. Researchers are also studying the effects of estrogen and administration of a drug at different points in a woman's monthly cycle.

STREAMLINING WOMEN'S HEALTH CARE

For years women have been frustrated by a fragmented approach to health care, cluttering their calendars with appointments with different doctors for reproductive, general, and mental health.

"When a woman goes to a doctor she wants to be seen as a total person," says Dr. Pinn. "A postmenopausal woman may think she doesn't need a pelvic exam or a Pap smear. An internist may assume she gets a Pap smear from her gynecologist. Or she may not go to a doctor at all, although with women more in tune with screening exams and wellness care, that is not as much the case any more. It is important that doctors recognize how important it is to do comprehensive exams. Most women don't have the luxury of seeing a specialist for everything."

Women's health advocates have helped drive health-care professionals toward a new awareness of women's needs as medical consumers. Primary care ob/gyn is a new specialty that acknowledges women's needs for one-stop shopping. The best doctors, says Dr. Pinn, "not only understand the importance of their practices to the lives and health of women, but the importance of women to their practices. Women play a major role in deciding on health care for their families."

FILLING IN THE GAPS

Of course, research must continue in heart disease, cancer, autoimmune disorders, and other areas that have gotten closer to their fair due in recent years. But many other areas remain woefully underexplored. Among those on Dr. Pinn's wish list are better understanding of endometriosis and fibroids, which contribute to the need for hysterectomies; exploration of sex-linked differences in gastrointestinal disorders, e.g., how hormones affect irritable bowel syndrome; better ways to detect ovarian and other cancers early.

Dr. Pinn is especially excited about the testing of a vaccine to prevent transmission of human papilloma virus, a sexually transmitted disease that increases a woman's risk of cervical cancer. She urges support of urogynecological research into key areas such as pelvic-floor disorders, including pelvic prolapse and its relationship to childbirth, exercise, obesity, and sexual dysfunction. Urinary and fecal incontinence also deserve more attention; for many women they make the difference between independent living or a nursing home.

TO A LONG LIFE

Now that the value, indeed the necessity, of including women in research is established, researchers are also reaffirming the importance of examining health issues within the context of the full life span, from the prenatal intrauterine environment, infancy, and childhood, through the teen years, the reproductive years, peri- and postmenopause, the elderly, and the frail elderly.

"With longer life expectancy,"says Dr. Pinn, "we must pay attention to women's health beyond the reproductive system. As women speak up to ask for information on preventing disease and improving the quality of life, they spur the medical community to come up with the answers."

Diane Hales

INTERVIEW BY TANIA KETENJIAN

Dianne Hales, Ph.D. is a journalist and the author of *Just Like A Woman: How Gender Science is Redefining What Makes Us Female.* This interview was conducted in April 1999.

TK: What have you observed about the acceptance of gender medicine?

DH: Like all new ideas, it captivates the imagination of some and is just dismissed by the inertia of others. Medicine is a very established, slow-moving science; there is a sense that everything has to be tested, everything has to be tried. That's the initial reaction. The intuitive response to gender medicine on the part of women in and out of science was: "This makes sense; we are different and we need to change the model to include our gender." In established medicine there was a sense of "Wait a second; women live longer than men, they've made tremendous gains in the last century; we must be doing something right. What is the added value of finding out more about women when male-based medicine seems to be good enough?" When some scientists started working on gender-specific medicine, their discoveries turned out to be so intriguing that it created contagious enthusiasm. When medical schools incorporate this into their curriculum, it will affect the new generation of researchers and doctors. Acceptance was slow to start but is accelerating rapidly.

TK: Does the lack of awareness or acceptance of gender medicine affect the care that patients receive or play a role in perpetuating diseases or ailments?
DH: It definitely plays a role, most dramatically with heart attacks. Heart attacks were basically seen as a male problem, which rallied attention because so many men were being killed in their prime by heart attacks. A decade ago, a talk on the female heart would draw one or two men and just a few women. Now you can't get into these sessions. Ultimately, heart disease is a number one killer for both sexes. Women develop heart disease a decade later, but when they get it, it's deadlier. More women die of heart attacks than men.

Heart attack is a different phenomenon in a woman, so women have called the emergency room or their doctors or a nurse and said, "I feel weak," or, "I feel flushed; I feel like something is really wrong." And they would be told to lie down and just check in the next day. Those symptoms are more characteristic of a female heart attack than the kind of elephant-on-the-chest pain that we know from the male model. This is a very dramatic example of how the lack of knowledge about gender difference has proven to be truly hazardous to health. A study that came out last year showed that women get to the hospital after a heart attack about an hour later than men. That delay results from their not understanding what is happening; the message is still not getting out. Once they get to the hospital, they get less aggressive treatment. Often, because doctors are assuming that the woman is not having a heart attack, they don't go into full battle mode and bring out the big guns to do whatever is needed to treat a heart attack. The response is just not the same for women as it is for men.

TK: What are some other key applications of gender medicine?

DH: There is a phenomenon now called "premenstrual exacerbation" that attributes everything that goes wrong with a woman in the week before her period to premenstrual syndrome. PMS is a charged term and is rather poorly understood. Through gender medicine, it was found that unisex diseases, like asthma and diabetes, actually have fluctuations in women that have to do with their menstrual cycles. The realization has been that perhaps women are not complaining because of PMS, but that their chronic medical conditions change with their cycles.

I think we are also going to see changes in diagnosis. Certainly with heart disease the gold standard has been the stress test, but that does not work as well with women. We must go back and look at everything. The cholesterol norms are different for women, the HDL/LDL—the measurements of HDL, LDL, and blood triglycerides are all lipids, they are all blood fats and they all play a role in very different ways in risk for coronary artery disease. All of these indications have to be gender-specific. Men develop more cancers and die more of cancer. There is a theory that, particularly in cancers that tend to metastasize, like melanoma, we can learn by studying gender differences that might lead to different treatment approaches. The potential is there across the board.

TK: Can you tell me about the 16-year ban of women from Food and Drug Administration testing? What was the reason for it and what were the consequences?

DH: The reasons for the ban were protective. It wasn't as if a group of guys in suits sat down and said, "We'll show these women; we're not going to put them in our studies." The thalidomide fear horrified everyone. Women who had been taking what they thought was an innocuous sleeping pill ended up having babies with truly terrible deformities. The idea was that the best way to protect women and their offspring would be to make sure that they were not given drugs that had not been thoroughly tested. As a result, however, researchers were just testing men; and testing was supposed to exclude women of reproductive age; that got expanded to include all women. It reached the point that, since human females were being left out, females of all species were excluded from studies. Funding began to go along with this, going more toward the diseases in which men were being studied. It kept perpetuating itself the way these things do, and it wasn't until the 1980s that everyone became aware of what a huge discrepancy there was in research on the genders and took steps to correct it. It was more than an oversight—a good intention run amok.

TK: What are some of the gender-biased methods of cure? For instance, in your book you mention the overprescription of Valium..

DH: Throughout history, women's wombs have been blamed for everything, any sort of insanity, almost anything that could go wrong. The assumption was that it must be that old rebel, the wandering uterus. Even though scientific observation that the uterus didn't move challenged that notion, the idea still remained that a woman's reproductive organs were capable of wreaking all sorts of havoc in her body and needed to be controlled, removed, or whatever. So, even earlier in this century in the 1920s there were medical school deans arguing that women couldn't study medicine because of their cycle. You can't have a woman menstruate and matriculate at the same time. That bias is very old, and we still see it in modern guises. PMS is an example of, "Oh, it must be her cycle that is making her depressed, or anxious, or moody." One of the treatments for PMS has been removal of the ovaries and shutting down the whole system. I think we're getting better about that, but we still don't really understand how the reproductive and central nervous systems really interact and why it is that antidepressants are an ineffectual treatment for PMS. The bias is old and the connections are far more complex than anyone had realized.

As for cures that are gender-specific for men, some of them have to do with blood pressure and the fact that the drugs that can help cardiac arrhythmia in a man can be fatal in a woman. There are some new heart medications that are actually more effective in women than men. A number of psychiatric drugs—Welbutrin is one of them—carry a risk of seizure, which is much more likely to happen in women, and even more likely in women who have eating disorders. That's the sort of instance where it's not a difference between good enough and excellent care, but the difference between good care and the wrong medicine for the wrong gender.

TK: Do you think that women didn't stand up and fight against this earlier because they were scared that discoveries might be used against them? Why do you think that they didn't say, "Wait a minute, we need to be paid attention to?"

DH: Women for the first time dealt with political realities in the 1970s. Before that, they weren't taken seriously, and the doctor's office was really no exception. But as women became more powerful and joined together to fight for political gains, we didn't want anybody telling us that we were different from men. In the 1970s, our idea of liberation was tied in with being just like men: we drank like men, we smoked like men, we (some of us) had the same kind of casual sexual relationships that men did. On the one hand, we had *Our Bodies, Ourselves,* and we were thrilled to get this recognition for our distinctive reproductive means, but we didn't push the issue. We didn't want people to come along and say, "You're different, so therefore you can't become a police officer, you can't become an astronaut." We were still scared that people would say "You can't menstruate and matriculate at the same time." We didn't know what science would find, and we had enough justification to think that it might not be good news.

TK: Turning to issues from your book, why is the liver "the sexiest organ in the body"?

DH: Even before birth, the quantity of sex hormones the liver is exposed to affects its development. A liver that is inside a male fetus develops in such a way that, throughout life, it is going to metabolize substances, including drugs and alcohol, in a way different than a liver that takes form in a female body. The liver breaks things down differently in men and than in women. Metabolic differences mean that a woman can end up a lot more drunk than a man, in part because of the liver, in part because she lacks some other enzymes in her intestinal tract.

TK: How does the bias of gender-specific medicine manifest in medical school?

DH: Biases against women in medical school come out in many forms. There's still just your plain old sexual harassment, but it also comes out in the lectures that traditionally defined "male" as "normal." Somebody might be talking about the female brain or heart but always there's the sense that the male heart and liver and everything else represent the norm. That is the kind of subliminal message that will be eliminated with gender-specific science being taught in medical schools.

A lot of women have had the same experience of going to a doctor and describing something kind of vague and being told, "It's all in your head." Basically, the woman patient didn't fit the male model. I think that's how the bias comes out.

TK: What are some of the ways that this research can become more prevalent and widely accepted?

DH: We need to find out what is known about gender differences and what is being done both in the Office of Women's Health and the Partnership for

Women's Health at Columbia University. We are doing basic literature searches in the databases such as the NIH's, Medline, and basically on-line computerized archives of all the medical literature, because a lot of times, even when women were included in a sample, the data wasn't broken down according to gender, and sometimes it's impossible to do a re-analysis and pinpoint the holes. For example, that search has been done with osteoporosis, and learning what's different about bone growth and development of bone deterioration in men may help us understand why these problems are so much more common in women. Another area for this re-analysis is nutrition. Obsessed as we are with diet and weight, women, even more so than men, become very intrigued by all these phyto-chemicals. I think women feel that they are more in the food-providing role in the house and yet they really don't know if men and women should be taking the same vitamins, the same supplements. Aspirin, for instance, does not protect both sexes against heart disease; it only protects men against stroke. It doesn't seem to have any effect on a woman's vulnerability to stroke. So I think all of these areas can be tested.

We need to have women included in trials, which is happening We need to ensure that products aren't just tested for safety or effectiveness for both sexes, but that products will actually be developed taking into account what we know about metabolism and disease processes. Treatments should be developed that are gender-specific. In ten years, there may well be gender-specific centers where a man and a woman with the same symptoms will go in with the same conditions—like diabetes or digestive ailments—and receive not off-the-wall different treatments, but treatments with precise and different approaches for both sexes.

TK: Do you think that women's health should be an area of specialization?

DH: No, actually I think there should be a specialty of gender-specific medicine. Everyone should be exposed and taught that health comes in male and female varieties. I worry about a designation of just women's health in that it will be about the bikini parts—the breasts and pelvis—and ignore all the other parts of the body. That is my concern: that a specialty of women's health would have too narrow a focus, and not be head to toe.

Women's Health Research Blossoms

CHARLES MANN

Excerpt by Charles Mann, from "Women's Health Research Blossoms," *Science magazine,* August 11, 1995. Excerpted with permission from Charles Mann and *Science* magazine. Copyright ©1995 American Academy for the Advancement of Science.

In 1957, journalist Barbara Seaman, in the hospital after the birth of her first child, asked what was in the pills they were feeding her. Medical personnel dismissed her questions. Only after her baby became very sick did she discover that the pills were laxatives, which she was inadvertently passing on to the child through her breast milk. The laxatives, she says, had been administered in the blithe assumption that no modern mother would choose breast feeding over formula.

Seaman's outrage over the laxatives led her to a crusade as medical muckraker that would eventually put her in the forefront of the women's health movement. By the early 1960s—soon after the drug company G. D. Searle began marketing Enovid, the first oral contraceptive—she was a health columnist for magazines such as *Brides* and *Ladies' Home Journal*. When readers deluged Seaman with questions about birth control pills, she began an investigation that culminated in *The Doctors' Case Against the Pill*, a 1969 exposé claiming that the Pill caused fatal strokes, heart disease, diabetes, depression, and a host of other ailments. The ensuing controversy cost Seaman her magazine jobs. But it also led then-Senator Gaylord Nelson to hold hearings on Pill safety in 1970.

Even as the hearings bared the Pill's defects, the dissent helped to launch a political movement focusing on women's health. "By 1975, nearly 2,000 [women's self-help medical] projects were scattered across the United States, many of them groups of volunteers without an institution," says Cynthia Pearson, program director of the National Women's Health Network, an advocacy clearinghouse founded by Seaman, [Alice] Wolfson, and three other women activists that year. The projects showed women how to examine their own breasts, cervixes, and vaginas for problems. Controversially, some promoted the Del-Em, a homemade device that let women perform abortions on themselves.

Although the movement centered on women, Pearson says, its targets—overuse of medical technology, insufficiently rigorous drug testing, and the refusal to listen to patients—affected both sexes. As today's clinicians and researchers readily concede, this nascent movement helped change medicine and medical research profoundly. A quarter century after *The Doctors' Case*, almost half of all U.S. medical students are female, universities have established programs in women's diseases, and governments across the world have created offices of women's health.

But as the women's health movement has expanded, it has divided into two diverse strains. In the industrialized world, women have changed their focus; they are less likely to criticize the attitudes of clinicians and more likely to argue that the male medical research hierarchy has historically mistreated them. Activists charge that scientists have neglected to include women in epidemiological studies and clinical trials, arguing that researchers mistakenly assumed that data from middle-aged white males apply equally well to women, minorities, and the elderly. And, feminists complain, while researchers have failed to fund research on women's diseases—breast cancer being the most notorious example—they have worked overtime on female contraception, neglecting comparable research on men. Partly because of these accusations, the new field of gender-based medicine has come into existence, concentrating on the fundamental differences in male and female responses to disease and treatment.

In the developing world, though, the concerns are different. Women in poor nations die at high rates from reproductive problems and diseases that can easily be cured or prevented, often at little additional cost. In some areas, rates of maternal mortality and morbidity are increased by cultural attitudes that block women's access to health services, especially if those services include abortion; in others, the problem has been exacerbated by the organizational failures of centralized economies. And, in the view of health professionals, some health-care promotion programs by industrialized nations have focused so intently on Third World children that they have ignored—or even added to—the problems of their mothers.

HAS MEDICAL RESEARCH NEGLECTED WOMEN?

"God knows male doctors have been rude and patronizing to women, but the idea that they have ignored them is ridiculous," scoffs one breast cancer specialist who requests anonymity. Nonetheless, advocates for women's health, many in high positions, often claim exactly that—with their greatest ire being reserved for inequalities in medical research. "When it comes to women's health, we are still playing catch-up," First Lady Hillary Rodham Clinton said on June 27, 1995, at the Women's Health Achievement Awards ceremony in Washington, D.C. "Illnesses that traditionally affect women have been ignored and still are ignored. Research has largely focused on men, and it still does," Indeed, the National Institutes of Health (NIH) admitted in a 1987 report that it had spent only 13.5 percent of its total research budget that year on diseases unique to women.

Clinical trials are a primary example of the neglect of women in medical research, according to Phyllis Greenberger, executive director of the Society for the Advancement of Women's Health Research. "All too often," she says, "no women have been included—look at MR FIT [the Multiple Risk Factor Intervention Trial] and the Physicians' Health Study." MR FIT examined the impact of losing weight, giving up cigarettes, and lowering cholesterol levels on the risk of heart attack in 12,866 men, whereas the Physicians' Health Study examined the effects of daily aspirin intake on the same risk in 22,071 men; neither experiment included a single woman.

But some experts point out that the same NIH inventory that established that 13.5 percent of its research budget was spent on female diseases found that only 6.5 percent of that budget went to diseases unique to men. On a per-fatality basis, more than four times as much research money is spent on the leading female-only cancer, breast cancer, as the leading male-only cancer, prostate cancer, according to data from the National Cancer Institute.

More men have been included in heart-disease trials than women, "but the criticisms are taken really out of context," says Maureen Henderson, head of cancer prevention research at the Fred Hutchinson Cancer Research Center in Seattle and one of the original principal investigators of MR FIT. In the 1960s and 1970s, she says, "heart disease was a national problem in middle-aged men, and MR FIT was an attempt to modify their risk factors to change the rate of heart attack in them. There's nothing to apologize for." In addition, according to [Curtis L.] Meinert [of the Johns Hopkins Center for Clinical Trials], heart attacks in middle-aged women are so rare that a female-only study with the same statistical power as MR FIT would have cost more than a billion dollars—almost 10 times the original trial's $115 million budget.

Similar logic applies to the Physicians' Health Study, in the view of its co-principal investigator, Julie Buring of Brigham and Women's Hospital in Boston. "We knew it would take 20,000 people to answer the question" of whether daily aspirin intake prevents heart attack, she says. Because the researchers wanted to conduct the trial by mail rather than through hospital visits—a far cheaper, although then-untested method—they decided to enlist doctors, an easily reached group of people who should be able to take pills every day without supervision. Unfortunately, Buring says, there were not enough middle-aged U.S. female physicians in 1982, when the trial began, to make their inclusion feasible.

In 1992, the Women's Health Study began, with Buring as principal investigator. Like the Physician's Health Study, it will examine the effects of aspirin on heart attack; it has now enrolled 38,000 female health-care professionals, doctors, nurses, dentists, and veterinarians among them. Preliminary results will not be available for a number of years; the exact length of time, according to Buring, depends on funding.

Pathologist Vivian Pinn, director of the NIH Office of Women's Health, says that, "Although it is true we can't document [bias], it is also true that as we focus more on gender issues we learn that there are a lot of conditions that affect men and women differently and that we should learn more about." From Pinn's point of view, it makes little difference whether bcollusion caused the lack of knowledge about the medical differences between men and women. "Whatever the cause," she says, "we don't know enough."

GENDER-BASED RESEARCH

Pinn's claim that "we don't know enough" is echoed by the medical establishment. Spurred partly by criticisms of past research practices, medical researchers are now aggressively examining medical differences between the sexes. Much research has focused on female hormones, which have wide-ranging effects that scientists are just beginning to unravel. Indeed, many researchers focusing on women's health find it difficult to believe that scientists have so long failed to appreciate the enormous medical implications of the sexes' diverse hormonal environments.

Roughly speaking, the explosion of new research is divided between studies examining the impact of endogenous hormones (those made by the body) on medical treatments and those examining the impact of exogenous hormones (those from outside sources, especially birth-control pills and menopause treatments) on diseases. Psychiatrist Margaret Jensvold, director of the Institute for Research in Women's Health in Washington, D.C., published one of the first studies of the cycle's impact on psychoactive drugs like anti-depressants. For many women, she discovered, a constant blood level of these drugs can only be achieved by varying the drug dose through the monthly estrogen-progesterone cycle. Unfortunately, she says, "many studies in the past didn't report data in a way that allowed us to make female-male comparisons."

Equally important—but more controversial—are exogenous hormones, especially estrogen replacement therapy, the widespread practice of administering estrogen supplements to relieve the symptoms of menopause. Even as many as a quarter of all postmenopausal women in industrialized nations take estrogen supplements, researchers are scrambling to understand their effects on those women. By means that are still poorly understood, menopausal estrogen loss apparently increases the risk of colon cancer, decreases the collagen that keeps skin moist and pliable, and worsens the ratio of high-to low-density lipoproteins ("good" and "bad" cholesterol). All these effects are apparently controlled by estrogen therapy. Yet it may also be that—as Seaman argued long ago in *Women and the Crisis in Sex Hormones* (1975)—"the estrogenizing of American women is a major factor in our rising rates of female cancers," especially endometrial cancer, breast cancer, and, possibly, ovarian and uterine cancer. The conflicting possibilities, Pearson says, men that women confront "an exceedingly complicated and unclear choice."

A good illustration of the complex scientific and social issues surrounding exogenous hormones is osteoporosis, the progressive loss of protein from bone, which causes bones to weaken and fracture easily. The problem arises much faster in women than in men—for reasons that remain unclear but that seem related to hormones. Nearly half of all women eventually develop osteoporosis; compared to men of the same ages, postmenopausal women are twice as likely to fracture their hips. In 10 percent to 20 percent of hip injuries, death follows within a year. According to a 1994 estimate by the Mayo Clinic, about 9.4 million postmenopausal white women in the United States have osteoporosis, making it a major public health problem.

Nonetheless, osteoporosis was not a hot research topic until recently, according to Joan M. Lappe of the Creighton University Osteoporosis Research Center in Omaha, Nebraska. The field began to open up in the 1980s as researchers gathered what Lappe calls "solid data" that estrogen replacement therapy forestalls bone loss. When these data came in, many women rushed to estrogen replacement therapy. Others, though, held back, as evidence gathered that the treatment apparently promotes breast cancer. In June, the estrogen-breast cancer link was supported by a major trial published in the *New England Journal of Medicine*. But the connection is not entirely clear; last month another big trial found no link. Meanwhile, other studies indicate that the risk of osteoporosis can be reduced by frequent exercise, proper diet, and the cessation of smoking.

Some answers may be provided by the 15-year, $650 million Women's Health Initiative, the largest clinical trial ever attempted. The trial will include 63,000 postmenopausal women and will test the impact of low-fat diets, estrogen, calcium, and vitamin D on the incidence of breast cancer, osteoporosis-induced hip fractures, and cardiovascular disease. In the estrogen wing of the trial, 27,500 women will be randomly assigned to hormone replacement therapy or placebo and followed for 8 years; initial results are expected in 2005.

POVERTY PRESENTS DIFFERENT PROBLEMS

Unlike the hormonal questions that vex women's health researchers in wealthy societies, what might be called "risks of motherhood" are the primary concerns of women in poor countries. Whereas the leading cause of death for First World women in their prime is breast cancer, the leading cause of death for their compatriots in the Third World is complications from pregnancy. Indeed, according to World Health Organization (WHO) figures, 99 percent of the women who die annually from the complications of pregnancy or childbirth live in the developing world.

Unfortunately, the WHO Safe Motherhood Initiative—a campaign launched in 1987 at an international conference in Nairobi, Kenya, to halve maternal mortality by the year 2000—has not reached its goal. Indeed, according to Carla Abou-Zahr of the maternal and child health division at WHO headquarters in Geneva, maternal mortality is actually rising in some parts of the world, like Francophone West Africa and the states carved from the former Soviet Union.

The reasons for the failure include a focus on prenatal rather than obstetric care, opposing cultural and political norms, and contrary government policies. But above all, the failure may stem from a lack of funding. The Safe Motherhood program received less than 0.1 percent of all health and population aid in 1990. That year, population-control and prenatal-care programs received 19 percent and 13 percent of that aid, respectively.

Even if better funded, better targeted programs existed, mothers would still face significant economic and political barriers. For example, many African governments had medical systems that provided free care. But the resulting quality of service, in Abou-Zahr's estimation, was "abysmal." Hospitals and clinics were frequently understaffed, without adequate supplies of drugs, or closed for much of the day. In recent years, African nations have begun to charge fees, the money from which helps to ensure funding for health-care facilities. The result, according to Patricio Rojas, a WHO representative in Maseru, Lesotho, has been improved health care for many. But it has also led to "a 10 to 20 percent decrease in consultations" for the very poorest. "And those are the ones who need more care," he says, "because they are most likely to eat less and live in poor conditions."

More important than economic barriers are social ones. According to Ann Way of Demographic and Health Surveys, a private research agency in Calverton, Maryland, "Women need to get permission from men in certain societies to seek health care. Generally, if a woman does not have free access to household funds, she will not have free access to health care." In Lesotho, for example, the majority of employed men work outside the country, in South Africa. Living alone, their wives face social barriers to leaving the house. "Women are effectively like minors in this country," Rojas says. "The constitution grants them equal rights, but comparing that to what they can do in real terms is night and day."

"There are lots of things that can be done," says Angel Kamara, deputy director of [a Columbia University–run] maternals mortality program, based in Accra, Ghana. "Yes, communities have various cultural quirks," Kamara concedes. "But the major deterrent was that even people in the most remote villages knew that even if they got to the facilities, drugs might not be available or they would have to search for the doctor because the hospital closed at three in the afternoon. Knowing this, they made no effort to go. When services are improved, women manage to get there."

CONTINUING ROLE FOR ACTIVISM

Although the existence of national offices of women's health and international women's health meetings might seem to indicate that the activists have accomplished their goals, the activists themselves don't think so. Seaman, for instance, has just produced a new, updated version of *The Doctors' Case against the Pill*, which details her reservations about the lower-dose birth-control pills that her previous work helped to put on the market.

Meanwhile, she has lost none of her skepticism about doctors. In December 1991, Seaman, Pearson, and three other activists protested the Women's Health Initiative's plan to test estrogen replacement therapy on women with intact uteruses, because it has been linked to endometrial cancer. Bernadine Healy, then-director of NIH, rejected their concerns, arguing that plans to monitor the test subjects with yearly biopsies would protect female subjects. Last January, though, when another trial revealed higher than expected rates of uterine cellular abnormalities in women on hormone therapy, the original plans were quietly dropped.

The National Women's Health Network has increasingly turned its attention to women who are not getting health-care services at all. The reasons include the controversy over abortion, which has effectively denied the procedure to many women, according to Stanley Henshaw, a researcher at the Alan Guttmacher Institute in New York City; a survey by the institute shows that 30 percent of U.S. women of reproductive age live in countries with no abortion provider. Women are also denied care because of the soaring costs of insurance, which has left greater numbers of the poor uninsured. Because women are disproportionately likely to be poor, Pearson says, they are disproportionately likely to be unprotected. "We have a lot to do," she says.

"Ultimately," [Mahmoud] Fathalla [a reproductive-health advisor to the Rockefeller Foundation in Egypt] says, "what is important is power—for women to gain power over their own bodies and their own lives." In his view, the only way the international community will address women's health issues completely in Beijing will be if women themselves demand it. Women in developed countries demanded attention to their concerns in the past, he says. "When people push, the world moves," he says. "That is what makes progress."

Chapter 73

Feminism for the 21st Century

A s we look backward and forward, assess our history, learn from our mistakes, wrestle with ambiguities, get knocked down, and stand up again for the same causes for the thousandth time, we give the last word in this collection to Susan Brownmiller, author of Against Our Will: Men, Women and Rape:

"I do not think we are not blaming the victim so much, but we're still not so far along in terms of ending the assaults. Someone once said to me, 'Well, if your book was so successful, why aren't there fewer rapes? Why are men still raping us?' Well, they're not the ones who are reading the book."

If rape is Susan's "signature" issue, mine is informed consent. Not to compare the AMA with rapists, exactly, but for 30 years, every time the FDA mandates full information to consumers on prescription drugs, the AMA sabotages and derails the plan. On February 14, 1996, at an FDA workshop entitled "Prescription drug information: What is a useful truth for the patient?" I pressed the AMA representatives for a truthful explanation of their stand, and got it to wit: Many prescriptions are written "off label," meaning that the drug in question has never been proven effective for the purpose at hand. The FDA wants all labeling to state the exact conditions for which the drug is indicated (to avoid prescription mix-ups, among other sound reasons), but the AMA dreads that patients may find out how many of their own remedies are scientifically unsound, exposing them as hypocrites in their stated contempt for alternative methods. (To be fair, the AMA by no means speaks for all physicians. Their membership has dropped from 45 percent of U.S. doctors in 1988 to 34 percent in 1999. The loss in dues makes them more reliant on drug ads in their journals, which bring in $54.7 million a year, 25 percent of their annual budget. Following the FDA workshop, the AMA did "read my book," and decided, 27 years after the fact, that they didn't like it. In the summer, JAMA published an excoriating review of the 25th anniversary edition of The Doctors' Case against the Pill by a physician whose laboratory happened to be bankrolled by Johnson & Johnson, the parent company of Ortho.)

As consumers take increasing responsibility for our own care, the judicial system, once guided by "medical paternalism" and prone to dismiss patient perspectives as "unscientific" are changing their views according to legal authority and author, Michael H. Cohen. In an important case, Texas patients challenged a Board of Medical Examiners ruling that acupuncture was experimental, its safety and effectiveness had not been demonstrated, and it would be applied by physicians only.

The U.S. District Court of Southern Texas scoffed at the Medical Examiners: "Acupuncture has been practiced for 2,000 to 5,000 years. It is no more experimental as a mode of medical treatment than is the Chinese language as a mode of communication. What is experimental is not acupuncture, but Westerners' understanding of it and their ability to use it properly."—B. S.

The Beauty Myth

NAOMI WOLF

Excerpted from Naomi Wolf, *The Beauty Myth: How Images of Beauty Are Used against Women, New York, Willi... Morrow, 1991. Reprinted by permission.*

During the past decade, women breached the power structure; meanwhile, eating disorders rose exponentially and cosmetic surgery became the fastest-growing medical specialty. During the past five years, consumer spending doubled, pornography became the main media category, ahead of legitimate films and records combined, and 33,000 American women told researchers that they would rather lose 10 to 15 pounds than achieve any other goal. More women have more money and power and scope and legal recognition than we have ever had before; but in terms of how we feel about ourselves physically, we may actually be worse off than our unliberated grandmothers. Recent research consistently shows that inside the majority of the West's controlled, attractive, successful working women, there is a secret "underlife" poisoning our freedom; infused with notions of beauty, it is a dark vein of self-hatred, physical obsessions, terror of aging, and the dread of lost control.

It is no accident that so many potentially powerful women feel this way. We are in the midst of a violent backlash against feminism that uses images of female beauty as a political weapon against women's advancement: the beauty myth. It is the modern version of a social reflex that has been in force since the Industrial Revolution. As women released themselves from the feminine mystique of domesticity, the beauty myth took over its lost ground, expanding as it waned to carry on its work of social control.

The contemporary backlash is so violent because the ideology of beauty is the last one remaining of the old feminine ideologies that still has the power to control those women whom second wave feminism would have otherwise made relatively uncontrollable: It has grown stronger to take over the work of social coercion that myths about motherhood, domesticity, chastity, and passivity no longer can manage. It is seeking right now to undo psychologically and covertly all the good things that feminism did for women materially and overtly.

The beauty myth tells a story: The quality called "beauty" objectively and universally exists. Women must want to embody it and men must want to possess women who embody it. This embodiment is an imperative for women and not for men, which situation is necessary and natural because it is biological, sexual, and evolutionary: Strong men battle for beautiful women, and beautiful women are more reproductively successful. Women's beauty must correlate to their fertility, and since this system is based on sexual selection, it is inevitable and changeless.

None of this is true. "Beauty" is a currency system like the gold standard. Like any economy, it is determined by politics, and in the modern age in the West it is the last, best belief that keeps male dominance intact. In assigning value to women in a vertical hierarchy according to a culturally imposed physical standard, it is an expression of power relations in which women must unnaturally compete for resources that men have appropriated for themselves.

Why Feminists Are in Such Good Shape

AMELIA RICHARDS

Amelia Richards, "Ask Amy," an on-line advice column at www.feminist.com. Reprinted by permission.

Amy fields approximately 20 questions per day on topics ranging from women's health, to research papers on feminism 101, to young women in need of a friend.

Q: Hello. I know that you do not know me but I would like to take only a moment of your time. I am 5 feet 4 inches and weigh approximately 107 pounds. I don't like to weigh over 103 pounds, but lately I have gotten lazy. I would like to know what my ideal weight is. I don't want to be extremely thin but I have this constant fear of becoming fat. I would like to also know what exercises will help me with my problem areas, which are my lower stomach and my thighs. If you will please reply and help me. Thank you for your time.

—Sincerely, Dawn

A: I am by no means a fitness expert or a physician, so I can't answer your questions from that level of expertise, but I can add personal insight.

First, I would hardly call 107 pounds "lazy"—if that's lazy then I am absolutely totally pathetic, and I know I'm not that. The thing about weight and body image is that there is no set formula. Every body—and everybody—is unique. By trying to fit yourself into a set pattern, you are ignoring that fact that life isn't that predictable—nor is your metabolism. As for weight, I am shorter than you (5 feet 1 inch) and I weigh a little more than you (110–115 pounds—I don't keep track). I run two times a week and walk whenever possible—for sanity of mind more than sanctity of body. Of course I have days where I think I am bordering on obese, but in general I am comfortable with my body and my health. Body image isn't as much about "poundage" as it is about a mental state—and false comparisons. It took me many years—with a little bulimia mixed in, although I didn't know that what me and my friends did after eating a pint of ice cream had a name—to realize that my body wasn't meant to be like Kate Moss's and my thighs would never look like those women in the Nike ads. What those years also taught me was that, thank goodness, I don't look like everyone else that's 5 feet 1 inch.

As for specific exercises—you need to figure out what you like to do, because the minute you start to do something purely to lose weight or stay in shape, it becomes a "must" and not a "want to," and therefore more drudgery than pleasure. So find out what you like—walking, swimming, running.

I've often thought of a comic: "why feminists are in such good shape.... " We work in a profession that doesn't pay that well, so we are forced to walk everywhere—good for the legs and the cardiovascular; we always have to defend ourselves and our beliefs, so we always have to have lots of literature on hand too—heavy bags help build up our arm muscles; we can't drink beer, because these ads are offensive to women, or eat Domino's pizza, because they support Operation Rescue; we can't eat dairy products, because we are educated enough to know that animal fat can cause cancer. I still need to work this out, but I hope you see my point.

If you think you might possibly have an eating disorder, it is best to speak to an expert. If you think this is the case, you can try using our database of women's services to find an eating disorder treatment center near you. Be well

—Amy

The Bra Story

LORI BARER

Bra, aka brassiere, undergarment, over-the-shoulder-boulder-holder, and pick-me-upper. Lingerie companies make them, we wear them. Since approximately 1913, bras have been marketed and sold in the United States; before this time "there was absolutely no interest in [the] uplift [of breasts]." Today, women of all ages, myself included, consider the bra an essential item in our wardrobe. As I lay awake each morning deciding what outfit I should pick out for the day, I cease to ponder whether or not I should wear a bra. I simply step out of bed, brush my teeth and turn directly toward my underwear drawer. To rid myself of this unfathomably uncomfortable norm I call a 'bra' was my idea of fun (or so I thought).

I woke up Friday, February 5th, with butterflies in my stomach, I couldn't move. I did not want to get out of bed; for today was my big day. I wore a tight shirt with a sweater over it, no bra. From the moment I stepped out of my room until the moment I reached it again, with all intentions of putting my bra on, I was miserable. I felt ugly, fat, weird, and all together brutish. There was not one point in the day in which I felt secure and proud that I was defying a societal norm, it was horrifying. No one said a word about my hanging breasts. Not one remark from my boyfriend, nor my roommates, nor strangers. I was shocked. What I did get were stares. All day long people stared at me, as if there was something to stare at; perhaps they thought I just had low-hanging breasts and I was, in fact, wearing a bra—what a stigma I might then have.

My boyfriend was the first to see me. He stared, he literally stared at my breasts while he spoke to me. No eye contact, no embarrassment that he wasn't looking at some other part of my body, he spoke directly to them. He was very, very confused. He didn't know whether I was wearing a bra and it for some reason or other wasn't "working" or if, heaven forbid, I didn't have one on. When he finally realized that there was just no way I was wearing one, he was almost embarrassed for me, he didn't know how to react, and never brought it up. My roommates all had the same reaction, they simply stared at my chest, then looked up at my face and down again to perhaps ponder whether my breasts had always been near my ankles or perchance gravity was beginning to take its toll.

When I finally ventured outside of my house where I was more likely to encounter people I didn't know (I went to several places, the pharmacy, food store), I was hoping to receive a different reaction. I don't know what I was looking for, I think I almost hoped someone would scream out *"Look at Her Sagging Breasts!"* so that this experiment I had planned for myself would, in fact, be worthwhile. They didn't. Again, no one said anything. They just looked... at my breasts. People commonly look at my breasts, this has been something I have had to deal with my entire postpubescent life, I have large breasts and people notice. The body of a woman was nearly exactly that of my own as a peripubescent 13-year-old, where full shapely breasts smothered my tiny torso and often seemed to block my innocent face. To have this body as a young girl meant having the repercussions that went along with it. This meant my eighth grade English teacher, who couldn't keep his eyes to himself. He often sent girls to the nurse's office because he said he could see their bra strap. He was known to seat the prettiest, shapeliest girls in the front and those less pleasing to the eye in the rear of the classroom. I still had my prepubescent figure and had gained my large breasts quickly and noticeably, putting me at center stage. What it was at this point in my life to have a female's body was to be stared at, to have all eyes on my chest, to have to go home and tell my mother, and my father, and ultimately the principal, that my teacher couldn't stop staring at my breasts. In summation, this meant sending my mother in a rage to my middle school to verbally beat the living shit out of this man. It also meant my embarrassment; telling the other children why I couldn't be in his class anymore, why I had to rearrange my schedule in the middle of the school year to get away from this very sick man.

This staring was different though. People were staring in disgust. It was as if they could not believe that a 'normal' looking, well-dressed woman would go out of the house like this. I was mortified and saddened by what I thought could have been a truly liberating feminist experience turning into one that was actually quite shameful. I'm disappointed in myself for, after studying gender and women for so long, still succumbing to societal pressures of bodily norms in accordance with gender.

Gender on a whole is socially constructed. This means that one is not born with gender, the individual's particular society molds gender and thus molds human beings to act or not act with certain gender-esque attributes. In our culture, for instance, people born with penises are acculturated to be aggressive and dominating, they should wear pants and suits and ties. On the other hand, people born with vaginas are should to be sensitive and emotional, to wear jewelry and high heels, and most certainly a bra. Unfortunately, this dichotomy of gender should look more like a continuum, but it does not. This therefore means that an individual is either "feminine" or "masculine," a "man" or a "woman." There are no in-betweens and there will be no crossing of boundaries. The "experiment" that I undertook did exactly that, I crossed the boundary. Wearing a bra in our society is distinctly feminine. This does not hold true for all societies and certainly not for everyone living in ours, but for the most part, it is upheld.

My rebellion against this particular aspect of gender norming was wildly successful. It showed that while the practice of wearing a bra is not "natural," we need to abide by it in order to be accepted within society. It also showed that this gendered bodily practice played an enormous role in self-concept. I have previously discussed how my self-image took a dramatic turn for the worse and my strength and power as an outspoken feminist was muted. While my sex was not altered, I was clearly less feminine. In the study "What is Beautiful is Good" it is concluded that "... attractive... persons are likely to secure more prestigious jobs than those of lesser attractiveness, as well as experiencing happier marriages, being better parents, and enjoying more fulfilling social and occupational lives" (Dion, et al.). This exemplifies the notion that my unattractiveness as a woman led to perceptions of me by others who perhaps thought the aforementioned conclusion. I was somehow not worthy of a prestigious job or a happy marriage, I was strange. Over time, our society has come to many conclusions about what is acceptable and unacceptable. Somehow, sagging breasts were seen to be unacceptable (most likely via media messages of WonderBras and Miracle Workers), thus my dissociation from society.

In actuality, we can all survive without wearing a bra ever again. If we raised our daughters without bras, they would be just as healthy as we are now (if not healthier according to new studies of a link between wearing bras and breast cancer). Therefore, there is nothing natural about the practice. What is natural, though, are the emotions felt from societies' reaction to breaking these gendered norms. To ostracize and isolate someone based upon a physical appearance, a way of dress, is abhorrent. The emotions felt now make the act of simply wearing something like a bra mandatory. I learned that it is perhaps a good idea to walk in the life of someone who does not abide by gender rules, if only for a day.

The kind of person that walks into a store, and you can't tell their sex, and it bothers you; and you might go home and think about that person all night, and wish you knew whether they were a man or a woman (because they could never be neither), but you would never think about why it matters in the first place, nor how any of those "signs" that you were looking for were ever construed. There is nothing natural about gender, thus nothing instinctive about gender norms.

"Tell Me More, Tell Me More": Young Women's Locker Room Talk as a Boomer-Feminist Legacy

PAULA KAMEN

Excerpted from Paula Kamen, *Her Way: Young Women's Evolving Sexual Choices*, New York, New York University Press, forthcoming. Reprinted by permission.

In college, one night there were six or seven girls, our same age, good friends, sitting in a bar and really talking, I mean just how we have orgasms," said Janine, 24. "And this happened to be a masturbation conversation. In the middle of the bar. There were [many] people around us, laughing and learning. It was unbelievable. I guess that's how we figure things out."

Recently, this Florida high school teacher and two of her friends again discussed this topic together in detail. One of them, Tammy, admitted that she never had an orgasm. "They told me how and now I can. I'm healed... ," Tammy said. "It's comforting to know that people have experienced similar things or that your friends know and that they understand that it's OK. I guess it's good to know that you're OK."

While all three women are generally open with their parents, their friends fill a distinct need for sexual information and openness—without judgment. "At age 16," said Janine, a Catholic from a Cuban-American family, "who was I going to talk to about having sex with my boyfriend? My friends."

While sex education from schools and parents give young women the information they should know, women's locker-room talk gives them what they really want to know. Women's locker-room talk today can be both edifying and trashy, therapeutic and ego-fanning. One's girlfriends are often a constant presence influencing sexual relationships in many roles: as a cheerleader, referee, Internet listserve, crisis hot line, absolving priest, Greek chorus, sister, mom, aunt, RA, RN, MSW, reference book, shameless voyeur, and, sometimes, feminist advocate.

As the rules about sex have changed, so have the rules for talking about it. Feeling less guilty about being sexual beings and taking advantage of strong and sharing friendships, women have cranked open their channels of communication. Instead of remaining silent, and serving only as subjects of conquest for men's "locker-room talk," as was the standard in the past, they have cultivated their own potent and shameless breed. By all accounts, women are even more likely than men to talk about sex, and in more vivid Technicolor detail and more critically.

The pervasiveness of locker-room talk among young women of all backgrounds also reflects the particular feminist legacy of the baby boomers. They opened the doors to free communication about the most intimate matters of one's life and promoted women's friendships as a nurturing, empowering force. The early personal consciousness-raising of the women's health movement, which was fringe work in the 1960s and 1970s, has now become a part of mainstream life. Like the radical message of the Sexual Revolution—to give women the permission to have sex outside of marriage—the feminists' ideologies of women breaking their silences have slowly been absorbed into the nation's collective psychic bloodstream. Today, although with less political emphasis, "third wave" feminists (along with women of color of all ages and safer-sex activists) build on their work advocating even more authentic and diverse conversations about the most unspoken aspects of women's lives.

Slut!: Growing Up Female with a Bad Reputation

LEORA TANENBAUM

Excerpted from Leora Tanenbaum, *Slut! Growing Up Female with a Bad Reputation*, New York, Seven Stories Press, 1999. Reprinted by permission.

When news broke that Monica Lewinsky had allegedly had consensual sexual relations with President Clinton, I was astounded by the torrent of nasty remarks, headlines, and public opinion polls picking apart her body, hair, psychological state, and sexuality. *New York* magazine reported that as an adolescent, Lewinsky had spent two summers at weight-loss camp, and that she had "paid particular attention to the guys. Jokes about Lewinsky's "big hair," and how she was sent home from the White House because she dressed too provocatively, became instant clichés. When *Vanity Fair* published photos of Lewinsky in glamorous poses, a female acquaintance of mine scrutinized the layout and decreed that the only reason Lewinsky looked so attractive was that the magazine gave her a great makeup job and airbrushed the photos. Clinton himself referred to Lewinsky as "that woman" ("I never had sexual relations with that woman"); with those two words alone he managed to portray her as a classic "slut," a throwaway woman he clearly didn't want to humanize by invoking her name.

A concerted effort to smear Lewinsky as an oversexed, hyperaggressive woman was under way. Speculation abounded that Lewinsky had invented the whole affair in a girlish fantasy; Representative Charles Rangel of New York said, "That poor child has serious emotional problems, She's fantasizing. And I haven't heard that she played with a full deck in her other experiences." In an editorial, *The Wall Street Journal* called her a "little tart." After being portrayed as a stalker who "used emotional blackmail to trap" a married lover by the *New York Post* and a "manipulative, sex-obsessed woman" by the *Daily News*, Fox News released a poll investigating whether the public thought she was an "average girl" or a "young tramp looking for thrills." Fifty-four percent rated her a tramp. Later it was revealed that President Clinton had referred to Lewinsky as a "stalker" with his staff. And all this was months before Independent Whitewater Counsel Kenneth Starr served up his own salacious report depicting Lewinsky as an exhibitionistic, sex-obsessed provocateur.

Personally I think Lewinsky is a good-looking woman who happens to have a voluptuous figure. Starstruck, she participated in an act that was reckless, foolish, and sad but hardly worthy of such national attention. Originally, she did not want to publicly advertise the affair (as Gennifer Flowers did in 1992 about her own extramarital relationship with the president); indeed, by lying about it initially in an affidavit, she demonstrated respectful discretion. (Her March 1999 interview with Barbara Walters and cooperation with the author of

Monica's Story were part of a defensive measure to try to counter her image as a tramp.) All in all, I believe, Lewinsky does not deserve to be written off as a *Melrose Place* bimbo.

But even as her name fades from late-night punch lines, there is no doubt that Lewinsky will spend the rest of her life in the shadow of her tarnished reputation. Obviously Clinton's own reputation has also suffered, but most Americans have been disappointed that he lied about the liaison for seven months, not because of the liaison itself. And even those who do find the liaison disturbing tend to describe Clinton as someone who has a "problem" or "disease," suggesting that his sexuality lies beyond his control. Meanwhile many Americans believe that an unmarried woman who capitalizes on her sexuality—to feel good about herself, to capture the attention of powerful men, for recreation—is debased.

But why should sex and femininity necessarily be at odds? Of course, sex is often used in ways that degrade women (rape, sexual harassment, forcible prostitution), and too many women mistakenly perceive that their sexuality is their only source of power. But sex is not always and inherently sexist, nor should it transform women into dirty tramps. When Clinton and Lewinsky participated in their liaison, the only people who got hurt, as I see it, were Hillary and Chelsea Clinton—and that's for them to decide.

Meanwhile, in the women's locker room at my local Y, semi- and fully naked women walk from their lockers to the showers and then back again every day. But when a repairman recently entered one circumscribed corner of the locker room for less than five minutes (all the while monitored by a female staffer), all hell broke loose. I had to pass that corner to get to the shower, and I didn't feel like waiting. I was wearing one of those gym towels that were clearly not intended for women, since they cover either the breasts or the hips, but not both. But what did I care? In the three years I've belonged to the Y, hundreds of different women had already seen me naked; why was I to be intimidated by the fact that one busy male might catch a quick glimpse of my flesh? Yet two clothed women "tsk-tsked" me as I padded by the repairman in my towel, telling me with a shake of their heads that I had committed some grave lapse in judgment. (He didn't even seem to notice.)

This is the sexual double standard: the idea that women are disgraced by sex outside of marriage, that sex transforms them into "sluts." The 1997 movie *Chasing Amy* illustrates how the sexual double standard effectively sidesteps men's concern about their own sexual abilities. In describing the film, reviewers said it was about the sorrows of a postcollege man who has the misfortune to fall in love with a young, cute lesbian. In fact, the movie says less about lesbianism than it does about the fear of "sluts." Holden is attracted to Alyssa, who is, it is true, a lesbian. When she falls for him too, he assumes he's the first man she's ever slept with. But Alyssa wasn't always a lesbian. It turns out that when she was in high school, Alyssa had considerable sexual experience with boys—including, once, a *ménage á trois* with two male classmates. Holden, who was infatuated with Alyssa when he knew that she had had sex with many women, is now disgusted. Having slept with men transforms Alyssa; it makes her a "slut" rather than a chic lesbian. And so Holden treats her like a "slut" by asking her to participate in a *ménage* with his best male friend. Deep down, he admits, he is intimidated by and fears her sexual experience with men. He feels inadequate and wants to even the score. Alyssa, who feels cheapened by the proposal, leaves him.

Likewise, in the 1986 Spike Lee movie *She's Gotta Have It,* Mars Blackman says, "Look, all men want freaks. We just don't want 'em for a wife." Blackman, played by Lee, is frustrated that his girlfriend, Nola, is sexually involved with two other men as well. All three men want Nola, but do they respect her? No. Boyfriend No. 2 sneers, "A nice lady doesn't go humping from bed to bed." Boyfriend No. 3 snickers, "Once a freak, always a freak." Then he rapes her. But it doesn't matter to Nola whether or not these men respect her: She respects herself. "I am not a one-man woman," she says with defiance.

You, too, might think that Alyssa's and Nola's casual attitude about sex is inappropriate, disgusting, or just wrong. You might be opposed to casual sex in principle, believing instead that sex should be reserved for a meaningful, romantic relationship. That's fine—but beside the point. There should be one sexual standard for both genders—and that applies to older teenagers and to adults over the age of twenty-one. If you think that sixteen-year-olds should not be having intercourse, that includes boys as well as girls. If you think that some sixteen-year-olds are mature enough to express their sexual longings, that includes girls as well as boys. Though sexually active girls alone carry the burden of potential pregnancy, both genders must be treated as equals since they share equally in the heterosexual act.

Holden's low opinion of Alyssa, and Mars's contempt for Nola, is indicative of the continued widespread prominence of the sexual double standard. Three quarters of young men and nearly 90 percent of young women surveyed by the Janus Report agreed that the sexual double standard prevails. Roughly half of American teenagers are sexually active—in 1997, 49 percent of boys aged fifteen to nineteen reported ever having had sexual intercourse, compared with 48 percent of girls—but when it comes to moralizing about the excesses of teenage sexuality, girls alone are ridiculed and made to feel cheap. As Steven, a Rhode Island high school junior, comments, his male friends always hang out with the freshman girls known as "sluts," not because they like those girls but because they can "get some." And like in the 1950s, it's usually girls, not boys, who are on the front lines of making fun of others as "sluts."

"In the eighth grade, I had a boyfriend and we sort of explored things sexually, though we never had intercourse," recalls Hanna Wallace, twenty-five, a magazine editor in New York. "I was quite honest with my best friend, Stacia, and told her about it. Her reaction was that she was disappointed in me. She and another friend got together and wrote me a letter that really upset me. It wasn't that they were worried about me, because everything I did with my boyfriend was consensual. They were chastising me for my behavior, which they thought was disgusting. They were moralizing. I felt: Did I have to hide my sexual relationship from my friends?"

Hannah's friend, Stacia Eyerly, vividly remembers the incident. "We did write her a note," she told me. "We were concerned about whether she was doing the right thing. A little of it was envy, but mostly it was the feeling that she shouldn't have done what she did, that it was inappropriate. But this feeling only applied to girls. It was definitely because she was a girl that I had a problem with it."

Despite humiliating encounters like Hanna's, sexually active "sluts" have an advantage over "good" girls. Once they are singled out for derision, they realize they have little to lose by living up to their reputations. And in defying the "good girl" rules, they develop a necessary critical perspective about love and sex. Unlike most girls, self-aware "sluts" perceive the unfairness of the sexual double standard. They know they are in a double bind: That boys like girls who are a little bit "slutty" but also look down on them as cheap and inferior. They are aware that girls as well as boys experience sexual pleasure; they know that if they are responsible, they can minimize their risk of disease, pregnancy, and emotional distress. And they recognize that most girls take adolescent romance much more seriously than boys do—too seriously. Sexually active "sluts" think of themselves as independent sexual agents and are less inclined to use sex as a bargaining chip for love and affection. As a result, I would argue, they, and not the "good" girls who call them insulting names, are more likely to have a healthy attitude about themselves and their futures.

Won by Love

NORMA McCORVEY

Norma McCorvey, with Gary Thomas, *Won By Love*, pub info TK

I had prepared a speech, just in case. I still couldn't believe that Jane Roe would not be asked to say something, even if she was blue-collar and didn't quite fit in with the Ivy League–educated feminists who ran the abortion movement. My pedigree, apparently, was an embarrassment to the Vassar-degreed lawyers. My grandmother had made a living as a prostitute and then, as she grew older, a fortune teller. My mother was an alcoholic Roman Catholic, my father a Jehovah's Witness and television repairmen. I'm part

Cajun and Cherokee Indian with a ninth-grade education. When people talk about "pump," I assume they're referring to gasoline, not shoes.

With this background, it's not so surprising that I had a difficult time fitting in with women who wore business suits and carried briefcases. Most of my friends were drug pushers or poor people or carnival workers. I met my closest friend, Connie, when she caught me shoplifting at her store.

Yet in spite of this background—or maybe because of it—I ended up being the lead plaintiff in the case that brought legalized abortion to the United States. Though I had recently begun letting people know that I was Jane Roe, there had never been a national "coming out." NBC had run a movie of my life, but they changed my name to protect my privacy.

In 1989 few recognized me or knew Jane Roe by the name Norma McCorvey. But the march organizers knew. Certainly Sarah Weddington, the lawyer who represented me in the case, knew. Yet most of the leaders didn't really care. That's how I could travel to the march and still be anonymous....

I hung up the phone and marveled at what had taken place. Finally, I had found a love that was all-encompassing. On many occasions, Sarah Weddington had made it clear that to her I was nothing more than a name in a class-action lawsuit. Jane Roe was all that mattered to Sarah; the real Norma McCorvey was irrelevant.

In Jesus, I realized it was exactly the opposite. God did not view me solely through the lens of what I had done or how I had been used. Now, after I had been forgiven, Jane Roe was irrelevant. The woman he loved—the woman he saved—was Norma Leah McCorvey....

All those years, I was wrong. Signing that affidavit, I was wrong. Working in an abortion clinic, I was wrong. No more of this first-trimester, second-trimester, third-trimester stuff. Abortion—at any point—was wrong. It was wrong. It was so clear. Painfully clear.

For many, many years, I always thought the worst thing I had done was to place my children for adoption (though one was placed against my will). I didn't want them to be hurt. I thought I couldn't care for them, and I did what I thought was best at the time; but even so, I always thought of this as my greatest failure.

But in one moment, I realize that placing a child for adoption could be an act of great courage. The real despicable act, the real blight on my life, was being Jane Roe and helping to bring legalized abortion this country. The very thing I was celebrated for on earth was the thing I would be most sorry for in heaven. The thing that brought me fame, notoriety, a movie deal, a couple of book contracts, media interviews galore—it was shameful. It was wrong. It was the worst thing I ever could have done.

Changing Concepts of Women's Health: Advocating for Change

JULIA SCOTT

Excerpted from a speech given at the Canada-U.S. Women's Health Forum, August 8, 1996, Ottawa, Canada. Reprinted by permission.

I want to reflect on the growth of the women's movement in the United States and its prospects for the future. I look at our current challenge as twofold. One is to get the word out about women's health status globally and not just in our own countries. The second, which is much harder, is getting past simply having the rhetoric and language about inclusiveness and diversity, and really getting down to the hard work for each of us and seeing how we hinder the expression and existence of that inclusiveness and diversity. It's very difficult to talk about these issues. Those of us who do are seen by the establishment as wild-eyed radicals, always bringing up things that might perhaps divide us. We want to be together in solidarity around gender issues. But we have to acknowledge that there are differences among us that impact our health. So if we raise these issues, it's not to be contentious or argumentative, although for some people that may be part of the reason, but to say that if we really believe in equality, we have to discuss what our differences are and not see them as ways that somehow make our effort less.

I always feel particularly challenged, particularly as a woman of color, to get up and speak on these issues. For the United States, I think we'll really be able to say that we have made progress in our movement when women other than women of color or poor women speak and work on these issues with the same fervor that they do on the issues of the so-called majority women.

Let's be clear that the women's health movement in the United States did not begin in the 1990s. The gains of the 1990s are directly related to and benefited from the organized women's movement of the 1970s and 1980s. The advances that we have been able to make in the 1990s, with the greater influx of women into positions of power, in legislation and administration, from the NIH to FDA, have been because of the hard work of women in the 1970s and 1980s. These women were not necessarily in the medical establishment, but they were activists and everyday women, who got sick and tired of not having answers and having all of our health problems labeled as hysterical or the results of our having our periods.

The woman's health movement also benefited from the struggles and the strategies of the civil rights movement. Many of the gains that the women's health movement has been able to make in the United States have been borne on the back of Black men and women who struggled for racial equality in the United States.

What we know from the many gains we have made is that, in spite of the valiant efforts of so many women, including President Clinton's appointment of many women throughout this administration, and the influx of women, especially women of color into our own legislatures, still have not afforded us the kind of access to health and health care that women so richly deserve. It's not enough simply to have women in place. We do have to question the philosophy of women who are appointed to these commissions and decision-making bodies, because very often some women who are not progressive have been some of our own worse enemies.

So, while it would not be possible to talk in detail about the all the women's groups and organizations who have pioneered this work in the United States, I can still say that it is recognized that the group of women who came together to prepare publication of *Our Bodies, Ourselves* gave us the first work that paved the way to confronting some of women's anger and frustration about the lack of information and control we had concerning our bodies and the lack of access to health-care treatment modalities. Also, the National Women's Health Network was and is the women's premier feminist health organization in the United States.

The National Black Woman's Health Project came out of that movement. Our founder Byllye Avery was on the board of that organization and became horrified when looking at the statistics and seeing the paucity of information

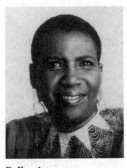

Byllye Avery

available about Black women's health. She was struck, especially, in 1979, by the National Health and Nutrition Examination Survey, conducted by the National Center for Health Statistics, Centers for Disease Control (NCHS/CDC), which showed that Black women, in a self-administered survey where they rated themselves, were in more psychological stress than White women who were institutionalized. It seemed to her—something that we have to acknowledge—even the best organizations that have the right kind of analyses in terms of race and class and their impact on our health status, they will never take the place of women of color having their own organizations and doing their own work. So, while we support and need the support of the broader White women's health movement, in our country and globally, we insist that work on these issues, especially issues that are critical to our health, are led by the women who are affected by them.

At the heart of our focus today is the fundamental question of how women can fully access good health and the best care that the United States, international leader in medical research, has to offer. We seek access for women who are poor or wealthy, married or single, migrant workers, office workers, homeless, differently abled, professionals, homemakers, heterosexual, bisexual or lesbian, This perspective was not in the mix when the women's health movement first began agitating. The first inkling of a women's health movement was the 1960s campaign where a few isolated women were fighting for natural childbirth. They wanted to decrease the use of anesthetics women were being given during delivery. And they started to banish from the delivery room practices which had developed, not to improve the overall well being of mother and infant, but to increase the convenience for doctors. In raising these issues, the small group began to insert a new dynamic into the doctor-patient relationship.

Let me take a moment to talk about some of the differences in health concerns, fully aware that sometimes such discussions will be seen as a way of dividing us. However, it's really important for us to acknowledge that there are differences.

I will give just a few examples of those differences. While breast cancer doesn't affect Black women at the same rates that it affects White women, it does affect us differently. We tend to get it at an earlier age, and the regulations which give an age at which women should get their first mammography is really problematic for us. That's why we have been fighting so valiantly to get those regulations changed. We would like it to be acknowledged that for Black women, getting our first mammography at age 40 or 50 is simply not good enough. We have also been fighting for more research on breast cancer to look at those differences. For instance, only last year a study came out suggesting that not only do we get it earlier but that we get a more virulent form of it. We, basically, have been told that the reason we die from breast cancer more frequently than other women is because of lack of access to such things as mammographies. While I'm sure that does have an impact on the situation, we have been struggling to make sure that we pay as much attention in our research agenda to the issues of the environment and of diet and how that relates to the different women of color communities.

The issue of AIDS is another area we have to look at differently. It's an issue that has been dealt with as a White male disease. But as the majority of the women who are being affected by this are minority women, mainly Black, Latino, and Native American women, we now find the money is starting to dry up. Also we find a lot of punitive legislation being aimed at women who are HIV-infected. Instead of funding treatment programs and research programs that would look at how women are differently affected by HIV, we find that legislatures and judges want to mandate that women take medications like AZT against their judgments and that there be mandatory HIV testing. These are all things that we have to be concerned about.

The area of reproductive technologies is a huge issue for all women, but especially for women of color in the U.S. These are the same women who have been targeted for unsafe contraception, for sterilization abuse—and this is not something that has simply happened in the past. This is something that is happening right now.

Let's also think about the work on identifying the breast cancer gene. This is something we have to be very concerned about. Now insurance companies have or will have the ability to get at information that identifies certain people as being at risk for chronic and debilitating diseases. Then those people are going to be excluded from getting health care. So, while we cannot minimize the opportunities that allow more choice to women, we have to look at the downside, and pay attention to it.

The women of color movement has been very forceful in the U.S. in looking at the use of long-acting contraceptives. We agree that this is something that is much needed in the very meager menu of choices that are available to women, but there are also serious problems with the discriminatory use of these methods aimed and targeted at poor women and women of color. We think it was the dragging of the feet of women and men in the health community, and in the women's health community itself not joining us in that struggle, that has brought us to a place now where we have a method that could be valuable for some women, but is now in jeopardy in our country. We cannot continue to hide our heads in the sand over this issue.

I think the women's health movement has grown to a place where it is starting to acknowledge, at least in rhetoric, that race, ethnicity, and class affect and impact the quality of health care for women; but I also think we have not gone that next step of working on how we can all very seriously talk together and address the racist practices in our institutions that keep us from working together. I hope we will spend more time talking about the issues and how we can address them. I hope we will come to a time when the broader women's community will be able to accept the leadership of women different from themselves, accept that we may have to change our strategies. Maybe we won't be able to get there the way everybody is used to getting there, but we will get there.

Women's Health and Government Regulation: 1980–1999

SUZANNE WHITE JUNOD

The last two decades have seen major developments in the detection and treatment of reproductive cancers, the development of new drugs, and greater legislative attention to women's health. Devices that caused problems in the past have been subject to greater regulation.

NEW DRUGS

In 1987, Prozac (fluoxetine) was approved as the first of a new type of antidepressants known as selective serotonin reuptake inhibitors (SSRIs). Prozac and other SSRIs have revolutionized the treatment of *mental disorders,* notably obsessive-compulsive disorder and depression.

In 1987, the FDA approved Retrovir (zidovudine, AZT) by Glaxo-Wellcome for treatment of *HIV infection.* In 1994, a preliminary study showed that only 8.3 percent of babies born to HIV-positive women taking Retrovir became infected, compared with 25.5 percent of babies born to women on placebo. The study was halted and FDA quickly approved new labeling for Retrovir, indicating the drug's safety and effectiveness in reducing the transmission of HIV from a pregnant woman to her fetus. The only other physical device remaining on the OTC market was the Reality female condom, approved in 1993.

In the 1990s a number of new *contraceptives* received FDA approval: Norplant (1990); Depo-Provera (1992); and Norplant 2 (1996). The vaginal sponge, which was approved in 1983, was withdrawn from the market in 1995 by the manufacturer, Whitehall Laboratories. The only other physical device was the Reality female condom, approved in 1993.

In 1995, the FDA approved two new treatments for *osteoporosis* for post-menopausal women with low bone density: Miacalcin Nasal Spray (calcitonin salmon) and Fosamax (alendronate), a bisphosphonate drug demonstrating a statistically significant increase in bone mass in the spine and hip.

In 1996, the FDA approved Redux (dexfenfluramine) for prolonged treatment of *obesity,* in conjunction with a reduced-calorie diet. Redux is a serotonin uptake inhibitor. There is some risk of pulmonary hypertension, so it is approved for use only with obese patients with a body mass index of at least 30. In 1997, shortly after physicians began combining fenfluramine and phentermine—two drugs that had been separately approved by the FDA—the FDA sent out a "Dear Doctor" letter warning doctors to carefully monito patients taking fen-phen combination. The FDA had received reports of 33 cases of heart valve abnormalities in women ages 30 to 72. A few months later, the FDA withdrew fen-phen for the treatment of obesity because documentation had shown that it caused a rare heart valve condition that allowed a backflow of blood into the heart chamber, leading to heart and lung di ... Subsequently, the U.S. Department of Health and Human Services issued preliminary recommendations for the medical management of people who took fenfluramine or dexfenfluramine; the guidelines were developed jointly by the FDA, the NIH, and the CDC.

OLD DEVICES

BREAST IMPLANTS The Public Citizen Health Research Group filed suit against the FDA in 1989 demanding that the agency release 30 years of research on the safety of implanted materials. The FDA argued that if voluntarily submitted documents were made public, manufacturers would be discouraged from doing safety studies and sharing the results with the government. Nevertheless, in 1990, a federal judge ordered the FDA to release Dow Corning's data summarizing the safety of silicone breast implants. A flurry of news reports followed. Finally, in November 1992, Dow Corning announced that it would make 300,000 documents available to the FDA without restriction within 30 days. This report acknowledged alteration of oven temperature charts dating from a 1992 inspection, but denied that these departures from Dow Corning's policies and procedures created any health risk. As of January 18, 1993, silicone inflatable breast prostheses, class III medical devices, required premarket approval.

TAMPONS In 1980, the American Society for Testing and Materials organized a task force to develop uniform absorbency testing and labeling at the FDA's request. The task force was disbanded in 1985 because no consensus on voluntary absorbency standards could be reached. That same year, in a lawsuit involving a death from TSS, the court awarded Playtex $10 million in punitive damages and then reduced the sum to $1.35 million when then company announced that it would no longer make tampons with polyacrylate fibers. Finally, in 1989, package labeling and absorbency testing regulations for tampons were published in the *Federal Register.*

PRENATAL RESEARCH

By the early 1980s amniocentesis could be used to assess the sex and maturity of the fetus and to diagnose around 90 prenatal health problems, including Down's syndrome, Tay-Sachs disease, and neural-tube defects.

In 1998, *The New England Journal of Medicine* published a study showing that a combination of two maternal blood indicators could predict the incidence of Down's syndrome in fetuses during the first trimester of pregnancy. That same year, manufacturers were allllowed to claim on the labels of grain products fortified with folate or folic acid that adequate intake of the nutrient has been shown to reduce the risk of neural-tube birth defects.

CANCER DETECTION AND TREATMENT

CERVICAL AND OVARIAN CANCER In 1992, problems of Pap smear classification were resolved by consensus recommendations of the American Cancer Society, the National Cancer Institute, the American Medical Association, and the American College of Obstetricians and Gynecologists. The so-called Bethesda system is the classification system accepted today in the United States. In 1995, the FDA approved new computer-assisted screening products to prepare specimens and select Pap smears for rereading. These devices can be used by laboratories as a quality-control tool to rescreen all normal Pap smears in order to detect cervical cancer more reliably. The system employs image processing and pattern-recognition techniques and can select the most suspicious cells for a second review by a cytotechnologist.

In July 1992, Taxol was approved for use by the FDA as an investigative new drug (IND) in the treatment of ovarian cancers. In a record-breaking five months, it was approved for general use in the treatment of advanced disease unresponsive to other therapies.

BREAST CANCER In 1986, the American Cancer Society and the American College of Radiation developed standards for physicians and technicians in mammography. In 1992 Congress passed the Mammography Quality Standards Act. As of October 1994, all mammography facilities have to be certified by FDA-approved accreditation bodies. To be certified, a facility must meet quality standards for x-ray images, equipment, and personnel and must be inspected annually. By early 1997, all U.S. facilities had been inspected at least once, and two-thirds had had their second annual inspection. Today there are over 10,000 certified mammography facilities in the United States.

In 1990, experts agreed that lumpectomy gave the same results as mastectomy in early-stage breast cancer if surgery was followed by radiation to kill any remaining cancer cells.

Two genes are linked to the occurrence of breast cancer: BrCa1 (discovered in October 1994) and BrCa2 (discovered in December 1996)(Breast Cancer 1).

In April 1996, the FDA approved the first blood test to help determine whether a woman's breast cancer has returned. The test measures a tumor marker that is found in the blood of patients with breast cancer and certain other types of cancer. In clinical studies, the new test accurately detected the breast cancer antigen in 60 percent of women who had a recurrence.

Also in April 1996, the FDA approved the use of Ultramark 9 High-Definition Imaging (HDI) ultrasound as an adjunct to mammography and physician breast exam. HDI enables doctors to distinguish solid tumors from fluid-filled ones and to judge whether the solid tumors are likely to be benign.

A year later, the National Cancer Institute announced that deaths from breast cancer had declined by 6.3 percent from 1991-1995, the first such decline since the 1930s.

In April 1998, the FDA approved Xeloda, a new oral treatment for advanced breast cancer patients who are resistant to other therapies.

WOMEN'S HEALTH EQUITY

In July 1977, the FDA issued its "Guidelines for the Format and Content of the Clinical Statistical Sections of New Drug Applications," which effectively precluded women's participation in the earliest stages of clinical drug trials. In the wake of the thalidomide crisis of the early 1960s, women had been routinely excluded from the earliest phases not only of new drug studies, but of other health research studies as well such as the Physicians' Health Study, which studied the effects of aspirin on heart disease in 22,000 male physicians. A major Rockefeller University study on the effects of estrogens on cancers of breast and uterus had even used male research subjects as their "normals." In 1982, the highly regarded Multiple Risk Factor Intervention Trial ("Mr. Fit") issued a report on the effect of lifestyle factors on cholesterol levels in 13,000 men. There is no corresponding study of women.

Representatives Patricia Schroeder, Olympia Snowe, and Henry Waxman set out to remedy this situation. In April 1990, they were instrumental in setting up hearings on women's health before the House Subcommittee on Health and the Environment. The hearings revealed that "the NIH has made little progress in implementing its policy to encourage the inclusion of women in research study populations." The policy had not been communicated to the scientific community and was not applied when reviewing grants for funding. NIH had also not collected any data on the actual inclusion of women in clinical studies. It acknowledged that only 13 percent of its funding was devoted to specific work on women's health issues. "NIH's attitude has been to consider over half the population as some kind of special case," Representative Snowe observed.

In the summer of 1990, the Women's Health Equity Act was introduced in Congress. Part of the legislation—the Breast and Cervical Cancer Mortality Prevention Act—was passed. The new law provided the states with funds through the Centers for Disease Control for Pap smears and mammography screening for low-income women. At the end of the summer, the NIH announced the creation of the Office of Research on Women's Health. The FDA established its Office of Women's Health in July 1994.

In February 1991, the NIH issued new policy requiring the inclusion of women and minorities in clinical research. All grant proposals for clinical studies must include women or have scientifically valid reasons for excluding them. That same month, Representatives Schroeder, Snowe, and Waxman request an investigation regarding the number of women included in FDA-regulated clinical studies of new drugs?

In October 1992, the Government Accounting Office issued a report on the inclusion of women in late-phase clinical drug trials ("Women's Health: FDA Needs to Ensure More Study of Gender Differences in Prescription Drug Testing"). The GAO concluded that FDA admonitions that new drugs be tested on "representative patient populations" were ill-defined and inconsistently applied by manufacturers. Although more than half of manufacturers surveyed reported that the FDA had asked them to include women in drug trials, one-quarter of drug manufacturers reported that they did not deliberately recruit women as participants. Hence, women were underrepresented in drug trials

In July 1993, the FDA issued "Guideline for the Study and Evaluation of Gender Differences in the Clinical Evaluation of Drugs," a revision of its 1977 guidelines, which were deemed to have discouraged women from taking part in the earliest stages of clinical investigation. The new guideline also called for an analysis of gender in judging the safety and effectiveness of drugs, biologics, and devices; it laid out broad areas for study, including the female hormonal environments, body size, body fat content and distribution, and metabolic phenotype.

In 1994, the Women's Health Initiative was launched, to increase spending on chronic diseases affecting females. As evidence showing the degree to which women had been excluded from basic research emerged, support for the initiative grew.

In September 1995, the FDA proposed a rule requiring clinical research sponsors to submitdata about gender, age, and race annually to the agency. Institutional review boards play a large role in regulating the balance of women and minorities in studies at universities and colleges. According to one board member, "Now if we see a study with only white men, we ask why before it ever gets started." The FDA conducted a workshop to clarify some basic concepts and principles pertaining to gender analysis entitled "Gender Studies in Product Development: Scientific Issues and Approaches."

In 1997, the Food and Drug Modernization Act was amended to encourage the inclusion of women in clinical trials. The era of considering the female population as a "special case" is over, at least for the moment.

Breaking the Walls of Silence: AIDS and Women in a Maximum State Prison

AIDS COUNSELING AND EDUCATION PROGRAM, BEDFORD HILLS CORRECTIONAL FACILITY

Excerpted from *Breaking the Walls of Silence: AIDS and Women in a New York State Maximum State Prison*. Woodstock, N.Y., Overlook Press, 1998Reprinted by permission.

I often ask myself how it is I came to be open about my status. For me, AIDS had been one of my best-kept secrets. I could not bring myself to say it out loud. As if not saying it would make it go away....

Somewhere behind the prison wall in Bedford Hills, a movement or community was being built. It was a diverse group of women teaming together to meet the needs and fears.... [They] believed that none of their peers should be discriminated against, isolated, or treated cruelly merely because they were ill.... They managed to build a community of women: Black, White, Hispanic, learned, illiterate, robbers, murderers, forgers, rich, poor, Christian, Muslim, Jewish, bisexual, gay, heterosexual—all putting aside their differences and egos for a collective cause.... Right before me a lay a model of how we, as a whole, needed to combat all the issues AIDS brought and we were building it from behind a wall, from prison. We were the community that no one thought would help itself....

AIDS IN PRISON

AIDS is the leading cause of death in prison in New York State prisons... [A]n estimated 17 to 20 percent of the 63,000 inmates in the Department of Correctional Services are infected with HIV; 8,000 have been definitely identified as HIV-positive....In [a] recent blind study of incoming inmates in New York State Correctional Facilities, the rate of HIV infection among women was twice that of men, 20.3 percent compared with 11.5 percent.

HOW ACE WAS CONCEIVED

We really didn't know a lot... Some of us leaned toward wanting the administration to be better about isolating people; others were concerned about supporting people who got sick. But the one thing we all shared was that we knew that our greatest enemy was fear and ignorance... We asked such things as was the laundry separated. There's a laundry where everyone sends their clothes to be washed. Although the clothes are in individual laundry bags, they are all washed together in one machine. One of the fears raised at the meeting was that maybe AIDS spread from clothes to clothes and what could be done about that?

THE BIRTH OF ACE

When Blackie first moved onto the floor, she could leave her cigarettes on a table and no one would touch them. And you know in here, people take things

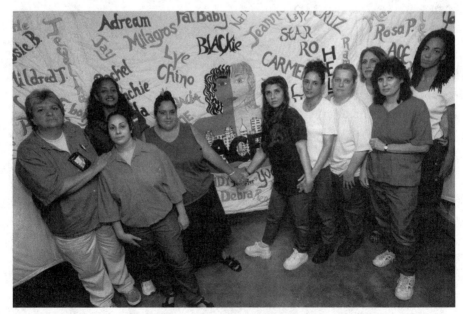

Members of the ACE staff at Bedford Hills Correctional Facility. [Carol Halebian]

that are left around, especially cigarettes—you can't ever forget a pack of cigarettes on a table because it won't be there when you go back for it. Then one day, Blackie came into the meeting so happy and told us, "They stole my cigarettes, they stole my cigarettes." She was so happy that now she was being treated like everyone else.

Women's Health Care in Prison

CASSANDRA SHAYLOR

Sherrie C. is a 41-year-old African-American woman who discovered a lump in her breast while in prison in 1984. Despite repeated requests for treatment, prison staff failed to diagnose her for ten years. By that point, the lump was visible through her clothes and the cancer had spread to her other breast and uterus. As a result of this medical neglect, Sherrie was forced to have a double mastectomy and a total hysterectomy. She has received no follow-up care and no pain medication.

Sherrie's story is not unique. Across the country women in prison face tremendous barriers to adequate health care and report a systematic pattern of medical neglect. Women's specific health needs, including routine gynecological care, are largely ignored. Serious illnesses, like Sherrie's cancer, often develop because prison officials fail to respond to complaints early. Pregnant women receive substandard prenatal care, and as a result experience avoidable complications and a high number of miscarriages; in many jurisdictions they are forced to give birth in shackles. Women do not receive regular treatment for chronic health problems like diabetes and heart disease, which often leads to serious complications and sometimes death. Prison officials are generally unwilling to address the spread and treatment of diseases like hepatitis and HIV, and as a result are creating a public health crisis inside.

The number of women effected by this medical mistreatment is growing rapidly. In this "tough on crime" political climate, with its increasing reliance on imprisonment as the catch-all solution to a wide range of social problems, women are the fastest growing population of people in prison. There are now approximately 150,000 women in prisons and jails in the U.S., compared to 10,000 only 20 years ago. More than 80 percent are serving time for nonviolent, property-, or drug-related crimes. Women of color are disproportionately represented in prison systems across the nation, comprising more than 60 percent of imprisoned women. As a result, a large number of the women who will suffer as a result of inadequate medical care will be women of color.

All of the problems confronting women generally are exacerbated by the prison system, which often fails to acknowledge even women's fundamental humanity. While women in general often feel alienated and infantilized by the medical care system, these feelings are even more profound in women in prison. While women on the outside (may) have a choice about their health care provider, women in prison do not. Furthermore, they are dependent on mostly male correctional officers for access to medical staff; these guards frequently disbelieve the women's assessments of their own health and accuse them of malingering. In addition, women prisoners often face sexual harassment and abuse by medical staff.

Mental health treatment inside is equally appalling; women are consistently over-medicated and ignored. Increasingly women are being confined for extended periods, sometimes for years, in solitary confinement, which often results in severe mental deterioration. Women prisoners are rarely provided any type of therapeutic counseling, though more than 60 percent have experienced some form of sexual or physical abuse at some point in their lives. They often report that the misogyny and abuse of the prison system amounts to a re-experience of that past trauma. In order for women's health care in prison to be adequately addressed, our definition of health must also include mental health and freedom from physical intimidation and violence.

People on the outside can provide vital links to women in prison. We can: provide information about women's health to prisoners; build grassroots campaigns to educate our communities about conditions inside; advocate for women's access to health care through legislatures and courts; and build coalitions with health care providers, student groups, women's groups, and human rights organizations to fight for women's rights to adequate health care, bodily integrity, and human dignity.

Putting Lesbian Health in Focus

VIVIEN LABATON

Vivien Labaton, "Putting Lesbian Health in Focus," *Ms.,* September/October 1998. Reprinted by permission.

During the heady days of the gay liberation movement in the early 1970s, Joan Waitkevicz, M.D., learned all too quickly that lesbians were not receiving adequate medical care despite gaining greater visibility: "Someone I knew of developed inoperable cancer of the cervix because she didn't feel she could go to a regular doctor for a Pap test."

Since 1974, when Waitkevicz and seven other lesbian health activists founded the St. Mark's Women's Health Collective in New York City—one of the first community-based clinics in the U.S. to offer care by and for lesbians—she has made it her priority as a physician to provide gay women with safe and comfortable medical environments. Today, she is the director of a first-of-its-kind hospital-based health center, the Gay Women's Focus (GWF) at Beth Israel Medical Center in New York City.

"Despite advances made in the private sector in the last 25 years, important barriers to health care for lesbians in the U.S. still persist," says Waitkevicz. Some include: homophobia and bias in doctors' offices and within institutions, fear and reluctance on the part of the patients to disclose their sexual orientation, and lack of training for health care providers on lesbians' particular health needs, such as donor insemination and treatment of sexually transmitted diseases. "For lesbians, the risk of sexually transmitted infections is different—not higher, but different," says Waitkevicz. "We have to ask a patient's sexual history in a nonjudgmental way, because ultimately, it's saving lesbian lives."

Run by three physicians and three staff members, GWF has seen approximately 2,000 patients since opening in 1997. On the future of GWF, Waitkevicz comments: "We're a little too new to start counting our successes, but I hope our work enables others to see its importance. I will be very happy when it's no longer needed, because that means we will have done our job educating our colleagues."

Lesbian Health Gains Long Due Attention from Institute of Medicine

AMY ALLINA

Amy Allina, "Lesbian Health Gains Long Due Attention from Institute of Medicine," *The Network News*, January/February 1999. Reprinted by permission.

In early January, the Institute of Medicine (IOM) released a study looking at the knowledge base and gaps in lesbian health research, *Lesbian Health: Current Assessment and Directions for the Future*. The IOM is a prestigious agency which carries great weight within the academic research community, and lesbian health advocates believe that the study will help establish the legitimacy of the field of lesbian health research. The fact that the IOM convened a committee to study lesbian health was in itself hailed as a breakthrough by lesbian health advocates. Though the committee's conclusion that more research into lesbian health is needed is not new to those who have followed the development of the lesbian health movement, it is ground-breaking for a mainstream institution to call for increased research attention to lesbian health.

HEIGHTENED RISK IS NOT ASSOCIATED WITH SEXUAL ORIENTATION ALONE

While noting that there is only limited research data available for a comparison of the health of lesbians with heterosexual women, based on the information that exists, "the committee did not find that lesbians are at higher risk for any particular health problem simply because they have a lesbian sexual orientation" (Executive Summary, p.5). Though some health problems may, in fact, be more prevalent among lesbians than heterosexual women, the committee asserts that increased incidence, where it exists, may be explained by other risk factors. The report cites several examples of this:

➤Breast cancer is more common in women who have not had children, and lesbians may be less likely than heterosexual women to bear children.

➤Lesbians often avoid seeking regular health care due to the homophobia they encounter from health care providers, and this reduced access could lead to an increased risk for some health problems.

➤As a result of their exposure to the stress effects of homophobia, lesbians may be more likely to experience stress-related health problems.

METHODOLOGICAL LIMITATIONS OF EXISTING LESBIAN HEALTH RESEARCH

The committee identified a number of methodological limitations with the research that has been done to date on lesbian health. First, and foremost, the lack of standard definition of what constitutes a lesbian limits the ability of researchers to compare findings from different studies. The IOM study notes that researchers working on lesbian health must consider the definition they will use in designing their studies and points out that "it should not be assumed that racial and ethnic minority cultures share views of lesbian sexual orientation identical with those of the dominant culture" (Executive Summary, p. 3.).

Another limitation of existing research on lesbian health is that most studies have been conducted using small samples of people who researchers found at bars, festivals, or through organizations. Most people in the studies have been white, middle-class, well-educated, and between 25 and 40 years old—not representative of the general lesbian population. Finally, very few studies have included control groups that would allow researchers to compare lesbian health to that of other subgroups of women, and there is almost no data tracking lesbian health over time.

HOMOPHOBIA CREATES ADDITIONAL CHALLENGES

In addition to the methodological challenges, the committee notes that homophobia creates another set of barriers to lesbian health research. Research institutions, research scientists, and research participants, all may fear being associated with a study that includes information about sexual orientation. Homophobia makes it difficult to find institutional support for lesbian health research, and there is very little money available for the work. There are few researchers working in the field, and those who are may have difficulty finding colleagues and mentors.

Researchers have reported political obstacles to conducting work on sexual behavior and have found it difficult to get their findings published. Homophobia also makes the confidentiality of research participants of critical importance, and lack of confidence in research confidentiality makes it harder to recruit people for studies.

PRIORITIES AND RECOMMENDATIONS FOR FUTURE RESEARCH

The committee established three priorities for future research on lesbian health. These are to gather more information about the physical and mental health status of lesbians, to determine how to define sexual orientation in general and lesbian orientation in particular, and to identify possible barriers to access to health care services for lesbians as well as ways to increase their access to these services.

Specifically, the committee recommended:
➤More public and private funding for lesbian health research, including a long-term federal commitment.
➤Finding for methodological research to improve the definition of lesbian sexual orientation.
➤The routine inclusion of questions about sexual orientations on data collection forms in relevant behavioral and biomedical studies, with pilot studies conducted first to assess the feasibility and impact of these types of questions.
➤When designing lesbian health research studies, researchers should consider the full range of racial, ethnic, and socioeconomic diversity among lesbians, include members of the study population in the development of the research, and give special attention to protecting the confidentiality and privacy of study participants.
➤Funding for a large-scale probability survey to determine the range of sexual orientation among all women and the prevalence of various risk and protective factors for health, by sexual orientation.
➤Increased dissemination of information about the conduct and results of lesbian health research.
➤The development and support by federal agencies, foundations, health professional associations, and academic institutions of mechanisms for information dissemination about lesbian health.
➤The development of strategies to train researchers in conducting lesbian health research.

You can obtain a copy of the IOM report by contacting the National Academy Press at 800-624-6242. Their Web site is www.nap.edu.

A Friend Indeed:
The Grandmother of Menopause Newsletters

SARI TUDIVER

IN THE BEGINNING...

A Friend Indeed was first conceived in 1983 by Janine O'Leary Cobb, a Canadian mother of five who taught sociology and humanities in Montreal. Approaching 50, Janine felt uncharacteristically tired, burned out, and increasingly unable to cope—symptoms that she finally realized were the effects of menopause. Her local medical library provided almost no helpful information. Janine vividly remembers coming across the printed lecture notes about menopause distributed to third-year medical students: "Well-adjusted women have no problem with menopause," it said. Just by asking a doctor about menopause, women would label themselves as maladjusted. Janine was outraged and decided to do something about it.

"I got the idea for a newsletter for menopausal women that could be both a source of information and a support group through the mail," Janine says. "Because menopause is a time when a woman often is in need, I called it *A Friend Indeed*. In April 1984, the first commercial issue of AFI was mailed to 40 women. A year later, word had spread and the newsletter had become a full-time occupation.

Demand grew and subscriptions have increased to thousands across North America and other parts of the world. While menopause has now become a popular topic in research and the press, AFI is recognized as "the grandmother of menopause newsletters." Offering helpful, well-researched, and balanced information about the litany of subjects that matter to women in mid-life—night sweats, gas and bloating, vaginal dryness, heart disease, menopausal migraine, hormone therapy, stress, and anger, among many others—AFI continues to flourish because it has a unique approach.

THE EXCHANGE

A key to the newsletter's success is its commitment that the voices of menopausal women be heard and taken seriously. "The Exchange" is a popular forum where women ask questions, receive responses from the editor or other readers, share concerns and personal experiences. Over the past 15 years, thousands of women have written to document their symptoms and feelings related to menopause and have described a variety of encounters with the health care system. The women's stories reveal frustrations, sometimes despair, along with creative approaches to solving problems. There is also a delightful and, at times, unexpected sense of humor.

The themes of the letters and inquiries have not changed dramatically over the years. For many women, there is relief at knowing others have felt the same way and that one's strange sensations... are not so strange after all:

"...With your help I feel that I have successfully navigated this particular 'sea of troubles.' I was fortunate that I was able to do so without additional help from the pharmaceutical companies, probably because I was aware that most of the strange things that were occurring were not unique to me. Others had gone through them and were still around to write about it. I now feel like a graduate with all the positive aspects of that term, and would like to thank you for your tutelage."

The women reveal a strong sense of respect for the normal, natural processes involved with the end of menstruation... a respect that is often lacking in the medical and research communities which commonly consider menopause a condition of hormone deficiency requiring treatment and manipulation. Women gain the courage to deal with care providers, to press for more details about a proposed test, hysterectomy, or a prescription, or to seek a second opinion.

"Several months have passed since I received your answer to my letter concerning my problem diagnosed as strophic vaginitis. I took your advice and made an appointment with a dermatologist. He advised me to stop using the cortisone and steroid creams. In his opinion the skin had become sensitive from prolonged use of the medications. He prescribed an anesthetic ointment. I followed those instructions and have had gradual but steady improvement... I very much appreciate your advice and especially for taking the time to write to me personally. I read every issue of *AFI* from cover to cover." (M.T.)

Over the years, women have posed many important questions that cannot be answered readily, given the limited state of research. These include queries on whether menopause might have unique effects on women with... chronic illnesses, cerebral palsy, or other disabilities. There are many questions from women who have experienced premature menopause (before the age of 40) and from women who have had severe menopausal symptoms induced by surgery, chemotherapy, or other treatments. These questions, grounded in women's complex medical and life histories, offer key insights into areas for future research. *AFI* offers a forum for women to share anecdotal insights and details about what therapies or approaches to self-care might have worked for them. As well, researchers and practitioners often write in with comments and suggestions.

Through "The Exchange" women are referred to other resources or are offered suggestions that they can explore on their own or with a care provider. While all letters are confidential, some women ask to be put in touch with others. If both agree, they correspond directly, and lasting friendships have emerged through *A Friend Indeed*. Each woman is seen as an individual who experiences menopause in her own unique way. This is in contrast to the blanket approach espoused by the pharmaceutical industry and many health providers who promote the latest pills for all, often unattuned to a woman's deeper concerns and needs.

Many women are able to solve some of their problems through research and reading. One woman described what she learned:

"I have found this publication to be extremely helpful and I have kept every issue so that I can share the information with my friends and doctors. While reading about other women and their problems, I began to realize that although we may all share some of the problems, every case is unique.

"I started feeling different when I was 52. My periods were regular, but I was very tired all the time and would get anxiety attacks while working at my job. I started hormone replacement therapy at that time and continued for six years. Although I tried various brands of estrogen, each and every one caused the same side effect—nausea. I can only describe it as having morning sickness every day of my life. About 18 months ago, I read your book *Understanding Menopause,* and there, on page 95, I discovered that every estrogen pill contains lactose. I am lactose intolerant. My doctors were totally unaware that lactose was used as a filler in these medications." (S.F.)

TRACKING THE RESEARCH

In addition to "The Exchange," there are lead articles and "Hot Flashes" (research updates) in each issue of AFI. These provide a more in-depth, documented look at a particular topic. Some of the most popular back issues focus on alternative, nonhormonal approaches to menopause and aging, as well as the pros and cons of hormone therapy.

A Friend Indeed also helps track and explain the many unresolved controversies surrounding the research into and treatment of menopause. It offers women critical tools to better understand the "hard" science of clinical trials and research about hormones, breast cancer, heart disease, and osteoporosis; to separate sound science from promotional hype; and to sift through what is currently known with some confidence from claims where evidence may be weak. *AFI* urges women to be informed, careful consumers whether considering more mainstream or alternative, complementary approaches and to read media and promotional information with great care.

AFI has often been on the "cutting edge' in identifying important research. As one reader recently noted, *AFI* "scooped the mainstream *New England Journal of Medicine*" by publishing an article almost a year earlier about alternative approaches to treatment of thyroid conditions for people not responding well to standard treatments. The newsletter also takes a critical "watchdog" approach to the pharmaceutical industry and its marketing practices. *AFI* takes no money from the pharmaceutical industry.

LOOKING AHEAD

> Menopause can be an interval,
> a closure, a threshold, a gateway...
> all of these things and more.
> —Janine O'Leary Cobb

Menopausal women have a tremendous capacity to widen their horizons and understandings. The menopausal years can be a time to reassess one's life, lay aside unresolved issues, and look forward to what the future may hold. Ideally it should be a time to share pleasures with those we care about and to find humor in the challenges of daily life.

Women are faced with pressures from many sources urging them "to make decisions about hormones" and a wide variety of other therapies. There is a vast amount of information to evaluate and absorb. The challenge is to remain afloat in the sea of information and heavily promoted products: to carefully evaluate the claims to what is known in order to develop strategies for good health and well being. There are many things we already know that are good for us all: nutritious food, pleasurable activity and exercise, a safe environment free from violence and poverty and satisfaction in our personal relationships. *A Friend Indeed* is a resource supporting women along this path to a deeper understanding of ourselves as we age.

To find out more about *A Friend Indeed: The Newsletter for Women in the Prime of Life,* write to PO Box 260, Pembina, ND 58271-0260; www.afriendindeed.ca

Out of Pain and Anger

MARILYN WEBB

Expanded from Marilyn Webb, "Out of Pain and Anger," which originally appeared in *Self,* March 1999. Reprinted by permission.

A t the White Hart Inn in Salisbury, Connecticut, a woman my mother's age hangs back from the departing crowd. She whispers to me, still stricken that she could do so little for her husband as he was dying. She felt powerless to get doctors to carry out his medical wishes, even to have them tell him the truth. "He knew he was dying, but he wanted information on what would happen," she said. "His doctors would all look away."

In New York City, another woman says her sister in a nursing home is physically threatened by the staff. If her sister were to go home, her children couldn't afford the help they'd need to give her the proper care. She pleads with me to help her find a good place; she can turn up nothing.

In Florida, a young man is weeping. He still has nightmares about how his partner died writhing in pain, his doctors unwilling, or unable, to give him the narcotic medication he needed. He and his family wonder why. And so do I.

All these people have come to hear talks I have been giving upon the publication of my book, *The Good Death,* a journalist's view, based on more than six years of research and cross-country reporting, of how we die in America. They have also come to tell stories of their own, most of them tales of personal tragedy, pain and fury. Talking about dying has been like lighting a match in a room filled with gas.

These are tales of ordinary Americans—mothers, fathers, grandparents, children, husbands, wives, sisters, brothers, and lovers—and in them I hear a new kind of anger, the voice of an enormous lack of empowerment in the face of modern medicine, the despair of having failed loved ones at a critical point in life, and not for lack of trying.

This is the terrible atmosphere in which many Americans now die. Yet as these stories have accumulated over the past year I have sensed the birth of a new grassroots movement for change, which in remarkably similar ways has the excitement of the early days of the women's movement.

Like that movement, this one is fueled by personal tales that, taken together, paint a much larger political picture. The members of this movement do not necessarily agree on how changes should be made, but together they are developing the language, tools, community programs, and networks to change the culture of dying.

The issues are ones of empowerment, the voices of patients and families struggling to change modern dying as natural childbirth has changed modern birth. By and large, this new movement rings out of the passions of women in their role as family caregivers, only now in later stages of life. This movement portends to be just as powerful as that one that went before it, generated often by the very same people, asking the very same questions. Now medicine has changed life at the end of life and this same generation has grown older.

FACING THE EVIDENCE

The way we die today is historically unprecedented, yet dying has changed so fast—in just one generation's time—that it has left us scrambling culturally to catch up. At the turn of the last century we died quickly of infectious or parasitic diseases and there wasn't much doctors could do to postpone life. Enter antibiotics, the watershed miracle born along with the baby boomers. Since then, a near avalanche of medical advances has added an extra generation of time to life, but it has also transformed dying into a long-term affair. Today's major killers—cancer, heart disease, stroke—are all illnesses with which we can live for many years, but these are years filled with difficult symptoms and choices.

No longer at issue is whether doctors are "doing everything possible," but when and how treatment should wind down, questions none of our religious, family, or medical institutions are prepared for. Research confirms what the public already knows: 70 to 90 percent of us now die when some decision is made either to withhold or withdraw such treatment as drugs, respirators, or feeding tubes. Yet, the questions remain: Who decides? And how?

Hospitals, once places to treat pneumonia or appendicitis or to go to die, are now just short stops in the turnstile of modern dying. This new path involves roller-coaster crises that take us in and out of medical centers, with long gaps in between. We stay home, grow weaker, and ultimately need more and more care.

Physicians are not fully trained to address the staggering symptoms of lengthy declines. In 1995, the sorry findings began to appear of an eight-year, $28 million study, dubbed Support, of 10,000 seriously ill patients—5,000 of whom eventually died—in five teaching hospitals across the United States. To researchers' shock, 50 percent of the dying suffered moderate to severe pain, 31 percent had signed documents saying they preferred that CPR be withheld, yet 53 percent of their doctors didn't know that.

Other studies have come up with similar findings. A world-renowned pain research team at the University of Wisconsin found in studies of cancer patients that more than 40 percent of them suffered long-term and undertreated pain. A study at Memorial Sloan-Kettering Cancer Center in New York City found undertreated pain in nearly 85 percent of AIDS patients. Almost half of this pain might have been alleviated with stronger drugs. And pain wasn't the only symptom. Other Sloan-Kettering research showed that hospitalized cancer patients suffered an average of 13 intolerable symptoms; AIDS patients averaged 18. Doctors weren't trained to address many of these symptoms.

These findings have since shaken the medical community into retraining doctors and nurses in better care for the dying and inspired state legislatures into initiatives on better pain management and improved ways of thinking about advanced directives.

Yet, a little-reported part of the Support study may be even more devastating to patients and families. More than half of the families studied suffered a major crisis in caring for a loved one. Thirty-four percent of the patients needed large amounts of family caregiving, causing 31 percent of the families to lose most of their savings, 29 percent to lose a major source of income, and 29 percent to require a major life change for another family member. In 12 percent, another family member became seriously ill from the stress of the intensive caregiving required.

Surprisingly, all these patients had health insurance, yet the impact of their illness on families was extreme. It should come as no shock to anyone that most of these caregivers were women who are now struggling to care for ill relatives, while at the same time bringing in much-needed family income, caring often for children at the same time they are now caring not just for one, but — as we live longer—of *two* generations of aging family members. This is a major women's issue of our time. It will peak into the next century as more boomers become chronically ill and aging themselves and, as their numbers mount, it becomes woefully obvious how inadequate the American health care system now is to address the way of life in long-term, modern dying.

Illness and dying are far more complicated than ever before, yet this is a generation that has already lived through the transformations of natural child-birth and the ongoing abortion wars. It believes in autonomy and choice. At the same time, the dying and their loved ones are beginning to look for answers beyond the clinic and the hospital, sometimes, in the bargain, land-ing in the international news.

In 1990, Jack Kevorkian, M.D., the notorious Michigan pathologist, helped Alzheimer's patient Janet Adkins die in the back of his rusty Volkswagen van. After he started a saline solution going, she activated his famous suicide machine, which first sent a sedative, then deadly potassium chloride to her heart. Since then and even after Dr. Kevorkian's medical license was taken away, after he resorted to using carbon monoxide for some of his patients, and finally in 1999 landed in jail for directly injecting lethal medications into Lou Gehrig's disease patient Thomas Youk on CBS's *60 Minutes,* polls have consis-tently shown that between 65 and 75 percent of the public supports physician-assisted suicide.

Those who oppose legalization of assisted suicide argue on ethical, reli-gious, or legal grounds, and say they fear it may lead to patient abuse. Some see redemption in suffering, or fear abuse should their care be compromised to the oppressive weight of medical cost-cutting. And of course there are oth-ers who believe the reverse: that it is a matter of choice, that abuse, like back alley abortion, will come from keeping assisted suicide illegal, or that legaliza-tion will prevent Lone Ranger tactics like Kevorkian's and create fail-safe guidelines for states and medical institutions to use to guard patients against private suffering.

Yet, those national studies cited above give clues to why there is strong public support for legalization. Government policy and the prickly atmos-phere surrounding the practice of medicine have only compounded the prob-lem. Drug laws in a "Just Say No" culture can prevent pain medications from reaching the dying. Doctors, fearing retaliation from medical licensing boards and federal agencies, tend to underprescribe. Medical insurance covers acute hospital care but not the very long-term care many ill people now require. Managed care has all too often taken medical decision-making away, not only from patients and families, but also from doctors. Doctors, patients, and fam-ilies are all suffering under the ironic burdens of medicine's great success.

CONSUMERS TAKE CHARGE

In Denver in May 1998, I attended a statewide meeting of the Colorado Collaboration on End-of-Life Care, a coalition of doctors, nurses, hospice volunteers, AIDS workers, clergy, and everyday people brought together by their common desire to change how Colorado cares for its dying.

This group is just one of many that has now begun organizing to address the critical state of end-of-life care. At their meeting I heard talk about the issues that are troubling many, many people across the country: how to improve hospitals and nursing homes, how to make living wills carry more weight in health care institutions, how to make hospice care, with its focus on pain management, comfort, and spiritual closure, available to more people.

Members of the clergy mused about how to address psycho-spiritual concerns, especially in an era of near-death-experience spirituality. Everyone wanted to change state drug laws that inhibit doctors' prescribing pain medications.

There were also private concerns. A member of the generation whose men never changed their children's diapers wept quietly, remembering how he changed his dying wife's bedding, how long this went on, how humiliated she was and how terribly lonely they both felt. A man who had AIDS said prisons are filled with men and women with AIDS and that hospices there are sorely needed. Both men wanted policies changed, as did the majority of women in attendance at that meeting, but they also wanted to create support groups that would provide the everyday help they wished had been given to them when they needed it.

One major reason such groups as the Colorado Collaboration are cropping up across the country is that their ideas have been funded over the past few years by a handful of generous charitable foundations, which share their vision of reshaping the American culture of dying. Since the late 1980s, when it gave $28 million to fund the Support study, the Robert Wood Johnson Foundation (RWJF), catalyzed by that national study's dismal findings, has spent nearly $50 million on changing end-of-life medical care, from education on proper pain management to raising public awareness through dialogue groups and media projects.

Beginning in 1999, another multi-million-dollar RWJF-funded initiative poured money into community-state partnership grantee coalitions in each state, adding to its Last Acts Campaign to mobilize American health care organizations nationally. A four-part, RWJF-funded Bill Moyers special on dying is scheduled for fall of the year 2000.

Philanthropist George Soros' Open Society Institute inaugurated the Project on Death in America in New York in 1994, and since then has given some $15 million to help transform the experience of dying through research, scholarship, the arts and humanities, and education.

The thousands of community projects now emerging will, in the end, have the most profound effect. Some are new consumer advocacy organizations such as Americans for Better Care of the Dying and the Partnership for Caring. Others are volunteer efforts, begun by people who brushed shoulders with grief and came away with a vision of change.

THE NEXT STEPS

If we can learn anything from the abortion wars, it will be that choice and diversity matter. We are a diverse nation with as many different cultural and religious views of dying as we have of living—and all of it matters! If we divide over this issue, fighting each other, we risk failing to alter a medical care system that has outlived its capacity to care for the ill under today's conditions for modern dying. Medicine has now given us the gift of time. It's how we make use of it that counts. Not to honor, legalize, support, or address the diverse ways each of us wants to make use of this time will only leave us flailing in battle, no one getting desperately needed care.

Dying is a sacred, not just a medical event. But medicine has so complicated our life at the end of life that we do not address or understand the complexities involved until we are in the midst of personal and family chaos. It behooves us all to think and plan ahead. Since the publication of *The Good Death*—and inspired by the voices and stories I have heard on my travels—I've helped begin a nonprofit organization, The Good Death Initiative Inc., to build an educational campaign to change how each of us understand and care for our own dying in the very villages and cities where we live.

We plan to hold public events called Town Meetings Across America on Death and Dying. My partners are Barbara Maltby, a movie producer, who helped make *Ordinary People,* and Paul Brenner, a New York hospice director, as well as other doctors, media people, attorneys, ethicists, and entertainers. We intend to go city to city, town to town, to explore what it means to make choices at the end of life, to empower communities to expand support to patients and families, to talk about the visionary programs we have heard about.

The following groups suggest a range of the enlightened resources now available. I hope that in addition to the political efforts now taking place to change state and national law, in addition to the retraining medical personnel are now receiving to reshape the way they give care, that these groups will inspire similar efforts in more communities around the country. If nothing else, what they are showing us is that a massive grassroots effort to change our healthcare system and how we all care for the dying is already here. Not surprisingly, much of is being led and/or inspired by women, often the same women who transformed American culture and healthcare once before.

LIVES RECORDED FOR POSTERITY

In the small university town of Missoula, Montana, the Missoula Demonstration Project's Life Story Task Force has instituted a pilot effort to focus the town's citizens on what might dramatically improve the care of the dying. Among its most welcomed programs is Gathering Life Stories, whose aim is to help those who are dying to leave a family legacy.

Volunteers are trained to sit down with people in hospitals, hospices, nursing homes, senior centers, and housing projects and interview them there, recording and writing their life stories. Preliminary studies show that these sessions not only engender a sense of meaning in the lives elders have led, but also reduce their sadness and stress.

LAUNDRY HELPERS

Auntie Helen's Fluff 'n' Fold, in San Diego, a free volunteer-run laundry service for men, women, and children who are ill with AIDS, was inspired by the simple idea that everyone should be able to die in a clean, dry bed. The service was named after the great-aunt of its founder, the late Gary Cheatham. "Gary had a friend named Ronnie," says executive director Bob Stanley, "who was so ill his laundry had piled up in a corner of his room. Gary picked it up, washed it and brought it back. After that he got a washing machine for his garage and began doing laundry for other people who were sick with AIDS."

That was in 1988. Now the nonprofit organization has eight commercial washers and nine dryers and does 1,500 loads of laundry a month for approximately 350 clients, with a 24-hour pickup and return time. "We have volunteers from every sector," Stanley says. "Senior citizens, people affected by HIV, the physically or emotionally challenged, college students. It makes everyone feel better to help others feel good. You know how a nice fresh pair of pajamas or clean sheets feel? Well, when you're so sick, they feel *really* great!"

PET VISITATION

I remember the day Maverick, a golden retriever, paid a visit to Hospice House, the residential unit of Hope Hospice in Fort Myers, Florida. He walked through the halls as though he owned them, greeting everyone as he wagged his tail. Then he lifted his leg and peed on the nurses' station. "Oh well," said the nurse to the dog's embarrassed human companion, "that's what hospice is all about." Maverick went on licking and nuzzling the dying, room by room, a working dog on a Wednesday afternoon.

Hope Hospice has six dog teams and one cat team. Some of these "therapy dogs" work in nursing homes; some visit in patients' homes. "There are studies that show that people who have pets live longer lives," says Melissa Mehlum, the volunteer coordinator. "It helps our patients, the touch, the smell, the company, the petting, the caregivers and our staff."

Deaths take a toll on the animals as well as the people they comfort, according to Deni Elliott, who runs S.T.A.R. Dogs, a similar program of volunteers in hospices, hospitals and nursing homes in Missoula, Montana. "Dogs understand death a lot better than people do," says Elliott. "We think dogs should be given a chance to see the person as dead, to go to the funeral so the dog understands that the person has died. There should be continuity with the hospice team so the dog does not feel a sense of continual loss."

Hope Hospice's dog and cat teams—all pets and their owners who want to volunteer by visiting at the hospice—are trained and certified locally. A national registration program is offered by Delta Society.

ASSISTED-SUICIDE SUPPORT

The terminally ill can buy Derek Humphry's bestseller, *Final Exit* (Dell), to find out what drugs to take to end life, but unless physician-assisted suicide is legalized in the state where they live, they, and any loved ones who help them, run the risk of criminal charges. Sadly, they and many others who suffer, whether or not they take such steps, are left to die alone.

Enter Compassion in Dying, founded in Seattle in 1993 by minister Ralph Mero, but now led by Barbara Coombs Lee, a former hospice nurse and now an attorney, and staffed by health care workers, volunteers, and clergy. Its philosophy: No one should have to die alone, no matter what she is dying of or how.

Compassion in Dying is best known for having brought the suits to legalize assisted suicide to the Supreme Court and for helping to pass the nation's first assisted-suicide law, in Oregon. The court battle was led by dynamo attorney Kathryn Tucker, and the Oregon law's most visible craftsman and public champion was Barbara Coombs Lee.

The group started as a nonprofit service organization to provide non-judgmental information and emotional support to the terminally ill, making house visits, bringing in professionals to assess whether additional pain medications or hospice support might be needed, and, if it is a patient's final choice, to give advice about lethal medications and sit with those who ultimately decide to take them.

Paradoxically, the strict guidelines covering assessment of need that Compassion helped draft for the Oregon assisted-suicide law have resulted in improved care of the dying throughout the state's health care system. Some 30 percent of all Oregonians now die with the help of a hospice, as opposed to 14 to 21 percent in the rest of the country; more die at home than in hospitals; and Oregon's medical use of morphine has increased by 70 percent, making it one of the states with the highest morphine use for treating the terminally ill.

For those who believe in assisted suicide as a rational choice for the terminally ill or when all other palliative care measures do not work, or for those who only want to help with assessment and service support groups, Compassion in Dying can provide start-up materials.

GOURMET DINNER FOR CAREGIVERS

Suzanne Mintz, president of the National Family Caregivers Association, says that 80 to 90 percent of all at-home caring for the chronically ill and disabled in the U.S. is provided by family members. This caregiving includes helping a loved one with cooking, cleaning, shopping, health care tasks, legal and financial matters, and giving huge amounts of emotional support. Studies show that the altruistic daughters, mothers, husbands, and partners of the dying who provide virtually round-the-clock care tend to suffer high levels of depression, frustration, and anxiety. When someone is dying, caregivers also grieve day by day. They need small respites. They need help.

The First Presbyterian Church in Annapolis, Maryland, like many churches and synagogues, has created a year-round caregivers program for its members, capped by an annual Caregivers Night Out. Often-isolated caregivers around town are invited to a gourmet dinner served by tuxedoed waiters. Someone is found to stay with the person who is ill, another to drive the caregiver to and from the event.

Church volunteers have also prepared a local resource guide for caregiver help, formed a support committee, and set up a squad of drivers to run errands for caregivers. All it takes is a car and a little time to help out a caregiver who might like to go out for a manicure or a long walk.

Good Mourning, America

AMY PAGNOZZI

Amy Pagnozzi, "Good Mourning, America," *MAMM,* October/November, 1998. Reprinted by permission.

When Betty Rollin's breast cancer recurred 14 years ago, she never seriously considered the possibility she might die. Oh, she was scared, all right. But it was a generalized terror, not one that manifested itself in the living wills, powers of attorney, or advanced directives she advocates now as the vice president of Death with Dignity National Center, a San Mateo, California based educational organization working to improve care for terminally ill patients and to decriminalize a patient's choice to die with a physician's aid. "I... never for myself," Rollin stammers, flummoxed, when asked if she considered it herself. "I mean, who wants to think about death unless they absolutely have to?" While recovering from each of her two bouts with cancer, her fears were usurped by a pure joy, unalloyed by mortal intimations. "I'm alive and I feel great and aren't I lucky and on with life" is how Rollin, newswoman for NBC for more than 25 years, describes this feeling.

But her utter lack of morbidity does set her apart, given that she's one of this country's leading physician-aid-in-dying advocates. Imagine the welcome Death with Dignity's executives must have given the much-respected and poised Rollin in 1994, knowing what wonders her authoritative and pleasant persona could bring to a debate that's veered toward the hysterical since Jack

Kevorkian took center stage. Bear in mind, even Derek Humphry's landmark right-to-die manual *Final Exit* was too much for some (chapter 19: "Self-Deliverance Via the Plastic Bag"). Death is a delicate subject, something that Rollin hadn't really considered before being forced to, 15 years ago, when her mother Ida was dying of ovarian cancer.

Her activism began accidentally. She was asked to help her mother and she did: It was no volunteer effort. "I've had a wonderful life, but now it's over," Ida Rollin told her daughter. Two and a half years after her diagnosis, she couldn't keep food down, walk, control her bladder or bowels. She'd been game enough to fight when there was hope—enduring eight months of punishing chemotherapy, then more, after a recurrence. Rather than wither away after her husband had died and her daughter was grown, she'd learned piano, joined a theater, made new friends, even taken a lover. "I'm not saying it couldn't be worse," she told Betty. "I know how some people suffer. But to me… life is taking a walk, visiting my children, eating! If I had life, I'd want it. I don't want this."

Betty and her mathematician husband, Harold M. Edwards ("Ed"), felt lost. It was 1983 and information about assisted dying was scarce. Humphry's *Final Exit* and its lethal-dosage charts were not yet available; there was no Internet to browse for cyanide recipes; and legislation suggesting doctors should help people die wasn't even pending.

Misinformation, on the other hand, was rampant. A doctor in New York City hinted, before hanging up abruptly, that Dalmane (flurazepam), a hypnotic agent used for insomnia, alone could be fatal—which was unlikely. A nurse had offered to show Betty's mother how to use a hypodermic, so she could create an air embolism—which might kill her or might merely blow out some brain cells. The Netherlands was one of the few places where assisted dying was permitted, and that's where they found the sole doctor who offered them accurate advice—an American-born friend-of-a-friend who provided drug information.

Luckily for Ida, Betty and Ed were only vaguely aware of the Kafkaesque scenarios that could befall her if they "botched" it, otherwise they might have put off acting until the matter was out of their hands. "People ask us, 'What was going through your mind?' But until the end, there was nothing," Betty says. "We were too afraid to be emotional, because if we got emotional it might upset her stomach, and then she wouldn't be able to keep the pills down and she'd wind up suffering more."

Wearing full makeup and a new flowered nightie, Ida Rollin downed two anti-anxiety drugs: one Compazine (prochlorperazine), prescribed for nausea, and then 20 Nembutal (pentobarbital sodium), the lethal part of the prescription cocktail. Then came five Dalmane. "I want you to know that I am a happy woman," she said before getting sleepy. "I made a man happy for 40 years, and I gave birth to the most wonderful child, and later in life I had another child [Ed] whom I love as if I had given birth to him too. No one has been more blessed than I. I've had a wonderful life, and this is my wish." She fell unconscious almost immediately, and hours later, Ida died peacefully in her own bed.

And her daughter Betty has "never had a bad moment" about what she did because "we pulled it off, we made this thing happen, she escaped from life." She thought she would write a book as a tribute to her mother and forget about it. But that's not how things turned out. Although death was neither a fascination nor her life's work, before and after the book, *Last Wish,* was published in 1985, she was up to her neck in it. (Public Affairs is reissuing the book in paperback this September.)

Rollin, you probably already know, was breast cancer's first-ever "It" girl, a title she's held since her breast cancer memoir, *First, You Cry,* was published in 1976. But even documenting her battle with breast cancer, her mastectomy, her leaving her first husband for a new love, and her unsuccessful search for the perfect prosthetic breast (she ended up cruising a drapery store with a pair of scissors, snipping off kitchen curtain pom-poms for nipples), didn't make Rollin flinch, even afterward. She's a boldly honest, resolute optimist. She gives a stock lecture on the "bright side" of breast cancer, which was not altered a whit by a recurrence and second mastectomy more than a decade ago. Rollin's attitude is rooted in an extraordinary sense of perspective that never lets her lose sight of others' misery. It would not be oversimplifying to state that *Last Wish,* similarly, is about the bright side of death, since it is the story of Rollin's mother's triumph over pain and suffering. However, not everyone sees it from that angle.

In some minds, the publication of *Last Wish* transformed Rollin overnight from a shining icon for survivors into "that woman who killed her mother." She even got disinvited from several hospitals where she'd been scheduled to do her cheery breast cancer lectures, after a board member or some such figure realized Rollin had written *Last Wish.* Nonetheless, the book shot up the bestseller lists, outdoing even *First, You Cry.* Ida Rollin the entrepreneur would have liked that. But no, for the notoriety, the Rollin the mother would have told her daughter that it wasn't worth it.

Betty expected a minor fuss over the fact that she'd researched guns, carbon monoxide, and poison on Ida's behalf—but not the storm she was facing, which has never completely settled. A review of her book on the front page of the *Washington Post* suggested she might soon be indicted for murder. It wasn't true—the most she could be charged with in New York was criminally assisting a suicide—but it was interesting enough for Barbara Walters to come calling. Magazines put her on their covers, and the book became a network TV movie.

But it was only after letters began pouring in by the thousands that Rollin realized she had hit a nerve and accomplished more than simply sharing "a powerful story about someone who happened to be my mother."

"Oh, I didn't think anyone else felt this way" or "I didn't think anyone went through this," wrote the daughters and sons, sisters and brothers, husbands and lovers. Their sense of relief that Rollin had again broken the silence on a taboo subject, as she had done with breast cancer, was palpable. "Me, too," said the letters. "My mother in County Clare is just like your mother." "My mother in Kyoto is just like your mother." Usually when they told their stories, Rollin says, "it didn't seem to me to be like my story at all," but she know she had struck a chord. The writers, most of them anguished over what they had or had not done, wanted desperately to share their experience, and Rollin had been chosen.

An activist was born, reluctantly. "Assisting my mother to die really worked for my family, but I now know that this is absolutely not something families should be doing," Betty, still startlingly youthful at 62, said recently in her sunny, Park Avenue penthouse. "You need a professional to help you, you need [to go to] a doctor. It's eminently sensible and merciful." Rollin continues to talk about death these days because "there are a lot of people in this country who think physician aid-in-dying is a bad idea, so I feel I am needed." Most of the people who feel that way "just don't get it," because it's never happened to them.

Her expectations for the movement are modest, and even if they weren't, this isn't exactly the sort of cause you wrap a ribbon around ("A nice noose-shaped twist of twine for that lapel, ma'am?"). Rollin reckons that it will be a long time before any kind of physician-assisted death is legal throughout the entire country, given that the U.S. Supreme Court has tossed the debate back to the state courts. She suspects California could be next to allow doctors to prescribe lethal prescriptions and Michigan might conceivably follow. So far, Oregon is still the only state where the dying can be helped by their doctors. Since November 4, 1997, 10 people have received lethal prescriptions, nine of whom were cancer patients. Eight used these prescriptions for self-deliverance and the other two died naturally of their diseases. Rollin wishes the act, basically limited to a prescription—"a piece of paper"—was a bit wider in scope so that it included some kind of provision for people who cannot swallow pills. But given that there wasn't even a Death With Dignity organization until 1994, the movement has come a long way. The public's consciousness has been raised.

"People don't have to go around thinking about death all the time to understand this issue," Rollin says. "I do think when they are called upon to vote on this issue, they might think how they would feel if they were at the end of life and suffering greatly and wanting to escape and not being able to." She's no zealot. Unlike some colleagues, she's "often thought that people who are against legal aid-in-dying are less cruel than inexperienced." As she wrote in a new introduction to *Last Wish*, "Many people, luckier than they know, have never had their bodies turned into torture chambers. Many people believe the myth that pain can (always) be stopped by drugs. Drugs are amazing, but they don't work equally well for everybody."

Before Ida Rollin actually asked her daughter for assistance in her death, she used this metaphor: "I'm locked in a room and I don't know where the key is." And Betty thinks that legislation addressing assisted suicide is "insurance" more than anything. "Look, intellectually, if I am ever in this situation, I want a choice," Rollin declares. "I just don't particularly expect to be in this situation."

Old Women Beware of Chemical Restraints

JOHN WYKERT

Excerpted from *Psychiatric News,* 1972.

Women, the principal consumers of mood-changing drugs, are more and more at risk as the years pass. In 1971, the American College of Neuropsychopharmacology published *Psychotropic Drugs in the Year 2000: Use by Normal Humans.* Reviewing the book for a sociology journal, I focused on the tranquilization and overmedication of (mostly female) nursing home residents. I wrote:

"The psychopharmacologists are dreaming of tomorrow and boy, have they ever got pharmaceutical plans for us! Their envisioned treatment may accomplish, within the next generation, what Aldous Huxley predicted in 1959: "a pharmacologic method of making people love their servitude and producing a dictatorship without tears, a kind of painless concentration camp of entire societies."

Older women, beware. One doctor proposes we find drugs that would give the elderly feelings of achievement. For the golden twilight years, he suggests putting them to sleep three to five times a week, feeding them small amounts of food and allowing them to wake up for one or two days. For waking days, he suggests a stimulant, perhaps a mild hallucinogen, to enhance their experiences (they might work or go to the opera) and keeping them alert.

Today, the inevitable nightmare is known as the "era of lifestyle drugs." Treatment goals have changed; it is no longer a matter of treating a disease, but of "enhancing life." Drugs are increasingly advertised directly to the public and, consequently, many doctors prescribe what patients think they need. Doctors prescribe drugs for uses not cleared by the FDA or keep prescribing after the first warning signals—witness fen-phen, a once-popular diet pill combination associated with fatal heart valve problems. Women were the victims there and females over 50 in particular remain entirely too vulnerable to medical malpractice in all forms of prescription writing.

In Defense of Shere Hite

SARAH J. SHEY

©1999 by Sarah J. Shey. Original for this publication.

In 1987, cultural historian and researcher Shere Hite presented results of a groundbreaking survey, *Women and Love: A Cultural Revolution in Progress,* to great animosity. It was her third of a trilogy, the first two being *The Hite Report on Female Sexuality* (1976) and *The Hite Report on Male Sexuality* (1981). Commenting on Hite's widespread influence, Naomi Weisstein, scientist and author of *How Psychology Constructs the Female* , wrote: "These books comprise complex and fascinating portraits of a crucial 15-year period in American culture—a period in which society came into an extraordinary confrontation with the traditional ideas of home and family."

The media scrutinized Hite's training, her methodology, her penmanship, her ringlet hair, but dismissed quite easily her findings collected from 4,500 women, who, by and large, yearned for independence, emotionally satisfying relationships with men, and equality at work and at home. In the following excerpt from *Backlash*, Pulitzer Prize-winning journalist Susan Faludi explores Hite's struggle with the press.

"The picture that has emerged of Shere Hite in recent weeks is that of a pop-culture demagogue," the November 23, 1987, issue of *Newsweek* informed its readers, under the headline "Men Aren't Her Only Problem." Shere Hite had just published the last installment of her national survey on sexuality and relationships, *Women and Love: A Cultural Revolution in Progress*, a 922-page compendium. The report's main findings: Most women are distressed and despairing over the continued resistance from the men in their lives to treat them as equals. Four-fifths of them said they still had to fight for rights and respect at home, and only 20 percent felt they had achieved equal status in their men's eyes. Their quest for more independence, they reported, had triggered mounting rancor from their mates.

This was not, however, the aspect of the book that the press chose to highlight. The media were too busy attacking Hite personally. Most of the evidence they marshaled against her involved tales, that as *Newsweek* let slip, "only tangentially involve her work." Hite was rumored to have punched a cabdriver for calling her "dear" and phoned reporters claiming to be Diana Gregory, Hite's assistant. Curious behavior, if true, but one that suggests a personality more eccentric than demagogic. Nonetheless, the nation's major publications pursued tips on the feminist researcher's peculiarities with uncharacteristic ardor. *The Washington Post* even brought in a handwriting expert to compare the signatures of Hite and Gregory.

Certainly, Hite's work deserved scrutiny; many valid questions could be raised about her statistical approach. But Hite's findings were largely held up for ridicule, not inspection. "Characteristically grandiose in scope," "highly improbable," "dubious," and "of limited value" was how *Time* dismissed Hite's report in its October 12, 1987, article "Back Off, Buddy"—leading one to wonder why, if the editors felt this way, they devoted the magazine's cover and six inside pages to the subject. The book is full of "extreme views" from "strident" women who are probably just "malcontents," the magazine asserted. Whether their views were actually extreme, however, was impossible to determine from *Time's* account: the lengthy story squeezed in only two two-sentence quotes from the thousands of women that Hite had polled and quoted extensively. The same article, however, gave plenty of space to Hite's critics—far more than to Hite herself.

When the media did actually criticize Hite's statistical methods, their accusations were often wrong or hypocritical. Hite's findings were "biased" because she distributed her questionnaires through women's right groups, some articles complained. But Hite sent her surveys through a wide range of women's groups, including church societies, social clubs, and senior citizens' centers. The press charged that she used a small and unrepresentative sample. Yet the results of many psychological and social science studies that journalists uncritically report are based on much smaller and nonrandom samples. And Hite specifically states in the book that the numbers are not meant to be representative; her goal, she writes, is simply to give as many women as possible a public forum to voice their intimate, and generally silenced, thoughts. The book is actually more a collection of quotations than numbers.

The reason for the cold shoulder turned toward Shere Hite by the press becomes further clouded when we consider that in the same year Hite's findings were being publicly trashed, psychologist Scrully Blotnick quickly became the darling of the news media. Susan Faludi considers the connection:

In 1987, the media had the opportunity to critique the work of two social scientists. One of them had exposed hostility to women's independence; the other had endorsed it....

At the same time the press was pillorying Hite for suggesting that male resistance might be partly responsible for women's grief, it was applauding another social scientist whose theory—that women's equality was to blame for contemporary women's anguish—was more consonant with backlash thinking. Psychologist Dr. Srully Blotnick, a *Forbes* magazine columnist and much quoted media "expert" on women's career travails, had directed what he called "the largest long-term study of working women ever done in the United States." His conclusion: success at work "poisons both the professional and personal lives of women." In his 1985 book, *Otherwise Engaged: The Private Lives of Successful Women,* Blotnick asserted that his 25-year study of 3,466 women proved that achieving career women are likely to end up without love, and their spinsterly misery would eventually undermine their careers as well. "In fact," he wrote, "we found that the anxiety, which steadily grows, is the single greatest underlying cause of firing for women in the age range of thirty-five to fifty-five." He took some swipes at the women's movement, too, which he called a "smoke screen behind which most of those who were afraid of being labeled egomaniacally grasping and ambitious hid."

The media received his findings warmly—he was a fixture everywhere from the *New York Times* to "Donahue"—and national magazines like *Forbes* and *Savvy* paid him hundreds of thousands of dollars to produce still more studies about these anxiety-ridden careerists. None doubted his methodology—even though there were some fairly obvious grounds for skepticism....

In the mid-'80s, Dan Collins, a reporter at *U.S. News & World Report,* was assigned to a story on that currently all-popular media subject: the misery of the unwed. His editors suggested he call the ever quotable Blotnick, who had just appeared in a similar story on the woes of singles in the *Washington Post.* After his interview, Collins recalls, he began to wonder why Blotnick had seemed so nervous when he asked for his academic credentials. The reporter looked further into Blotnick's background and found what he thought was a better story: the career of this national authority was built on sand. Not only was Blotnick not a licensed psychologist, almost nothing on his résumé checked out; even the professor cited as his current mentor had been dead for fifteen years.

But Collins's editors at *U.S. News* had no interest in that story... and the article was never published. Finally, a year later, after Collins had moved to the *New York Daily News* in 1987, he persuaded his new employer to print the piece. Collins's account prompted the state to launch a criminal fraud investigation against Blotnick, and Forbes discontinued Blotnick's column the very next day. But the news of Blotnick's improprieties and implausibilities made few waves in the press; it inspired only a brief news item in *Time,* nothing in *Newsweek.* And Blotnick's publisher, Viking Penguin, went ahead with plans to print a paperback edition of his latest book anyway. As Gerald Howard, then Viking's executive editor, explained at the time, "Blotnick has some very good insights into the behavior of people in business that I continue to believe have an empirical basis."

Since then, professors and scholars—men and women—have come out in support of Hite's innovative essay methodology, which depends on thousands of anonymous responses. To quote Barbara Seaman, "Even if the survey was not representative, it was probably representative of what was coming down the turnpike. The rest of the culture is in the process of catching up with the forerunners and pioneers who responded to Hite's questionnaires." Below are some examples of those who lauded this forward thinker.

> When analyzing emotions and attitudes in depth, it has been customary
> in the social/psychological sciences to use extremely small samples;
> indeed, Freud based whole books on a handful of subjects. Thus for Hite

to have used the small samples typical of psychological studies would have been quite legitimate. However, she took on the more difficult goal of trying to develop a larger and more representative sample, while still retaining the in-depth qualities of smaller studies. She does the latter by allowing thousands of people to speak freely instead of forcing them to choose from preselected categories—in essence, predefining them and prepackaging them, as with so many studies. It is a method that is hard on the researcher, requiring analysis of thousands of individual replies to hundreds of open-ended questions, an analysis that involves many steps.—Gladys Engel Lang, Professor of Communications, Political Science and Sociology, University of Washington

To call Shere Hite's monumental work "surveys is" to use an inadequate label. The ground-breaking questionnaires she designed... became the underpinnings of a new and most illuminating frame of reference for analyzing power and the relationship between the sexes.... Until the modern women's movement it was accepted practice for men to speak for women in everything from marriage ceremonies to anthropological studies and research findings. No questions were asked about the validity of the "male only" opinions. But when Shere Hite presented women speaking for themselves, she was denounced for use of flawed methodology!—Dale Spender, Feminist theorist and writer

The Hite Reports are a medium that has made it possible for a large number of human beings to speak openly and candidly about needs the expression of which society has tended to censor or limit, and the satisfaction of which society has often condemned and punished.... *The Hite Reports* are essays in knowledge of others and also in knowledge of ourselves. In them we have a classic example of how science and morality go hand in hand: they offer a knowledge of human beings that lead at a future in which we may better fulfill each other because we better understand each other.—Joseph P. Fell, Presidential Professor of Philosophy, Bucknell University

Hite's 127 questions that sparked fury ranged from "Do you have a daughter? How do you feel about her? Have you talked to her about menstruation and sexuality? What did you say? What did she say? (#120)" to "What is the biggest problem in your relationship? How would you like to change things, if you could? (#31)" From the thousands of women's answers, Hite culled data about women's attitudes toward relationships, marriage, and monogamy:

➤ *On Affairs:* The majority of women having affairs say they feel alienated, emotionally closed out, or harassed in their marriages; for 60 percent, having an affair is a way of enjoying oneself, reasserting one's identity, having one person appreciate you in a way that another doesn't.... "I am a homemaker, raising two children going back to school at fifty-five. Do I believe in monogamy? Yes, but I am not monogamous. The reason for my affair for three years now has been hunger for affection. I told my husband several times I could not live without affection. But I plan to stay married."

➤ *On Love in Marriages:* Most of the women in this study do not marry the men they have most deeply loved.... Women, as seen here, hope that by avoiding the highs and lows of being "in love," they can make a relationship more secure, if not inspired, and a better setting for living and raising children.

➤ *On Marriage and Divorce:* Fifty percent of women leave their marriages, 50 percent stay, even if not emotionally satisfied. We are clearly at a turning point, half in and half out of a new time. The picture is striking—almost as if women were pausing, stopping a moment for reflection, halfway out of a door, still turning to look back, bidding goodbye to the past, before setting out on a journey.

➤ *On Gender:* Gender may be the basic, original split that needs to be healed to alter society, to lessen aggression as a way of life. Women are re-integrating "female" identity, leaving behind the double-standard split that began at the beginning of patriarchy, with Eve, followed by Mary as her opposite— and beyond this, trying to end/overcome the opposition between "male" and "female" emphasized by our culture.

➤ *On Relationships:* Ninety-eight percent of the women in this study say they want to make basic changes in their relationships and marriages, improve their emotional relationships they have with men.

"Our biggest problem is not being able to talk. He talks at me, and what he says is law."...

As women think about [why relationships are so difficult]—first asking themselves if there is something wrong with them, then trying to decipher the personal history of the man they love, asking themselves about his childhood, his family, why he is silent, why he behaves the way he does—when women are asking themselves these things, they frequently go on to question the whole system that has made relationships the way they are, and ask, "Why does it have to be this way?"

At least 88 percent of the women in this study, whether married or single, are now asking themselves these questions on a more or less daily basis.... [Women are,] unavoidably, changing who they are—and the more distant they are (ironically) becoming from the very men they want to be closer to—the men with whom they can't even discuss these questions.

Sifting through the women's responses to Shere Hite's questions in *The Hite Report*, Susan Faludi found little to scorn. In her book, *Backlash*, she wrote:

> While the media widely characterized these women's stories about their
> husbands and lovers as "man-bashing diatribes," the voices in Hite's

book are far more forlorn than vengeful: "I have given heart and soul of everything I am and have... leaving me with nothing and lonely and hurt, and he is still requesting more of me. I am tired, so tired." "He hides behind a silent wall." "Most of the time I just feel left out—not his best friend." "At this point, I doubt that he loves me or wants me.... I try to wear more feminine nightgowns and do things to please him." "In daily life he criticizes me for trivial things, cupboards and doors left open.... I don't like him angry. So I just close the cupboards, close the drawers, switch off the lights, pick up after him, etc., etc., and say nothing."...

That the media find this data so threatening to men is a sign of how easily hysteria about female "aggression" ignites under an antifeminist backlash. For instance, should the press really have been infuriated—or even surprised—that the women's number-one grievance about their men is that they "don't listen"?

If anything, the media seemed to be bearing out the women's plaint by turning a deaf ear to their words. Maybe it was easier to flip through Hite's numerical tables at the back of the book than to digest the hundreds of pages of rich and disturbing personal stories. Or perhaps some journalists just couldn't stand to hear what these women had to say; the overheated denunciations of Hite's book suggest an emotion closer to fear than fury—as do the illustrations accompanying *Time* 's story, which included a woman standing on the chest of a collapsed man, a woman dropping a shark in a man's bathwater, and a woman wagging a viperish tongue in a frightened male face.

The impact of Hite's research is evident not only in the voluminous, heart-felt responses to her questionnaires but in the transformation of traditional psychology and of women's perceptions about their lives.

"We seem to be living in a time of a radical shift: we are in the midst of a very real revolution," wrote Naomi Weisstein in her introduction to Shere Hite's 1993 book, *Women as Revolutionary Agents of Change*. "Despite the cultural backlash, despite the media blitz and the mocking feminism, what the modern women's movement started continues its explosive growth. Women all over the United States have come to some very important conclusions; indeed, their whole perspective on the world seems to be changing. What we see in *Women and Love* (*The Hite Report on Love, Passion, and Emotional Violence*) is women defining themselves emotionally, defining themselves on their own terms, leaving behind a 'male' view of the world, saying goodbye to an allegiance to 'male' cultural values which define women as second-class emotionally or any other way, and which insist that competition and aggression are the basic realities of 'human nature.'"

Dale Spender agrees: "The chorus of women whom Shere Hite has brought together is taking on a new role and insisting on new words. They are voicing ideas, possibilities, and criticisms that many men (and some women) do not want to hear. Their speaking out is one reason that Shere Hite and her reports have received a backlash press over the years. Disliking the message, some individuals have tried to shoot the messenger.... Shere Hite's essays have broken the silence so that women now know what's happening in relationships other than their own. They are beginning to appreciate that they are not alone with their 'problems.'"

The climate of the late 1980s had been such that the "messenger"—Hite—chose to sell her New York apartment. Having undoubtedly inspired generations of American women, Shere Hite moved to Paris with her husband in 1989, and has continued to publish books and articles in Europe and other parts of the world, actively campaigning for women's rights in many areas.

Looking Back on Our Bodies, Ourselves

EDITED BY JOANNA PERLMAN AND SARAH SHEY

Excerpted from *Our Bodies, Ourselves for the New Century,* New York, Simon & Schuster, 1998; Judy Norsigian et al., "The Boston Women's Health Book Collective and *Our Bodies, Ourselves," Journal of American Medical Women's Association,* Winter 1999; and Joanna Perlman's interview with Judy Norsigian, conducted in March 1999. Reprinted by permission.

JP: What are some of the early issues *OBOS* picked up on that are now taken for granted?

JN: We included a chapter on sexually transmitted diseases in the 1973 edition, and we were among the first to talk about the fact that women were largely asymptomatic when we had STDs. We encouraged safer-sex practices before the term had even been coined. We saw the transition from when STDs couldn't be talked about to now when they're more frequently addressed.

Another issue we raised early on was out-of-hospital birth, home birth and greater utilization of midwives. We raised questions about... the best place for birth and... the best caregivers. We now know that out-of-hospital birth can be as safe as hospital birth, and sometimes even safer.

JP: What are some of the issues that *OBOS* has not been able to overcome or tackle?

JN: From our very earliest editions we did mention violence in women's lives as a major threat to women's health. When we first began, we talked about rape. Subsequent editions add other forms of violence against women: for example, incest, domestic partner abuse, sexual harrassment. Although there are many more resources like shelters and rape programs, this is the one area where statistics seem to get worse year by year.

JP: When the collective first set out, were there any unanticipated roadblocks?

JN: I don't think we gave much attention to the profound effect of technology, especially reproductive technology, on women's lives—for example, the possibility of women giving birth well past menopause. There are women who have undergone repeated attempts at in vitro fertilization who say they wish they had never done it because it made their lives so miserable for so long. Very small percentages of women actually succeed with these methods in having biological children of their own. We hear about the successes but we don't often hear about the failures and the emotional struggle that women and their partners feel. These technologies have brought limited benefits and serious drawbacks.

CHANGING DIAGNOSIS AND TREATMENTS

New causes of infertility will be discovered as our environment becomes more toxic. Names and kinds of drugs change rapidly. New techniques and treatments appear regularly; few are studied in a controlled, randomized fashion.... You have a right to know whether your treatment is new, or part of an experimental study. (*OBOS*, 1999, p. 533)

JP: How have women's economic situations played into the quality of medical and health care they receive?

JN: In a climate where profit looms large and companies want to make a fast buck, we see advertising and the promotion of products that have not been adequately assessed from a scientific point of view. A recent example is the promotion of tamoxifen, which in some studies has been shown to reduce breast cancer risk. We saw a very misleading advertising campaign by Zeneca, which produces and distributes tamoxifen under a brand name. The National Women's Health Network successfully protested the misleading nature of Zeneca's ads, and as a result the FDA sent Zeneca a very strongly worded letter to remove these ads from magazines. Because pharmaceutical companies can now advertise prescription products directly to consumers, consumers must be more wary than ever. Silicone breast implants represent a good example of putting profit before safety. We still don't know whether the silicone implants are really and truly safe. But we do know that for 30 years no good quality data were collected by plastic surgeons or the implant manufacturers, despite repeated requests by the FDA. Is this a statement on how we, as a society, have valued women's health? There shouldn't be products on the market not adequately tested.... If we don't have a strong FDA and strong government controls we will see unethical behavior time and time again.

JP: Another economic concern is funding for women's health research. In recent years, the amount of funding for breast cancer research has increased a great deal. Do you think there's a particular reason breast cancer is getting so much of the attention, and do you think we'll see a spillover into increased funding and research for other areas of women's health—or does breast cancer stand out for a particular reason?

JN: In this country, the squeaky wheel gets the grease more often than not. There are a number of women with breast cancer who are articulate, middle-class, and able to organize around this issue.... For example, they gathered 600,000 signatures to pressure Congress for more research. We can learn a lot from both the breast cancer and AIDS activists of the past decade or so.

JP: With all the funding going toward breast cancer and the attention women's health issues have been getting because of the squeaky wheel, do you think we could see a backlash against the women's health movement or women's health activists, who might be perceived as somewhat leftist or radical?

JN: I don't think so. What has happened is that the pharmaceutical companies have begun defining the women's health terrain, and they want to promote drugs for prevention as well as therapy because of the potential market and profits. They don't necessarily want to emphasize lifestyle practices that promote prevention. Take our sexual experiences, for example. Drug companies are pursuing Viagra-like drugs for women to go along with their increasingly medicalized view of female sexual "dysfunction." For women without particular medical problems, we could just as well promote greater knowledge of our sexuality—how to masturbate, for example—as another approach to improving our sexual experience.

Ironically, it is because of Viagra and the way it allowed us to expose a double standard, that we finally were able to obtain insurance and HMO coverage for prescription contraceptives. If having sexual experiences wasn't considered essential to women's health and well-being, then how could it be argued that having erections was essential for men's health?

JP: Since you mention not having basic contraceptive coverage and women's limited access to primary health care, do you think that somehow that detracts from or downplays the progress the women's health movement has made over the past 30 years?

JN: We've made a lot progress in many areas but many women still don't have access to health and medical care, don't have even the most basic insurance or HMO coverage. That problem has only been exacerbated as we've seen the profit motive become a dominant force in health and medical care. It doesn't belong there, and we've long advocated strongly for a government-funded model. There should be universal coverage that is not tied to employment. Health care is a right, not a privilege. We liken it to the police department and fire department—essential services in our communities.

JP: Barbara Seaman says that *OBOS* became one of the most powerful debriefing documents of patriarchy. What is your response to that?

JN: Feminism is about creating a society that recognizes capabilities in everyone and opportunities for everyone.... The book tries to point out the ways in which women are shortchanged and the ways in which women could be more fulfilled human beings. *OBOS* tries to create a picture, a critique, that isn't so adversarial, and that doesn't portray men as necessarily being the enemy. We challenge institutions and traditional patriarchal values, and even invite men to join up in this effort—ultimately everyone benefits from eliminating sexism and other forms of oppression.

JP: Why hasn't the collective come out with a book that is more accessible and more friendly to men so that men can start to be incorporated into this movement of women's health?

JN: The point of *OBOS* is to reach *women* and help *women* to think about the particulars of our lives. We have encouraged men to do a similar book for men, and in fact there have been some books like *OBOS* for men. Many men have found *OBOS* to be helpful, especially in better understanding the issues their women partners face.

JP: Do you think that some women might not find the book very accessible because of its leftist position?

JN: It might be a deterrent. However, the practical information is so accessible and so well-written that most women who disagree with the politics simply decide to put the politics aside and concentrate on the material they find most useful. Hopefully, we are able to reach those unconnected with the women's movement to adopt a more feminist perspective.

JP: What do you see coming to the foreground of the women's health movement in the next few years?

JN: Because there are now so many places where you can get women's information, it will become increasingly important to identify sources and distinguish quality information from material that is largely commercial hype.

JP: With all the rapid changes in the medical and health fields as well as the increasing amount of new information, how does *OBOS* keep up to date?

JN: It's extremely difficult. In the book we included information on Web sites that are constantly updated with new information and at our own Web site we constantly offer updated resources.

JP: How could you measure the impact of *OBOS*?

JN: We know from the tremendous amount of mail we get that the book is relevant and useful to many women. In other countries women have translated and adapted the book to suit their own needs, maintaining the essential feminist perspective that has become a universal theme in so many parts of the world. We are committed to updating this book and keeping it alive as a tool for social change.

THE IMPACT OF OBOS ON ONE WOMAN'S LIFE

I think you would have been proud of the way I handled the situation with the surgeon. Despite a fair amount of crying on my part, I was able to demand a second opinion for my diverticulosis treatment and the most conservative treatment possible. My surgeon was appalled when I balked at surgery… without what I felt was adequate time to discuss the situation or get another opinion. I really think that if it wasn't for my experience with the Women's Health Collective and the support of my friends and family, I would have a temporary colostomy right now. (*OBOS*, 1999, p. 681)

JP: When the Boston collective celebrates the book's fiftieth anniversary, in 2020, what would you have to see as its greatest accomplishment?

JN: With over 3.5 million copies in print, the book has heightened awareness among so many women and even pushed the health and medical care system to be more responsive to women's needs. At our fiftieth anniversary, maybe we will be able to say that health and medical care has become less driven by profits, and more science-based and accessible to all. Maybe we will be able to say that we are finally rid of the sexism, racism, and other forms of discrimination that are still so common today. I think these are things we would be very happy to say have happened.

LOOKING BACK AT OUR BODIES, OURSELVES

The following excerpt, from an article published in the *Journal of American Medical Women's Association,* looks at *OBOS*'s transition from a small, grassroots collective to a nonprofit organization working at both the domestic and international levels.

RECENT GROWTH AND DEVELOPMENT

Over the nearly three decades since the first edition of *OBOS*, we have continued to develop our awareness of the injustices that prevent women from experiencing full and healthy lives. As we approach the millennium, such causes of poor health as poverty, racism, hunger, and homelessness continue to disproportionately affect Black and Brown populations in this country and around the world.

We continue to believe that effective strategies for mitigating these problems require all of us to reject the assumptions that so often have hurt women of color and women who are poor. Over the years we have collaborated with women's groups both in the United States and abroad to ensure that the priorities for the women's health movement reflect the needs and concerns of all women. We also recognize the importance of supporting the leadership of women of color and low-income women within our own organization as well as in the larger women's health movements. Although this is a difficult challenge for many groups founded originally by white women, we believe that our ultimate success as a movement depends on respectful collaboration at many levels.

The structure of the Boston Women's Health Book Collective (BWHBC) has evolved over the years. We began as a collective, a circle of 12 women.... We took no profits from sales of the books, using the royalties to support women's health projects and eventually to start our own WHIC and advocacy work. As soon as we hired staff who were not authors of the book, the BWHBC was not formally a collective any more, although the board (mostly original authors for many hears) and the paid staff each worked in a largely collaborative manner.

BWHBC'S ROLE IN THE GLOBAL WOMEN'S HEALTH MOVEMENT

Over the years, we have developed a number of fruitful collaborations with women's groups in different countries and have attended almost all the international women and health meetings that have been convened since the first

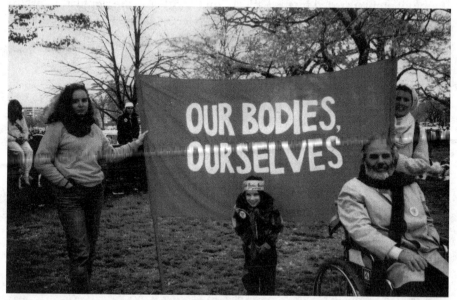

Left to right: Boston Women's Health Book Collective staff member and cofounder Sally Whelan; Kyra Zola Norsigian; Irving Kenneth Zola, longtime friend and contributor to OBOS; Cynthia Pearson, now executive director of the National Women's Health Network. [Courtesy of Judy Norsigian]

International Conference on Woman and Health held in Rome in 1977. At the 1995 NGO Women's Forum in Beijing, many of the women working on these translation/adaptation projects came together to compare notes and to share strategies for dealing with problems such as government censorship and fundraising.

One continuing concern of the current global women's health movement has been the growing trend, especially among environmental groups, to label population growth as a primary cause of environmental degradation. It would be a serious step back if this trend were to lead to more overly zealous family planning programs' driven by demographic goals rather than by women's reproductive health needs. We believe that the unethical and growing use of quinacrine, a sclerosing agent, as a means of nonsurgical sterilization in countries such as Indonesia, India, Pakistan, and Vietnam, represents the very "population control" mentality that has so often been destructive to women's health. Thus, we have joined activists around the globe in protesting the use of quinacrine.

We also collaborated with such other groups as the Women's Global Network for Reproductive Rights (Amsterdam), the International Reproductive Rights and Research Action Group (IRRRAG), and WomanHealth Philippines to sponsor "The Double Challenge," a well-attended workshop series at the Beijing NGO Forum in September 1995. The brochure for this series stated: "Women from around the world face a formidable challenge. On one side are the fundamentalists led by the Vatican; on the other is the population establishment. Both are vying for control over women's sexual and reproductive lives. While the fundamentalists outlaw contraception and abortion, the populationists push new reproductive and contraceptive technologies."

THE CONTINUED NEED FOR A WOMEN'S HEALTH MOVEMENT

The concerns that brought women together several decades ago to form women-controlled health centers, advocacy groups, and other educational and activist organizations largely remain. Women are still the major users of health and medical services, for example, seeking care for themselves even when essentially healthy (birth control, pregnancy and childbearing, and menopausal discomforts). Because women live longer than men, we have more problems with chronic diseases and functional impairment, and thus require more community and home-based services. Women usually act as the family "health broker": arranging care for children, the elderly, spouses, or relatives, and are also the major unpaid caregivers for those around them.

Although women represent the great majority of health workers, we still have a relatively small role in policy making in all arenas. Despite increases in the number of women physicians, we also have a limited leadership role in U.S. medical schools, where women represent less than 10 percent of all tenured faculty. Women face discrimination on the basis of sex, class, race, age, sexual orientation, and disability in most medical settings. Many continue to experience condescending, paternalistic, and culturally insensitive treatment. Older women, women of color, fat women, women with disabilities, and lesbians routinely confront discriminatory attitudes and practices, and even outright abuse.

Women usually find it difficult to obtain the good health and medical information necessary to ensure informed decision making, especially for alternatives to conventional forms of treatment. This problem is intensified for poor women and for those who do not speak English, in part because their class, race, and culture increasingly differ markedly from those of their health care providers.

Many women are subjected to inappropriate medical interventions, such as overmedication with psychotropic drugs (especially tranquilizers and antidepressants), questionable hormone therapy, and unnecessary cesarean sections and hysterectomies, although managed care has reduced the rates of unnecessary surgery in some places.

Despite enormous advances for women over the past two decades, ongoing gender bias in public and private settings continues to relegate women to a separate and unequal place in society. We must have a strong community of women's organizations to assist women individually, to articulate women's needs, to advocate for policy reform, and to resist the more destructive aspects of corporate medicine. Organizations such as the National Women's Health Network, the National Black Women's Health Project, the National Latino Health Organization, the National Asian Women's Health Organization, and the Native American Women's Health Education Resource Center, to name just a few, could play a key role in ensuring that lay and consumer voices are part of any larger women's health debate. The inclusion of such groups by the Office of Women's Health Research at the National Institutes of Health already has enriched discussions concerning research affecting women.

Ironically, except in a handful of states, poor women on Medicaid can obtain a federally funded sterilization but not a federally funded abortion. This limitation has led some women to "choose" sterilization because we have so few options. As the women's health movement continues to emphasize, without access to all reproductive health services, there can be no real choice in matters of childbearing.

Over the years, the BWHBC has collaborated with physicians who have shared the feminist perspective represented in *OBOS*. One such colleague, Mary Howell, M.D. (more recently known as Mary Raugust), died from breast cancer in February 1998. The author of a popular 1972 book entitled *Why Would a Girl Go into Medicine?* and the first woman dean at Harvard Medical School, Mary contributed to the research that resulted in a legal ruling forcing medical schools to eliminate female quotas. These informal quotas had kept the female presence in medical schools no more than 8 percent of the total number of students since the turn of the century. She remains for us one of the finest role models for women in medicine, and we hope that her speeches and writings will be published to inspire the younger generations of female physicians. Another physician, Alice Rothchild, M.D., has written and spoken eloquently about her experience as a feminist obstetrician-gynecologist, and we have made her 1998 AMWA speech available at our website (www.ourbodiesourselves.org).

Members of the media often ask us if we think that progress has been made in addressing the concerns women have had about medicine. We believe that physician awareness of condescending and paternalistic behaviors that are now generally regarded as disrespectful elsewhere in society has been heightened. It also appears that more women feel that their physicians take their concerns seriously, rather than dismissing complaints with, "It's all in your head." But other problems have been exacerbated, and although not unique to women, women's more frequent contact with the medical care system means that women confront these issues much more regularly than men do. Many managed care plans have contributed to reductions in access to care, especially good quality care, for some women. They have, for example, not allowed some physicians to provide needed treatments. Sometimes, physicians have not had the time to adequately assess the plethora of new drugs and medical technologies that they regularly recommend to patients. Cutbacks in local community services and public health programs make it harder to sustain an emphasis on preventive health care.

The BWHBC has a special interest in such problems as the increasing influence of right-wing organizations over public policies affecting women's health, the explosion of health and medical technologies marketed primarily to women, the objectification of women's bodies in the media, the exclusion of consumers from policy setting and oversight functions in many managed care plans, and the relatively few sources of noncommercial information about women and health, especially with a well-informed consumer perspective. We recognize institutional racism as a continuing problem exacerbated by the fact that most caregivers and health care administrators come from economic, social, racial, and ethnic backgrounds quite different from those of the people they are serving. Finally, we believe it is critical to challenge the tendency to overmedicalize women's lives and turn normal events such as childbearing and menopause into disabling conditions requiring medical intervention.

As the women's health movement moves into the next century, the ability to build broad coalitions will largely determine the political effectiveness of women's health care advocates. We can learn much, for example, from the passage of the Americans with Disabilities Act, which succeeded in large part because of the disability rights community reached out to form broad alliances with other groups not initially aware of the universal impact of this legislation. Finding common ground and ways to bridge racial, ethnic, and class differences in particular, will be among the great challenges we face.

Dr. Susan Love

INTERVIEW BY TANIA KETENJIAN

Susan Love, M.D. is the author of *Dr. Susan Love's Breast Book* and *Dr. Susan Love's Hormone Book*. This interview was conducted in April 1999.

TK: Rose Kushner was a major pioneer for breast cancer. How did she influence you?

SL: Rose Kushner was one of the first real breast cancer activists. She didn't stop at being dissatisfied with her own treatment. She continued to lobby and advocate until things were changed for everybody. I think there are greater things than just your personal issues. One person actually *can* change how a disease is approached. And Rose worked pretty much by herself. She inspired a lot of people. She didn't have a huge grassroots organization behind her, and she did great. So I think her chutzpah was a great example of what one person can do.

TK: Who else was a great influence on you?

SL: Eleanor Roosevelt [laughs]. She's another example of how you really can make a difference on a broader stage if you just try. People like Mary Howell and Barbara Seaman. Both were among the very early workers looking at health and women, who said, "Wait a minute, we don't just have to do what doctors say we have to do. We can actually take some action ourselves and change the way things are done." They were a strong influence. I was coming up through medical school at that time to residency, where I would get just the opposite message crammed into my head. Internship and residency and even medical school are a little bit like a cult. You're sleep deprived and overworked, and then they're giving you all these messages, so it's very important to have a countermessage out there. For me it was people like those at *Our Bodies, Ourselves*, people like Mary Howell, people like Barbara Seaman, who changed the balance.

TK: Dr. Mary Howell declined cancer treatment because she didn't want to destroy the quality of her life at that time. What do you think of that?

SL: Oh, I think she was a smart person. She knew a lot about what therapy—as far as we could tell—could do, and she was a grownup, and I think you have to let grownups make their own decisions. We don't cure all breast cancers, and we do indeed spend a lot of energy and time giving people treatment that destroys their lives and the lives of the people close to them. She wasn't being totally crazy. According to the data, we have about twelve thousand bone marrow transplants per year in this country, and there is no evidence that they work. She knew that once you get sucked into the medical system, you're going to get lots of treatment, and it may or may not be worth doing. Now the other side of the question—and I don't know the answer, because I didn't take care of her—involves whether she was really in a situation where nothing would work. That's hard to know, and it's hard to dispute, too. In the long run I give her credit for being honest and making the decisions that were good for her.

TK: I understand you were in a convent. Then, after medical school, you became a general surgeon, and then you focused on breast surgery. How did that whole process happen?

SL: Well, even when I was in the convent, which wasn't for a huge amount of time, I was still planning on becoming a doctor. So that part was pretty firm in my mind. But then I went to medical school and decided that what I liked best was surgery. At that time there were still quotas for women. It was ten percent where I went to school, but five percent at other New York schools, and many of the schools that I applied to said, "Sorry, we're not interested." The amazing thing to me is that I didn't think that was abnormal. I just said, "Oh well." It never occurred to me that that wasn't fair and they shouldn't be allowed to do it.

When I was in the middle of medical school things opened up. But there were very few women applying, so the process turned around in our favor. I went to Harvard Medical School and trained in surgery at Beth Israel, which is one of Harvard's hospitals, and I was the second woman in my program. When I was finishing I said, "I am not going to do breast surgery," because in those days people who did breast surgery were basically old and tapering down—they just were not very capable. But very soon I went into practice and started being sent patients who had breast problems—they weren't going to send me male patients, God forbid. It was still very strange to have a woman surgeon—it was considered very brave to be a patient with a female surgeon. But it became very clear to me [that these women with breast cancer] were not being treated very well and that I had much more to offer. I could really change their thinking, since the way you think about your breast is a lot different from the way you think about your gallbladder. At the time people said, "Oh, you can never make a living as a breast surgeon, there's not enough work, blah, blah, blah." Of course none of that was true, and before I knew it I became part of a mission. And here I am, still doing it, still on a mission.

TK: Do you see yourself as an activist?

SL: Oh there's no question that I have been an activist from the beginning. When I was first going into practice, there was good randomized, controlled data about radiation being as good as mastectomies, and yet surgeons were offering mastectomies as the only option. So the first thing I did was start yelling and screaming about that. It became clear to me that doctors were not talking to women and not giving them the information they needed to make their own decisions about breast cancer, so I wrote my book about breast cancer, and it did very well. But doctors believed that you shouldn't share information with the public, God forbid, they might find out we don't know everything.

Then, as I was doing my book tour, it became very clear that the moment had arrived to politicize breast cancer. The AIDS movement, which had been around for a couple of years, was the model for people with a disease lobbying for greater medical information. Three or four groups popped up, almost like spontaneous combustion, in different parts of the United States: Berkeley, California, Cambridge, Massachusetts, Washington, D.C. I thought, "Boy, somebody's gotta pull this all together, it's really the moment to be doing it." Then I was in Salt Lake City giving a talk to about six hundred people in the middle of the day, middle of the week, mostly older women who were not working. I was looking for a laugh in a long talk about breast cancer, and I said, "I don't know what it's going to take to eradicate breast cancer, but maybe we need to march topless on the White House." The image of George Bush dealing with all those topless women was a great one, and everybody laughed. But then I thought, "If they're ready to march on the White House in Salt Lake City, Utah, the time has come to really politicize the issue."

So I went back home and called a couple of people. Within a year we had the National Breast Cancer Coalition. Within a couple of years we not only increased the funding for breast cancer, but made sure that people with breast cancer were involved in the decision making at all levels, how the money is spent. We really changed the landscape. Now you won't see a medical program or a conference that does not include sympathy for a layperson's needs. So am I an activist? Yeah, a troublemaker.

TK: What are some of the greatest misconceptions about breast cancer?

SL: One is that if it's not in your family, you're not going to get it. Only 5 percent of women with breast cancer have a history of it in their family. People think somehow they are immune because it's not in their family. Another is that if you're diagnosed with breast cancer, you have to have surgery, something has to be done, it's an emergency. The truth is that most breast cancers have been there 8 to 10 years, and if you're doing something this week or next week, it really isn't a critical factor. Those two are big ones. Another one is that coffee has something to do with lumpy breasts or cancer. That was disproved a long time ago.

TK: For 70 percent of women with breast cancer the cause is unknown.

SL: Right.

TK: What do you think causes it?

SL: Well, I think we know some of the reasons. We're awash in hormones in our society, whether environmental hormones from pesticides or all the drugs we take. Think about what we do to women these days. We start out taking birth control pills early on and take them until we're ready to get pregnant. By then we need fertility drugs—and God knows how bad they are—and next we go on postmenopausal hormones until we die. What is this doing to and saying about women's bodies? Some very provocative recent studies show that women who take birth control pills and then take HRT have a much higher risk of breast cancer. We're just pumping up our bodies with these hormones, with this notion that we need high-level hormones to be healthy. But the data for that are really not very strong.

Diet, exercise, lifestyle changes probably do have something to do with breast cancer. We don't know exactly what, but we know that in Japan there are very low percentages of women with breast cancer, and when Japanese women emigrate to this country, their breast cancer rates increase significantly, and so do their daughters'. What is the reason for that? Lifestyle, diet—right now the in thing is soy. We don't know exactly what the reason is, but it's something we need to investigate because not enough has been established. Breast cancer is much more common among women at a high socioeconomic level than among poor women. It's higher in White women than in Black women. That speaks to something environmental or genetic.

TK: Some people were very disturbed by how your hormone book was treated. Do you feel your books accomplished what you wanted them to?

SL: Well, the breast book certainly accomplished what I wanted it to. In fact, I'm now working on the third edition. It's a heavy thing. It's the bible on breasts, and I feel a greater responsibility to make sure everything is right. But I think the hormone book touched a nerve, and if you're going to touch a nerve, you have to put up with the consequences. I think there's no question that the way we have prescribed HRT in this country for menopause is short-sighted and not based on a lot of data. When you point that out to people, it's like saying the emperor has no clothes. They get very defensive because they know at some level that there really isn't that much data, yet here they've been pushing the treatment.

I feel that the way that book was treated shows that this really is an area we need to shine some more light into. The data are not as strong as people would like, and since the book came out, that's become obvious. The first study on HRT and heart disease showed no benefit. So all these people who said, "Oh well, it reduces heart disease by fifty percent and that trumps breasts cancer" are now saying, "Oops, no benefits. What does that mean?" and going back to the drawing board. I think my book and other books played a role in this, they've made people say, "Well, you know, she's right, we don't have all that data," and maybe they don't come on quite as strong as they before.

People who are very quick to believe in science and some popular notions tend to forget that we don't have the data to support HRT. Observational data are very good for generating hypotheses. So we compare the women who are not on HRT to the women who are on HRT, and indeed the women who are on it have 50 percent less heart disease. But they also are women at higher socioeconomic levels, so they go to the doctor more often, they exercise more often, they are more likely to treat their high blood pressure. The question is not so much, "Do hormones make you healthy?" The question is, "Do healthy women need hormones?" Until you do a study with a good number of couch potatoes in each group, you won't be able to answer that. What happened was that we took that kind of data, which is nice and interesting, but only enough to say, "Gee, we really ought to look into this," and we extrapolated from that as if it meant that HRT worked, and you can't say that. It's like saying lung cancer is more common among people who carry cigarette lighters in their pocket. That's probably true, but you can't then assume that cigarette lighters cause lung cancer, and reducing the use of cigarette lighters is not necessarily going to reduce the rates of lung cancer.

People start believing all this observational data, not questioning it, and before you know it they forget that they actually haven't proven what they're saying. My job is to be the annoying kid who says, "Hey, the emperor has no clothes." I think that's an important job. But if you do that, you can't expect people to love you because they don't like having it pointed out to them; it makes them feel like fools. So I was not surprised by the reception the hormone book got. I would have been surprised if people had embraced it as a great thing. When the breast book first came out, it wasn't embraced either. I'll be interested to see the data becoming clearer over the next few years. Already my points are being validated. I don't care if I get credit for it, but it does make me feel like I at least contributed to asking questions.

TK: You have accomplished so many things, and these books are just an example of that. What are some of them?

SL: We made a model of how to treat breast cancer at UCLA. It says we need a multidisciplinary approach: patients need to see the medical oncologist, plastic surgeon, and mental health specialist. In the way we used to do it, you'd see a surgeon, be diagnosed, be sent to an oncologist and then to a radiation therapist, but none of them ever talked to the others, there was no coordination. At UCLA people were seen by a panel all at once, and it was done for the convenience of the woman rather than the physician. Everybody sat down together with the slides and the mammograms, reviewed the case, decided what to do, and then as a team took care of the patient. That model and variations of it

HEALTH EMPOWERMENT FOR WOMEN   **1475**

have been picked up in many places around the country. It's now considered the way that women with breast cancer should be treated. They're not always treated that way, but it's certainly the model, and that was one of the major contributions. The whole concept that women have the right to information, second opinions, and all that didn't exist before.

Some of these things are not uniquely mine. What happened was that I said a combination of my ideas and things that various other people had said in a loud voice. Other people—and this goes full circle to what you asked about Rose Kushner—may be saying and doing the same things. But having the chutzpah or whatever to say it out loud, to publish it, to say it in a bigger forum is what I think helps to get things changed. When I was doing the hormone book, I interviewed some of the people who were doing all the science—Deborah Gren, Elizabeth Barrett-Connor. Elizabeth said, "I'm so glad you're doing this. Somebody has to do it, and I don't want to have to do the talk shows and all that stuff." Deborah said, "I don't want to have to answer all the patients' questions that will come up, but I'm glad you're doing it, because somebody needs to." It wasn't always me who came up with these ideas, but maybe it was that I was brazen enough to talk about it out loud.

TK: What are some things other activists are doing now that are helpful?

SL: They're still questioning, and there was no questioning before we started the coalition. People running a group like the Breast Cancer Coalition had to be activists. Having providers like myself do it would just be continuing the traditional model like the American Cancer Society, which is run by doctors, or the American Heart Association, which is run by doctors, and that really was not what we wanted to be. Fran Visco, an attorney and the head of the National Breast Cancer Coalition, Pat Barr, who is in Vermont, and some of the other advocates against breast cancer are taking things well beyond what I could have possibly done myself. That has been critical if we're going to be success-ful. I'm sort of a catalyst. The coalition turned out fantastically well, which I attribute to all the activists who were in involved in it. The National Women's Health Network, Cindy Pearson, and that group, in spite of changing winds in popularity and everything else, have continued to be a voice for women against all the forces that are trying to diminish the influence of the women's health movement—against hospitals, against the FDA. These advocates for women started out being enormously popular and now are considered to be a more of a radical fringe. Yet they have enormous power because they are always there and they're always willing to step up to the plate. That is really crucial in how things have evolved.

TK: What projects are you working on now?

SL: Right now I'm eradicating breast cancer [laughs]. That's the plan. I'm not seeing patients, I'm doing research. I founded a startup company to commercialize my research because doing it in the academic setting just didn't work. There's not enough money, and it's too hard to get the money that there is. It takes too long and they don't like innovation, they just want to do the same old thing. So I have fifteen employees in Menlo Park, a kind of venture capital company. We have a new device that we hope is going to be a Pap smear for breast cancer so that you can find it really fast, and that will make a difference.

TK: Do you agree that many changes have happened in the last twenty years in the field of breast cancer?

SL: Yes and no. I think we are actually on the verge of the real changes. The changes that have happened up to now are changes in the quality of people's lives. Certainly doing lumpectomy and radiation instead of mastectomy, doing reconstruction immediately instead of delaying it, and being able to give chemotherapy without destroying people's lives in the process are major changes. But we really have to reduce mortality. The first year there was any decrease in mortality was 1998, and it was only about one to two percent. That's good, but far from perfect. My real concern is that we haven't found the Big Cure.

But I think we're on the verge of some major paradigm shifts that will lead us toward that. Right now, we're at a crossroads. We've treated breast cancer as if it were a foreign invader and our job was to kill every cancer cell, stamp it out. Chemotherapy, bone marrow transplants, all of that is based on that idea of a bigger, stronger, harder attack—kill every cell. What we're starting to learn is that killing every cell may not be necessary. We may be able to reverse the cancer, we may be able to control it, sort of like mental health. These are not foreign invaders, they're just cells that are going kind of crazy. If they've gone too far psychotic, we may not be able to intervene, but otherwise we probably can reverse the process and rehabilitate them. That's really where people are moving at the moment in terms of treatment and perception, and some of the new biological treatments are opening that door.

The flip side of that is the part I am working on, which goes along both with identifying the chain of causation for breast cancer and with some prevention tactics. I don't think we're quite there yet—I'm not sure tamoxifen is the right drug for prevention—but I think the paradigm will be prediction and prevention rather than diagnosis and treatment—that is, being able to figure out at a much earlier stage who is going to get the disease and then reverse it so that they never get it, much as we do with Pap smears. If you're getting regular Pap smears, it's rare to get cervical cancer. We discover it in an early stage and then we do something to fix it. I think that's where we're heading. Those two changes are going to make an amazing difference, so that the next generation just won't know breast cancer.

Map of the Women's Health Movement

SHERYL BURT RUZEK

Excerpted from Sheryl Burt Ruzek, "The Map of the Women's Health Movement," paper presented at the Seminar on the History and Future of Women's Health, Washington, D.C., June 11, 1998; Sheryl Burt Ruzek and Julie Becker, "The Women's Health Movement in the United States: From Grass-Roots Activism to Professional Agendas," *Journal of the American Medical Women's Association,* Winter 1999. Reprinted by permission.

Women's health activists have generated public debate and spearheaded social action in a number of waves throughout U.S. history, waves that University of Michigan Sociologist Carol Weisman views as part of a women's health "megamovement" that has spanned two centuries. The U.S. women's health movement grew rapidly through the 1970s; broadened its base with women of color and others in the early 1980s; and contracted, was co-opted, and became institutionalized during the late 1980s and 1990s. The general feminist movement of the 1960s and 1970s spawned dozens of specific movements and hundreds of movement organizations, shaping public consciousness.

RISE AND DEVELOPMENT OF THE WOMEN'S HEALTH MOVEMENT

Looking back now at the early days of the women's health movement in the late 1960s, it seems almost incredible how hard it was to get access to medical information unless you were a doctor—and most doctors were men. Few books on women's health could be found in bookstores, except for books on childbirth. The assumption was simply that physicians were the experts and women were to do as instructed. Breaking open this closed system, laywomen asserted that personal, subjective knowledge of one's own body was a valid source of information and deserved recognition, not scorn. The idea of women creating "observational" data out of their own health and body experiences was truly "revolutionary."

From demonstrations during the Senate hearings on the Pill—to gynecological self-help groups in homes, the women's health movement grew rapidly through the early 1970s. This activism didn't emerge in a vacuum, but out of a social environment in which a wide array of social movements was reshaping the landscape.

The women's health movement grew rapidly through the leadership of several grassroots groups with strong ties to other social change movements, particularly the abortion rights, prepared childbirth, and consumer health movements. As the general feminist movement of the 1960s and 1970s sought equal rights and the full participation of women in all public spheres, many believed that without control over reproduction, all other rights were in jeopardy. Thus in the early years, reproductive issues defined many branches of the movement and shaped group consciousness and social action. Reproductive rights remain central to feminist health agendas worldwide.

Feminist health writers such as Barbara Seaman, Barbara Ehrenreich, Deirdre English, Ellen Frankfort, Gena Corea, Claudia Dreifus, and columnists for prominent feminist newspapers galvanized women to explore their own health, providing critical momentum for the emerging grassroots movement. The Boston Women's Health Book Collective produced the enormously popular *Our Bodies, Ourselves,* which has had numerous U.S. and foreign language printings. The Federation of Feminist Women's Health Centers "invented" and championed gynecological self-help and woman-centered reproductive health services. The National Women's Health Network (NWHN) linked a wide array of local groups to provide a voice for women in Washington. Monitoring legislation, Food and Drug Administration actions, and informing the public about women's health issues continue to be central to this organization's mission. A few nationally prominent groups focused on specific diseases or condition (e.g., DES Action, the Endometriosis Association). Members of pivotal groups and other health activists traveled, spoke, and published widely, and used contacts with the media effectively, becoming spokespeople for the rapidly growing movement.

Movement activists also sought a number of reforms: regulation of drugs and devices; out of hospital birthing centers and midwifery; alternative and complementary therapies; lay access to medical information; and better communication between patients and health providers. Activists have also questioned medical orthodoxies—particularly birth practices, hormone replacement therapies, and cancer prevention and treatment.

An important achievement of the women's health movement was transferring women's health from the domain of largely male experts to women themselves. Developing in parallel with self-help medical care movements, consciousness-raising and gynecological self-help became strategies for empowering women to define their own health and create alternative services. Local movement groups in all 50 states were providing gynecological self-help, women-controlled reproductive health clinics, clearinghouses for health information and referral services and producing their own health educational materials. Advocacy ranged from accompanying individual women seeking medical care to advising and influencing state and local health departments.

By the mid-1970s, more than 250 formally identifiable groups provided education, advocacy, and direct service in the United States. Nearly 2,000 informal self-help groups and projects provided additional momentum to the movement Although ideologically committed to being inclusive, the leadership of the women's health movement remained largely white and middle class in North America during the early years. Sterilization abuse mobilized women of color to seek government protection during the 1970s, and groups such as the Committee to End Sterilization Abuse (CESA) were founded.

The women's health movement grew visibly global, with groups such as ISIS in Geneva creating opportunities for worldwide feminist health activism. By the mid-1970s, there were more than 70 feminist health groups in Canada, Europe, and Australia. Today, there are growing efforts to make connections with feminist health activists, both in industrialized and developing countries.

As the women's health movement evolved in the United States, the distinct health needs of diverse women emerged, and women of color formed their own movement organizations such as the National Black Women's Health Project, the National Latina Women's Health Organization, the Native American Women's Health Education and Research Center, and the National Asian Women's Health Organization. Women of color health organizations gained national recognition and developed agendas to protect women against racist sterilization and contraceptive practices; to widen access to medical care for lower income women, including abortions no longer covered by Medicaid; and to focus on diseases and conditions affecting women of color such as lupus, fetal alcohol syndrome, hypertension, obesity, drug addiction, and stress related to racism and poverty that were ignored or misunderstood by largely white movement groups. By the late 1980s, the National Black Women's Health Project had established local chapters with more than 150 self-help groups for African-American women. Women's health agendas also grew within organizations that addressed a broad range of issues for both men and women of color.

Other women added distinct health agendas in the 1970s and 1980s. Lesbians (the Lesbian Health Agenda), rural women, and women with disabilities (the Dis-Abled Women's Network) joined older women's groups (the Older Women's League) and women with specific health concerns to broaden constituencies and issues. With the rise of environmental health concerns, groups such as the Women's Environmental Development Organization (WEDO) built bridges between feminist health activism and other movements for social change.

Of course social movements never retain their peak levels of participation, and like other movements, grassroots feminist health organizations declined in the 1980s, apparently as a result of changes in movement adherents and the social context in which movement groups operated. For example, many founders of movement organizations returned to school, began families, or entered the paid labor force, as have the next generation of women who increasingly juggle careers and families, thus reducing the traditional volunteer labor pool. Much of organized feminism, as it evolved both in media imagery and academe, came to be seen as distant or disconnected from ordinary women's lives.

The success of single-issue groups, particularly acquired immune deficiency syndrome (AIDS) organizations, to secure funding for direct services, education, and research presented new models for health activism. And the discovery of mainstream health institutions that "marketing to women" could increase profits led to the designation of a wide array of clinical services as "women's health clinics." By the 1990s, women's health services were widespread, although most were now part of larger medical institutions. In her recent national survey of women's health services, Weisman found that most centers founded in the 1960s and 1970s claimed a commitment to a feminist ideology; those founded later or sponsored by hospitals were significantly less likely to report this commitment. Within the movement, concerns emerged over whether new interest in women's health reflected co-optation or institutionalization. One price of "success" is that it is increasingly difficult for women to know whether particular "women's health centers" are truly woman-centered or simply marketed as such.

By the end of the 1980s, most alternative feminist health clinics had ceased to exist, and the survivors had broadened their range of services and affiliated with larger health systems. Gynecological self-help has virtually disappeared. The surviving grassroots movement advocacy and education groups such as the NWHN must work hard to retain support from both individuals and foundations as they compete with newer organizations for members and resources. Thus, grassroots groups contracted internally as they were diluted externally by the growing prominence of both mainstream women's support groups (on a wide array of health issues ranging form alcohol problems to breast cancer) and disease-focused health advocacy groups whose efforts supported the growing federal initiatives for greater equity in women's health research.

FROM GRASSROOTS IDEOLOGIES TO PROFESSIONAL INSTITUTIONAL AGENDAS

The impact of the women's health movement is reflected in the extent to which mainstream organizations and institutions, particularly federal agencies, have incorporated or adopted core ideas and created new opportunities for women's health advocates. By 1990, the reform wings of feminism had made significant claims for gender equity in all social institutions and federal equity agendas emerged. With a growing number of women in Congress, in the biomedical professions, and in health advocacy communities, organizations that had pursued very different paths to improving women's health coalesced around the 1989 General Accounting Office (GAO) report. This report, showing that the National Institutes of Health (NIH) had failed to implement its policy of including women in study populations, proved to be a catalyst for pressuring Congress and the NIH to take action and by the end of 1990, the Women's Health Equity Act was passed, and the NIH established the Office of Research on Women's Health. In 1991, the NIH undertook the Women's Health Initiative, the largest project of its kind, seeking data on prevention and treatment of cancer, cardiovascular disease and osteoporosis. Scientific and professional interest in women's health burgeoned. Spurred by growing federal investment in women's health and by the "cold-war dividend" funding of women's research through the Department of Defense, health activists saw opportunities to collaborate with scientists and professionals who were eager to take advantage of these new research priorities.

Although grassroots women's health groups have criticized many aspects of federally funded research, and have attempted to rectify perceived problems in consent procedures and inclusion criteria, they have largely supported greater federal funding of biomedical and psycho-social research on women's health. Thus after two decades of activism, the health movement's critique of biomedicine and the call for demedicalizing women's health care was largely reframed into a bipartisan agenda for parity in funding for women's and men's healt-related research.

The 1990s became a period of heightened activism. To maximize the likelihood of obtaining federal funding for research on women's health, scientists and their consumer allies focused on specific diseases—from AIDS to breast cancer. This narrowing of focus was critical for navigating federal funding streams that are tied to specific diseases and organ systems. The new "disease-oriented" organizations reflect the interests of women who expect a high level of professionalism. Facing dual roles as workers outside the home and traditional caretakers inside the home, the highly educated women who support the new single-issue groups may find that their interests lie in organizations that dispense professionally endorsed information, solicit donations, and carry out advocacy efforts on behalf of women. Thus the success of women's entry into the labor force, changes in cultural ethos, and women's own commitment to specialization and professionalism may explain why the narrower, highly professionalized women's health organizations that emphasize parity for women's health research attract women who do not identify either with broader movements for social change or with feminism per se.

AIDS advocacy groups also raised a new standard of effectiveness for health activists. They not only successfully increased funding for education and research, but gained a voice in how these added appropriations from government and foundations would be spent. Julie Becker, a public health advocate, observes that thereafter, breast cancer advocates and others (ovarian cancer advocates, Parkinson patients and their families, etc.) adopted many of the AIDS organizations' strategies, albeit with a more professional and less confrontational style. A growing willingness to own illness and become "poster people" for cancer, as people with AIDS had done effectively, put a face on diseases that women privately and pervasively feared. Creating strong alliances between consumers, medical professionals, and researchers, breast cancer advocates rallied behind a specific cause that affected many of them directly or through family and friends. Many activists who threw their energy into propelling the such as the national breast cancer coalition into national prominence left behind older-style support groups and feminist health organizations with broader agendas.

Using well-established letter-writing and advocacy strategies, breast cancer activists testified at hearings, held press conferences, and took their case to the NIH. In collaboration with growing bipartisan support in Congress and the scientific community, advocates succeeded in increasing federal funding for breast cancer research from $84 million to more than $400 million in 1993. Breast cancer advocates also insisted that survivors be involved in shaping research agendas and educational efforts and aligned themselves more consistently and collaboratively with scientists than had some AIDS activists or earlier grassroots movement leaders.

The success of breast cancer advocacy quickly created a "disease *du jour*" climate, where professionals rallied people directly or indirectly affected by particular diseases to lobby for increased funding. Ovarian cancer was the next women's disease to achieve national prominence. While this approach secures more resources or particular groups in the short run, it pits diseases against each other, turning research funding into a "popularity contest" or war of each against all—to be won by the group that can make the most noise or wield the greatest political pressure. A result may be overfunding some diseases without regard for their prevalence, contribution to overall population health, or likelihood of scientific value. In this environment, orphan diseases will join orphan drugs as unfortunate, but probably unavoidable downsides of market-driven research and medicine.

A question that both Ruzek and Weissman have pondered together is the extent to which these newer groups are part of the women's health movement—or represent, at least in part, a separate and distinct, although overlapping, wave of activism.

DIFFERENCES BETWEEN GRASSROOTS AND PROFESSIONALIZED WOMEN'S HEALTH ORGANIZATIONS

Many grassroots women's health movement groups see themselves as different from what they perceive to be more professional mainstream organizations, although these differences are not always clearly articulated. After observing a wide range of groups for three decades, Ruzek argues that surviving grassroots advocacy groups can be differentiated from most professionalized, disease-focused groups in the following six ways:

➤*Social movement orientation.* The founders of many grassroots feminist groups had ties to progressive or radical social movements that emphasized social justice and social change, to which many remain committed. In contrast, the newer professionalized support and advocacy organizations are typically more narrowly focused on a single disease or health issue, and except for environmentally focused groups such as WEDO, few are integral to broader social movements for social change (although some individual members may have such commitments).

➤*Leadership.* Although some women physicians who were critical of medical education, training, and practice were leaders of the grassroots women's health movement, lay leadership was the norm. The role of physicians relative to others remains a point of contention among some feminist groups. In contrast, the professionalized support and advocacy groups formed in the 1990s had a growing pool of women physicians, scientists, and other highly trained professionals to turn to for leadership.

➤*Attitude toward biomedicine.* A recurring theme in the grassroots women's health movement has been the demand for "evidence-based medicine," long before this term came into vogue. Major feminist advocacy groups aligned themselves with scientists and physicians who sought to put medical practice on a more scientific basis at a time when it was resisted by many clinicians. Grassroots health activists were critical of the side effects of inadequately tested drugs and devices, particularly early high-dose oral contraceptives, diethylstilbestrol, and intrauterine devices. They also questioned the number of unnecessary hysterectomies and radical mastectomies performed. In short, consumer groups sought to protect women from unsafe or unnecessary biomedical interventions. The professionalized advocacy groups founded in the 1990s focus more on ensuring women an "equal" share of biopsychosocial science and treatment a stance that concerns many grassroots activists who fear overmedicalization and overtreatment of both men and women. The growing number of women physicians and scientists also facilitates alliances with women consumers because perceived interests in safety and effectiveness make these relationships seem mutually beneficial to many women.

➤*Relationships with corporate sponsors.* Older grassroots advocacy groups remain deeply concerned about the effects of drug and device manufacturers sponsoring journals and organizational activities. In fact, this issue is a pivotal source of strain between grassroots groups and highly professional women's health organizations. While organizations of women physicians and professional advocacy groups rely heavily on corporate sponsorships, older grassroots groups avoid such relationships on grounds that financial ties affect the willingness of groups to criticize sponsors, promote competitors' products, or address alternative or complementary therapies that might undermine conventional prescribing patterns. Research confirms that sponsorship has this effect. Refusing support from corporate sponsors remains a hallmark of grassroots movement groups, but they struggle financially as a result. Because professional groups accept corporate support from drug and device manufacturers, they have more resources for education and advocacy.

➤*Goals of education.* Both older and newer women's health organizations share the goal of educating women to improve their own health and make decisions about their own care. Grassroots feminist groups, particularly through the 1970s, focused on demystifying medicine and encouraging women to trust their subjective experience of their own health. Having access to larger number of women physicians may have reduced the perceived need to demystify medicine, and professional organizations appear largely concerned with making their highly educated constituencies aware of medical and scientific information.

➤*Lay versus professional authority.* Grassroots health groups remain committed to substantial lay control over health and healing and to expanding the roles of such nonphysician healers as midwives, nurses, and counseling professionals. They would involve consumers in all aspects of health policy making, not simply transfer legitimate authority from male to female physicians. In largely professional organizations, women physicians are viewed as the primary societal experts on women's health matters.

The grassroots women's health movement organizations leave a legacy of making health an important social concern and educating women to take responsibility for their own health and health care decision making. The movement as a whole has made substantial efforts to influence powerful social institutions—organized medicine, the pharmaceutical industry, and regulatory agencies. In partnership with newer, professionalized equity organizations, health movement activists have taken up mainstream reform efforts that will become increasingly important as medical care is dominated by market forces. Thus the current episode of women's health activism overlaps with, but is, in many ways, different from the activism of the 1960s and 1970s. These distinct episodes of women's health activism need to be differentiated and understood in the specific historical contexts in which they emerged, recognizing the distinct roles that their history may lead them to play in the future. Because of the complexity of assessing the safety, effectiveness and cost effectiveness of medical technologies worldwide, social justice demands ways to include women's health advocates who are committed to good science that is free from conflict of interest in patient education and health system coverage decisions. Finding ways to ensure women access to such information needs to be a priority for both grassroots and professionalized advocacy organizations.

The next challenge: who will speak for women in the electronic age? The electronic communication technologies foster a climate in which researchers and consumers expect to find information instantaneously and effortlessly. The reliability of information in electronic media is often questionable, however. Until data can be transformed into usable knowledge that can shape human action, the information age will not fulfill its promise. Neither grassroots women's health movement organizations nor newer professionalized disease agenda groups have adequately grappled with how to communicate with their constituencies effectively. Both types of groups as well as government and mainstream health organizations NEED to assess, manage, and distribute what each sees as "reliable" health information. Organizational survival may depend increasingly on teaching both "customers" and staff how to use reliable information effectively.

Because of the role of advocacy groups in health policy making in the United States, it is important how they present themselves and are perceived. As electronic media provide all comers the opportunity to claim organizational status in an increasingly "virtual" world, and the number of groups claiming to speak for women increases, how will the public differentiate among them? As we navigate the uncharted "information age," the ability of the grassroots women's health movement to remain nationally recognized as critical spokespersons may become problematic because the technology allows anyone with a computer and minimal skill to "create" an organization with worldwide visibly. Most movement organizations are just beginning to move from hard copy resource centers and clearinghouses to electronic purveyors of information. Newer professional advocacy groups that are better funded and more attuned to technological advancements are likely to gain because those who position themselves in electronic media will be perceived as speaking for women. In an effort to address the complexity of electronic media, the boston women's health book collective included a section on how to assess the adequacy of electronic sources of information in the 1998 edition of *Our Bodies, Ourselves.*

Who speaks for women's health in the electronic age very much depends on where one looks—Yahoo, for instance, or Healthfinders, the electronic database the Department of Health and Human Services unveiled for public use in May 1999—and how willing one is to sift through hundreds of self-characterized "women's health organizations." Becker, who is researching how Web sites present reliable information, emphasizes that women need to be vigilant in assessing information gleaned from the Internet, because it is so "easy" to log on and "find something."

Both grassroots and professionalized women's health advocates need new strategies for remaining key information-brokers in an increasingly complex sea of women's health information. Grassroots health movement groups remain important forces for increasing awareness of women's health issues and are viewed as trustworthy sources of information by feminist groups in the United States and worldwide. But the cacophony of often contradictory and conflicting medical advice—from all sorts of journals, newsletters, Internet "chat rooms," and government and private health organizations—is likely to strain the individual's ability to sort out fact from fiction, established scientific evidence from snake oil, and hypotheses from hype. As it becomes more complex to be a well-informed consumer, the divide between information "haves" and "have nots" will widen. However, professionalized equity organizations, too, face competition from a growing array of institutions that claim expertise in matters of women's health. The challenge for both types of women's health groups will be to differentiate themselves for others whose interests lie more in marketing than in meeting diverse women's health needs.

As we enter the new millennium we must address growing disparities in wealth and access to health insurance among women. Women's health advocates need to find ways to widen access and equity to care for all women.

Interview with Cindy Pearson

TANIA KETENJIAN

Cindy Pearson is the executive director of the National Women's Health Network. This interview was conducted in May 1999.

TK: What is the central belief of the National Women's Health Network?

CP: We believe that women need a watchdog organization to look out for their health interests because too many women have received health care based either on someone's unproven opinion about what works, or on someone's interest in making a profit. We try to provide information to women who don't have a source they can trust and, because we don't take any money from drug companies or companies that manufacture medical devices, we believe we can present an independent voice that isn't influenced by anything other than what women would consider in making decisions for themselves.

TK: How are women at a disadvantage when they enter the doctor's office?

CP: Women interact with the health care system much more often than men do. We go when we're young and healthy for reproductive health services and, because we live longer than men, we're more likely to have chronic health conditions. So whatever is wrong with the health care system, women experience it more. Over the years that's led to all kinds of abuses and unnecessary and inappropriate treatment. Because of the lingering effects of sexism in the health care system, women's true needs are ignored by their health care providers. Women are given the brush-off or are thought of as "just another complaining woman," so women are at a real disadvantage when it comes to the health care system.

TK: I've realized in talking to leaders in the women's health movement that doctors intervene too much. Can you talk about that a bit?

CP: American life is overmedicalized, especially for women, although also for men. My hope is that our women's health movement, to the extent that it succeeds in improving health care and making it more humane for women, will apply to men as well. Basically, we have paid a price in this country for making great technological improvements. Personally, I'm delighted that if my body is broken in a car crash there is high-tech medical care available to put me back together. Similarly, acute, raging infections can be treated by wonderful antibiotics. But what I don't like, and what I'm part of a movement to oppose, is the complete medicalization of the normal aspects of life. For example, we schedule our children to be seen by pediatricians in the first couple years of life more than they're seen by their grandparents. Those pediatricians prescribe unnecessary drugs, maybe as often as every third or fourth visit, leading these kids, some would say, to more health problems in their future than they would have had in the first place and making those drugs less effective when you really need them. I'm also part of a movement working against turning pregnancy and childbirth into a medical procedure, which happened decades ago in this country. It doesn't need to happen, and if it weren't that way, if there were a midwife instead of an obstetrician for every woman, we would have healthier women and babies in the United States. I certainly don't like it that there's an entire profession telling women that menopause is the beginning of an estrogen deficiency disease that lasts the rest of their lives and will cause them all kinds of ill health if they don't take drugs to stop it. Menopause, which is the reverse side of the coin of puberty, is a time of hormonal transition, turmoil, and turbulence; but it's no more the beginning of ill health than puberty is the beginning of ill health. Each of the examples that I could give you about the medicalization of women's lives is not supported by scientific medicine, but by a veneration of physicians that, in some instances, is appropriate, but not in this instance. If we can challenge that which I think we have started to do in this country and take back our health from the medical realm altogether, we're going to be much better off.

TK: What do you think of the current state of medical practice as a whole?

CP: A lot of women think that finding a nice woman doctor is the answer to their problems with health care, but you know what? Women doctors are more doctor than they are woman. Now, I don't mean to be insulting at all because there are plenty of wonderful women physicians who I respect and love, but the fact is that going through training as a physician in the United States is so intensive and so weighted toward a certain viewpoint, that most people, whether male or female, can only come out with that viewpoint. For the most part our advice to women is to bring knowledge and a questioning attitude to their doctors. You can't just search for the right kind of doctor or a woman doctor and think that guarantees you the right kind of treatment. One thing that's particularly frustrating to women who don't like the medicalization of normal life processes like childbirth and menopause, is how incredibly medicalized most female OBGYNs are. They're just as likely to do cesarean sections as men; they're just as likely to intervene in slow labors; they're just as likely to push hormone replacement therapy to women going through the menopause; and, even though there may be an empathy factor, they may take a little more time, they may listen a little more, they're—for the most part—still going to offer you the same tried and true techniques that though tried and true, aren't actually good for our health.

TK: So what changes would you like to see in women's health care?

CP: When I think of the world as I would like it to be for women's health, I think of a world in which women start to learn about their health at home: they learn about their bodies; they're familiar with self-examination techniques; they know home remedies that have been passed down through their family; and they really have a sense of, "I'm the one who knows my body best." They go on from there to get well-woman care whenever possible from either lay health workers, peer education counselors, nurse practitioners, certified nurse midwives, allied health professionals who are like the people they care for, and who work from an holistic perspective. I would like to see a world in which profit and patentability driving what gets approved by the FDA no longer causes problems. Then the long-standing remedies that we now call "alternative," but that have been used in many cultures for millennia, the ones that actually work, can be marketed. This would differ from today when no one will invest in these products because they can't get the return they get from manufacturing a brand name prescription drug. I would like to see the use of physician specialists for primary care fade away so that when women are seeing physicians for primary care, they are seeing someone who supports the healthy-person approach, rather than supporting this test and that procedure, the let's-dive-in-and-intervene approach. Then we'd certainly have a less expensive, all-around healthier approach to women's health.

TK: What are some issues that need to be addressed but aren't always recognized?

CP: Some of the issues that don't get recognized as women's health issues have a big impact on younger women who should expect the best of health. One, for example, is the health effect of domestic violence. It's only in recent years that domestic violence has been pushed out of the closet that violent men would like to keep it in, and brought out, not only as a social problem, or a problem of violence, but also as a problem that effects women's health. Domestic violence is one of the leading reasons women go to the emergency room. Another issue, for example, is women's work in reducing the rate of deaths and injuries caused by drunk drivers through Mothers Against Drunk Drivers. You wouldn't think of drunk driving as a women's health issue, but the fact that women got active and came up with an effective prevention strategy of tighter rules for blood alcohol levels has lowered the rate of these accidents and led to better health and longer lives. So you can look at important women's health issues from a general, public health perspective and find a very broad approach to women's health.

TK: What do you think of demystifying patients' health issues?

CP: Thirty years ago if anyone talked about a bad experience they had with the health care system, if they found a friendly ear, the response would usually be, "You need a better doctor, let me give you my doctor's number," or "Let me tell you about the person I heard speak." The response was "Find a better professional" not "Take charge yourself." The movements—the feminist health movement, the patient's rights movement, the AIDS movement, and the emphasis on alternative health have all started to shift that to, instead of finding a better professional or a good doctor, educating yourself, taking charge and being the decision maker for yourself as much as possible. It's interesting to me that, in this time when many individual consumers and patients are trying to have more power, we're seeing more groups focused on health care that are really just trying to change practitioners to different or better professionals, like nicer doctors or more female doctors and researchers. In reality, the core of being in charge of your own health is taking control yourself. There's a subtle but important difference between groups that say, "We need better, nicer doctors, more female doctors, doctors that know more about alternative medicine," and groups or movements that say, "Patients and consumers need to be in control." That's where the women's health movement started. People talked about finding a good doctor, but then realized, good doctors aren't the answer, informed patients are the answer.

TK: So what do you think can be done to give patients a stronger voice and more power when dealing with their doctors?

CP: If you believe in a health care movement with the goal of putting power in the hands of patients, you have to believe in information being freely available to everybody, and the source of information being visible, identified. This means no hidden, sneaky drug company information that masquerades as an educational effort by a non-profit group, and no fake web sites named as if they're nonprofit and represent the patient's perspective, but in fact are financed by drug companies. You know, to really make a movement that changes things around so that people are in control of their own health, people must have information from a trustworthy source.

TK: How does one judge whether or not the information provided by an expert physician or scientist in a medical journal is biased? In other words, how can a lay person be sure that the information from these prominent people isn't tainted by outside influences from politics or drug manufacturers?

CP: One of the things we always advise consumers is to watch for the source of the information they're getting, and to see if there's any potential bias that might be subtly influencing its recommendations. You can hear an eminent researcher or scientist on a morning talk show, or on the nightly news, or you can read a newspaper account of an article that's been published in a prestigious journal; what you may not hear is that that researcher's results have been funded by the manufacturer whose product they're talking about. It's starting to be possible to occasionally find that information in written disclosures in medical journals. If you have access to a medical journal, you can see who funds the work. It's very rare to get that kind of disclosure in average, mainstream, broadcast media. The morning talk shows put people on all the time giving their opinion about certain health issues; we activists know just how tightly connected these people are to the companies that make the products they're talking about. There's no way you would know that from watching the TV shows. Similarly, the people who are turned to to give their 10 seconds of august opinion in broadcast news almost never disclose their connections. We encourage anyone who sees experts with connections to drug or medical or insurance companies acting as if they're a neutral source to report them, to just call back the media source that's featured this person and say, "Look, I know that X, Y, and Z companies support this person's research, and I think you should have put that into your coverage." The National Women's Health Network is trying to get a campaign going for a data bank journalists could use to check the financial ties of medical spokespeople that are often in the media. But it's a challenge because uncovering that information is hard going.

TK: Is overprescription of drugs common?

CP: Years ago we used to complain that the only drugs women could get out of their doctors were tranquilizers; that if women came in with anything from arthritis to back trouble to endometriosis they would get a literal or verbal pat on the head, and a prescription for tranquilizers. I think that's changed somewhat, although there are still lots of prescriptions written for mood-altering drugs. Drug companies have realized that women are a fabulous market for prescription drugs: women are concerned about their health; they're used to seeing the doctor frequently; they like to stay informed; and now they're being targeted in the same way that Nike targets young adults for their shoe ads. Women are being targeted with drug ads to convince them that it would be a good idea to take any number of drugs on an ongoing basis.

TK: So what are the main consequences of that targeting by pharmaceutical companies?

CP: "There's no drug safe enough to be worth taking if you don't need it." That axiom comes from Dr. Philip Corfman, a Food and Drug Administration medical officer with a lot of years of experience in women's health. The basic point is that if you're in dire straits, and a drug has been shown to work, it's probably worth taking, even if it has some pretty serious side effects. But if you're healthy to start with, and what you need from the medical system is a way in which to manage your reproduction, or a way to go through the menopausal transition more comfortably, you don't want to deal with any extra risks.

TK: What are the effects of pharmaceutical industries advertising directly to the public?

CP: Unless you're a hermit, you know that the rules have changed about advertising brand name prescription drugs. There are ads on TV that name drugs, and there are ads that don't have any of the long list of warnings and details that used to be in tiny fine print in the back of magazine ads. For consumer groups, that means a mixed blessing. Thirty years ago, we were fighting desperately for people to get information about the drugs they were taking. How can we say that it's bad to get information about drugs through an ad? Shouldn't we be for information? But what is information that's in an ad; is it actually informative, or is it really a sales technique? Our experience so far with direct-to-consumer ads on television is that it's much more of a sales technique than it is informative or educational in any way. Ads naming the drug have been allowed on television for a little less than two years now. In that time, the FDA has found that over half of the pharmaceutical companies that advertise their drugs on television have been breaking the rules: they exaggerate the benefits; they minimize or don't mention the risks; they try to claim that the drug works for groups of people in whom it hasn't been studied; and they try to mislead the public in other ways. The trouble is that the FDA has no power to preview these ads before they're on the air. They don't have nearly the staff or resources they need to watch all these ads. Many times they take action after receiving a complaint from a group like ours; all they can do is tell the company to pull the ad. Maybe the drug company was likely to change that ad anyway to get a fresh image out before people's minds. But the damage has already been done when a consumer sees a misleading ad on television, even if it's later pulled by the FDA. We're concerned that in the long run, something needs to change in terms of laws and regulations so that at a minimum, the FDA has the power and the resources to review ads before they go on TV. In the short term, patients and consmers need to insist that if they even have the faintest glimmer of talking to their doctor about a drug because of direct advertising, they need to insist that they get written medication guides produced by the government, or by an independent consumer group, before they swallow their first pill. It's vitally important that people see the contraindications to taking a drug in writing. The women's health movement that in the 1970s held a memorial service in front of the FDA proved that if women could get their hands on information, they could make the use of a drug safer by ruling themselves out if it was too risky for them, or quickly getting off it if they had any complications. If patients and consumers would insist on that kind of written information now, we could counterbalance the hard sell that's going on with television ads for brand name drugs.

TK: The Network has had some major successes in the past few years involving the National Institutes of Health, the FDA, the National Cancer Institute, to give some examples. Can you discuss some of these?

CP: Some of the things the network has tried to accomplish in the last few years have really been about the misuse of research that puts healthy women at much higher risks than necessary. We've been concerned that too many research trials have been designed by short-sighted doctors used to dealing with dangerous medications, day in and day out. They don't seem to realize that, in designing a prevention study with healthy volunteer subjects, they should be starting with the safest approach possible. We have complained bitterly about the design of the tamoxifen trial for healthy women. We got the consent forms changed and women really listened to us; many that were at low risk actually stayed out of that trial. Another accomplishment was that we told the National Institutes of Health that they were making a mistake in the design of their estrogen replacement therapy study in healthy women. They originally wanted to ask women to volunteer to take estrogen, which is known to cause cancer of the uterus. We told them, "This is wrong, this is ethically wrong; even in a research environment, you shouldn't be asking women to put themselves at risk with a known cancer-causing agent." They finally listened to us, although not until two years later, and after much cost and bureaucratic hassle. But they did change the way they organized that trial. So I think those are some of the accomplishments that have really made a difference in the last few years: protecting healthy people from unnecessary risks in government-funded research.

TK: There are many controversies surrounding breast cancer; can you tell me what some of the most prominent ones are?

CP: Breast cancer has been controversial since the first courageous women started talking to each other about it. Even now that it's a big, justice-based social movement that has mobilized millions of women to agitate for more funding for research, for better treatment, for more respect for survivors, all those things; so many issues related to breast cancer are controversial. One example is that even a good ten years after it's been accepted by leading researchers and policymakers that removing the cancer itself, in a lumpectomy, is as likely to lead to the woman's survival as removing her whole breast, many doctors still routinely do mastectomies. Many hundreds of thousands of women are having mastectomies, having their breasts removed, who don't need that procedure. That's one area that's still controversial. Another area is how to treat advanced disease, because in contrast to women who are diagnosed with their breast cancer early and have good odds of surviving as long as women have been followed so far (about fifteen or twenty years), women whose cancer is diagnosed in an advanced state, or whose cancer recurs in another part of their body, don't have any treatment that's been shown to work for any considerable length of time. A few women do survive for many years; but most women who have advanced breast cancer face continued progression of the disease to the point where it kills them. These women want to live, and their doctors want to help them find a way to live. And all they've been able to offer so far is more of the same: literally, more chemotherapy. If some chemotherapy can't stop advanced cancer, well maybe lots of chemotherapy could. The trouble is that lots of chemotherapy by itself can kill you because it kills the cells in the bone marrow which produce new blood cells and new infection-fighting cells. A very expensive, elaborate procedure designed several years ago has been shown to be effective in cancers based in the blood: high-dose chemotherapy followed by a bone marrow transplant. Very soon after that was shown to be effective in cancers based in the blood, it was offered to women with breast cancer, mostly out of a feeling of "We've got nothing else, so let's give it a try." It became very controversial: it's extremely expensive (in the realm of $100,000), it has fatal side effects itself. Even in the best centers that do it frequently, a percentage of women die within the following couple of weeks as a result of this treatment. Yet women were told, "This is your only chance; this has a twenty-five percent chance of creating a complete remission as opposed to a three percent chance if you just have regular chemotherapy." So women fought for it: sued their insurance companies, lobbied Congress, got state laws passed to mandate that this be covered. In the last several years, about twelve thousand women in the United States have had this procedure, but sadly, only about a thousand of them received it in a clinical trial, so it's taken all this time and all this fighting to find out that it's not a better treatment. We now have five studies that, with the exception of one, have found the high-dose chemotherapy approach is no better than regular chemotherapy. So we're really left back where we were eight, nine, or ten years ago. It's a sad commentary on the way our medical system approaches diseases like cancer. They keep trying the same approaches even when they haven't worked. We've wasted a lot of time that could have been spent looking for approaches that do work.

TK: In the magazine *MAMM,* you were quoted as saying, "What makes it harder for the breast cancer movement than for other movements (such as the AIDS movement) is women's issues about putting themselves first." Can you comment on this?

CP: You know, over the years, there have been so many different kinds of health movements and when people ask me to comment on the women's health movement, or women-specific disease movements like the breast cancer movement, I'm always struck by how much harder it is for women to sustain the kind of energy that men feel so free to give to the causes that effect them. The AIDS movement, for example, liberated tremendous amounts of energy from individuals who gave several nights a week to be part of Act Up or other AIDS projects. On the other hand, the breast cancer movement sparked the same kind of fire in women, but so many women found themselves paying a terrible cost in terms of their families. There were the judgments about them not spending time with their kids because they were gone every night at these meetings; they weren't with their boyfriends or husbands. Women are so much less free to put themselves first, even when their own lives depend on it. So it's really been impressive to me that, fighting against such odds, the breast cancer movement has strongly sustained itself throughout this decade. Because it's not easy to be a woman feminist health activist, let me tell you.

TK: To what do you attribute the success of the National Women's Health Network?

CP: The National Women's Health Network is small, poor, and beleaguered. We're often in a David-versus-Goliath situation; the only reason we have existed for nearly 25 years is because we represent the heartfelt wishes of a strong constituency of individual women (and some of the men who support them) who want a more humane health care system for both women who receive healthcare and women who provide it. They keep us alive with their support and their input, and we go out and try to take their words and make them heard by the people in power. We do a good enough job for our members to keep us alive.

Alice Wolfson

INTERVIEW BY TANIA KETENJIAN

Alice Wolfson is a founding member of the National Women's Health Network. This interview was conducted in May 1999.

TK: I know that you've accomplished a tremendous amount for the women's movement, and that you sparked Carol Downer and so many other women. What would you say are the accomplishments in these last twenty or thirty years of which you are the most proud?

AW: I'm proud of the fact that women feel like they have a right to question what goes into their bodies. I'm proud of the fact that abortion is legal, although clearly a right that we have to constantly be vigilant about. I'm very proud of the fact that more and more people are questioning the medications that they take. Women have been experimented on by the drug companies for years; some of the real medical atrocities have been perpetrated on women, such as diethylstilbestrol, or DES; the Dalkon shield; the birth control pill; estrogen replacement therapy. It was only after the FDA and the pharmaceutical industry were forced to admit that ERT caused endometrial cancer that it finally stopped being automatically prescribed. There are new combinations now—HRT, or, hormone replacement therapy—but back then unopposed estrogen was the drug that women were being given, without being told of its dangers. They had no idea it caused endometrial cancer and that was the risk they were taking. It's not clear to me today how long the FDA, or the pharmaceutical industry, or the medical establishment knew, before women were finally told of its dangers. There was a time when ERT was considered the magic youth pill, a panacea that would protect women against the physical effects of aging: "Worried about wrinkles? Take estrogen!!" There was a book called *Feminine Forever*, which was about taking the pill and staying young forever. Doctors would just say to women as they came into their forties, "Start to take this pill." In fact, my own doctor, just a few years ago, said the same thing to me. I said to her, "Just a minute here," and I handed her the National Women's Health Network booklet on hormones and hormone replacement; so, as an activist, even when you think you've made a lot of changes, you find you haven't. The system is hard to buck.

TK: I'm sure you had a vision for women's health thirty years ago. Does what's happening now match that vision?

AW: It does in some ways, and in some ways it doesn't. What sparks the vision? When I was late in my pregnancy with my first child, I was in the examining room, waiting for the doctor. My ex-husband was with me. The doctor, who was a man and enlightened for the times, came in—and instead of coming over to me, walked right over to my husband and said, "Hello Dr. Wolfson, it's nice to see you." And I thought, "Hey, wait a second; *I'm* the one who's pregnant, *I'm* the one with the big belly lying here in stirrups." I don't think that would happen anymore. I think women are treated with more respect now and no doctor would do that—at least not one who wanted to keep his patients. And that's another thing. You probably won't find many male gynecologists. I don't know a single woman who would go to a male gynecologist. But when I was having kids, you couldn't find a woman in the profession.

TK: What changes in women's health would you like to see today?

AW: Under managed care, allowing only twenty-four hours of hospital care for the birth of a baby or 48 hours after a mastectomy was an outrageous apportionment of care that women were successful in turning around. I think if you get angry enough and the issue means enough to you, you realize that if you become public and large, in the sense of many small voices coming together, you can truly effect change. When we started, we never had any plan whatsoever to demonstrate about the birth control pill. All of us had taken the pill. It looked like something we really wanted. Remember, abortion was illegal and finally we had what we thought was safe and effective birth control. Nobody told us we were going to be paying a very big price for that. We were at a time in our lives when social change was happening all around us and it wasn't so frightening to think of doing something like disrupting Senate hearings and getting arrested for what we believed in. It's much more frightening now because there is less of a climate for social change and less belief that you can effect social change. I think people in some ways have to be braver now.

TK: How did you decide to become a lawyer?

AW: I decided to become a lawyer because, increasingly, all of the issues I was working on as a women's health feminist were ending up in court: sterilization abuse, abortion rights, issues around equal access and the Hyde Amendment; informed consent and products liability. I was able to take the issues just so far and then had to leave them. I had been working for a small community-based women's health organization for 10 years and felt that it was time for a change, and decided to apply to law school, and got in and went.

TK: Do you feel feminism died down in the 1980s?

AW: I don't know that it did because I was in a feminist women's health group throughout the entire 1980s. I didn't go to law school till 1986, so I was surrounded by the feminist movement through the mid-1980s. I would say that the sense of really being able to effect the larger picture probably diminished. We really thought we were going to change the entire system. We really thought that in order to win on our issues, legalized abortion, home births, alternative birth centers, universal day care and after care and all of the different things that made up the great crux of women's movement were really going to change the system. Instead, the system kind of expanded—not completely, obviously, but enough so that enough women had the perception that they had more rights. And then we all got a little older, had kids, and we also had to work and we had less time, and we were not willing to live on the meager salaries you got in the movement if you were lucky enough to be paid at all. So we drifted off into other arenas.

TK: What is it like to look back on your beliefs and ardent forwardness at that time, and how have your concerns changed?

AW: For me, feminism defined my life in a way that political activism I had participated in previously did not. Up until the beginning of my time in the feminist movement, which really started about 1968, I had taken part in political movements, but they were always movements about somebody else: the civil rights movement, the antiwar movement. In those early days, feminism suddenly gave us such a feeling, I think, of belonging and of community, and of something larger than ourselves, that I believe that it continues to inform my life. I believe that the values of those early feminist days stay with me.

TK: How do you think 1960s and 1970s feminism is different from 1990s feminism?

AW: Young women today—depending, obviously, on their socioeconomic class, and what advantages they have—have so much more. They can expect to be true about their lives. Simply being a woman isn't the same kind of problem it was for people in my generation. I think of myself in many ways as part of a transitional generation: on the one hand, growing up in a nice, secure, middle-class way with the expectation that I would go to college, but with the lesson and the constant message that your job is to get married. So, having to weigh the two required me to make choices that today I wouldn't have to make.

TK: A major complaint in the 1960s and 1970s was that women were not really involved in medicine, that medicine was dominated by men. Do you think it has made a big difference that women are now more involved?

AW: It's true that women are more involved in medicine; there are far more women doctors than there were back when we were beginning to demonstrate. But I think that you'll find that, at the top, medicine is still pretty heavily dominated by men. My guess is that managed care is going to change everything. As medicine becomes less desirable in terms of the amount of money you can make, you'll see more and more women coming into the profession. Most young women now prefer, for instance, women gynecologists.

TK: Do you think there are groups now, apart from the National Women's Health Network, that can be effective in bringing forward a woman's voice? Furthermore, can groups that take pharmaceutical money be effective?

AW: It's clear, if you take money from any sector, pharmaceutical, tobacco, whatever, you're beholden to that sector. I don't think, however, that it necessarily means you can't be effective.

TK: What are the different ways that the health groups get funding and support?

AW: That's the ancient question of how to fundraise: membership, a membership base of major donors, foundations. I've spent many years fundraising for women's health groups, and it's a never-ending process. The problem is, if you take a major part of your money from a sector that then wants to use you, you're pretty compromised about what you can do and how independent your voice can be.

TK: It's less common now for groups of women or even men to stand up and protest against something they don't feel comfortable with. What would you say to those people that feel discouraged? What should they do to be effective?

AW: Maybe we made the changes that were possible because there was room for the system to give. My sense is that for significant social change to happen now, we will have to develop a unified social vision. I was in that part of the women's movement that felt, not that we wanted a piece of the pie, but rather that the whole pie had to change. In that sense, I don't think that we've been that successful, because I don't think the whole pie has changed. But in the sense that there's been much more of the pie available to us, we have been successful.

TK: If you were to be part of a feminist health group now, as the century is turning, would you find yourself asking for things similar to what you asked for in the past?

AW: I would see us having to wage some of the same struggles if I were to go back into a feminist group at the turn of the century. I see the fight for quality child care as so important and integral to women's rights. And we certainly don't have that. I also consider access to information, access to health care, access to education for women as very primary and important issues. I loved having children and loved having the luxury of being with them and working as much or as little as I had to, but that, again, is a question of choice. If you're going to be really able to have the choice, then you have to have so many societal supports in place to make that a true choice. We just don't have it. I don't see these things as having improved at all.

Belita Cowan

INTERVIEW BY TANIA KETENJIAN

Belita Cowan is president of the Lymphoma Foundation of America and a founder and former executive director (1978-83) of the National Women's Health Network. This interview was conducted in September 1999.

TK: When you started the feminist newspaper *Her-Self,* I imagine it was a more receptive time. What would you suggest for people today who would like to start a newspaper like yours?

BC: We live in a different age now. It's almost unnecessary to mail out specialized newspapers because of the Internet. Almost every news story can be found on-line today. Of course, you still have to consider the source of the news story and whether or not you trust that source. That was a big question when we started the National Women's Health Network: Who do you trust to give you the whole truth about medical treatments? Drug companies? Hospitals? A government agency? It was clear that the most trustworthy source of information was us!

TK: What should people do if they encounter a situation similar to the one in Ann Arbor—they know the results of an experiment are false, and they know that the subjects may not even know they were in an experiment?

BC: Because of the work I did to expose the Ann Arbor study in the 1970s, I doubt there is a college or university today that would test a drug on students without the proper protocol, or signed consent forms, or an ethics review board.

TK: How has your work with the DES experiments manifested in other areas?

BC: In general, I think my work on DES has taught us all a good lesson: Don't be afraid to challenge researchers, scientists, and medical authorities if you have good reason to think they are wrong.

TK: What have you been working on now?

BC: For the past 10 years, I have served as president of the Lymphoma Foundation of America, a nonprofit charity that I started because I disagreed with the politics of the cancer establishment. I wanted to create an organization that welcomes controversial issues and carves out new health rights for cancer patients. For example, we filed a freedom of information request with the National Cancer Institute on behalf of a cancer patient whose doctor wouldn't let him read the research protocol for the experimental drugs he was taking. NCI ruled in our favor, and as a result all cancer patients enrolled in government-funded studies now have the right to see the protocols for their particular experiment.

Although many national cancer organizations were approached, my lymphoma organization was the only one in the country willing to participate with the ACLU in a reproductive rights case on behalf of a pregnant patient who was denied life-saving leukemia drugs because she was pregnant. The patient was forced by the hospital against her will to have a c-section, causing the death of both her and her baby. The settlement resulted in a new policy that guarantees the right of a cancer patient to receive cancer treatments while pregnant.

We also filed a lawsuit against the U.S. Drug Enforcement Agency to change marijuana from a class I drug to a class II drug, thus allowing doctors to prescribe marijuana to relieve nausea in cancer patients undergoing chemotherapy. The Lymphoma Foundation of America was the only cancer organization that would participate in this important lawsuit.

Currently I am working on a research project to see if pesticides cause lymphoma.

Before starting the Lymphoma Foundation of America, I served for 5 years as the health policy advisor to the attorney general of Maryland. I worked on patients' rights issues in the Consumer Protection Division. While there, I wrote two books, one of which became the most popular consumer publication in 1988 and 1989: *Health Care Shopper's Guide: 59 Ways to Save Money!* and won a national award. I also directed a project for the chief of consumer protection, publishing first-of-its-kind consumer price lists of individually-named doctors and what they charged patients for their services. This data, formerly kept secret by the government, was obtained through the Medicare program.

TK: You've had so many accomplishments. What would you say that you're most proud of?

BC: Starting the National Women's Health Network, starting the Lymphoma Foundation of America, helping Byllye Avery start the National Black Women's Health Project, and writing the *Health Care Shopper's Guide.*

TK: How did you help Byllye Avery establish the National Black Women's Health Project?

BC: With my good friend Byllye Avery, I had the pleasure and privilege of becoming her mentor, teaching her fundraising skills, publicity techniques, and introducing her to some important people—all needed to start the NBWHP. I helped her plan the first national Black women's health conference in Atlanta, and raised funds for it. I was delighted when her project separated from the National Women's Health Network in order to become an independent health advocacy organization.

TK: What would you say to emerging activists about how to organize and make a voice for themselves?

BC: I would urge people to become familiar with the National Women's Health Network, become involved in its work, and be passionate about your beliefs. Don't compromise your ideals. And don't feel discouraged if others become petty or jealous. With the national Women's Health Network, we had, from the very beginning, a policy forbidding the organization from accepting drug company or industry money. To this day, 25 years later, that policy allows the Network to speak out on controversial women's health issues with a clear conscience and no conflict of interest.

I became an activist and have been one for so long because of my sense of justice. You see injustice and you're motivated to do something about it. That's why I became involved in social activism. Who is going to advocate for people who don't have a voice? That's what I want to do.

Susan Brownmiller: Memoir of a Revolutionary

CARRIE CARMICHAEL

Susan Brownmiller's most recent book is *In Our Time: Memoir of a Revolution* (Dial Press, 1999). This interview was conducted in May 1999. ©1999 by Carrie Carmichael. Reprinted by permission.

Antirape activist and feminist author Susan Brownmiller shares her thoughts with writer and stand-up comic Carrie Carmichael about women's progress since the heady days of the 1970s women's movement, and about her life as a feminist today.

CC: When did you get into the movement?

SB: In 1968. By 1970, I was full-time. But the feeling was that there would be a revolution within five years. Whatever the feeling was then was that revolution wouldn't take more than 5 years. And I never felt that way. You know, I was older. Most of the public space people and leaders of the movement were older than that group of twenty-somethings that made the revolution. So I knew it wasn't going to happen in five years. They got very upset at the institutionalization of our ideas. For example, we were talking about rapists, political crimes against women, you had to stop the rapists. And then it became a social work strategy with the rape crisis centers. That's something else. Same thing with battered women. The whole idea was to stop the batterers, and to help the women too, of course. But now it's become institutionalized with the battered women's shelters, which were an idea from the movement. But the taking over of radical causes, and then dropping the feminist politics and just going with the social concern, is inevitable. Although a lot of people would say that it has made them unhappy. I mean, where is the politics in all this anymore? I don't know. But what does bother me is that we have lived through enormous changes, and young people don't seem to know that all these changes were hard-won; that people fought for them, that a whole generation of women fought for these changes. They don't know about it. They just know this is the way the world is now. So that makes me sad. But the changes have been enormous, particularly the transformation of the workplace. It's absolutely enormous.

CC: I feel that tinge of sadness when I see the huge changes in the workplace. Women aren't Fortune 500 CEOs yet, but there are these short-skirted executives, throwing out their IPOs, who are now multizillionaires, who have absolutely no sense of historical perspective—who they owe or who helped get them there. Do I expect something from them? Not that I was that active in the movement that way, but as a generation member, as a political supporter, I would expect them to at least know the history and to acknowledge it. And it saddens me. Is that vanity on my part or is it that I'm so afraid that women's power and rights will just get sucked away again?

SB: It's possible because there are certainly those out there who would like that to happen. But I guess they haven't known the history because they haven't been given the history *as history*. While it was happening, there was no need to say anything. We were all doing it. Everybody knew. Then there was that decade or so when people just said, "Shut up, already, would you?" Nobody wanted to talk about it. And now we're all starting to write our books and try to get our programs on television and say, "Hey, look—this was a revolution! We did it; We ought to know about it."

CC: I wanted to talk about aging and taking care of our aging bodies both as political women and as—

SB: It's tough. It's tough to see the changes to your body and know that they are not attractive. Being attractive is so important to a woman's sense of identity. It's not pleasant.

CC: Do you think it's easier to be aging and older and still attractive as a woman now?

SB: Yes. For sure. We don't have to wear old-lady clothes.

CC: And it's a function of...?

SB: It's a function of the women's movement. And it's a function of the whole loosening up of conformity, which led to so much rigidity in attire and clothing. You can be in your sixties and wear jeans, and people don't think you're weird. You can wear a T-shirt. You don't have to look like what they always used to say, "A little old lady in tennis shoes," which was such a hostile image. You don't have to look that way anymore....

CC: When you were in your twenties and you thought about someone in her sixties, what did she look like in your mind's eye? Was she healthy? I mean, she certainly wasn't in jeans.

SB: Well, it seemed like it was the end of the line. But it's not now, because we all are living longer and we all are healthier.... There are all sorts of problems that our parents' generation and our grandparents' generation faced in terms of health that we do not face in terms of health. So our problems now include face lifts. Because people feel, "Hey, I'm still alive and I'm still sexual, and I can look a little better."

CC: There's a terrible pressure to maintain a false sense of youth.

SB: You know, it's funny. I read a section from my book out loud and it was from our *Ladies' Home Journal* sit-in. And one of our demands was, "We demand that the magazine stop publishing all articles geared to the preservation of youth, implying that age has no graces of its own"—something that young women could say. Now I'm trying to figure out, what are the graces, I don't know any. I got so upset a few years ago.... I hadn't done anything athletic in years. And also I noticed all of these terrible things happening to my body that I know can be fixed by plastic surgery: A little liposuction here, a little moving the breasts back up to where they used to be here. And when I began to realize I was thinking of these things, I was terrified. I was absolutely horrified that even I had fallen into a consideration of these procedures. And then I remembered that... if I wanted to do something positive for my body at this stage of my life, I should find a sport and do it. So I took up competitive Ping-Pong. And it's wonderful. It didn't take away those problems, but I'm thinking about other things. I'm thinking about how to whop that ball, really wallop it.

CC: How different are we now from the way we were 30 years ago and—for young women—in terms of seeing ourselves as the world sees us… choosing to extend the time of aging, and changing our appearance to be more beautiful?

SB: I don't know, because aging is a whole other thing. You can't just ask that generation that was militant in the 1970s, you can't ask them in the 1990s if they have reevaluated some of the things they thought they'd never do, because they would say yes. But it's not fair. You have to talk to young women and find out if things are different for them. And I don't think they are so different—I think that no one ever thinks they're going to age. And certainly our movement was a Peter Pan and Wendy movement. I don't think we ever thought we'd age. And I don't think we ever thought that we would have to deal with these problems. But you notice how many women who were feminists, or who still are feminists, write a final book about aging. It's no accident that the list includes Beauvoir, Friedan, Germaine Greer. There you are. If you are a person who has been dissatisfied in life with the condition of women, and then you find that you are an old woman, you're going to be latching on to that issue. But it is a slightly different issue.

CC: Your second class status is now compounded by your elderly status. When men may, for the first time in their lives, maybe upon retirement or infirmity, suddenly get a sense of "I'm not as powerful as I was before."

SB: Getting older has certainly made me understand why older men choose younger women. It gives them that illusion that they are young again. It must be wonderful for them.

CC: Does it make you want to take up with a younger man?

SB: I did.

CC: And did it do the same thing for you?

SB: At the time. Yes, it did. I still see him a bit. But I'm too realistic. I can't delude myself into thinking I'm that age. And also it's not what I need. I need that, yes. You can't think of that as a life partnership for the rest of your life.

CC: My own personal theory is that older men take up with bimbos that they would never take home to Mom because, by the time they are older, mothers are dead.

SB: Now they can literally play.

CC: I think that in the last 10 years, menopause has come out of the closet.

SB: I don't know, has it?

CC: I think people talk about it. I think women who were feminists learned how to fight in the medical women's movement field, and I think they fought in the menopause area pretty well too. What's your take on that, or your experience with friends who've gone through menopause and the hormonal replacement issue?

SB: But hormonal replacement is so debatable. I don't know. I had such an easy menopause that it wasn't a concern. Friends who had a tougher one and chose to do estrogen replacement, I wish they hadn't chosen that. That's just my feeling, that it's not a good thing. And we haven't talked at all about breast cancer.

CC: That's totally out of the closet. We don't even refer to it as "the big C" anymore. We're very clear about it: there are pink ribbons, there are marches.

SB: That was fascinating because it seemed to be the result of all the AIDS activism. Women with breast cancer said, "Hey, what about us?" There are a lot more women with breast cancer than men with AIDS. Once they became militant, now there's this movement of men with prostate cancer. It's all very positive.

CC: What all these movements tell me, as a mortal person subject to disease, is that you've got to be in a constant state of diligence and advocacy for yourself because the model of the medical community is not going to help you out unless you scream. It's the squeaky wheel syndrome. And I think that women learned that early on and now various diseases in groups have taken that up. Abortion rights wouldn't have changed if it hadn't been for the screaming. Breast cancer treatment wouldn't have changed if it hadn't been for the screaming. We'd like to think that the medical community could help us out. One of the things that I think that is difficult for the unsophisticated and the non-insiders to figure out is what health experts to pay attention to. Which ones are really being paid by the drug companies to promote something. Do you have any sense of how we can judge who we should listen to? I can't find a doctor who is not trying to push hormone replacement on me. It's almost like brainwashing. I do not believe in it. I think if you have bad symptoms, short-term hormonal replacement is okay to get you through.... How do you judge a health expert's independence? How can you trust them?

SB: I don't know. I don't know what job the women's magazines are doing in sorting it all out. There are so many kooks out there with health regimens for people.

CC: Herbal colonics.

SB: Right. It's hard to know. You just have to go with what sounds right to you and what sounds very wrong to you is wrong....

CC: I have a friend who is really smart, and she self-diagnosed a couple of conditions and she took a copy of *Harvard Women's Health Watch* [a health newsletter] to her internist. And she has a fairly young female internist who is of a different mind who said, "You know, you're right." This is a sea change in a medical practitioner who, because of youth, or experience, or gender, could see herself in a partnership with the patient. That's an enormous difference.

SB: And also they're not first-naming you and treating you like a child anymore either.

CC: What about abortion? How do we evaluate the direction we're going in?

SB: There's a problem with abortion rights. Because when abortion was illegal, the movement could speak with one voice and say, "We demand our right, we demand access to good and legal medical attention. We need the procedure. We need the right to abortion." And it was a very simple articulation. And as soon as abortion became legal, unfortunately, in a movement led largely by women—people like Lynda Bird Franke and others—they began to express their doubts, they began to talk about the trauma of having an abortion, they began to say, "Oh God, I really wish I didn't have to. It's a memory I'm going to have to live with for the rest of my life." I think that's been very, very negative. And it's not anything that I've ever thought. I've had three abortions and I never had a moment of doubt that what I was doing was anything but absolutely right and necessary. So in a strange way, the success of *Roe v. Wade* opened a whole new dialogue. There was another reason for it, and that was that reproductive technology itself became much more sophisticated so that you could save the life of the fetus outside the womb earlier than you could before. But it's almost impossible now to say "I had an abortion, and you know what, I didn't suffer any ambivalence or any emotional trauma here, I was just very glad that I was unpregnant." It's impossible to say that aloud now. Because the conventional discourse says that you must suffer in some way. It has to have been an agonizing decision. And I can tell you that for a lot of us, it wasn't. By putting that new element into the public dialogue, it has prevented a lot of women from having an abortion. They're not so afraid of the physical procedure, it's that they have been conditioned to expect emotional repercussions. And I think that's nonsense. I really do.

CC: Do you think that that is a sadistic or manipulative plot from those who fight choice?

SB: Well, it becomes that.... The right to abortion is such a fundamental right for women that the anti-abortion movement is fueled by those who wish that women would not have equal rights in society. They convince themselves that they are so obsessed about saving lives. There are lots of lives out there to save if they want to save lives. But they know that it's the crucial issue to women's evolving. They must have the right to an abortion.

CC: Where do you think we are in terms of maintaining the security of that right? Is it threatened if women take it for granted?

SB: They take it for granted until it happens to them and then they don't take it for granted any more. It's hard.

CC: You've done a lot with not only the way we move our bodies around, but with how they are invaded and assaulted against our will in your study of rape. Where are we now as a society in terms of dealing with rape, the medical consequences of it for the victims?

SB: There have been enormous changes. When we started talking about rape, it was shrouded in silence, it was the subject of frightening, hysterical rumors, and also giggles. It was not a subject you could talk about without nervous laughter. And that has certainly disappeared. And I think more women than ever before in history are aware of their right not to be violated physically. And if they are, they get much more sympathetic treatment by the police, by the hospitals, and in the courts. There have been famous cases. Like the Tupac Shakur case, [which] was extraordinary, and Mike Tyson. That's just amazing.

CC: On a scale from 0 to 100 percent, where are we in terms of removing the victim as blame object?

SB: That still crops up from time to time, because you've still got defense lawyers out there who want to win at any cost. So they'll keep bringing it up. And if it's an interracial case, people are still afraid to challenge a defense that tries to play with it. That's a tough area, because you're pitting race against sex. I do think we are not blaming the victim so much, but we're still not so far along in terms of ending the assaults. Someone once said to me, "Well, if your book was that successful, why aren't there fewer rapes? Why are men still raping us?" Well, they're not the ones who are reading the book.

Contributor Biographies

MARGOT ADLER is a correspondent for National Public Radio and the author of *Drawing Down the Moon*, the classic study of contemporary paganism, *Goddess Spirituality* and *Heretic's Heart*, a memoir of the 1960s.

AMY ALLINA is program director at the National Women's Health Network, an independent, member-supported organization dedicated to safeguarding women's health rights and interests by providing accurate, unbiased health information to women and advocating for national health policies that address women's health needs. They accept no money from pharmaceutical companies, medical device manufacturers, or tobacco companies, and have been an independent voice for women's health since their founding in 1974. The Network was founded by Barbara Seaman, Belita Cowan, Alice Wolfson, Mary Howell, and Phyllis Chesler.

CHARON ASETOYER is currently the executive director and founder of the Native American Women's Health Education Resource Center and the Native American Community Board. Prior to founding the Resource Center, Charon developed a Native American Health Education Project for the American Friends Service Committee and worked to improve community health in San Francisco through the Urban Indian Health Clinic. Ms. Asetoyer has served on the board of directors for the Indigenous Women's Network, the Honor the Earth Campaign, and the National Women's Health Network.

BYLLYE Y. AVERY founded the National Black Women's Health Project in 1981, and has been a women's health care activist for more than 20 years. Ms. Avery co-founded the Gainsville Women's Health Center and co-founded Birthplace, an alternative birthing center in Gainsville, Florida.

She moved to Atlanta in 1981 to begin the NBWHP, a non-profit organization committed to defining, promoting, and maintaining the physical, mental, and emotional well-being of African-American women.

A dreamer, "visionary," and grassroots realist, Byllye Avery has combined activism and social responsibility in developing a national forum for the exploration of health issues of African-American women, the gathering and documenting of the African-American woman's health experiences in America, and the provision of a supportive atmosphere for African-American women.

Byllye Avery has received the MacArthur Foundation Fellowship for Social Contribution, the Essence Award for community service, and many other awards and honors.

LORI BARER, originally from New Jersey, is a graduate of the University of Michigan. She plans on attending public health school in the fall, where she will study women's health.

PAULINE B. BART is professor emerita of sociology and women's studies in the department of psychiatry at the University of Illinois. Her most recent books are *Stopping Rape: Successful Survival Strategies,* co-authored with Patricia O'Brien, and *Violence Against Women: The Bloody Footprints,* co-authored with Eileen Moran. As an activist in issues of violence against women and women's health, fields which have recently substantially converged, she considers her task to demystify the world for women.

JENNIFER BAUMGARDNER is a New York–based writer and activist. Once an editor at *Ms.,* she now writes for *Bust,* the *Nation, Jane, Out, HUES, Glamour, Marie Claire, Z,* and *Ms.,* among other magazines. She has also written for the book *Alt.culture* and contributed a chapter with Judy Blume to *Letters of Intent.* Her essay "Desperately Seeking Farrah" is featured in the recent book *The Bust Guide to the New Girl Order,* and she is the co-author of a book on the state of feminism called *Manifesta: Young Women, Feminism, and the Future,* forthcoming in Y2K from Farrar, Straus & Giroux.

JULIE BECKER, M.P.H., is a Ph.D. candidate at the department of health studies, Temple University. Having founded the Women's Environmental Health Network, she is currently researching the quality and accessibility of health information on the internet.

KAREN BEKKER studied Judaic studies and art at Oberlin College. She is on the board of New York NOW, and has been actively involved in the feminist movement for several years. Her writing includes several articles in *Lilith*.

LOUISE BERNIKOW is the author of six books and currently lectures on college campuses on "The Shoulders We Stand On: Women As Agents of Change."

JOEL BLEIFUSS is the editor of *In These Times*, an independent newsweekly based in Chicago with which he has been affiliated since 1986. As author for many years of "The First Stone" column in *In These Times*, Bleifuss regularly covered public health issues. His series of articles on carcinogens in cosmetics was honored as Project Censored's No. 2 "most censored" story of 1997.

SUSAN BROWNMILLER is the author of *Against Our Will* (1975), *Femininity* (1984), *Waverly Place* (1989), and *Seeing Vietnam* (1994). Her most recent book is *In Our Time: Memoir of a Revloution*, published by Dial Press in 1999.

DIAN DINCIN BUCHMAN, PH.D., is an internationally published expert on preventive medicine. Her books include *Herbal Medicine, Ancient Healing Secrets, The Complete Herbal Guide to Natural Health and Beauty, The Complete Guide to Natural Sleep*, and *The Complete Book of Water Therapy*, to be republished as *The Complete Guide to Water Healing* in December 2000.

CAEDMON MAGBOO CAHILL, a native Bostonian, is currently a student of anthropology at Barnard College in New York City.

PAULA J. CAPLAN, PH.D., is a clinical and research psychologist and author of the *New Don't Blame Mother: Mending the Mother-Daughter Relationship* (Routledge, 2000); *The Myth of Women's Masochism; They Say You're Crazy: How the World's Most Powerful Psychiatrists Decide Who's Normal;* and six other books. She is a Visiting Scholar at Brown University's Pembroke Center for Research and Teaching on Women.

CARRIE CARMICHAEL is a writer and performer living in New York City. She is the author of the classic *Non-Sexist Childraising* (Beacon Press), *How to Relieve Menstrual Cramps and Other Menstrual Problems* with Marcia L. Storch, M.D., and three other books. Ms. Carmichael won broadcast awards for her work on the NBC Radio Network, and has contributed to numerous magazines and broadcasts. Now she acts and does standup comedy. "Geriatric Obstetrics" grew out of her comedy act and was first published in the *East Hampton Star*. Currently she is finishing her one-woman show, *The Carmichael Crumb Theory*.

San Francisco-based medical journalist MICHAEL CASTLEMAN is "one of the nation's top health writers" (*Library Journal*). He is the author of 10 books, most recently: *There's Still a Person in There* (Putnam), a comprehensive guide to Alzheimer's disease, and *Blended Medicine* (Rodale), a home medical guide that combines mainstream and complementary approaches to treating more than 100 conditions. Castleman has written for dozens of magazines, among them: *Reader's Digest, Family Circle, New Woman, Redbook, Cosmopolitan, Men's Health,* and *Healthy Living.* He has also taught medical writing at the University of California, Berkeley, Graduate School of Journalism. He is the husband of a breast cancer survivor.

DEBORAH CHASE is the author of seven books, including *Terms of Adornment* (HarperCollins) and *The Extend Your Life Diet* (Pocket Books). She is an alumnus of Bronx High School of Science, a winner of the Westinghouse Science Talent Search, and graduated from New York University with a dual degree in science and journalism. She has done research at the National Cancer Institute, New York University School of Medicine and is currently writing a book on the prevention of diabetes.

ARIEL CHESLER is in his senior year at Brandeis University. He is an English major with a minor in Judaic Studies and has also completed the women's studies program. He plans to attend law school after graduation, and hopes to begin a career in the law as well as becoming an author.

PHYLLIS CHESLER, PH.D., is professor emerita of psychology and women's studies, a co-founder of the Association for Women in Psychology (1969) and the National Women's Health Network (1974). She is the author of nine books including *Women and Madness,* and most recently, *Letters to a Young Feminist.* She is an expert courtroom witness and psychotherapist.

SUZANNE CLORES is the author of a children's book, *Native American Women* (Chelsea House, Inc., 1995) and a forthcoming book about Generation X women and the pursuit of spirituality (Conari Press, 2000).

MARCIA COHEN is an editor and writer whose work has appeared in the *New York Times Magazine* as well as many other national newspapers and magazines. She is the author of *The Sisterhood,* a Book of the Month Club Featured Alternate. She is also co-author, with Dr. Gilbert Simon, of *The Parents' Pediatric Companion.*

VICTOR COHN is a former science editor of the *Washington Post* whose long-time coverage of science and medicine won him many of journalism's highest honors, as well as an honorary doctorate of science from Georgetown University.

His contribution here is drawn from his book *News & Numbers: A Guide to Reporting Statistical Claims and Controversies in Health and Other Fields* (Iowa State University Press, 1989, rev. 1994), now in an eighth printing and in use at many journalism schools. *Nieman Reports* called it a "classic."

GENA COREA is a writer, dancer, co-founder of the Feminist International Network of Resistance to Reproductive and Genetic Engineering (FINRRAGE), and a certified focusing trainer. She gives workshops on creating a first person science of reproduction and also on developing a relationship with body symptoms. Her books include *The Hidden Malpractice* (Jove Publications), *The Mother Machine,* and *The Invisible Epidemic* (HarperCollins). She lives in Cambridge, Massachusetts.

PHILIP CORFMAN, M.D., a graduate of Oberlin College, Harvard Medical School, and obstetrics and gynecology residencies at Harvard Hospital, practiced his specialty at one of the first HMOs in the county, the Rip Van Winkle Clinic in upstate New York. He was appointed a Macy Foundation research fellow at Columbia-Presbyterian and, following the fellowship, Dr. Corfman joined the National Institute of Child Health and Human Development as a consultant in obstetrics and gynecology". In 1968 he became the first Director of the Center for Population Research. During this period, he was at the World Health Organization and served on several of its advisory committees. In 1984, he was detailed full time by NIH to the Human Reproduction Programme to reorganize and direct its research and development activities. In 1987, at the end of his WHO assignment, Dr. Corfman moved to the FDA to be in charge of the medical review of drugs for contraception, fertility, obstetrics, and gynecology. He retired from the FDA in late 1997 and is now doing consulting work.

BELITA COWAN is president of the Lymphoma Foundation of America, Inc., and previously was Health Policy Advisor to the attorney general (1985-89), a consultant to The American Prevention Council, Inc. (1992-95) and a founder and executive director of the National Women's Health Network (1978-83). She is also the author of *Health Care Shoppers Guide: 59 Ways to Save Money* (1987), *Nursing Homes: What You Need to Know* (1990), and *Women's Health Care: Resources, Writings, and Bibliographies* (1977). She has testified before the U.S. Senate, the U.S. House of Representatives, the U.S. Food and Drug Administration, and the District of Columbia, City Council.

ANGELA Y. DAVIS is known internationally for her ongoing work to combat all forms of oppression in the U.S. and abroad. Over the years she has been active as a student, teacher, writer, scholar, and activist/organizer. She is a living witness to the historical struggles of the contemporary era.

In 1969 she came to national attention after being removed from her teaching position in the philosophy department at UCLA as a result of her social activism and her membership in the Communist Party. In 1970 she was placed on the FBI's Ten Most Wanted List on false charges, and was the subject of an intense police search that drove her underground and culminated in one of the most famous trials in recent U.S. history. During her sixteen-month incarceration, a massive international "Free Angela Davis" campaign was organized, leading to her acquittal in 1972.

During the last twenty-five years, Professor Davis has lectured in all of the fifty United States, as well as in Africa, Europe, the Caribbean, and the former Soviet Union. Her articles and essays have appeared in numerous journals and anthologies, and she is the author of five books, including *Angela Davis: An Autobiography; Women, Race & Class;* and the recently published *Blues Legacies and Black Feminism: Gertrude "Ma" Rainey, Bessie Smith and Billie Holiday. The Angela Y. Davis Reader,* a collection of Professor Davis's writings that spans nearly three decades, will be forthcoming from Blackwell Publishers in late 1998 or early 1999.

ANSELMA DELL'OLIO is a writer, lecturer, founder and director of the New Feminist Theater, and associate producer of *Woman* on WCBS-TV in New York.

MAGDA DENES was a postgraduate professor of psychoanalysis and psychotherapy at Adolph University and New York University, and a supervisor in the department of psychiatry at the Mount Sinai School of Medicine. She was also a psychoanalyst in private practice in New York. Her other book is *Castles Burning: A Child's Life in War.*

CAROL DOWNER has become a legendary figure in the women's health movement. In the early '70s she pioneered the concept of vaginal and cervical self-examination as a key to self-empowerment, A lawyer, she is the founding executive director of the Federation of Feminist Women's Health Centers.

MARTA DRURY is a donor-activist with a focus on women and children of color. She has also been active with women's groups in the Balkans. She lives in California and opens her home to non-profit groups for rest and recreation or board meetings.

OPHIRA EDUT is the editor of *Adios, Barbie: Young Women Write About Body Image and Identity* (Seal Press), and the founding publisher of *HUES* magazine. She is currently associate editor of *Ms.,* and lives in New York.

BARBARA EHRENREICH is the author of *Blood Rites: Origins and History of the Passions of War.*

MARVIN S. EIGER, M.D., is a nationally known pediatrician who practiced in New York City for 30 years; most of his patients were breastfed. Educated at Harvard University, Dr. Eiger received medical training at New York University School of Medicine and served his residency in pediatrics at Bellevue Hospital. Dr. Eiger is the father of two children and lives in Manhattan with his wife, Carol.

ARLENE EISENBERG is the author of several bestselling books, including *What to Expect When You're Expecting, What to Eat When You're Expecting, What to Expect the First Year,* and *What to Expect the Toddler Years.* For several years she has written an informative column with her daughter Heidi Murkoff for *Parenting* and *Baby Talk* magazines. Updated every six weeks, the "expect" books are in their 75th printing. Together they have sold nearly 17 million copies and have been translated in 21 different languages.

VICTORIA ENG lives and works in New York City. She is currently enrolled at Columbia University, earning her MFA in Creative Nonfiction.

BARBARA FINDLEN, editor-at-large for *Ms.,* is the editor of the anthology *Listen Up: Voices From the Next Feminist Generation* (Seal Press), and co-author, with Kristen Golden, of *Remarkable Women of the Twentieth Century: 100 Portraits of Achievement* (Friedman/Fairfax).

PHYLLIS L. FINE is a psychotherapist in private practice and the co-founder of Midwest Support, an organization formed specifically to work with victims of professional abuse. She is also a founder of Families Against Sexually-abusive Therapists and other professionals (FAST).

SHULAMITH FIRESTONE was a founder of the Women's Liberation Movement in the late '60s and author of the classic *The Dialectic of Sex: The Case for Feminist Revolution* (William Morrow, 1970). More recently she has been writing fiction, notably *Airless Spaces* (Semiotext(e), 1998)

AUDREY FLACK is one of the world's leading photorealist painters. Her work is in the collections of many great museums. In recent decades she has turned to sculpture, where, in particular, she has been "searching for the Goddess." Her books, such as *Art and Soul,* have also been bestsellers. Flack has been called the feminist conscience of the College Art Association.

ANNE ROCHON FORD has worked in Canada as a writer and activist on women's health issues for the past 16 years. She co-founded several national, provincial and local women's health groups, including the Canadian Women's Health Network and DES Action Toronto. A particular focus of her work has remained the issue of women and pharmaceuticals.

ELLEN FRANKFORT was the health columnist for the *Village Voice* and the author of several books. She was one of the key journalists who popularized the women's health movement. In the early 1970s, she served as a trustee at the Women's Medical Center on Irving Place in New York City, the first freestanding legal abortion clinic in the Western world.

LUCINDA FRANKS is a winner of the Pulitzer Prize for National Reporting, 1972, and many other awards. She has written for the *New York Times,* the *New Yorker,* and *Talk* magazine.

MARLENE GERBER FRIED is director of the Civil Liberties and Public Policy Program at Hampshire College, and president of the National Network of Abortion Funds. She is a long-time activist in the reproductive right movement and editor of *From Abortion to Reproductive Freedom: Transforming A Movement* (South End Press, 1990).

CHARLOTTE PERKINS GILMAN (1860–1935) was born in Hartford, Connecticut. After *The Yellow Wallpaper,* her most famous book, came *Women and Economics,* published in 1898. From 1909 to 1916 she edited and wrote *The Forerunner,* a monthly feminist magazine.

STEPHANIE GOLDEN is an independent scholar, journalist, and medical writer. Her most recent book is *Slaying the Mermaid: Women and the Culture of Sacrifice* (1998). She is also the author of *The Women Outside: Myths and Meanings of Homelessness* (1992), which was a finalist for the Robert F. Kennedy Book Award, and co-author (with Yamuna Zake) of a fitness/exercise book, *Body Rolling: An Experiential Approach to Complete Muscle Release* (1997). She has written for *Brooklyn Bridge,* the *San Francisco Chronicle, New York Newsday,* and *Yoga Journal,* among other publications.

JENNIFER GONNERMAN has been a staff writer for the *Village Voice* since 1997. She covers the criminal justice beat and has reported on prisons, drugs, gangs, domestic violence, and the courts. Her stories have also appeared in *Vibe, Ms., Glamour, The Source,* the *New York Observer,* and the *Nation.* In January 1999, she won a Media Fellowship from the Center on Crime, Communities & Culture of the Open Society Institute.

LOIS GOULD has written eight novels, two works of non-fiction, two satires posing as children's fables, and a collection of personal essays. A frequent contributor of articles and reviews to the *New York Times,* she created that newspaper's personal column "HERS." Her memoir about her mother, the fashion designer Jo Copeland, titled *Mommy Dressing: A Love Story,* was published in 1998 by Anchor/Doubleday.

TARA GREENWAY is an actress and playwright in New York City. With collaborator/ director Ariane Brandt, Tara has written and performed *Missionary Position*, a play about one woman's fight for sexual and spiritual freedom, which premiered off-Broadway at the Grove Street Playhouse in New York after its original workshop production at the HERE Arts Center.

GERMAINE GREER was born in Melbourne, Australia in 1939. She is the author of several books, including *The Female Eunuch* (1969) and *The Whole Woman* (1999).

CATHERINE GUND is a film/videomaker, writer, teacher and activist. Her media work—which focuses on the radical right, art and culture, HIV/AIDS, and gay and lesbian issues—has screened around the world in festivals, on public and cable television, at community-based organizations, universities and museums. Her productions include *Hallelujah! Ron Athey: A Story of Deliverance; When Democracy Works; Positive: Life with HIV; Sacred Lies Civil Truths; Not Just Passing Through; Among Good Christian People; I'm You You're Me—Women Surviving Prison Living With AIDS;* and *Keep Your Laws Off My Body;* as well as work with the collectives DIVA TV (co-founder) and Paper Tiger Television. She was the founding director of BENT TV, the video workshop at the Hetrick-Martin Institute for gay, lesbian, bisexual and transgender youth. She currently serves on the boards of Third Wave Foundation (co-founder), Reality Dance Company, V era List Center for Art and Politics at The New School, and the George Gund Foundation.

DORIS B. HAIRE is best known for *The Cultural Warping of Childbirth*, a well-referenced analysis of worldwide obstetric practices published by the International Childbirth Education Association in 1972, while she was president of ICEA. This booklet marked a turning point in international obstetric care.

Haire, a consumer activist and pioneer in the area of informed consent, has also authored *The Pregnant Patient's Bill of Rights*, (1974), *How the FDA Determined the "Safety" of Drugs: Just How Safe is Safe* (1984), and *Drugs in Labor and Birth* (1987). She has observed obstetric care in 72 countries and continues to lecture worldwide.

DIANNE HALES, one of the most widely published and honored freelance writers in the country, is author of *Just Like a Woman: How Gender Science Is Redefining What Makes Us Female* (1999). She also is a contributing editor for *Parade, Ladies Home Journal* and *Working Mother* and has written more than 1,000 articles for national publications, including *American Health, Family Circle, Glamour, Good Housekeeping, Mademoiselle, McCall's,* the *New York Times, Readers' Digest, Redbook, Seventeen,* the *Washington Post* and *Woman's Day.*

MICHELLE HARRISON, M.D. is a physician, writer, teacher, and leader in women's health. She consults and lectures internationally about women's health and other related health policy issues. Harrison is the author of *A Woman in Residence* (Random House 1982; Ballantine 1993), The *Pre-teen's First Book About Love, Sex, and AIDS* (American Psychiatric Press Inc., 1995), and *Self-Help for Premenstrual Syndrome* (Third Edition Random House, 1998).

THOMAS PAZ-HARTMAN is a writer, teacher, and computer consultant living in New York City.

MOLLY HASKELL is a film critic and has written for the *New York Times*, the *New York Times Book Review*, the *Nation*, and *Film Comment*, among other publications. She lectures on film at numerous universities, and is a member of the New York Film Critics Circle and the National Society of Film Critics.

JUDITH LEWIS HERMAN, M.D. is associate clinical professor of psychiatry at the Harvard Medical School and director of training at the Victims of Violence Program at Cambridge Hospital.

JEANNE HIRSCH and her mother LOLLY HIRSCH (1922–1986), the self-proclaimed "first feminist mother-daughter team since the Pankhursts," founded New Moon Publications, Inc. in 1969 (later changed to New Moon Communications, inc.) to publish the truth about women, starting with the first and only issue of *Women: To, By, Of, For, and About* commemorating the 50th anniversary of women's suffrage, August 26, 1970.

New Moon also produced *The Proceedings of the First International Childbirth Conference; The Witch's Os; Directions for a Non-Traumatic Abortion;* and *The World Women and Children's Culture Caravan Herstory.*

SHERE HITE's groudbreaking Hite Reports have had a profound and lasting influence on generations of readers—countless millions all over the world. Hite grew up in Missouri, and left America to live in Europe because of a fundamentalist political backlash after the publication of her works. She renounced her U.S. citizenship in 1996 and became a German citizen.

Hite's initial research grew out of her involvement with a feminist group in New York, and it was with the publication of *The Hite Report on Female Sexuality* in 1976 that she shot to international acclaim.

The four Hite Reports, showing an increasing depth to her controversial theories, have been translated into fifteen langugages and published in thirty-five countries, receiving numerous academic and professional awards and honors. The initial Hite Report was named as one of the 100 key books of the twentieth century by the *Times* in 1998. The latest Hite Report also includes future predictions of new cultural trends worldwide.

She is now a professor of gender and culture at Nikon University.

LINDA JANET HOLMES, executive director of the office of minority health, New Jersey Department of Health and Senior Services, is a long-time women's health activist and writer. Her previous work with the nurse-midwifery program at the University of Medicine and Dentistry of New Jersey sparked her interest in celebrating the age-old wisdom of traditional African American midwives. Through oral history, multi-media exhibitions, print, and video, Ms. Holmes has spent more than two decades documenting the southern black midwifery experience. She continues to collect information about the healing roles of women in African-American communities today.

MARY HOWELL (RAUGUST), A.K.A. MARGARET CAMPBELL, was a co-founder of the National Women's Health Network and a contributor to the Boston Women's Health Book Collective. She had a law degree as well as a medical degree, and a Ph.D. in child development, besides being the author of many books. In 1973 she was the first woman ever hired as a dean at Harvard Medical School.

LEAH HYDER was a National Women's Health Network interm in the summer of 1998.

JANE WEGSCHEIDER HYMAN, PH.D. is a researcher and writer on women's health. Her latest book is *Women Living with Self-Injury* (Temple University Press, 1999).

ERICA JONG is one of the liveliest and most influential women writing today. When her landmark first novel *Fear of Flying* appeared in 1973, Henry Miller cheered it as "a female *Tropic of Cancer*," opening the door for women to "find their own voices and give us great sagas of sex, life, joy and adventure." In her six subsequent novels, prize-winning collections of poetry, and countless articles, Jong has continued to celebrate women's strengths and possibilities with energy and passion.

SUSAN JORDAN is a former partner of Dresner, Sykes, Jordan and Townsend, a nationally known political and commercial research consulting firm. She currently sits on the board of the League for Coastal Protection, an environmental organization based in California. A lifelong feminist, she worked on a successful seven-year campaign to legalize the cervical cap in the U.S. The birth of her son, Jedd Benjamin Levine, led her to reassess societal assumptions about motherhood and to fight to protect the declining rights of all mothers.

SUZANNE WHITE JUNOD is a medical historian with a Ph.D. from Emory University, and she is employed by the U.S. Food and Drug Administration. She has a special interest in women's health issues and is currently working on a published history in the field.

PAULA KAMEN is the author of what is widely noted as the first and still the only journalistic book on young women and feminism, *Feminist Fatale: Voices from the "Twentysomething" Generation Explore the Future of the "Women's Movement"* (Donald I. Fine/Penguin, 1991). Her second book, *Her Way: Young Women's Evolving Sexual Choices*, the first "big picture" book on postboomer women's sexual attitudes and behaviors, is forthcoming from NYU Press. Her writing has appeared in about a dozen anthologies, the *New York Times, Washington Post, Chicago Tribune, Salon* and many other publications. In 1999, her play, *Jane: Abortion and the Underground*, about the legendary pre-Roe abortion service, premiered in Chicago. A Chicago writer, she has been a visiting research scholar with the women's studies program at Northwestern University since 1994.

DR. STEPHEN KANDALL retired in 1998 as chief of neonatology at Beth Israel Medical Center in New York and professor of pediatrics at the Albert Einstein College of Medicine. During his professional career he lectured widely nationally and internationally, served on many advisory committees, and published more than 90 articles and book chapters, most dealing with substance abuse. His book, *Substance and Shadow*, grew from his advocacy efforts on behalf of women prosecuted for drug use during pregnancy.

ANNE S. KASPER, PH.D., is a pioneer in understanding the social contexts of women's health, particularly breast cancer. Dr. Kasper is a founding member of the U.S. women's health movement, and has been an advocate, sociologist, researcher, and public policy expert on women's health for more than 20 years. As the first co-chair of the National Women's Health Network. She was instrumental in gaining national attention for women's health. From 1990 to 1994, Dr. Kasper was the director of the Campaign for Women's Health, a coalition of more than 100 national, state, and grassroots organizations convened to advance women's health in health care reform. Dr. Kasper is a Senior Research Scientist at the Center for Research on Women and Gender at the University of Illinois at Chicago and a recipient of the Center's Women's Health Policy Research Fellowship.

TANIA KETENJIAN is a graduate of Bard College and an associate editor at Seven Stories Press. She was named after the famed "urban terrorist" Patty Hearst (alias "Tania") who was freed from the Symbionese Liberation Army on Septemeber 30, 1975, the day of Tania's birth.

FRANCINE KLAGSBRUN, an author and lecturer, is a columnist for *The Jewish Week* and *Moment* magazine. Her most recent book is *Jewish Days: A Book of Jewish Life and Culture Around the Year* (Farrar, Straus & Giroux).

JUDITH RAPHAEL KLETTER spent 18 years working as an associate art editor managing the International Art Distribution Center at *Reader's Digest* after graduating Emerson College. Currently she is a freelance researcher who is also writing a self-help book based on her life as a survivor of her father's suicide.

VIVIEN LABATON is director of the Third Wave Foundation, the only national organization for young feminist activists between the ages of 15 and 30. She is also a research associate to Gloria Steinem.

BERNARD LEFKOWITZ is the author of *Our Guys: The Glen Ridge Rape and the Secret Life of the Perfect Suburb*. He has written three previous books on social issues.

BARRON H. LERNER, M.D., PH.D. is a medical historian and internist at the College of Physicians and Surgeons of Columbia University. Dr. Lerner, who is the Angelica Berrie Gold Foundation assistant professor of medicine and public health, is author of *Contagion and Confinement: Controlling Tuberculosis Along the Skid Road* (Johns Hopkins, 1998). He is currently writing a history of breast cancer screening and treatment in the United States, 1945 to the present.

CHARLOTTE LIBOV is an award-winning author and professional speaker specializing in women's health issues. She is the author of *Beat Your Risk Factors: A Woman's Guide to Reducing Her Risk for Cancer, Heart Disease, Stroke, Diabetes and Osteoporosis* and *The Woman's Heart Book*, and lives in Bethlehem, Connecticut.

E. JAMES LIEBERMAN is clinical professor of psychiatry at George Washington University School of Medicine and author of *Acts of Will: The Life and Work of Otto Rank*.

BETTY JEAN LIFTON, PH.D. is an author and psychologist, and has an adoption counseling practice with all members of the triad in New York City. Her adoption books include: *Twice Born: Memoirs of An Adopted Daughter; Lost and Found: The Adoption Experience; Journey of the Adopted Self: A Quest For Wholeness*, and the picture book *Tell Me A Real Adoption Story*. Among her other books are: *The King of Children: The Life and Death of Janusz Korczak* and *A Place Called Hiroshima*. Dr. Lifton is a member of the Ethics Committee of the Donaldson Institute, and a former board member of the American Adoption Congress.

SUSAN LOVE, M.D. is an author, teacher, surgeon, lecturer, researcher and activist. Dr. *Susan Love's Breast Book* has been termed the bible for women with breast cancer; released in 1997, *Dr. Susan Love's Hormone Book* provides an equally authoritative range of information about menopause. Her website, SusanLoveMD.com, will provide an in-depth internet site for women with breast cancer and women at midlife.

KRISTIN LUKER, PH.D. is professor of sociology and a professor in the Jurisprudence and Social Policy Program (Boalt Hall School of Law) at the University of California, Berkeley. She is the author of many scholarly articles, as well as three books: *Taking Chances: Abortion and the Decision Not to Contracept* (1975), *Abortion and the Politics of Motherhood* (1984) and *Dubious Conceptions: The Politics of Teenage Pregnancy* (1996). She is currently at work on her fourth book, tentatively entitled *Bodies and Politics*, which is about sex education controversies in the United States.

Professor Luker has been elected to the American Academy of Arts and Sciences and the Sociological Research Association, and was invited to the White House by President Clinton to discuss issues of politics and social policy. She has been awarded grants from the Spencer and Ford Foundations, as well as the Commonwealth Fund, and has won fellowships from the Guggenheim Foundation and the National Endowment for the Humanities.

She has written for the *New York Times, Harper's* and *The American Prospect.*

HARRIET LYONS was an original editor of *Ms.,* where she was responsible for identifying Marilyn Monroe's life and career as a subject for feminist interpretation and where she coordinated investigative reports. She was a recipient of the Women in Communications' Clarion Award for "The Decade of Women: A *Ms.* History of the '70s in Words & Pictures."

In 1980, she joined the *Daily News* to edit lifestyle sections, and was from 1990 to 1993 editor of the *Sunday Magazine.* As a *McCall's* and *Redbook* senior editor, from 1993 to 1997, she edited cover profiles, articles concerning social issues and human interest stories. In 1994, the American Legion Auxiliary awarded her the Heart of America Award for Best Magazine Article, about a woman who adopted two children from a mother dying of AIDS. She is currently Special Sections editor at the *Daily News.*

CAROLYN MACKLER, 26, published her first young-adult novel with Delacourte Press in fall 2000. A contributing editor of *Ms.,* her articles and essays have also appeared in publications including the *Los Angeles Times, HUES,* and *New Moon.* Carolyn has compiled an anthology for *George* magazine entitled *250 Ways to Make America Better* (Villard Books). She lives in New York City, where she is at work on her next young-adult novel.

THOMAS MAEDER is the author of six non-fiction books, including *Children of Psychiatrists* and *Adverse Reactions,* and has published articles in the *Atlantic Monthly,* the *New York Times Magazine,* and elsewhere. In collaboration with Cathy Crimmins he has written seven humor books, including *Newt Gingrich's Bedtime Stories for Orphans,* and develops traveling interactive science museum exhibits. He lives in Narberth, PA.

CHARLES C. MANN is a correspondent for the *Atlantic Monthly* and *Science* magazine. He has written or co-written four books and was the editorial coordinator for the *Material World* series of photography books. His writing has received awards from the American Bar Association, the American Institute of Physics, the Alfred P. Sloan Foundation, and the Margaret Sanger Foundation.

CARLA MARCELIS is a naturopathic physician and long-time women's health activist. She has channeled her concerns fro safe medicines and a women-friendly health-care system through her work with organizations such as Women's Health Interaction, the Canadian Women's Health Network, and D.E.S. Action Canada.

HELEN MARIESKIND has been active in women's health issues since the early 1970s. She is author of the landmark *Evaluation of Caesarean Section in the United States* (DHEW, 1979), *Women in the Health System: Patients, Providers and Programs* (C.V. Mosby, 1980), and the founder and editor for six years of *Women & Health* (Haworth Press). She lives in Washington, D.C. and works as a writer/editor for the Office of Juvenile Justice and Delinquency Prevention, Office of Justice Programs, U.S. Department of Justice.

APRIL MARTIN is a clinical psychologist in private practice in New York City, and the author of *The Lesbian and Gay Parenting Handbook.* She and her partner of 21 years have had two donor insemination children together, Emily, 18, and Jesse, 15. Their family also includes two grandchildren, Jamelin and Chiandra, and an adopted dog named Ixey.

NORMA FOX MAZER is the author of 26 novels for children and young adults, plus two collections of short stories. She has edited an anthology of womens poetry and contributed articles, essays, and short stories to numerous journals and anthologies. Among her awards are a Newbery Honor, the California Young Readers Medal, a Christopher Medal, and an Edgar. Her newest book is *Goodnight Maman* (Harcourt Brace).

NORMA MCCORVEY has worked as a crisis counselor in a Dallas women's clinic. She is a frequent speaker on abortion rights and women's issues. She lives in Dallas, Texas.

JEAN BAKER MILLER, M.D., is a Clinical Professor of Psychiatry at Boston University School of Medicine, Director of the Jean Baker Miller Training Institute at the Stone Center, Wellesley College. She has written *Toward a New Psychology of Women*, co-authored *The Healing Connection: How Women Form Relationships in Therapy and in Life; Women's Growth in Connection;* and edited *Psychoanalysis and Women*, as well as numerous articles on depression, dreams, and the psychology of women. A practicing psychiatrist and psychoanalyst, she is a fellow of the American Psychiatric Association, the American College of Psychiatrists, the American Orthopsychiatric Association, the American Academy of Psychoanalysis, and has been a member of the board of trustees of the last two. She is also member, consultant to, and teacher of several women's groups.

Congresswoman PATSY T. MINK (D, Hawaii) is a third generation Japanese-American graduate of University of Chicago Law School (1951). Title IX was her work product as a member of the Education and Labor Committee, as was WEEA, and many sex equity provisions of law. Her law suit, *Mink vs. EPA et al,* established the core principles of the Freedom of Information Act. An environmentalist, advocate of consumer rights, individual rights and civil rights, Mink made her mark first as an opponent of the Vietnam War. The Surface Mining and Reclamation Act (1977) was written under her management of the Subcommittee on Mines and Mining and remains intact today 20 years later to protect against the ravages of strip-mining.

STEVEN MOSHER is director of the Claremont Institute's Asian Studies Center: One of the nation's foremost China scholars, Mr. Mosher was the first Western social scientist permitted to carry out a full-length study of a Chinese village since the Communist revolution. He found forced abortions, abortions in the third trimester of pregnancy, and officially sanctioned infanticide occurring in the countryside where he lived.

Mr. Mosher now serves as director of the Claremont Institute's Asian Studies Center, a post he has held since 1986. He is the author of several books, including *Broken Earth: The Rural Chinese; Journey to the Forbidden China; China Misperceived: American Illusions and Chinese Reality*, and the recently released *A Mother's Ordeal.*

MARYANN NAPOLI is a co-founder and the associate director of the Center for Medical Consumers in New York City. She writes *Health Facts,* the Center's monthly newsletter.

JUDY NORSIGIAN is co-author of *Our Bodies, Ourselves for the New Century.*

SALLY WENDKOS OLDS has written extensively about relationships, health, and personal growth, and has won national awards for both her book and magazine writing. Her college textbooks on child and adult development, *A Child's World* and *Human Development*, co-authored with psychologist Diane E. Papalia, Ph.D., have been read by more than two million students and are the leading texts in their fields. She is also the author of *The Working Parents' Survival Guide* and *The Eternal Garden: Seasons of Our Sexuality*, and the co-author of *Helping Your Child Find Values to Live By, Psychology*, and *Raising a Hyperactive Child* (winner of the Family Service Association of America National Media Award).

A former president of the American Society of Journalists and Authors, Ms. Olds is also a member of La Leche League International, International Childbirth Education Association, the Authors Guild, and other professional and civic organizations.

Ms. Olds lives on Long Island with her husband, Mark. She nursed her own three daughters and is now the proud grandmother of four breastfed children.

LESYLE E. ORLOFF founded Ayuda's unique domestic violence program, dedicated to serving the interrelated legal and social service needs of battered Latina and immigrant women and children. She has written local and national training curricula and manuals for battered women's advocates, attorneys, police, judges, and health professionals on domestic violence, cultural competency, The Violence Against Women's Act's immigration provisions, welfare rights of battered immigrant women and the nexus between domestic violence and immigration law. Ms. Orloff published a 400 page law review article analyzing civil protection order statutes, case law and practice in the 50 states, D.C. and Puerto Rico.

Ms. Orloff was a co-founder of the National Network on Behalf of Battered Immigrant Women and is the Washington, D.C. spokesperson for that organization. In that capacity she was involved in drafting the Protection for Battered Immigrant Women Provisions of the Violence Against Women Act and is leading the effort to secure further law reforms for battered immigrant women in VAWA II 1999. In September of 1999, Ms. Orloff joined NOW Legal Defense and Education Fund's Washington, D.C. office as the Director of the Immigrant Women Program and Senior Staff Attorney.

AMY PAGNOZZI writes for *New York, Vanity Fair, Glamour*, and *Penthouse*.

CINDY PEARSON is executive director of the National Women's Health Network. She is responsible for representing the Network's position in Congress and Federal agencies such as the Food and Drug Administration and the National Institutes of Health. In addition, Ms. Pearson represents the Network on the Board of Directors of the National Breast Cancer Coalition, and the

Steering Committee of the National Action Plan on Breast Cancer, where she is co-chair for the Etiology Working Group. In the past, Ms. Pearson served as Executive Director at Womancare, a community-based clinic in San Diego, California. In the past 12 years she has presented addresses on women's health care at many symposia, conferences, and annual meetings throughout the United States.

MARK PENDERGRAST is an investigative journalist and independent scholar who writes in Vermont. He is the author of *For God, Country and Coca-Cola*; *Victims of Memory*, and *Uncommon Grounds: The History of Coffee and How it Transformed Our World*.

DIANA PETITTI, M.D. is a nationally and internationally recognized expert in reproductive epidemiology and women's health.. She is currently Director of Research and Evaluation, Southern California Permanente Medical Group. Dr. Petitti received her M.D. degree from Harvard Medical School in 1975. After an internship in Medicine at the University of Colorado Affiliated Hospitals, she spent two years as an Epidemic Intelligence Service Officer with the Centers for Disease Control. She first joined Kaiser Permanente in 1978 as an Epidemiologist in the Division of Research in Northern California. In 1981, she received her M.P.H. in epidemiology from the Berkley School of Public Health. In 1984, she left Kaiser Permanente to join the full-time faculty at the University of California, San Francisco School of Medicine, where she stayed until rejoining Kaiser Permanente Southern California in 1993 as the Director of Research and Evaluation.

LETTY COTTIN POGREBIN is a writer and lecturer. Among her books are *Growing Up Free* (1980), *Stories for Free Children* (1982), and *Getting Over Getting Older: An Intimate Journey* (1996). She was a founding editor of *Ms.*, and is presently the president of the Author's Guild.

AMY RICHARDS is a writer, researcher, organizer, and fundraising consultant. A co-founder and executive committee member of the Third Wave Foundation, Richards was profiled by *Ms.* in 1997 in "21 for the 21st: Leaders for the Next Century." Her writings can be found in *The Nation, Ms., The New Internationalist*, and *Bust*, and her work has been anthologized in *Listen Up! Voices from the Next Feminist Generation* (Seal Press 1994), *Adios, Barbie* (Seal Press 1998), *Letters of Intent* (The Free Press 1999), and *The Bust Guide to the New Girl Order* (Penguin 1999). Richards is currently co-authoring *Manifesta: Young Women/Feminism/The Future*, a book about the state of feminism.

CAROL EISEN RINZLER graduated from Goucher College and received her law degree from Yale University. Her legal practice began at Cahill Gordon &

Reindel and she was of counsel to Rembar & Curtis until her untimely death in 1990. Mrs. Rinzler wrote for many publications and was the author of many books: *Nobody Said You Had to Eat Off the Floor* (1971); *The Girl Who Got All the Breaks* (1980); *Your Adolosscent: An Owner's Manual* (1981); and, (with J. Gelman) *How to Set Up for a Mah-Jongg Game and Other Lost Arts* (1987). Mrs. Rinzler's children, Jane Rinzler Buckingham and Michael Rinzler, live in New York City and London respectively.

ESTHER (SEIDMAN) ROME was a founding member of the Boston Women's Health Book Collective and co-author of its best-selling book *Our Bodies, Ourselves.*

Esther was one of a group of women that first met at a women's liberation conference in Boston in 1969. The group continued as a self help and support group, meeting weekly for over ten years. They researched and wrote a number of articles on women's health issues that evolved into the book *Our Bodies, Ourselves.* Over the many editions of the book, Esther wrote about anatomy, menstruation, food and nutrition, and cosmetic surgery. It was her belief that many so called "medical" issues in women's health were, in reality, much broader issues requiring social, economic, and political solutions.

In her 25 years of working with the Boston Women's Health Book Collective, Esther made unique contributions in two areas. In response to the serious issue of women becoming severely ill and even dying from toxic shock syndrome, Esther began a campaign to require uniform labeling of tampons. For most of the 1980s she served as a consumer representative to a task force of the American Society for Testing Materials, which after many years of meetings, and due largely to Esther's persistence, finally enacted a uniform standard for tampon labeling.

When confronted with breast cancer, Esther persistently and energetically researched treatment options and shared what she had learned with all who were interested.

She died at home on June 24, 1995, surrounded by her family.

JUDITH ROSSNER is the author of such best-selling novels as *Looking for Mr. Goodbar, August,* and *Emmaline,* on which the opera by Tobias Picker is based.

BETTY ROTHBART, M.S. W. is a health columnist for *Hadassah* magazine and the author of a number of books on health and parenting, including *Multiple Blessings: From Pregnancy Through Childhood, a Guide for Parents of Twins, Triplets or More* (Hearst). She is the author of four curricula on HIV/AIDS and abuse prevention for the New York City Board of Education, where she conducts teacher trainings on health and sexuality education. She has taught at the graduate schools of Hunter College and the Bank Street College of Education, and been a consultant to Planned Parenthood Federation of

America, the Sexuality Information and Education Council of the United States (SIECUS), and others.

LORRAINE ROTHMAN, M.S.co-founded the women's self-help movement with Carol Downer in 1971. She invented and patented a home health kit used in menstrual extractions, and is a major researcher and author of *Menopause Myths and Facts, What Every Woman Should Know About Hormone Replacement Therapy.*

SHERYL BURT RUZEK, PH.D. is professor of health studies at Temple University. She is currently working on a second edition of her 1978 book, *The Women's Health Movement, Feminist Alternatives to Medicine Control* and is a consultant to numerous public health organizations. Her recent publications include *Women's Health: Complexities and Differences* (with Virginia Olesen and Adele Clarke) and articles on the future of health reform.

MEI HWEI ASTELLA SAW graduated from Northwestern University and is now an associate editor at Seven Stories Press. A daughter of two fine doctors, she doesn't think members of the medical profession are gods.

HAGAR SCHER is a journalist and writer living in New York City. Her articles about politics, feminism, sex, women's health, fitness, sports, and first-person experiences have appeared in *Ms., Glamour, New Woman, Fitness, Ladies' Home Journal,* and *Latina* magazines. She has also published pieces in *2sexE: Urban Tales of Love, Liberty, and The Pursuit of Gettin' In On* (North Atlantic Books, 1999), and the *North Atlantic Review,* a literary journal. A woman-of-the-world, Hagar was raised in Israel and Canada, and has resided in Italy and England, too.

JULIA R. SCOTT, president of the Black Woman's Health Project, has a long history as a leader and activist in preventive health and in the struggle for the advancement of people of color. Her professional life spans three decades of community activism as an administrator, advocate, trainer and nurse-practitioner. The Black Women's Health Project is a Washington-based national organization focused on self help and health advocacy. The project develops and administers projects bringing about more equitable distribution of health care resources. Prior to becoming president, Julia Scott was director of public education and policy for that project. She has held a variety of other posts, including director of training for the Boston Family Planning Project, and reproductive rights field coordinator and executive director of the Foundation of Women. She has received the Gloria Steinem Women of Vision award.

SHERRILL SELLMAN is an international author, lecturer, health writer and psychotherapist. She has extensively researched the most vital and up-to-date information necessary for women's hormonal health and well-being. Through her writing, lecturing and seminars, she has empowered women all over the world to make more educated and informed health choices.

CASSANDRA SHAYLOR is a staff attorney with Legal Services for Prisoners with Children in San Francisco, CA. She is also a Ph.D. candidate in the History of Consciousness Department at the University of California, Santa Cruz, where she is working on a dissertation entitled, "The Abject of the Nation: Women of Color, Citizenship, and Solitary Confinement." Ms. Shaylor was a co-founder of Critical Resistance and is an active member of several grassroots organizations committed to social and economic justice.

SARAH J. SHEY received her M.F.A. in nonfiction writing from Columbia University in October 1999. She has been published in such publications as the *Christian Science Monitor*, the *Philadelphia Inquirer*, and *This Old House Magazine*.

ALIX KATES SHULMAN's eleven books include two books on the anarchist Emma Goldman, three books for children, four novels *(Memoirs of an Ex-Prom Queen, Burning Questions, On the Stroll, In Every Woman's Life...)*, and two memoirs (the award winning *Drinking the Rain* and *A Good Enough Daughter*). Hailed by the *New York Times* as "the voice that has for three decades provided a lyrical narrative of the changing position of women in American society," her works have been translated into eleven languages. In 1997 Penguin issued her pioneering feminist novel *Memoirs of an Ex-Prom Queen* in a 25th anniversary edition. She divides her time between New York City and Maine.

KATIE SINGER is certified to teach Fertility Awareness by the Ovulation Method Teachers' Association. She teaches at Women's Health Services in Santa Fe, NM. Her first novel *The Wholeness of a Broken Heart*, has recently been published by Riverhead Books.

MARGOT SLADE is deputy editor, special sections, of the *New York Times* and the mother of twins, Emma and Jacob.

MARGARET CHARLES SMITH is one of the few remaining traditional southern black midwives with thousands of birthing stories to share. This life-long resident of Eutaw, Alabama, now in her 90s, practiced as a midwife for more than 40 years before she was forced to retire when Alabama eliminated lay midwife practices. Her resilient spirit prevails as she continues to be a leading voice in efforts to strengthen midwifery in Alabama.

ELIZABETH CADY STANTON, the boldest and most brilliant of the nineteenth-century American feminists, was born in 1815 in upstate New York. For more than 50 years, there seemed to be no impediment to women's full equality that Elizabeth did not notice and attempt to route: besides suffrage, she campaigned for birth control, property rights for wives, custody rights for mothers, equal wages, cooperative nurseries, co-education, and "deliverance from the tyranny of self styled medical, religious and legal authorities." Through it all Elizabeth was a doting, hands-on mother of five sons and two daughters.

JOHN STAUBER founded the Center for Media & Democracy and edits its journal *PR Watch*, which investigates the propaganda strategies of business and government. He co-authored (with Sheldon Rampton) *Toxic Sludge is Good for You: Damn Lies and the Public Relations Industry* (Common Courage Press, Monroe, ME), an expose of the public relations field.

GLORIA STEINEM is one of the most influential writers, editors, and activists of our time. She travels worldwide as a lecturer and feminist organizer, and is a frequent media spokeswoman on issues of equality. In the words of her biographer, Carolyn Heilbrun, "Steinem has rarely laced courage in grappling with the world, or with herself.... She is most honored and most cherished by people throughout the country who remember her speaking, her helping to start their rape-crisis center, her timely support for their various burgeoning organizations."

Gloria co-founded *Ms.* in 1971 and was one of its editors for fifteen years. She recently brought together a group of women investors to form Liberty Media for Women and re-purchase *Ms.*, where she will serve as consulting editor.

KOFI TAHA is a writer, activist, entrepreneur, and renowned broke philanthropist. His poems, essays and articles have been published in various forms, ranging from academic journals to newspapers to hip hop tabloids, and he is currently completing a book of poetry entitled *Postdiluvian America: Drought of Humility*.

LEORA TANENBAUM is the author of *Slut! Growing Up Female with a Bad Reputation* (Seven Stories Press, 1999). Her writing has appeared in *Newsday, Seventeen, Ms.*, and other newspapers and magazines. She lives in New York City.

NOY THRUPKAEW is the news editor of *Sojourner: The Women's Forum*, a national feminist newspaper based in Boston. She has lived in Japan and Thailand, and frequently writes on international women's human rights, welfare policy, and Southeast and East Asian literature and film.

LEONORE TIEFER, PH.D. is a psychologist in New York City who has special-ized in sexuality in research, theory, teaching, and clinical work. Her ideas are presented in *Sex is Not a Natural Act, and Other Essays* (Westview Press, 1995).

SOJOURNER TRUTH was born into slavery in New York State. She won her free-dom in 1827, when that state emancipated its slaves. Sojourner Truth consis-tently and actively identified herself with the cause of women's rights. She was the only Black woman present at the First National Woman's Rights Convention in Worcester, Massachusetts, in 1850.

SARI TUDIVER, PH.D., is the Resource Coordinator at the Women's Health Clinic, a community health center in Winnipeg, Manitoba and the Editor of *A Friend Indeed*, an international newsletter for women on menopause and midlife. An anthropologist by training, she has been involved in research, writ-ing, education and advocacy on many aspects of women's health, including reproductive technologies and the international pharmaceutical industry. She is a founding member of the Canadian Women's Health Network.

REBECCA WALKER is a writer currently living in Berkeley, CA.

DR. LILA A. WALLIS, M.D. is clinical professor of Medicine at Cornell University Medical College and Attending Physician at the New York Hospital in New York City. Dr. Wallis is an internationally recognized expert on estrogen replacement therapy, menopause, and osteoporosis. She is also celebrated for her contributions to women's health and medical education through her orga-nizational activities, lectures, and publications, including the *Textbook of Women's Health*, a 1044-page volume with 150 contributors, published by Lippincott-Raven in 1998.

Called by her colleagues the "Godmother of Women's Health," Dr. Wallis has received many awards and honors, including the Woman of the Century Award in women's health from the Women's Medical Association of New York City.

Dr. Wallis is senior author of *The Whole Woman—Take Charge of Your Health in Every Phase of Your Life*, published by Avon Books in May 1999.

ELIZABETH SIEGEL WATKINS has her Ph.D. in the history of science from Harvard University, from which her book *On the Pill* is derived. She is an his-torian with the Historical Society of Western Pennsylvania in Pittsburgh, and writes, teaches, and consults in Pennsylvania.

KATHRYN WATTERSON, who teaches writing at Princeton University, has written several prize-winning nonfiction books, including most recently, *Not by the Sword* (Simon & Schuster), which won the 1996 Christopher Award. Her first book, *Women in Prison* (1996 edition, Northeastern University Press), is considered a classic on the subject and was the basis for an ABC documentary *Women In Prison. You Must Be Dreaming* (basis for the NBC movie *Betrayal of Trust*), which tells the story of co-author Barbara Noël, singer and psychiatric patient, who battled to bring her world-renowned psychiatrist to justice for his sexual and ethical betrayals, galvanized the American Psychiatric Association to issue a public apology and undertake a yearlong review of their ethical policies and procedures for reporting professional misconduct.

MARILYN WEBB is one of the early founders of the Second Wave of the women's movement. An organizer, speaker and writer, she also began *Off Our Backs*, one of the first feminist newspapers, the nation's first college-based women's studies program—at Goddard College in Vermont—and Sagaris, a feminist think-tank. She was subsequently a journalist—a senior editor at *Woman's Day* and *McCall's*—a writer for many national magazines and editor-in-chief of *Psychology Today*. Most recently she has become a leader of a new movement-to improve the care of the dying. She is the author of the influential book, *The Good Death: The New American Search to Reshape the End of Life* (Bantam 1997 and 1999) and founder of a non-profit organization to hold town meetings across America on death and dying.

ELAINE WEISS has conducted dozens of domestic violence training sessions around the country. She contributed to the development of a domestic abuse awareness web site and is a member of an international task force on domestic abuse prevention, which is currently developing a career development program to help battered women achieve economic justice. Her writings about domestic abuse have appeared in local and national publications and are used as teaching resources in a number of battered women's shelters. She is currently working on a book about women who have survived domestic violence.

EDITH WHITE, the author of *Breastfeeding and HIV/AIDS: The Research, the Politics, the Women's Responses*, spent more than 25 years teaching breastfeeding management to health professional and was one of the founders of the International Board of Lactation Consultants. In 1996 she was selected by UNICEF to be one of two breastfeeding trainers to represent the United States at the First International Training Colloquium on Breastfeeding in Bangkok. She is now executive director of the South Shore AIDS Project, Inc. in Plymouth, Massachusetts.

FRANCES CERRA WHITTELSEY is an award-winning journalist, magazine editor and author.

NAOMI WOLF was born in San Francisco in 1962. She was educated at Yale University and at New College, Oxford University where she was a Rhodes Scholar.

Her essays have appeared in various publications including: *The New Republic, Wall Street Journal, Glamour, Ms., Esquire*, the *Washington Post*, and the *New York Times*. She also speaks widely on college campuses.

The Beauty Myth was her first book. *Fire With Fire: The New Female Power And How It Will Change The 21st Century* was published by Random House in 1993. Her latest book, *Promiscuities: The Secret Struggle for Womanhood*, was published by Random House in 1997. At present, Ms. Wolf is writing a book which will focus on mothering, entitled *You Walk That Bridge Alone*, to be published by Anchor Books in early 2000.

Naomi Wolf has joined with a board of remarkable young women who are putting their common ideals into action, in the form of The Woodhull Institute. This Institute, of which Ms. Wolf is president of the board, has been created to cultivate ethical leadership for the 21st century. Its special focus is a Fellowship Program to teach professional development in business, law, arts and the media to young women ages 21–28. She lives in New York City.

ALICE WOLFSON is an attorney specializing in defending the rights of insurance policy holders for the firm Bourhis, Wolfson, and Schlichtmann in San Francisco, California.

JOHN WYKERT is a prize-winning New York journalist who was the long-time New York correspondent for *Psychiatric News*, the official newspaper of the American Psychiatric Association. His best-known work is *The Book of Alfred Kantor*, a major source book on the Holocaust, published in six languages and eight countries.

LAURA YAEGER's stories have appeared in *Beacon, Kaleidoscope, The Paris Review* and *The Missouri Review*. She's won awards at *Seventeen* and *Cosmopolitan* and was the recipient of the Louis Sudler Prize in the Arts. She received degrees from Oberlin College, Iowa State University and the University of Iowa. She is currently working on a novel about interracial relationships.

Index

AIDS Counseling and Education Program (ACE), 1066, 1432-1434
Alcohol, , 669-670, 750-751, 762, 764, 1002-1003, 1020, 1036, 1041, 1152, 1221, 1262, 1339, 1403, 1479-1480, 1489
    addiction to, 6–7
    breast cancer and, 108
    ovarian cancer and, 152, 153
Alcoholism, 665, 670, 1252, 1259, 1322
Alcoholics Anonymous, 7
Alexander technique, 474–476, 580, 590
Alfalfa
    anemia and, 44
    arthritis and, 57
    menopause and, 358
    vaginal infection, 569
Ali, Dr. Majid, 164, 165, 167, 168 169, 170, 173, 180, 182
Allergies
    arthritis and, 57, 62, 73–78
    carpal tunnel syndrome and, 506
    chronic fatigue syndrome and, 165–167
    dairy, 57
    detoxification and, 4
    diabetes and, 213
    eating disorders and, 238
    environmental, 73–78, 405
    food, 73–78, 88, 90, 404–405
    hormone imbalance and, 327
    lupus and, 344
    migraines and, 402–403, 404–405
    multiple sclerosis and, 417–418
    urinary tract infections and, 549
Allina, Amy, 1436, 1507
Aloe vera, 45
    breast cancer and, 122
    dysmenorrhea and, 367
    lupus and, 344
    sexually transmitted diseases and, 522
    vaginal infection, 569
Alpha carotene, infertility and, 337
Alpha-linolenic acid, 115
Alpha lypoic acid
    arthritis and, 90
    caffeine and, 6
    eating disorders and, 226
Alternative therapies, 666-667, 1394
Alumina, vaginal infection and, 570
Alzheimer's disease, 34
AMA. See American Medical Association.
Amenorrhea, 369–373
American Cancer Society (ACS), 683, 774, 1007, 1035, 1240-1241, 1245, 1393-1394, 1430, 1475

American College of Obstetrics and Gynecology, 698, 709, 1330
American Medical Association (AMA), 644, 647, 656, 660, 664, 666, 668-669, 671, 691, 710, 714, 727, 729-731, 747-748, 768, 778, 964-965, 1085, 1329-1330, 1332, 1383, 1390, 1430
American Medical Women's Association (AMWA), 703, 1331, 1382, 1384, 1461, 1466, 1469, 1477
American medical profession, 640, 646
American Nursing Association, 651
American Psychiatric Association, 681, 771, 790, 1175, 1249, 1318-1319, 1321, 1519, 1525-1526
American Way of Death, The, 717
AMWA. See American Medical Women's Association.
Amyl nitrate, menopause and, 360
Amytal, 1249-1250, 1252-1254, 1256
Ancient Gorgon, The, 623
Anderson, Nina, 29
Anemia, 41–46
    ayurveda and, 44–45
    blood cell destruction in, 41
    blood loss and, 41
    causes, 41–43
    diagnosis, 43
    diet and, 43–44
    herbs for, 44, 45
    hypoprolactin, 337
    lupus and, 344
    nutrition and, 41–42
    in pregnancy, 42, 43
    sickle cell, 104, 434
    supplements and, 42, 44
    symptoms, 43, 45
Angina pectoris, 277
Angioplasty, 303, 304
Ankylosing spondylitis, 49
Anorexia, 233–235. See also Eating disorders
Anshen bu nao pien, 286
Anthony, Susan B., 608
Anti-inflammatory agents, 636
Antibiotics, 671, 905, 908, 916, 1212, 1444, 1487
Antioxidants
    aging and, 20–22, 35
    breast cancer and, 121–122
    chronic fatigue syndrome and, 166, 173
    endometriosis and, 248
    environmental illness and, 260
    fibrocystic breast disease and, 136
    heart disease and, 281, 283

Aurum metallicum
    depression and, 396–397
    pregnancy and, 487
Aurum muriaticum, fibroids and, 151
Austin, Donald, 755
Avery, Byllye, 604, 689, 981, 1044-1045, 1425, 1500, 1508
Ayurveda, 591
    anemia and, 44–45
    chronic fatigue syndrome and, 183–185
    menopause and, 362
AZT, 1027, 1427-1428
Babes, Aurel, 671
Bach Flower remedy, 591
Baoxin wan, 286
Barberry
    heart disease and, 283
    sexually transmitted diseases and, 519
    urinary tract infections and, 576
    vaginal infection, 573, 575
Barber-surgeons, 610, 639, 654-655, 657
Barer, Lori, 1280, 1415, 1508
Barium sulfide, 671
Barnard, Dr. Neil, 430–431, 432, 434, 435, 437
Barnes, Broda, 283, 533, 542
Bar-Shalom, Dr. Ruth, 135, 136, 137, 369
Bart, Pauline, 698, 713, 894, 901, 909, 912
Baths, 663, 667-668, 762, 1041, 1131
Batt, Sharon, 683, 1238
Baumgardner, Jennifer, 974, 1076, 1213, 1508
Bayberry, sexually transmitted diseases and, 516
Bearberry, vaginal infection and, 569
Becker, Julie, 1389, 1477, 1482, 1508
Beechwood, urinary incontinence and, 548
Bee propolis, herpes and, 320
Bekker, Karen, 683, 1508
Belladonna, 636
    menopause and, 360
    premenstrual syndrome and, 497
    urinary incontinence, 548
Bellevue Hospital, 648, 1512
Bellis perennis, pregnancy and, 483
Benson, Dr. Herbert, 289
Bentonite, 29
Berberine, vaginal infection and, 567
Bergin, Judge Eugene, 1349
Bernikow, Louise, 1071-1072, 1508
Bernini, 620-621
Berro
    depression and, 396
    menopause and, 363

migraines and, 413
Bertarelli, Fabio, 332
Berwick, Ann, 425, 481, 513, 558
Beta carotene
    aging and, 21
    breast cancer and, 121
    cervical cancer and, 154
    cervical dysplasia and, 144
    chronic fatigue syndrome and, 166, 168, 173, 174, 176
    endometriosis and, 248
    environmental illness and, 260
    fibrocystic breast disease and, 137
    heart disease and, 281
    herpes and, 320
    infertility and, 337
    lupus and, 345
    osteoporosis and, 423
    repetitive strain injury and, 504
    sexually transmitted diseases and, 521
    vaginal infection, 571, 574
Biofeedback, 31, 251, 407, 591–592
Bioflavonoids, 23
    arthritis and, 90
Biology, 673, 689, 704-705, 712, 763, 784, 917, 950, 956, 1001, 1077, 1202-1203, 1221
Birth control, 96–106, 603, 606, 612, 642, 665, 673, 700, 708, 711, 717-718, 720-721, 723-725, 727, 730-731, 733, 735, 738, 742, 745, 749, 757, 760, 762-764, 767-768, 779, 799, 801, 814, 833, 893, 904, 939-947, 950-951, 953-954, 956-957, 959-961, 963, 967-968, 1023-1024, 1026-1027, 1030, 1053, 1068, 1076, 1115-1119, 1125, 1243-1244, 1261, 1281, 1306, 1363, 1372, 1405, 1468, 1473, 1495-1496, 1523
    Billings method, 96–98
    bodily changes and, 97
    cervical cap, 98, 100–101
    condoms, female, 99–100
    condoms, male, 98–99
    contraceptive film, 98, 102–103
    diabetes and, 208
    diaphragm, 98, 101–102
    fertility awareness and, 96–98
    mucus observation in, 96–98
    natural family planning, 96–98
    Norplant, 105
    pills, 103–105
    spermicide, 99, 100, 102, 103
    sterilization, 105–106
    temperature and, 97
Birth defects, 466
    folic acid and, 42

Bryonia
  arthritis and, 81
  menstruation and, 361
  pregnancy and, 482
Bucci, Dr. Luke, 55, 56, 436
Bucci, Susan, 32, 33, 34
Buchman, Dian Dincin, 666-667, 1509
Buchu, urinary tract infections and, 556,
  557
Buckwheat, 23
Buffalo gourd
  depression and, 396
  menopause and, 363
Bugleweed, heart disease and, 283
Bulimia, 233–235. *See also* Eating disorders
Bulvodynia, 251
Bupleurum
  premenstrual syndrome and, 495
  sexually transmitted diseases and,
  523
Burdock
  sexually transmitted diseases and,
  516, 517, 522
  urinary tract infections and, 557
Butcher's broom
  heart disease and, 283
  varicose veins and, 578
Butternut, infertility and, 342
BWHBC. *See* Boston Women's Health
  Book Collective.
Cabbage extract, 23
Cadmium, 27
Caffeine
  addiction to, 3
  anxiety and, 5
  arthritis and, 59
  blood pressure and, 5
  detoxification and, 5–6
  fibrocystic breasts and, 6
  fibroids and, 145
  infertility and, 333
  withdrawal from, 6
Cahill, Caedmon Magboo, 1271, 1509
Calapai, Dr. Christopher, 16, 18
Calcarea phosphoric, osteoporosis and,
  428
Calcium
  absorption, 177
  aging and, 24
  alcohol and, 7
  anxiety and, 382
  arthritis and, 59, 70, 93
  breast cancer and, 122
  caffeine and, 5, 6
  channel blockers, 1389

chronic fatigue syndrome and, 168,
  173
  heart disease and, 288, 302
  infertility and, 336
  lupus and, 345
  menopause and, 357
  pregnancy and, 470, 477
  repetitive strain injury and, 504
  temporomandibular joint dysfunction
  and, 530
Calendula, sexually transmitted diseases
  and, 517, 518, 519
Califilum, pregnancy and, 484
Call, Dr. Hyla, 532
Calomel, 629, 641-643, 645
Calvin, John, 628
Campbell, Margaret A., 919, 1515
Camu-camu
  depression and, 396
  herpes and, 322
  infertility and, 342
  migraines and, 413
Cancer, 671-672, 676, 683-685, 690-691,
  698, 715, 725, 740, 744-746, 750-755,
  760, 762-763, 773-775, 805, 821, 873,
  918, 947, 955, 965, 967-969, 975-977,
  995, 1004-1007, 1025, 1027-1028,
  1033, 1035-1039, 1043, 1047, 1049-
  1050, 1055, 1071, 1079, 1085, 1092,
  1095-1101, 1110, 1125-1127, 1134,
  1137, 1212, 1217-1219, 1237-1247,
  1251, 1270, 1273-1276, 1279, 1281,
  1293, 1295-1297, 1353, 1357, 1363,
  1367, 1372, 1375-1376, 1378-1379,
  1385-1386, 1389, 1391-1394, 1398-
  1399, 1401, 1405-1410, 1415, 1417,
  1426-1427, 1430-1431, 1434, 1436-
  1437, 1442, 1444, 1450-1453, 1462-
  1463, 1469-1478, 1480-1482, 1492-
  1495, 1499-1500, 1504, 1509, 1515-
  1517, 1520-1521
  aging and, 18
  breast, 354
  caffeine and, 6
  cervical, 128, 142, 153–154, 520
  coffee enemas and, 156
  Coley's toxins and, 157–158
  colorectal, 19, 230
  diet and, 152–153, 155–156, 229–230
  emotional healing, 127–129
  endometrial, 154, 351
  environmental factors, 84
  exercise and, 31
  fluoroscopy and, 112–113
  free radicals and, 20
  hormones and, 154

hyperbaric oxygen and, 157
liver, 118, 119
lung, 128
metastisization of, 116
nutrition and, 155–156
ovarian, 103, 128, 152–153
plastics and, 111–112
risk factors, 154
survival rates, 155
tobacco and, 116
uterine, 103, 117, 119
Cancer, breast, 104, 107–141
antioxidants and, 121–122
bras and, 111–113, 120
causes, 108–116
diet and, 114–115, 119–125
enzymes and, 124–125
essential fatty acids and, 125
estrogen and, 108–109, 116–117
exercise and, 125–126
herbs and, 123–124
immune system and, 126–127
immunoaugmentive therapy and,
126–127
lumpectomy, 121
lymphatic drainage and, 110–113
massage and, 126
mastectomy, 121
nutrition and, 109–110
pesticides and, 110
plastics and, 111–112
prevention, 119–132
protection against, 109
psychoneuroimmunology and,
127–129
symptoms, 116
tamoxifen and, 116–119
xenoestrogens and, 109–110
x-rays and, 112–113
Candida, 167, 169–171, 260–261, 564, 565
Candidiasis, 9, 377, 379, 564 673
Cannabis, 677
Cantharis, urinary tract infections and,
557
Capitalism, 633, 705, 943, 1060, 1122,
1284
Caplan, Paula J., 1162, 1509
Capsicum, aging and, 26
Carbohydrates
complex, 19, 211, 279, 307, 493
diabetes and, 211
digestion, 177
eating disorders and, 226
heart disease and, 301–302
refined, 89, 229, 261, 446
slow-acting, 355

sources, 19
Carcinogens, 109–110, 118
Carmichael, Carrie, 986, 1008, 1298, 1501,
1509
Carnegie, 646, 769
Carnivora, breast cancer and, 123
Carob, infertility and, 342
Carotid artery, 28
Carpal tunnel syndrome, 51, 80, 505–508
allergies and, 506
alternative treatments, 507–508
causes, 505–507
conventional treatment, 507
diabetes and, 506
hormones and, 506
risk factors, 505
Cartilage, 49
Cass, Dr. Hyla, 237, 238, 540, 544–545
Cassia
infertility and, 342
lupus and, 347
vaginal infection, 573
Castleman, Michael, 1387, 1509
Catachin, chronic fatigue syndrome and,
166
Cataracts, 21, 38
tamoxifen and, 117
Catheter, 850, 905-906
Catheterization, 656, 1085
Cat's claw
breast cancer and, 122, 123
chronic fatigue syndrome and, 107
lupus and, 344
Caustic Poison Act, 671
Causticum, urinary incontinence, 548
Cayce, Edgar, 136
Cayenne
arthritis and, 90
caffeine and, 6
chronic fatigue syndrome and, 170
heart disease and, 283–284, 296
migraines and, 413
CDC. *See* Centers for Disease Control
Cellini, 622-623
Center for Population Research, 955,
1280, 1510
Centers for Disease Control (CDC), 777,
955, 1020, 1030, 1047, 1425, 1429,
1431, 1520
Certner, Roberta, 358–359
Cervical cancer, 672, 774, 1035, 1125,
1217-1219, 1281, 1293, 1399, 1430-
1431, 1477
Cervical caps, 98, 100–101
Cervical dysplasia, 142–159
causes, 142–143

conventional treatment, 143–144
diagnosis, 143
diet and, 144
herbs and, 144–145
immunoaugmentive therapy and, 145
naturopathic treatment, 144
prevention, 143
smoking and, 142–143
symptoms, 143
Cervicitis, 142
Chaitow, Dr. Leon, 576, 577, 579
Chalker, Rebecca, 100, 510, 511, 796-798, 804
Chambers, Veronica, 604, 995
Chamomile, 677
Chamomilla, dysmenorrhea and, 368
Chaparral, sexually transmitted diseases and, 517, 522
Chase, Deborah, 1000, 1509
Chaste berry
endometriosis and, 248
hormone imbalance and, 330
menopause and, 360
premenstrual syndrome and, 498
Chaya, infertility and, 342
Chelation therapy, 592
aging and, 20, 27–28, 38
arthritis and, 38, 92
heart disease and, 27–28, 287–288
lupus and, 345
varicose veins and, 579
Chemotherapy, 128, 181
Chesler, Ariel, 1141, 1509
Chesler, Dr. Phyllis, 698
Chichoke, Dr. Anthony, 525
Chickpea, menopause and, 363
Chicory, diabetes and, 220
Childbirth, 610, 616-617, 628-629, 636, 653, 669, 697, 699, 704, 726, 731, 766-767, 777, 789, 797, 800-801, 805-806, 808, 817-818, 834, 836, 838, 844, 846, 849, 851, 853-855, 857-858, 863, 870-871, 873, 893, 955, 967-968, 1021-1023, 1036-1037, 1049, 1090-1091, 1208, 1228, 1275, 1280, 1305-1306, 1310-1311, 1399, 1409, 1426, 1443, 1445, 1477-1478, 1487-1488, 1514, 1520
anesthesia during, 455
birth defects, 466
birth positions, 459–460
breast-feeding, 462–463
cesareans at, 460–461
labor, 475–476, 483–484
national practices, 455–456
natural, 456–459
painkillers and, 458–459

water birth, 484
Children Afflicted with Toxic Substances Foundation, 201
Chinese cabbage
depression and, 396
heart disease and, 293, 295
migraines and, 413
Chinese foxglove, infertility and, 342
Chiropractic, 592
arthritis and, 60
Chlamydia, 517–519
infertility and, 333
pelvic inflammatory disease and, 517, 518
symptoms, 517–518
treatment, 518–519
Chloral hydrate, 677
Chloroform, 655, 1005
Chlorophyll, 44
chronic fatigue syndrome and, 181
fibroids and, 150
heart disease and, 280
vaginal infection, 568
Cholesterol
aging and, 18
detoxification and, 4
diet and, 19
exercise and, 280–281
heart disease and, 280–281
reduction, 278, 286
Choline
aging and, 20, 38
premenstrual syndrome and, 495
Chondroitin
arthritis and, 56, 57, 64, 90, 94
repetitive strain injury and, 504
Christian theology, 637
Chromium
aging and, 20, 24
alcohol and, 7
breast cancer and, 122
chronic fatigue syndrome and, 168
diabetes and, 214
eating disorders and, 227
heart disease and, 282, 302
Chronic fatigue syndrome, 22, 37, 160–189
acupuncture and, 182
allergies and, 165–167
ayurveda and, 183–185
candida and, 167
causes, 163–169
Chinese herbal therapy, 178–179
Coxsackie virus and, 164
diagnosis, 169–171
diet and, 180–181, 185–186

temporomandibular joint dysfunction
and, 529
urinary tract infections and, 573–574
varicose veins and, 578–579
weight training, 31, 424
yoga, 31
Exfoliative cytology, 672
Expulsion of Adam and Eve from the Garden, The, 617-618
FA. *See* Fertility awareness.
False unicorn root
endometriosis and, 249
fibroids and, 149
Faludi, Susan, 1455-1456, 1460
fasting, 627, 1064
Fat
arthritis and, 91
breast cancer and, 108
cancer and, 114–115
estrogen and, 148
heart disease and, 307–309
monounsaturated, 279, 301
polyunsaturated, 279
reduction, 278–279
saturated, 89, 154
unsaturated, 115, 279
FDA. *See* Food and Drug Administration.
Feldenkrais method, 31, 593
Feldman, Dr. Martin, 15, 16, 19, 163, 170, 173
Female Eunuch, The, 970, 1213-1216, 1220, 1513
Female circumcision (FC), 1223-1224
Female deity, 625
Female genital mutilation (FGM), 1115, 1223, 1225, 1227, 1306
Female healers, 631, 637, 639, 652
Female sexuality, 628, 634, 678-679, 681-682, 697, 796, 810, 815-816, 823-829, 910, 929, 992, 1019, 1455, 1515
Feminism, 604, 644, 717, 727, 809-810, 813, 910, 926, 943, 1008-1009, 1064-1065, 1114, 1143, 1202, 1214, 1217, 1220-1221, 1261, 1302-1303, 1306, 1313-1314, 1412-1414, 1461, 1464, 1480-1481, 1496-1497, 1508, 1511, 1516, 1521-1522
Feminist Women's Health Center (FWHC), 797-798, 807-808, 963
Feminists, 605, 608, 612, 625, 633, 643, 650, 684, 689, 698, 707-710, 713, 717, 719, 721-722, 726-728, 732-733, 757, 778, 800-801, 807-808, 812-814, 834-836, 885, 902, 931, 939, 942-943, 946, 961, 984, 1063, 1076, 1112, 1118, 1121-1122, 1139, 1162, 1203, 1205-1207, 1213-

1216, 1219, 1227, 1261-1264, 1277, 1302-1303, 1306, 1353, 1405, 1414-1415, 1419, 1423, 1503-1504, 1523
Fennel
endometriosis and, 249
menopause and, 358
premenstrual syndrome and, 498
urinary tract infections and, 557
vaginal infection, 569
Fenugreek, menopause and, 363
Ferguson, Dr. John Henry, 743
Fertility, 662, 665, 669, 710, 724, 758, 761, 763, 803-806, 862, 888, 892, 936, 948, 956, 1012, 1016, 1021, 1023, 1032, 1053, 1069-1070, 1115-1119, 1201, 1233, 1299-1300, 1372-1373, 1375, 1413, 1473, 1510, 1523
Fertility awareness (FA), 1115-1119, 1523
Fetal movement, 661
Fetus, 654-655, 665, 673, 710-711, 749, 773, 838, 847-850, 855-858, 864, 868, 908, 941, 1019-1020, 1141, 1162, 1199, 1206, 1403, 1428-1429, 1505
Feudalism, 632-633
Feverfew
detoxification and, 14
migraines and, 406
Fiber
dietary, 19
endometriosis and, 247
Fibroids, 6, 109, 145–152
acupuncture and, 151
causes, 145–146
Chinese herbals and, 150
conventional treatment, 146–147
diet and, 148–150
exercise and, 148–150
homeopathy and, 151–152
hysterectomy and, 146–147
laparoscopy for, 147
myoma coagulation and, 146, 147–148
myomectomy for, 146
naturopathic treatment, 150
symptoms, 146
Fibromyalgia, 49, 403–404
breast implants and, 198, 207
homeopathy and, 62, 79–80
symptoms, 79–80
Fibrositis. *See* Fibromyalgia
Fine, Phyllis L., 604, 1256, 1512
Finkbine, Sherri, 689, 692
Finkle, William, 754
Finman-Nahman, Tovah, 569
Firestone, Shulamith, 604, 689, 704, 1202, 1265, 1512

Firman, Dr. Joel, 229
Flack, Audrey, 604, 616, 624, 1167, 1512
Flavonoids, 279
Flax
    diabetes and, 220
    heart disease and, 296
Flaxseed, 29
    aging and, 25, 35
    breast cancer and, 122
    fibrocystic breast disease and, 137
    lupus and, 344
    menopause and, 358
    multiple sclerosis and, 418
    tea, 28
    urinary tract infections and, 557
Fleckenstein, Al, 288
Fleming, Alexander, 671
Flexner report, 646-647
Flexner, Abraham, 646
Flucocorticoids, 66
Fluoroscopy, 112–113
Folic acid
    aging and, 24
    anemia and, 41–42, 44
    arthritis and, 59
    birth defects and, 42
    breast cancer and, 121
    cervical cancer and, 154
    cervical dysplasia and, 144
    chronic fatigue syndrome and, 175, 176
    deficiencies, 42
    heart disease and, 283
    infertility and, 332, 336
    osteoporosis and, 423
    pregnancy and, 478
    sexually transmitted diseases and, 521
Folliculinum, premenstrual syndrome and, 496
Food and Drug Act, 670-672, 727, 776, 1432
Food and Drug Administration (FDA), 668, 671-672, 691-692, 708-709, 713-714, 716, 718, 721, 725, 727-733, 740, 746-749, 751, 755, 760, 774-779, 834, 935, 939, 953-954, 956-958, 960-961, 964, 966-969, 1004-1007, 1026, 1123-1125, 1279, 1292, 1368, 1401, 1478, 1491, 1511, 1515, 1520
Food, Drug, and Cosmetic Act, 727, 776
Forceps, 611, 639-640, 654, 656, 665, 803, 848, 859-861
Ford, Anne Rochon, 1371, 1512
Formaldehyde, 263–264
Fo-ti
    aging and, 25

chronic fatigue syndrome and, 178
Frankfort, Ellen, 697, 714, 770, 797-798, 806, 1478, 1512
Frankincense, 285
Franks, Lucinda, 1071, 1103, 1512
Free and Female, 765, 815, 909, 1522
Free radicals, 36
    aging and, 16, 18, 20
    breast cancer and, 124
    chronic fatigue syndrome and, 166
    fats and, 115
    scavengers of, 93
    stress and, 289
Freedom of Information Act, 729, 731, 1519
Freud, Sigmund, 622, 682, 708, 781-783, 811, 823, 886, 1162, 1174-1175, 1211, 1264, 1458
Friedman, Richard, 288, 289
Furman, Dr. Joel, 228, 230, 231, 232, 346
FWHC. *See* Feminist Women's Health Center
GABA, 38
Gage, Frances D., 674
Gage, Suzanne, 802
Galante, Dr. Michele, 166, 167, 171, 180, 181, 188, 398–399
Galen, 637, 640, 681
Gamma-linolenic acid
    pain and, 437
    premenstrual syndrome and, 493–494
    sexual dysfunction and, 512
Gammalinolinic acid, menopause and, 357
Gard, Dr. Zane, 262, 275
Gardenia, dysmenorrhea and, 366
Garden sorrel, lupus and, 347
Gardnerella vaginalis, 562, 563
Garlic
    aging and, 26
    arthritis and, 59
    chronic fatigue syndrome and, 181, 186
    heart disease and, 283–284
    herpes and, 320
    lupus and, 345
    premenstrual syndrome and, 498
    repetitive strain injury and, 505
    sexually transmitted diseases and, 522
    urinary tract infections and, 556
    vaginal infection, 567, 568, 571
Garry, Dr. Robert, 204
Garson, Barbara, 502
Gelinas, Denise, 1322
Gelsemium, pregnancy and, 484
Gender

chronic fatigue syndrome and, 167–168, 175
endometriosis and, 246
estradiol, 66, 67, 349
estrogen, 22–23, 38, 326, 348–349
follicle-stimulating, 103, 246, 333
gender, 168
gonadotropin-releasing, 246
growth, 312
imbalances, 37, 326–330
infertility and, 332
lupus and, 343
luteinizing, 168, 246, 333
migraines and, 403, 405
natural, 38
osteoporosis and, 423
pregnancy and, 489
progesterone, 22–23, 38, 326
progestin, 105
prolactin, 337
replacement therapy (HRT), 247, 351–354, 731, 956-958, 1038-1039, 1051-1057, 1084-1085, 1219, 1221, 1366, 1368-1370, 1409, 1441, 1473-1474, 1488, 1495, 1522
sex, 66
temporomandibular joint dysfunction and, 527–528
testosterone, 22–23, 38, 66, 67
thyroid stimulating, 542
urinary tract infections and, 549–551
Horse chestnut
herpes and, 322
varicose veins and, 578
Horsetail, osteoporosis and, 423
House of Representatives, 669, 967, 1111, 1511
Howell, Mary, 604, 781, 918-920, 964, 968, 1469-1471, 1507, 1515
HRT. *See* hormone replacement therapy
Huang li, 575
Huang po
urinary tract infections and, 576
vaginal infection, 575
Hudson, Dr. Tori, 44, 119, 142, 143, 144, 147, 248, 249, 512, 575, 579
Hufnagel, Dr. Vicki, 147, 205–206, 246, 369–370, 511
Huggins, Charles, 673, 775
Huggins, Dr. Hal, 17
Human papilloma virus, 142, 520–522
treatment, 521–522
Humors, 638, 645
Hutchinson, Ann, 641
Hyde Amendment, 949, 962, 1032, 1034, 1054, 1496

Hydergine, 35–36
Hydrochloric acid, 42, 44, 177, 344
hydropaths, 666
hydrotherapy, 666-667, 682
Hygiene
arthritis and, 58–60
endometriosis and, 254–255
natural, 341, 594
sexual, 338
Hyman, Jane Wegscheider, 1068, 1515
Hyperglycemia, 22, 209
Hypertension, 179
birth control and, 104
heart disease and, 277–278
homeopathy and, 290
treatment, 310–313
Hypnosis, for addiction, 3, 10–13
Hypoglycemia, 167
anxiety and, 378
detoxification and, 5
Hypothyroidism, 16–17, 532
symptoms of, 16
Hysterectomy, 751, 935-936, 982, 1030-1032, 1036, 1039, 1114, 1125, 1131, 1137-1139, 1175, 1217, 1219, 1233, 1434, 1440
cancer and, 155
fibroids and, 146–147
Hysteria, 633, 679-682, 708, 1013, 1189, 1261, 1322-1323, 1325, 1460
Ibuprofen, 50
Ignatia
depression and, 397
pregnancy and, 486
premenstrual syndrome and, 497
Immigrants, 645, 647, 656, 662, 665, 679, 943, 1052, 1097, 1226
Immigration, 662, 665, 945, 1227, 1314, 1520
Immune system
AIDS and, 166
breast cancer and, 126–127
chronic fatigue syndrome and, 163
endometriosis and, 244, 248
environmental illness and, 261
medications and, 53
steroids and, 169
thymus gland and, 17
urinary tract infections and, 551
Immunoaugmentive therapy, 126–127, 145
In vitro fertilization, 673, 773, 1199-1201, 1204, 1462
Indian fig, diabetes and, 220
Indian Health Service, 1058-1061
Infant mortality, 648, 710, 844-851, 888,

Lomatium, sexually transmitted diseases and, 523
Lombardi, Susan, 26, 31–32
Lonsdorf, Dr. Nancy, 183
Lordosis, 202
Lotson, Anita, 28
Love, Dr. Susan, 119, 1079, 1470, 1517
L-tryptophan, obsessive-compulsive disorder and, 384
L-tyrosine, temporomandibular joint dysfunction and, 530
Luffa, lupus and, 347
Lumpectomies, 121, 691, 1100, 1246, 1430, 1476
Luncheon on the Grass, 622
Lupus, 49, 52, 343–347
   allergies and, 344
   causes, 343
   diet and, 345–346
   exercise and, 346
   herbs and, 344–345, 346–347
   intravenous therapies, 345
   natural therapies, 344–347
   stress and, 346
   supplements and, 344–345
   symptoms, 343–344
   traditional treatment, 344
Lutaigou, 338
Lycopene, chronic fatigue syndrome and, 166
Lyme disease, 37
Lymphatic system, 110–111
   manual lymphatic drainage massage, 126
Lymphedema, 111, 126, 139–141
   symptoms, 140
Lyons, Harriet, 991, 993, 1517
Lysine
   environmental illness and, 261
   herpes and, 320, 321
MacDonald, Paul, 753
MacEoin, Beth, 151
Mack, Thomas, 754
Mackenzie, Dr. Ian, 112, 113
Mackler, Carolyn, 987, 1518
Maeder, Thomas, 1175, 1518
Magnesium
   aging and, 24
   alcohol and, 7
   anxiety and, 382
   arthritis and, 52, 55, 56, 59, 70
   breast cancer and, 122
   caffeine and, 5, 6
   chronic fatigue syndrome and, 168, 173
   depression and, 389–390

   diabetes and, 214
   dysmenorrhea and, 366
   eating disorders and, 227
   endometriosis and, 246
   fibrocystic breast disease and, 136
   heart disease and, 282, 302, 303
   lupus and, 345
   migraines and, 403–404, 406
   osteoporosis and, 423
   pain and, 436, 437
   premenstrual syndrome and, 493, 495
   repetitive strain injury and, 504
   sexual dysfunction and, 512
   temporomandibular joint dysfunction and, 530
Magnet therapy, 32–34, 61, 441–443
Maines, Rachel, 679-680
Makeup, 649, 783, 809, 979, 994, 1002, 1008-1009, 1335, 1419, 1452
Malabsorption syndrome, 21
Malaria, 606, 1290
Malleus Maleficarum, 633, 635
Malleus, 633-636, 639
Mammography, 114, 121
Mandell, Dr. Marshall, 62, 73–78, 259
Manet, 622
Manganese
   arthritis and, 55, 59
   breast cancer and, 122
   osteoporosis and, 423
   repetitive strain injury and, 504
Manganum, menopause and, 360
Mann, Charles, 1404
Mao dong qing, 286
Maracuya, 220
Margolies, Marjorie, 1180-1181
Marigold, sexually transmitted diseases and, 518
Marieskind, Helen, 609, 1518
Marijuana, 1499-1500
Marriage, 608, 627-628, 675, 692-693, 787, 799, 810, 823, 828-829, 836, 842, 882, 886-888, 942, 977, 1066, 1078, 1118, 1144, 1150, 1190, 1193, 1227, 1229, 1232, 1261, 1303-1305, 1314, 1336-1339, 1344, 1347, 1350-1351, 1417, 1419, 1421, 1458-1459
Marsh mallow
   diabetes and, 220
   urinary tract infections and, 556, 558
Masaccio, 617-618
Mason Clinic, University of Washington, Seattle, 754
Massage, 31, 39–40, 596
   breast cancer and, 126
   infertility and, 337

Muscle spasms, 680
Myoma coagulation, 146, 147–148
Myomectomy, 146
Myrrh
    arthritis and, 58
    heart disease and, 285
    pain and, 436
    sexually transmitted diseases and, 516
    vaginal infection, 573
Nader, Ralph, 258, 717, 731, 966
Napoli, Maryann, 1387, 1519
Nasturtium, lupus and, 347
National Black Women's Health Project
    (NBWHP), 1015-1016, 1019, 1021-
    1023, 1026-1028, 1031-1032, 1034,
    1036-1037, 1039-1042, 1044-1045,
    1048, 1061, 1468, 1479, 1500, 1507-
    1508
National Cancer Institute (NCI), 672, 744,
    774, 1005-1007, 1098, 1100, 1240,
    1245, 1392, 1406, 1430-1431, 1492,
    1499, 1509
National Coalition Against Domestic
    Violence, 582
National Institutes of Health (NIH), 702,
    748, 755, 764, 953-956, 958, 1005,
    1042, 1100, 1247, 1365, 1370, 1391,
    1397-1398, 1406-1407, 1410, 1425,
    1429, 1431, 1469, 1481-1482, 1492,
    1510, 1520
National Latina Health Project, 1061, 1479
National Organization for Nonparents
    (NON), 885
National Organization for Women (NOW),
    732, 976, 1043-1044, 1508, 1520
National Wholesale Druggists
    Association, 669
National Women's Health Network
    (NWHN), 685, 689, 720, 733, 740, 778,
    781, 834, 956, 959, 963-964, 966-968,
    1027, 1045-1046, 1051, 1057, 1061,
    1080, 1275, 1279, 1293, 1353, 1368,
    1374, 1382, 1384, 1386, 1405, 1410,
    1425, 1462, 1467-1468, 1475, 1478,
    1480, 1486, 1490, 1494-1495, 1497-
    1500, 1507, 1510, 1515-1516, 1520
National Women's Industrial League, 669
Natmur
    pregnancy and, 486
    premenstrual syndrome and, 496
Natrum muriaticum
    herpes and, 323
    menstruation and, 361
    migraines and, 409
Natural family planning (NFP), 1115,
    1117-1118

Naturopathy, 595
    chronic fatigue syndrome and,
    185-187
NBWHP. See National Black Women's
    Health Project.
Nelson, Senator Gaylord, 717, 722, 757,
    957
Nembutal, 677, 1452
Neonatal ophthalmia, 647
Nervousness, 680, 751, 895, 1153, 1275
Nettle, anemia and, 44
Neurasthenia, 678
Neurotransmitters, 176, 384, 386
New England Journal of Medicine, The,
    673, 745-746, 753, 958, 965, 1287,
    1289, 1388, 1409, 1429, 1442
NFP. See natural family planning
Niacin
    caffeine and, 6
    depression and, 393
    heart disease and, 282
Nightingale nurse, 649
Nightingale, Florence, 648-649
NIH. See National Institutes of Health
Nineteenth Amendment, 670, 684
Nitric acid
    menstruation and, 361
    vaginal infection, 570
NON. See National Organization for
    Nonparents.
Noninflammatory pelvic problems, 668
Norepinephrine, 386
Norman, Laura, 362, 499, 500
Norplant, 105, 733, 958, 1025, 1027-1028,
    1061, 1273-1278, 1428
Norsigian, Judy, 689, 698-699, 964, 1461,
    1467, 1519
Nose straighteners, 671-672
Novak, Dr. Edmund R., 698
Novello, Antonia, 1330
NOW. See National Organization for
    Women.
Null, Gary, 605
Nurse's aide, 630, 707
nurses, 604, 610, 629-630, 640, 648-652,
    659, 672-673, 678, 771, 791, 844, 852,
    868, 871, 905, 926, 1018, 1078, 1088,
    1091, 1112, 1128, 1155, 1203, 1259,
    1273, 1366, 1407, 1445-1446, 1449,
    1484
nursing school, 649
nursing, 606, 610, 640, 648-651, 653, 693,
    707, 767, 845, 865, 868, 877, 925, 1088-
    1089, 1092-1095, 1162, 1176, 1275-
    1276, 1293, 1307, 1399, 1443, 1446,
    1448-1449, 1454, 1510

exercise and, 437
guided imagery and, 444
herbs and, 435–436
joint, 58, 344, 518
laughter and, 443–444
magnet therapy, 441–443
management, 429–444
menstrual, 433
migraines and, 440
mind-body connection, 443–444
premenstrual syndrome, 435–436
relievers, 627-628, 636, 1293
rolfing, 441
sciatica, 437
shiatsu and, 438–439
sickle cell anemia, 434
sleep and, 437
Trager technique, 440
urinary, 518
Pancreatin, stroke and, 525
Pansy, herpes and, 322
Pantethine, chronic fatigue syndrome
and, 173
Pantothenic acid
anxiety and, 382
arthritis and, 52, 59
chronic fatigue syndrome and, 175,
176
temporomandibular joint dysfunction
and, 530
Papain
multiple sclerosis and, 419
pain and, 437
stroke and, 525
Pap smears, 143, 144, 520, 672, 774, 902,
1039, 1043, 1047, 1140, 1218, 1270,
1399, 1430, 1476
Papanicolaou, George, 671-672
Paracelsus, 638
Paraphenylene diamine, 671
Parasites, 445–453
causes, 447–448
chlamydia, 517–519
constipation, 447
contaminated water and, 447–448
diet of, 446–447
herbs and, 453
hookworms, 445
pinworms, 445
prevention, 449–451
protozoa, 445, 446, 447
ringworms, 445
roundworms, 445
sugar and, 8
symptoms, 448
tapeworms, 445

treatment, 449–451
Parathyroid, osteoporosis and, 428
Partnership of Women's Health, 1077,
1397
Passion flower
hormone imbalance and, 330
pain and, 437
Patient package insert (PPI), 727, 730-731,
778, 957, 960
Patient stories
aging, 39–40
anemia, 46–46
anxiety, 399–401
arthritis, 71–73, 75–78
breast cancer, 132–135
cervical cancer, 158–159
depression, 399–401
diabetes, 217–219
eating disorders, 240–241
endometriosis, 252–255
environmental illness, 272–275
fibrocystic breast disease, 139
heart disease, 314–315
lymphedema, 141
menstruation, 375
migraines, 413–414
ovarian cancer, 159
pregnancy, 488–489
premenstrual syndrome, 500
Reiki massage, 39–40
thyroid disease, 537–538, 542–545
trichomona, 574–575
vaginal infection, 572, 574–575
Patriarchal system, 626, 727, 1202
Pau d'arco, 27
chronic fatigue syndrome and, 187
lupus and, 344
sexually transmitted diseases and, 516
vaginal infection, 567, 568, 569
Paz-Hartman, Thomas, 1353, 1514
Pearson, Cynthia (Cindy), 1080, 1275,
1382, 1405, 1467, 1475, 1486, 1520
Peat, Dr. Ray, 279, 283, 340, 341
Pelton, Dr. Ross, 34, 35, 36
Pelvic inflammatory disease, 103, 516,
517, 518, 519–520
birth control and, 519
causes, 519
symptoms, 519–520
treatment, 520
Pendergrast, Mark, 1162, 1520
Penepent, Dr. Anthony, 150, 254, 341, 370
Penicillin, 671, 1024
Pepsin, 177
Perejil, 347
Perimenopause, 348

Rape of the Sabine Woman, 620-621
Rape in great art, 604, 616
Rape, 604, 616, 618-621, 623-624, 707,
    779, 791, 796, 899, 909-917, 949, 1018-
    1019, 1026, 1046, 1215, 1251, 1258-
    1259, 1261-1264, 1281, 1306, 1320,
    1330-1331, 1335, 1343-1345, 1420,
    1462, 1501, 1506, 1508, 1516
Rapp, Dr. Doris, 238, 388
Raymond, Jennifer, 435
Raynaud's disease, 344
Reach to Recovery, 683, 690
Red clover
    chronic fatigue syndrome and, 178
    menopause and, 358
    premenstrual syndrome and, 498
    vaginal infection, 569
Red mangrove, herpes and, 322
Red raspberry leaf
    anemia and, 44
    hormone imbalance and, 330
    menopause and, 358
    pregnancy and, 468–469
    premenstrual syndrome and, 494
Redstockings, 732
Reflexology, 596
    menopause and, 362
    migraines and, 410–413
    premenstrual syndrome and, 498–499
Reflex therapy, 61
Reichenberg-Ullman, Judyth, 557, 558
Reid, Dr. Susanna, 152, 153, 154, 215, 216,
    489
Reiki, 31, 39–40, 596
Renaissance, 681, 1090, 1132, 1163
Rennin, 177
Repetitive strain injury, 501–508
    diet and, 503
    herbs and, 504–505
    homeopathy and, 505
Reproduction, 630, 693, 704-707, 710-713,
    757, 761-763, 797, 799-800, 901, 905,
    939, 947, 950, 958, 1016-1018, 1026,
    1029, 1199, 1202, 1204, 1207, 1258,
    1478, 1491, 1510
Retinyl, chronic fatigue syndrome and,
    174
Reubens, 621
Rheingold, Paul, 741
Rheumatism, 58, 79, 85
Rhubarb
    arthritis and, 57
    urinary tract infections and, 576
    vaginal infection, 575
Rhus tox, 83
    arthritis and, 80, 81

carpal tunnel syndrome and, 80
migraines and, 409
Ribner, Dr. Rich, 55
Rich, Adrienne, 628
Richards, Amelia, 1414
Right-to-life movement, 661
Rinchen dragjor-rilnag chenmo, 58
Rinzler, Carol, 977
Ringworms, 445
Rist-Podrecca, Abigail, 146, 151, 359, 422,
    513, 590
Robbins, Dr. Frederick, 708
Robins, Dr. Howard, 21, 55, 297–298, 424
Rock, Dr. John, 762
Rodin, 620-621
Rodriguez-Trias, Helen, 604, 981, 1051
Roe v. Wade, 604, 796, 894-895, 900, 940,
    1053, 1505
Rolfing, 250, 441, 596–597
Rollin, Betty, 683, 885-886, 1450
Roman Empire, 661
Roosevelt, Eleanor, 668, 671, 1470
Rosemary
    breast cancer and, 124
    pregnancy and, 470
    vaginal infection, 569
Rosenblatt, Rebecca, 991, 993
Rossner, Judith, 1196, 1522
Rothbart, Betty, 1397, 1522
Rothblatt, Henry, 68, 69
Rothman, Barbara Katz, 604, 834, 870,
    1199, 1284, 1295, 1302
Rothman, Lorraine, 796-797, 800, 802,
    1522
Rouges, 671
Roundworms, 445
RU-486, 953, 958, 1371
Russian olive, heart disease and, 296
Rusty-gate syndrome, 80, 81
Ruta, 83
Rutin, 23
Sabina, menopause and, 361
Safe Motherhood Initiative, 1409
Safflower, diabetes and, 220
St. John's wort, 83
    pain and, 436
    sexually transmitted diseases and, 523
Sanger, Margaret, 642, 724-725, 733, 757,
    768, 944-946, 950, 1024, 1518
Sanitary pads, 672
Sarnoff, Dr. Debra, 191–192, 193, 194, 195,
    196
Sarsaparilla
    dysmenorrhea and, 367
    menopause and, 358
    premenstrual syndrome and, 498

Tang kuei, 58
Tanzer, Dr. Deborah, 697, 767
Tapeworms, 445
Tarragon, herpes and, 322
Tattoo removal, 194
Tatz, Shmuel, 61
Taurine, heart disease and, 283
Tea, green
    aging and, 23
    detoxification and, 14
    dysmenorrhea and, 367
    heart disease and, 286
Tea, herbal, 29
Tea tree oil, sexually transmitted diseases
    and, 519
Teich, Dr. Morton, 57
Temporomandibular joint dysfunction,
    527–530
    body rolling and, 529
    causes, 527–528
    craniosacral therapy and, 528–529
    hormones amd, 527–528
    implants, 201
    isotonic exercise and, 529
    nutrition and, 529–530
    symptoms, 528
Terr, Lenore, 1321
Testing
    aging and, 18
    arthritis, 53
    chronic fatigue syndrome, 169–171
    hormone imbalance, 329
    parasite, 448–449
    "provocative," 74
    thyroid disease, 533–534
Testosterone, 22–23, 67
    aging and, 38
    arthritis and, 66
Tew, Marjorie, 457
Thalidomide, 691-692, 779, 882, 1372,
    1401, 1431
Thallium acetate, 671
Theodosakis, Dr. Jason, 49, 51, 62, 63–65
Three Snakes Formula, 58
Thrupkaew, Noy, 1223, 1524
Thuja occidentalis, 409
Thyme, diabetes and, 220
Thymic involution, 17
Thymus extract, aging and, 24
Thymus gland, 21
    aging and, 17, 34
Thyroid
    aging and, 16–17
    dysfunction, 18
    importance of, 532
    supplements, 16–17

underactive, 13
Thyroid disease, 531–545
    alternative therapies, 541–542
    causes, 535–537
    environmental factors, 536
    symptoms, 532, 533
    thyroiditis, 532, 539–545
    treatment, 537
Tien ma, 58
Titian, 618-619
Title IX, 918–920, 1071, 1109, 1111-1113,
    1519
Tobacco, 120, 121
    cancer and, 116
    cervical dysplasia and, 142–143
    depression and, 390–391
    infertility and, 333
    ovarian cancer and, 152
Tokuyama, Dr. I., 762
Tolle, Roger, 440
Toxic Discovery Network, 200, 203
Toxic home syndrome, 37
Toxic shock syndrome, 373–374
    diet and, 374
    herbs and, 374
    naturopathy and, 373–374
    prevention, 374
Trager technique, 440, 597
Trahan, Dr. Christopher, 439
Tranquilizers, 175, 792, 917, 977, 1244,
    1468, 1490
Trans-fatty acids, 89
Traut, Herbert, 672
Trichomona, 562, 563, 572–575
    symptoms, 572–573
    treatment, 573–575
Triglycerides, 167
    aging and, 18
Trillium, for fibroids, 151
Truth, Sojourner, 604, 674, 1524
Trypsin, 177
    pain and, 437
    stroke and, 525
Tryptophan
    anxiety and, 382
    chronic fatigue syndrome and, 175
    depression and, 395
Tuberculosis, 197, 523
Tudiver, Sari, 1439, 1524
Turmeric, 58
    breast cancer and, 124
Tyramine, migraines and, 402–403
Tyrosine
    aging and, 20, 24, 37
    anxiety and, 382
    chronic fatigue syndrome and, 175

depression and, 394, 395
eating disorders and, 227
Ubiquinone, environmental illness and, 260
Ulcers
fiber and, 19
peptic, 53
Ullman, Dana, 62, 78–83, 497, 548
Ullman, Robert, 557, 558
Unsafe at Any Speed, 717
Uric acid, 57
Urinary tract infections/inflammation, 549–576
acupuncture and, 558
Asian perspective, 575
causes, 549–552
constipation and, 552
conventional treatment, 552–555
cystitis, 551, 557, 559–575
diagnosis, 552
diet and, 555, 558–559
exercise and, 573–574
herbs and, 556–557, 558
high-risk factors, 550
homeopathy and, 557
hormones and, 549–551
hydrotherapy and, 557
immune system and, 551
incontinence, 546–548
naturopathic treatment, 555–557
prevention, 558–575
structural problems in, 551–552
symptoms, 552
Urokinase, stroke and, 526
Uterine infections, 647
Uterus
bleeding in, 145–152
cancer of, 103, 117, 119
contractions of, 244–245
endometriosis and, 243–255
fibroid tumors, 6, 109, 145–152
Uva-ursi, urinary tract infections and, 556, 557
Vagina, 622, 655, 681, 740, 744, 746, 750, 764, 778, 804, 808, 811, 816-822, 833, 937, 982, 1005, 1028, 1116, 1134, 1210, 1212, 1215-1218, 1228, 1268-1272
Vagina, inflamation/infection
alternative therapies, 566–572
bacterial vaginosis, 563, 575
candidiasis, 564–572
causes, 562, 564–565
colon therapy and, 569
diagnosis, 566
diet and, 566–567
discharge, 117, 518, 520, 562

dryness, 361
homeopathy and, 570
stress and, 565
supplements and, 567–569, 574
symptoms, 562–563, 565–566, 572–573
treatment, 563, 573–575
trichomona, 562, 563, 572–575
vaginitis, 562–563
yeast infection, 563, 564–572
Vaginal Politics, 697, 714, 770, 797-798, 806, 909
Vaginal intercourse, 679
Vaginal orgasm, 682, 694, 811, 815-817, 821-823, 826
Vaginal smears, 671-672
Valerian
chronic fatigue syndrome and, 178
dysmenorrhea and, 367
pain and, 437
repetitive strain injury and, 504–505
Valium, 677, 1076, 1388, 1402
Vanadium
chronic fatigue syndrome and, 168
eating disorders and, 226
Vanadyl sulfate, diabetes and, 214
Varicose veins, 576–580
causes, 576–577
chelation therapy and, 579
exercise and, 578–579
herbs and, 578
nutrition and, 578
symptoms, 577
Vegetarianism. *See* Diet, vegetarian
Venus of Willendorf, 616-617
Vergara, Nilsa, 39
Vesselago, Dr. Michael, 169, 188
Vestibulitis, 251
Viburnum, dysmenorrhea and, 368
Vibrator, 679-680, 682, 831-832, 979
Victorian era, 678
Vinespinach
lupus and, 347
menopause and, 363
migraines and, 413
Violence, sexual and physical, 581–588
Virtue, Dr. Doreen, 223, 224, 225
Visualization therapy, 11, 13
infertility and, 337
Vitamin A
aging and, 21
arthritis and, 21, 59, 70, 92–93
breast cancer and, 121
cataracts and, 21
cervical dysplasia and, 144
chronic fatigue syndrome and, 173, 174, 176

endometriosis and, 249
environmental illness and, 260
heart disease and, 21, 302
herpes and, 320
lupus and, 345
sexually transmitted diseases and, 522
urinary tract infections and, 556
Vitamin B$_1$
anxiety and, 381, 382
arthritis and, 59
breast cancer and, 121
depression and, 393
endometriosis and, 246
heart disease and, 283
Vitamin B$_2$
arthritis and, 59
pain and, 436
Vitamin B$_3$
anxiety and, 381
arthritis and, 56
depression and, 393
Vitamin B$_5$
chronic fatigue syndrome and, 175
lupus and, 345
Vitamin B$_6$
anxiety and, 382
arthritis and, 59
breast cancer and, 121
chronic fatigue syndrome and, 175, 176
depression and, 393
fibrocystic breast disease and, 136
heart disease, 302
herpes and, 320
infertility and, 332
migraines and, 405
obsessive-compulsive disorder and, 385
pain and, 436, 437
pregnancy and, 487
premenstrual syndrome and, 493, 495
temporomandibular joint dysfunction and, 530
Vitamin B$_{12}$
aging and, 24
anemia and, 41–42, 44
anxiety and, 382
arthritis and, 59
caffeine and, 6
chronic fatigue syndrome and, 176, 187
environmental illness and, 260
heart disease and, 283
herpes and, 320
infertility and, 332
lupus and, 345

multiple sclerosis and, 419
pregnancy and, 478
sources of, 44
Vitamin B complex
alcohol and, 7
anxiety and, 381
chronic fatigue syndrome and, 187
depression and, 393, 394
endometriosis and, 247, 249
fibrocystic breast disease and, 136
herpes and, 320
lupus and, 345
menopause and, 356
sexually transmitted diseases and, 521
temporomandibular joint dysfunction and, 530
vaginal infection, 568, 571
Vitamin C
aging and, 21
alcohol and, 7
anxiety and, 382
arthritis and, 52, 56, 59, 61, 70, 93
breast cancer and, 121
caffeine and, 6
cervical cancer and, 154
cervical dysplasia and, 144
chronic fatigue syndrome and, 166, 168, 172, 173, 174, 176, 186
endometriosis and, 246, 247, 248, 249
environmental illness and, 260, 261
fibroids and, 149
heart disease and, 281, 283, 302, 303
herpes and, 320, 321
infertility and, 337
lupus and, 345
osteoporosis and, 423
pregnancy and, 478
sexual dysfunction and, 512
sexually transmitted diseases and, 520, 521, 522
temporomandibular joint dysfunction and, 530
urinary tract infections and, 556
vaginal infection, 568, 571, 574
varicose veins and, 578
Vitamin D
arthritis and, 59, 70
menopause and, 357
osteoporosis and, 423
Vitamin E
aging and, 20, 21
AIDS and, 21
arthritis and, 56, 59, 70, 93
caffeine and, 6
cervical cancer and, 154

Women's National Labor League, 669
Women's health movement, 613, 632, 644,
    651, 717, 731, 733, 777-779, 797-798,
    806, 918, 939, 953, 955, 963, 965-966,
    1001, 1080, 1096, 1098-1099, 1268,
    1271, 1372, 1376, 1405, 1419, 1425-
    1427, 1463-1464, 1466, 1468-1470,
    1476-1480, 1482-1485, 1487, 1489,
    1492, 1494, 1511-1512, 1516, 1522
Women's nervous diseases, 675-676
Women's rights, 643, 674-675, 726, 942,
    954, 964, 1051, 1223, 1227, 1277, 1435,
    1461, 1498, 1507, 1519, 1524
Workingmen's Party, 642
World Health Organization (WHO), 954,
    956, 958, 1115, 1207, 1223-1224, 1228-
    1229, 1276, 1287-1291, 1371, 1409-
    1510
World War II, 679, 731, 794, 1029
Wormwood, infertility and, 338
Wright, Dr. Johnathan, 344
Wunderlich, Dr. Ray, 51, 52, 505, 506, 507
Wu-wei, 359
Wyeth-Ayerst Laboratories, 1381
Wykert, John, 1454, 1526
Xenoestrogens, 109–110, 335, 336
Xiao yao wan, 286
    breast cancer and, 123
    dysmenorrhea and, 366–367
    fibrocystic breast disease and, 137
X-rays, cancer and, 112–113
Yang, Dr. Yuan, 61
Yans shen jia jiao wan, 285
Yarrow
    hormone imbalance and, 330
    urinary tract infections and, 557
    varicose veins and, 578
Yaryura-Tobias, Dr. José, 236–237, 383,
    384, 385
Yeager, Laura, 1146
Years of Potential Life Lost, 1367
Yeast
    infections, 9
    vaginal, 100
Yellow dock
    anemia and, 44
    vaginal infection, 569
Yellow gential, heart disease and, 294
Yellow Wallpaper, The, 604, 675-676, 1513
Yoga, 31
    arthritis and, 62
    depression and, 398–399
    fibrocystic breast disease and, 138
    infertility and, 337
    osteoporosis and, 425–426
Yunnan Pain yao, 367

Yutsis, Dr. Pavel, 445, 446
Zake, Yamuna, 427, 529
Zand, Janet, 44, 330, 494, 495
Zann, Dr. Alfred, 263
Zeneca Pharmaceuticals, 1353, 1394
Ziel, Harry, 754
Zinc
    aging and, 20, 21
    anxiety and, 381
    arthritis and, 52, 55, 70
    breast cancer and, 122
    chronic fatigue syndrome and, 174,
    176
    depression and, 395
    diabetes and, 214
    eating disorders and, 227, 238–239
    endometriosis and, 246, 247
    herpes and, 320, 321
    infertility and, 342
    lupus and, 345
    menopause and, 356
    osteoporosis and, 423
    pregnancy and, 478
    repetitive strain injury and, 504
    sexually transmitted diseases and,
    520, 521
    thyroid disease and, 535, 537
    urinary tract infections and, 556
    vaginal infection, 571, 574

About the Authors

GARY NULL, Ph.D. is one of America's leading health and fitness writers and alternative practitioners. Trained as a nutritionist, he is the author of dozens of books and hundreds of medical articles. His one-hour health radio program airs daily on WBAI in New York City, and is carried weekly to 32 stations natiowide over the Virtual Radio Network. Null is a former faculty member of the New School for Social Research and a National TAC Master Champion Racewalker. Among his many best-selling books are *Get Healthy Now!*, *Healing Your Body Naturally*, and *The Ultimate Anti-Aging Program.* He lives in New York City.

BARBARA SEAMAN has been cited by the Library of Congress as the author who raised sexism and health care as a worldwide issue. Her *The Doctors' Case against the Pill* is credited with influencing the FDA to require informational inserts in packages of oral contraceptives and other medicines. She also wrote *Free and Female* and *Women and the Crisis in Sex Hormones.* The *New York Times* wrote that these three books "triggered a revolution, fostering a willingness among women to take issues of health into their own hands." A founder of the National Women's Health Network and a contributing editor to *Ms.*, Seaman lives in New York City.